NUTRITION IN THE PREVENTION AND TREATMENT OF ABDOMINAL OBESITY

NUTRITION IN THE PREVENTION AND TREATMENT OF ABDOMINAL OBESITY

Edited by

RONALD ROSS WATSON, BS, PhD

University of Arizona, Division of Health Promotion Sciences, Mel and Enid Zuckerman College of Public Health, and School of Medicine, Arizona Health Sciences Center, Tucson, AZ, USA

ELSEVIER

AMSTERDAM • BOSTON • HEIDELBERG • LONDON
NEW YORK • OXFORD • PARIS • SAN DIEGO
SAN FRANCISCO • SINGAPORE • SYDNEY • TOKYO

Academic Press is an imprint of Elsevier

Academic Press is an imprint of Elsevier
32 Jamestown Road, London NW1 7BY, UK
225 Wyman Street, Waltham, MA 02451, USA
525 B Street, Suite 1800, San Diego, CA 92101-4495, USA

Medicine is an ever-changing field. Standard safety precautions must be followed, but as new research and clinical experience broaden our knowledge, changes in treatment and drug therapy may become necessary or appropriate. Readers are advised to check the most current product information provided by the manufacturer of each drug to be administered to verify the recommended dose, the method and duration of administrations, and contraindications. It is the responsibility of the treating physician, relying on experience and knowledge of the patient, to determine dosages and the best treatment for each individual patient. Neither the publisher nor the authors assume any liability for any injury and/or damage to persons or property arising from this publication.

Notice

No responsibility is assumed by the publisher for any injury and/or damage to persons or property as a matter of products liability, negligence or otherwise, or from any use or operation of any methods, products, instructions or ideas contained in the material herein. Because of rapid advances in the medical sciences, in particular, independent verification of diagnoses and drug dosages should be made

British Library Cataloguing-in-Publication Data
A catalogue record for this book is available from the British Library

Library of Congress Cataloging-in-Publication Data
A catalog record for this book is available from the Library of Congress

ISBN: 978-0-12-407869-7

Typeset by Scientific Publishing Services
www.sps.co.in

Printed and bound in United States of America
Transferred to Digital Printing, 2014

Contents

PART E

DIETARY FOODS AND VISCERAL FAT ACCUMULATION AND REMOVAL

22. Fermented Soypastes, *Doenjang* and *Cheonggukjang*, and Obesity

MYOUNGSOOK LEE AND YONGSOON PARK

23. Alcohol Intake and Hormonal Dysregulation of Food Intake in Visceral Fat Accumulation

GUSTAVO D. PIMENTEL AND THAYANA O. MICHELETTI

24. Coffee Intake and Obesity

GUSTAVO D. PIMENTEL, THAYANA O. MICHELETTI, AND ASTRID NEHLIG

25. Bread Intake and Abdominal Fat

INMACULADA BAUTISTA-CASTAÑO, ALMUDENA SANCHEZ-VILLEGAS, AND LUIS SERRA-MAJEM

26. Role of the Immune System in Obesity-Associated Inflammation and Insulin Resistance

YOSHINORI NAGAI AND KIYOSHI TAKATSU

27. Metabolic Effects of Abdominal Fats in Animal Models and Humans

MICHAL M. MASTERNAK

28. Appetite and Reward Signals in the Brain: Sugar Intake Effects on Brain Activity as Measured by Functional Magnetic Resonance Imaging

SAMANTHA M. HUDGINS, ANNA SCHLAPPAL, AND THOMAS W. CASTONGUAY

PART F

DIETARY SUPPLEMENTS AND VISCERAL OBESITY

29. Flaxseed Secoisolariciresinol Diglucoside and Visceral Obesity

JAE B. PARK

30. Carotenoids as a Nutraceutical Therapy for Visceral Obesity

KAZUO MIYASHITA AND MASASHI HOSOKAWA

31. Nutritional Deficiencies in Obese Sleeve Gastrectomy Patients

ANTJE DAMMS-MACHADO AND STEPHAN C. BISCHOFF

PART G

MACROMOLECULES IN FOODS AND DIETS AND ABDOMINAL OBESITY

32. Dairy Whey Proteins and Obesity

SEBELY PAL, SIMONE RADAVELLI-BAGATINI, SULEEN HO, JENNY-LEE MCKAY, MARTIN HAGGER, AND MONICA JANE

33. Probiotics to Treat Visceral Obesity and Related Liver Disease

PIETRO VAJRO, MARCO POETA, LUCA PIERRI, CRISTINA PIZZA, ROBERTA D'ANIELLO, MARIA SANGERMANO, GRAZIA MASSA, AND GIULIA PAOLELLA

34. Beta-Cryptoxanthin, a Novel Carotenoid Derived from Satsuma Mandarin, Prevents Abdominal Obesity

KATSUHIKO TAKAYANAGI AND KATSUYUKI MUKAI

35. A Diet with Carbohydrates Eaten Primarily at Dinner: an Innovative, Nutritional Approach to End the Vicious Cycle of Abdominal Obesity

SIGAL SOFER, ALIZA STARK, GERSHON FINK, AND ZECHARIA MADAR

PART H

MICROMOLECULES AND NUTRIENTS AS MODULATORS OF VISCERAL FAT

36. Effects of Different Dietary Fatty Acids on Human Energy Balance, Body Weight, Fat Mass, and Abdominal Fat

SZE YEN TAN

37. Conjugated Linoleic Acid in Human Health Effects on Weight Control

YEONHWA PARK

38. Essential Amino Acid Supplementation for the Prevention and Treatment of Obesity

GIUSEPPE D'ANTONA

PART I

ACTIVITY OF ADIPOCYTES: ROLE IN GROWTH AND ACCUMULATION OF FAT

39. Fibroblast Growth Factor 21 is a Regulator of Energy Metabolism in the Liver and Adipose Tissue

NIINA MATIKAINEN

40. Genetics of Abdominal Obesity

MIN XU AND LU QI

41. The Role of Site-Specific Adipose Tissue Fatty Acid Composition in Obesity

FÁTIMA PÉREZ DE HEREDIA AND MARTA GARAULET

PART J

FIBER AND VISCERAL OBESITY

42. Using Psyllium to Prevent and Treat Obesity Comorbidities

SEBELY PAL, SIMONE RADAVELLI-BAGATINI, SULEEN HO, JENNY-LEE MCKAY, AND MONICA JANE

43. Whole Grains in the Prevention and Treatment of Abdominal Obesity

J. PHILIP KARL AND NICOLA M. MCKEOWN

Preface

Abdominal or visceral fat comprises fat deposits between the liver and kidneys that are packed into the abdominal cavity. This fat is distinct from subcutaneous and intramuscular fat because it is primarily visceral and includes several adipose depots. Historically, such fat has a played a key role in survival in times of famine. As described in the book, such fat is subject to lifestyle management as well as to accumulation.

EPIDEMIOLOGY AND CLINICAL MANAGEMENT OF ABDOMINAL OBESITY

Appetite-regulating gut hormones, work, diet, and physical activity in adults, children, and adolescents have all been described as factors that affect abdominal fat accumulation. Tarantino describes the efficacy of physical activity in treating nonalcoholic fatty liver disease. Its actions in specific populations, for example the elevated hypertension of African-Americans, are defined and explained by Hornbuckle. Von Gruenigen shows how fat plays a role in cancer survivorship, while Clement reviews massive obesity and its consequences. Clearly, and historically, lifestyle factors are major factors that affect abdominal fat; these are defined by Suliga with Gomez-Martinez in their review of the role of physical activity in abdominal obesity in adolescents. Therapies including surgery and sleeve gastrostomy are reviewed by Ruiz-Tovar, while the beneficial effects of supplemental magnesium are defined by Kokot.

Fat is constantly being stored and released from adipose tissue. Storage in adipose tissue is regulated by insulin and stimulated by high serum glucose. Thus, fat cells have an important role in maintaining triglyceride and free fatty acid levels. However, abdominal fat is more prone to inducing insulin resistance; therefore, central obesity is a marker of impaired glucose tolerance as a risk factor for many obesity-related diseases. Gasevic et al. show that adipose tissue affects insulin resistance and is further modified by ethnicity. In addition, Rossi and colleagues describe visceral fat as key to ectopic fat accumulation, while Leblanc and Poirier discuss how high blood pressure risk is lessened by reducing visceral obesity. Finally, Prasad defines the problems of advanced glycation end-products in relation to adiposity.

DIET, SUPPLEMENTS, AND FOODS IN THE MANAGEMENT OF VISCERAL OBESITY

Understanding abdominal obesity will promote its modification and prevention, thus reducing chronic disease levels. Under standard conditions, adipose depots provide feedback on hunger and dietary needs to the central nervous system. A variety of biochemical, physiological, and food-regulated mechanisms that alter abdominal obesity and thus disease risk are reviewed. Maeda identifies glucagon-like peptide 1 as an agonist of visceral fat adiposity and appetite. Castonguay defines the role of fructose in hypertriglyceridemia and obesity. Dietary foods play key roles in visceral fat accumulation and its removal. The effects of intermittent fasting versus daily calorie restriction on visceral fat loss are compared by Trepanowski and Varady. Laurant and colleagues show that gender and exercise, which both modulate cytokines, affect obesity and thus heart disease. Stress-induced eating also affects obesity, and Finch and Tomiyama describe relevant physiological and behavioral stress responses. Campbell and coworkers review fructose-induced hypertriglyceridemia as a cause of abdominal obesity that can be modified by changes in food intake. Yoshinaga describes how the gender and lifestyle of individuals and their parents combine to modify obesity.

Adipose tissues play important roles in health; their primary role is as a reserve of lipids needed to provide energy. Fat tissues consist of about 86% fat, and a variety of different cell types regulate fat accumulation. Lipolysis is modulated by lipolytic β-adrenergic receptors and antilipolysis is regulated by α2A adrenergic receptors. Dietary foods and supplements can play critical roles in modifying and preventing such fat accumulation. Park describes several types of soy protein and fermented soypastes that can reduce visceral obesity. Reviews by the Pimentel and Bautista-Castaño groups describe the roles of alcohol, coffee, and bread in modifying obesity through various mechanisms, including immunomodulation of inflammation, which is obesity induced. As Nagai and Takatsu review in humans and Masternak in animal models, these mechanisms are important in metabolic disorders associated with chronic diseases. Castonguay and coauthors describe appetite and reward signals in the brain, with sugar being a major mediator, as shown by magnetic resonance imaging.

Additionally, the effects of dietary supplements on fat regulation and thus visceral obesity are an important focus of this book. A stringent vegan diet with dietary restriction produces significant weight loss. A supplement containing flaxseed components changes visceral obesity, inflammation, lipids, and chronic hypertension, as Park summarizes. Damms-Machado shows that nutritional deficiencies in obese patients are a common condition, which are additionally impacted by bariatric operations, like sleeve gastrectomy. Miyashita and Hosokawa show the importance of plant carotenoids as nutraceutical therapies for visceral obesity.

Other macromolecules and foods are modulators of visceral fat and play a key role in a host of diseases, including diabetes, insulin resistance, cardiovascular disease, inflammation, and other obesity-related health problems. Pal and coauthors describe a role for psyllium as a therapy for obesity comorbidities. Karl and McKeown describe the role of whole grain (with its intrinsic fiber) in obesity prevention, while Pal defines a similar role for dietary whey protein. Vajro and coworkers describe the role of other complex carbohydrates known as probiotics in treating hepatic obesity and related diseases. Dinner carbohydrates, if used as described by Madar and colleagues, produce weight loss and have other effects on visceral fat. Citrus is a food that, as Mukai describes in animal models and humans, changes visceral fat accumulation. Lipids are the major modulators of fat. Tan describes the effects of dietary fatty acids on weight, fat mass and abdominal fat. Park shows that conjugated linoleic acid benefits human health by controlling weight. Finally, D'Antona reviews the current evidence that amino acid supplementation affects obesity. Free fatty acids are released from lipoproteins by enzymes and enter adipocytes to be reassembled into triglycerides for storage. Through regulating adipose tissues in visceral fat, different cell types (primarily adipocytes, fibroblasts, macrophages, lymphocytes, and endothelial cells) can have wide-ranging effects on health. Matikainen describes the role of fibroblast growth factor 21 in regulating energy metabolism in adipose tissues to promote health. Qi discusses how polymorphisms in the gene encoding neuropeptide Y (and other genes) affect central obesity. Finally, Garaulet defines site-specific adipose tissue fatty acid composition and its role in the regulation of abdominal obesity.

In conclusion, the authors describe how factors that affect the current abdominal obesity epidemic will provide major benefits by preventing chronic diseases, especially heart, vascular, and diabetic diseases. A broad range of disciplines are involved in dealing with the consequences of excessive abdominal fat, including cardiology, diabetes research, endocrinology, exercise physiology, and studies focusing on lipids, metabolism, nutrition, and obesity. We describe how abdominal obesity, a major cause of mortality and morbidity in much of the world through its associated diseases, can be regulated by food and dietary therapies.

Acknowledgments

The work of Dr. Watson's editorial assistant, Bethany L. Stevens, and the project managers, Megan Wickline and Jeffrey Rossetti, in communicating with authors and working on the manuscripts was critical to the successful completion of the book. It is very much appreciated. Support for the work of Ms. Stevens and Dr. Watson was graciously provided by the Natural Health Research Institute (www.naturalhealthresearch.org), an independent, nonprofit organization that supports science-based research into natural health and wellness. It is committed to promoting scientific evidence for the usefulness and cost-effectiveness of diet, supplements, and a healthy lifestyle in improving health and wellness, and reducing disease. Finally, the work of Mari Stoddard, the librarian of the Arizona Health Science Library, was vital and very helpful in identifying key researchers who participated in the book.

Contributors

Machiko Aoki, MD, PhD Department of Pediatrics, Aoki Clinic of Internal Medicine, Cardiovascular Medicine & Pediatrics, Fukuoka, Japan.

Inmaculada Bautista-Castaño, MD, PhD Department of Clinical Sciences, University of Las Palmas de Gran Canaria, Las Palmas de Gran Canaria, Spain Biomedical Research Center Network on Obesity and Nutrition (CIBERobn) Physiopathology of Obesity and Nutrition, Institute of Health Carlos III, Madrid, Spain.

Paolo Bertassello, MD Division of Geriatric Medicine, University of Verona, Ospedale Maggiore, Verona, Italy.

Stephan C. Bischoff, MD, Prof. Institute of Nutritional Medicine, University of Hohenheim, Stuttgart, Germany.

Rafael Calpena, MD, PhD Department of Surgery, Bariatric Surgery Unit, General University Hospital Elche, Alicante, Spain.

Eric Campbell Department of Nutrition and Food Science, University of Maryland, College Park, MD, USA.

Raquel Canuto, PhD Department of Nutrition, University of Vale do Rios dos Sinos, RS, Brazil.

Department of Nutrition, University of Caxias do Sul, RS, Brazil.

Thomas W. Castonguay, PhD Department of Nutrition and Food Science, University of Maryland, College Park, MD, USA.

Karine Clément, MD, PhD Institute of Cardiometabolism and Nutrition, ICAN, Pitié-Salpêtrière Hospital; Assistance Publique-Hôpitaux de Paris, CRNH-Ile de France, Paris, France.

Anderson da Silva Garcez, MD Postgraduate Program in Collective Health, University of Vale do Rios dos Sinos, RS, Brazil.

Antje Damms-Machado, PhD Institute of Nutritional Medicine, University of Hohenheim, Stuttgart, Germany.

Roberta D'Aniello, MD Department of Medicine and Surgery, Medical School of Salerno, Baronissi, Salerno, Italy.

Giuseppe D'Antona, MD, PhD Department of Molecular Medicine and the Laboratory for the Study of Motor Activities in Rare Diseases, University of Pavia, Voghera, Italy.

Sylwia Dzięgielewska-Gęsiak Department of Internal Diseases, Silesian Medical University, Katowice, Poland.

Magdy El-Salhy, MD, PhD Section for Gastroenterology, Department of Medicine, Stord Helse-Fonna Hospital, Norway.

Section for Gastroenterology, Department of Clinical Medicine, University of Bergen, Norway.

Francesco Fantin, MD, PhD Division of Geriatric Medicine, University of Verona, Ospedale Maggiore, Verona, Italy.

Laura E. Finch, B.S. Cornell University Department of Psychology, Los Angeles, CA, USA.

Carmine Finelli, MD, PhD INT "Fondazione Pascale" - Cancer Research Center of Mercogliano, Mercogliano (AV), Italy.

Gershon Fink, MD Kaplan Medical Center, Rehovot, Israel.

Yuya Fujishima, MD Department of Metabolic Medicine, Graduate School of Medicine, Osaka University, Osaka, Japan.

Marta Garaulet, PhD, Full Professor of Physiology, Department of Physiology, Faculty of Biology, University of Murcia, Murcia, Spain.

Danijela Gasevic, MD Department of Biomedical Physiology and Kinesiology, Simon Fraser University, Burnaby, British Columbia, Canada.

Eliana Geller Department of Nutrition and Food Science, University of Maryland, College Park, MD, USA.

Sonia Gómez-Martínez, PhD, Research officer Department of Metabolism and Nutrition, Institute of Food Science, Technology and Nutrition, Spanish National Research Council, Madrid, Spain.

Doris Gundersen, PhD Department of Research, Helse-Fonna, Haugesund, Norway.

Martin Hagger School of Public Health; Curtin Health Innovation Research Institute; Curtin University of Technology, Perth, Western Australia, Australia.

Takashi Hamajima, MD Department of Endocrinology and Metabolism, Aichi Children's Health and Medical Center, Motiokamachi, Obu, Aichi, Japan.

Jan Gunnar Hatlebakk, MD, PhD Section for Gastroenterology, Institute of Medicine, University of Bergen, Norway.

Trygve Hausken, MD, PhD Section for Gastroenterology, Department of Clinical Medicine, University of Bergen, Norway.

Section for Gastroenterology, Department of Medicine, Haukland University Hospital, Bergen, Norway.

Suleen Ho, PhD, Hons School of Public Health, Curtin Health Innovation Research Institute, Curtin University of Technology, Perth, Western Australia, Australia.

Lyndsey M. Hornbuckle, PhD, RD Department of Exercise Science and Sport Management, Kennesaw State University, Kennesaw, Georgia, USA.

Masashi Hosokawa Faculty of Fisheries Sciences, Hokkaido University, Hakodate, Japan.

Samantha M. Hudgins Department of Nutrition and Food Science, University of Maryland, College Park, MD, USA.

Gary R. Hunter, PhD Department of Human Studies, University of Alabama at Birmingham, Birmingham, Alabama, USA.

Monica Jane, BSc School of Public Health, Curtin Health Innovation Research Institute, Curtin University of Technology, Perth, Western Australia, Australia.

J. Philip Karl, MS, RD Jean Mayer USDA Human Nutrition Research Center on Aging, Tufts University, Boson, MA, USA.

Nadia Khan MD, MSc Department of Medicine, University of British Columbia, Vancouver, British Columbia, Canada.

Simi Kohli, MD, MSc Department of Biomedical Physiology and Kinesiology, Simon Fraser University, Burnaby, British Columbia, Canada.

Teresa Kokot, MD, PhD Department of Internal Diseases, Silesian Medical University, Katowice, Poland.

Pascal Laurant, PhD Laboratoire Pharm-Ecologie Cardio-vasculaire, UFRip Sciences Technologies Santé, Université d'Avignon et des Pays du Vaucluse, Avignon, France.

Scott A. Lear, PhD Faculty of Health Sciences, Simon Fraser University, Vancouver, British Columbia, Canada.

Marie-Ève Leblanc, RN, MSc Faculty of Pharmacy, Université Laval and Institut Universitaire de Cardiologie et de Pneumologie de Québec, Quebec City, Quebec, Canada.

Myoungsook Lee, PhD Department of Food and Nutrition, and Research Institute of Obesity Sciences, Sungshin Women's University, Seoul, Korea.

Zecharia Madar Kaplan Medical Center, Rehovot, Israel.

Norikazu Maeda, MD, PhD Department of Metabolic Medicine, Graduate School of Medicine, Osaka University, Osaka, Japan.

Ascensión Marcos Department of Metabolism and Nutrition, Institute of Food Science, Technology and Nutrition, Spanish National Research Council, Madrid, Spain.

David Martínez-Gómez, PhD, Associate lecturer Department of Physical Education, Sports and Human Movement, Faculty of Teacher Training and Education, Universidad Autónoma de Madrid, Madrid, Spain.

Grazia Massa, RD Department of Medicine and Surgery, Medical School of Salerno, Baronissi, Salerno, Italy.

Michal M. Masternak, PhD University of Central Florida, Burnett School of Biomedical Sciences, College of Medicine, Orlando, FL, USA.

Niina Matikainen, MD, PhD Department of Endocrinology and Cardiovascular Research Unit, Heart and Lung Center, Helsinki University Central Hospital, University of Helsinki, Helsinki, Finland.

Michele L. McCarroll, PhD Department of Obstetrics and Gynecology, Summa Health System, Akron, Ohio, USA.

Jenny-Lee McKay, BSc School of Public Health, Curtin Health Innovation Research Institute, Curtin University of Technology, Perth, Western Australia, Australia.

Nicola M. McKeown, PhD Jean Mayer USDA Human Nutrition Research Center on Aging, Tufts University, Boson, MA, USA.

Thayana O. Micheletti Department of Internal Medicine, Faculty of Medical Sciences, University of Campinas (UNICAMP), São Paulo, Brazil.

Kazuo Miyashita Faculty of Fisheries Sciences, Hokkaido University, Hakodate, Japan.

Ayumi Miyazaki, MD, PhD Department of Pediatrics, Japan Community Health Care Organization Takaoka-Fushiki Hospital, Takaoka, Toyama, Japan.

Małgorzata Muc-Wierzgoń Department of Internal Diseases, Silesian Medical University, Katowice, Poland.

Katsuyuki Mukai R&D Center, UNITIKA Ltd, Uji, Kyoto, Japan.

Yoshinori Nagai, MD, PhD, FAHA Department of Immunobiology and Pharmacological Genetics, Graduate School of Medicine and Pharmaceutical Science for Research, University of Toyama, Toyama-shi, Toyama, Japan.

Masami Nagashima, MD, PhD, FAHA Department of Rehabilitation, Aichi Saiseikai Rehabilitation Hospital, Nishi-ku, Nagoya, Japan.

Astrid Nehlig French Medical Research Institute, INSERM U 663, Faculty of Medicine, Strasbourg, France.

Ewa Nowakowska-Zajdel Department of Internal Diseases, Silesian Medical University, Katowice, Poland.

Maria Teresa Anselmo Olinto, PhD Postgraduate Program in Collective Health, University of Vale do Rios dos Sinos, RS, Brazil.

Department of Nutrition, Federal University of Health Science of Porto Alegre, RS, Brazil.

Sebely Pal, PhD, Hons School of Public Health, Curtin Health Innovation Research Institute, Curtin University of Technology, Perth, Western Australia, Australia.

Giulia Paolella, MD Department of Medicine and Surgery, Medical School of Salerno, Baronissi, Salerno, Italy.

Jae B. Park Diet, Genomics, and Immunology Laboratory, Beltsville Human Nutrition Research Center, United States Department of Agriculture Agricultural Research Service, Beltsville, MD, USA.

Yeonhwa Park Department of Food Science, University of Massachusetts, Amherst, MA, USA.

Yongsoon Park, PhD Department of Food and Nutrition, Hanyang University, Seoul, Korea.

Zdenka Pausova, MD The Hospital for Sick Children, University of Toronto, Toronto, Canada.

Fátima Pérez de Heredia, PhD Lecturer in Physiology, School of Natural Sciences and Psychology, Liverpool John Moores University, Liverpool, United Kingdom.

Luca Pierri, MS Department of Medicine and Surgery, Medical School of Salerno, Baronissi, Salerno, Italy.

Gustavo D. Pimentel Department of Internal Medicine, Faculty of Medical Sciences, University of Campinas (UNICAMP), São Paulo, Brazil.

Cristina Pizza, MS Department of Medicine and Surgery, Medical School of Salerno, Baronissi, Salerno, Italy.

Marco Poeta, MS Department of Medicine and Surgery, Medical School of Salerno, Baronissi, Salerno, Italy.

Paul Poirier, MD, PhD, FRCPC, FACC, FAHA Faculty of Pharmacy, Université Laval and Institut Universitaire de Cardiologie et de Pneumologie de Québec, Quebec City, Quebec, Canada.

Christine Poitou, MD, PhD Institute of Cardiometabolism and Nutrition, ICAN, Pitié-Salpêtrière Hospital; Assistance Publique-Hôpitaux de Paris, CRNH-Ile de France, Paris, France.

Lu Qi, MD, PhD Department of Nutrition, Harvard School of Public Health, Boston, MA, USA.

Channing Division of Network Medicine, Department of Medicine, Brigham and Women's Hospital and Harvard Medical School, Boston, MA, USA.

Simone Radavelli-Bagatini, PhD, Hons School of Public Health, Curtin Health Innovation Research Institute, Curtin University of Technology, Perth, Western Australia, Australia.

Catherine Riva, PhD Laboratoire Pharm-Ecologie Cardiovasculaire, UFRip Sciences Technologies Santé, Université d'Avignon et des Pays du Vaucluse, Avignon, France.

Andrea P. Rossi, MD, PhD Division of Geriatric Medicine, University of Verona, Ospedale Maggiore, Verona, Italy.

G. Dante Roulette, MD Department of Obstetrics and Gynecology, Summa Health System, Akron, Ohio, USA.

Jaime Ruiz-Tovar, MD, PhD Department of Surgery, Bariatric Surgery Unit, General University Hospital Elche, Alicante, Spain.

Almudena Sanchez-Villegas DPharm, PhD Department of Clinical Sciences, University of Las Palmas de Gran Canaria, Las Palmas de Gran Canaria, Spain Biomedical Research Center Network on Obesity and Nutrition (CIBERobn) Physiopathology of Obesity and Nutrition, Institute of Health Carlos III, Madrid, Spain.

Maria Sangermano, MD Department of Medicine and Surgery, Medical School of Salerno, Baronissi, Salerno, Italy.

E. Sartori, MD Division of Geriatric Medicine, University of Verona, Ospedale Maggiore, Verona, Italy.

Anna Schlappal, PhD Department of Nutrition and Food Science, University of Maryland, College Park, MD, USA.

Luis Serra-Majem MD, PhD Department of Clinical Sciences, University of Las Palmas de Gran Canaria, Las Palmas de Gran Canaria, Spain Biomedical Research Center Network on Obesity and Nutrition (CIBERobn) Physiopathology of Obesity and Nutrition, Institute of Health Carlos III, Madrid, Spain.

Masaki Shinomiya, MD, PhD Department of Internal Medicine, Nishifuna Naika, Funabashi, Chiba, Japan.

Sigal Sofer, MSc, RD Institute of Biochemistry, Food Science and Nutrition, The Robert H. Smith Faculty of Agriculture, Food and Environment, The Hebrew University of Jerusalem, Jerusalem, Israel.

Aliza Stark, PhD, RD Institute of Biochemistry, Food Science and Nutrition, The Robert H. Smith Faculty of Agriculture, Food and Environment, The Hebrew University of Jerusalem, Jerusalem, Israel.

Edyta Suliga, PhD Department of the Prevention of Alimentary Tract Diseases, Faculty of Health Sciences, Jan Kochanowski University, Kielce, Poland.

Kiyoshi Takatsu, PhD Toyama Prefectural Institute for Pharmaceutical Research, Imizu City, Toyama, Japan.

Katsuhiko Takayanagi R&D Center, UNITIKA Ltd, Uji, Kyoto, Japan.

Sze Yen Tan, PhD, APD University of South Australia, School of Pharmacy and Medical Sciences, Adelaide, Australia.

Giovanni Tarantino, MD Department of Clinical Medicine and Surgery, Federico II University Medical School of Naples, Naples, Italy and INT "Fondazione Pascale" - Cancer Research Center of Mercogliano, Mercogliano (AV), Italy.

A. Janet Tomiyama, PhD Department of Psychology, University of California, Los Angeles, CA, USA.

John F. Trepanowski, MS Department of Kinesiology and Nutrition, University of Illinois, Chicago, Chicago, IL, USA.

Pietro Vajro, MD Department of Medicine and Surgery, Medical School of Salerno, Baronissi, Salerno, Italy.

European Laboratory for the Investigation of Food-Induced Diseases, University of Naples Federico II, Naples, Italy.

Krista Varady, PhD Department of Kinesiology and Nutrition, University of Illinois, Chicago, Chicago, IL, USA.

Camille Vatier, MD Institute of Cardiometabolism and Nutrition, ICAN, Pitié-Salpêtrière Hospital; Assistance Publique-Hôpitaux de Paris, CRNH-Ile de France, Paris, France.

Agnes Vinet, PhD Laboratoire Pharm-Ecologie Cardiovasculaire, UFRip Sciences Technologies Santé, Université d'Avignon et des Pays du Vaucluse, Avignon, France.

Vivian E. von Gruenigen, MD Department of Obstetrics and Gynecology, Summa Health System, Akron, Ohio, USA.

Min Xu, MD, PhD Department of Nutrition, Harvard School of Public Health, Boston, MA, USA. Shanghai Clinical Center for Endocrine and Metabolic Diseases, Shanghai Institute of Endocrine and Metabolic Diseases, Ruijin Hospital Affiliated to Shanghai Jiao Tong University School of Medicine, Shanghai, China.

Masao Yoshinaga, MD, PhD Department of Pediatrics, National Hospital Organization Kagoshima Medical Center, Kagoshima, Japan.

Mauro Zamboni, MD Division of Geriatric Medicine, University of Verona, Ospedale Maggiore, Verona, Italy.

Valeria Zanandrea, MD Division of Geriatric Medicine, University of Verona, Ospedale Maggiore, Verona, Italy.

SECTION 1

EPIDEMIOLOGY AND CLINICAL MANAGEMENT OF VISCERAL OBESITY

PART A

EPIDEMIOLOGY AND PATHOPHYSIOLOGY OF ABDOMINAL OBESITY

CHAPTER

1

Diet and Irritable Bowel Syndrome, with a Focus on Appetite-Regulating Gut Hormones

Magdy El-Salhy[a,c], *Doris Gundersen*[b], *Jan Gunnar Hatlebakk*[c], *and Trygve Hausken*[c]

[a]Section for Gastroenterology, Department of Medicine, Stord Helse-Fonna Hospital, Norway; [b]Department of Research, Helse-Fonna, Haugesund, Norway; [c]Section for Gastroenterology, Institute of Medicine, University of Bergen, Norway

INTRODUCTION

Irritable bowel syndrome (IBS) is a common chronic gastrointestinal disorder with a prevalence of 5–20% and a reported incidence of 200 cases per 100,000 in the adult population [1–9]. IBS patients are often young and predominantly female, and IBS is associated with abnormal gastrointestinal motility and visceral hypersensitivity [2,6,10–25]. Patients with IBS complain of abdominal pain or discomfort, altered bowel habits, and bloating and/or abdominal distension [1]. The severity of symptoms varies from tolerable to severe, with some patients suffering from daily symptoms while others report intermittent symptoms at intervals of weeks or months [1].

Although IBS is not known to be associated with the development of serious disease or increased mortality, it does considerably reduce the patients quality of life by an amount comparable to that reported for patients with inflammatory bowel disease, diabetes, congestive heart failure, renal insufficiency, and hepatic cirrhosis [1,6,26–31]. In addition to the morbidity caused by IBS, this disorder represents an economic burden to society [1]. Although most IBS patients ignore their symptoms and regard them as a normal part of everyday life, they generate a substantial workload in both primary and secondary health care [32,33]. It has been reported that IBS patients are responsible for 12–14% of primary healthcare visits and constitute 28% of referrals to gastroenterologists [34–43]. Added to this are the costs associated with diagnostic tests, medication, hospitalization, and the reduced productivity of IBS patients [36,41,42].

IBS diagnosis is based mainly on symptom assessment since there are no biochemical, radiological, or morphological diagnostic tests for the condition. The Rome criteria III are widely accepted and applied for the diagnosis of IBS [44]. Patients are subdivided further on the basis of differences in the predominant bowel pattern into diarrhea predominant (IBS-D), constipation predominant (IBS-C), or a mixture of both diarrhea and constipation (IBS-M). These three subtypes have a similar prevalence [34,45–49]. Although several biomarkers for the diagnosis of IBS have been considered, the only reproducible test is gut transit measured by radioisotope markers, and this test has a limited availability [50]. Duodenal chromogranin A cell density has been proposed as a good marker for the diagnosis of IBS, with high sensitivity and specificity, but needs to be confirmed in a large cohort of IBS patients [51]. Postinfectious IBS is a subset of IBS that occurs in a considerable number of patients and is defined as a sudden onset of IBS symptoms following gastroenteritis in individuals who have not previously had any gastrointestinal complaints [52]. However, postinfectious IBS has also been reported following nongastrointestinal infections such as respiratory, urinary tract, and skin infections [53]. It is reported that 6–17% of IBS patients believe that their symptoms began with an infective illness, and 7–31% of patients who suffer an acute episode of infectious gastroenteritis go on to develop postinfectious IBS despite clearance of the inciting pathogen [54–56].

There are both nonpharmacological and pharmacological options for the treatment of IBS. The

Nutrition in the Prevention and Treatment of Abdominal Obesity
http://dx.doi.org/10.1016/B978-0-12-407869-7.00001-5

nonpharmacological approach comprises the provision of information, reassurance, dietary guidance, regular exercise, probiotic intake, gut-directed hypnotherapy, cognitive therapy, acupuncture, and herbal therapy. Pharmacological treatment depends upon the symptoms and mainly includes antidiarrheal drugs, prokinetics, laxatives, antispasmodics, antidepressants, antianxiety drugs, and antibiotics [1].

DIET INTAKE IN IRRITABLE BOWEL SYNDROME PATIENTS

IBS patients tend to avoid certain food items that they associate with onset of their symptoms such as milk and dairy products, wheat products, caffeine, certain meat, cabbage, onion, peas/beans, hot spices, fried food, and smoked food products [57,58]. It has been reported that 62% of IBS patients limit or exclude food items from their daily intake, with 12% of them making such drastic changes to their diet that long-term nutritional deficiencies are possible [59]. Despite such food avoidance, the dietary composition of IBS patients does not differ from the background population in terms of energy, carbohydrate, protein, and fat intake [60–66]. A common belief among IBS patients is that lactose is the main cause of their symptoms; they consequently reduce their intake of milk and dairy products, which in turn results in a low daily intake of calcium, vitamin B2, and phosphorus [59,63,65,67].

IBS patients have a lower consumption of food items known to be rich in fermentable oligo-, di-, and monosaccharides, and polyols (i.e. FODMAPs) such as buns, couscous, millet, pasta, spaghetti, rice, and some vegetables (e.g. raw broccoli, cabbage, garlic, green beans, leeks, mushrooms, onion, peppers, and tomatoes) [63]. However, they have a higher consumption of other FODMAP-rich vegetables such as grapes, mango, melon, peaches, pears, peas, and plums [63].

THE ROLE OF DIET IN THE DEVELOPMENT OF IBS SYMPTOMS

Food Allergy or Intolerance

There is no convincing evidence for an allergic response to, or an intolerance for, any specific foodstuff in IBS [1,68–73]. In absence of a typical immunoglobulin E (IgE) reaction, another antibody class (IgG) has been suggested to be implicated in food-related allergies in IBS [74,75]. However, this suggestion is controversial, probably because the tests used are not sufficiently sensitive or specific [65,68,73,75–83]. Nevertheless, food allergy mediated by mucosal mechanisms may occur in patients with atopic and postinfectious IBS [1,55,84].

The triggering of IBS symptoms by the ingestion of wheat products is thought to be caused by the sugar polymers, fructans and galactans [85,86],. The occurrence of nonceliac gluten sensitivity in IBS patients is widely debated [87]. The existence of nonceliac gluten intolerance was advocated following a randomized, double-blind, placebo-controlled rechallenge trial [88]. It has been suggested that IBS patients with wheat intolerance who possess genotypes associated with celiac disease (*HLA DQ2* or *DR3*) but do not have typical serological markers or changes in small intestine histology exhibit other immunologic evidence of gluten reactivity and respond to a gluten-free diet [89]. The role of gluten intolerance in IBS remains to be clarified. Celiac disease and IBS have overlapping clinical presentations, resulting in some patients with celiac disease being mistakenly diagnosed as having IBS [90,91]. The number of patients with celiac disease among those with IBS is reported to vary between 0.04% and 4.7% [92–102].

Poorly Absorbed Carbohydrates and Fibers

FODMAPs are short-chain carbohydrates that are poorly absorbed, and a significant portion of these ingested carbohydrates enter the distal small bowel and colon [103]. These sugars include fructose, lactose, sugar alcohols (sorbitol, maltitol, mannitol, xylitol, and isomalt), fructans, and galactans. Fructose and lactose are present in apples, pears, watermelon, honey, fruit juices, dried fruits, and milk and milk products. Polyols are used in low-calorie food products. Galactans and fructans are present in wheat, rye, artichokes, asparagus, broccoli and Brussels sprouts, cabbage, garlic, leeks, onions, legumes, lentils, and soy [90,91,104].

FODMAPs increase the osmotic pressure within the large intestine and provide a substrate for bacteria fermentation, leading to gas production and distension of the large intestine. An increase in the intraluminal pressure can stimulate the release of serotonin and substance P into the interstitial fluid. Serotonin activates the submucosal sensory branch of the enteric nervous system (ENS), which conveys the sensation to the central nervous system (CNS), probably causing abdominal pain and discomfort [105–107]. Furthermore, serotonin controls gastrointestinal motility and chloride secretion via interneurons and motor neurons, which may result in motility and secretion disturbances [105–107]. Although increasing dietary fiber intake is still recommended for patients with IBS, especially those with IBS-C, clinical practice shows that this increases abdominal pain, bloating, and distension [108]. However, it has been shown that soluble fiber intake is effective in improving overall IBS symptoms and has fewer side effects than insoluble fiber [44–46,109–111].

The fermentation of FODMAPs and insoluble fiber to produce gas and intraluminal distention depends upon the composition of the intestinal flora. A dominance of *Clostridium* spp. in the intestinal flora over beneficial bacteria such as *Lactobacillus* and *Bifidobacterium* spp., which do not produce gas upon fermenting carbohydrates, would worsen the IBS symptoms [1]. On the other hand, consuming foods supplemented with probiotics that contain these latter bacteria would increase tolerance to both FODMAPs and fiber [1].

ABNORMALITIES IN THE ENDOCRINE SYSTEM OF THE GUT IN IRRITABLE BOWEL SYNDROME

The Endocrine System of the Gut

The field of endocrinology originated in 1902 following the discovery of secretin by Bayliss and Starling [112,113]. Despite the dominance of the concept of nervism in controlling the gut function, which was introduced by Pavlov in the nineteenth century, it has now been established that the gut is an endocrine organ that controls its own function [114]. This was possible due to the development of novel techniques for the isolation, purification, and measurement of a large number of recently discovered gut hormones [115]. It is currently believed that the gut is controlled by a complicated integrated mechanism that includes both endocrine and nervous components, which interact with each other [1]. This regulatory system—which lies within the gut and communicates with the CNS—is called the neuroendocrine system (NES) of the gut [1,107].

The gut NES is a local regulatory system that controls the primary gut functions (i.e. the digestion and absorption of nutrients) by regulating gut motility, secretion, absorption, microcirculation, local immune defense, and cell proliferation [1,107]. Moreover, to optimize the digestion and absorption processes, the gut NES regulates appetite and the secretion of many gut hormones in order to reduce food intake and limit meal size [115].

The NES of the gut consists of two parts: (1) endocrine cells that are spread between the epithelial cells of the mucosa facing the gut lumen; and (2) peptidergic and serotonergic as well as nitric oxide-containing nerves of the ENS in the gut wall. The NES of the gut comprises a large number of bioactive messengers that act via endocrine, paracrine, or neuroendocrine pathways, or by synaptic signaling. The different components of this system interact and are integrated both with each other and with the afferent and efferent nerve fibers of the CNS [1]. The gut intraluminal content of carbohydrates, proteins, or fat triggers the release of different signaling substance of the NES of the gut (Fig. 1.1) [1,107].

Abnormalities in Gut Endocrine Cells in Patients with Irritable Bowel Syndrome

There seems to be a general depletion of gut endocrine cells in patients with sporadic IBS [51,116,117]. Several abnormalities in the density of gut endocrine cells have been described in both sporadic and postinfectious IBS patients (Tables 1.1 and 1.2) [55,118–132]. It is noteworthy that the abnormalities observed are structural and not merely changes in hormone concentration. Changes

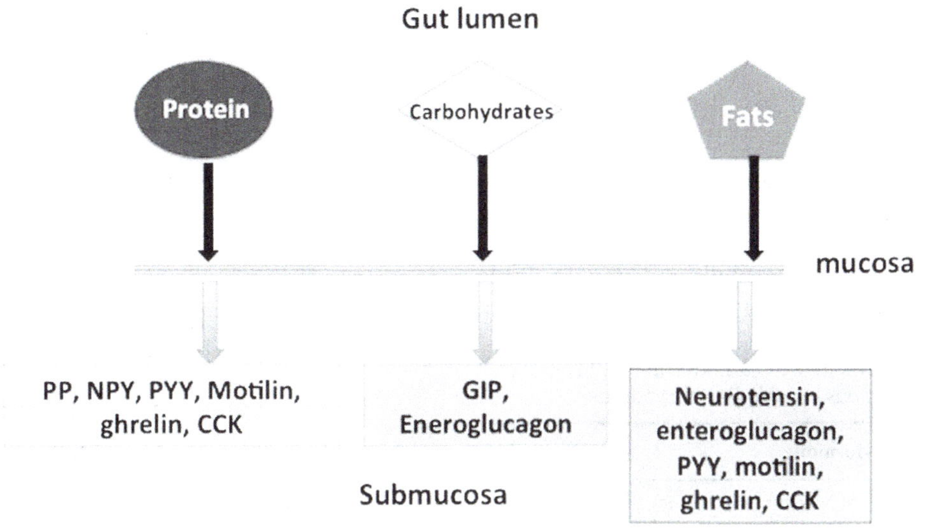

FIGURE 1.1 Schematic drawing of triggering the release of different gut hormones by the intraluminal of nutrient content. Depending upon the intraluminal content of proteins, carbohydrates, or fat, a particular gut hormone is released into the interstitial fluid, where it may act via endocrine/paracrine action or as a neurotransmitters/neuromodulators on the neurons in the enteric nervous system. CCK, cholecystokinin; GIP, gastric inhibitory polypeptide; NPY, neuropeptide Y; PP, pancreatic polypeptide; PYY, peptide YY.

TABLE 1.1 Abnormalities in Gut Endocrine Cells in Patients with Sporadic Irritable Bowel Syndrome

Gastrointestinal structure	Hormone	Cell Density	Hormone Mode of Action
Stomach	Ghrelin	Increased in IBS-D Decreased in IBS-C	Increases appetite and feeding; stimulates gastric and intestinal motility
Duodenum	Gastric inhibitory polypeptide	Decreased	Incretin; inhibits gastric acid secretion
	Somatostatin	Decreased	Inhibits intestinal contraction and exocrine and neuroendocrine secretion
	Secretin	Decreased in IBS-D	Stimulates pancreatic bicarbonate and fluid secretion; inhibits gastric and intestinal motility
	Cholecystokinin	Decreased in IBS-D	Inhibits gastric motility; stimulates gallbladder contraction and intestinal motility; stimulates pancreatic exocrine secretion and growth; inhibits food intake
Ileum	Serotonin	Decreased	Stimulates gastric and intestinal motility; activates the submucosal sensory branch of the enteric nervous system
	Peptide YY	Increased in IBS-C	Delays gastric emptying; inhibits gastric and pancreatic secretion; major ileal brake mediator; regulates appetite
Colon	Serotonin	Decreased	Stimulates gastric and intestinal motility; activates the submucosal sensory branch of the enteric nervous system
	Peptide YY	Decreased	Delays gastric emptying; inhibits gastric and pancreatic secretion; major ileal brake mediator; regulates appetite
Rectum	Peptide YY	Decreased	Delays gastric emptying; inhibits gastric and pancreatic secretion; major ileal brake mediator; regulates appetite
	Enteroglucagon (oxyntomodulin)	Decreased	Reduces gastric motility and secretion; regulates appetite.
	Somatostatin	Increased	Inhibits intestinal contraction and exocrine and neuroendocrine secretion

IBS-C, irritable bowel syndrome, constipation predominant; IBS-D, irritable bowel syndrome, diarrhea predominant.

in hormone levels reflect hormone synthesis and release in response to a physiologic condition, while structural changes represent a longstanding condition with long-term consequences. The abnormalities listed in Table 1.1 may explain the abnormal gastrointestinal secretion, motility, and visceral hypersensitivity seen in patients with IBS.

TABLE 1.2 Abnormalities in the Gut Endocrine Cell Densities in Patients with Postinfectious Irritable Bowel Syndrome

Gastrointestinal Structure	Hormone	Cell Density
Duodenum	Cholecystokinin	Increased
	Serotonin	Increased
Large intestine	Serotonin	Increased
	Peptide YY	Increased

IRRITABLE BOWEL SYNDROME AND APPETITE-REGULATING GUT HORMONES

Appetite regulation is complex and involves a large number of peptide hormones, several of which are gut hormones [115]. Many gut hormones act on the hypothalamic centers of appetite control [115]. The arcuate nucleus (ARC), which acts as the center for integrating neurological and blood-borne signals, lies in the median eminence. This region lacks a complete blood-brain barrier and is thus susceptible to factors circulating in the blood [133–135]. Similarly, the brainstem is proximal to other regions with an incomplete blood-brain barrier, allowing it to receive blood-borne signals [115,135]. The intake of palatable foods (hedonic feeding) is controlled by the brain reward system in the midbrain, which is modulated by blood-borne signals [135].

The function of five hormones known to be involved in appetite regulation are altered in the gut of IBS patients: ghrelin, cholecystokinin (CCK), peptide YY (PYY), enteroglucagon (oxyntomodulin), and serotonin. Ghrelin is an orexigenic hormone, while CCK, PYY, enteroglucagon, and serotonin are anorexigenic hormones.

Ghrelin is a 28-amino-acid peptide hormone that was first isolated from the stomach [124,136–138]. The major source of circulating ghrelin is endocrine cells of the oxyntic mucosa of the stomach, but small amounts are expressed in the small intestine, the large intestine, and the ARC of the hypothalamus [136–139]. Ghrelin has several functions, including regulating the release of somatotropin/growth hormone (GH) from the pituitary gland, where it acts synergistically with the GH-releasing hormone [136–139]. Moreover, ghrelin accelerates gastric and intestinal motility [140–153]. Ghrelin also increases appetite and feeding and plays a major role in energy metabolism [115,135]. Thus, both central and peripheral administration of ghrelin stimulates food intake and body weight gain [136]. Ghrelin is involved in meal initiation: ghrelin plasma levels rise during fasting and fall upon eating, and are inversely correlated with body weight. Moreover, basal ghrelin levels rise after weight loss [154–164]. As mentioned above, patients with IBS-D have a high density of ghrelin-producing cells, while in IBS-C the density of these cells is low (Fig. 1.2) [118]. However, the plasma ghrelin level in these patients does not appear to differ from that of healthy controls [118,119,165]. It has been postulated that the change in the number of ghrelin units (cells) is compensated by a change in synthesis and/or release of this hormone and that symptoms develop when there is fatigue in this compensation mechanism [118]. This change in ghrelin implies an increase in appetite and food intake in IBS-D, and a corresponding decrease in IBS-C.

In addition to the functions of CCK shown in Table 1.1, this hormone has an anorexigenic action [166–177]. There are two receptors for CCK: CCK-A and CCK-B (or CCK-1 and CCK-2, respectively) [178–182]. Both receptor subtypes are distributed throughout the CNS and gut, although CCK-A receptors predominate in the gut and CCK-B receptors predominate in the brain [178–182]. The density of duodenal CCK cells is reported to be reduced in sporadic IBS (Fig. 1.3) and increased in postinfectious IBS [120,121]. An increase in food intake

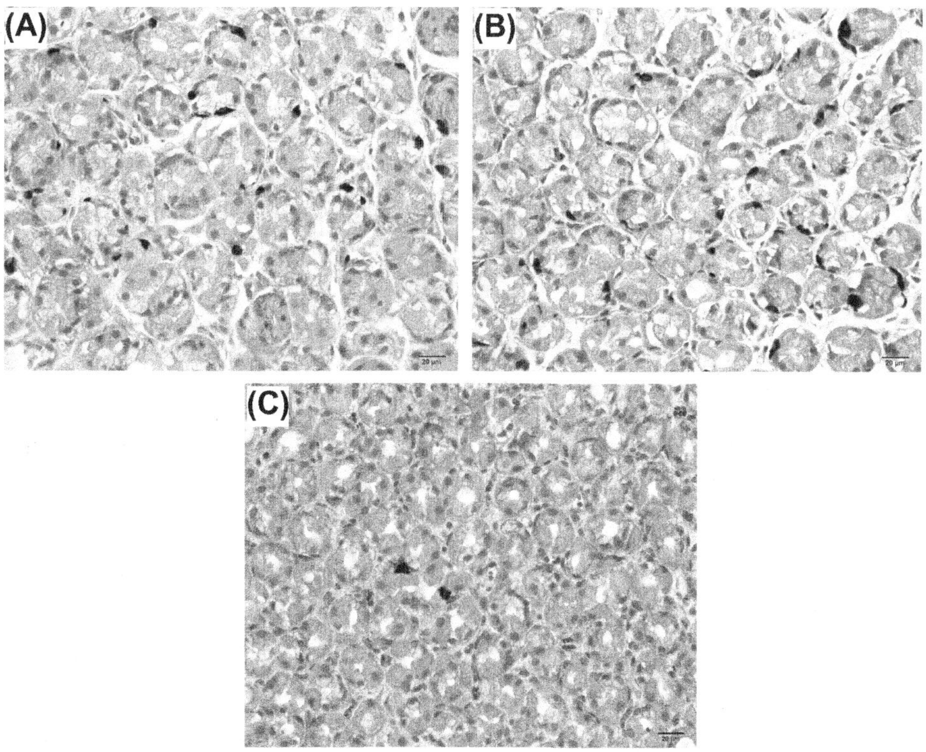

FIGURE 1.2 Ghrelin-immunoreactive cells in the oxyntic mucosa of a healthy subject (A), a patient with irritable bowel syndrome, diarrhea predominant (B) and a patient with irritable bowel syndrome, constipation predominant (C).

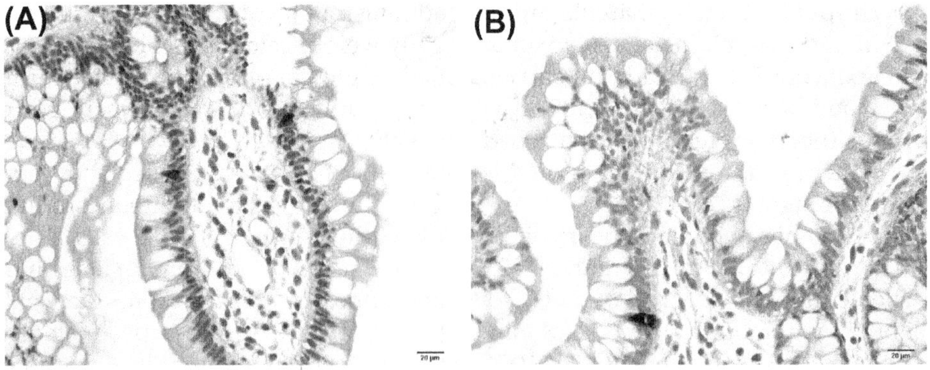

FIGURE 1.3 Cholecystokinin-producing cells in the duodenum of a healthy subject (A) and a patient with irritable bowel syndrome (B).

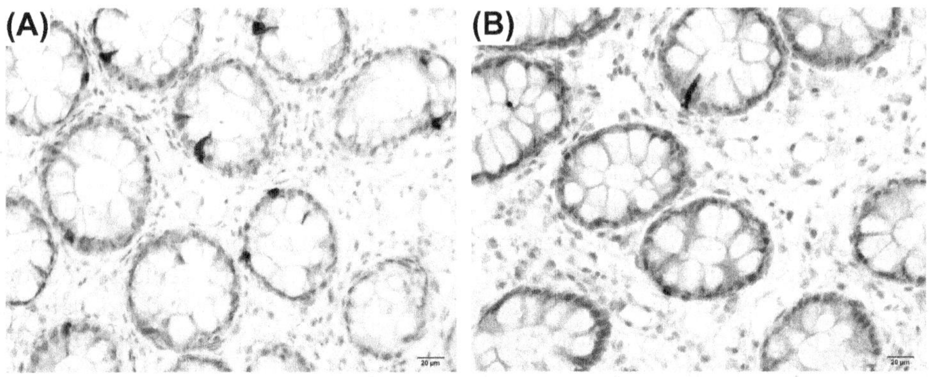

FIGURE 1.4 Peptide YY-immunoreactive cells in the colon of a healthy subject (A) and a patient with irritable bowel syndrome (B).

in sporadic IBS and decreased food intake in postinfectious IBS is therefore to be expected.

PYY is released into the circulation following a meal in proportion to the calories ingested and the meal composition [183]. Infusion of $PYY_{3\text{-}36}$ reduced food consumption during test meals, and obese subjects had a low PYY plasma level [184,185]. Circulating $PYY_{3\text{-}36}$ binds to Y2 receptors on the presynaptic terminals of hypothalamic neuropeptide Y (NPY) and agouti-related protein (AgRP) neurons, and inactivation of these neurons is associated with the induction of anorexia [186]. PYY is a major regulator of the ileal brake in that it acts to inhibit further food intake once nutrients, and especially lipids, have reached the distal small intestine (ileum) [187–196]. The density of PYY cells is generally decreased in sporadic IBS (Table 1.1 and Fig. 1.4). However, whether this increases food intake and appetite in IBS patients remains to be established.

Enteroglucagon is released into the blood circulation following food ingestion in proportion to the amount of calories ingested [197,198]. It has some effect on incretin and reduces gastric motility and secretion [199–204]. However, enteroglucagon is considered to have only a modest anorexigenic effect [135]. Serotonin is also known to exert an anorexigenic effect [205]. The densities of enteroglucagon- and serotonin-producing cells are reduced in patients with IBS, which might have an impact on their food intake and appetite.

While several appetite-regulating gut hormones are altered in patients with IBS, body mass index (BMI) and appetite have not been studied in detail, and the few available data are controversial. Thus, while Simrén et al. reported that most of the 330 IBS patients they examined were normal or overweight, Kubo et al. found that low BMI was associated with IBS in the 367 patients they investigated [57,206]. It is noteworthy that several studies found that food intake in IBS patients did not differ from that of the normal control population [60–66]. It has yet to be determined whether IBS patients have increased appetite or whether the avoidance of eating because of worsening of symptoms upon eating prevents excessive food intake and therefore excessive weight gain. Further studies are needed to clarify this issue.

EFFECT OF DIETARY GUIDANCE

Dietary guidance should include information regarding the importance of regular meals and healthy eating habits, the avoidance of dietary FOODMAPs, and the insoluble fiber content of the dietary components and to avoid them. This guidance should also include helping patients to identify the food items that they do not tolerate well [63,66]. the provision of dietary guidance to IBS patients resulted in the consumption of a better diet with respect to vitamins and minerals. In addition, patients were made aware of FODMAP-rich food items so that these could be avoided or consumed in low quantities, ultimately resulting in reduced symptoms and an improved quality of life [63]. Patients also consumed more food items supplemented with *Lactobacillus* and *Bifidobacterium* spp. which in turn increased their tolerance to FOODMAPs [63].

CONCLUSION

IBS is a common gastrointestinal disorder. Although it does not develop into a serious disease or increase mortality, it does considerably reduce the quality of life of the patients and is an economic burden to society. Diet plays an important role in the development of IBS symptoms. IBS symptoms can be caused by the intake of FODMAP-rich foods, the dominance of *Clostridium spp.* in the intestinal flora, and abnormalities in gut endocrine cells. Guidance aimed at establishing healthy eating habits, the avoidance of FODMAP-rich food and insoluble fiber, and adjusting the dietary composition reduces symptoms and improves the quality of life in IBS patients. Several of the endocrine cells that produce anorexigenic gut hormones are depleted in IBS patients. However, the possible impact on appetite and BMI in IBS patients is unknown; further studies are therefore urgently needed to clarify this issue.

References

[1] El-Salhy M, Gundersen D, Hatlebakk JG, Hausken T. Irritable bowel syndrome: diagnosis, pathogenesis and treatment options. New York: Nova Science Publishers, Inc.; 2012.
[2] Ford AC, Vandvik PO. Irritable bowel syndrome. Clin Evid 2012;01:410.
[3] Quigley EM, Locke GR, Mueller-Lissner S, et al. Prevalence and management of abdominal cramping and pain: a multinational survey. Aliment Pharmacol Ther 2006;24:411–9.
[4] Vandvik PO, Lydersen S, Farup PG. Prevalence, comorbidity and impact of irritable bowel syndrome in Norway. Scand J Gastroenterol 2006;41:650–6.
[5] Drossman DA, Li Z, Andruzzi E, et al. U.S. householder survey of functional gastrointestinal disorders. Prevalence, sociodemography, and health impact. Dig Dis Sci 1993;38:1569–80.
[6] Wong RK, Drossman DA, Weinland SR, et al. Partner burden in irritable bowel syndrome. Clin Gastroenterol Hepatol 2013;11:151–5.
[7] Saito YA, Schoenfeld P, Locke 3rd GR. The epidemiology of irritable bowel syndrome in North America: a systematic review. Am J Gastroenterol 2002;97:1910–5.
[8] Locke 3rd GR, Yawn BP, Wollan PC, Melton 3rd LJ, Lydick E, Talley NJ. Incidence of a clinical diagnosis of the irritable bowel syndrome in a United States population. Aliment Pharmacol Ther 2004;19:1025–31.
[9] Lovell RM, Ford AC. Global prevalence of and risk factors for irritable bowel syndrome: a meta-analysis. Clin Gastroenterol Hepatol 2012;10:712–21.
[10] Whorwell PJ, Clouter C, Smith CL. Oesophageal motility in the irritable bowel syndrome. BMJ 1981;282:1101–2.
[11] Caballero-Plasencia AM, Valenzuela-Barranco M, Herrerias-Gutierrez JM, Esteban-Carretero JM. Altered gastric emptying in patients with irritable bowel syndrome. Eur J Nucl Med 1999;26:404–9.
[12] Evans PR, Bak YT, Shuter B, Hoschl R, Kellow JE. Gastroparesis and small bowel dysmotility in irritable bowel syndrome. Dig Dis Sci 1997;42:2087–93.
[13] van Wijk HJ, Smout AJ, Akkermans LM, Roelofs JM, ten Thije OJ. Gastric emptying and dyspeptic symptoms in the irritable bowel syndrome. Scand J Gastroenterol 1992;27:99–102.
[14] Cann PA, Read NW, Brown C, Hobson N, Holdsworth CD. Irritable bowel syndrome: relationship of disorders in the transit of a single solid meal to symptom patterns. Gut 1983;24(5):405–11.
[15] Kellow JE, Phillips SF. Altered small bowel motility in irritable bowel syndrome is correlated with symptoms. Gastroenterology 1987;92(6):1885–93.
[16] Kellow JE, Phillips SF, Miller LJ, Zinsmeister AR. Dysmotility of the small intestine in irritable bowel syndrome. Gut 1988;29(9):1236–43.
[17] Mertz H, Naliboff B, Munakata J, Niazi N, Mayer EA. Altered rectal perception is a biological marker of patients with irritable bowel syndrome. Gastroenterology 1995;109(1):40–52.
[18] Lembo T, Munakata J, Mertz H, et al. Evidence for the hypersensitivity of lumbar splanchnic afferents in irritable bowel syndrome. Gastroenterology 1994;107(6):1686–96.
[19] Munakata J, Naliboff B, Harraf F, et al. Repetitive sigmoid stimulation induces rectal hyperalgesia in patients with irritable bowel syndrome. Gastroenterology 1997;112(1):55–63.
[20] Van Ginkel R, Voskuijl WP, Benninga MA, Taminiau JA, Boeckxstaens GE. Alterations in rectal sensitivity and motility in childhood irritable bowel syndrome. Gastroenterology 2001;120(1):31–8.
[21] Verne GN, Robinson ME, Price DD. Hypersensitivity to visceral and cutaneous pain in the irritable bowel syndrome. Pain 2001;93(1):7–14.
[22] Kanazawa M, Hongo M, Fukudo S. Visceral hypersensitivity in irritable bowel syndrome. J Gastroenterol Hepatol 2011;26(Suppl. 3):119–21.
[23] Nozu T, Okumura T. Visceral sensation and irritable bowel syndrome; with special reference to comparison with functional abdominal pain syndrome. J Gastroenterol Hepatol 2011;26(Suppl. 3):122–7.
[24] Manabe N, Wong BS, Camilleri M, Burton D, McKinzie S, Zinsmeister AR. Lower functional gastrointestinal disorders: evidence of abnormal colonic transit in a 287 patient cohort. Neurogastroenterol Motil 2010;22:293-e82.
[25] Sadik R, Bjornsson E, Simren M. The relationship between symptoms, body mass index, gastrointestinal transit and stool frequency in patients with irritable bowel syndrome. Eur J Gastroenterol Hepatol 2010;22:102–8.
[26] Whitehead WE, Burnett CK, Cook 3rd EW, Taub E. Impact of irritable bowel syndrome on quality of life. Dig Dis Sci 1996;41:2248–53.
[27] Gralnek IM, Hays RD, Kilbourne A, Naliboff B, Mayer EA. The impact of irritable bowel syndrome on health-related quality of life. Gastroenterology 2000;119:654–60.
[28] Pace F, Molteni P, Bollani S, et al. Inflammatory bowel disease versus irritable bowel syndrome: a hospital-based, case-control study of disease impact on quality of life. Scand J Gastroenterol 2003;38:1031–8.

[29] Sloth H, Jorgensen LS. Chronic non-organic upper abdominal pain: diagnostic safety and prognosis of gastrointestinal and non-intestinal symptoms. A 5- to 7-year follow-up study. Scand J Gastroenterol 1988;23:1275–80.
[30] Harvey RF, Mauad EC, Brown AM. Prognosis in the irritable bowel syndrome: a 5-year prospective study. Lancet 1987;1:963–5.
[31] Norgaard M, Farkas DK, Pedersen L, et al. Irritable bowel syndrome and risk of colorectal cancer: a Danish nationwide cohort study. Br J Cancer 2011;104:1202–6.
[32] Mitchell CM, Drossman DA. Survey of the AGA membership relating to patients with functional gastrointestinal disorders. Gastroenterology 1987;92:1282–4.
[33] Schuster MM. Defining and diagnosing irritable bowel syndrome. Am J Manag Care 2001;7:S246–51.
[34] Hungin AP, Whorwell PJ, Tack J, Mearin F. The prevalence, patterns and impact of irritable bowel syndrome: an international survey of 40,000 subjects. Aliment Pharmacol Ther 2003;17:643–50.
[35] Talley NJ, Gabriel SE, Harmsen WS, Zinsmeister AR, Evans RW. Medical costs in community subjects with irritable bowel syndrome. Gastroenterology 1995;109:1736–41.
[36] Jones R, Lydeard S. Irritable bowel syndrome in the general population. BMJ 1992;304:87–90.
[37] Bordie AK. Functional disorders of the colon. J Indian Med Assoc 1972;58:451–6.
[38] O'Keefe EA, Talley NJ, Zinsmeister AR, Jacobsen SJ. Bowel disorders impair functional status and quality of life in the elderly: a population-based study. J Gerontol A Biol Sci Med Sci 1995;50:M184–9.
[39] Everhart JE, Renault PF. Irritable bowel syndrome in office-based practice in the United States. Gastroenterology 1991;100:998–1005.
[40] Wilson S, Roberts L, Roalfe A, Bridge P, Singh S. Prevalence of irritable bowel syndrome: a community survey. Br J Gen Pract 2004;54:495–502.
[41] Harvey RF, Salih SY, Read AE. Organic and functional disorders in 2000 gastroenterology outpatients. Lancet 1983;1(8325):632–4.
[42] Peery AF, Dellon ES, Lund J, et al. Burden of gastrointestinal disease in the United States: 2012 update. Gastroenterology 2012;143:1179–87. e1-3
[43] Sandler RS, Everhart JE, Donowitz M, et al. The burden of selected digestive diseases in the United States. Gastroenterology 2002;122:1500–11.
[44] Longstreth GF, Thompson WG, Chey WD, Houghton LA, Mearin F, Spiller RC. Functional bowel disorders. Gastroenterology 2006;130:1480–91.
[45] Guilera M, Balboa A, Mearin F. Bowel habit subtypes and temporal patterns in irritable bowel syndrome: systematic review. Am J Gastroenterol 2005;100:1174–84.
[46] Mearin F, Balboa A, Badia X, et al. Irritable bowel syndrome subtypes according to bowel habit: revisiting the alternating subtype. Eur J Gastroenterol Hepatol 2003;15:165–72.
[47] Mearin F, Baro E, Roset M, Badia X, Zarate N, Perez I. Clinical patterns over time in irritable bowel syndrome: symptom instability and severity variability. Am J Gastroenterol 2004;99:113–21.
[48] Drossman DA, Morris CB, Hu Y, et al. A prospective assessment of bowel habit in irritable bowel syndrome in women: defining an alternator. Gastroenterology 2005;128:580–9.
[49] Tillisch K, Labus JS, Naliboff BD, et al. Characterization of the alternating bowel habit subtype in patients with irritable bowel syndrome. Am J Gastroenterol 2005;100:896–904.
[50] Spiller RC. Potential biomarkers. Gastroenterol Clin North Am 2011;40:121–39.
[51] El-Salhy M, Lomholt-Beck B, Hausken T. Chromogranin A as a possible tool in the diagnosis of irritable bowel syndrome. Scand J Gastroenterol 2010;45:1435–9.
[52] Ghoshal UC, Park H, Gwee KA. Bugs and irritable bowel syndrome: the good, the bad and the ugly. J Gastroenterol Hepatol 2010;25:244–51.
[53] McKeown ES, Parry SD, Stansfield R, Barton JR, Welfare MR. Postinfectious irritable bowel syndrome may occur after non-gastrointestinal and intestinal infection. Neurogastroenterol Motil 2006;18:839–43.
[54] Longstreth GF, Haweekey CJ, Mayer EA, et al. Characteristics of patients with irritable bowel syndrome recruited from three sources: implications for clinical trials. Aliment Pharmacol Ther 2001;15:959–64.
[55] Spiller R, Campbell E. Post-infectious irritable bowel syndrome. Curr Opin Gastroenterol 2006;22:13–17.
[56] Spiller R, Garsed K. Infection, inflammation, and the irritable bowel syndrome. Dig Liver Dis 2009;41:844–9.
[57] Simren M, Mansson A, Langkilde AM, et al. Food-related gastrointestinal symptoms in the irritable bowel syndrome. Digestion 2001;63:108–15.
[58] Nanda R, James R, Smith H, Dudley CR, Jewell DP. Food intolerance and the irritable bowel syndrome. Gut 1989;30:1099–104.
[59] Monsbakken KW, Vandvik PO, Farup PG. Perceived food intolerance in subjects with irritable bowel syndrome—etiology, prevalence and consequences. Eur J Clin Nutr 2006;60:667–72.
[60] Jarrett M, Heitkemper MM, Bond EF, Georges J. Comparison of diet composition in women with and without functional bowel disorder. Gastroenterol Nurs 1994;16:253–8.
[61] Saito YA, Locke 3rd GR, Weaver AL, Zinsmeister AR, Talley NJ. Diet and functional gastrointestinal disorders: a population-based case-control study. Am J Gastroenterol 2005;100:2743–8.
[62] Williams EA, Nai X, Corfe BM. Dietary intakes in people with irritable bowel syndrome. BMC Gastroenterol 2011;11:9.
[63] Ostgaard H, Hausken T, Gundersen D, El-Salhy M. Diet and effects of diet management on quality of life and symptoms in patients with irritable bowel syndrome. Mol Med Rep 2012;5:1382–90.
[64] Bohn L, Storsrud S, Simren M. Nutrient intake in patients with irritable bowel syndrome compared with the general population. Neurogastroenterol Motil 2013;25:23-e1.
[65] Ligaarden SC, Lydersen S, Farup PG. Diet in subjects with irritable bowel syndrome: a cross-sectional study in the general population. BMC Gastroenterol 2012;12:61.
[66] El-Salhy M, Ostgaard H, Gundersen D, Hatlebakk JG, Hausken T. The role of diet in the pathogenesis and management of irritable bowel syndrome (Review). Int J Mol Med 2012;29:723–31.
[67] Vesa TH, Seppo LM, Marteau PR, Sahi T, Korpela R. Role of irritable bowel syndrome in subjective lactose intolerance. Am J Clin Nutr 1998;67:710–5.
[68] Zar S, Benson MJ, Kumar D. Food-specific serum IgG4 and IgE titers to common food antigens in irritable bowel syndrome. Am J Gastroenterol 2005;100:1550–7.
[69] Dainese R, Galliani EA, De Lazzari F, Di Leo V, Naccarato R. Discrepancies between reported food intolerance and sensitization test findings in irritable bowel syndrome patients. Am J Gastroenterol 1999;94:1892–7.
[70] Uz E, Turkay C, Aytac S, Bavbek N. Risk factors for irritable bowel syndrome in Turkish population: role of food allergy. J Clin Gastroenterol 2007;41:380–3.
[71] Park MI, Camilleri M. Is there a role of food allergy in irritable bowel syndrome and functional dyspepsia? A systematic review. Neurogastroenterol Motil 2006;18:595–607.
[72] Bischoff S, Crowe SE. Gastrointestinal food allergy: new insights into pathophysiology and clinical perspectives. Gastroenterology 2005;128:1089–113.

[73] Murch S. Allergy and intestinal dysmotility—evidence of genuine causal linkage? Curr Opin Gastroenterol 2006;22:664–8.

[74] Tobin MC, Moparty B, Farhadi A, DeMeo MT, Bansal PJ, Keshavarzian A. Atopic irritable bowel syndrome: a novel subgroup of irritable bowel syndrome with allergic manifestations. Ann Allergy Asthma Immunol 2008;100:49–53.

[75] Petitpierre M, Gumowski P, Girard JP. Irritable bowel syndrome and hypersensitivity to food. Ann Allergy 1985;54:538–40.

[76] Gui XY. Mast cells: a possible link between psychological stress, enteric infection, food allergy and gut hypersensitivity in the irritable bowel syndrome. J Gastroenterol Hepatol 1998;13:980–9.

[77] Zar S, Kumar D, Benson MJ. Food hypersensitivity and irritable bowel syndrome. Aliment Pharmacol Ther 2001;15:439–49.

[78] Atkinson W, Sheldon TA, Shaath N, Whorwell PJ. Food elimination based on IgG antibodies in irritable bowel syndrome: a randomised controlled trial. Gut 2004;53:1459–64.

[79] Whorwell PJ. The growing case for an immunological component to irritable bowel syndrome. Clin Exp Allergy 2007;37:805–7.

[80] Hunter JO. Food elimination in IBS: the case for IgG testing remains doubtful. Gut 2005;54:1203. [author reply]

[81] Teufel M, Biedermann T, Rapps N, et al. Psychological burden of food allergy. World J Gastroenterol 2007;13:3456–65.

[82] Beyer K, Teuber SS. Food allergy diagnostics: scientific and unproven procedures. Curr Opin Allergy Clin Immunol 2005;5:261–6.

[83] Ortolani C, Bruijnzeel-Koomen C, Bengtsson U, et al. Controversial aspects of adverse reactions to food. European Academy of Allergology and Clinical Immunology (EAACI) reactions to food subcommittee. Allergy 1999;54:27–45.

[84] Walker MM, Talley NJ. Functional gastrointestinal disorders and the potential role of eosinophils. Gastroenterol Clin North Am 2008;37:383–95. [vi]

[85] Heizer WD, Southern S, McGovern S. The role of diet in symptoms of irritable bowel syndrome in adults: a narrative review. J Am Diet Assoc 2009;109:1204–14.

[86] Carroccio A, Mansueto P, Iacono G, et al. Non-celiac wheat sensitivity diagnosed by double-blind placebo-controlled challenge: exploring a new clinical entity. Am J Gastroenterol 2012;107:1898–906. [quiz 907]

[87] Aziz I, Sanders DS. Emerging concepts: from coeliac disease to non-coeliac gluten sensitivity. Proc Nutr Soc 2012;71:576–80.

[88] Newnham ED. Does gluten cause gastrointestinal symptoms in subjects without coeliac disease? J Gastroenterol Hepatol 2011;26(Suppl. 3):132–4.

[89] Wahnschaffe U, Schulzke JD, Zeitz M, Ullrich R. Predictors of clinical response to gluten-free diet in patients diagnosed with diarrhea-predominant irritable bowel syndrome. Clin Gastroenterol Hepatol 2007;5:844–50. [quiz 769]

[90] Morcos A, Dinan T, Quigley EM. Irritable bowel syndrome: role of food in pathogenesis and management. J Dig Dis 2009;10:237–46.

[91] Eswaran S, Tack J, Chey WD. Food: the forgotten factor in the irritable bowel syndrome. Gastroenterol Clin North Am 2011;40:141–62.

[92] Frissora CL, Koch KL. Symptom overlap and comorbidity of irritable bowel syndrome with other conditions. Curr Gastroenterol Rep 2005;7:264–71.

[93] El-Salhy M, Lomholt-Beck B, Gundersen D. The prevalence of celiac disease in patients with irritable bowel syndrome. Mol Med Rep 2011;4:403–5.

[94] Fasano A, Berti I, Gerarduzzi T, et al. Prevalence of celiac disease in at-risk and not-at-risk groups in the United States: a large multicenter study. Arch Intern Med 2003;163:286–92.

[95] Catassi C, Kryszak D, Louis-Jacques O, et al. Detection of Celiac disease in primary care: a multicenter case-finding study in North America. Am J Gastroenterol 2007;102:1454–60.

[96] van der Wouden EJ, Nelis GF, Vecht J. Screening for coeliac disease in patients fulfilling the Rome II criteria for irritable bowel syndrome in a secondary care hospital in The Netherlands: a prospective observational study. Gut 2007;56:444–5.

[97] Locke 3rd GR, Murray JA, Zinsmeister AR, Melton 3rd LJ, Talley NJ. Celiac disease serology in irritable bowel syndrome and dyspepsia: a population-based case-control study. Mayo Clin Proc 2004;79:476–82.

[98] Hin H, Bird G, Fisher P, Mahy N, Jewell D. Coeliac disease in primary care: case finding study. BMJ 1999;318:164–7.

[99] Shahbazkhani B, Forootan M, Merat S, et al. Coeliac disease presenting with symptoms of irritable bowel syndrome. Aliment Pharmacol Ther 2003;18:231–5.

[100] Korkut E, Bektas M, Oztas E, Kurt M, Cetinkaya H, Ozden A. The prevalence of celiac disease in patients fulfilling Rome III criteria for irritable bowel syndrome. Eur J Intern Med 2010;21:389–92.

[101] Sanders DS, Patel D, Stephenson TJ, et al. A primary care cross-sectional study of undiagnosed adult coeliac disease. Eur J Gastroenterol Hepatol 2003;15:407–13.

[102] Verdu EF, Armstrong D, Murray JA. Between celiac disease and irritable bowel syndrome: the "no man's land" of gluten sensitivity. Am J Gastroenterol 2009;104:1587–94.

[103] Barrett JS, Gibson PR. Fermentable oligosaccharides, disaccharides, monosaccharides and polyols (FODMAPs) and nonallergic food intolerance: FODMAPs or food chemicals? Ther Adv Gastroenterol 2012;5:261–8.

[104] Biesiekierski JR, Rosella O, Rose R, et al. Quantification of fructans, galacto-oligosacharides and other short-chain carbohydrates in processed grains and cereals. J Hum Nutr Diet 2011;24:154–76.

[105] Kuwahara A, Kuramoto H, Kadowaki M. 5-HT activates nitric oxide-generating neurons to stimulate chloride secretion in guinea pig distal colon. Am J Physiol 1998;275:G829–34.

[106] Gershon MD. Plasticity in serotonin control mechanisms in the gut. Curr Opin Pharmacol 2003;3:600–7.

[107] El-Salhy M, Seim I, Chopin L, Gundersen D, Hatlebakk JG, Hausken T. Irritable bowel syndrome: the role of gut neuroendocrine peptides. Front Biosci (Elite Ed) 2012;4:2783–800.

[108] Bijkerk CJ, Muris JW, Knottnerus JA, Hoes AW, de Wit NJ. Systematic review: the role of different types of fibre in the treatment of irritable bowel syndrome. Aliment Pharmacol Ther 2004;19:245–51.

[109] Ford AC, Talley NJ, Spiegel BM, et al. Effect of fibre, antispasmodics, and peppermint oil in the treatment of irritable bowel syndrome: systematic review and meta-analysis. BMJ 2008;337:a2313.

[110] Francis CY, Whorwell PJ. Bran and irritable bowel syndrome: time for reappraisal. Lancet 1994;344:39–40.

[111] Bijkerk CJ, de Wit NJ, Muris JW, Whorwell PJ, Knottnerus JA, Hoes AW. Soluble or insoluble fibre in irritable bowel syndrome in primary care? Randomised placebo controlled trial. BMJ 2009;339:b3154.

[112] Bayliss WM, Starling EH. The mechanism of pancreatic secretion. J Physiol 1902;28:325–53.

[113] Chey WY, Chang TM. Secretin, 100 years later. J Gastroenterol 2003;38:1025–35.

[114] Modlin IM, Champaneria MC, Bornschein J, Kidd M. Evolution of the diffuse neuroendocrine system—clear cells and cloudy origins. Neuroendocrinology 2006;84:69–82.

[115] Chaudhri O, Small C, Bloom S. Gastrointestinal hormones regulating appetite. Philos Trans R Soc Lond B Biol Sci 2006;361:1187–209.

[116] El-Salhy M, Mazzawi T, Gundersen D, Hausken T. Chromogranin A cell density in the rectum of patients with irritable bowel syndrome. Mol Med Rep 2012;6:1223–5.
[117] El-Salhy M, Wendelbo I, Gundersen D. Reduced chromogranin A cell density in the ileum of patients with irritable bowel syndrome. Mol Med Rep 2013;7(4):1241–4.
[118] El-Salhy M, Lillebo E, Reinemo A, Salmelid L. Ghrelin in patients with irritable bowel syndrome. Int J Mol Med 2009;23:703–7.
[119] El-Salhy M. Ghrelin in gastrointestinal diseases and disorders: a possible role in the pathophysiology and clinical implications (review). Int J Mol Med 2009;24:727–32.
[120] El-Salhy M, Vaali K, Dizdar V, Hausken T. Abnormal small-intestinal endocrine cells in patients with irritable bowel syndrome. Dig Dis Sci 2010;55:3508–13.
[121] Dizdar V, Spiller R, Singh G, et al. Relative importance of abnormalities of CCK and 5-HT (serotonin) in Giardia-induced post-infectious irritable bowel syndrome and functional dyspepsia. Aliment Pharmacol Ther 2010;31:883–91.
[122] El-Salhy M, Gundersen D, Ostgaard H, Lomholt-Beck B, Hatlebakk JG, Hausken T. Low densities of serotonin and peptide YY cells in the colon of patients with irritable bowel syndrome. Dig Dis Sci 2012;57:873–8.
[123] Spiller RC, Jenkins D, Thornley JP, et al. Increased rectal mucosal enteroendocrine cells, T lymphocytes, and increased gut permeability following acute *Campylobacter* enteritis and in post-dysenteric irritable bowel syndrome. Gut 2000;47:804–11.
[124] Dunlop SP, Jenkins D, Neal KR, Spiller RC. Relative importance of enterochromaffin cell hyperplasia, anxiety, and depression in postinfectious IBS. Gastroenterology 2003;125:1651–9.
[125] Lee KJ, Kim YB, Kim JH, Kwon HC, Kim DK, Cho SW. The alteration of enterochromaffin cell, mast cell, and lamina propria T lymphocyte numbers in irritable bowel syndrome and its relationship with psychological factors. J Gastroenterol Hepatol 2008;23:1689–94.
[126] Wang SH, Dong L, Luo JY, et al. Decreased expression of serotonin in the jejunum and increased numbers of mast cells in the terminal ileum in patients with irritable bowel syndrome. World J Gastroenterol 2007;13:6041–7.
[127] Park JH, Rhee PL, Kim G, et al. Enteroendocrine cell counts correlate with visceral hypersensitivity in patients with diarrhoea-predominant irritable bowel syndrome. Neurogastroenterol Motil 2006;18:539–46.
[128] Van Der Veek PP, Biemond I, Masclee AA. Proximal and distal gut hormone secretion in irritable bowel syndrome. Scand J Gastroenterol 2006;41:170–7.
[129] Kim HS, Lim JH, Park H, Lee SI. Increased immunoendocrine cells in intestinal mucosa of postinfectious irritable bowel syndrome patients 3 years after acute Shigella infection—an observation in a small case control study. Yonsei Med J 2010;51:45–51.
[130] Coates MD, Mahoney CR, Linden DR, et al. Molecular defects in mucosal serotonin content and decreased serotonin reuptake transporter in ulcerative colitis and irritable bowel syndrome. Gastroenterology 2004;126:1657–64.
[131] El-Salhy M, Gundersen D, Hatlebakk JG, Hausken T. Abnormal rectal endocrine cells in patients with irritable bowel syndrome, Regul Pept 2013, in press.
[132] El-Salhy M, Gundersen D, Hatlebakk JG, Hausken T. Abnormal endocrine cells in the ileum of patients with irritable bowel syndrome, World J Gastroenterol 2013, in press.
[133] Peruzzo B, Pastor FE, Blazquez JL, et al. A second look at the barriers of the medial basal hypothalamus. Exp Brain Res 2000;132:10–26.
[134] Cone RD, Cowley MA, Butler AA, Fan W, Marks DL, Low MJ. The arcuate nucleus as a conduit for diverse signals relevant to energy homeostasis. Int J Obes Relat Metab Disord 2001;25(Suppl. 5):S63–7.
[135] Yu JH, Kim MS. Molecular mechanisms of appetite regulation. Diabetes Metab J 2012;36:391–8.
[136] Kojima M, Hosoda H, Date Y, Nakazato M, Matsuo H, Kangawa K. Ghrelin is a growth-hormone-releasing acylated peptide from stomach. Nature 1999;402:656–60.
[137] Kojima M, Hosoda H, Kangawa K. Purification and distribution of ghrelin: the natural endogenous ligand for the growth hormone secretagogue receptor. Horm Res 2001;56(Suppl. 1):93–7.
[138] Kojima M, Hosoda H, Matsuo H, Kangawa K. Ghrelin: discovery of the natural endogenous ligand for the growth hormone secretagogue receptor. Trends Endocrinol Metab 2001;12:118–22.
[139] Date Y, Kojima M, Hosoda H, et al. Ghrelin, a novel growth hormone-releasing acylated peptide, is synthesized in a distinct endocrine cell type in the gastrointestinal tracts of rats and humans. Endocrinology 2000;141:4255–61.
[140] Masuda Y, Tanaka T, Inomata N, et al. Ghrelin stimulates gastric acid secretion and motility in rats. Biochem Biophys Res Commun 2000;276:905–8.
[141] Fujino K, Inui A, Asakawa A, Kihara N, Fujimura M, Fujimiya M. Ghrelin induces fasted motor activity of the gastrointestinal tract in conscious fed rats. J Physiol 2003;550:227–40.
[142] Asakawa A, Ataka K, Fujino K, et al. Ghrelin family of peptides and gut motility. J Gastroenterol Hepatol 2011;26(Suppl. 3):73–4.
[143] Dornonville de la Cour C, Lindstrom E, Norlen P, Hakanson R. Ghrelin stimulates gastric emptying but is without effect on acid secretion and gastric endocrine cells. Regul Pept 2004;120:23–32.
[144] Fukuda H, Mizuta Y, Isomoto H, et al. Ghrelin enhances gastric motility through direct stimulation of intrinsic neural pathways and capsaicin-sensitive afferent neurones in rats. Scand J Gastroenterol 2004;39:1209–14.
[145] Edholm T, Levin F, Hellstrom PM, Schmidt PT. Ghrelin stimulates motility in the small intestine of rats through intrinsic cholinergic neurons. Regul Pept 2004;121:25–30.
[146] Levin F, Edholm T, Schmidt PT, et al. Ghrelin stimulates gastric emptying and hunger in normal-weight humans. J Clin Endocrinol Metab 2006;91:3296–302.
[147] Tack J, Depoortere I, Bisschops R, et al. Influence of ghrelin on interdigestive gastrointestinal motility in humans. Gut 2006;55:327–33.
[148] Ariga H, Tsukamoto K, Chen C, Mantyh C, Pappas TN, Takahashi T. Endogenous acyl ghrelin is involved in mediating spontaneous phase III-like contractions of the rat stomach. Neurogastroenterol Motil 2007;19:675–80.
[149] Ariga H, Nakade Y, Tsukamoto K, et al. Ghrelin accelerates gastric emptying via early manifestation of antro-pyloric coordination in conscious rats. Regul Pept 2008;146:112–6.
[150] Tumer C, Oflazoglu HD, Obay BD, Kelle M, Tasdemir E. Effect of ghrelin on gastric myoelectric activity and gastric emptying in rats. Regul Pept 2008;146:26–32.
[151] Tebbe JJ, Mronga S, Tebbe CG, Ortmann E, Arnold R, Schafer MK. Ghrelin-induced stimulation of colonic propulsion is dependent on hypothalamic neuropeptide Y1- and corticotrophin-releasing factor 1 receptor activation. J Neuroendocrinol 2005;17:570–6.
[152] Fujimiya M, Ataka K, Asakawa A, Chen CY, Kato I, Inui A. Regulation of gastroduodenal motility: acyl ghrelin, des-acyl ghrelin and obestatin and hypothalamic peptides. Digestion 2012;85:90–4.
[153] Ogiso K, Asakawa A, Amitani H, Inui A. Ghrelin: a gut hormonal basis of motility regulation and functional dyspepsia. J Gastroenterol Hepatol 2011;26(Suppl. 3):67–72.

[154] Callahan HS, Cummings DE, Pepe MS, Breen PA, Matthys CC, Weigle DS. Postprandial suppression of plasma ghrelin level is proportional to ingested caloric load but does not predict intermeal interval in humans. J Clin Endocrinol Metab 2004;89:1319–24.
[155] Cummings DE. Ghrelin and the short- and long-term regulation of appetite and body weight. Physiol Behav 2006;89:71–84.
[156] Cummings DE, Foster-Schubert KE, Overduin J. Ghrelin and energy balance: focus on current controversies. Curr Drug Targets 2005;6:153–69.
[157] Cummings DE, Frayo RS, Marmonier C, Aubert R, Chapelot D. Plasma ghrelin levels and hunger scores in humans initiating meals voluntarily without time- and food-related cues. Am J Physiol Endocrinol Metab 2004;287:E297–304.
[158] Cummings DE, Overduin J. Gastrointestinal regulation of food intake. J Clin Invest 2007;117:13–23.
[159] Cummings DE, Purnell JQ, Frayo RS, Schmidova K, Wisse BE, Weigle DS. A preprandial rise in plasma ghrelin levels suggests a role in meal initiation in humans. Diabetes 2001;50:1714–9.
[160] Cummings DE, Shannon MH. Roles for ghrelin in the regulation of appetite and body weight. Arch Surg 2003;138:389–96.
[161] Cummings DE, Weigle DS, Frayo RS, et al. Plasma ghrelin levels after diet-induced weight loss or gastric bypass surgery. N Engl J Med 2002;346:1623–30.
[162] Foster-Schubert KE, McTiernan A, Frayo RS, et al. Human plasma ghrelin levels increase during a one-year exercise program. J Clin Endocrinol Metab 2005;90:820–5.
[163] Foster-Schubert KE, Overduin J, Prudom CE, et al. Acyl and total ghrelin are suppressed strongly by ingested proteins, weakly by lipids, and biphasically by carbohydrates. J Clin Endocrinol Metab 2008;93:1971–9.
[164] Overduin J, Figlewicz DP, Bennett-Jay J, Kittleson S, Cummings DE. Ghrelin increases the motivation to eat, but does not alter food palatability. Am J Physiol Regul Integr Comp Physiol 2012;303:R259–69.
[165] Sjolund K, Ekman R, Wierup N. Covariation of plasma ghrelin and motilin in irritable bowel syndrome. Peptides 2010;31:1109–12.
[166] Corwin RL, Gibbs J, Smith GP. Increased food intake after type A but not type B cholecystokinin receptor blockade. Physiol Behav 1991;50:255–8.
[167] Gibbs J, Falasco JD, McHugh PR. Cholecystokinin-decreased food intake in rhesus monkeys. Am J Physiol 1976;230:15–18.
[168] Gibbs J, Smith GP. Satiety: the roles of peptides from the stomach and the intestine. Fed Proc 1986;45:1391–5.
[169] Gibbs J, Smith GP. Cholecystokinin and satiety in rats and rhesus monkeys. Am J Clin Nutr 1977;30:758–61.
[170] Smith GP, Falasco J, Moran TH, Joyner KM, Gibbs J. CCK-8 decreases food intake and gastric emptying after pylorectomy or pyloroplasty. Am J Physiol 1988;255:R113–6.
[171] Smith GP, Gibbs J. Role of CCK in satiety and appetite control. Clin Neuropharmacol 1992;15(Suppl. 1 Pt A):476A.
[172] Smith GP, Gibbs J. Gut peptides and postprandial satiety. Fed Proc 1984;43:2889–92.
[173] Smith GP, Gibbs J. Cholecystokinin: a putative satiety signal. Pharmacol Biochem Behav 1975;3:135–8.
[174] Smith GP, Tyrka A, Gibbs J. Type-A CCK receptors mediate the inhibition of food intake and activity by CCK-8 in 9- to 12-day-old rat pups. Pharmacol Biochem Behav 1991;38:207–10.
[175] Stallone D, Nicolaidis S, Gibbs J. Cholecystokinin-induced anorexia depends on serotoninergic function. Am J Physiol 1989;256:R1138–41.
[176] Weller A, Smith GP, Gibbs J. Endogenous cholecystokinin reduces feeding in young rats. Science 1990;247:1589–91.
[177] Woods SC, Gibbs J. The regulation of food intake by peptides. Ann N Y Acad Sci 1989;575:236–43.
[178] Huppi K, Siwarski D, Pisegna JR, Wank S. Chromosomal localization of the gastric and brain receptors for cholecystokinin (CCKAR and CCKBR) in human and mouse. Genomics 1995;25:727–9.
[179] Silvente-Poirot S, Wank SA. A segment of five amino acids in the second extracellular loop of the cholecystokinin-B receptor is essential for selectivity of the peptide agonist gastrin. J Biol Chem 1996;271:14698–706.
[180] Tarasova NI, Stauber RH, Choi JK, et al. Visualization of G protein-coupled receptor trafficking with the aid of the green fluorescent protein. Endocytosis and recycling of cholecystokinin receptor type A. J Biol Chem 1997;272:14817–24.
[181] Tarasova NI, Wank SA, Hudson EA, et al. Endocytosis of gastrin in cancer cells expressing gastrin/CCK-B receptor. Cell Tissue Res 1997;287:325–33.
[182] Wank SA. Cholecystokinin receptors. Am J Physiol 1995;269:G628–46.
[183] Adrian TE, Ferri GL, Bacarese-Hamilton AJ, Fuessl HS, Polak JM, Bloom SR. Human distribution and release of a putative new gut hormone, peptide YY. Gastroenterology 1985;89:1070–7.
[184] Batterham RL, Cohen MA, Ellis SM, et al. Inhibition of food intake in obese subjects by peptide YY3-36. N Engl J Med 2003;349:941–8.
[185] Batterham RL, Cowley MA, Small CJ, et al. Gut hormone PYY(3–36) physiologically inhibits food intake. Nature 2002;418:650–4.
[186] Michel MC, Beck-Sickinger A, Cox H, et al. XVI International Union of Pharmacology recommendations for the nomenclature of neuropeptide Y, peptide YY, and pancreatic polypeptide receptors. Pharmacol Rev 1998;50:143–50.
[187] Lin HC, Zhao XT, Wang L. Jejunal brake: inhibition of intestinal transit by fat in the proximal small intestine. Dig Dis Sci 1996;41:326–9.
[188] Lin HC, Zhao XT, Wang L. Intestinal transit is more potently inhibited by fat in the distal (ileal brake) than in the proximal (jejunal brake) gut. Dig Dis Sci 1997;42:19–25.
[189] Lin HC, Zhao XT, Wang L, Wong H. Fat-induced ileal brake in the dog depends on peptide YY. Gastroenterology 1996;110:1491–5.
[190] Van Citters GW, Lin HC. The ileal brake: a fifteen-year progress report. Curr Gastroenterol Rep 1999;1:404–9.
[191] Ohtani N, Sasaki I, Naito H, Shibata C, Matsuno S. Mediators for fat-induced ileal brake are different between stomach and proximal small intestine in conscious dogs. J Gastrointest Surg 2001;5:377–82.
[192] Pironi L, Stanghellini V, Miglioli M, et al. Fat-induced ileal brake in humans: a dose-dependent phenomenon correlated to the plasma levels of peptide YY. Gastroenterology 1993;105:733–9.
[193] Van Citters GW, Lin HC. Ileal brake: neuropeptidergic control of intestinal transit. Curr Gastroenterol Rep 2006;8:367–73.
[194] Maljaars J, Peters HP, Masclee AM. Review article: the gastrointestinal tract: neuroendocrine regulation of satiety and food intake. Aliment Pharmacol Ther 2007;26(Suppl. 2):241–50.
[195] Maljaars PW, Peters HP, Mela DJ, Masclee AA. Ileal brake: a sensible food target for appetite control. A review. Physiol Behav 2008;95:271–81.
[196] Maljaars PW, Symersky T, Kee BC, Haddeman E, Peters HP, Masclee AA. Effect of ileal fat perfusion on satiety and hormone release in healthy volunteers. Int J Obes (Lond) 2008;32:1633–9.
[197] Ghatei MA, Uttenthal LO, Christofides ND, Bryant MG, Bloom SR. Molecular forms of human enteroglucagon in tissue and plasma: plasma responses to nutrient stimuli in health and in disorders of the upper gastrointestinal tract. J Clin Endocrinol Metab 1983;57:488–95.
[198] Le Quellec A, Kervran A, Blache P, Ciurana AJ, Bataille D. Oxyntomodulin-like immunoreactivity: diurnal profile of a new potential enterogastrone. J Clin Endocrinol Metab 1992;74:1405–9.

[199] Dubrasquet M, Bataille D, Gespach C. Oxyntomodulin (glucagon-37 or bioactive enteroglucagon): a potent inhibitor of pentagastrin-stimulated acid secretion in rats. Biosci Rep 1982;2:391–5.

[200] Dubrasquet M, Roze C, Ling N, Florencio H. Inhibition of gastric and pancreatic secretions by cerebroventricular injections of gastrin-releasing peptide and bombesin in rats. Regul Pept 1982;3:105–12.

[201] Schjoldager B, Mortensen PE, Myhre J, Christiansen J, Holst JJ. Oxyntomodulin from distal gut. Role in regulation of gastric and pancreatic functions. Dig Dis Sci 1989;34:1411–9.

[202] Schjoldager BT, Baldissera FG, Mortensen PE, Holst JJ, Christiansen J. Oxyntomodulin: a potential hormone from the distal gut. Pharmacokinetics and effects on gastric acid and insulin secretion in man. Eur J Clin Invest 1988;18:499–503.

[203] Dakin CL, Small CJ, Batterham RL, et al. Peripheral oxyntomodulin reduces food intake and body weight gain in rats. Endocrinology 2004;145:2687–95.

[204] Wynne K, Park AJ, Small CJ, et al. Subcutaneous oxyntomodulin reduces body weight in overweight and obese subjects: a double-blind, randomized, controlled trial. Diabetes 2005;54:2390–5.

[205] Fang XL, Shu G, Yu JJ, et al. The anorexigenic effect of serotonin is mediated by the generation of NADPH oxidase-dependent ROS. PloS One 2013;8:e53142.

[206] Kubo M, Fujiwara Y, Shiba M, et al. Differences between risk factors among irritable bowel syndrome subtypes in Japanese adults. Neurogastroenterol Motil 2011;23:249–54.

CHAPTER

2

Work and Abdominal Obesity Risk

Maria Teresa Anselmo Olinto[a,b], *Raquel Canuto*[c,d], *and Anderson da Silva Garcez*[a]

[a]Postgraduate Program in Collective Health, University of Vale do Rios dos Sinos, RS, Brazil;
[b]Department of Nutrition, Federal University of Health Science of Porto Alegre, RS, Brazil;
[c]Department of Nutrition, University of Vale do Rios dos Sinos, RS, Brazil;
[d]Department of Nutrition, University of Caxias do Sul, RS, Brazil

Understanding the determinants of obesity is important for global public health and the global economy. The etiology of obesity is multifaceted, involving interactions between individuals and their social, cultural, and physical environments. Traditionally, the causes of general obesity (as well as abdominal obesity) have been linked to an imbalance between caloric intake and physical activity [1]. However, modern life has led to other changes in human behavior, such as those influenced by work and the workplace.

Therefore, several researchers have focused on occupational health to investigate the role of certain work characteristics as possible risk factors for abdominal obesity. In these studies, an increased prevalence of abdominal obesity has been associated with working position, job strain, physical activity at work, shift work, and unemployment. Thus, this section focuses on how such work characteristics influence the occurrence of abdominal obesity, with the aim of advancing our understanding of factors associated with abdominal obesity among workers.

OCCUPATIONAL STATUS

An individual's occupation indicates certain levels of status and power, which reflect the material and symbolic capital related to the conditions at work. Occupation-based indicators may be related to health not only through issues such as differential accessibility to health care but also by reflecting social networks or psychosocial processes that are associated with health outcomes. Thus, several studies have investigated the relationship between employment grade and changes in cardiometabolic factors worldwide.

Two studies conducted in European countries (the United Kingdom and Norway) investigated the relationship between occupational status and waist circumference (WC) in both sexes: they concluded that participants at higher employment grades had smaller WCs [2,3]. A study in Portugal examined the gender-specific prevalence of variations in WC across occupational levels. Among women, there was an inverse correlation between occupation and abdominal obesity. However, abdominal obesity was not associated with occupation among men [4].

The gender-specific association between occupational status and abdominal obesity is more evident among Asian workers. Two studies conducted in Japan and China reported higher levels of abdominal obesity among management-level males compared with other male workers. In contrast, a higher waist-hip ratio (WHR) was recorded in female laborers compared with female engineers [5,6]. Similarly, a Cameroon study found that, in men only, the risk of abdominal obesity was significantly higher for those at high compared with low occupational levels [7].

Therefore, the influence of occupational status on the occurrence of abdominal adiposity is gender dependent. Women with higher status positions are protected from abdominal obesity; men in the same positions are at an increased risk.

In addition to gender, abdominal obesity may be influenced by social position, which is represented by three characteristics: occupational status, education, and income. Occupational status is both a consequence of educational level and a determinant of income level. In investigations of the influence of social position on health outcomes, these three characteristics should be considered simultaneously. Accordingly, we conducted

Nutrition in the Prevention and Treatment of Abdominal Obesity
http://dx.doi.org/10.1016/B978-0-12-407869-7.00002-7

a brief review of the scientific literature (from the last 5 years) concerning studies of the relationships among education, income, and obesity in men and women.

We retrieved 21 studies that examined the relationship between educational status and abdominal obesity. Of the 19 studies with male participants, nine found a positive association between educational status and abdominal obesity [6,8–15], whereas seven demonstrated a negative association [16–22]. However, 15 of 21 studies found higher rates of abdominal obesity among women with lower educational status [9,10,13,14,17–27], and the other five found no association between these two factors in women.

Nine articles regarding the relationship between income and abdominal obesity were retrieved. Of these, five studies reported that income level was positively associated with abdominal obesity in men [6,9,10,12,21]. In women, income was negatively associated with income, according to seven studies [6,9,10,12,21,22,28].

These data provide strong evidence for an association between low social status (income, education, and occupational status) and abdominal obesity in women. Moreover, abdominal obesity is linked to higher social positions in men, although this finding is more controversial than the results for women.

The consequences of social inequality have been more conclusively established for women than for men. However, the link between occupational status (i.e. social position) and abdominal obesity is partly mediated by individual behavioral characteristics (dietary habits, leisure time physical activity, smoking, and physiologic stress). This link is also strongly related to work characteristics, such as job strain and physical activity at work.

JOB STRAIN

Employees throughout the world are currently facing immense challenges, such as an increasingly fast-paced business environment and growing demands for increased productivity [29]. Since 2000, many companies located in industrialized countries have been attempting to dynamically outrun other firms in the global economic race by introducing various managerial innovations, such as just-in-time production and total quality management. As a result, we can expect profound changes in the amount of work stress experienced by employees.

The impact of job stress on health outcome has been studied since the publication of Karasek's model in 1981. According to this model, a combination of a heavy workload (defined as high job demands) and low job control may be experienced by an individual as job strain. Four different types of psychological work experiences were generated by combining high or low job demands with high or low job control (decision latitude). These experiences were divided into four job categories: high-strain jobs, low-strain jobs, active jobs, and passive jobs. Thus, individuals with high job demands and low job control may have an increased risk of mental job strain, which can eventually lead to fatigue, depression, sleeping difficulties, burnout, substance abuse, or other physical ailments. Active jobs with both high demands and high levels of control are considered to be stimulating jobs with fewer negative psychological effects or health risks. Passive jobs, in contrast, do not allow individuals to use their skills; such occupations may lead to psychological strain and diseases [30].

Stress at work is linked to coronary heart disease, according to retrospective and prospective studies, as well as meta-analyses [16,31,32]. Stress may contribute to coronary heart disease via psychological effects on behavior and metabolism; these metabolic changes could directly increase abdominal adiposity. Furthermore, abdominal obesity is an important component of metabolic syndrome [33] and a risk factor for vascular diseases [34,35]. Therefore, several studies have found that work stress is linked to the development of abdominal obesity.

Most studies that investigated this relationship measured work stress using Karasek's Job Strain Questionnaire; they provided evidence that job strain is an independent risk factor for abdominal obesity [36,37]. Major life events and periods of acute stress appear to play a greater role in the onset of general obesity for men than for women, as has been previously reported [38]. Nonetheless, an association between perceived stress and abdominal obesity is present in both sexes [39,40].

Workload stress is a potential determinant of central adiposity that deserves considerable attention. One explanation for the association between workload stress and central adiposity is that the waist-hip circumference ratio and the abdominal sagittal diameter are estimations of body fat centralization that are highly dependent on endocrine status. The central accumulation of fat is a consequence of long-term activation of the hypothalamic-pituitary-adrenal (HPA) axis due to stress. Cortisol, other steroid hormones, and growth are involved in this process. Cortisol activates lipoprotein lipase (LPL), the gatekeeper of lipid accumulation in adipocytes. Furthermore, in the presence of insulin, cortisol inhibits the lipid mobilization system. Because these events are mediated by central glucocorticoid receptors, which are present at a higher density in intra-abdominal visceral fat than in other depots, cortisol activity and the consequent accumulation of fat are accentuated in this adipose tissue [41,42].

Additionally, stress affects the behavior of workers. Almost 50% of the members of a representative sample from the USA who were concerned about the amount of stress in their lives coped by engaging in unhealthy behaviors, such eating to relieve stress [43]. Stress affects eating in a bidirectional fashion: a subset of stressed individuals (approximately 30%) decrease their food intake and lose weight during or after stress, whereas most stressed individuals increase their food intake [44] and exhibit an intensified preference for higher-fat, energy-dense foods [43,45]. Stress has also been shown to reduce leisure time physical activity [46], again potentially favoring a positive energy balance.

Another unhealthy behavior with a high prevalence among workers under stress is smoking [47]. Population-based studies have demonstrated that smokers have a larger WC and WHR than former smokers and never smokers; WHR is positively associated with the number of cigarettes smoked per day [48]. Studies of workers who smoke have demonstrated the same association [36]. For example, in a cross-sectional study in Great Britain, Kwok found that cigarette smoking, particularly smoking >20 cigarettes per day, was associated with a larger WC and WHR [49].

OCCUPATIONAL PHYSICAL ACTIVITY

In recent decades, occupational physical activity levels have been broadly affected by changes in society and in the economy. These changes have been accompanied by a substantial decrease in physically active occupations and an increase in sedentary activities [50,51]. Furthermore, changes in the workplace such as computerization and mechanization may cause workers to be more vulnerable to weight gain; daily occupation-related energy expenditure has exhibited a decreasing trend [50,52]. Thus, occupational physical activity plays an important role in total energy expenditure, i.e. occupation-related physical activity has a significant impact on daily caloric expenditure [50,53].

Because occupational physical activity is an important factor in daily energy expenditure, physically active occupations may help protect against abdominal obesity. Correspondingly, studies have shown an inverse association between the activity level of an occupation and abdominal obesity: workers in high-activity occupations have a reduced risk of abdominal obesity compared with workers in low-activity or sedentary occupations [5,54–60].

Steeves et al. showed that the association between occupational physical activity and abdominal obesity was independent of leisure time, transportation, and domestic activity levels and sociodemographic factors among citizens of the USA [54]. In addition, Chu and Moy showed that occupational physical activity was more strongly associated with abdominal obesity than were household, transportation, and leisure time physical activities among middle-aged adults in a middle-income country [56]. These findings indicate that occupational physical activity level is linked to central adiposity and has an impact on the risk of abdominal obesity that is independent of other types of physical activity.

The association between occupational physical activity and abdominal obesity is also dependent on socioeconomic status (education and income). Individuals with a lower socioeconomic position are more likely to hold jobs with a higher level of occupational physical activity, whereas individuals with a higher socioeconomic position engage in more leisure time physical activity [55,61]. Interestingly, socioeconomic status has a significant impact on the tendency for individuals with higher levels of occupational physical activity to engage in less leisure time activity: subjects from lower socioeconomic levels were less active during leisure time compared with those from higher socioeconomic levels, even after controlling for occupational physical activity [62,63]. Furthermore, occupational and leisure time physical activities may affect each other: most people who classified their jobs as active reported being sedentary in their leisure time [64–66].

In summary, technological and economic factors contribute to low energy expenditures in people's daily routines, including decreases in physical activity levels at work. However, occupational physical activity has been demonstrated to be a protective factor against abdominal obesity: high-activity occupations are associated with a reduced risk of abdominal obesity.

Physical activity behaviors have been demonstrated to provide significant protection against multiple health problems and are associated with a longer life expectancy [67,68]. In recognition of the importance of physical activity for health, a series of recommendations was developed to increase daily physical activity levels in different areas of life, including recreation and leisure time, transportation (e.g. walking or cycling), household chores and work [69].

SHIFT WORK

The prevalence of shift work is increasing in modern society as an important mechanism for greater flexibility in the organization of work schedules. The term *shift work* refers to a work schedule that involves irregular or unusual hours, such as night work or rotating shift work, in contrast to normal daytime work [70]. According to the results of a survey conducted in 2005, more than 17% of European Union workers are employed in the night-shift, with significant variations among the countries (from 6.4% to 30.0%) [71]. Shift work is associated with a higher incidence of several health disorders, including cardiovascular, metabolic, gastrointestinal, and psychiatric disorders [72–75].

Some studies have also reported effects of shift work on abdominal obesity. Amelsvoort et al. found a positive association between the duration of shift work and the WHR [76]. Ishizaki et al. showed that a larger WHR is associated with night work [59]. Another study comparing Japanese male shift workers with day workers showed a greater tendency toward central obesity among the shift workers [77]. De Bacquer et al. evaluated the relationship between employment in rotating shifts and the incidence of metabolic syndrome. By separately analyzing the components of metabolic syndrome, the authors observed that the risk of abdominal obesity was greater among rotating shift workers compared with dayshift workers [72]. Among Iranian drivers, shift work was also associated with the occurrence of abdominal obesity: shift workers were 49% more likely to exhibit abdominal obesity compared with day workers [78]. A Brazilian study of employees of a 24-h poultry processing plant found nightshift work to be associated with abdominal obesity: nightshift workers were 45% more likely to exhibit abdominal obesity compared with dayshift workers [79]. Furthermore, a recent systematic review found strong evidence for an association between shift work and weight gain [75].

The precise mechanisms that link shift work to abdominal obesity and metabolic disturbances are not well understood. Shift workers experience desynchronized circadian rhythms because they work at a time that is physiologically better suited to sleep [80]. Moreover, these workers are prone to sleep deprivation as a direct consequence of shift work [81,82]. Thus, the scientific literature has explained the independent impacts of these two risk factors on the occurrence of metabolic disorders.

All metabolic processes are related to the circadian system. In adipose tissue, for example, adipocytes must adjust the rates of triglyceride synthesis, storage, and breakdown over a period of 24 h. Adipocytes also express certain factors, such as leptin, adipsin, resistin, and adiponectin, in a rhythmic fashion. Additionally, disruption of the circadian system leads to the dysregulation of glucose metabolism. This dysfunctional response can also contribute to the pathophysiology of metabolic disorders such as visceral obesity [80,83].

Chronic sleep deprivation in humans is associated with changes in thermoregulation, i.e. reductions in overall energy expenditure. Furthermore, sleep deprivation may increase an individual's total caloric intake by affecting peripheral regulators of satiety. Studies have linked sleep deprivation to decreases in leptin levels and increases in ghrelin levels; consequently, increases in appetite and weight gain are observed [84–88].

Moreover, shift workers have irregular eating habits due to the temporal reorganization of food consumption. Most studies have found no association between total energy intake and dietary nutrient content. However, studies have found a redistribution of food consumption among shift workers; i.e. these workers eat larger numbers of smaller meals throughout the day compared with individuals who work day shifts [88–91]. Lennernas et al. reported that such reorganization resulted in a higher consumption of food among nightshift workers [88]. A higher consumption of food during the night may contribute to desynchronization of the rhythmicity of glucose and triglycerides, resulting in increased abdominal fat deposits and dyslipidemias [92,93].

UNEMPLOYMENT

As detailed above, several characteristics of work are strongly linked to worker morbidities, such as abdominal obesity. However, an individual must be relatively healthy to be employable, and both morbidity and mortality rates are usually lower within the workforce than in the general population. Thus, although increased morbidity may occur due to harmful exposures at work, unemployment is also associated with health problems.

Accordingly, the study of unemployment and its relationship with health has expanded over the last four decades. Unemployment has also been linked to a higher prevalence of risky health behaviors, including problematic alcohol consumption and smoking [40,94]; a higher rate of all-cause mortality [95]; and higher rates of cardiovascular illnesses [96] and metabolic disturbances [97], including general obesity [97–99] and abdominal obesity [40,100].

Unemployment is a state, whereas job loss is an event that leads to unemployment unless a new job is obtained immediately. The state of unemployment emerged largely as a product of the machine age and the exchange of goods. With the introduction of wage rates that allowed individuals to purchase (rather than produce) the goods that they needed and wanted, maintaining a viable wage rate became critical to an individual's survival. As a result, individuals depend on various occupations and can no longer provide for themselves. Thus, unemployment has become a problem for many individuals, often in both economic and psychological terms [101].

We demonstrated in the previous sections that abdominal obesity is associated with the gender and

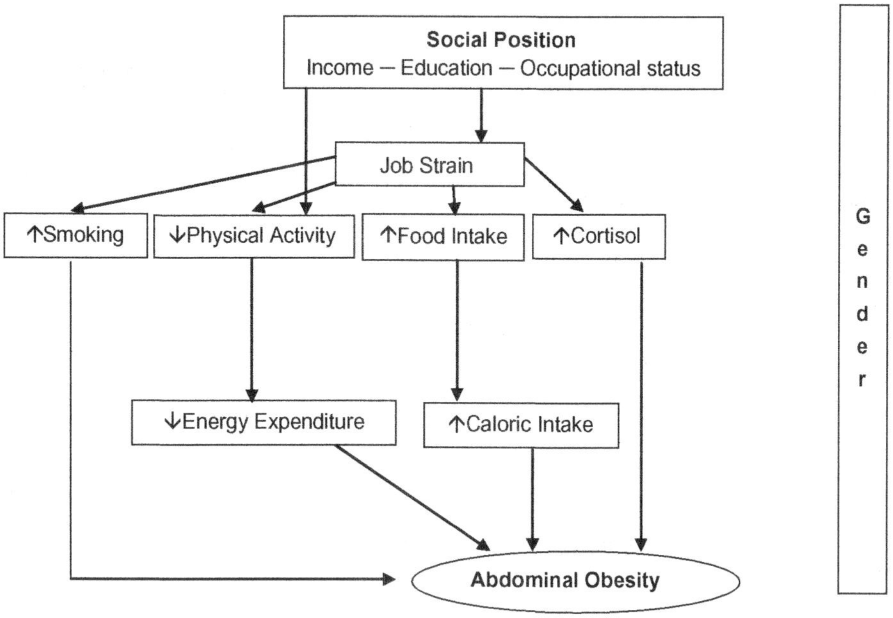

FIGURE 2.1 Causal pathway between social position and abdominal obesity.

social position of workers. The direction of this association is more evident in women than in men: a lower social position is associated with a higher prevalence of abdominal obesity [9,100]. Similarly, studies have reported that unemployment produces different health consequences for men and women [100–103].

European, Canadian, Mexican, and Brazilian population studies have demonstrated a clear association between employment status and abdominal obesity in women: employed women had smaller WCs and WHRs than their unemployed counterparts [39,100,104–106]. However, this association has not been found in men [40].

CONCLUSION

In this chapter, we have shown how work characteristics influence the occurrence of abdominal obesity. Changes in the occupational environment may directly contribute to the epidemic of abdominal obesity. The rapid shift toward more sedentary work with less physical activity is an obvious risk factor for abdominal obesity. There is also evidence that psychosocial factors, such as job strain, occupational position, and shift work, may contribute to abdominal obesity; however, the temporal trends of these potential risk factors are less obvious. Unemployment is another important risk factor for abdominal obesity because it is linked to a higher prevalence of risky health behaviors, including problematic alcohol consumption and smoking.

Therefore, abdominal obesity is influenced by gender and socioeconomic factors. Fig. 2.1 depicts the causal pathway between social position and abdominal obesity. Occupational status or unemployment, education, and income constitute a group of characteristics that represent the social position of an individual. Thus, the influence of work characteristics on the occurrence of abdominal adiposity should be investigated in terms of the gender and social position of individuals. The consequences of social inequality are more deleterious for women than for men. Women of low socioeconomic status (i.e. low educational and income levels) have a higher prevalence of abdominal obesity compared with women of higher socioeconomic status. Likewise, women who are unemployed, who work at a low occupational level, or who experience job strain are at a greater risk of abdominal obesity. However, independent of gender and social position, the pathway that leads from work characteristics to abdominal obesity is mediated by risk behavior characteristics, such as smoking, dietary habits, occupational and leisure time physical activity, and/or metabolic disturbances.

Ultimately, an examination of the causes of abdominal obesity with a focus on occupational health will improve our understanding of the multifactorial nature of this important health problem. Thus, further studies employing novel methodologies should be conducted to elucidate how work characteristics may represent an important risk factor for abdominal obesity.

References

[1] Cohen DA. Obesity and the built environment: changes in environmental cues cause energy imbalances. Int J Obes (Lond) 2008;32(Suppl. 7):S137–42.

[2] Elovainio M, Ferrie JE, Singh-Manoux A, Shipley M, Batty GD, Head J, et al. Socioeconomic differences in cardiometabolic factors: social causation or health-related selection? Evidence from the Whitehall II Cohort Study, 1991–2004. Am J Epidemiol 2011;174(7):779–89.

[3] Kjollesdal MR, Holmboe-Ottesen G, Mosdol A, Wandel M. The relative importance of socioeconomic indicators in explaining differences in BMI and waist:hip ratio, and the mediating effect of work control, dietary patterns and physical activity. Br J Nutr 2010;104(8):1230–40.

[4] Alves L, Azevedo A, Silva S, Barros H. Socioeconomic inequalities in the prevalence of nine established cardiovascular risk factors in a southern European population. PLoS One 2012;7(5):e37158.

[5] Ishizaki M, Yamada Y, Morikawa Y, Noborisaka Y, Ishida M, Miura K, et al. The relationship between waist-to-hip ratio and occupational status and life-style factors among middle-aged male and female Japanese workers. Occup Med (Lond) 1999;49(3):177–82.

[6] Wang H, Wang J, Liu MM, Wang D, Wang D, Liu YQ, et al. Epidemiology of general obesity, abdominal obesity and related risk factors in urban adults from 33 communities of Northeast China: the CHPSNE study. BMC Public Health 2012;12:967.

[7] Fezeu L, Minkoulou E, Balkau B, Kengne AP, Awah P, Unwin N, et al. Association between socioeconomic status and adiposity in urban Cameroon. Int J Epidemiol 2006;35(1):105–11.

[8] Qin L, Stolk RP, Corpeleijn E. Motorized transportation, social status, and adiposity: the China health and nutrition survey. Am J Prev Med 2012;43(1):1–10.

[9] Yoo S, Cho H-J, Khang Y-H. General and abdominal obesity in South Korea, 1998–2007: gender and socioeconomic differences. Prev Med 2010;51(6):460–5.

[10] Subramanyam MA, Diez-Roux AV, Hickson DA, Sarpong DF, Sims M, Taylor Jr HA, et al. Subjective social status and psychosocial and metabolic risk factors for cardiovascular disease among African Americans in the Jackson Heart Study. Soc Sci Med 2012;74(8):1146–54.

[11] Stewart-Knox B, E Duffy M, Bunting B, Parr H, Vas de Almeida MD, Gibney M. Associations between obesity (BMI and waist circumference) and socio-demographic factors, physical activity, dietary habits, life events, resilience, mood, perceived stress and hopelessness in healthy older Europeans. BMC Public Health 2012;12:424.

[12] Schumann B, Kluttig A, Tiller D, Werdan K, Haerting J, Greiser KH. Association of childhood and adult socioeconomic indicators with cardiovascular risk factors and its modification by age: the CARLA Study 2002–2006. BMC Public Health 2011;11:289.

[13] Rehkopf DH, Dow WH, Rosero-Bixby L. Differences in the association of cardiovascular risk factors with education: a comparison of Costa Rica (CRELES) and the USA (NHANES). J Epidemiol Community Health 2010;64(9):821–8.

[14] Boissonnet C, Schargrodsky H, Pellegrini F, Macchia A, Marcet Champagne B, Wilson E, et al. Educational inequalities in obesity, abdominal obesity, and metabolic syndrome in seven Latin American cities: the CARMELA Study. Eur J Cardiovasc Prev Rehabil 2011;18(4):550–6.

[15] Ford ES, Li C, Zhao G, Tsai J. Trends in obesity and abdominal obesity among adults in the United States from 1999–2008. Int J Obes 2011;35(5):736–43.

[16] Kivimäki M, Nyberg ST, Batty GD, Fransson EI, Heikkilä K, Alfredsson L, et al. IPD-work consortium. Job strain as a risk factor for coronary heart disease: a collaborative meta-analysis of individual participant data. Lancet 2012;380(9852):1491–7.

[17] Hermann S, Rohrmann S, Linseisen J, May AM, Kunst A, Besson H, et al. The association of education with body mass index and waist circumference in the EPIC-PANACEA study. BMC Public Health 2011;11:169.

[18] Gupta R, Deedwania PC, Sharma K, Gupta A, Guptha S, Achari V, et al. Association of educational, occupational and socioeconomic status with cardiovascular risk factors in Asian Indians: a cross-sectional study. PLoS One 2012;7(8):e44098.

[19] Kestila P, Magnussen CG, Viikari JS, Kahonen M, Hutri-Kahonen N, Taittonen L, et al. Socioeconomic status, cardiovascular risk factors, and subclinical atherosclerosis in young adults: the cardiovascular risk in Young Finns Study. Arterioscler Thromb Vasc Biol 2012;32(3):815–21.

[20] Marques-Vidal P, Bochud M, Mooser V, Paccaud F, Waeber G, Vollenweider P. Prevalence of obesity and abdominal obesity in the Lausanne population. BMC Public Health 2008;8:330.

[21] Kavanagh A, Bentley RJ, Turrell G, Shaw J, Dunstan D, Subramanian SV. Socioeconomic position, gender, health behaviours and biomarkers of cardiovascular disease and diabetes. Soc Sci Med 2010;71(6):1150–60.

[22] Schulz AJ, House JS, Israel BA, Mentz G, Dvonch JT, Miranda PY, et al. Relational pathways between socioeconomic position and cardiovascular risk in a multiethnic urban sample: complexities and their implications for improving health in economically disadvantaged populations. J Epidemiol Community Health 2008;62(7):638–46.

[23] Yala SM, Fleck EM, Sciacca R, Castro D, Joseph Z, Giardina EG. Metabolic syndrome and the burden of cardiovascular disease in Caribbean Hispanic women living in northern Manhattan: a red flag for education. Metab Syndr Relat Disord 2009;7(4):315–22.

[24] Shahraki M, Shahraki T, Ansari H. The effects of socio-economic status on BMI, waist:hip ratio and waist circumference in a group of Iranian women. Public Health Nutr 2008;11(07):757–61.

[25] Hajian-Tilaki KO, Heidari B. Association of educational level with risk of obesity and abdominal obesity in Iranian adults. J Public Health 2010;32(2):202–9.

[26] Gronner MF, Bosi PL, Carvalho AM, Casale G, Contrera D, Pereira MA, et al. Prevalence of metabolic syndrome and its association with educational inequalities among Brazilian adults: a population-based study. Braz J Med Biol Res 2011;44:713–9.

[27] de Sousa TF, Nahas MV, Silva DA, Del Duca GF, Peres MA. Factors associated with central obesity in adults from Florianopolis, Santa Catarina: a population based-study. Rev Bras Epidemiol 2011;14(2):296–309.

[28] Sousa TF, Nahas MV, Silva DAS, Del Duca GF, Peres MA. Factors associated with central obesity in adults from Florianópolis, Santa Catarina: a population based-study. Brazilian Journal of Epidemiology 2011;14:296–309.

[29] Kirsten W. Making the link between health and productivity at the workplace—a global perspective. Ind Health 2010;48(3):251–5.

[30] Karasek R, Baker D, Marxer F, Ahlbom A, Theorell T. Job decision latitude, job demands, and cardiovascular disease: a prospective study of Swedish men. Am J Public Health 1981;71(7):694–705.

[31] Chandola T, Brunner E, Marmot M. Chronic stress at work and the metabolic syndrome: prospective study. BMJ 2006;332(7540):521–5. Mar 4

[32] Kivimaki M, Virtanen M, Elovainio M, Kouvonen A, Vaananen A, Vahtera J. Work stress in the etiology of coronary heart disease—a meta-analysis. Scand J Work Environ Health 2006;32 (6):431–42.

[33] Alberti KG, Eckel RH, Grundy SM, Zimmet PZ, Cleeman JI, Donato KA, et al. Harmonizing the metabolic syndrome: a joint interim statement of the International Diabetes Federation Task Force on Epidemiology and Prevention; National Heart, Lung, and Blood Institute; American Heart Association; World Heart Federation; International Atherosclerosis Society; and International Association for the Study of Obesity. Circulation 2009;120(16):1640–5.

[34] Cornier MA, Després JP, Davis N, Grossniklaus DA, Klein S, Lamarche B, et al. American heart association obesity committee of the council on nutrition; physical activity and metabolism; council on arteriosclerosis; thrombosis and vascular biology; council on cardiovascular disease in the young; council on cardiovascular radiology and intervention; council on cardiovascular nursing, council on epidemiology and prevention; council on the kidney in cardiovascular disease, and stroke council. assessing adiposity: a scientific statement from the American heart association. Circulation 2011;124(18):1996–2019.

[35] Klein S, Allison DB, Heymsfield SB, Kelley DE, Leibel RL, Nonas C, et al. Association for weight management and obesity prevention; NAASO, the obesity society; American Society for Nutrition; American Diabetes Association. Waist circumference and cardiometabolic risk: a consensus statement from Shaping America's Health: association for weight management and obesity prevention; NAASO, the obesity society; the American society for nutrition; and the American diabetes association. Am J Clin Nutr 2007;85(5):1197–202.

[36] Brunner EJ, Chandola T, Marmot MG. Prospective effect of job strain on general and central obesity in the Whitehall II Study. Am J Epidemiol 2007;165(7):828–37.

[37] Ishizaki M, Nakagawa H, Morikawa Y, Honda R, Yamada Y, Kawakami N. Influence of job strain on changes in body mass index and waist circumference—6-year longitudinal study. Scand J Work Environ Health 2008;34(4):288–96.

[38] Torres SJ, Nowson CA. Relationship between stress, eating behavior, and obesity. Nutrition 2007;23(11–12):887–94.

[39] Rosmond R, Bjorntorp P. Psychosocial and socio-economic factors in women and their relationship to obesity and regional body fat distribution. Int J Obes Relat Metab Disord 1999;23(2):138–45.

[40] Rosmond R, Lapidus L, Bjorntorp P. The influence of occupational and social factors on obesity and body fat distribution in middle-aged men. Int J Obes Relat Metab Disord 1996;20(7):599–607.

[41] Bjorntorp P. Do stress reactions cause abdominal obesity and comorbidities? Obes Rev 2001;2(2):73–86.

[42] Drapeau V, Therrien F, Richard D, Tremblay A. Is visceral obesity a physiological adaptation to stress? Panminerva Med 2003;45(3):189.

[43] Adam TC, Epel ES. Stress, eating and the reward system. Physiol Behav 2007;91(4):449–58.

[44] Stone AA, Brownell KD. The stress-eating paradox: multiple daily measurements in adult males and females. Psychol Health 1994;9(6):425–36.

[45] Mikolajczyk R, El Ansari W, Maxwell A. Food consumption frequency and perceived stress and depressive symptoms among students in three European countries. Nutr J 2009;8(1):31.

[46] Kouvonen A, Kivimaki M, Cox SJ, Cox T, Vahtera J. Relationship between work stress and body mass index among 45,810 female and male employees. Psychosom Med 2005;67(4):577–83.

[47] Kouvonen A, Kivimaki M, Virtanen M, Pentti J, Vahtera J. Work stress, smoking status, and smoking intensity: an observational study of 46,190 employees. J Epidemiol Community Health 2005;59(1):63–9.

[48] Berlin I. Smoking-induced metabolic disorders: a review. Diab Metab 2008;34(4, Part 1):307–14.

[49] Kwok S, Canoy D, Soran H, Ashton DW, Lowe GD, Wood D, et al. Body fat distribution in relation to smoking and exogenous hormones in British women. Clin Endocrinol (Oxf) 2012;77(6):828–33.

[50] Church TS, Thomas DM, Tudor-Locke C, Katzmarzyk PT, Earnest CP, Rodarte RQ, et al. Trends over 5 decades in U.S. occupation-related physical activity and their associations with obesity. PloS One 2011;6(5):e19657.

[51] Brownson RC, Boehmer TK, Luke DA. Declining rates of physical activity in the United States: what are the contributors? Annu Rev Public Health 2005;26:421–43.

[52] Shimotsu ST, French SA, Gerlach AF, Hannan PJ. Worksite environment physical activity and healthy food choices: measurement of the worksite food and physical activity environment at four metropolitan bus garages. Int J Behav Nutr Phys Act 2007;4:17.

[53] Dong L, Block G, Mandel S. Activities contributing to total energy expenditure in the United States: results from the NHAPS study. Int J Behav Nutr Phys Act 2004;1(1):4.

[54] Steeves JA, Bassett Jr DR, Thompson DL, Fitzhugh EC. Relationships of occupational and non-occupational physical activity to abdominal obesity. Int J Obes (Lond) 2012;36(1): 100–6.

[55] Choi B, Schnall PL, Yang H, Dobson M, Landsbergis P, Israel L, et al. Sedentary work, low physical job demand, and obesity in US workers. Am J Ind Med 2010;53(11):1088–101.

[56] Chu AH, Moy FM. Associations of occupational, transportation, household and leisure-time physical activity patterns with metabolic risk factors among middle-aged adults in a middle-income country. Prev Med 2012;57(Suppl.):S14–7.

[57] Duncan BB, Chambless LE, Schmidt MI, Szklo M, Folsom AR, Carpenter MA, et al. Correlates of body fat distribution. Variation across categories of race, sex, and body mass in the atherosclerosis risk in communities study. The Atherosclerosis Risk in communities (ARIC) study investigators. Ann Epidemiol 1995;5(3):192–200.

[58] Hajian-Tilaki KO, Heidari B. Prevalence of obesity, central obesity and the associated factors in urban population aged 20–70 years, in the north of Iran: a population-based study and regression approach. Obes Rev 2007;8(1):3–10.

[59] Ishizaki M, Morikawa Y, Nakagawa H, Honda R, Kawakami N, Haratani T, et al. The influence of work characteristics on body mass index and waist to hip ratio in Japanese employees. Ind Health 2004;42(1):41–9.

[60] Barengo NC, Kastarinen M, Lakka T, Nissinen A, Tuomilehto J. Different forms of physical activity and cardiovascular risk factors among 24–64-year-old men and women in Finland. Eur J Cardiovasc Prev Rehabil 2006;13(1):51–9.

[61] Beenackers MA, Kamphuis CB, Giskes K, Brug J, Kunst AE, Burdorf A, et al. Socioeconomic inequalities in occupational, leisure-time, and transport related physical activity among European adults: a systematic review. Int J Behav Nutr Phys Act 2012;9:116.

[62] Drygas W, Kwasniewska M, Kaleta D, Pikala M, Bielecki W, Gluszek J, et al. Epidemiology of physical inactivity in Poland: prevalence and determinants in a former communist country in socioeconomic transition. Public Health 2009;123(9):592–7.

[63] Kaleta D, Jegier A. Occupational energy expenditure and leisure-time physical activity. Int J Occup Med Environ Health 2005;18(4):351–6.

[64] Vioque J, Torres A, Quiles J. Time spent watching television, sleep duration and obesity in adults living in Valencia, Spain. Int J Obes Relat Metab Disord 2000;24(12):1683–8.
[65] Caban-Martinez AJ, Lee DJ, Fleming LE, LeBlanc WG, Arheart KL, Chung-Bridges K, et al. Leisure-time physical activity levels of the US workforce. Prev Med 2007;44(5):432–6.
[66] Chau JY, van der Ploeg HP, Merom D, Chey T, Bauman AE. Cross-sectional associations between occupational and leisure-time sitting, physical activity and obesity in working adults. Prev Med 2012;54(3–4):195–200.
[67] WHO. Global health risks: mortality and burden of disease attributable to selected major risks. Geneva: World Health Organization; 2009. <http://www.who.int/healthinfo/global_burden_disease/GlobalHealthRisks_report_full.pdf> [accessed 10.09.13].
[68] Lee IM, Shiroma EJ, Lobelo F, Puska P, Blair SN, Katzmarzyk PT. Effect of physical inactivity on major non-communicable diseases worldwide: an analysis of burden of disease and life expectancy. Lancet 2012;380(9838):219–29.
[69] WHO. Global recommendations on physical activity for health. Geneva: World Health Organization; 2010. <http://www.who.int/dietphysicalactivity/factsheet_recommendations/en/> [accessed 10.09.13].
[70] Morshead DM. Stress and shiftwork. Occup Health Saf 2002;71(4):36–8.
[71] Straif K, Baan R, Grosse Y, Secretan B, Ghissassi FE, Bouvard V, et al. Carcinogenicity of shift-work, painting, and fire-fighting. Lancet Oncol 2007;8(12):1065–6.
[72] De Bacquer D, Van Risseghem M, Clays E, Kittel F, De Backer G, Braeckman L. Rotating shift work and the metabolic syndrome: a prospective study. Int J Epidemiol 2009;38(3):848–54.
[73] Wang XS, Armstrong ME, Cairns BJ, Key TJ, Travis RC. Shift work and chronic disease: the epidemiological evidence. Occup Med (Lond) 2011;61(2):78–89.
[74] Knutsson A, Boggild H. Shiftwork and cardiovascular disease: review of disease mechanisms. Rev Environ Health 2000;15(4):359–72.
[75] van Drongelen A, Boot C, Merkus S, Smid T, van der Beek A. The effects of shift work on body weight change—a systematic review of longitudinal studies. Scand J Work Environ Health 2011.
[76] van Amelsvoort LG, Schouten EG, Kok FJ. Duration of shiftwork related to body mass index and waist to hip ratio. Int J Obes Relat Metab Disord 1999;23(9):973–8.
[77] Nakamura K, Shimai S, Kikuchi S, Tominaga K, Takahashi H, Tanaka M, et al. Shift work and risk factors for coronary heart disease in Japanese blue-collar workers: serum lipids and anthropometric characteristics. Occup Med (Lond) 1997;47(3):142–6.
[78] Mohebbi I, Shateri K, Seyedmohammadzad M. The relationship between working schedule patterns and the markers of the metabolic syndrome: comparison of shift workers with day workers. Int J Occup Med Environ Health 2012;25(4):383–91.
[79] Macagnan J, Pattussi MP, Canuto R, Henn RL, Fassa AG, Olinto MT. Impact of nightshift work on overweight and abdominal obesity among workers of a poultry processing plant in southern Brazil. Chronobiol Int 2012;29(3):336–43.
[80] Garaulet M, Ordovas JM, Madrid JA. The chronobiology, etiology and pathophysiology of obesity. Int J Obes (Lond) 2010;34(12):1667–83.
[81] Biggi N, Consonni D, Galluzzo V, Sogliani M, Costa G. Metabolic syndrome in permanent night workers. Chronobiol Int 2008;25(2):443–54.
[82] Karlsson B, Knutsson A, Lindahl B. Is there an association between shift work and having a metabolic syndrome? Results from a population based study of 27,485 people. Occup Environ Med 2001;58(11):747–52.
[83] Garaulet M, Madrid JA. Chronobiology, genetics and metabolic syndrome. Curr Opin Lipidol 2009;20(2):127–34.
[84] Ogawa Y, Kanbayashi T, Saito Y, Takahashi Y, Kitajima T, Takahashi K, et al. Total sleep deprivation elevates blood pressure through arterial baroreflex resetting: a study with microneurographic technique. Sleep 2003;26(8):986–9.
[85] Gangwisch JE, Heymsfield SB, Boden-Albala B, Buijs RM, Kreier F, Pickering TG, et al. Short sleep duration as a risk factor for hypertension: analyses of the first National Health and Nutrition Examination Survey. Hypertension 2006;47(5):833–9.
[86] Meier-Ewert HK, Ridker PM, Rifai N, Regan MM, Price NJ, Dinges DF, et al. Effect of sleep loss on C-reactive protein, an inflammatory marker of cardiovascular risk. J Am Coll Cardiol 2004;43(4):678–83.
[87] Stamatakis KA, Punjabi NM. Effects of sleep fragmentation on glucose metabolism in normal subjects. Chest 2010;137(1):95–101.
[88] Lennernas M, Hambraeus L, Akerstedt T. Shift related dietary intake in day and shift workers. Appetite 1995;25(3):253–65.
[89] Sudo N, Ohtsuka R. Nutrient intake among female shift workers in a computer factory in Japan. Int J Food Sci Nutr 2001;52(4):367–78.
[90] de Assis MA, Nahas MV, Bellisle F, Kupek E. Meals, snacks and food choices in Brazilian shift workers with high energy expenditure. J Hum Nutr Diet 2003;16(4):283–9.
[91] Reinberg A, Migraine C, Apfelbaum M, Brigant L, Ghata J, Vieux N, et al. Circadian and ultradian rhythms in the feeding behaviour and nutrient intakes of oil refinery operators with shift-work every 3–4 days. Diab Metab 1979;5(1):33–41.
[92] Lennernas M, Akerstedt T, Hambraeus L. Nocturnal eating and serum cholesterol of three-shift workers. Scand J Work Environ Health 1994;20(6):401–6.
[93] Salgado-Delgado R, Angeles-Castellanos M, Saderi N, Buijs RM, Escobar C. Food intake during the normal activity phase prevents obesity and circadian desynchrony in a rat model of night work. Endocrinology 2010;151(3):1019–29.
[94] Hammarström A, Gustafsson PE, Strandh M, Virtanen P, Janlert U. It's no surprise! Men are not hit more than women by the health consequences of unemployment in the Northern Swedish Cohort. Scand J Public Health 2011;39(2):187–93.
[95] Roelfs DJ, Shor E, Davidson KW, Schwartz JE. Losing life and livelihood: a systematic review and meta-analysis of unemployment and all-cause mortality. Soc Sci Med 2011;72(6):840–54.
[96] Anand SS, Yusuf S, Jacobs R, Davis AD, Yi Q, Gerstein H, et al. Risk factors, atherosclerosis, and cardiovascular disease among Aboriginal people in Canada: the Study of Health Assessment and Risk Evaluation in Aboriginal Peoples (SHARE-AP). Lancet 2001;358(9288):1147–53.
[97] Laitinen J, Nayha S, Kujala V. Body mass index and weight change from adolescence into adulthood, waist-to-hip ratio and perceived work ability among young adults. Int J Obes (Lond) 2005;29(6):697–702.
[98] Olinto MTA, Nácul LC, Dias-da-Costa JS, Gigante DP, Menezes AMB, Macedo S. Distribution of general and abdominal obesity in adults in a city in southern Brazil. Reports in Public Health 2006;22:1207–15.
[99] Tavassoli AA, Gharipour M, Khosravi A, Kelishadi R, Siadat ZD, Bahonar A, et al. Gender differences in obesogenic behaviour, socioeconomic and metabolic factors in a population-based sample of Iranians: the IHHP study. J Health Popul Nutr 2010;28(6):602–9.
[100] Sarlio-Lahteenkorva S, Silventoinen K, Lahti-Koski M, Laatikainen T, Jousilahti P. Socio-economic status and abdominal obesity among Finnish adults from 1992 to 2002. Int J Obes 2006;30(11):1653–60.

[101] Hanisch KA. Job loss and unemployment research from 1994 to 1998: A review and recommendations for research and intervention. J Vocat Behav 1999;55(2):188–220.
[102] Bambra C, Eikemo TA. Welfare state regimes, unemployment and health: a comparative study of the relationship between unemployment and self-reported health in 23 European countries. J Epidemiol Community Health 2009;63(2):92–8.
[103] Garcy AM, Vågerö D. The length of unemployment predicts mortality, differently in men and women, and by cause of death: a six year mortality follow-up of the Swedish 1992–1996 recession. Soc Sci Med 2012;74(12):1911–20.
[104] Ayala GX, Elder JP, Campbell NR, Slymen DJ, Roy N, Engelberg M, et al. Correlates of body mass index and waist-to-hip ratio among Mexican women in the United States: implications for intervention development. Women's Health Issues 2004;14(5): 155–64.
[105] Teichmann L, Olinto MTA, Costa JSDD, Ziegler D. Risk factors associated with overweight and obesity in women living in São Leopoldo, RG. Brazilian Journal of Epidemiology 2006;9:360–73.
[106] Olinto MT, Costa JS, Kac G, Pattussi MP. Abdominal obesity epidemiology amongst adult women resident in Southern Brazil. Arch Latinoam Nutr 2007;57(4):349–56.

CHAPTER

3

Effects of Dietary Patterns and Physical Activity on the Establishment of Abdominal Obesity in Adolescents

Fátima Pérez de Heredia[a], David Martínez-Gómez[b], Sonia Gómez-Martínez[c], and Ascensión Marcos[c]

[a]School of Natural Sciences and Psychology, Liverpool John Moores University, Liverpool, United Kingdom; [b]Department of Physical Education, Sports and Human Movement, Faculty of Teacher Training and Education, Universidad Autónoma de Madrid, Madrid, Spain; [c]Dept. Metabolism and Nutrition, Institute of Food Science, Technology and Nutrition, Spanish National Research Council, Madrid, Spain

ABDOMINAL OBESITY IN ADOLESCENTS

Tackling Obesity in Children and Adolescents

At the beginning of the twenty-first century, the World Health Organization declared obesity to be a global epidemic [1]. Its prevalence is rapidly growing worldwide, with perhaps little chance for improvement, as evidenced by the concerning increase of its incidence in young people of many countries [2]. So far, this trend predicts a further rise in adult obesity and also implies the appearance of obesity-related diseases at earlier ages. Due to the high economic and social impact of obesity and its comorbidities [3,4], prevention is a priority, as is understanding the factors leading to obesity in younger ages. Although there is a genetic component in the susceptibility to obesity and related disorders, the final outcome will depend on the interaction of each individual's genetic background with their exposure to more or less obesogenic environments that encourage inadequate eating habits or sedentary behaviors [5,6].

Therefore, the need for multidisciplinary approaches in the management of pediatric obesity has been recognized, involving the participation of pediatricians, experts in nutrition and physical activity, and even psychologists working as a single, multidisciplinary team [7]. Dietary treatments for obese children and adolescents must ensure adequate growth and development by reducing excessive fat mass accumulation but avoiding loss of lean mass, improving well-being and self-esteem, and preventing cyclical weight regain. Any nutritional intervention addressed to children and adolescents should be based on foods to eat rather than foods to exclude, thus ensuring variety and avoiding nutritional deficiencies and excess. Sensible meal planning and energy distribution through the day also helps to improve eating behavior.

Physical activity is the other key pillar for preventing and treating overweight and obesity. Despite cross-sectional studies having found only moderate relationships between levels of physical activity and weight status, prospective studies have linked low levels of physical activity with greater weight gain over time [8]. In addition, exercise programs have been shown to reduce percentage body fat in overweight children and adolescents [9].

Abdominal Obesity in Children and Adolescents: A Matter of *Where*, not Just *How Much*

Alongside general obesity trends, the prevalence of abdominal obesity is also increasing in children and adolescents in both developed and developing countries [10–13]. Similar to the case for adults, this feature has been identified as an independent risk factor for disease in young people, in particular for metabolic alterations leading to insulin resistance and for cardiovascular risk [14]. Indeed, the International Diabetes Federation (IDF) adapted the criteria to define metabolic syndrome in

Nutrition in the Prevention and Treatment of Abdominal Obesity
http://dx.doi.org/10.1016/B978-0-12-407869-7.00003-9

adults, including that of abdominal obesity, to be used in children over 10 years of age and in adolescents [15].

It is important to note that diagnosing abdominal obesity in pediatric populations is not without controversy. According to a systematic review on prevalence of central obesity in children and adolescents (10–19 years), there is a lack of agreement on both the outcome measure(s) and the cutoff points to use as indicators of abdominal obesity [16]. Although waist circumference is the most frequently employed parameter, not all studies use the same anatomical position to measure this. Also, cutoff values can vary between the 70th, 75th, 90th (this one the most common [17–20]) and 95th percentiles, and even the references for these percentiles are variable—sometimes it is the population to which the sample belongs (also the most common case), sometimes it is the studied sample itself, and sometimes the reference value belongs to a population from a different country (mainly the USA) [16,18,19,21]. Partly for this reason, there is considerable disparity in the data on prevalence of abdominal obesity among studies: values range between 10% and 20% or more according to country and study, and there is not a general gender-related pattern, with some studies showing a higher prevalence in boys and others in girls [16,21]. In contrast, authors consistently observe an association between lower socioeconomic backgrounds and a higher prevalence of abdominal obesity, and also (in those studies that present results from different years) describe a trend toward increased prevalence with time [16]. In fact, it has been reported that the relative raise in central fat accumulation can even surpass that of the body mass index (BMI) [12].

Despite the different measurements that can be found in the literature, waist circumference seems to be the most adequate indicator of abdominal obesity, and is a better predictor of cardiovascular risk than the BMI [22–24]. Among the criteria established by the IDF to diagnose metabolic syndrome in children and adolescents, waist circumference is included as the gold standard to define abdominal obesity, and different cutoff values have been established according to age. For individuals between 10 and 15 years, this value corresponds to the 90th percentile in the reference population, unless it is higher than the adult cutoff, in which case the latter will be used. For adolescents over 15 years, adult values are used [15]; for example, these correspond to a waist circumference of ≥94 cm for Caucasian males and of ≥80 cm for females. Also, waist-derived indexes, in particular the waist-height ratio, are gaining popularity for determining abdominal obesity in children and adolescents [25–27].

Regardless of the marker used, once abdominal obesity and metabolic syndrome are established, treatment becomes a challenging question. As a recent review explains in further detail, evidence is lacking to support the effectiveness and even safety of currently available pharmacological therapies to tackle both abdominal obesity and related metabolic alterations in pediatric populations [28]. Therefore, for the time being it is clear that the pathway to follow is that of lifestyle modification, aimed particularly at improving eating and physical activity habits. Pharmacological options should be kept only for the most severe cases, and always as a complement to lifestyle intervention. In this chapter we will present and discuss the available evidence on the relationships between eating habits and physical activity and abdominal fat accumulation in adolescents.

MEAL PATTERNS, FOODS, AND ABDOMINAL OBESITY IN ADOLESCENTS

Particular foods or food patterns—which makes us fatter? In recent years, the concepts of *functional food* and *nutraceuticals* have become familiar to a growing audience beyond the scientific community, including the food industry and consumers. Specific foods, nutrients, and ingredients are gaining greater attention as potential therapeutic tools for the amelioration of nutrition-related problems, and obesity is not an exception. However, along with this functional ingredient craze, there is a trend toward increasing recognition of the importance of eating patterns as a whole, rather than of single dietary components. As we will see, data from observational studies can actually provide support for all the different hypotheses, presenting evidence for relationships between abdominal obesity and meal patterns, food groups, and even some nutrients.

Impact of Meal Patterns on Markers of Abdominal Obesity

The Importance of Meal Frequency

Studies from our group and others are demonstrating the importance of meal frequency in the management of body weight and abdominal obesity in adolescents, reaching a generalized conclusion that a higher number of meals over the day protects from total and central fat accumulation.

Within the AVENA (Alimentación y Valoración del Estado Nutricional en Adolescentes) study, our group conducted a cross-sectional study on a nationally representative sample of over 3000 Spanish adolescents (13–18.5 years). This project aimed to evaluate dietary patterns, anthropometry, lifestyle habits, and health markers in the young population in order to detect risk factors for future disease, among other objectives. In 1978 of these adolescents, we analyzed the interactions between dietary patterns and measures of obesity [29]. Participants were asked about different aspects of their eating habits: consumption of different meals (breakfast, mid-morning snack, lunch, afternoon snack, dinner, and evening snack), ready-to-eat foods, and soft drinks (excluding sugar-free beverages): data were categorized as "yes" or "no". Waist circumference was the marker used for determining abdominal obesity, and differences in relation to dietary habits were analyzed, controlling for age and the practice of physical activity during leisure time (as self-reported). We did not find any significant differences in waist circumference in relation to intake of particular foods (i.e. soft drinks or ready-to-eat foods), but we did observe that adolescents who reported eating more than four meals per day presented with smaller waist circumference values than did those who ate fewer meals. Significant associations were found between the consumption of certain meals and central fat accumulation: adolescents who regularly had mid-morning snacks (only boys) and afternoon snacks (boys and girls) had lower waist circumference values than those who usually did not. Breakfast skipping did not seem to have a significant influence on waist circumference in the whole sample. Nevertheless, an interesting aspect of consuming breakfast arose in a subsequent analysis: it was significantly associated with the practice of physical activity (although only in boys). According to our data, male adolescents who reported taking part in physical activity had a lower waist circumference than those who did not, regardless of skipping or consuming breakfast regularly. However, in boys who did not take part in physical activity, regular breakfast consumption was accompanied by lower waist circumference, matching the values seen in active adolescents [29].

Other studies have also looked at the relationship between meal frequency and markers of abdominal obesity, obtaining results similar to ours. For example, Jääskeläinen and colleagues analyzed this relationship in a cohort of over 6200 Finnish adolescents. In particular, they looked at the differences between three different meal patterns: five meals a day; four or fewer meals a day including breakfast (≤four meals including breakfast); and four or fewer meals without breakfast (≤four meals skipping breakfast). They assessed abdominal obesity according to IDF criteria. In agreement with our findings, these authors found that adolescents who had ≤four meals (including breakfast) or five meals a day were less likely to present with abdominal obesity than those skipping breakfast, independent of lifestyle habits, pubertal stage, and BMI [30].

Breakfast in particular is considered to be a reference for healthy dietary and lifestyle habits [31–33]. Although some studies have not found positive associations between skipping breakfast and body weight in children and adolescents [34–36], evidence is accumulating in favor of an inverse association between breakfast consumption and the risk of becoming obese, despite the fact that breakfast consumers may have a greater daily energy intake [37–40]. In the HELENA (Healthy Lifestyle in Europe by Nutrition in Adolescence) study, in which our group has also participated, associations were analyzed between breakfast consumption and several markers of cardiovascular risk, including waist circumference, in a representative sample of European adolescents (12.5–17.5 years) [41]. Results showed that, in boys, skipping breakfast was significantly associated with greater waist circumference (controlling for age, country, and indicators of sociodemographic status). No significant difference was found, however, for girls [41]. Similarly, Nurul-Fadhilah and colleagues studied 236 Malaysian adolescents (12–19 years) in two groups: those who had breakfast at least 5 days/week and those who had breakfast fewer than 5 days/week. Breakfast eaters had a significantly lower waist circumference, independent of age, pubertal maturation, income, physical activity levels, and dietary factors (such as frequency of eating out, snacking, and total daily energy intake). Interestingly, this significant difference was observed in both female and male adolescents [42]. Another study on nearly 3000 Saudi adolescents again found significant differences in breakfast frequency according to BMI and abdominal obesity (as estimated from waist-height ratio with the cutoff point set at 0.50); again, these differences were gender specific. As such, breakfast frequency decreased with greater degrees of overweight and obesity only in boys, while in girls there was a U-shaped trend, with the highest breakfast frequency observed in obese and the lowest in overweight adolescents [27].

Results from the National Health and Nutrition Examination Survey (NHANES; 1999–2004), comprising data from over 5800 American adolescents (12–18 years) send us a similar message in relation to snacking. Although snack consumption showed a positive relationship with energy intake, it was negatively related to body weight, BMI, and waist circumference (after adjusting for sex, age, ethnicity, income, physical activity, television and computer use, smoking, and having ever tried to lose weight). Also, the prevalence of both obesity and abdominal obesity showed a negative association with the number of snacks per day. Similar results were obtained when the percentage of daily energy intake derived from snacks was considered. According to the study, the risk of presenting with abdominal obesity dropped to approximately one-third in adolescents who consumed ≥ four snacks pr day, compared to those who did not have snacks. In relation to energy intake, adolescents who consumed ≥ 40% of their daily energy intake from snacks had a 39% likelihood of abdominal obesity; this rose to 80% in those who had <10% of their energy from snacks [17].

The Importance of Meal Patterns

Apart from the number of meals a day, dietary pattern as a whole—i.e. a particular combination of food groups—has been reported to have an effect on central fat accumulation in adolescents [18,43,44].

In a population with a tradition of Mediterranean diet, e.g. Tunisia, food intake was assessed from 1000 adolescents by a semiquantitative frequency questionnaire. From the answers, the conductors of the study derived two different dietary patterns: the "modern" and the "meat-and-fish" patterns. The modern pattern was characterized by a reduced consumption of cereals and grains in favor of white bread and sugars (the latter due in great part to sweet drinks), a higher intake of butter and other added fats to the detriment of oils, a marked reduction of vegetable and pulses intake (although with an elevated fruit intake), and increases in the intake of dairy products (mainly milk and yogurt), eggs, canned fish, and processed turkey (although the intake of chicken decreased). Of interest, this modern diet pattern also showed reduced consumption of tea and increased consumption of coffee. The meat-and-fish diet basically included a higher consumption of meat and fish. Adoption of a more "modern" diet or a "meat-and-fish" diet was linked to a greater BMI and waist circumference values in male adolescents, while no such relationships were observed in the females [44].

Similarly, Moschonis and colleagues analyzed dietary patterns in 2000 Greek children and adolescents (9–13 years), with the aid of 24-h recall interviews. They identified five lifestyle profile components, three of which were directly and exclusively associated with eating patterns: (1) adequate breakfast, more frequent meals, and a higher consumption of dairy products; (2) a higher consumption of fiber-rich foods (fruit, vegetables, and whole grains); and (3) a higher consumption of red meat along with a lower consumption of fish. The first two components were inversely associated with the sum of skinfolds, but only the first was significantly associated with BMI, percentage body fat, and waist circumference. The researchers then divided the sample into quartiles according to the different components, and found that adolescents in the 2nd, 3rd, and 4th quartiles of component 1 were 15%, 24%, and 8% less likely, respectively, to present with abdominal obesity than those in the 1st quartile [18].

Modifying Dietary Habits

As with all observational studies, no cause-and-effect relations can be determined between dietary patterns and the development of abdominal obesity. Interventions are necessary to confirm the probable conclusions we derive from cross-sectional observations. However, there are practically no studies that aimed to ameliorate abdominal obesity in youth populations, with the exception (to our knowledge) of that of Singhal and colleagues [45]. This group showed how a school-based lifestyle and nutritional education intervention for 6 months in adolescents (15–17 years) could improve dietary habits and also ameliorate markers of abdominal obesity. As a control, the authors studied another school with similar sociodemographic characteristics, which received no intervention of any kind. The intervention covered different aspects of lifestyle, from encouraging the practice of physical activity in school and in everyday life to allowing the subjects to plan their own diets, and providing information on health. In addition, individual counseling was provided by the nutritionists, school menus were adapted to offer healthy alternatives, and parents and teachers were also engaged through nutritional counseling. At baseline, the two schools presented similar average values for all parameters measured. At the end of the intervention period, adolescents in the target school had significantly changed some of their eating habits by increasing their consumption of milk and decreasing that of white bread, fizzy drinks, and fast food, as well as bringing fruit for their lunch more often. There were no significant differences between schools in body weight or BMI, but waist circumference, sagittal abdominal diameter, and waist-hip ratio were significantly smaller in the target school at the end of the intervention period [45].

Heroes and Villains: Impact of Food Groups, Individual Foods, and Nutrients in Abdominal Obesity in Adolescents

Contributions of Foods and Food Groups to the Establishment of Abdominal Obesity

If it is complicated to determine the influence of dietary habits on the development of obesity and abdominal obesity, drawing conclusions about the role of particular foods or ingredients is an even more intricate task. Efforts have been made to highlight the importance of total energy balance but, as we have already discussed, energy intake alone may not be so important. In addition, the consumption of some foods has been suggested to affect the establishment of obesity in adolescents [46–48], and this could also be the case for abdominal obesity.

We have commented on the potentially protective role of certain dietary patterns, like the Mediterranean diet, against central fat accumulation. These patterns are usually characterized by a higher consumption of whole grains, legumes, vegetables, fruits, nuts, and sources of unsaturated fat, like olive oil and fish. However, evidence is lacking for the positive effects of these individual food groups on abdominal obesity in adolescents. For example, we could not find studies analyzing the relationships between legumes, nuts, or fish intake and abdominal obesity in adolescents, and found only one (the third NHANES youth study) in which the consumption of grains was analyzed. According to this study, adolescents (12–16 years) in the top quartile for waist circumference had a significantly lower frequency of grain intake than those in the other quartiles [48]. In addition, a few studies have found no association at all between markers of abdominal obesity and the consumption of fruits and vegetables [21,27].

In contrast, several studies point out the beneficial effects of other food groups, in particular dairy products [18,19,46–49]. They found significant negative associations between abdominal obesity and absolute calcium consumption [19], milk intake [49], and dairy product consumption [19,27,48]. In the study by Al-Hazzaa and colleagues on Saudi adolescents, the relationship between abdominal obesity (defined as a waist-height ratio of $\geq$0.5) and the frequency of milk and dairy consumption was gender specific, being negative in girls but positive in boys [27]. It is important to mention that this study did not analyze absolute intakes (either as energy or as mass) of the different food categories, but only the frequency of consumption according to the number of days per week, with possible answers ranging from "never" (0 days/week) to "every day" (7 days/week) [27]. Although other authors failed to find negative associations between dairy consumption and obesity [44,50], there seems to be a rationale for a protective effect of calcium against fat accumulation through the modulation of fat absorption and oxidation and adipocyte metabolism [51,52].

Finally, in relation to the traditional enemies of nutritional health, such as sugary drinks, confectionary, or potato chips, no wide consensus can be extracted from the available literature. For example, Ferreira de Moraes and Falcão analyzed the contributions of different food groups to abdominal obesity in Brazilian adolescents aged 14–18 years, using a qualitative weekly frequency consumption questionnaire to estimate dietary habits. They observed a higher prevalence of abdominal obesity in female adolescents who drank fizzy drinks more than four times per week than in those who did not (a similar trend, although not statistically significant, was found in males) [21]. Unlike these authors, we did not find any significant differences in waist circumference in relation to soft drinks in the AVENA study [29]; even more surprising, Al-Hazzaa and colleagues found that the frequency of consumption of sugar-sweetened drinks was higher in adolescents without abdominal obesity [27]. Similarly, markers of abdominal obesity were also found to be lower in adolescents who reported eating sweets more often [21,27]; in Saudi adolescents, this was also the case for baked goods and potato chips [27].

Although these results appear to refute the widely accepted negative view of these types of food, they must be interpreted with care. It is important to remember that in all studies cited, no absolute amounts were recorded or computed, and only the frequency of consumption was considered. Also, causality cannot be derived from cross-sectional studies; therefore, the authors suggested that overweight or obese adolescents could be less prone to eating energy-dense foods in an attempt to control their body weight or because they go on diets more often [21].

Food Ingredients of Particular Interest

Even less conclusive information is available with regards to specific nutrients and central obesity, although recent work suggests the involvement of two particular nutrients in the development of abdominal obesity. We will briefly comment on this.

On the *villains* side, data have been presented to indicate that higher fructose consumption is implicated in enhanced central fat accumulation [53]. The authors explain that since the end of the twentieth century fructose consumption has increased due, on the one hand, to a general rise in sucrose intake and, on the other, to the use of corn syrup as the predominant sweetener used by the food industry, mainly in processed foods and soft drinks [54,55]. They also note that fructose consumption is particularly popular among adolescents [56,57]. Therefore, they studied fat distribution in relation to fructose consumption in 559 white and black American adolescents (14–18 years) using 24-h dietary recalls, dual X-ray absorptiometry (DEXA) for fat distribution, and magnetic resonance imaging to measure visceral and subcutaneous fat area. No significant differences were found between tertiles of fructose intake for BMI distribution and, although there was a tendency toward higher fat mass and subcutaneous fat area in the upper tertile, they were only marginally significant. However, there was a significant positive linear trend toward higher visceral fat area with greater fructose consumption. It is interesting to point out that there were no significant differences in total energy or macronutrient intake between the fructose consumption groups: the only dietary differences were that higher fructose consumption was accompanied by a greater percentages of energy derived from added sugars (both fructose and sucrose) and fiber intake was lower. It is also worth mentioning that when the authors looked at the relative contributions of different fructose sources, the proportion of sugars obtained from vegetables and fruits decreased significantly across fructose tertiles, while that obtained from juices and sugar-sweetened foods and beverages increased. Moreover, higher fructose intake was also associated with features of metabolic risk, such as a higher systolic blood pressure, fasting glucose, and homeostasis model assessment index for insulin resistance and C-reactive protein (CRP), and a lower plasma high-density lipoprotein cholesterol and adiponectin. These associations seemed to be mediated by visceral fat [53].

On the *heroes* side, evidence is increasing in favor of a protective role of vitamin D against obesity; again, the

NHANES study has provided data to support this [20]. Serum levels of 25-hydroxyvitamin D [25(OH)D] were measured in more than 3500 adolescents who participated in the 2001–2004 NHANES, and found to be related to waist circumference. When analyses were adjusted for age, gender, ethnicity, economic status, and physical activity, there was a significant linear decrease in waist circumference with increasing quartiles of 25(OH)D concentration. The prevalence of abdominal obesity increased from 9.7% (in the top quartile) to 26.9% (in the bottom quartile), representing 7.2-fold higher risk with the lowest 25(OH)D levels. The relationship between vitamin D and obesity is unclear. Some authors have suggested that low circulating vitamin D levels could be actually a consequence of obesity because its lipophilic nature means that it would be sequestered within adipose tissue [58,59]. However, it has also been proposed that vitamin D deficiency leads to increased parathyroid hormone levels, which in turn raises intracellular calcium content in adipocytes leading to enhanced lipogenesis [60]. This last hypothesis contradicts the antiobesity potential of calcium mentioned earlier, indicating that further research is needed to clarify the effects of particular nutrients on central fat accumulation.

Similarly, it would be of interest to analyze the role of other allegedly antiobesity nutrients and food compounds, such as fish oils or polyphenols, in the development of abdominal obesity in children and adolescents.

PHYSICAL ACTIVITY AND ABDOMINAL OBESITY IN ADOLESCENTS

Physical Activity: Definition, Characteristics, and Assessment

In the field of health-related research, physical activity is commonly defined as "any bodily movement produced by skeletal muscles that results in energy expenditure" [61]. Related terms that sometimes are incorrectly used as synonyms are *exercise* and *physical fitness*. *Exercise* is defined as a "physical activity that is planned, structured, and repetitive, and results in improvements and maintenance of one or more components of physical fitness" [61]. On the other hand, *physical fitness* is defined as "a set of attributes that people have or achieve that relates to the ability to perform physical activity" [61]. The health-related components of physical fitness are: (1) cardiorespiratory fitness; (2) muscular endurance; (3) muscular strength; (4) body composition; and (5) flexibility.

Physical activity can be described by its intensity, duration, frequency, mode, and continuity [62]. Intensity is the rate of energy expenditure while an activity is being performed (e.g. light, moderate, vigorous). Duration is defined as the length of time that an activity is performed. Frequency is usually given in the number of times per day, week, or month that an activity is performed, but can be expressed in any time unit (e.g. 6 days/week). Mode refers to the type of specific activity that is performed (e.g. soccer, martial arts, or basketball) and to the circumstances or domains under which the activity is carried out (e.g. active commuting to school or extracurricular physical activity). Continuity refers to the period of time during which the activity has been carried out (e.g. continuous or intermittent). All of these different characteristics mean that the assessment of physical activity is a challenge for researchers in health-related research, especially involving young people [62,63].

An accurate assessment of physical activity in young people is necessary to identify their physical activity levels as well as the effectiveness of intervention programs designed to increase their physical activity [63,64]. There are many methods for assessing physical activity but it must be noted that precision and economic costs are tightly related, whereas feasibility is inversely associated with these two features. Hence, advantages and disadvantages related to these factors must be considered in the design of any study [62–64].

The scientific literature reports several methods that facilitate the assessment of physical activity in children and adolescents in free-living conditions [64]. The doubly labeled water method is the standard criterion for assessing physical activity in free-living conditions, but the technique is relatively costly, which reduces the possibility of using it for large groups or epidemiological samples. Subjective methods such as diaries and recall instruments (i.e. questionnaires, interviews, and parent interviews) are easy to use but have clear limitations for using with young people. Despite the limitations for accurate estimations, there is renewed interest in the value of these instruments in providing valuable contextual information. Activity monitors (e.g. pedometers, accelerometers, and heart-rate monitors) have been increasingly used to provide objective information about physical activity in young people.

Physical Activity Recommendations for Adolescents and Current Practice

Many years have passed between the first recommendation of physical activity for children and adolescents provided by the American College of Sports Medicine in 1988 [65], and the more recently launched physical activity guidelines for young people from the U.S. Department of Health and Human Services in December 2008 [66]. To date, only one physical activity recommendation (from 1994) has been specifically developed for adolescents; this states that adolescents should participate in moderate-to-vigorous physical activity for at least 20 min/day [67]. After this, physical activity recommendations have considered children and adolescents together [66]. These evidence-based recommendations suggest that young people should engage in moderate-to-vigorous physical activity for at least 60 min/day [66].

Overall, the prevalence of adolescents meeting the current recommendation of 60 min/day in moderate-to-vigorous physical activity is low. In a recent report by Hallal and colleagues [68] using self-reported data from 105 countries, the proportion of 13–15-year-olds meeting the recommendation was 19.7%, with boys being more active than girls. Using objectively measured instruments, these figures change slightly. For example, recent data from European adolescents shows that the proportion of adolescents meeting this recommendation is 41% (56.8% of boys and 27.5% of girls) [69]. In USA adolescents, however, these figures are lower (11% for boys and 4% for girls) [70]. Differences between countries and methods for assessing physical activity have been considered in these studies [68–71].

Physical Activity and Abdominal Body Fat in Adolescents

Many studies have investigated the effect of physical activity on body fat levels in adolescence. However, most have only included measures of total body fat (e.g. BMI and skinfolds) and little is known about abdominal body fat. In this section, we are going to present relevant cross-sectional, longitudinal, and intervention studies that examined the associations between physical activity and abdominal body fat in adolescents. For simplicity and in line with the importance of using accurate assessments of physical activity, we have only included studies with objective measures of physical activity.

Cross-Sectional Studies

Cross-sectional studies provide a cost-effective way of testing potential associations between variables. However, as mentioned earlier in this chapter, we cannot establish the causal direction between the variables under study in a cross-sectional design. Many studies in the scientific literature have examined whether physical activity might prevent an excess of abdominal body fat in adolescents.

One of the first international studies to objectively measure physical activity to examine its association with abdominal body fat was the EYHS (European Youth Heart Study) in young people. The EYHS was initially designed to be a cross-sectional survey of children and adolescents conducted in five countries—Denmark, Estonia, Norway, Portugal, and Sweden—but it has since been extended to include Iceland and Spain. More countries are also planning to join the study. A minimum of 1000 boys and girls aged 9 and 15 years were recruited from each study location. Although most research questions in this study were answered using merged data from children and adolescents, the Swedish part presented one study on the association between physical activity and abdominal body fat in adolescents alone. Ortega and colleagues found that only vigorous physical activity was inversely associated with a high-risk waist circumference [72].

AFINOS

The AFINOS (La Actividad Física como Agente Preventivo del Desarrollo de Sobrepeso, Obesidad, Alergias, Infecciones y Factores de Riesgo Cardiovascular en Adolescentes, Physical Activity as a Preventive Agent of the Development of Overweight, Obesity, Infections, Allergies and Factors of Cardiovascular Risk in Adolescents) was a surveillance study done in the region of Madrid (Spain) in which health status and lifestyle indicators were assessed by questionnaire in a representative adolescent sample aged 13 to 17 years ($n \approx 2000$). A set of measurements including anthropometry, objectively measured physical activity by accelerometer, physical fitness, and blood analysis were performed in a subsample of 232 adolescents. We found that physical activity of different intensities was not significantly associated with waist circumference; however, cardiorespiratory fitness was inversely associated with waist circumference, and both vigorous and moderate-to-vigorous physical activity were positively associated with cardiorespiratory fitness. Hence, these results suggest that physical activity, especially vigorous physical activity, might have a key role in determining abdominal body fat levels through cardiorespiratory fitness [73].

HELENA

The HELENA study (which we have already mentioned in relation to eating habits) was a multicenter investigation carried out in 10 European cities: Athens (Greece), Dortmund (Germany), Ghent (Belgium), Heraklion (Greece), Lille (France), Pécs (Hungary), Rome (Italy), Stockholm (Sweden), Vienna (Austria), and Zaragoza (Spain). The main aim of this study was to obtain reliable and comparable data in >3000 adolescents on a broad battery of relevant lifestyles and health outcomes. Some analyses from the HELENA study have examined important issues related to the role of physical activity on abdominal body fat. For example, in a subsample of 1025 adolescents we found that only objectively measured vigorous physical activity was significantly associated with waist circumference. Interestingly, we also found that vigorous physical activity, as measured by the International Physical Activity Questionnaire for Adolescents, was not significantly associated with waist circumference [74].

In a subsample of 365 Spanish adolescents from the same study, Moliner-Urdiales and colleagues included abdominal adiposity measured by DEXA to examine the same outcome [75]. Abdominal adiposity was assessed at three different regions: R1, with the upper border parallel to the end of the lowest rib; R2, with the upper border parallel to the junction between the twelfth thoracic and the first lumbar vertebrae; and R3, with the upper border parallel to the middle of the cost-vertebrae articulation of the last rib. All had the lower horizontal border on the top of the iliac crest. In addition, waist circumference was included as a measure of abdominal adiposity. These researchers also found that only vigorous physical activity was significantly associated with waist circumference. Vigorous physical activity was also significantly associated with R1, R2, and R3 adiposity, but the authors found that moderate-to-vigorous physical activity and total physical activity were also significantly associated with R1, R2, and R3 body fat. In the same sample, España-Romero and coworkers examined the effect of cardiorespiratory fitness on the association between physical activity and abdominal body fat [76]. This study hypothesized that only adolescents with low levels of cardiorespiratory fitness might benefit from engaging in physical activity to prevent abdominal fatness. Although the percentage of variance in abdominal body fat by DEXA explained by physical activity was slightly higher in adolescents with low cardiorespiratory fitness (3–8%) compared to those with high cardiorespiratory fitness (2–4%), these findings indicated that there is not a clear effect of cardiorespiratory fitness on the association between physical activity and abdominal body fat. Another analysis by Ruiz and colleagues within the HELENA study tested gene-lifestyle interactions in abdominal body fat [77]. They examined whether physical activity attenuates the effect of the *FTO* rs9939609 polymorphism on waist circumference in 752 adolescents, and detected a borderline gene × physical activity interaction ($P=0.10$). The effect of the *FTO* rs9939609 polymorphism on abdominal body fat was much lower in adolescents who met the daily physical activity recommendations (i.e. >60 min/day of moderate-to-vigorous physical activity) compared with those who did not (+0.60 cm vs. +1.15 cm of waist circumference per risk allele). These findings were confirmed by a posterior meta-analysis of 19,268 children and adolescents that also included data from the HELENA study ($P_{interaction}=0.002$) [78].

One of the more important collaborative works that examined the cross-sectional associations between objectively measured physical activity and abdominal body fat was conducted using data from the International Children's Accelerometer Database (ICAD). Ekelund and colleagues presented a meta-analysis of data pooled from 14 studies between 1998 and 2009 comprising 20,817 children and adolescents (aged 4–18 years). In this study, both total and moderate-to-vigorous physical activity was significantly associated with waist circumference [79].

Longitudinal Studies

Few studies have examined longitudinal associations between physical activity and abdominal body fat using objective measures of physical activity. A recent review by Jimenez-Pavón and colleagues [80] found that only seven studies have examined associations between objectively measured physical activity and body fat in a longitudinal design, although none included measures of abdominal fat. Ekelund and colleagues [79] examined this research question with the ICAD database. For this additional analysis, the authors included 6413 participants in a 2.1-year follow-up: moderate-to-vigorous physical activity was not associated with waist circumference at follow-up; and a higher waist circumference at baseline was not associated with lower amounts of physical activity at follow-up.

Interventions

Not many studies have explored the effectiveness of physical activity interventions in decreasing abdominal fat in adolescents. The recent Cochrane review on this topic showed that the effectiveness of interventions based exclusively on physical activity had little or no effect on decreasing abdominal fat measures in adolescent samples [81]. This fact can be explained by the difficulty of increasing physical activity levels in adolescents. For example, a recent review by Metcalf and colleagues [82] provides strong evidence that physical activity interventions have had only a small effect on overall activity levels, as measured by accelerometers in young people. These findings may partially explain why interventions have had limited success in reducing abdominal fat in this population [81].

CONCLUSIONS

- The prevalence of abdominal obesity is increasing among children and adolescents, and will lead to a double health burden if uncorrected.: a further raise

in the incidence of adult obesity in the future; and the diagnosis of metabolic diseases typical for adults and a prematurely higher cardiovascular risk in young people.
- The best approach so far for the management of pediatric obesity is based on lifestyle modification and aimed at encouraging healthier food choices and the practice of physical activity in an everyday setting.
- Research is now showing that higher meal frequency, snacking included, helps maintain a healthier body weight. In addition, not enough stress can be put on the importance of consuming breakfast every day. These practices (higher meal frequency, snacking, and consuming breakfast) can be beneficial for preventing abdominal obesity, despite implying a greater daily energy intake.
- Dietary pattern as a whole seems to be more influential in the development of abdominal obesity in adolescents than particular foods. The inclusion of processed foods as major components of the usual diet, the so-called *Westernized* pattern, is currently contributing to central fat accumulation. It is crucial to reinstate more traditional diets that provide a combination of fresh, natural foods.
- Milk and dairy products deserve special attention. Having been stigmatized for a long time due to their fat content, they could in fact be key food items for the healthy growth and development of young people, thus helping prevent abdominal fat accumulation.
- Cross-sectional studies indicate a role for vigorous physical activity in reducing the risk of abdominal fat accumulation, and some suggest a similar role, although to a lesser extent, for moderate-to-vigorous physical activity. However, this has not yet been confirmed by longitudinal studies.
- Interventions focused solely on physical activity have proven to have little effect in preventing abdominal fat accumulation in adolescents. It is therefore necessary to conduct more long-term interventions targeting eating and physical activity habits within the context of a more comprehensive approach.

References

[1] World Health Organization. Obesity: preventing and managing the global epidemic. Report of a WHO consultation on obesity. Geneva:World Health, Organization; 2000.

[2] Lobstein T, Baur L, Uauy R. IASO International Obesity Task Force: Obesity in children and young people: a crisis in public health. Obes Rev 2004;5(Suppl. 1):5–85.

[3] Coldiz GA, Mariani A. The cost of obesity and sedentarism in the United States. In: Bouchard C, editor. Physical activity and obesity. Champaign, IL: Human Kinetics; 2000. p. 55–65.

[4] Katzmarzyk PT, Janssen I. The economic costs associated with physical inactivity and obesity in Canada: an update. Can J Appl Physiol 2004;29:90–115.

[5] Campion J, Milagro FI, Martinez JA. Individuality and epigenetics in obesity. Obes Rev 2009;10:383–92.

[6] Marti A, Ordovas J. Epigenetics lights up the obesity field. Obes Facts 2011;4:187–90.

[7] Martinez-Gomez D, Gomez-Martinez S, Puertollano MA, Nova E, Wärnberg J, Veiga OL, et al. Design and evaluation of a treatment program for Spanish adolescents with overweight and obesity. The EVASYON study. BMC Public Health 2009;9:414.

[8] Dishman RK, Washburn RA, Health GW. Physical activity epidemiology. In: Dishman RK, editor. Champaign, IL: Human Kinetics; 2004.

[9] Strong WB, Malina RM, Blimkie CJR, Daniels SR, Dishman RK, Gutin B, et al. Evidence based physical activity for school-age youth. J Pediatr 2005;146:732–7.

[10] Wang Y, Monteiro C, Popkin B. Trends of obesity and underweight in older children and adolescents in the United States, Brazil, China, and Russia. Am J Clin Nutr 2002;75:971–7.

[11] Liang YL, Xi B, Song AQ, Liu JX, Mi J. Trends in general and abdominal obesity among Chinese children and adolescents 1993–2009. Pediatr Obes 2012;7:355–64.

[12] Mindell JS, Dinsdale H, Ridler C, Rutter HR. Changes in waist circumference among adolescents in England from 1977–1987 to 2005–2007. Pub Health 2012;126:695–701.

[13] Ogden CL, Carroll MD, Kit BK, Flegal KM. Prevalence of obesity and trends in body mass index among US children and adolescents, 1999–2010. JAMA 2012;307:483–90.

[14] Bacha F, Saad R, Gungor N, Janosky J, Arslanian SA. Obesity, regional fat distribution, and syndrome X in obese black versus white adolescents: race differential in diabetogenic and atherogenic risk factors. J Clin Endocrinol Metab 2003;88:2534–40.

[15] Zimmet P, Alberti KG, Kaufman F, Tajima N, Silink M, Arslanian S, et al. IDF Consensus Group. The metabolic syndrome in children and adolescents—an IDF consensus report. Pediatr Diabetes 2007;8(5):299–306.

[16] De Moraes ACF, Fadoni RP, Ricardi LM, Souza TC, Rosaneli CF, Nakashima ATA, et al. Prevalence of abdominal obesity in adolescents: a systematic review. Obes Rev 2011;12:69–77.

[17] Keast DR, Nicklas TA, O'Neil CE. Snacking is associated with reduced risk of overweight and reduced abdominal obesity in adolescents: National Health and Nutrition Examination Survey (NHANES) 1999–2004. Am J Clin Nutr 2010;92:428–35.

[18] Moschonis G, Kalliora AC, Costarelli V, Papandreou C, Koutoukidis D, Lionis C, et al. On behalf of the Healthy Growth Study Group. Identification of lifestyle patterns associated with obesity and fat mass in children: the Healthy Growth Study. Pub Health Nutr 2013:1–10 http://dx.doi.org/10.1017/S13689800130 00323.

[19] Abreu S, Santos R, Moreira C, Vale S, Santos PC, Soares-Miranda L, et al. Association between dairy product intake and abdominal obesity in Azorean adolescents. Eur J Clin Nutr 2012;66:830–5.

[20] Reis JP, von Mühlen D, Miller 3rd ER, Michos ED, Appel LJ. Adolescent population vitamin D status and cardiometabolic risk factors in the United States. Pediatrics 2009;124:e371–9.

[21] Ferreira de Moraes AC, Falcão MC. Lifestyle factors and socioeconomic variables associated with abdominal obesity in Brazilian adolescents. Ann Hum Biol 2013;40(1):1–8.

[22] Karelis AD, St-Pierre DH, Conus F, Rabasa-Lhoret R, Poehlman ET. Metabolic and body composition factors in subgroups of obesity: what do we know? J Clin Endocrinol Metab 2004;89:2569–75.

[23] Després J, Lemieux I. Abdominal obesity and metabolic syndrome. Nature 2006;444:881–7.

[24] De Almeida CA, Pinho AP, Ricco RG, Elias CP. Abdominal circumference as an indicator of clinical and laboratory parameters associated with obesity in children and adolescents: comparison between two reference tables. J Pediatr 2007;83:181–5.
[25] Taylor RW, Jones IE, Williams SM, Goulding A. Evaluation of waist circumference, waist-to-hip ratio, and the conicity index as screening tools for high trunk fat mass, as measured by dual-energy X-ray absorptiometry, in children aged 3–19 y. Am J Clin Nutr 2000;72:490–5.
[26] McCarthy HD, Ashwell M. A study of central fatness using waist-to-height ratios in UK children and adolescents over two decades supports the simple message—"keep your waist circumference to less than half your height". Int J Obes 2006;30:988–92.
[27] Al-Hazzaa HM, Abahussain NA, Al-Sobayel HI, Qahwaji DM, Musaiger AO. Lifestyle factors associated with overweight and obesity among Saudi adolescents. BMC Public Health 2012;12:354.
[28] Pacifico L, Anania C, Martino F, Poggiogalle E, Chiarelli F, Arca M, et al. Management of metabolic syndrome in children and adolescents. Nutr Metab Cardiovasc Dis 2011;21:455–66.
[29] Gómez-Martínez S, Martínez-Gómez D, Pérez de Heredia F, Romeo J, Cuenca-Garcia M, Martín-Matillas M, et al. Eating habits and total and abdominal fat in Spanish adolescents: influence of physical activity. The AVENA Study. J Adolesc Health 2012;50:403–9.
[30] Jääskeläinen A, Schwab U, Kolehmainen M, Pirkola J, Järvelin MR, Laitinen J. Associations of meal frequency and breakfast with obesity and metabolic syndrome traits in adolescents of Northen Finland Birth Cohort 1986. Nutr Metab Cardiovasc Dis 2012. Available from http://www.nmcd-journal.com/article/S0939-4753%2812%2900179-2/abstract. Accessed 11 September 2013.
[31] Keski-Rahkonen A, Kaprio J, Rissanen A, Virkkunen M, Rose RJ. Breakfast skipping and health-compromising behaviors in adolescents and adults. Eur J Clin Nutr 2003;57:842–53.
[32] Matthys C, De Henauw S, Bellemans M, De Maeyer M, De Backer G. Breakfast habits affect overall nutrient profiles in adolescents. Public Health Nutr 2007;10:413–21.
[33] Deshmukh-Taskar PR, Nicklas TA, O'Neil CE, Keast DR, Radcliffe JD, Cho S. The relationship of breakfast skipping and type of breakfast consumption with nutrient intake and weight status in children and adolescents: the National Health and Nutrition Examination Survey 1999–2006. J Am Diet Assoc 2010;110:869–78.
[34] Abalkhail B, Shawky S. Prevalence of daily breakfast intake, iron deficiency anaemia and awareness of being anaemic among Saudi school students. Int J Food Sci Nutr 2002;53:519–28.
[35] William P. Breakfast and the diets of Australian children and adolescents: an analysis of data from the 1995 National Nutrition Survey. Int J Food Sci Nutr 2007;58:201–16.
[36] Mota J, Fidalgo F, Silva R, Ribeiro JC, Santos R, Carvalho J, et al. Relationship between physical activity, obesity and meal frequency in adolescents. Ann Hum Biol 2008;35:1–10.
[37] Rampersaud GC, Pereira MA, Girard BL, Adams J, Metzl JD. Breakfast habits, nutritional status, body weight, and academic performance in children and adolescents. J Am Diet Assoc 2005;105:743–60.
[38] Harding S, Teyhan A, Maynard MJ, Cruickshank JK. Ethnic differences in overweight and obesity in early adolescence in the MRC DASH study: the role of adolescent and parental lifestyle. Int J Epidemiol 2008;37:162–72.
[39] Szajewska H, Ruszczynski M. Systematic review demonstrating that breakfast consumption influences body weight outcomes in children and adolescents in Europe. Crit Rev Food Sci Nutr 2010;50:113–9.
[40] Tin SP, Ho SY, Mak KH, Wan KL, Lam TH. Breakfast skipping and change in body mass index in young children. Int J Obesity 2011;35:899–906.
[41] Hallström L, Labayen I, Ruiz JR, Patterson E, Vereecken CA, Breidenassel C, et al. On behalf of the HELENA Study Group. Breakfast consumption and CVD risk factors in European adolescents: the HELENA (Healthy Lifestyle in Europe by Nutrition in Adolescence) Study. Public Health Nutr 2013;16(7):1296–305.
[42] Nurul-Fadhilah A, Teo PS, Huybrechts I, Foo LH. Infrequent breakfast consumption is associated with higher body adiposity and abdominal obesity in Malaysian school-aged adolescents. PLoS ONE 2013;8(3):e59297. http://dx.doi.org/10.1371/journal.pone.0059297.
[43] Striegel RH, Ritchie LD, Spector P, Stevens MJ, Schmidt MM, Schreiber GB, et al. Dietary patterns in adolescence are related to adiposity in young adulthood in black and white females. J Nutr 2007;137:399–406.
[44] Aounallah-Skhiri H, Traissac P, El Ati J, Eymard-Duvernay S, Landais E, Achour N, et al. Nutrition transition among adolescents of a south-Mediterranean country: dietary patterns, association with socio-economic factors, overweight and blood pressure. A cross-sectional study in Tunisia. Nutr J 2011;10:38.
[45] Singhal N, Misra A, Shah P, Gulati S. Effects of controlled school-based multi-component model of nutrition and lifestyle interventions on behavior modification, anthropometry and metabolic risk profile of urban Asian Indian adolescents in North India. Eur J Clin Nutr 2010;64:364–73.
[46] Novotny R, Daida YG, Acharya S, Grove JS, Vogt TM. Dairy intake is associated with lower body fat and soda intake with greater weight in adolescent girls. J Nutr 2004;134:1905–9.
[47] Moore LL, Singer MR, Qureshi MM, Bradlee ML. Dairy intake and anthropometric measures of body fat among children and adolescents in NHANES. J Am Coll Nutr 2008;27:702–10.
[48] Bradlee ML, Singer MR, Qureshi MM, Moore LL. Food group intake and central obesity among children and adolescents in the Third National Health and Nutrition Examination Survey (NHANES III). Public Health Nutr 2010;13:797–805.
[49] Abreu S, Santos R, Moreira C, Santos PC, Vale S, Soares-Miranda L, et al. Relationship of milk intake and physical activity to abdominal obesity among adolescents. Pediatr Obes 2013. doi: 10.1111/j.2047-6310.2012.00130.x. Epub ahead of print].
[50] Phillips SM, Bandini LG, Cyr H, Colclough-Douglas S, Naumova E, Must A. Dairy food consumption and body weight and fatness studied longitudinally over the adolescent period. Int J Obes Relat Metab Disord 2003;27:1106–13.
[51] Zemel MB. Role of calcium and dairy products in energy partitioning and weight management. Am J Clin Nutr 2004;79(5):907S–12S.
[52] Dougkas A, Reynolds CK, Givens ID, Elwood PC, Minihane AM. Associations between dairy consumption and body weight: a review of the evidence and underlying mechanisms. Nutr Res Rev 2011;24:72–95.
[53] Pollock NK, Bundy V, Kanto W, Davis CL, Bernard PJ, Zhu H, et al. Greater fructose consumption is associated with cardiometabolic risk markers and visceral adiposity in adolescents. J Nutr 2012;142:251–7.
[54] Park YK, Yetley EA. Intakes and food sources of fructose in the United States. Am J Clin Nutr 1993;58:S737–47.
[55] Bray GA, Nielsen SJ, Popkin BM. Consumption of high-fructose corn syrup in beverages may play a role in the epidemic of obesity. Am J Clin Nutr 2004;79:537–43.
[56] Marriott BP, Cole N, Lee E. National estimates of dietary fructose intake increased from 1977 to 2004 in the United States. J Nutr 2009;139:S1228–35.
[57] Vos MB, Kimmons JE, Gillespie C, Welsh J, Blanck HM. Dietary fructose consumption among US children and adults: the Third National Health and Nutrition Examination Survey. Medscape J Med 2008;10:160.

[58] Liel Y, Ulmer E, Shary J, Hollis BW, Bell NH. Low circulating vitamin D in obesity. Calcif Tissue Int 1988;43(4):199–201.
[59] Reinehr T, de Sousa G, Alexy U, Kersting M, Andler W. Vitamin D status and parathyroid hormone in obese children before and after weight loss. Eur J Endocrinol 2007;157(2):225–32.
[60] McCarty MF, Thomas CA. PTH excess may promote weight gain by impeding catecholamine-induced lipolysis-implications for the impact of calcium, vitamin D, and alcohol on body weight. Med Hypotheses 2003;61(5–6):535–42.
[61] Caspersen CJ, Powell KE, Christenson GM. Physical activity, exercise, and physical fitness: definitions and distinctions for health-related research. Public Health Rep 1985;100:126–31.
[62] Welk GJ. Physical activity assessment in health-related research. In: Welk GJ, editor. Champaign, IL: Human Kinetics; 2002.
[63] Welk GJ, Corbin CB, Dale D. Measurement issues in the assessment of physical activity in children. Res Q Exerc Sport 2000;71(Suppl. 2):S59–73.
[64] Sirard JR, Pate RR. Physical activity assessment in children and adolescents. Sports Med 2001;31:439–54.
[65] American College of Sports Medicine . Opinion statement on physical fitness in children and youth. Med Sci Sports Exerc 1988;20:422–3.
[66] U.S. Department of Health and Human Services . Physical activity guidelines for Americans. Be active, healthy and happy!. Washington, DC: U.S. Department of Health and Human Services; 2008.
[67] Sallis JF, Patrick K. Physical activity guidelines for adolescents: consensus statement. Pediatr Exerc Sci 1994;6:302–14.
[68] Hallal PC, Andersen LB, Bull FC, Guthold R, Haskell W, Ekelund U. Physical Activity Series Working Group. Global physical activity levels: surveillance progress, pitfalls, and prospects. Lancet 2012;380(9838):247–57.
[69] Ruiz JR, Ortega FB, Martínez-Gómez D, Labayen I, Moreno LA, De Bourdeaudhuij I, et al. Objectively measured physical activity and sedentary time in European adolescents: the HELENA study. Am J Epidemiol 2011;174(2):173–84.
[70] Troiano RP, Berrigan D, Dodd KW, Mâsse LC, Tilert T, McDowell M. Physical activity in the United States measured by accelerometer. Med Sci Sports Exerc 2008;40:181–8.
[71] Ekelund U, Tomkinson G, Armstrong N. What proportion of youth are physically active? Measurement issues, levels and recent time trends. Br J Sports Med 2011;45(11):859–65.
[72] Ortega FB, Ruiz JR, Sjöström M. Physical activity, overweight and central adiposity in Swedish children and adolescents: the European Youth Heart Study. Int J Behav Nutr Phys Act 2007;19(4):61.
[73] Martínez-Gómez D, Eisenmann JC, Moya JM, Gómez-Martínez S, Marcos A, Veiga OL. The role of physical activity and fitness on the metabolic syndrome in adolescents: effect of different scores. The AFINOS Study. J Physiol Biochem 2009;65(3):277–89.
[74] Martinez-Gomez D, Gomez-Martinez S, Ruiz JR, Diaz LE, Ortega FB, Widhalm K, et al. Objectively-measured and self-reported physical activity and fitness in relation to inflammatory markers in European adolescents: the HELENA Study. Atherosclerosis 2012;221(1):260–7.
[75] Moliner-Urdiales D, Ruiz JR, Ortega FB, Rey-Lopez JP, Vicente-Rodriguez G, España-Romero V, et al. Association of objectively assessed physical activity with total and central body fat in Spanish adolescents; the HELENA Study. Int J Obes 2009;33(10):1126–35.
[76] España-Romero V, Ortega FB, Ruiz JR, Artero EG, Martínez-Gómez D, Vicente-Rodríguez G, et al. Role of cardiorespiratory fitness on the association between physical activity and abdominal fat content in adolescents: the HELENA study. Int J Sports Med 2010;31(10):679–82.
[77] Ruiz JR, Labayen I, Ortega FB, Legry V, Moreno LA, Dallongeville J, et al. Attenuation of the effect of the *FTO* rs9939609 polymorphism on total and central body fat by physical activity in adolescents: the HELENA study. Arch Pediatr Adolesc Med 2010;164(4):328–33.
[78] Kilpeläinen TO, Qi L, Brage S, Sharp SJ, Sonestedt E, Demerath E, et al. Physical activity attenuates the influence of *FTO* variants on obesity risk: a meta-analysis of 218,166 adults and 19,268 children. PLoS Med 2011;8(11):e1001116 http://dx.doi.org/10.1371/journal.pmed.1001116.
[79] Ekelund U, Luan J, Sherar LB, Esliger DW, Griew P, Cooper A. International Children's Accelerometry Database (ICAD) Collaborators. Moderate to vigorous physical activity and sedentary time and cardiometabolic risk factors in children and adolescents. JAMA 2012;307(7):704–12.
[80] Jiménez-Pavón D, Kelly J, Reilly JJ. Associations between objectively measured habitual physical activity and adiposity in children and adolescents: Systematic review. Int J Pediatr Obes 2010;5(1):3–18.
[81] Waters E, de Silva-Sanigorski A, Hall BJ, Brown T, Campbell KJ, Gao Y, et al. Interventions for preventing obesity in children. Cochrane Database Syst Rev 2011;7(12):CD001871.
[82] Metcalf B, Henley W, Wilkin T. Effectiveness of intervention on physical activity of children: systematic review and meta-analysis of controlled trials with objectively measured outcomes (EarlyBird 54). BMJ 2012;345:e5888.

CHAPTER

4

Lifestyle Factors Affecting Abdominal Obesity in Children and Adolescents: Risks and Benefits

Edyta Suliga

Department of the Prevention of Alimentary Tract Diseases, Faculty of Health Sciences, Jan Kochanowski University, Kielce, Poland

Abbreviations

BMI, body mass index; CRF, cardiorespiratory fitness; DEXA, dual-energy X-ray absorptiometry; IAAT, intra-abdominal adipose tissue; MVPA, moderate-to-vigorous physical activity; SAT, subcutaneous adipose tissue; VPA, vigorous physical activity; VAT, visceral adipose tissue; WC, waist circumference; WHtR, waist-height ratio; WHR, waist-hip ratio

INTRODUCTION

The mechanisms that determine the type of adipose tissue distribution in humans are complex and have not yet been satisfactorily explained. An important role is played by genetic factors, ethnicity, the body's hormone levels, growth, and maturation, as well as "modifiable" factors related to lifestyles [1]. The latter mainly include diet; recreation, including physical activity; sleep duration; and the use or avoidance of stimulants, such as alcohol and cigarettes. The following section presents the results of research on the risks and benefits associated with the lifestyles of children and adolescents in relation to abdominal obesity.

PHYSICAL ACTIVITY AND ABDOMINAL OBESITY

Physical Activity in Leisure Time

Limiting physical activity has a significant impact on direct and indirect processes conducive to excess body weight. Decreased energy expenditure resulting from a lack of activity directly affects the body's energy balance. An appropriate level of physical activity is an important factor in maintaining normal insulin sensitivity and protects the organism from the occurrence of chronic cardiovascular and hormonal diseases, whereas insufficient amounts result in insulin resistance and increased fat deposition in the body [2,3].

In determining the relationship between physical activity in leisure time and abdominal obesity, the most important results are those of studies that include both direct measurements of visceral adipose tissue (VAT) and the objective assessment of physical activity using an accelerometer. Saelens and colleagues [4] demonstrated in 8-year-old children with obesity risk factors that increased physical activity, measured using an accelerometer, was associated with lower VAT levels ($r = -0.43$). The dependence was significant even after adjustment for whole-body fat. No analogous relationship with subcutaneous adipose tissue (SAT) and whole-body fat was found. The study also showed a statistically significant relationship only in the analysis of the objective measurement of physical activity and not in a parallel assessment by questionnaire.

In subsequent studies, abdominal obesity was evaluated by DEXA (dual-energy X-ray absorptiometry). In children aged 8–11 years, the time devoted to intense physical activity (> 6 metabolic equivalents) significantly negatively correlated with total abdominal fat ($r = -0.35$) and the proportion of abdominal fat to total body fat ($r = -0.22$) [5]. In adolescents aged 12.5–17.5 years, all indicators of central adiposity (i.e. the amount of abdominal fat measured by DEXA in three regions and the WC) were negatively associated with vigorous physical activity (VPA; $P < 0.01$) [6]. Moreover, abdominal fat was negatively associated with both moderate-to-vigorous physical activity (MVPA; $P \leq 0.001$) and counts per minute ($P < 0.01$). Adolescents that met the recommendations for MVPA, i.e. at least 60 min/day of activity [7],

Nutrition in the Prevention and Treatment of Abdominal Obesity
http://dx.doi.org/10.1016/B978-0-12-407869-7.00004-0

showed not only a lower overall fat content ($P<0.05$) but also a lower central fat content ($P \leq 0.01$). The authors found that intense physical activity may have a greater impact on the prevention of obesity than lower intensity activity, while both the average and at least moderate physical activity can have an effect on abdominal adiposity in adolescents.

Roemmich and colleagues [8], using a direct measurement of VAT and a 7-day assessment of physical activity (with the help of a questionnaire) in healthy children aged 10–14 years, reported that only for boys did the overall level and intensity of physical activity significantly correlate with VAT ($r=-0.43$ and $r=-0.39$, respectively). However, Stallman-Jorgensen and colleagues [9] found no significant association for physical activity, determined on the basis of a 24-h self-assessment of VAT amount in adolescents aged 14–18 years.

A relationship between physical activity and obesity is also confirmed by the majority of cross-sectional studies, which made an objective assessment of physical activity and an indirect assessment of abdominal obesity, usually based on waist circumference (WC) measurements. Ortega and colleagues [10] found that children aged 9.5 years and adolescents aged 15.6 years with the lowest VPA levels (first tertile) exhibited twice the risk of having a high WC measurement compared with their peers from the highest tertile; this relationship remained significant even after correction for sedentary activities. However, neither gross nor moderate physical activity was significantly associated with WC. Chaput and colleagues [11] demonstrated that MVPA is inversely related to the size of waist-height ratio (WHtR) (adj. $\beta=-0.071$; $P<0.001$) in 8–10-year-old children, regardless of the time spent on sedentary activities. Steele and colleagues [12] found an inverse relationship between the time dedicated to physical activity (measured by an accelerometer) and WC in 9–10-year-old children, but the relationship was strongest for VPA. These relationships were independent of objectively measured time spent in sedentary activities, as well as sleep duration, energy consumption, and other variables. Duncan and colleagues [13], by examining physical activity by a pedometer, found that 5–12-year-old children in a group with high WC ($\geq$ 80th percentile) had lower activity levels both during the weekend and during weekdays when compared with their peers with lower WC (<80th percentile). Hussey and colleagues [14] observed in children aged 7–10 years a significant correlation between WC and both moderate ($r=-0.47$) and intense physical activity ($r=-0.37$), but only in boys. Similarly, Purslow and colleagues [15] found a significant inverse relationship between WC (waist standard deviation score) and total physical activity ($\beta=-0.26$, $P=0.002$) and MVPA ($\beta=-0.031$, $P<0.001$) in boys, whereas in girls this relationship was not significant. The only study that demonstrated a negative correlation between WC and physical activity, even one of a low intensity, was made by Butte and colleagues [16], who examined children and adolescents aged 4–19 years. This relationship was significant when corrected for the percentage of body fat.

Relationships between objectively measured physical activity and obesity indicators were not found by Ekelund and colleagues [17], Hussey and colleagues [14]—in the case of girls; and Fisher and colleagues [18] in a prospective annual study of 8–10-year-old children. It was also not shown in a meta-analysis of prospective studies conducted by Ekelund and colleagues [19]. A combined analysis showed, however, that WC differences between individuals from the lowest and highest MVPA tertiles was 5.6 cm.

Studies in which physical activity was assessed by questionnaire yielded less conclusive results regarding relationships with abdominal obesity. In children and adolescents aged 6–16 years, activity in leisure time significantly correlated with abdominal obesity ($r=-0.258$), as measured by WC [20]. Similar results were also obtained by Klein-Platat and colleagues [21] in 12-year-olds; Dos Santos Cavalcanti and colleagues [22] in 14–19-year-old adolescents; and Collison and colleagues [23] in 10–19 year-old adolescents, but only in cases of boys. At the age of 14–19 years, the risk of abdominal obesity, defined on the basis of WHtR values ($\geq$0.50) was highest in the group that allocated less time to intense physical activity [24]. The relationship between physical activity (assessed by questionnaire) and abdominal obesity has not been confirmed in several other studies [25–28], including some long-term studies [29].

Cardiorespiratory Fitness

Although cardiorespiratory fitness (CRF) is determined by a number of nonmodifiable factors, such as gender, age, and genetic factors, it has also been considered in recent years an objective indicator of physical activity and used to assess the relationship between physical activity and health status [30,31]. Therefore, relationships observed between indicators of abdominal obesity and CRF may indirectly prove a relationship between physical activity and abdominal obesity. Of particular importance are the results of studies that made direct measurements of VAT. The earliest study on the subject reported CRF to show a significant correlation only with the amount of total abdominal adipose tissue and SAT, but not with VAT [32]. In another study, however, CRF was observed to negatively correlate with VAT in 13-year-old girls ($r=-0.45$) and boys ($r=-0.43$) [33]. Similar results were obtained in a study of white and black young people aged 8–17 years ($r=-0.43$ and $r=-0.68$, respectively) [34].

In 8-year-olds within the same BMI category, children with high CRF (assessed using a maximal multistage 20-m shuttle run test), had a significantly lower WC ($P = 0.001$) and a lower fat percentage in the abdominal region, as measured by DEXA ($P < 0.001$), compared to children with low CRF [35]. A similar relationship between CRF and WC in children and adolescents has been shown in many other studies [14,28,36–38], although some were no longer statistically significant after adjusting for the amount of fat [39]. CRF explained 9–26% of the variance of WC in children and adolescents of all ages [10,40]. A long-term study of children aged 6–12 years showed that the risk of continuation of abdominal obesity after 2 years was highest among those who had a high WC (1.9-fold) and low CRF (4.3-fold) at baseline [41]. Ortega and colleagues [37] also found that CRF appears to modify the relationship between objectively measured physical activity and abdominal obesity, and that the time devoted to intense activity is likely to be a key factor associated with abdominal obesity in children and adolescents with low fitness.

Effect of Aerobic Exercise

The majority of randomized controlled trials conducted in children and adolescents confirm the positive impact of interventions involving the use of aerobic exercise on VAT amount determined on the basis of both direct measurements [42–45] and WC measurements [46]. Similar results are also obtained in nonrandomized studies using VAT measurements [47] and WC measurements [48,49]. Owens and colleagues [42], after a 4-month period of training conducted in obese children aged 7–11 years (five times/week, 40 min/day, at 70–75% maximal heart rate), reported a significant SAT reduction ($-16.2\,cm^3$ vs. $48.9\,cm^3$) and a smaller VAT increase ($1.3\,cm^3$ vs. $20.9\,cm^3$) in the intervention group, despite body weight gain, compared with the control group. In turn, in obese adolescents aged 13–16 years who participated in an 8-month program involving both exercise (5 days/week) and lifestyle education, SAT ($-69.7\,cm^3$ vs. $40.4\,cm^3$) and VAT ($-42.0\,cm^3$ vs. $-11.0\,cm^3$), reduction was reported in relation to their peers who received only lifestyle education [44]. However, the authors were unable to determine whether high intensity training was more effective for improving body composition than moderate intensity training. A 10-month training program (including 30 min of MVPA, >150 beats/min) in black girls (8–12 years; subjects from the entire adiposity range) contributed to a reduction in the increment of VAT ($0.8\,cm^3$ vs. $16.1\,cm^3$), SAT ($65.2\,cm^3$ vs. $130.0\,cm^3$), and WC (1.4 cm vs. 2.9 cm) in comparison with the control group [45]. Davies and colleagues [50] showed that a 16-week training program (aerobic + strength training, twice a week, 60–90 min/session) had a positive effect on the reduction of body fat in adolescents (15.8 ± 1.1 years) who were overweight or obese. Compared with the control group, a significant reduction in waist size (−3% vs. 3%) and VAT (−10% vs. 6%) was observed. They also found that additional use of motivational interview behavioral therapy in one of the surveyed groups did not have much effect. In order to determine the effect of an aerobic training dose on health status indicators and adiposity, including VAT, in overweight children (mean age 9.4 years), Davies and colleagues [51] allocated them randomly to one of two training groups: low dose (20 min/day) or high dose (40 min/day). Aerobic training lasted 13 weeks (5 days/week). In both groups a significant improvement in adiposity indicators was found. Changes in VAT amount dependent on exercise dose were $-3.9\,cm^3$ ($P < 0.001$) and $-2.8\,cm^3$ ($P = 0.01$) in the high- and low-dose groups vs. the control groups, respectively.

In a nonrandomized study, a 12-week intervention involving the use of exercise (30 min, 4 days/week) contributed to a significant VAT reduction (54.7 ± 6.0 to $49.6 \pm 5.5\,cm^2$) in obese adolescents without body weight loss or BMI change [47]. In nonobese boys aged 15–17 years with previously sedentary lifestyle, an endurance-type training program (5 times/week, 120–150 min/day) lasting for 5 weeks contributed to a significant reduction in abdominal subcutaneous fat (−1.8% vs. 1.8%) and prevented an increase in visceral fat (−0.2% vs. 4.5%), despite the absence of weight loss, compared with the control group [43]. Kim and colleagues [46], after the application of a 6-week intervention (5 days/week, 40 min/day) to obese 17-year-old boys, reported an improvement in WC (92.1 ± 2.2 cm vs. 89.6 ± 2.0, $P < 0.05$) as well as a reduction in BMI and other indicators of fatness. Similar results were obtained in nonrandomized studies by Lazar and colleagues [48] and Kelishadi and colleagues [49]. Relationships between aerobic exercise and WC or VAT amount in children and adolescents were not seen in only a few cases [32,52,53].

SEDENTARY ACTIVITIES

A meta-analysis conducted in 2004 showed a statistically significant relationship between watching television and adiposity among children and adolescents, but it seemed too small to be of clinical importance [54]. The authors also found that single activity markers, such as watching television or videos or playing computer games, were unlikely to explain the relationship between a sedentary lifestyle and health. Research carried out in the following years did not provide a clear explanation for these issues, particularly for abdominal obesity. Purslow and colleagues [15] found no significant relationship between objectively measured time devoted to sedentary activities and WC in 8–9-year-old children. Similarly, Chaput and colleagues [11], using an objective measurement of the time spent in sedentary activities for children aged 8–10 years, did not find it to be associated with indicators of general or abdominal obesity. The relationship was demonstrated only in the case of MVPA. In a long-term annual study of 13-year-old adolescents Altenburg and colleagues [55] also did not report a relationship between time spent in front of the screen and obesity: they stated that time spent watching TV was a predictor of BMI and WC only in boys, and not in girls. A meta-analysis conducted by Ekelund and colleagues [12] showed that in prospective studies the objectively measured time spent in sedentary activities for children and adolescents was not associated with WC during the observation period, but a higher WC at baseline was associated with an increasing number of sedentary activities during the observation period. However, Butte and colleagues [16], using an objective measurement of activity by an accelerometer in children and adolescents aged 4–19 years, reported a weak ($r=0.07$) but significant correlation between sedentary activities and WC.

In a survey of Brazilian adolescents, screen time (i.e. time spent watching television, playing video games, and using the computer) grew beginning with 60 min/day for 11 year-olds, and changes of this time in the period between ages 11 and 15 years showed a positive correlation with adiposity indexes, including WC [56]. Chinapaw and colleagues [57], who studied Dutch and Hungarian children aged 10–12 years, confirmed that WC was significantly higher in children from the fourth quartile of time spent in sedentary activities compared with children in the lowest, first quartile (70 ± 8 cm vs. 66 ± 8 cm). A positive correlation between time spent in sedentary activities and WC, found by Steele and colleagues [12] in 9–10-year-old children, decreased significantly after adjustment for MVPA, which suggests that the VPA level has a greater impact on children's obesity rates than the time spent in sedentary activities. However, Ortega and colleagues [10] reported that, in 15-year-old adolescents only, sedentary activities and not physical activity during leisure time were significantly associated with abdominal obesity; this explained 18% of WC variance in girls and 10% in boys.

Further studies that confirmed the existence of a relationship between sedentary activities and abdominal obesity suggest that among different sedentary activities a particularly negative factor is the amount of play time devoted to watching TV. A positive correlation between sedentary activities, i.e. mainly watching TV, and WC was found in a group of 12-year-old girls and boys [21]. In adolescents aged 12–18 years, after adjusting for age, gender, annual household income, and MVPA, each additional hour of watching TV and each additional hour devoted to computer and video games was significantly associated with a higher risk of abdominal adiposity (OR = 1.27 and OR = 1.20, respectively) [58]. Carson and Jansen [59], on the basis of cross-sectional data from the U.S. National Health and Nutrition Examination Survey (NHANES), found that in children and adolescents aged 6–19 years, watching TV ≥4 h/day, the risk of having a high WC was significantly greater (OR = 2.35), compared with the reference time (<1 h/day). However, no significant relationships was found between WC and the time spent in computer use and other objectively measured sedentary activities. In addition, one reference study found that the amount of time spent watching television is more strongly associated with general obesity in children and adolescents than the time spent using a computer [60]. This may be associated with the fact that the energy expenditure of children and adolescents watching TV is even lower than their energy expenditure during sleep [61]. In addition, watching TV is a time when young people are particularly vulnerable to increased food intake without feeling hungry [62], making long-term wrong choices concerning food [63], and consuming high-energy snacks and beverages [64,65].

SLEEP DURATION

A survey of studies on sleep duration in humans shows a fairly consistent pattern of increased risk of obesity in people with a limited duration of sleep [66–69]. Experimental studies describe a number of chronic physiological and behavioral responses of the body to sleep disorders that may contribute to weight increments. Sleep greatly affects the secretion of various hormones, such as cortisol, insulin, thyroid stimulating hormone, and human somatotropin/growth hormone [70], which play important roles in the regulation of body weight, including fat distribution. Sleep limitation can lead to a reduction in the concentration of leptin and increased ghrelin, which affect hunger and regulate appetite, motivation to eat, and food intake [68]. Shorter sleep duration in children and adolescents was associated with a 58% greater risk of being overweight or obese, compared with longer sleep duration, and each additional hour of sleep reduced the risk by an average of 9% [67]. However, there are still far too few studies into the relationship between sleep duration and abdominal obesity in younger age groups. Yu and colleagues [71] showed that females aged 10–20 years with either long or short sleep duration had greater adiposity compared with females with an average sleep duration. This relationship was stronger for truncal fat, as measured by DEXA, and WC ($P<0.05$) than for BMI ($P=0.06$). A similar relationship was not found in boys, however. Likewise, in a study conducted in subjects aged 6–20 years, in which short sleep was defined as <10 h/day for children <10 years and <9 h/day for others, sleep duration was negatively correlated with WC z-score in both boys ($r=-0.20$, $P<0.01$) and girls ($r=-0.19$, $P<0.05$), but only in girls was short sleep duration associated with a 2.3-fold increased risk of abdominal obesity [72]. Garaulet and colleagues [73], in a study of adolescents aged 12.5–17.49 years from 10 European cities, found that in individuals who had a shorter sleep duration (<8 h) WCs and other indicators of adiposity were higher, compared to those with adequate sleep duration (≥8 h), particularly in the group of girls. However, in studies conducted by Collison and colleagues [23], the number of hours of night sleep negatively correlated with WC in a multivariate regression model, but only for boys. Bawazeer and colleagues [74] showed that in adolescents aged 10–19 years sleep that lasts ≤7 h significantly increased the risk of obesity in both girls and boys, but the risk of having abdominal obesity (WC>90th percentile) was also statistically significant only in boys (OR=1.25). However, Al-Hazzaa and colleagues [75] found that in adolescents aged 15–19 years both general and abdominal obesity inversely correlated with sleep duration, regardless of gender.

Studies conducted in children and adolescents indicate a clear relationship between sleep duration and other lifestyle factors that may also increase the risk of obesity. Von Kries and colleagues [76] reported that short sleep duration was associated with rare participation in sports. Although Garaulet and colleagues [73] found no relationship between sleep duration and physical activity; however, they showed that young people with short sleep duration devoted more time to sedentary activities. A shorter sleep duration was associated with frequent consumption of fast foods and sugar-sweetened beverages [72,73], and longer sleep duration was linked to a healthier diet, i.e. an adequate consumption of fruit, vegetables, fish, skim milk, and breakfast cereal [73]. A positive correlation between sleep duration and resting energy expenditure adjusted for fat-free mass was also found in boys, and this could also result in a positive energy balance [72]. At the age of 9–16 years, late bedtimes and late wake-up times were associated with poorer quality diets, irrespective of sleep duration [77].

NUTRITION

The consumption of different amounts and types of food can affect the fat content in both direct and indirect ways [78]. Different types of food may not only have a diverse energy values but they may also affect satiety in various ways due to differences in volume consumed, i.e. the degree of stomach filling, and differences in the rate of gastric emptying. Individual products may regulate body weight also indirectly through their influence on thermogenesis, energy storage, lipogenesis, and insulin sensitivity.

Intake of Nutrients

The literature survey described above showed that the impact of diet on the development of visceral obesity in children and adolescents has not been well studied so far, and most of the results obtained by various authors have not led to significant conclusions [1]. Casazza and colleagues [79], by analyzing the independent contributions of dietary variables to body composition parameters in children aged 7–12 years, found that the percentage of energy derived from protein in the diet significantly affected (1) the amount of intra-abdominal adipose tissue (IAAT; $\beta=0.15$, $P=0.04$), and SAT ($\beta=0.40$, $P=0.04$) in the total sample; and (2) IAAT ($\beta=0.26$, $P=0.02$) in African-Americans, but with no effect on SAT. Studies conducted in young overweight adults (17–35 years) showed that the energy value of diet in women correlated only with the amount of SAT ($r=0.36$), whereas the best predictor of VAT in both men and women was total fat intake [80].

Among the dietary factors associated with abdominal obesity in children and adolescents, the beneficial effects of dietary fiber was best documented in a series of studies of overweight Latino children with a familial risk of the common type 2 diabetes. Ventura and colleagues [81], in a cross-sectional study of adolescents aged 10–17 years, showed an inverse correlation between the content of various fractions of dietary fiber (total, soluble, and insoluble) and WC ($r=-0.21$ to -0.27). Increasing the amount of soluble fiber in the diet by the value of one standard deviation (1.91 g) was equivalent to a reduction in WC by 0.022 cm. Subjects, who did not have risk factors for metabolic syndrome, consumed an average of 5.2 g/day of soluble fiber, while their peers with ≥3 metabolic syndrome symptoms consumed 4.1 g daily, i.e. 27% more (1.1 g daily). This amount is the equivalent of one item of fresh fruit, such as an apple, or one portion of legumes.

The next 16-week randomized controlled trial of adolescents aged 15.5 years, in which VAT amount was determined by direct magnetic resonance imaging (MRI), showed that in subjects who increased fiber intake by 5 g/day (an amount that is equivalent of half a cup of legume seeds) during the experiment the amount of VAT was reduced to 10%, regardless of the applied intervention related to physical activity [82]. Davies and colleagues [83], during a 2-year study of Latino adolescents aged 11–17 years, found that an increased intake of overall dietary fiber (g/1000 kcal) and insoluble fiber (g/1000 kcal) was associated with a significant reduction in the amount of VAT ($r = -0.29$, and $r = -0.27$ for total and insoluble fiber, respectively), regardless of changes in SAT. In subjects who lowered their total fiber intake (mean decrease of 3 g/1000 kcal/day), a significant increase in visceral fat was found, compared to those who significantly increased its consumption (21% vs. −4%). The authors emphasize that this phenomenon is observed in the absence of significant changes in the energy value of the diet. No other dietary variable, including the energy value of the diet, the amount of fat, protein, and sugar, and the glycemic index and glycemic load was associated with changes in adiposity. This study also found no significant relationship between the number of food servings and beverages consumed during the day and the size of the indicators of abdominal obesity, but it is known that the increase in dietary fiber during the period considered was mainly a result of an increased consumption of nonfried vegetables (by 1.3 servings/day), mixed food containing fruit and vegetables (by 2 servings/day), and legumes (by 0.5 portions/day).

Another study that directly measured VAT also showed that a higher intake of dietary fiber by adolescents aged 14–18 years was associated in both boys and girls with a smaller amount of visceral fat ($P < 0.03$) after adjustment for age, race, Tanner stage, fat-free soft tissue mass, physical activity, and energy intake [84]. The mechanism linking increased fiber intake with reduced amounts of VAT has not yet been fully explained, although several possible factors are indicated. First, fiber increases stool weight and shortens the time of passage of gastric contents, thus reducing the time available for the digestion and absorption of nutrients [85,86]. Second, fiber has a direct effect on the regulation of glucose and insulin [87], and insulin is known to affect both lipid metabolism and appetite. Third, high-fiber foods, particularly fruits and vegetables, often contain phytoestrogens (isoflavones and lignans), the levels of which are inversely correlated with both abdominal obesity [88] and insulin resistance [89].

The Impact of Dietary Pattern

Dietary components are not, however, consumed in isolation. In assessing the impact of diet on the occurrence of abdominal obesity, an analysis of dietary patterns, or at least the frequency of consumption of specific groups of food products (as normal nutritional behavior is a component of lifestyle) seems to be useful. There are few studies into the relationship between dietary patterns and directly measured VAT amount in children and adolescents; the vast majority of studies have analyzed abdominal obesity as measured by WC.

In a long-term cohort study of more than 2000 girls between the ages of 9–10 and 18–19 years, Ritchie and colleagues [90] found that those who adhered to the healthy pattern, characterized by a high intake of vegetables, fruit, dairy products, cereals without added fat, as well as fiber, vitamins, and minerals (in addition to low intake of sodium and fast food, soft drinks, and other sweet or fried foods) and the lowest amounts of both total and saturated fat, showed significantly lower values of WC at the final follow-up and smaller increases in WC ($P = 0.037$) compared with girls with the sweets-and-snack-type food pattern. A similar effect was not found, however, in female African-Americans. Bradlee and colleagues [78], who conducted a cross-sectional study on a representative sample of children and adolescents in the USA, showed that individuals meeting the criteria for abdominal obesity (WC ≥ 85th percentile for age and sex) declared a significantly lower intake of dairy products, all cereals, and fruit and vegetables. However, there was no relationship between abdominal obesity and the consumption of meat. Collison and colleagues [23] noted negative correlations between the consumption of fruits, vegetables, milk, and fish and WC. These relationships, however, occurred only in boys. Other cross-sectional studies showed that university students with abdominal obesity consumed significantly more fast food and sweets, compared with nonobese students [91]. The consumption of fast food, however, was not significantly associated with abdominal obesity in a representative group of adolescents aged 15–19 years from Jamaica [92].

Studies conducted in Asian countries confirm that increased incidence of obesity in children and adolescents is accompanied by the use of "Western" dietary patterns compared with patterns based on traditional diet. An analysis carried out on more than 12,000 Korean adolescents showed that the prevalence of obesity was higher in the group with the Western pattern diet, characterized by the highest consumption of flour and bread, fast foods, sugars and sweets, meat, and carbonated beverages, compared with the traditional Korean dietary pattern, based on a high consumption of rice and kimchi, fish and seaweed, and legumes [93]. Overall caloric intake and the percentage of energy from protein and fat was highest in boys and girls using the standard Western diet.

Studies carried out in China on more than 5000 elementary school children showed that the prevalence of abdominal obesity was lowest among children for whom a "healthy dietary pattern" was typical (13.1%) [94]. This was characterized by high intake of milk and yogurt, fruits, vegetables, and eggs and a low intake of meat such as pork, poultry, organ meat, and other red meat. There was a slightly lower incidence of obesity in children with a transitive dietary pattern (17.3%), while the largest incidence of obesity was found in children with a Western dietary pattern (20.7%), characterized by a high consumption of red meat, eggs, and refined grain products. Both children with the transitive dietary pattern and children with the Western dietary pattern had a greater risk of abdominal obesity (1.31 and 1.71, respectively), compared with those with a healthy dietary pattern, after the adjustment for age, sex, family socioeconomic status, and other lifestyle factors. Research carried out in Iran on a representative sample of children and adolescents aged 6–18 years showed that the dietary pattern characterized by junk foods (including fast foods, salty and fatty snacks, carbohydrates, and sweets) increased the odds of having a hypertriglyceridemic waist phenotype (OR = 1.426), whereas the other dietary pattern including healthy foods (fruits, vegetables, and dairy products) decreased this odds ratio (OR = 0.874) [95]. The risk of the hypertriglyceridemic waist phenotype rose with the consumption of solid hydrogenated fat as well as white-flour bread. A 6-month education program aimed at changing lifestyle and diet among students aged 15–17 years in India contributed to a significant improvement in fruit consumption and a reduction in the consumption of carbonated beverages and foods with high energy density [96]. It also resulted in a significant decrease in the value of the indicators of abdominal obesity [WC, sagittal abdominal diameter, and waist-hip ratio (WHR)] with unchanged BMI, as compared with the control group.

Some researchers have found that an excessive consumption of food portions and frequent away-from-home eating foods may have contributed to the epidemic of obesity in children and adolescents [97]. Chiang and colleagues [98] found that a high availability of "junk food" in the vicinity of the school significantly increased the risk of both general (BMI) and abdominal (WC) obesity in boys aged 6–13 years. Research carried out in Australia has also shown that eating takeaway food at least twice a week is associated with a poorer quality diet and an increased risk of moderate obesity in young men and women [99]; however, a subsequent analysis of the relationship between abdominal obesity and the level of involvement in the preparation of meals did not show a significant association [100].

Milk and Dairy Products

Studies described above on the relationship between dietary patterns and obesity in children and adolescents also suggest a beneficial effect for a higher content of milk and dairy products in the diet on WC [78,90]. Spence and colleagues [101], based on an analysis of the literature, showed that studies done so far do not generally confirm that a higher consumption of milk and dairy products is associated with weight reduction and favorable changes in body composition; however, some prospective studies have reported clear associations.

A randomized clinical trial designed to investigate the long-term impact of a diet rich in dairy products on generalized and abdominal obesity in 5–6-year-old children was carried out by Kelishadi and colleagues [102]. In addition to participating in educational sessions on healthy lifestyle (control group), children in a second group received an isocaloric dairy-rich diet (>800 mg calcium/day), while a calorie-restricted diet was applied in the third group. The groups were then observed for 3 years. In all groups, BMI and WC decreased significantly after 6 months; after a follow-up period continued until the end of the study, a significant increase in the value of these indicators was reported. Increase in WC was found to be considerably lower in the group that consumed dairy products than in the other two groups (4.1 cm vs. 4.8 cm and 5.2 cm). Poddar and colleagues [103], examining 19-year-old college students, found that individuals who consumed more low-fat dairy products were generally characterized by a higher quality diet. In this group, after 6 months there was a reduction in WC as well as the total amount of body fat, compared with the group that consumed less low-fat dairy products. Hirschler and colleagues [104], in a cross-sectional study, also reported that increased milk consumption was associated with a lower WC in children under the age of 10 ± 2.3 years.

However, the beneficial effects of milk and dairy products on WC or the amount of VAT in children and adolescents were not confirmed in many other studies. In a randomized trial, St-Onge and colleagues [105] evaluated whether a high consumption of milk during 16 weeks of a healthy diet leads to a greater weight loss compared to a low consumption of milk. In this study, it is important that both indirect (WC) and direct (VAT) measures of abdominal obesity were taken into account. In overweight children aged 8–10 years, an intake of 4 servings of milk a day as part of a healthy diet did not lead to an increased loss of body weight or to changes in body composition, as compared with peers who consumed 1 serving of milk per day. One possible reason for the lack of effect of a higher consumption of milk on weight loss and change in body composition may have been the relatively short duration of the study (16 weeks), and the small number of individuals participating in the study ($n = 45$). Similarly, Keller and colleagues [106], in a cross-sectional study of twins aged 3–7 years found that the amount of milk (or calcium) consumption was associated with WC.

It follows from a survey of the literature by Major and colleagues [107] that the consumption of calcium and dairy products in general, if linked with making healthier food choices, has the potential to replace other foods (high in calories and fat), which can result in a higher positive energy balance. In addition, higher intakes of calcium and dairy products may contribute to an earlier feeling of fullness as well as a reduction in fat absorption, increased fat oxidation, and the promotion of fat cell apoptosis; thus, it may lead to a decrease in or maintenance of the appropriate amount of body fat tissue over time. As shown in some studies, the effect of dairy products on maintaining the proper balance of energy and fat is greater than calcium supplementation alone, which suggests that other components of milk (peptides and proteins) may also be involved in this process. The effect of calcium on obesity appears to be particularly important for visceral fat because it is more metabolically active and sensitive to lipolysis than are other fat tissue deposits [108]. It was found that increased consumption of calcium changes the concentration of 1,25-dihydroxyvitamin D_3 in serum, which in turn positively affects the local concentration of cortisol and may thus lead to a preferential loss of visceral fat [109].

Sugar-Sweetened Beverages

Many studies suggest that a significant risk factor for obesity is a high consumption of sugar-sweetened beverages. In a literature review, Wolff and Dansinger [110] found that out of 25 cross-sectional studies and prospective cohort studies, 12 indicated significant correlations between the consumption of nonalcoholic beverages (soft drinks) and weight gain. One of the hypothetical mechanisms to explain the effect of sugar-sweetened beverages on obesity is that liquid calories, i.e. taken as beverages, are consumed in addition to the usual diet. This means that people do not take into account calories received in drinks in their consumption structure and do thus not reduce the amount of calories in their diet by the amount provided in drinks. The result is an excessive energy intake [111].

Cohort studies in children have confirmed a relationship between the consumption of sugar-sweetened beverages and the risk of obesity, but did not show a consistent relationship between other indicators of the consumption of sugars and adiposity [112]. One of the few studies on associations between the consumption of sugar-sweetened drinks and the percentage of body fat and abdominal obesity in children and adolescents was conducted by Fiorito and colleagues [113]: this was a long-term study in girls between 5 and 15 years of age. A higher intake of sweetened beverages at age 5 years ($\geq$ 2 servings/day) was associated with a higher percentage of body fat and a greater WC at ages 5–15 years. Girls who drank $\geq$2 servings/day of sweetened beverages at age 5 years had a significantly higher percentage of their total energy intake from sugar-sweetened beverages during the entire study period. According to the authors, a high content of fructose in many sweetened beverages may explain their association with obesity, based on differences in digestion and absorption between glucose and fructose [114].

Studies cited above into the relationship between dietary patterns and abdominal obesity in children and adolescents also suggested that a high consumption of sweetened beverages is associated with a higher WC [90,93,96]. Keller and colleagues [106] also noted in their studies of twins at ages 3–7 years that the consumption of sweetened beverages, after adjusting for milk intake, was not associated with a BMI *z*-score, but did show a significant correlation with WC. The cross-sectional results of subsequent studies confirmed a positive correlation between the consumption of sugar-sweetened carbonated beverages, BMI, and WC, but only in boys [23]. Francis and colleagues [92] found that in adolescents aged 15–19 years the consumption of sweetened beverages was significantly associated only with being overweight and not with WC. Increased consumption of soda in girls was associated with abdominal obesity; an inverse relationship was found in boys [115]. A lower consumption of sweetened beverages in obese adolescents in cross-sectional studies may, however, be due to the fact that obese girls and boys are more likely to declare reduced intakes of these beverages [75,115].

Confirmation of the impact of soft drinks on the development of abdominal obesity can be found in studies of overweight and obese adults who, in the course of a 10-week trial, consumed beverages providing 25% of daily calories that were sweetened with either glucose or fructose [116]. Although both groups showed a similar increase in body weight during the intervention, the volume of VAT increased significantly only in subjects consuming fructose. Increased VAT in individuals consuming fructose and an increased expression of lipogenic genes in SAT in subjects consuming glucose suggests that the type of sugar consumed (i.e. glucose or fructose) causes the differences in body fat distribution. VAT accumulation in response to fructose consumption was more pronounced in men than in women.

The results of these investigations, however, highlight another important finding associated with the risk of obesity, both generalized and abdominal, linked to the increased consumption of sweetened beverages: a high intake of these drinks has a negative association with the amount of milk in the diet of children and adolescents, as well as with the content of calcium and vitamin D. Reduced intake of these food components can further enhance the adverse effects of sweetened beverages on body weight, including abdominal obesity [106,113,117–119].

Meal Frequency

Less frequent meals throughout the day are considered to be one of the factors that contributes to obesity. This relationship has been demonstrated in studies of both adults [120,121] and children [122,123], although some analyses do not confirm this [124,125]. This issue has been investigated only sporadically in relation to obesity in children and adolescents. In a long-term study of girls aged between 9–10 and 19–20 years, Ritchie [126] found that a lower frequency of eating meals during the first 2 years of the study was associated with greater WC increments over 10 years. In addition, a cross-sectional study found that female students with abdominal obesity at age 19–24 years consumed some meals less regularly, i.e. they missed lunches and dinners significantly more often than did nonobese female students [91].

It is suggested that the usual consumption of a greater number of meals increases 24-h fat oxidation and reduces the fluctuation of glucose and insulin levels, which positively affects the feeling of satiety [127,128]. By eating less frequent meals, people tend to eat more food overall. A large meal causes a greater stomach stretch, which is followed by faster gastric emptying. This phenomenon, together with the higher initial load of calories, results in a faster absorption of nutrients [129,130]. A higher concentration of nutrients leads, through the action of insulin, to their faster oxidation and faster triacylglycerol synthesis in adipose tissue, which may cause a greater likelihood of obesity. Individuals who consume fewer daily meals may also have lower thermogenesis, which leads to a further positive energy balance [131].

Skipping Breakfast

The beneficial effect of regular breakfast consumption on reducing the risk of obesity in children and adolescents is fairly well established in the literature [132,133]. Skipping breakfast is suggested to be associated with the consumption of food of low nutritional value accompanied by high energy density [134,135]. It can also lead to an increased feeling of hunger, and thus to the consumption of larger portions in subsequent meals during the day [136,137]. A study of Latino adolescents aged 10–17 years, in which breakfast was defined as any food or beverage consumed between 0500 and 1000 h with a combined total energy $\geq$100 kcal, showed that participants who skipped breakfast were characterized by a greater amount of IAAT ($47.2 \pm 3.8\,cm^2$), compared to patients who ate breakfast occasionally ($32.1 \pm 2.7\,cm^2$) or regularly ($32.0 \pm 3.0\,cm^2$), after controlling for covariates [138]. This difference remained significant after adjusting for SAT. The results of this study suggest, therefore, that even the occasional consumption of breakfast by adolescents is associated with lower visceral adiposity. Data from the U.S. NHANES 1999–2006 confirmed that children and adolescents (aged 9–18 years) who skipped breakfast had a greater WC compared to their peers who ate breakfast [139]. A study of Saudi adolescents aged 14–19 years also showed that a less regular consumption of breakfast (<3 days/week) was significantly associated with a higher risk of abdominal adiposity, defined on the basis of WHtR values [75].

The regular intake of breakfast may be associated with a higher frequency of food intake during the day and may favor appetite regulation [132] and energy balance [140]. In addition, a proper selection of products consumed for breakfast can help improve the nutritional density of the diet [139], including increasing the calcium content [141], which can play a positive role in the reduction of body fat [78,102,142].

ALCOHOL CONSUMPTION

Studies into the risk factors for general obesity in adolescents have shown a positive relationship between alcohol consumption and the prevalence of overweight in girls and boys [143], as well as the percentage of body fat in girls [144]. These results were confirmed in prospective studies. After a year of observation, a positive relationship was confirmed between alcohol consumption and body weight gains during that time [145]. During a 9-year study of teenage twins, Pajari and colleagues [146] found that increases in BMI were lower in men who were alcohol abstainers ($-0.62\,kg/m^2$) and women who drank less than once a month ($-0.38\,kg/m^2$), compared with those who drank from 0.25 to 0.5 drinks/week.

Many studies conducted in adults have identified alcohol consumption as a risk factor not only for general obesity but also for abdominal obesity [147–150] and visceral obesity [151,152]. In some studies, WC showed a U- or V-shaped dependence associated with the intensity of total alcohol consumption [153], or a J-shaped dependence associated with drinking wine [154]. Analysis of the different types of alcohol has shown that abdominal obesity may be related particularly to a high consumption of beer [147,155,156] and spirits [147].

Studies have shown that the frequency of alcohol use by young people is quite high in several countries. Alcohol was drunk at least once a week by 4% of 11-year-olds, 8% of 13-year-olds, and 21% of 15-year-olds, and at least 2% of 11-year-olds, 9% of 13 year-olds, and 32% of 15-year-olds from European countries, the USA, and Canada had experienced alcohol intoxication at least twice in their lives [157]. Despite this, very few studies on the association between alcohol consumption by young people and abdominal obesity have been published. The only analysis of the impact of alcohol consumption on the amount of VAT and SAT measured directly showed that it was not associated with the amount of the two body fat depots in girls 4 years after menarche [158]. It was noted, however, that a higher intake of alcohol (on ≤2 days vs. ≥3 days in the past month) was associated with 4-year changes in VAT, both before and after adjusting for changes in total body fat ($P=0.016$ and $P=0.021$, respectively). There was no such dependence in the case of SAT.

Studies into abdominal obesity based on indirect measurements, such as WC, conducted among Brazilian adolescents aged 14–18 years [115] and Greek adolescents aged 13–19 years [159] showed no association with alcohol consumption in both girls and boys. In a long-term study, Van Lenthe and colleagues [160] also found no significant relationship between WC and alcohol. Slattery and colleagues [155] found that WHR was directly related to the overall alcohol consumption in young men aged 18–30 years, and with the consumption of beer in all investigated men and women. Laitinen and colleagues [148] demonstrated that the declared alcohol consumption at age 14 was significantly associated with later abdominal obesity, but only in women and only in a model adjusted for BMI and other confounding variables. Pajari and colleagues [146] found that alcohol drinking by teenagers (i.e. adolescents aged 16–18 years) had little effect on the development of abdominal obesity at age 23–27 years.

Research carried out in adults has shown that alcohol can contribute to the formation of obesity in many ways. First, it can be a significant source of calories in the diet because there is no reduction in other food ingredients in response to energy supplementation from alcohol [161]. Alcohol cannot be stored in the body, so it is quickly metabolized using a variety of mechanisms, such as increased thermogenesis and reduced lipolysis [161–163]. Alcohol also causes increased cortisol secretion as well as high levels of androgens in women and androgen reduction in men, which contributes to increased visceral fat accumulation [164–168].

SMOKING

Studies conducted in adults have shown that smokers generally tend to have a lower body weight than nonsmokers [169]. Exposure to nicotine derived from cigarette smoke can alter the regulation of food intake in the brain to reduce appetite through both the mechanisms of energy homeostasis (homeostatic energy) of the body and reward mechanisms, which contributes to a negative energy balance, i.e. reduced energy consumption and its increased expenditure, which leads to a low weight [170]. Smoking is, however, considered to be a factor predisposing to obesity [169,171,172] and excess VAT [152,173,174] in adults, although in some studies this association has not been confirmed [175]. In recent studies, it was found that both WC and VAT in adults showed a J- or U-shaped relationship with the intensity of smoking, determined as both the number of cigarettes smoked and the duration of smoking over the course of the lives of the respondents, while measures of total body fat, such as BMI, percentage body fat, and SAT, did not show such a relationship [176].

To the best of our knowledge, there is only one published study on the effects of smoking on the amount of VAT (determined by a direct method) in adolescents [158]. This study found that VAT was significantly associated with smoking in girls 4 years after the onset of menarche ($P=0.043$), after adjusting for the total fat amount and physical activity. The regression model explained 69% of VAT variance. When, however, the model also included drinking alcohol, these variables were no longer predictors of VAT amount. In none of the models under consideration was a significant correlation found between smoking and SAT amount. Smoking was also an important predictor of a 4-year change in VAT amounts, both in the crude model (i.e. not adjusted to other factors; $P=0.034$) and after adjusting for the total amount of body fat ($P=0.004$). The model, which took drinking alcohol and smoking into account in addition to the total amount of fat and physical activity, also explained 60% of variance in VAT changes with age. Four-year changes in SAT were not associated with smoking in the unadjusted model. Only in the model that took into account the total amount of fat were SAT changes associated with smoking ($P=0.013$). However, after adjustment for alcohol, this dependence was no longer statistically significant. The authors concluded, therefore, that both VAT and SAT changes are associated with smoking, but the degree to which this relationship is applied to each of the two depots of fatty tissue separately remains undetermined. It is worth mentioning that statistically significant effects were observed even when a small amount of cigarettes were smoked (<5 vs. ≥5 cigarettes/month) [158].

An analysis of the impact of lifestyle on abdominal obesity, measured by WC, in a representative group of Brazilian adolescents aged 14–18 years showed no such relationship, in either girls or boys [115]. In a study of Greek adolescents aged 13–19 years, Tzotzas and colleagues [159] noted that although smoking was associated with an increased risk of overweight and obesity only in girls, it had no significant effect on abdominal obesity measured by WC. In female students aged 19–24 years, it was found, however, that there were significantly more smokers (67.2%) in the group with abdominal obesity than in the nonobese group (15.0%) [91]. It is difficult to determine which effect was the result and which the cause because smoking is a strategy often used to reduce excess body weight [177–179]. In young adults aged 18–30 years, WHR was directly related to smoking, but this association was not found in black men [155].

An HBSC (Health Behaviour in School-Aged Children) survey, which included European countries, as well the countries of the Russian Federation, Israel, the USA, and Canada, showed that 13% of 15-year-olds, 3% of 13-year-olds, and 1% of 11-year-olds smoke cigarettes every day, and that 24% of the 15-year-olds had started smoking at the age of ≤13 years [157]. Therefore, a group with a 5-year or longer period of smoking can be distinguished among 18-year-olds. Research in adults indicates that in so-called "heavy" smokers, or those with a long period of smoking and a greater number of smoked cigarettes, WC and VAT reach much higher levels than in "light" smokers [176]. The negative effects of smoking during teenage years can be extended to the later stages of life. Laitinen and colleagues [148] found that smoking at age 14 years is associated with abdominal obesity at age 31 years, but only in women; Saarni and colleagues [180] have shown that smoking at least 10 cigarettes/day at age 16–18 years significantly increased the risk of obesity in adulthood (OR = 1.77) for both sexes. After adjusting for current BMI and other factors that confound risk, this was reduced (OR = 1.34). Only Van Lenthe and colleagues [160], in a long-term study of subjects between 13 and 27 years of age, found no significant association between WC and smoking.

The effect of smoking on body fat distribution is not yet fully understood. Studies conducted in adults have shown that this is due to the impact on the metabolism of sex hormones that may regulate directly the distribution of body fat [181,182].

CONCLUSION

A literature review of the risks and benefits of lifestyle in relation to abdominal obesity in children and adolescents indicates that many issues have not yet been exhaustively studied and explained. Some of these are a result of methodological problems. It is in fact assumed that WC is the best predictor of VAT, which explains 64.8–67.4% of the VAT variance; however, both of these measures are also highly correlated with indicators of overall body fat and BMI, as well as with percentage body fat [1,4,183,184]. A lack of adjustment of measures of abdominal obesity for general adiposity indicators is a weakness of many of the studies analyzed in this chapter.

The results of this analysis indicate a clear relationship between physical activity and abdominal obesity in children and adolescents; this is confirmed primarily by studies in which an objective assessment of activity was made. In accordance with observations already presented, self-assessment of physical activity is not in many cases a sufficiently accurate method for evaluating the association with adiposity [185]. In surveys, overweight adolescents can in fact overestimate their level of physical activity [186]. Issues that require further study include determining the minimum or optimal amount of exercise that will help reduce body fat in children and adolescents with abdominal obesity, as well as reducing age-related increases in visceral fat in healthy children. Clarification is especially needed to determine which intensity of exercise is most effective in physical activity. Most studies show that intense activity is most effective; however, some suggest that even moderate activity may have a beneficial effect on abdominal fat in adolescents. Different results obtained in observational studies concerning the intensity of physical activity may depend on the gender and age of the observed group, as well as the level of activity in the studied populations. Many of the studies cited indicate that relationships between physical activity and abdominal obesity are reported more frequently in boys than in girls [8,14,15,23], This may be due to the fact that girls are generally less active [157,187] and that therefore the differences between analyzed categories of activity is weaker in girls than in boys. Purslow and colleagues [15] reported that in the group covered by their study as many as 72% of boys and 30% of girls complied with current recommendations for physical activity, i.e. ≥60 min/day of MVPA [7], whereas Fisher and colleagues [188] found that these recommendations were applied by only 1% of respondents.

The benefits resulting from the guidelines for physical activity (i.e. ≥60 min/day of MVPA) are confirmed by research into genetic determinants of obesity. These indicate that the level of physical activity in line with current guidelines can overcome the effect of having negative versions of some genes. Ruiz and colleagues [189], in their analysis of the *FTO* gene polymorphism in adolescents in the HELENA (Healthy Lifestyle in Europe by Nutrition in Adolescence) cross-sectional study, showed that the rs9939609 allele of the *FTO* gene was significantly associated not only with higher BMI and percentage body fat but also with a greater WC (0.85 cm per risk allele). The effect of the *FTO* rs9939609 polymorphism on WC was significantly lower in individuals who followed the physical activity recommendations, compared with those who did not (0.60 cm vs. 1.15 cm per risk allele, respectively). Physical activity should therefore be included in any strategy for the reduction and prevention of abdominal obesity in children and adolescents.

There is little evidence for an increased risk of abdominal obesity resulting from long periods spent in sedentary activities. So far this association has not been proven sufficiently by studies that used objective sedentary activities measurement, and underestimation of sedentary activities in the surveys should be taken into account, as is done for food intake [190]. Studies conducted so far have shown that the level of physical activity plays the most important role here. There is, however, some evidence that of the various classes of sedentary activities, long periods of television watching can significantly increase the risk of development of abdominal obesity. Most studies, however, show quite clearly that too short sleep duration may be a risk factor for abdominal obesity in children and adolescents. Some studies have shown that very long sleep duration may also be associated with abdominal obesity, although to a lesser extent. Therefore, further research is required to determine the optimal duration of sleep for the prevention of abdominal obesity in different age groups of children and adolescents.

It has been proven that a lower risk of abdominal obesity is linked to the application of "healthy" patterns of diet, based on a high intake of fruits, vegetables, fish, milk, and dairy products. Elevated risk is associated with increased consumption of fast food, sugar, sweets, and sweetened beverages. In studies conducted in Asian countries, high meat intake was also associated with a higher risk of abdominal obesity. The literature highlights the negative effect of sugar-sweetened beverages, but some studies suggest that an increased risk of abdominal obesity may be particularly associated with the consumption of fructose-sweetened beverages. Reducing the consumption of sweetened beverages and promoting healthier alternatives can help optimize the diet of children and adolescents in terms of nutrient content, including calcium and vitamin D, and can thereby also reduce the risk of obesity.

Less frequent meals are also among the dietary risk factors for abdominal obesity, but there is little research supporting this association in children and adolescents. Abdominal obesity is undoubtedly associated, however, with breakfast skipping. It was found that even the occasional consumption of breakfast by adolescents was associated with lower visceral fatness. It is difficult to point to the effect of individual nutrients on abdominal obesity, but it may be associated with the fact that individuals with excess body weight underestimate their actual food consumption [190]. Only the beneficial effects of a high intake of dietary fiber have been proven, although there is some evidence that calcium also has a beneficial effect.

So far, very little research has been done into the effect of alcohol on the development of abdominal obesity in adolescents; the cause of ambiguous results obtained by different authors may be that the intensity of alcohol drinking by adolescents is too low to reveal a significant impact on abdominal obesity; some studies conducted in adults demonstrate that the relationship between alcohol consumption and abdominal obesity is revealed only in heavy drinkers [191]. Similarly, it is difficult to draw clear conclusion about the impact of cigarette smoking on the distribution of body fat in adolescents. It was found, however, that smoking in adolescence may increase the risk of obesity in adulthood. Therefore, efforts to reduce alcohol consumption and smoking by young people because of their potential to be risk factors for abdominal obesity seems reasonable.

In the development of prevention programs aimed at reducing the risk of abdominal obesity, attention should be paid to the co-occurrence of different adverse health behaviors in the same individuals. It was found that making wrong food choices is often associated with less physical activity, more time spent in sedentary activities, and a shorter sleep duration [62,63,73].

Children have very little visceral fat tissue in proportion to total body fat; therefore, as some researchers state, the risk of cardiovascular disease and type 2 diabetes in children results from general adiposity [184,192]. However, the risk of abdominal obesity could be signaled at the age of at least 7 years: it was found that over 62% of boys and 51% girls with abdominal distribution of body fat at age 7 years remain in the same category of adiposity throughout adolescence [193]. Other long-term studies also showed that each additional year of abdominal obesity was associated with a 4% higher risk of developing diabetes [194]. As the amount of VAT in humans tends to rise with age, a better knowledge of the mechanisms of abdominal fat distribution in children and adolescents and the factors determining it would enable appropriate early intervention to more effectively prevent the excessive development of abdominal obesity and its metabolic consequences later in life.

References

[1] Suliga E. Visceral adipose tissue in children and adolescents: a review. Nutr Res Rev 2009;22:137–47.
[2] Antonogeorgos G, Papadimitriou A, Panagiotakos DB, Priftis KN, Nikolaidou P. Physical activity patterns and obesity status among 10- to 12-year old adolescents living in Athens. J Phys Act Health 2010;7:633–40.
[3] Fernandes RA, Zanesco A. Early physical activity promotes lower prevalence of chronic diseases in adulthood. Hypertens Res 2010;33:926–31.
[4] Saelens BE, Seely RJ, van Schaick K, Donnelly LF, O'Brien KJ. Visceral abdominal fat is correlated with whole-body fat and physical activity among 8-y-old children at risk of obesity. Am J Clin Nutr 2007;85:46–53.
[5] Dencker M, Thorsson O, Karlsson MK, Lindén C, Wollmer P, Andersen LB. Daily physical activity related to aerobic fitness and body fat in an urban sample of children. Scand J Med Sci Sports 2008;18:728–35.
[6] Moliner-Urdiales D, Ruiz JR, Ortega FB, Rey-Lopez JP, Vicente-Rodriguez G, España-Romero V, et al. Association of objectively assessed physical activity with total and central body fat in

Spanish adolescents; the HELENA Study. Int J Obes (Lond) 2009;33:1126–35.
[7] Strong WB, Malina RM, Blimkie CJ, Daniels SR, Dishman RK, Gutin B, et al. Evidence based physical activity for school-age youth. J Pediatr 2005;146:732–7.
[8] Roemmich JN, Clark PA, Walter K, Patrie J, Weltman A, Rogol AD. Pubertal alterations in growth and body composition. V. Energy expenditure, adiposity, and fat distribution. Am J Physiol Endocrinol Metab 2000;279:1426–36.
[9] Stallmann-Jorgensen IS, Guttin B, Hatfield-Laube JL, Humphries MC, Johnson MH, Barbeau P. General and visceral adiposity in black and white adolescents and their relation with reported physical activity and diet. Int J Obes 2007;31:622–9.
[10] Ortega FB, Ruiz JR, Sjöstrom M. Physical activity, overweight and central adiposity in Swedish children and adolescents: the European Youth Heart Study. Int J Behav Nutr Phys Act 2007;4:61. http://dx.doi.org/10.1186/1479-5868-4-61.
[11] Chaput JP, Lambert M, Mathieu ME, Tremblay MS, O'Loughlin J, Tremblay A. Physical activity vs. sedentary time: independent associations with adiposity in children. Pediatr Obes 2012;7:251–8.
[12] Steele RM, van Sluijs EMF, Cassidy A, Griffin SJ, Ekelund U. Targeting sedentary time or moderate- and vigorous-intensity activity: independent relations with adiposity in a population-based sample of 10-y-old British children. Am J Clin Nutr 2009;90:1185–92.
[13] Duncan JS, Schofield G, Duncan EK. Pedometer-determined physical activity and body composition in New Zealand children. Med Sci Sports Exerc 2006;38:1402–9.
[14] Hussey J, Bell C, Bennett K, O'Dwyer J, Gormley J. Relationship between the intensity of physical activity, inactivity, cardiorespiratory fitness and body composition in 7–10- year-old Dublin children. Br J Sports Med 2007;41:311–6.
[15] Purslow LR, Hill C, Saxton J, Corder K, Wardle J. Differences in physical activity and sedentary time in relation to weight in 8–9 year old children. Int J Behav Nutr Phys Act 2008;5:67. http://dx.doi.org/10.1186/1479-5868-5-67.
[16] Butte NF, Puyau MR, Adolph AL, Vohra FA, Zakeri I. Physical activity in nonoverweight and overweight Hispanic children and adolescents. Med Sci Sports Exerc 2007;39:1257–66.
[17] Ekelund U, Anderssen SA, Froberg K, Sardinha LB, Andersen LB, Brage S. Independent associations of physical activity and cardiorespiratory fitness with metabolic risk factors in children: the European youth heart study. Diabetologia 2007;50:1832–40.
[18] Fisher A, Hill C, Webber L, Purslow L, Wardle J. MVPA is associated with lower weight gain in 8–10 year old children: A Prospective Study with 1 Year Follow-Up. PLoS ONE 2011;6:e18576. http://dx.doi.org/10.1371/journal.pone.0018576.
[19] Ekelund U, Luan J, Sherar LB, Esliger DW, Griew P, Cooper A, et al. Moderate to vigorous physical activity and sedentary time and cardiometabolic risk factors in children and adolescents. J Am Med Assoc 2012;307:704–12.
[20] Haas GM, Liepold E, Schwandt P. Metabolic risk factors, leisure time physical activity, and nutrition in German children and adolescents. Cholesterol, Article ID 370850, 2012, http://dx.doi.org/10.1155/2012/370850.
[21] Klein-Platat C, Oujaa M, Wagner A, Haan MC, Arveiler D, Schlienger JL, et al. Physical activity is inversely related to waist circumference in 12-y-old French adolescents. Int J Obes (Lond) 2005;29:9–14.
[22] Dos Santos Cavalcanti CB, Gomes de Barros MV, Lins Menêses A, Menêses Santos C, Pires Azevedo AM, de Sá Pereira Guimarães FJ. Abdominal obesity in adolescents: prevalence and association with physical activity and eating habits. Arq Bras Cardiol 2010;94:350–6.
[23] Collison KS, Zaidi MZ, Subhani SN, Al-Rubeaan K, Shoukri M, Al-Mohanna FA. Sugar-sweetened carbonated beverage consumption correlates with BMI, waist circumference, and poor dietary choices in school children. BMC Public Health 2010;10:234.<http://www.biomedcentral.com/1471-2458/10/234>
[24] Al-Hazzaa HM, Abahussain NA, Al-Sobayel HI, Dina M, Qahwaji DM, Musaiger AO. Lifestyle factors associated with overweight and obesity among Saudi adolescents. BMC Public Health 2012;12:354.
[25] Ortega FB, Tresaco B, Ruiz JR, Moreno LA, Martin-Matillas M, Mesa JL, et al. Cardiorespiratory fitness and sedentary activities are associated with adiposity in adolescents. Obesity 2007;15:1589–99. [Silver Spring]
[26] Kelishadi R, Razaghi EM, Gouya MM, Ardalan G, Gheiratmand R, Delavari A, et al. Association of physical activity and the metabolic syndrome in children and adolescents: CASPIAN Study. Horm Res 2007;67:46–52.
[27] Chou YC, Pei JS. Risk factors of adolescent obesity in Taiwan and its association with physical activity, blood pressure and waist circumference. Asian J Sports Med 2010;1:214–22.
[28] Santos Silva DA, Pelegrini A, Ferreira de Lima e Silva JM, Petroski EL. Epidemiology of abdominal obesity among adolescents from a Brazilian state capital. J Korean Med Sci 2011;26:78–84.
[29] Garnett SP, Cowell CT, Baur LA, Shrewsbury VA, Chan A, Crawford D, et al. Increasing central adiposity: the Nepean longitudinal study of young people aged 7–8 to 12–13 y. Int J Obes (Lond) 2005;29:1353–60.
[30] Paffenbarger RS, Blair SN, Lee IM, Hyde RT. Measurement of physical activity to assess health effects in free living populations. Med Sci Sports Exerc 1993;25:60–70.
[31] LaMonte MJ, Blair SN. Physical activity, cardiorespiratory fitness, and adiposity: contributions to disease risk. Curr Opin Clin Nutr Metab Care 2006;9:540–6.
[32] Eliakim A, Burke GS, Cooper DM. Fitness, fatness, and the effect of training assessed by magnetic resonance imaging and skinfold-thickness measurements in healthy adolescent females. Am J Clin Nutr 1997;66:223–31.
[33] Winsley RJ, Armstrong N, Middlebrooke AR, Ramos-Ibañez N, Williams CA. Aerobic fitness and visceral adipose tissue in children. Acta Paediatr 2006;95:1435–8.
[34] Lee SJ, Arslanian SA. Cardiorespiratory fitness and abdominal adiposity in youth. Eur J Clin Nutr 2007;61:561–5.
[35] Stigman S, Rintala P, Kukkonen-Harjula K, Kujala U, Rinne M, Fogelholm M. Eight-year-old children with high cardiorespiratory fitness have lower overall and abdominal fatness. Int J Pediatr Obes 2009;4:98–105.
[36] Carnethon MR, Gulati M, Greenland P. Prevalence and cardiovascular disease correlates of low cardiorespiratory fitness in adolescents and adults. J Am Med Assoc 2005;294:2981–8.
[37] Ortega FB, Ruiz JR, Castillo MJ, Sjöström M. Physical fitness in childhood and adolescence: a powerful marker of health. Int J Obes 2008;32:1–11.
[38] Ostojic SM, Stojanovic MD, Stojanovic V, Maric J, et al. Correlation between fitness and fatness in 6–14-year old Serbian school children. J Health Popul Nutr 2011;29:53–60.
[39] Shaibi GQ, Cruz ML, Ball GD, Weigensberg MJ, Kobaissi HA, Salem GJ, et al. Cardiovascular fitness and the metabolic syndrome in overweight Latino youths. Med Sci Sports Exerc 2005;2005(37):922–8.
[40] Klasson-Heggebo L, Andersen LB, Wennlof AH, Sardinha LB, Harro M, Froberg K, et al. Graded associations between cardiorespiratory fitness, fatness, and blood pressure in children and adolescents. Br J Sports Med 2006;40:25–9.

[41] Psarra G, Nassis GP, Sidossis LS. Short-term predictors of abdominal obesity in children. Eur J Public Health 2006;16:520–5.
[42] Owens S, Gutin B, Allison J, Riggs S, Ferguson M, Litaker M, et al. Effect of physical training on total and visceral fat in obese children. Med Sci Sports Exerc 1999;31:143–8.
[43] Eliakim A, Makowski GS, Brasel JA, Cooper DM. Adiposity, lipid levels, and brief endurance training in nonobese adolescent males. Int J Sports Med 2000;21:332–7.
[44] Gutin B, Barbeau P, Owens S, Lemmon CR, Bauman M, Allison J, et al. Effects of exercise intensity on cardiovascular fitness, total body composition, and visceral adiposity of obese adolescents. Am J Clin Nutr 2002;75:818–26.
[45] Barbeau P, Johnson MH, Howe CA, Allison J, Davis CL, Gutin B, et al. Ten months of exercise improves general and visceral adiposity, bone, and fitness in black girls. Obesity 2007;15:2077–85. (Silver Spring)
[46] Kim ES, Im JA, Kim KC, Park JH, Suh SH, Kang ES, et al. Improved insulin sensitivity and adiponectin level after exercise training in obese Korean youth. Obesity 2007;15:3023–30. (Silver Spring)
[47] Van der Heijden GJ, Wang ZJ, Chu Z, Toffolo G, Manesso E, Sauer PJJ, et al. Strength exercise improves muscle mass and hepatic insulin sensitivity in obese youth. Med Sci Sports Exerc 2010;42:1973–80.
[48] Lazaar N, Aucouturier J, Ratel S, Rance M, Meyer M, Duche P. Effect of physical activity intervention on body composition in young children: influence of body mass index status and gender. Acta Paediatr 2007;96:1315–20.
[49] Kelishadi R, Hashemi M, Mohammadifard N, Asgary S, Khavarian N. Association of changes in oxidative and proinflammatory stages with chages in vascular function after a lifestyle modification trial among obese children. Clin Chem 2008;54:147–53.
[50] Davies JN, Gyllenhammer LE, Vanni AA, Meija M, Tung A, Schroeder ET, et al. Startup circuit training program reduces metabolic risk in Latino adolescents. Med Sci Sports Exerc 2011;43:2195–203.
[51] Davies CL, Pollock NK, Waller JL, Allison JD, Dennis BA, Bassali R, et al. Exercise dose and diabetes risk in overweight and obese children: a randomized controlled trial. J Am Med Assoc 2012;308:1103–12.
[52] Watts K, Beye P, Siafarikas A, Davis EA, Jones TW, O'Driscoll G, et al. Exercise training normalizes vascular dysfunction and improves central adiposity in obese adolescents. J Am Coll Cardiol 2004;43:1823–7.
[53] Resnicow K, Taylor R, Baskin M, McCarty F. Results of go girls: a weight control program for overweight African-American adolescent females. Obes Res 2005;13:1739–48.
[54] Marshall SJ, Biddle SJH, Gorely T, Cameron N, Murdey I. Relationships between media use, body fatness and physical activity in children and youth: a meta-analysis. Int J Obes 2004;28:1238–46.
[55] Altenburg TM, Singh AS, van Mechelen W, Brug J, Chinapaw MJW. Direction of the association between body fatness and self-reported screen time in Dutch adolescents. Int J Behav Nutr Phys Activ 2012;9:4.
[56] Dumith SC, Garcia LM, da Silva KS, Menezes AM, Hallal PC. Predictors and health consequences of screen-time change during adolescence –1993 Pelotas (Brazil) birth cohort study. J Adolesc Health 2012;51:16–21.
[57] Chinapaw MJM, Yildirim M, Altenburg TM, Singh AS, Kovács E, Molnár D, et al. Objective and self-rated sedentary time and indicators of metabolic health in Dutch and Hungarian 10–12 year olds: The ENERGY-Project. PLoS ONE 2012;7:e36657. http://dx.doi.org/10.1371/journal.pone.0036657.
[58] Byun W, Dowda M, Pate RR. Associations between screen-based sedentary behavior and cardiovascular disease risk factors in Korean youth. J Korean Med Sci 2012;27:388–94.
[59] Carson V, Jansen I. Volume, patterns, and types of sedentary behavior and cardio-metabolic health in children and adolescents: a cross-sectional study. BMC Public Health 2011;11:274.
[60] Rey-Lopez JP, Vicente-Rodriguez G, Biosca M, Moreno LA. Sedentary behaviour and obesity development in children and adolescents. Nutr Metab Cardiovasc Dis 2008;18:242–51.
[61] Klesges RC, Shelton ML, Klesges LM. Effects of television on metabolic rate: potential implications for childhood obesity. Pediatrics 1993;91:281–6.
[62] Chaput JP, Klingenberg L, Astrup A, Sjödin AM. Modern sedentary activities promote overconsumption of food in our current obesogenic environment. Obes Rev 2011;12:12–20.
[63] Bar-Anderson DJ, Larson NI, Nelson MC, Neumark-Sztainer D, Story M. Does television viewing predict dietary intake five years later in high school students and young adults? Int J Behav Nutr Phys Act 2009;30:7. http://dx.doi.org/10.1186/1479-5868-6-7.
[64] Pearson N, Ball K, Crawford D. Mediators of longitudinal associations between television viewing and eating behaviours in adolescents. Int J Behav Nutr Phys Act 2011;30:23. http://dx.doi.org/10.1186/1479-5868-8-23.
[65] Rey-Lopez JP, Vicente-Rodríguez G, Répásy J, Mesana MI, Ruiz JR, Ortega FB, et al. Food and drink intake during television viewing in adolescents: the Healthy Lifestyle in Europe by Nutrition in Adolescence (HELENA) study. Publ Health Nutr 2011;14:1563–9.
[66] Cappucio FP, Taggart FM, Kandala NB, Currie A, Peile E, Stranges S, et al. Meta-analysis of short sleep duration and obesity in children and adults. Sleep 2008;31:619–26.
[67] Chen X, Beydoun MA, Wang Y. Is sleep duration associated with childhood obesity? A systematic review and meta-analysis. Obesity 2008;16:265–74. [Silver Spring]
[68] Hart CN, Cairns A, Jelalian E. Sleep and obesity in children and adolescents. Pediatr Clin North Am 2011;58:715–33.
[69] Knutson KL. Does Inadequate Sleep Play a Role in Vulnerability to Obesity? Am J Hum Biol 2012;24:361–71.
[70] Copinschi G. Metabolic and endocrine effects of sleep deprivation. Essent Psychopharmacol 2005;6:341–7.
[71] Yu Y, Lu BS, Wang B, Wang H, Yang J, Li Z, et al. Short sleep duration and adiposity in Chinese adolescents. Sleep 2007;30:1688–97.
[72] Hitze B, Bosy-Westphal A, Bielfeldt F, Settler U, Plachta-Danielzik S, Pfeuffer M, et al. Determinants and impact of sleep duration in children and adolescents: data of the Kiel Obesity Prevention Study. Eur J Clin Nutr 2009;63:739–46.
[73] Garaulet M, Ortega FB, Ruiz JR, Rey-López JP, Béghin L, Manios Y, et al. Short sleep duration is associated with increased obesity markers in European adolescents: effect of physical activity and dietary habits. The HELENA study. Int J Obes 2011;35:1308–17.
[74] Bawazeer NM, Al-Daghri NM, Valsamakis G, Al-Rubeaan KA, Sabico SLB, Huang TTK, et al. Sleep duration and quality associated with obesity among Arab children. Obesity 2009;17:2251–3.
[75] Al-Hazzaa M, Al-Hazzaa HM, Musaiger AO, Abahussain NA, Hana I, Al-Sobayel HI, et al. Prevalence of short sleep duration and its association with obesity among adolescents 15- to 19-year olds: a cross-sectional study from three major cities in Saudi Arabia. Ann Thorac Med 2012;7:133–9.
[76] Von Kries R, Toschke AM, Wurmser H, Sauerwald T, Koletzko B. Reduced risk for overweight and obesity in 5- and 6-y-old children by duration of sleep: a cross-sectional study. Int J Obes Relat Metab Disord 2002;26:710–6.

[77] Golley RK, Maher CA, Matricciani L, Olds TS. Sleep duration or bedtime? Exploring the association between sleep timing behaviour, diet and BMI in children and adolescents. Int J Obes 2013:8. http://dx.doi.org/10.1038/ijo.2012.212.

[78] Bradlee ML, Singer MR, Qureshi MM, Moore LL. Food group intake and central obesity among children and adolescents in the third national health and nutrition examination survey (NHANES III). Publ Health Nutr 2010;13:797–805.

[79] Casazza K, Beasley TM, Fernandez JR. Beyond thriftiness: Independent and interactive effects of genetic and dietary factors on variations in fat deposition and distribution across populations. Am J Phys Anthropol 2011;145:181–91.

[80] Bailey BW, Sullivan DK, Kirk EP, Donnelly JE. Dietary predictors of visceral adiposity in overweight young adults. Br J Nutr 2010;103:1702–5.

[81] Ventura EE, Davis JN, Alexander KE, Shaibi GQ, Lee W, Byrd-Williams CE, et al. Dietary intake and the metabolic syndrome in overweight Latino children. J Am Diet Assoc 2008;108:1355–9.

[82] Ventura E, Davis J, Byrd-Williams C, Alexander KE, McClain A, Lane CJ, et al. Reduction in risk factors for type 2 diabetes mellitus in response to a low-sugar, high-fiber dietary intervention in overweight Latino adolescents. Arch Pediatr Adolesc Med 2009;163:320–7.

[83] Davies JN, Alexander KE, Ventura EE, Toledo-Corral CM, Goran MI. Inverse relation between dietary fiber intake and visceral adiposity in overweight Latino youth. Am J Clin Nutr 2009;90:1160–6.

[84] Parikh S, Pollock NK, Bhagatwala J, Guo DH, Gutin B, Zhu H, et al. Adolescent fiber consumption is associated with visceral fat and inflammatory markers. J Clin Endocrinol Metab 2012;97:1451–7.

[85] Jenkins DJ, Jenkins AL, Wolever TM, Rao AV, Thompson LU. Fiber and starchy foods: gut function and implications in disease. Am J Gastroenterol 1986;81:920–30.

[86] Kimm SY. The role of dietary fiber in the development and treatment of childhood obesity. Pediatrics 1995;96:1010–4.

[87] Lundin EA, Zhang JX, Lairon D, Tidehag P, Aman P, Adlercreutz H, et al. Effects of meal frequency and high-fibre rye-bread diet on glucose and lipid metabolism and ileal excretion of energy and sterols in ileostomy subjects. Eur J Clin Nutr 2004;58:1410–9.

[88] De Kleijn MJ, van der Schouw YT, Wilson PW, Grobbee DE, Jacques PF. Dietary intake of phytoestrogens is associated with a favorable metabolic cardiovascular risk profile in postmenopausal U.S. women: the Framingham study. J Nutr 2002;132:276–82.

[89] Pan A, Demark-Wahnefried PA, Ye X, Yu Z, Li H, Qi Q, et al. Effects of a flaxseed-derived lignan supplement on C-reactive protein, IL-6 and retinol-binding protein 4 in type 2 diabetic patients. Br J Nutr 2009;101:1145–9.

[90] Ritchie LD, Spector P, Stevens MJ, Schmidt MM, Schreiber GB, Striegel-Moore RH, et al. Dietary patterns in adolescence are related to adiposity in young adulthood in black and white females. J Nutr 2007;137:399–406.

[91] Suliga E, Wronka I, Pawlińska-Chmara R. The prevalence and correlates of abdominal obesity in female students. Pediatr Endocrinol Diabetes Metab 2011;17:201–5.

[92] Francis DK, Van den Broeck J, Younger N, Shelly McFarlane S, Rudder K, et al. Fast-food and sweetened beverage consumption: association with overweight and high waist circumference in adolescents. Publ Health Nutr 2009;12:1106–14.

[93] Kim JA, Kim SM, Lee JS, Oh HJ, Han JH, Song Y, et al. Dietary patterns and the metabolic syndrome in Korean adolescents. Diabetes Care 2007;30:1904–5.

[94] Shang X, Li Y, Liu A, Zhang Q, Hu X, Du S, et al. Dietary pattern and its association with the prevalence of obesity and related cardiometabolic risk factors among Chinese children. PLoS ONE 2012;7:e43183. http://dx.doi.org/10.1371/journal.pone.0043183.

[95] Alavian SM, Motlag MEh, Ardalan G, Motaghian M, Davarpanah AH, Kelishadi R. Hypertriglyceridemic waist phenotype and associated lifestyle factors in a national population of youths: CASPIAN Study. J Trop Pediatr 2007;54:169–77.

[96] Singhal N, Misra A, Shah P, Gulati S. Effects of controlled school-based multi-component model of nutrition and lifestyle interventions on behavior modification, anthropometry and metabolic risk profile of urban Asian Indian adolescents in North India. Eur J Clin Nutr 2010;64:364–73.

[97] Kant AK, Graubard BI. Predictors of reported consumption of low-nutrient-density foods in a 24-h recall by 8–16 year old US children and adolescents. Appetite 2003;41:175–80.

[98] Chiang PH, Wahlqvist ML, Lee MS, Huang LY, Chen HH, Huang ST. Fast-food outlets and walkability in school neighbourhoods predict fatness in boys and height in girls: a Taiwanese population study. Publ Health Nutr 2011;14:1601–9.

[99] Smith KJ, McNaughton SA, Gall SL, Blizzard L, Dwyer T, Venn AJ. Takeaway food consumption and its associations with diet quality and abdominal obesity: a cross-sectional study of young adults. Int J Behav Nutr Phys Act 2009;6:29. http://dx.doi.org/10.1186/1479-5868-6-29.

[100] Smith KJ, McNaughton SA, Gall SL, Blizzard L, Dwyer T, Venn AJ. Involvement of young Australian adults in meal preparation: cross-sectional associations with abdominal obesity and body mass index. J Am Diet Assoc 2011;111:1187–91.

[101] Spence LA, Cifelli CJ, Miller GD. The role of dairy products in healthy weight and body composition in children and adolescents. Curr Nutr Food Sci 2011;7:40–9.

[102] Kelishadi R, Zemel MB, Hashemipour M, Hosseini M, Mohammadifard N, Poursafa P. Can a dairy-rich diet be effective in long-term weight control of young children? J Am Coll Nutr 2009;28:601–10.

[103] Poddar KH, Hosig KW, Nickols-Richardson SM, Anderson ES, Herbert WG, Duncan SE. Low-fat dairy intake and body weight and composition changes in college students. J Am Diet Assoc 2009;109:1433–8.

[104] Hirschler V, Oestreicher K, Beccaria K, Hidalgo M, Maccalini G. Inverse association between insulin resistance and frequency of milk consumption in low-income Argentinean school children. J Pediatr 2009;154:101–5.

[105] St-Onge MP, Goree LLT, Gower B. High-milk supplementation with healthy diet counseling does not affect weight loss but ameliorates insulin action compared with low-milk supplementation in overweight children. J Nutr 2009;139:933–8.

[106] Keller KL, Kirzner J, Pietrobelli A, St-Onge MP, Faith MS. Increased sweetened beverage intake is associated with reduced milk and calcium intake in 3–7 y. old children at multi-item laboratory lunches. J Am Diet Assoc 2009;109:497–501.

[107] Major GC, Chaput JP, Ledoux M, St-Pierre S, Anderson GH, Zemel MB. Recent developments in calcium-related obesity research. Obes Rev 2008;9:428–45.

[108] Wajchenberg BL, Gianella-Neto D, da Silva ME, Santos RF. Depot-specific hormonal characteristics of subcutaneous and visceral adipose tissue and their relation to the metabolic syndrome. Horm Metab Res 2002;34:616–21.

[109] Morris KL, Zemel MB. 1,25-dihydroxyvitamin D3 modulation of adipocyte glucocorticoid function. Obes Res 2005;13:670–7.

[110] Wolff E, Dansinger ML. Soft drinks and weight gain: how strong is the link? Medscape J Med 2008;10:189–98.

[111] Birch LL, Fisher JO. Development of eating behaviors among children and adolescents. Pediatrics 1998;101:539–49.

[112] Te Morenga L, Mallard S, Mann J. Dietary sugars and body weight: systematic review and meta-analyses of randomised

controlled trials and cohort studies. Br Med J 2012;345:e7492. http://dx.doi.org/10.1136/bmj.e7492.

[113] Fiorito LM, Marini M, Francis LA, Smiciklas-Wright H, Birch LL. Beverage intake of girls at age 5 y predicts adiposity and weight status in childhood and adolescence. Am J Clin Nutr 2009;90:935–42.

[114] Bray GA, Nielsen SJ, Popkin B. Consumption of high fructose corn syrup in beverages may play a role in the epidemic of obesity. Am J Clin Nutr 2004;79:537–43.

[115] Ferreira de Moraes AC, Falcão MC. Lifestyle factors and socioeconomic variables associated with abdominal obesity in Brazilian adolescents. Ann Hum Biol 2013;40:1–8.

[116] Stanhope KL, Schwarz JM, Keim NL, Griffen SC, Bremer AA, Graham JL, et al. Consuming fructose-sweetened, not glucose-sweetened, beverages increases visceral adiposity and lipids and decreases insulin sensitivity in overweight/obese humans. J Clin Invest 2009;119:1322–34.

[117] Harnack L, Stang J, Story M. Soft drink consumption among U.S. children and adolescents: nutritional consequences. J Am Diet Assoc 1999;99:436–41.

[118] Bowman SA. Beverage choices of young females: changes and impact on nutrient intakes. J Am Diet Assoc 2002;102:1234–9.

[119] Marshall TA, Eichenberger Gilmore JM, Broffitt B, Stumbo PJ, Levy SM. Diet quality in young children is influenced by beverage consumption. Am J Clin Nutr 2005;24:65–75.

[120] Kant A, Schatzkin A, Graubard B, Ballard-Barbash R. Frequency of eating occasions and weight change in the NHANES I Epidemiologic Follow-up Study. Int J Obes Relat Metab Disord 1995;19:468–74.

[121] Ma Y, Bertone ER, Stanek 3rd EJ, Reed GW, Hebert JR, Cohen NL, et al. Association between eating patterns and obesity in a free-living US adult population. Am J Epidemiol 2003;158:85–92.

[122] Toschke AM, Küchenhoff H, Koletzko B, von Kries R. Meal frequency and childhood obesity. Obes Res 2005;13:1932–8.

[123] Toschke AM, Thorsteindottir KH, von Kries R. GME Study Group. Meal frequency, breakfast consumption and childhood obesity. Int J Pediatr Obes 2009;4:242–8.

[124] La Bounty PM, Campbell BI, Wilson J, Galvan E, Berardi J, Kleiner SM, et al. International Society of Sports Nutrition position stand: meal frequency. J Int Soc Sports Nutr 2011;16:4. http://dx.doi.org/10.1186/1550-2783-8-4.

[125] Kim JH, So WY. Association between frequency of breakfast eating and obesity in Korean adolescents. Iran J Publ Health 2012;41:50–7.

[126] Ritchie LD. Less frequent eating predicts greater BMI and waist circumference in female adolescents. Am J Clin Nutr 2012;95:290–6.

[127] Jenkins DJ. Carbohydrate tolerance and food frequency. Br J Nutr 1997;77(Suppl. 1):71–81.

[128] Smeets AJ, Westerterp-Plantenga MS. Acute effects on metabolism and appetite profile of one meal difference in the lower range of meal frequency. Br J Nutr 2008;99:1316–21.

[129] Jenkins DJ, Wolever TM, Vuksan V, Brighenti F, Cunnane SC, Rao AV, et al. Nibbling versus gorging: metabolic advantages of increased meal frequency. N Engl J Med 1989;321:929–34.

[130] Tai MM, Castillo P, Pi-Sunyer FX. Meal size and frequency: effect on the thermic effect of food. Am J Clin Nutr 1991;54:783–7.

[131] Bellisle F, McDevitt R, Prentice AM. Meal frequency and energy balance. Br J Nutr 1997;77(Suppl. 1):57–70.

[132] Timlin MT, Pereira MA, Story M, Neumark-Sztainer D. Breakfast eating and weight change in a 5-year prospective analysis of adolescents: project EAT (eating among teens). Pediatrics 2008;121:638–45.

[133] Tin SP, Ho SY, Mak KH, Wan KL, Lam TH. Breakfast skipping and change in body mass index in young children. Int J Obes (Lond) 2011;35:899–906.

[134] Nicklas TA, Reger C, Myers L, O'Neil C. Breakfast consumption with and without vitamin-mineral supplement use favorably impacts daily nutrient intake of ninth-grade students. J Adolesc Health 2000;27:314–21.

[135] Niemeier HM, Raynor HA, Lloyd-Richardson EE, Rogers ML, Wing RR. Fast food consumption and breakfast skipping: Predictors of weight gain from adolescence to adulthood in a nationally representative sample. J Adolesc Health 2006;39:842–9.

[136] Miech RA, Kumanyika SK, Stettler N, Link BG, Phelan JC, Chang VW. Trends in the association of poverty with overweight among US adolescents, 1971–2004. J Am Med Assoc 2006;295:2385–93.

[137] Lioret S, Volatier JL, Lafay L, Touvier M, Maire B. Is food portion size a risk factor of childhood overweight? Eur J Clin Nutr 2009;63:382–91.

[138] Alexander KE, Ventura EE, Spruijt-Metz D, Weigensberg MJ, Goran MI, Davis JN. Association of breakfast skipping with visceral fat and insulin indices in overweight Latino youth. Obesity 2009;17:1528–33.

[139] Deshmukh-Taskar PR, Nicklas TA, O'Neil CE, Keast DR, Radcliffe JD, Cho S. The relationship of breakfast skipping and type of breakfast consumption with nutrient intake and weight status in children and adolescents: The National Health and Nutrition Examination Survey 1999–2006. J Am Diet Assoc 2010;110:869–78.

[140] Drummond S, Crombie N, Kirk T. A critique of the effects of snacking on body weight status. Eur J Clin Nutr 1996;50:779–83.

[141] Song WO, Chun OK, Kerver J, Cho S, Chung CE, Chung S-J. Ready-to-eat breakfast cereal consumption enhances milk and calcium intake in the US population. J Am Diet Assoc 2006;106:1783–9.

[142] Zemel MB, Richards J, Milstead A, Campbell P. Effects of calcium and dairy on body composition and weight loss in African-American adults. Obes Res 2005;13:1218–25.

[143] Croezen S, Visscher TLS, Ter Bogt NCW, Veling ML, Haveman-Nies A. Skipping breakfast, alcohol consumption and physical inactivity as risk factor for overweight and obesity in adolescents: results of the E-MOVO project. Eur J Clin Nutr 2009;63:405–12.

[144] Vígstrand K, Barkeling B, Forslund HB, Elfhag K, Linné Y, Rössner S, et al. Eating habits in relation to body fatness and gender in adolescents—results from the "SWEDES" study. Eur J Clin Nutr 2007;61:517–25.

[145] Berkey CS, Rockett HRH, Colditz GA. Weight gain in older adolescent females: the internet, sleep, coffee, and alcohol. J Pediatr 2008;153:635–9.

[146] Pajari M, Pietiläinen KH, Kaprio J, Rose FJ, Saarni S. The effect of alcohol consumption on later obesity in early adulthood—a population-based longitudinal study. Alcohol 2010;45:173–9.

[147] Halkjær J, Sørensen TIA, Tjønneland A, Togo P, Holst C, Heitmann BL. Food and drinking patterns as predictors of 6-year BMI-adjusted changes in waist circumference. Br J Nutr 2004;92:735–48.

[148] Laitinen J, Pietilainen K, Wadsworth M, Sovio U, Jarvelin MR. Predictors of abdominal obesity among 31-y-old men and women born in Northern Finland in 1966. Eur J Clin Nutr 2004;58:180–90.

[149] Schröder H, Morales-Molina JA, Bermejo S. Relationship of abdominal obesity with alcohol consumption at population scale. Eur J Nutr 2007;46:369–76.

[150] Lourenço S, Oliveira A, Lopes C. The effect of current and lifetime alcohol consumption on overall and central obesity. Eur J Clin Nutr 2012;66:813–8.

[151] Cignolini M, Targher G, Bergamo Andreis IA, Tonoli M, Filippi F, Muggeo M, et al. Moderate alcohol consumption and its relation to visceral fat and plasma androgens in healthy women. Int J Obes Relat Metab Disord 1996;20:206–12.
[152] Molenaar EA, Massaro JM, Jacques PF, Pou KM, Ellison RC, Hoffmann U, et al. Association of lifestyle factors with abdominal subcutaneous and visceral adiposity. Diabetes Care 2009;32:505–10.
[153] Wakabajashi I. Cross-sectional relationship between alcohol consumption and prevalence of metabolic syndrome in Japanese men and women. J Artherioscler Thromb 2010;17:695–704.
[154] Halkjær J, Tjønneland A, Thomsen BL, Overvad K, Sørensen TIA. Intake of macronutrients as predictors of 5-y changes in waist circumference. Am J Clin Nutr 2006;84:789–97.
[155] Slattery ML, McDonald A, Bild DE, Caan BJ, Hilner JE, Jacobs Jr DR, et al. Associations of body fat and its distribution with dietary intake, physical activity, alcohol, and smoking in blacks and whites. Am J Clin Nutr 1992;55:943–9.
[156] Bergmann MM, Schütze M, Steffen A, Boeing H, Halkjær J, Tjonneland A, et al. The association of lifetime alcohol use with measures of abdominal and general adiposity in a large-scale European cohort. Eur J Clin Nutr 2011;65:1079–87.
[157] Currie C, Zanotti C, Morgan A, Currie D, de Looze M, Roberts C, et al, editors. Social determinants of health and well-being among young people. Health Behaviour in School-aged Children (HBSC) study: international report from the 2009/2010 survey. Copenhagen, WHO Regional Office for Europe (Health Policy for Children and Adolescents, No. 6); 2012.
[158] Must A, Bandini LG, Tybor DJ, Janssen I, Ross R, Dietz WH. Behavioral risk factors in relation to visceral adipose tissue deposition in adolescent females. Int J Pediatr Obes 2008;3(Suppl. 1):28–36.
[159] Tzotzas T, Kapantais E, Tziomalos K, Ioannidis I, Mortoglou A, Bakatselos S, et al. Epidemiological survey for the prevalence of overweight and abdominal obesity in Greek adolescents. Obesity 2008;16:1718–22. [Silver Spring]
[160] Van Lenthe F, van Mechelen W, Kemper HCG, Post GB. Behavioral variables and development of a central pattern of body fat from adolescence into adulthood in normal-weight whites: the Amsterdam Growth and Health Study. Am J Clin Nutr 1998;67:846–52.
[161] Yeomans MR, Caton S, Hetherington MM. Alcohol and food intake. Curr Opin Clin Nutr Metab Care 2003;6:639–44.
[162] Buemann B, Astrup A. How does the body deal with energy from alcohol? Nutrition 2001;17:638–41.
[163] Suter PM. Is alcohol consumption a risk factor for weight gain and obesity? Crit Rev Clin Lab Sci 2005;42:197–227.
[164] Khaw KT, Barrett-Connor E. Lower endogenous androgens predict central adiposity in men. Ann Epidemiol 1992;2:675–82.
[165] Eriksson CJ, Fukunaga T, Lindman R. Sex hormone response to alcohol. Nature 1994;369:711.
[166] Sarkola T, Fukunaga T, Mäkisalo H, Peter Eriksson CJ. Acute effect of alcohol on androgens in premenopausal women. Alcohol Alcohol 2000;35:84–90.
[167] Björntörp P. Do stress reactions cause abdominal obesity and comorbidities? Obes Rev 2001;2:73–86.
[168] Blouin K, Boivin A, Tchernof A. Androgens and body fat distribution. J Steroid Biochem Mol Biol 2008;108:272–80.
[169] Canoy D, Wareham N, Luben R, Welch A, Bingham S, Day N, et al. Cigarette smoking and fat distribution in 21,828 British men and women: a population-based study. Obes Res 2005;13:1466–75.
[170] Chen H, Sonia Saad S, Shaun L, Sandow SL, Bertrand PP. Cigarette smoking and brain regulation of energy homeostasis. Front Pharmacol 2012;3:147.
[171] Ball K, Brown W, Crawford D. Who does not gain weight? Prevalence and predictors of weight maintenance in young women. Int J Obes Relat Metab Disord 2002;26:1570–8.
[172] Akbartabartoori M, Lean ME, Hankey CR. Relationships between cigarette smoking, body size and body shape. Int J Obes (Lond) 2005;29:236–43.
[173] Komiya H, Mori Y, Yokose T, Tajima N. Smoking as a risk factor for visceral fat accumulation in Japanese men. Tohoku J Exp Med 2006;208:123–32.
[174] Yun JE, Heejin Kimm H, Choi YJ, Jee SH, Huh KB. Smoking is associated with abdominal obesity, not overall obesity, in men with type 2 diabetes. J Prev Med Publ Health 2012;45:316–22.
[175] Onat A, Ayhan E, Hergenc G, Can G, Barlan MM. Smoking inhibits visceral fat accumulation in Turkish women: relation of visceral fat and body fat mass to atherogenic dyslipidemia, inflammatory markers, insulin resistance, and blood pressure. Metabolism 2009;58:963–70.
[176] Kim JH, Shim KW, Yoon YS, Lee SY, Kim SS, Oh SW. Cigarette smoking increases abdominal and visceral obesity but not overall fatness: an observational study. PLoS ONE 2012;7:e45815. http://dx.doi.org/10.1371/journal.pone.0045815.
[177] Neumark-Sztainer D, Story M, French SA. Covariations of unhealthy weight loss behaviors and other high-risk behaviors among adolescents. Arch Pediatr Med 1996;150:304–8.
[178] Fulkerson JA, French SA. Cigarette smoking for weight loss or control among adolescents: gender and racial/ethnic differences. J Adolesc Health 2003;32:306–13.
[179] Saarni K, Silventoinen K, Rissanen A, Sarlio-Lähteenkorva S, Kaprio J. Intentional weight loss and smoking in young adults. Int J Obes 2004;28:796–802.
[180] Saarni SE, Pietiläinen K, Kantonen S, Rissanen A, Kaprio J. Association of smoking in adolescence with abdominal obesity in adulthood: a follow-up study of 5 birth cohorts of Finnish twins. Am J Publ Health 2009;99:348–54.
[181] Tziomaios K, Carcoulis F. Endocrine effects of tobacco smoking. Clin Endocrinol 2004;61:664–74.
[182] Pölkki M, Rantala MJ. Smoking affects womens' sex hormone-regulated body form. Am J Publ Health 2009;99:1350. http://dx.doi.org/10.2105/AJPH.2009.163485.
[183] Brambilla P, Bedogni G, Moreno LA, Goran MI, Gutin B, Fox KR, et al. Crossvalidation of anthropometry against magnetic resonance imaging for the assessment of visceral and subcutaneous adipose tissue in children. Int J Obes 2006;30:23–30.
[184] Benfield LL, Fox KR, Peters DM, Blake H, Rogers I, Grant C, et al. Magnetic resonance imaging of abdominal adiposity in a large cohort of British children. Int J Obes 2008;32:91–9.
[185] Rowlands AV, Ingledew DK, Eston RG. The effect of type of physical activity measure on the relationship between body fatness and habitual physical activity in children: a meta-analysis. Ann Hum Biol 2000;27:479–97.
[186] Slootmaker SM, Schuit AJ, Chinapaw MJ, Seidell JC, van Mechelen W. Disagreement in physical activity assessed by accelerometer and self-report in subgroups of age, gender, education and weight status. Int J Behav Nutr Phys Act 2009;6:17. http://dx.doi.org/10.1186/1479-5868-6-17.
[187] Spittaels H, Van Cauwenberghe E, Verbestel V, De Meester F, Van Dyck D, Verloigne M, et al. Objectively measured sedentary time and physical activity time across the lifespan: a cross-sectional study in four age groups. Int J Behav Nutr Phys Act 2012;9:149. <http://www.ijbnpa.org/content/9/1/149>
[188] Fisher A, Hill C, Webber L, Purslow L, Wardle J. MVPA is associated with lower weight gain in 8–10 year old children: a prospective study with 1 year follow-up. PLoS ONE 2011;6:e18576. http://dx.doi.org/10.1371/journal.pone.0018576.
[189] Ruiz JR, Labayen I, Ortega FB, Legry V, Moreno LA, Dallongeville J, et al. Attenuation of the effect of the *FTO* rs9939609 polymorphism on total and central body fat by physical activity in adolescents: The HELENA Study. Arch Pediatr Adolesc Med 2010;164:328–33.

[190] Maffeis C, Schutz Y, Zaffanello M, Piccoli R, Pinelli L. Elevated energy expenditure and reduced energy intake in obese prepubertal children: paradox of poor dietary reliability in obesity? J Pediatr 1994;124:348–54.

[191] Sayon-Orea C, Martinez-Gonzalez MA, Bes-Rastrollo M. Alcohol consumption and body weight: a systematic review. Nutr Rev 2011;69:419–31.

[192] Lawlor DA, Benfield L, Logue J, Tilling K, Howe LD, Fraser A, et al. Association between general and central adiposity in childhood, and change in these, with cardiovascular risk factors in adolescence: prospective cohort study. BMJ 2010;341:c6224. http://dx.doi.org/10.1136/bmj.c6224.

[193] Chrzanowska M, Suder A, Kruszelnicki P. Tracking and risk of abdominal obesity in the adolescence period in children aged 7–15. The Cracow Longitudinal Growth Study. Am J Hum Biol 2012;24:62–7.

[194] Reis JP, Hankinson AL, Loria CM, Lewis CE, Powell-Wiley T, Wei GS, et al. Duration of abdominal obesity beginning in young adulthood and incident diabetes through middle age: The CARDIA Study. Diabetes Care 2012:17. http://dx.doi.org/10.2337/dc12-1714.

CHAPTER

5

Female Cancer Survivorship and Obesity

Michele L. McCarroll, G. Dante Roulette, and Vivian E. von Gruenigen

Department of Obstetrics and Gynecology, Summa Health System, Akron, Ohio, USA

OBESITY AND FEMALE CANCER

Obesity is an epidemic in the developed world. As of 2012, in the United States the prevalence of overweight and obese individuals in the population approaches 60%, as measured by a body mass index (BMI) greater than 25 kg/m^2 [1]. Obesity has long been recognized as a risk factor for many chronic diseases, chief among these being diabetes and disorders of the cardiovascular system. The link between obesity and the risk of cancer has been known since as early as 2002, when the International Agency for Research on Cancer (IARC) concluded there was adequate evidence for an association between obesity and several types of cancer [2].

Obesity contributes to 11% of colon cancers, 9% of breast cancer in postmenopausal women, 39% of gynecological cancers, 37% of esophageal cancers, and 25% of renal cancers, as published by the IARC in 2011 [3]. It is estimated that <90,000 deaths could be avoided each year in the United States if the adult population maintained a normal BMI [4]. The exact mechanisms leading to the elevation in cancer risk are incompletely understood, although several plausible mechanisms have been proposed. These mechanisms center on derangements of metabolism and endocrine signaling. Obesity is marked by an increase in the amount of subcutaneous and visceral adipose tissue, with visceral adipose tissue being more metabolically active [5]. This adipose tissue, through several mechanisms, alters the synthesis and bioavailability of endogenous sex steroids (estrogens, androgens, and progesterone). Adipose tissue itself is an active endocrine gland and can have wide-ranging effects on metabolism.

In 2004, Calle et al. summarized these effects succinctly by demonstrating that adipose tissue responds to signaling by increasing or decreasing the levels of circulating free fatty acids [6,7]. In addition, peptide hormones including leptin, adiponectin, resistin, and tumor necrosis factor (TNF-α) are released. Insulin resistance is mediated by the release of these hormones. A relative increase in insulin resistance by peripheral tissue leads to compensatory hyperinsulinemia. Insulin acts as a growth factor, and chronically elevated levels of insulin have been associated with tumor growth both directly and indirectly via effects on insulin-like growth factor I (IGF-I) in animal models. Tumor tissues generally have increased levels of IGF-I and insulin receptors. Adipose tissue also expresses various sex steroid-metabolizing enzymes, which ultimately increase the levels of endogenous estrogens through the conversion of androstenedione to estrone and the aromatization of androgens to estradiol. The levels of circulating estrogens are therefore directly related to the amount of adipose tissue.

A secondary effect is a decrease in the level of sex hormone-binding globulin (SHBG) by the liver due to increases in insulin and IGF-I. As estrogens normally circulate in the bloodstream in a bound (and biologically inactive) form, this leads to a relative increase in the amount of estrogens in the bloodstream. Together, these two increases are thought to account for most of the increased amount and bioavailability of estrogen seen by target tissues [6–8]. Increased androgen synthesis and hyperestrogenism is also seen in polycystic ovary syndrome (PCOS), a disorder specific to women. The condition is seen in 4–6% of women and is characterized by obesity, hyperinsulinemia, and the subsequent relative increase in estrogen via previously discussed mechanisms.

Obesity is one of the only risk factors that is modifiable throughout life. Cancers specific to women present an interesting opportunity to discuss mechanisms and treatment. Herein, we discuss these hormonally driven cancers, specifically breast, endometrial, and ovarian

Nutrition in the Prevention and Treatment of Abdominal Obesity
http://dx.doi.org/10.1016/B978-0-12-407869-7.00005-2

cancer, as well the impact of obesity on treatment and quality of life outcomes.

Gynecological Cancers

Endometrial cancer was among the first to be recognized as related to obesity. Cancer of the uterine lining, or endometrial cancer, is the fourth most common cancer among women, with an estimated 47,130 new diagnoses in 2012 [9]. It is the second most common cause of death from gynecological cancer, with an estimated 8120 deaths in 2011. Women have a 2.6% lifetime risk of this malignancy. The incidence of endometrial cancer has been increasing, more than doubling from 1987 to 1998, in the face of plateauing incidence and mortality for several other cancers over the same time period. Among the recognized risk factors for the development of endometrial cancer include unopposed estrogen therapy, increasing age, diabetes, nulliparity, and obesity (Table 5.1). It is estimated that approximately 90% of type 1 (hormone-mediated) endometrial cancer patients are obese [10]. There is a significant increased risk of endometrial cancer with higher BMI categories and higher body fat measurements using skinfold calipers [11]. Of all women diagnosed with endometrial cancer, 25% will be premenopausal, with obesity and nulliparity shown to be the strongest risk factors in a retrospective series [12].

Women diagnosed with endometrial cancer are typically treated with surgical staging, and in some cases with adjuvant radiotherapy and/or chemotherapy. Surgical treatment can be technically challenging in this cohort of patients, given the frequency of obesity. These patients may also present with medical comorbidities that make desirous a shortened surgical time and duration of anesthesia. Numerous studies have made it clear that minimally invasive procedures can be performed in this population without compromise in oncologic outcomes [13–15]. Giugale et al. recently reported a decrease in the percentage of minimally invasive procedures from obese to morbidly obese to super obese women. There was also a concomitant increase in blood loss, rising with the degree of obesity, and a decrease in the number of nodes retrieved during lymph node dissection [16].

TABLE 5.1 Risk Factors for Endometrial Cancer

Obesity (relative risk of 2–11)
• Relative risk of 3.0 in women 21–50 lb overweight and 10 in women more than 50 lb overweight
Nulliparity (relative risk of 2–3)
Late menopause, i.e., occurring in women older than 52 years (relative risk of 2.4)
Exogenous unopposed estrogen (relative risk of 1.6–12)
Tamoxifen (relative risk of 1.7–2.5)
Diabetes (relative risk of 1.3–2.7)
Hypertension (relative risk of 1.2–2.1)
High dietary fat consumption (relative risk of 1.1–2.0)
Radiation therapy (relative risk of 8)
Hereditary Non-polyposis Colorectal Cancer (HNPCC; 39–60% lifetime risk of EC)

Source: Ref. [10]. *Modified from: Smith RA et al. American Cancer Society Guidelines for Early Endometrial Cancer Detection: Update 2001.*

Fortunately, with treatment, the expectation is that the majority of women with endometrial cancer will live longer than 5 years after diagnosis; however, many studies do reveal in increase in mortality from causes unrelated to cancer in obese endometrial cancer patients [17,18]. While weight has been shown to impact cancer recurrence in breast, colorectal, and prostate cancers, it has not been shown to impact endometrial cancer recurrence [19–21]. A 2013 study shows a 5-year, all-cause mortality hazard ratio (HR) of 1.84 [95% confidence interval (CI) = 1.17–2.88] for BMI of 30–35 kg/m^2, and 2.35 (95% CI = 1.48 to 3.73) for BMI $\geq$35 kg/m^2 [22]. Furthermore, while HR estimates for 10-year all-cause and endometrial cancer-specific mortality, as related to BMI, were similar to 5-year HR estimates, 10-year cardiovascular disease mortality was significantly higher for BMI > 35 kg/m^2 (HR = 4.08, 95% CI = 1.56–10.71).

Comparable studies have demonstrated parallel correlations with ovarian cancer and obesity. In a meta-analysis by the Collaborative Group on Epidemiological Studies of Ovarian Cancer, ovarian cancer risk significantly increased with increasing height and increasing BMI ($P = 0.001$ for each) [23]. In short, the heavier/more obese women were, the greater the risk of ovarian cancer. Conversely, in a large population-based study of $n = 1423$ invasive epithelial ovarian cancer survivors, there were no significant associations between height, weight, or BMI and ovarian cancer-specific mortality [24]. Thus, for ovarian cancer risk related to obesity more research is needed to identify continued associations of risk and mortality.

Breast Cancer

Breast cancer is the most common female cancer diagnosed among all demographic groups, and the second most common cause of death from cancer among women in the United States [25]. Since as early as 1992, obesity has been known to be significantly associated with breast cancer. A meta-analysis at the time estimated that being overweight (BMI of 25–29.9 kg/m^2) or obese (BMI > 30 kg/m^2) was significantly associated with a 78% and 91% risk of recurrence, respectively, and an increased risk of mortality [26]. Subsequently, this was confirmed in numerous studies in both pre- and postmenopausal women. In 2004, using data from the Nurses' Health Study in which 5204 participants were diagnosed with breast cancer, Kroenke et al. were able to conclude that weight before diagnosis was associated with recurrence of breast cancer and with death [27]. Furthermore, in women whose BMI increased by 0.5–2.0 kg/m^2, the relative risk of breast cancer death was 1.35 (95% CI = 0.93–1.95). For women with a BMI increase of >2.0 kg/m^2, the relative risk of breast cancer death further increased to 1.64 [28]. Several other large cohort studies have corroborated this association between obesity and breast cancer prognosis [29,30].

FEMALE CANCER SURVIVORSHIP

Cardiovascular disease (CVD) is the leading cause of death in female cancer survivors, and CVD comorbidities are the leading cause of death among gynecological and breast cancer survivors secondary to obesity. Specifically, the risk of death from CVD-related causes in gynecological cancer begins to exceed the risk from cancer-related causes 3.5 years after diagnosis (Figure 5.1) [31]. In a prospective study by Ward et al., researchers examined the relationship between cancer, BMI, and risk of death, demonstrating a significantly increased risk of death in obese women with endometrial cancer. From the current data, we know the majority of obese cancer survivors are not meeting public health exercise and/or nutrition recommendations. Unfortunately, gynecological cancer survivors are not likely to engage in exercise without supervision or direct intervention [32].

According to the Institute of Medicine, survivorship care plans should be crafted to focus on four goals: prevention of recurrent cancer, surveillance, intervention to treat the consequences of cancer, and coordination of survivorship care [33,34]. Today, the increasing population of women diagnosed with obesity-driven female cancers underscores the need for health-care providers to provide health promotion interventions in this population [35]. The majority of research on exercise programs for gynecological and breast cancer patients support mixed interventions to improve aerobic fitness, strength, dietary compliance, weight loss, and quality of life. The National Cancer Institute (NCI) recognizes the need to specifically define patterns of weight, physical activity, and nutrition that contribute to cancer survivorship [36]. Since cardiovascular comorbidities are the leading cause of death for most gynecological and breast cancer survivors, interventions addressing cardiac risk factors (physical activity, nutrition quality, and weight loss) are essential for improving both short-term and long-term cancer survivorship.

PHYSICAL ACTIVITY

One historical approach to improving cardiovascular comorbidities is the implementation of physical activity or rehabilitation programs using a multidisciplinary, medically supervised, and risk factor reduction strategy to assist adherence to lifestyle changes, including exercise, in cancer survivorship. Exercise is therapeutic but has the literature defined the dosage for a specific diagnosis, symptom, and sign?

Definitions

Exercise and physical activity are important for the prevention and control of several chronic diseases. Exercise and physical activity are encouraged in overweight and obese cancer survivors to encourage energy

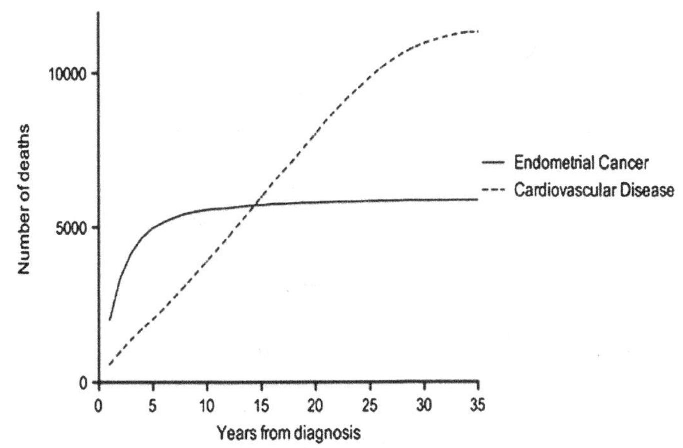

FIGURE 5.1 Endometrial cancer cardiovascular death rates after diagnosis. *Source: Ref.* [31].

balance for weight loss. According to the World Health Organization (WHO), physical activity is defined as any bodily movement produced by skeletal muscles that requires energy (caloric) expenditure, whereas exercise is a subcategory of physical activity that is planned, structured, repetitive, and purposeful [37]. Energy balance for weight control is defined as a balance of caloric intake and expenditure (Figure 5.2) [38]. Exercise and physical activity are promoted to maintain energy balance or to create an energy deficit for weight loss. Interestingly, total caloric energy intake ≥1972.1 kcal/day among endometrial cancer patients was significantly higher compared to women without endometrial cancer [39]. Consequently, it appears that an energy imbalance among endometrial cancer survivors is the leading cause of obesity.

Overall, exercise can be beneficial to gynecological oncology patients at any place on the spectrum of survivorship in various settings of outpatient or inpatient venues [40]. The Society of Gynecologic Oncology (SGO) recently developed recommendations for physical activity for cancer survivors to help guide survivorship treatment [41]. The SGO recommends exercise and lifestyle programming to improve survivorship. Specifically, they encourage a healthy lifestyle that engages a healthy diet, stress management, tobacco cessation, and whole-system approaches to wellness. In particular, supervised exercise programs have produced promising outcomes in reducing symptoms and improving physical and psychosocial functioning [42,43]. A recent Cochrane review on the effects of exercise and cancer-related fatigue [44] reviewed a total of 56 studies that demonstrated a significant impact on the aerobic system and in reducing fatigue for cancer patients compared to controls. In addition, a systematic review by Ballard-Barbash et al. [45], identified cancer survivors with higher levels of activity as being more likely to reduce risk of death from any cause, and there may even be a dose-related response to physical activity. However, the question still remains as to whether the exercise programming actually reduces cardiovascular risk factors such as obesity.

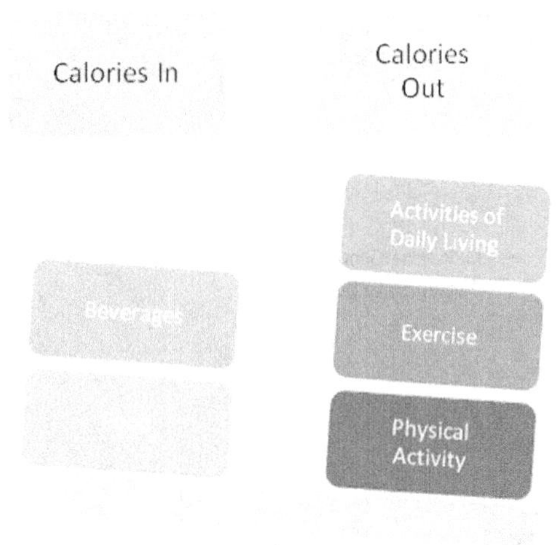

FIGURE 5.2 Energy balance for weight loss.

Interventions

Several studies cite the benefits of physical activity in survivorship, yet the optimal frequency, intensity, type, and timing of exercise for patients undergoing treatment or in survivorship remain unclear. The American College of Sports Medicine (ACSM) and the American Cancer Society (ACS) have joint guidelines that establish detailed exercise prescriptions for cancer survivorship during and after treatment [46]. The ACSM follows the 2008 Federal Physical Activity Guidelines for Americans, which encourage at least 150 min/week of moderate intensity aerobic activity [47]. Generally, studies have determined that moderate intensity aerobic exercise, resistance exercise, neurocognitive training, and/or combined programs lead to improved functional capacity, quality of life, and reduced chronic fatigue; however, the effects of regular physical activity alone on weight regulation and weight loss in survivorship are complex.

Consequently, obese women appear to have more barriers to exercise adherence than do women of normal weight. Similarly, correlations of physical activity and obesity in gynecological cancer survivors have been further verified by Blanchard et al., who found that only 30% of endometrial cancer patients met physical activity recommendations and most exhibited a BMI >30 kg/m^2 [48]. Even with these startling correlations of obesity, weight gain, and physical inactivity commonly found in gynecological cancer patients before and after a cancer diagnosis, there is still a lack of participation in exercise programming [49].

Courneya et al. found significant negative correlations between BMI and the number of minutes per week of moderate-to-strenuous exercise in 386 endometrial and ovarian cancer survivors [50]. Moreover, Courneya and colleagues demonstrated that cancer survivors who met exercise guidelines were more likely to be of normal weight. Continued work by von Gruenigen et al. [51] provides further support by showing that 90% of obese endometrial cancer survivors had dangerous amounts of abdominal obesity as well as poor physical activity patterns—80% reported no strenuous exercise and 54% did not even participate in moderate exercise. Likewise, a 6-month physical activity intervention in cancer survivors demonstrated that women with higher BMI and larger waist circumference adhered to fewer minutes of physical activity and did not meet the prescribed 150 min/week of moderate intensity exercise [52].

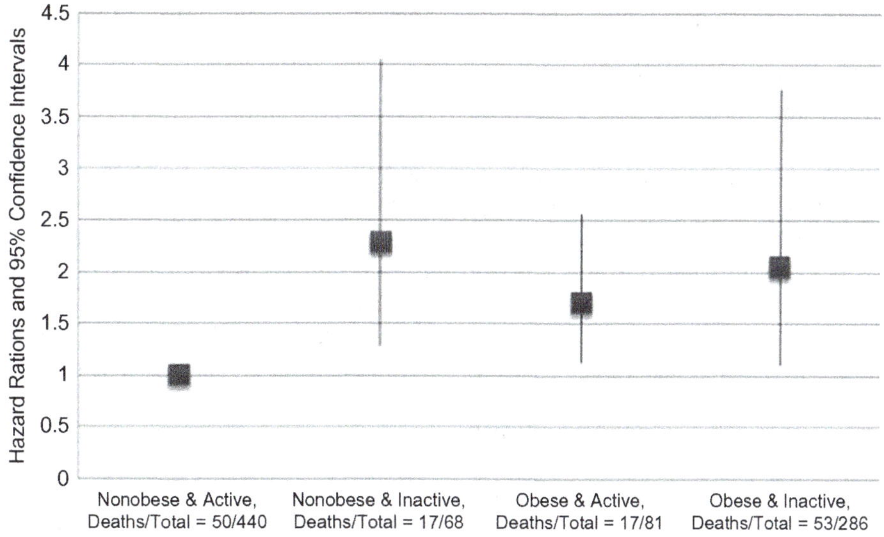

FIGURE 5.3 Joint effects of prediagnosis physical activity and obesity (n = 875) on 5-year all-cause mortality rate in the National Institutes of Health AARP Diet and Health Study. Cox proportional hazards models were used with age as the underlying time metric (age at diagnosis and age at death or censoring). Nonobese was defined as a body mass index of <30kg/m2 and active was defined as >1 h/week of moderate-to-vigorous physical activity. Pinteraction = 0.14 for obesity and physical activity. *Source: Ref.* [56].

Other publications have reported associations between physical activity after diagnosis and prognosis among breast cancer survivors. In 2987 women from the Nurses' Health Study diagnosed with stage I-III breast cancer between 1984 and 1998 and followed until death or 2002, the relative risk of death from breast cancer for activity equivalents of walking was 0.80 for 1–3 h/week, 0.50 for 3–5 h/week, 0.56 for 5-8 h/week, and 0.60 for 8 h/week, compared with inactive women [53]. Similar outcomes have also been reported in other studies [54]. A new study, the ENERGY (Exercise and Nutrition to Enhance Recovery and Good Health for You) trial, aims to be part of a fully powered trial of women who will be evaluated for breast cancer recurrence and disease-free survival [55]. The trial is underway and results are forthcoming.

In a cohort of 1400 women diagnosed with invasive epithelial endometrial cancer, combined BMI and physical activity had an effect on endometrial cancer survival [56]. Specifically, Arem and colleagues found beneficial effects of physical activity to be more pronounced in overweight or obese patients compared to those of normal weight (Figure 5.3). Nevertheless, evidence on physical activity and weight loss in endometrial cancer survival is sparse. Indeed, a number of gynecological cancer patients gain weight after diagnosis.

An example of the conundrum of physical activity and weight loss effect on survivorship stems from a randomized clinical trial incorporating a 12-week, home-based, moderate intensity exercise program, where some cancer survivors believed that physical activity was helping to improve body image and functional capacity but weight loss was less impressive (Figure 5.4) [57]. Von Gruenigen et al. [58] validated a lifestyle intervention program with exercise and diet modifications for obese endometrial cancer patients in which the intervention group lost 3.5 kg compared to a 1.4 kg gain in controls, with no significant decrease in intake of calories.

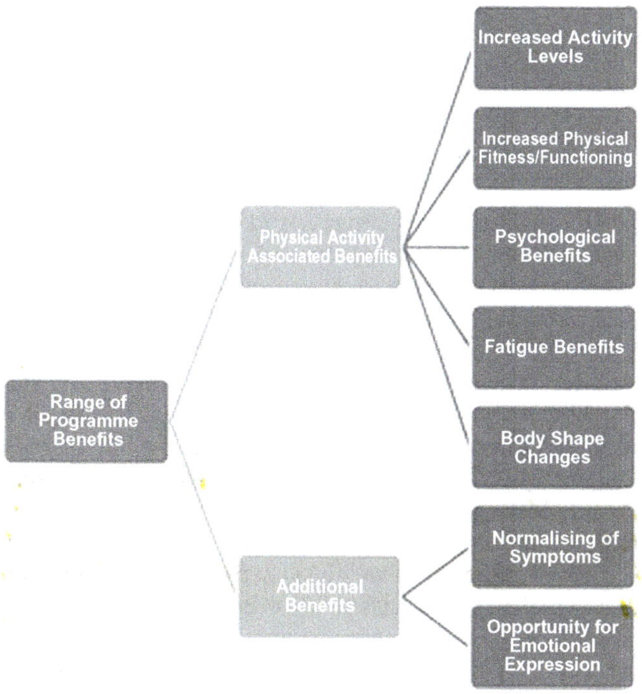

FIGURE 5.4 A focus group study exploring gynecological cancer survivors' experiences and perceptions of participating in a randomized controlled trial (RCT) testing the efficacy of a home-based physical activity intervention. *Source: Ref.* [57].

Encouraging patients to be physically active can improve glucose metabolism, digestive function, immune function, and cardiovascular risk factors [59,60]. However, according to Gary Taubes, the energy balance concept of *calories in* versus *calories out* for weight loss and/or weight management falls short of supporting evidence via clinical trials [61]. Furthermore, Taubes demonstrates in his book that exercise may actually increase appetite and cause people to be carbohydrate (i.e. the fuel for making people fat) hungry.

From these studies, we can determine that obesity appears to be related to physical inactivity; however, the question remains as to whether exercise helps with weight loss regardless of diet. This is not to diminish the documented benefits of exercise also found in a self-reported cohort study of 126 gynecological cancer survivors, where 43 women reported that exercising for more than 6-months led to significant improvements in weight, sleep, feeling better, and a perceived reduction of other chronic diseases compared to nonexercisers [62]. Thus, the debate continues.

There are few studies showing an association between cancer survivors meeting physical activity guidelines and eating a healthy diet (including five-a-day fruit or vegetable servings) and successful weight loss. Moreover, there are fewer studies related to long-term survivorship of endometrial cancer, particularly in the areas of lifestyle modifications to reduce cardiovascular risk factors such as obesity [63]. Most studies published on any lifestyle programming in gynecological cancer patients including endometrial, uterine, and ovarian are limited to 1-year follow-up and still require further study.

DIET CONSIDERATIONS

As described above, many studies have explored the relationship between obesity and physical inactivity in gynecological malignancies, yet evidence for the effects of nutrition and diet remain inconclusive. For example, a cohort study of gynecological cancer cases and controls reported no significant differences in physical activity status; however, cases with higher recent weight and BMI were associated with significantly increased risks [64]. Remarkably, Nagle et al. discovered that women who intentionally lost weight (approximately 9 kg) and maintained this weight loss were not at increased risk. This provides further evidence that weight loss reduces risk, yet how does a patient accomplish this task in cancer survivorship?

Definitions

Diets are synonymous with weight loss. There are various types of diets, paradigms, and hypotheses to answer the conundrum of the obesity epidemic. To date, there is no overwhelming evidence that one specific plan works for any single overweight/obese individual. We previously mentioned that the caloric theory is the mainstay of maintaining energy balance and is endorsed by the United States Department of Agriculture (USDA), which recommends a daily intake of approximately 1600–2000 calories for those women who are not physically active. Also, the USDA states that a "healthy diet" for women is one containing daily portions of 1.5–2 cups of fruit, 2–2.5 cups of vegetables, 3 ounce equivalents of whole grains, 5–5.5 ounce equivalents of protein, 3 cups of dairy, and 5–6 teaspoons of oils [65].

Interventions

Diet plays an important role in survivorship, especially during chemotherapy treatments. A cross-sectional mail survey from 802 gynecological cancer survivors evaluated health behaviors revealed no association between quality of life and fruit consumption, vegetable consumption, or BMI class [66]. In parallel to the self-reported survey study, an interventional lifestyle study of 27 ovarian cancer patients receiving chemotherapy treatment revealed minimal changes in fruit, vegetable, and low-fat dairy consumption—although this did not meet the recommended guidelines by the ACS [67]. Ovarian cancer patients with high-nutrient diets showed significantly longer survival rates with increased fruits and vegetables, in particular, yellow and cruciferous vegetables significantly favored survival [68,69]. With respect to protein intake, few prospective studies have investigated meat intake as a potential determinant of gynecological cancer risks in survivorship. In a case-cohort analysis of 39,614 women, a nonsignificant increase in survival was associated with an increased consumption of red meat, processed meat, and all meat combined, but with no clear patterns for poultry or fish only [70]. In 1994, the Canadian National Breast Screening Study reported on a subsample of 678 patients who completed a diet history prior to diagnosis. In the study, the risk of dying from breast cancer increased by 50% (HR = 1.50, 95% CI = 1.08–2.08) for every 5% increase in energy from saturated fat. Thus, lower saturated fat intake was associated with survival [71]. Unfortunately, these studies do not relate improved nutritional content to weight loss, even after diagnosis and during treatment.

In a recent study using the Health Eating Index, ovarian cancer patients scored very similar to controls: no differences in the consumption of whole fruit, dark green and orange vegetables, and whole grains were identified [72]. The only significant difference between groups was related to meat and bean intake, which were slightly higher in controls.

Given the linkage between obesity, breast cancer, risk of recurrence, and mortality, observational studies evaluating dietary interventions were undertaken. Two subsequent randomized controlled trials, the Women's Intervention Nutrition Study (WINS) and the Women's Healthy Eating and Living (WHEL) study reduced the amount of energy from dietary fat, with WHEL primarily focused on increasing vegetable, fruit, and fiber in the diet. Among early stage breast cancer patients, the WHEL study revealed no difference in breast cancer recurrence (HR = 0.96, 95% CI = 0.80–1.14) or mortality (HR = 0.91, 95% CI = 0.72–1.15) [73]. Among the 2437 women in the WINS trial, there were a total of 277 relapse events (local, regional, distant, or ipsilateral breast cancer recurrence or new contralateral breast cancer) reported: 96 (9.8%) out of 975 women in the dietary group and 181 (12.4%) out of 1462 women in the control group [74]. The discrepancy in results between the trials was initially explained by a lack of change in body weight in the WHEL trial; however, there were differences in the eligibility criteria for each study. The WHEL study enrolled both pre- and postmenopausal patients, and those patients were enrolled within 4 years of diagnosis, as opposed to 1 year in the WINS study. Furthermore, patients with relatively worse prognoses may have been excluded from the WINS trial, compared to WHEL [75]. Taken as a whole, the evidence tends toward a negative effect of dietary fat consumption, and the potential for other dietary interventions.

FUTURE DIRECTIONS

In summary, a multidisciplinary approach highlighting nutrition and physical activity appears to be the combination required for successful survivorship. Von Gruenigen et al. [76] used a whole systems approach in a 6-month lifestyle intervention program supporting physical activity, dietary compliance of fruits and vegetables, and counseling to improve self-efficacy and quality of life. As a result, significant increases in physical activity, daily intake of fruits and vegetables, and significant weight loss were achieved, thus providing evidence that a combination of lifestyle changes leads to improved weight loss [77,78]. Nevertheless, dietary and exercise recommendations for cancer survivorship and weight loss remain controversial. We hope that results from the NCI evaluating nutrition, energetics, and physical activity, and the Transdisciplinary Research on Energetics and Cancer (TREC) initiative will be able to identify more specifically the time, dose, and type of substrate required by gynecological and breast cancer patients to improve long-term survivorship [79].

Ultimately, studies may show that physical activity and obesity predict overall cancer survivorship. It is important to engage survivors in supervised exercise and lifestyle programs because most female cancer survivors do not make spontaneous lifestyle changes. Accordingly, physicians have a responsibility to ensure that patients receive referrals to rehabilitation programs to improve their well-being and provide support on the journey of survivorship. We conclude that obesity is linked to prognosis and overall survival in gynecological cancer survivors and that medically supervised programs to encourage weight loss are essential.

References

[1] Flegal KM, Carroll MD, Kit BK, Ogden CL. Prevalence of obesity and trends in the distribution of body mass index among US Adults, 1999–2010. J Am Med Assoc 2012;307(5):491–7. http://dx.doi.org/10.1001/jama.2012.39.

[2] Basen-Engquist K, Chang M. Obesity and cancer risk: recent review and evidence. Curr Oncol Rep 2011;13:71–6. http://dx.doi.org/10.1007/s11912-010-0139-7.

[3] International agency for research on cancer. world cancer Report. <http://www.iarc.fr/>. Retrieved April 25, 2013.

[4] Calle EE, Rodriguez C, Walker-Thurmond K, Thun MJ. Overweight, obesity, and mortality from cancer in a prospectively studied cohort of US adults. N Engl J Med 2003;348:1625–38.

[5] Doyle SL, Donohoe CL, Lysaght J, Reynolds JV. Visceral obesity, metabolic syndrome, insulin resistance and cancer. Proc Nutr Soc 2002;71:181–9. http://dx.doi.org/10.1017/S002966511100320X.

[6] Celle EE, Kaaks R. Overweight, obesity and cancer: epidemiological evidence and proposed mechanisms. Nat Rev Cancer 2004;4:579–91. http://dx.doi.org/10.1038/nrc1408.

[7] Hajamor S, Després JP, Couillard C, Lemieux S, Tremblay A, Prud'homme D, et al. Relationship between sex hormone-binding globulin levels and features of the metabolic syndrome. Metabolism 2003;52:724–30. http://dx.doi.org/10.1016/S0026-0495(03)00066-0.

[8] Fader AN, Arriba LN, Frasure HE, von Gruenigen VE. Endometrial cancer and obesity: epidemiology, biomarkers, prevention and survivorship. Gynecol Oncol 2009;114:121–7.

[9] Arem H, Irwin ML. Obesity and endometrial cancer survival: a systematic review. Int J Obes May 2013;37(5):634–9.

[10] von Gruengen VE, Gil KM, Frasure HE, Jenison EJ, Hopkins MP. The impact of obesity and age on quality of life in gynecologic surgery. Am J Obstet Gynecol 2005;193:1369–75.

[11] Austin HJ, Austin Jr M, Partridge EE, et al. Endometrial cancer, obesity, and body fat distribution. Cancer Res 1991;51:568–72.

[12] Soliman PT, Oh JC, Schmeler KM, Sun CC, Slomovitz BM, Gershenson DM, et al. Risk factors for young premenopausal women with endometrial cancer. Obstet Gynecol 2005;105:575–80.

[13] Everett E, Tamimi H, Greer B, Swisher E, Paley P, Mandel L, et al. The effect of body mass index on clinical/pathologic features, surgical morbidity, and outcome in patients with endometrial cancer. Gynecol Oncol 2003;90:150–7.

[14] Fader AN, Michener CM, Giannios N, Frasure H, Belinson JL, Zanotti KM. Total laparoscopic hysterectomy versus laparoscopic-assisted vaginal hysterectomy in endometrial cancer: surgical and survival outcomes. J Min Inv Gynecol 2009;16(3):333–9.

[15] Gehrig PA, Cantrell LA, Shafer A, Abaid LN, Mendivil A, Boggess J. What is the optimal minimally invasive surgical procedure for endometrial cancer staging in the obese and morbidly obese woman? Gynecol Oncol 2008;111:41–5.

[16] Giugale LE, DiSanto N, Smokin ME, Havrilesky LJ, Modesitt SC. Beyond mere obesity: Effect of increasing obesity classifications on hysterectomy outcomes for uterine cancer/hyperplasia. Gynecol. Oncol. 2012;127:326–31.

[17] von Gruenigen VE, Tian C, Frasure HE, Waggoner SE, Barakat RR. Treatment effects, disease recurrence and survival as related to obesity in women with early endometrial carcinoma: a Gynecologic Oncology Group study. Cancer 2006;107:2786–91.
[18] Chia VM, Newcomb PA, Trentham-Dietz A, Hampton JM. Obesity, diabetes, and other factors in relation to survival after endometrial cancer diagnosis. Int J gynecol Cancer 2007;17:441–6.
[19] Kroenke CH, Chen WY, Rosner B, Holmes MD. Weight, weight gain, and survival after breast cancer diagnosis. J Clin Oncol 2005;23:1370–8.
[20] Meyerhardt JA, Catalano PJ, Haller DG, Mayer RJ, Benson 3rd AB, Macdonald RS, et al. Influence of body mass index on outcomes and treatment-related toxicity in patients with colon carcinoma. Cancer 2003;98:484–95.
[21] Amling CL, Riffenburgh RH, Sun L, Moul JW, Lance RS, Kusuda L, et al. Pathologic variables and recurrence rates as related to obesity and race in men with prostate cancer undergoing radical prostatectomy. J Clin Oncol 2004;22:439–45.
[22] Arem H, Park Y, Pelser C, Ballard-Barbash R, Irwin ML, Hollenbeck A, et al. Prediagnosis body mass index, physical activity, and mortality in endometrial cancer patients. J Natl Cancer Inst 2013;105:342–9. http://dx.doi.org/10.1093/jnci/djs530.
[23] Collaborative Group on Epidemiological Studies of Ovarian Cancer. Ovarian cancer and body size: individual participant meta-analysis including 25,157 women with ovarian cancer from 47 epidemiological studies. PLoS Med. 2012;9(4):e1001200 (Epub 2012 April 3).
[24] Kotsopoulos J, Moody JR, Fan I, Rosen B, Risch HA, McLaughlin JR, Sun P, Narod SA. Height, weight, BMI and ovarian cancer survival. Gynecol Oncol 2012 Oct;127(1):83–7.
[25] United States Cancer Statistics (USCS). Centers for Disease Control and Prevention, 08 January 2013. Web 28 April 2013. <http://www.cdc.gov/Features/CancerStatistics/>. Accessed 13 September 2013.
[26] Goodwin PJ, Esplen MJ, Winocur J. Development of a weight management program in women with newly diagnosed locoregional breast cancer. In: Bitzer JSM, editor. Psychosomatic Obstetrics and Gynecology. Bologna, Italy: Monduzzi Editore, International Proceedings Division; 1995. p. 491–6.
[27] Kroenke CH, Chen WY, Rosner B, Holmes MD. Weight, weight gain, and survival after breast cancer diagnosis. J Clin Oncol 2005;23:1370–8. http://dx.doi.org/10.1200/JCO.2005.01.079.
[28] Zhang S, Folsom AR, Sellers TA, et al. Better breast cancer survival for postmenopausal women who are less overweight and eat less fat: The Iowa Women's Health Study. Cancer 1995;76:275–83.
[29] Carmichael AR. Obesity and prognosis of breast cancer. Obesity Reviews: An Official Journal of the International Association for the Study of Obesity 2006;7:333–40.
[30] Protani M, Coory M, Martin JH. Effect of obesity on survival of women with breast cancer: systematic review and meta-analysis. Breast Cancer Res Treat 2010;123:627–35. http://dx.doi.org/10.1007/s10549-010-0990-0.
[31] Ward KK, Shah NR, Saenz CC, Mchale MT, Alvarez EA, Plaxe SC. Cardiovascular disease is the leading cause of death among endometrial cancer patients. Gynecol Oncol 2012 Aug;126(2):176–9.
[32] von Gruenigen VE, Gil KM, Frasure HE, et al. Complementary medicine use, diet and exercise in endometrial cancer survivors. J Cancer Integr Med 2005;3:3–18.
[33] Ganz P. Quality of care and cancer survivorship: the challenge of implementing the Institute of Medicine recommendations. J Oncol Pract 2009;5:101–5.
[34] Hewitt MGS, Stovall E. From Cancer Patient to Cancer Survivor: Lost In Transition. Washington DC: National Academy Press; 2005.
[35] Campo RA, Rowland JH, Irwin ML, et al. Cancer Prevention after Cancer: Changing the Paradigm—a Report from the American Society of Preventive Oncology. Cancer Epidemiol Biomarkers Prev 2011;20:2317–24.
[36] National Cancer Institute. Research-Tested Intervention Program (RTIPs). Moving Science Into Programs For People. <http://Rtips. Cancer. Gov/Rtips/>. Retrieved 19 February 2013.
[37] World Health Organization. Health Topics: Physical Activity. <http://www.who.int/topics/physical_activity/en/> Retrieved 25 April 2013.
[38] Healthy Weight—it's not a diet, it's a lifestyle! Available at <http://www.cdc.gov/healthyweight/calories/#Striking> Retrieved 25 April 2013.
[39] Reeves KW, Carter GC, Rodabough RJ, Lane D, McNeeley G, Stefanick ML, et al. Obesity in relation to endometrial cancer risk and disease characteristics in the Women's Health Initiative. Gynecol Oncol. 2011;121:376–82.
[40] Shin KY, Guo Y, Konzen B, Fu J, Yadav R, Bruera E. Inpatient cancer rehabilitation: the experience of a national comprehensive cancer center. Am J Phys Med Rehabil 2011;90(Suppl):S63YS68.
[41] Society of Gynecological Oncology. Survivorship Toolkit. <https://www.sgo.Org/Clinical-Practice/Management/Survivorship-Toolkit/>. Retrieved 19 February 2013.
[42] Courneya KS, Segal RJ, Mackey JR, et al. Effects of aerobic and resistance exercise in breast cancer patients receiving adjuvant chemotherapy: a multicenter randomized controlled trial. J Clin Oncol 2007;25:4396Y404.
[43] Courneya KS, Mackey JR, Bell GJ, et al. Randomized controlled trial of exercise training in postmenopausal breast cancer survivors: cardiopulmonary and quality of life outcomes. J Clin Oncol 2003;21:1660Y8.
[44] Cramp F, Byron-Daniel J. Exercise for the management of cancer-related fatigue in adults. Cochrane Database Syst Rev 2012 Nov 14;11:CD006145.
[45] Ballard-Barbash R, Friedenreich CM, Courneya KS, Siddiqi SM, McTiernan A, Alfano CM. Physical activity, biomarkers, and disease outcomes in cancer survivors: a systematic review. J Natl Cancer Inst 2012 Jun 6;104(11):815–40.
[46] American Cancer Society. <http://Www. Cancer. Org/Cancer/News/News/Guidelinesaddress-Diet-Exercise-And-Weight-Control-For-Cancer-Survivors>. Retrieved 19 February 2013.
[47] Physical Activity Guidelines for Americans 2008 . <http://Health. Gov/Paguidelines/Pdf/Paguide. Pdf> Retrieved 19 February 2013.
[48] Blanchard CM, Courneya KS, Stein K. American Cancer Society's SCS-II. Cancer survivors' adherence to lifestyle behavior recommendations and associations with health-related quality of life: results from the American Cancer Society's SCS-II. J Clin Oncol 2008;26:2198–204.
[49] Irwin ML, McTiernan A, Bernstein L, Gilliland FD, Baumgartner R, Baumgartner K, et al. Physical activity levels among breast cancer survivors. Med SciSports Exerc 2004;36:1484–91.
[50] Courneya KS, Karvinen KH, Campbell KL, Pearcey RG, Dundas G, Capstick V, et al. Associations among exercise, body weight, and quality of life in a population-based sample of endometrial cancer survivors. Gynecol Oncol 2005;97(2):422–30.
[51] von Gruenigen VE, Waggoner SE, Frasure HE, Kavanagh MB, Janata JW, Rose PG, Courneya KS, et al. Lifestyle challenges in endometrial cancer survivorship. Obstet Gynecol Jan 2011;117(1):93–100.
[52] Latka RN, Alvarez-Reeves M, Cadmus L, Irwin ML. Adherence to a randomized controlled trial of aerobic exercise in breast cancer survivors: the Yale exercise and survivorship study. J Cancer Surviv 2009;3:148–57.
[53] Holmes MD, Chen WY, Feskanich D, Kroenke CH, Colditz GA. Physical activity and survival after breast cancer diagnosis. J Am

Med Assoc 2005;293(20):2479–86. http://dx.doi.org/10.1001/jama.293.20.2479.
[54] McTiernan A, Irwin M, Vongruenigen V. Weight, physical activity, diet, and prognosis in breast and gynecologic cancers. J Clin Oncol 2010;28(26):4074–80.
[55] Rock CL, Byers TE, Colditz GA, Demark-Wahnefried W, Ganz PA, WOLIN KY, et al. Reducing breast cancer recurrence with weight loss, a vanguard trial: the Exercise and Nutrition to Enhance Recovery and Good Health for You (ENERGY) Trial. Contemp Clin Trials 2013;34(2):282–95. http://dx.doi.org/10.1016/j.cct.2012.12.003.
[56] Arem H, Park Y, Pelser C, Ballard-Barbash R, Irwin ML, et al. Prediagnosis body mass index, physical activity, and mortality in endometrial cancer patients, Obstet Gynecol 2011;117:93–100.
[57] Donnelly CM, Lowe-Strong A, Rankin JP, Campbell A, Blaney JM, Gracey JH. A focus group study exploring gynecological cancer survivors' experiences and perceptions of participating in a RCT testing the efficacy of a home-based physical activity intervention. Support Care Cancer Jun 2013;21(6):1697–708.
[58] von Gruenigen VE, Courneya KS, Gibbons HE, Kavanagh MB, Waggoner SE, Lerner E. Feasibility and effectiveness of a lifestyle intervention program in obese endometrial cancer patients: A randomized trial. Gynecol Oncol 2008;19:19–26.
[59] U.S. Department Of Health And Human Services Office of the Assistant Secretary For Planning And Evaluation. Physical Activity Fundamental to Preventing Disease. June 20, 2002.
[60] U.S. Department of Health and Human Services. 2008 Physical Activity Guidelines For Americans Be Active, Healthy, And Happy! Fact Sheet. <http://www.health.gov/paguidelines/factsheetprof.aspx> Retrieved 9 February 2013.
[61] Taubes, G. Why We Get Fat: And What to Do About It. Anchor Books, A Division of Random House, Inc. New York. 2011 eISBN: 978-0-307-59551-5.
[62] Lukowski J, Gil KM, Jenison E, Hopkins M, Basen-Engquist K. Endometrial cancer survivors' assessment of the benefits of exercise. Gynecol Oncol 2012;124:426–30.
[63] Fader AN, Arriba LN, Frasure HE, von Gruenigen VE. Endometrial cancer and obesity: Epidemiology, biomarkers, prevention and survivorship. Gynecol Oncol 2009;114:121–7.
[64] Nagle CN, Marquart L, Bain CJ, O'Brien S, Lahmann PH, Quinn M, et al. On behalf of the Australian National Endometrial Cancer study group impact of weight change and weight cycling on risk of different subtypes of endometrial cancer European. J Cancer Aug 2013;49(12):2717–26.
[65] Choose My Plate, United States Department of Agriculture. <http://www.choosemyplate.gov/food-groups/>. Retrieved 25 April 2013.
[66] Beesley VL, Eakin EG, Janda M, Battistutta D. Gynecological cancer survivors' health behaviors and their associations with quality of life. Cancer Causes Control 2008;19:775–82.
[67] von Gruenigen VE, Frasure HE, Kavanagh MB, Lerner E, Waggoner SE, Courneya KS. Feasibility of a lifestyle intervention for ovarian cancer patients receiving adjuvant hemotherapy. Gynecol Oncol 2011;122:328–33.
[68] Dolecek TA, McCarthy BJ, Joslin CE, Peterson CE, Kim S, Freels SA, et al. Prediagnosis food patterns are associated with length of survival from epithelial ovarian cancer. J Am Diet Assoc 2010;110:369–82.
[69] Nagle CM, Purdie DM, Webb PM, Green A, Harvey PW, Bain CJ. Dietary influences on survival after ovarian cancer. Int J Cancer 2003;106:264–9.
[70] van Lonkhuijzen L, Kirsh V, Kreiger N, Rohan T. Endometrial cancer and meat consumption: a case-cohort study. Eur J Cancer Prev Jul 2011;20(4):334–9.
[71] Jain M, Miller AB, To T. Premorbid diet and the prognosis of women with breast cancer. JNatl Cancer Inst 1994;86(18):1390–7.
[72] Chandran U, Bandera EV, Williams-King MG, Paddock LE, Rodriguez-Rodriguez L, Lu SE, et al. Healthy eating index and ovarian cancer risk. Cancer Causes Control Apr 2011;22(4):563–71.
[73] Pierce JP, Natarajan L, Caan BJ, Parker BA, Greenberg ER, Flatt SW, et al. Influence of a diet very high in vegetables, fruit, and fiber and low in fat on prognosis following treatment for breast cancer. J Am Med Assoc 2007;298(3):289–98.
[74] Chlebowski RT, Blackburn GL, Thomson CA, Nixon DW, Shapiro A, Hoy MK, et al. Dietary fat reduction and breast cancer outcome: interim efficacy results from the Women's Intervention Nutrition Study. J Natl Cancer Inst 2006;98(24):1767–76.
[75] Pierce JP. Diet and breast cancer prognosis: making sense of the WHEL and WINS trials. Curr Opin Obstet Gynecol 2009;21(1):86.
[76] von Gruenigen V, Frasure H, Kavanagh MB, Janata J, Waggoner S, Rose P, et al. Survivors Of Uterine Cancer Empowered By Exercise And Healthy Diet (SUCCEED): A Randomized Controlled Trial. Gynecol Oncol Jun 2012;125(3):699–704.
[77] von Gruenigen VE, Waggoner SE, Frasure HE, Kavanagh MB, Janata JW, Rose PG, et al. Lifestyle challenges in endometrial cancer survivorship. Obstet Gynecol 2011;117:93–100.
[78] von Gruenigen VE, Courneya KS, Gibbons HE, Kavanagh MB, Waggoner SE, Lerner E. Feasibility and effectiveness of a lifestyle intervention program in obese endometrial cancer patients: a randomized trial. Gynecol Oncol 2008;109:19–26.
[79] Patterson RE, Colditz GA, Hu FB, Schmitz KH, Ahima RS, Brownson RC, Carson KR, et al. The 2011–2016 Transdisciplinary Research on Energetics and Cancer (TREC) initiative: rationale and design. Cancer Causes Control. Apr 2013;24(4):695–704. http://dx.doi.org/10.1007/s10552-013-0150-z. Epub 2013 Feb 3

CHAPTER

6

Evaluation of Visceral Fat in Massive Obesity

Camille Vatier, Christine Poitou, and Karine Clément

Institute of Cardiometabolism and Nutrition, ICAN, Pitié-Salpêtrière Hospital, Assistance Publique-Hôpitaux de Paris, CRNH-Ile de France, Paris, France

Abbreviations

BIA, bioelectrical impedance analysis; BMI, body mass index; CT, computed tomography; DEXA, dual-energy X-ray; absorptiometry; MRI, magnetic resonance imaging; NAFLD, nonalcoholic fatty liver diseases; SAT, subcutaneous adipose tissue; T2DM, type 2 diabetes mellitus; TNF-α, tumor necrosis factor; VAT, visceral adipose tissue; WC, waist circumference; WHR, waist-hip ratio

Obesity is associated with a major prevalence of cardiometabolic diseases, which include alterations in glucose homeostasis, nonalcoholic fatty liver diseases (NAFLD), and increased cardiovascular risks and some cancers. As shown by the Prospective Studies Collaboration, cardiovascular risk factors increase with increasing body mass index (BMI) [1]. In a French study conducted on the general population, the proportion of subjects treated for cardiovascular risk factors (dyslipidemia, diabetes, and hypertension) was 14-fold higher in obese subjects compared to those of normal weight [2]. There is a wealth of epidemiological and clinical evidence indicating that total body fat accumulation contributes to obesity comorbidities. Beyond fat mass per se, the pattern of fat distribution has a profound influence on cardiometabolic risk. The prevalence of obesity (i.e. subjects with $BMI \geq 30\,kg/m^2$) has markedly increased in the past few decades, and the increase of the prevalence of morbid or massive obesity (i.e. subjects with $BMI \geq 40\,kg/m^2$) is even more important [3], with a 400% [4] increase in Canada in the last two decades and a 40% increase in France between 1997 and 2012 [2]. Given the rise in morbid obesity rates, the need to better identify personal cardiometabolic risk is an important challenge for the medical care of this population. Another challenge in this field is to better define the patient phenotypic characteristics; accurate stratification should help to improve patient treatment and the prediction of complication risks.

Body fat tissue is distributed into two main compartments with different metabolic characteristics: subcutaneous adipose tissue (SAT) and visceral adipose tissue (VAT). SAT represents ≈85% of total fat mass, and about 15% of total fat mass is intra-abdominal. Abdominal SAT is separated by a membranous layer into superficial and deep SAT, and recent studies have shown strong links between deep SAT, VAT, and blood parameters of metabolic complications [5–7]. The contribution of abdominal fat mass to total fat mass is at least partially influenced by gender, age, physical activity level, and total adiposity. Abdominal obesity, which is characterized by increased adipose tissue surrounding the intra-abdominal organs (VAT), is also referred to as visceral or central obesity. VAT includes intraperitoneal fat mass (mesenteric and omental), which drains directly into the portal system of the liver, and retroperitoneal fat mass, which drains into the systemic circulation. VAT-derived molecules can affect liver functions [5].

The accumulation of VAT in obese subjects is strongly implicated in the pathogenesis of insulin resistance [8], type 2 diabetes mellitus (T2DM), and ischemic heart diseases [9], but is also linked to an increased predisposition to cancers of the colon [10], breast [11], and prostate [12]; prolonged hospital stays; and increased mortality in hospital [13]. The pathogenic role of VAT has been shown in previous studies, in which individuals of normal weight but with excess VAT have a significantly higher risk of developing insulin resistance and T2DM [8].

Although associations between visceral adiposity and various medical pathologies are well established, few studies have included subjects with World Health Organization grade III obesity. It is unclear whether the

Nutrition in the Prevention and Treatment of Abdominal Obesity
http://dx.doi.org/10.1016/B978-0-12-407869-7.00006-4

relative distribution of adipose tissue is important and clinically relevant to massively obese subjects, as only few reports address the issue of VAT and its significance in massive obesity.

As visceral obesity is associated with a poor prognosis, metabolic disturbances, and the pathological evolution of several chronic diseases, it is of great importance to identify methods that explore adipose tissue accurately and, more specifically, VAT. Modern concepts in obesity medicine, including grading of diseases, indicate that key determinants of phenotypes other than BMI may be effective measures of the global risk to patients. The concept of going beyond BMI to phenotype accurately obese subjects has been proposed [14,15]. Therefore, it is important to explore the distribution of adipose tissue, and particularly its perivisceral deposition. The corpulence imposed by severe obesity poses a tremendous challenge to the measurement of body composition and the evaluation of abdominal fat mass.

Herein, we report on the different methods to measure body composition, especially abdominal fat mass, and discuss how these can be interpreted in morbidly obese subjects.

ANTHROPOMETRIC ASSESSMENTS

Body Mass Index

Weight and height are base indicators of fat mass, but the BMI, defined by Quetelet in 1835 [16] and now used worldwide in clinical practice, is a good reflection of fat mass because it is positively correlated with it. However, despite its frequent use, it cannot be used to distinguish between lean and fat body mass, and it does not clearly differentiate between subcutaneous and visceral fat compartments [17]. In the context of massive obesity, an accurate scale has to be used combining BMI and other anthropometric and/or biological parameters to more precisely define abdominal fat repartition.

Waist-Hip Circumference Ratio

Other clinical measurements (hip and waist circumference) have been proposed to be superior to BMI for predicting cardiovascular risk. The waist-hip ratio (WHR) is a simple technique for determining body fat distribution. Guidelines have been proposed to accurately measure waist and hip circumference but there is still no uniformly accepted protocol. Waist circumference (WC) must be measured midway between the lower rib and the iliac crest on the midaxillary line, and hip circumference at the level of the widest circumference over the great trochanters. Both circumferences must be measured on standing subjects at the end of a gentle expiration. The WHR has been found to be more strongly related to visceral fat than to subcutaneous fat [18,19]. Nevertheless, WHR has limitations because it cannot distinguish between subcutaneous and visceral abdominal fat [18,20], which makes this index inappropriate for estimating VAT [18,21,22].

The central adiposity marker has been studied in nonobese population, first by Ashwell et al., who found significant correlation between WHR and the ratio of VAT to SAT cross-sectional area [quantified by computed tomography (CT) images of the abdominal region]. The validity of this anthropometric marker and others, with positive correlations between WHR and visceral fat, ranges between 0.55 and 0.85 in women [18,21,23] and between 0.60 and 0.88 in men [21,24–26]. Nevertheless, there is high interindividual variability in fat mass distribution, which can be partially explained by factors such as gender, race, and age. For this reason, a given WC measurement does not always mean the same content of abdominal visceral fat [27,28]. In obese populations, there is very little evidence of a correlation between WC and VAT [29]. Indeed previous observations show that as BMI increases, WC became a weaker marker of VAT [29]. In obese subjects, Ferland et al. have shown that the ability of the WHR to predict the percentage of deep abdominal fat is quite weak [23], and these data have been more confirmed recently [30].

One study revealed that prediction of intra-abdominal fat by the WHR was highly dependent on gender and did not seem to be a good marker for obese men [31]. The magnitude of WC is influenced by measurement techniques and standardization issues. Whereas the impact of the measurement method on cardiovascular risk estimation is unclear [32,33], the corpulence of morbidly obese subjects is another technical issue for applying a standardized protocol: severe obesity is often associated with a large hanging abdominal apron, which may make it difficult to clearly define and measure the hip circumference.

Abdominal Diameter

Abdominal diameters, in particular the sagittal diameter, which measures the anteroposterior diameter of the abdomen, are good estimators for the amount of VAT [21], as subcutaneous fat is displaced inferiorly by gravity. The transverse abdominal diameter is the largest spanned width, whereas the sagittal abdominal diameter is the largest spanned height of the abdomen [21]. A correlation has been found between the transverse abdominal diameter and SAT [21,34,35], and this correlation persists in obese subjects [36]. Interestingly, in this group, sagittal abdominal diameter shows a better correlation with visceral obesity compared with other measures, such as WC or BMI [35,36]. It has also been shown that changes in visceral fat with weight loss are more strongly correlated with changes in sagittal diameter than with changes in WC or WHR in men [34]. Nevertheless, the validity of these indicators depends on gender. Van der Kooy et al. found that sagittal abdominal diameter was not a bad indicator for women compared to WHR or WC (where BMI ranged from 28 to 38 kg/m^2). Technical measurement of the abdominal diameter should be easier than measuring the waist in severe obesity because these measurements are made on resting patients. One study evaluated the predictive value of the sagittal abdominal diameter on the cardiovascular risk and found a good correlation, but in this case the sagittal abdominal diameter was measured by CT [37].

Neck Circumference

Neck circumference has been described as a valid marker for identifying obese individuals, and is known to correlate well with other anthropometric measurements [38]. In the Framingham Study, neck circumference was also a better anthropometric marker of homeostasis model assessment of insulin resistance (HOMA-IR) than WC, and was associated with risk factors for cardiovascular disease even after adjustment for VAT and BMI [39]. This circumference is measured at mid-neck, between the midcervical spine and the midanterior neck, on subjects standing upright and facing forwards, with shoulders relaxed. In men with a laryngeal prominence (Adam's apple), it must be measured just below the prominence [38]. A study of 18 morbidly obese subjects (BMI of 50.6 ± 6 kg/m^2) showed that neck circumference correlated closely with VAT area, indicating that it could represent a powerful, selective marker for visceral adiposity [40] in extreme obesity forms. Nevertheless, sometimes the difficulty in locating the osseous structures causes a technical difficulty in measuring the neck circumference in morbidly obese persons and could limit the usefulness of this parameter in clinical practice.

Skinfold Measurement

Skinfolds provide an estimate of body fat [41], and some skinfold ratios have been proposed for use in evaluating fat distribution. Some skinfolds (subscapular and tricipital) have been described as markers of the central distribution of fat mass [42] and others have been correlated with subcutaneous abdominal fat [43]. However, measurements of skinfold thickness are inaccurate in obese subjects [34,44] because in general skinfold thickness exceeds the width of the caliper. Although an equation using skinfold measurement to predict the different compartments of abdominal fat has been validated in populations with a BMI $<$ 30 kg/m^2 [45], correlations between skinfold measures and intra-abdominal fat area become weaker with increasing age [22] and ~~no~~ there are no data available to validate these measures for the evaluation of abdominal fat in severely obese persons.

In summary, the assessment of abdominal obesity in massively obese subjects using anthropometric measurements is technically difficult, but can be performed according to the guidelines. An option could be to use a combination of the different measurements already discussed, including sagittal diameter in men and WHR in women: these have been described as the best predictors of VAT in severely obese subjects. However, although these anthropometric measurements are simple, inexpensive, quick, and easy to perform, their accuracy differs according to gender and age. Results vary from one ethnic population to another [46]. They can only provide indirect, approximate information on the amount of visceral fat and have not been thoroughly evaluated in morbid obesity. The ability to predict visceral fat from anthropometry is limited in patients with extremely high BMIs.

PHYSICAL METHODS TO ASSESS MASSIVE ABDOMINAL OBESITY

CT and magnetic resonance imaging (MRI) are considered the gold standards for assessing VAT and have been validated using direct morphometric methods on cadavers [47,48]; however, these techniques are expensive, are often not readily available, and CT has non-negligible radiation exposure, which limits kinetic studies. However, dual-energy X-ray absorptiometry (DEXA) is a widely available technique that requires only a minimal radiation dose and is relatively inexpensive. In this section, we explore the different advantages and disadvantages of a number of techniques for assessing abdominal adiposity and their accuracy and feasibility in massively obese subjects.

Bioelectrical Impedance Analysis

Bioelectrical impedance analysis (BIA) is a safe and cost-efficient method that avoids exposure to radiation and is used to measure body composition [49]. It is based on the difference in resistance when an electrical current is conducted through fat or lean components of the body. It can estimate whole-body fat content based on the determination of total body water content. An impedancemetry-specific equation for determining obesity has been developed [50,51]. However, in massively obese subjects, this technique results in the overestimation of lean mass and underestimation of fat mass [52]. The percentage of fat-free mass hydration in obese individuals is higher than in normal subjects [53], and the obese have expanded extracellular space in adipose tissue, so the reference hydration factor used in the equations for fat-free mass results in the underestimation of fat mass in obese subjects, and the error becomes greater with increasing BMI.

Recent studies on nonobese healthy subjects have attempted to assess the amount of abdominal SAT and VAT using BIA, and have indicated significant correlations when compared with precise imaging techniques such as CT [54,55]. However, caution should be taken when interpreting these results as they are based on measurements of fat-free tissue, and BIA calculates total fat mass by subtracting fat-free mass from body weight. If lean tissue measurements by BIA are imprecise (in general, these are strongly influenced by hydration status), then these errors will also confound fat measures. Moreover, no data are available concerning the validity of BIA to measure VAT in obese populations.

Dual-Energy X-Ray Absorptiometry

DEXA is a technique that can determine the whole-body and regional distribution of fat and lean mass; however, its ability to determine abdominal fat compartments is limited. Although some studies have found significant correlations between VAT as evaluated by CT scans and percentage of trunk fat obtained by DEXA [56,57], other studies have not confirmed these results [58]. Moreover, there is an increased bias when using DEXA to assess abdominal fat with increased body weight [59]. The DEXA software identifies the composition of lean, fat, and bone tissue over each individual pixel. Given that fat tissue is the least dense and bone the most dense, pixels containing fat and bone tissues may be identified as lean tissue, which can thus influence the estimation of trunk fat in obese individuals. These factors raise concerns regarding the accuracy with which DEXA can predict the quantity of intra-abdominal fat tissue in obese patients [60].

A new DEXA method for assessing VAT has recently been reported and can effectively assess VAT using a CT scan at L4-L5 [61]. A recent study has validated this technique based on changes in grayscale values and special modeling techniques to assess abdominal fat compartments, including VAT, in premenopausal women across a weight spectrum ranging from 15.6 to 47.5 kg/m^2 [62].

It should be kept in mind that in obese subjects the quality of the image and the data obtained with DEXA can be a significant issue because it is impossible to scan the entire body, especially the arms and legs. In very obese patients, it is sometimes useful to perform half-body DEXA for determination of whole body composition. However it is not validated in large cohorts and for abdominal fat assessment.

Ultrasound

Ultrasound is another technique suitable for estimating subcutaneous and intra-abdominal fat tissue; it has been used since 1993 [63], but its reproducibility and accuracy are generally poor [64]. It estimates the ratio of the thickness of the preperitoneal fat layer (extending from the anterior surface of the liver to the linea alba) to the thickness of subcutaneous fat in the abdomen, termed the abdominal-wall fat index. Nevertheless, several studies have shown a good correlation between abdominal ultrasound measurement and the amount of intra-abdominal adipose tissue on CT, as well as its usefulness in diagnosing intra-abdominal obesity [43]. Concerning morbid obesity, of the few studies that have used this measurement, none report any difficulties in obese populations, and some interesting results have been obtained [65,66]. Thus, this approach should be evaluated more precisely in obese and extremely obese subjects.

Computed Tomography

CT measurements are based on the specific range of attenuation values associated with adipose, muscle, and bone tissues. This technique allows the whole or specific parts of the body to be scanned; it clearly distinguishes the three tissues and calculates their respective cross-sectional areas [23,67,68]. Tokunaga et al. showed for the first time that it is possible to distinguish adipose tissue located in the abdominal cavity (VAT) from abdominal adipose tissue located subcutaneously [68]. However, due to the amount of radiation involved, the number of scans performed on subjects is limited: most subsequent studies performed with CT have used single-scan measurements obtained at either L4-L5 or the umbilicus [68]. Cross-sectional areas of VAT measured at various abdominal levels strongly correlate with each other [69,70–72]. Studies that have used multiple slices show that there is substantial variation in the absolute cross-sectional area of VAT, depending on the location of the scan (for example, from L1-L2 or L4-L5) [69,73]. Although this method may be the gold standard for measuring visceral fat, its possible limitations in severe obesity have not been explored.

Magnetic Resonance Imaging

MRI is well suited for imaging severely obese patients because the radio frequency used does not have difficulty in penetrating large amounts of adipose tissue, unlike ionizing radiation or sound waves [74]. Previously, conventional MRI devices were limited by the gantry size and the table weight limit. However, the development of open-configuration magnetic resonance scanners has allowed improved patient access and near real-time imaging. Further, the newer low-field magnetic resonance imagers, with a larger gantry size and greater weight capacity, have opened up the potential to image severely obese subjects [74,75] who could not be evaluated previously by standard MRI or CT.

CT or MRI is often used to determine body fat distribution in visceral and subcutaneous deposits [66,76]. In practice, multiple-slice MRI is one of the preferred options for volume calculation, but its use is limited by accessibility and cost. Along with CT imaging, multislice-volume MRI is generally considered a gold standard reference for measuring total and regional adipose-tissue volumes [26,77]. With multislice imaging for volumetric analysis, single cross-sectional images can be used as representative measures of VAT, and provide a compromise between accuracy and cost [78]. Similar to CT imaging, the correlation varies between VAT cross-sectional area in a single slice and VAT volume measured with multiple slices; however, strong correlations are generated ($r=0.82$-0.99) regardless of sample size [21,26,79]. Shen et al. [80] showed that single abdominal adipose tissue slice areas obtained by MRI at 5 cm superior to the L4-L5 level revealed the highest correlation with total body adipose tissue. Furthermore, the influence of age, gender, ethnicity, imaging position (prone or supine), BMI, and WC on the relationship between single adipose-tissue areas and corresponding total body adipose-tissue volume were insignificant [80,81]. However, it should be emphasized that, despite being a reliable technique that can be also used to assess abdominal fat distribution, MRI equipment is expensive and less widely available than CT equipment.

In conclusion, CT and MRI seem to be the best techniques for assessing abdominal obesity and for distinguishing between SAT and VAT. However, imaging tables often have a weight limit and the abdominal diameter of massively obese patients can limit their access to the MRI tunnel or scanner. This is an important issue when considering abdominal obesity in cases of massive obesity.

BIOLOGICAL PARAMETERS

Although many biological parameters of glucose and lipid metabolism and of inflammation have been correlated with abdominal fat in normal-weight or obese populations, and have been confirmed in a fundamental study on SAT and VAT secretion [82], no specific study has yet been conducted on subjects with severe obesity to confirm this correlation.

Lipid and Glucose Homeostasis

Subjects with large amounts of VAT have higher fasting plasma triglyceride levels and higher plasma glucose responses following an oral glucose challenge [83]. Hypertriglyceridemia correlates with visceral obesity and has been associated with the presence of atherogenic small, dense, low-density lipoprotein particles [84,85]. Therefore, viscerally obese patients have a very atherogenic plasma lipoprotein-lipid profile.

In glucose homeostasis, visceral adiposity is independently associated with impaired plasma glucose homeostasis and with insulin resistance [86–88]. A close relationship between the accumulation of VAT and plasma insulin or apolipoprotein B (ApoB) has been reported [89]. Viscerally obese people have the highest glycemic and insulinemic responses to an oral glucose challenge and are at the highest risk of developing T2DM [86,90,91].

Adipokines and Inflammation Markers

As a hormonally active organ, adipose tissue releases different bioactive molecules named *adipokines* and inflammation-related proteins, such as adiponectin, leptin, tumor necrosis factor (TNF-α), resistin, and interleukin-6 (IL-6), whose secretions differ between visceral and subcutaneous depots. Whereas some of these adipose tissue-derived molecules are mostly produced by adipocytes (i.e. leptin and adiponectin), the majority are produced by the nonadipocyte fraction (i.e. the stroma vascular fraction).

Among the adipokines, circulating adiponectin has been inversely correlated with the amount of VAT [92]. Obese individuals, particularly those with accumulated visceral fat, have reduced plasma levels of adiponectin [93,94]. Nevertheless, there are controversial data concerning the correlation between VAT or SAT and adiponectin concentration [94–97]. The negative correlation between adiponectin and VAT seems to be stronger than that between adiponectin and SAT [98,99]. Leptin expression and secretion has been found to be higher in SAT than in VAT [100–102]. Data from clinical studies relating serum leptin to fat distribution in obese patients are conflicting: some studies have found a relationship with both deposits [103] or with SAT alone [104–106], whereas no relationship was found between leptin and fat distribution in two other studies [107,108]. In morbidly obese patients, Monocci et al. found a correlation between leptin and SAT [106]. Circulating visfatin and its expression in adipose tissue is increased in severe obesity. Recently, visfatin has been found to be strongly related to the proinflammatory cytokines, which suggests a relationship with visceral adiposity [109].

Insulin-like growth factor-binding protein-1 (IGFBP-1), uric acid, and hepatic enzymes are other biological markers that have been studied in normal-weight populations and can predict body fat distribution [110].

Visceral obesity is also associated with a low-grade inflammatory state characterized by chronic increases in TNF-α [111], IL-6 [34] and C-reactive protein (CRP) [112], and their circulating concentrations are correlated with VAT. Another inflammatory marker, plasma plasminogen activator inhibitor 1 (PAI-1), is closely correlated with intra-abdominal fat deposits in humans [113], suggesting that its significance in the development of vascular disease.

As we have shown, no one unique biological marker is directly associated with VAT. Furthermore, systemic inflammation of obese subjects takes its origin not only in VAT but also in other cells (e.g. monocytes and lymphocytes) and tissues (such as the intestine and endothelium). Particularly, in morbidly obese subjects, who are characterized by relatively high levels of chronic inflammation, the use of biological parameters alone is questionable. However, the combination of all of these parameters in an adipo-inflammation score, plus CT or MRI quantification of VAT, could be an interesting strategy to stratify massively obese subjects according to the importance of abdominal obesity.

HISTOLOGICAL MARKERS IN ADIPOSE TISSUE

SAT and VAT differ in their physiological metabolic properties and their potential contribution to disease risk factors. Subcutaneous fat is organized into tightly packed lobules, whereas fat in visceral depots is found in lobules that are more irregular and less well organized. SAT is relatively stable metabolically compared to visceral fat compartments [114]. Nevertheless, histological markers of VAT cannot be used in clinical practice, because its confirmation requires taking an invasive intra-abdominal sample. However, sampling SAT is simple and easy to perform and has no serious adverse effects.

If the histopathological analysis of SAT can provide sufficient information to reflect fat distribution and its contribution to abdominal obesity, then this tool could significantly improve the deciphering of phenotypes of obesity. However, to date, no study has reported an association between the histological aspects of adipose tissue in severe obesity and abdominal fat repartition.

Adipocyte Size

For an identical BMI value, adipocyte size in SAT and VAT can be very variable. For normal-weight individuals and for those who are overweight or have grade I obesity, regional differences are relatively constant for any adiposity level: omental adipocyte diameter is most strongly associated with VAT, whereas abdominal subcutaneous adipocyte size is correlated with total body-fat mass [12,82]. In severe obesity, adipocyte hypertrophy in SAT has been associated with altered metabolic profiles, especially with diabetes [115]. However, no study has been conducted on adipocyte size and abdominal obesity in severe obesity.

Adipose Tissue Inflammation

In obesity, adipose white tissue is the target of major cellular and structural modification. Macrophages are major components of the stromal vascular fraction of adipose tissue and contribute to the low-grade inflammation that occurs with obesity. The abundance of adipose-tissue macrophages differs among fat depots: there are twice as many macrophages in VAT than in SAT [116,117]. Through the release of proinflammatory mediators, macrophages may be associated, at least in part, with VAT mass [118]. However, in morbidly obese subjects, no clear association has been found between glucose homeostasis parameters and adipose-tissue macrophage counts in SAT or VAT [116,119]. Another interesting study, in a severely obese population, showed that VAT area is an independent and significant predictor of macrophage infiltration, as assessed by the percentage macrosialin-positive ($CD68^+$) cells in both omental and subcutaneous fat [120]. Mast-cell number and their inflammatory phenotypes are associated with diabetes parameters: thus, this parameter could be linked with visceral adiposity [121].

Adipose Tissue Fibrosis

The nature of adipose tissue fibrosis in humans and its clinical relevance are both very poorly documented and are new areas of interest. There are no data concerning the association of adipose tissue fibrosis and abdominal fat repartition, but omental adipose tissue fibrosis has been found to be related to blood lipid parameters (negative correlation with triglycerides and a positive correlation with high-density lipoprotein cholesterol and ApoA-I) [122]: thus, we could expect VAT fibrosis to be associated with visceral fat accumulation.

The discovery that the structure of adipose tissue is altered in obesity, and especially in chronic inflammation, opens up perspectives for research on the physiopathological mechanisms that link adipose tissue and obesity-related complications. Adipocyte size or macrophage counts in adipose tissue represent interesting tools to assess obesity phenotypes. Further research is therefore needed to explore the possible links between adipose tissue analysis and VAT in massive obesity.

OTHER METHODS USED TO ASSESS ABDOMINAL FAT REPARTITION

Liver Fat

As liver fat levels strongly increase with glycemia, the evaluation of liver fat could reflect abdominal fat repartition [123].

Hepatic Histology

Very few studies have looked into the relationship between adipose tissue and liver histology, and the results are controversial: some have found a correlation between VAT and the histological severity of liver steatosis [124], whereas others have found a correlation between SAT and hepatic steatosis [125]. Recently, Bedossa et al. proposed a histopathological algorithm and scoring system to evaluate liver lesions in morbidly obese patients. The new SAF score [based on steatosis (S), inflammation activity (A), and fibrosis (F)] can identify special subgroups of patients and allows the precise phenotyping of liver lesions that could be linked to abdominal fat repartition [126]. This score is currently under evaluation in different cohorts.

Epicardial Fat Volume

Measurements of epicardial fat can be made by 3-tesla (3-T) cardiovascular MRI and by proton magnetic resonance spectroscopy (which evaluates myocardial triglyceride content). Interestingly, Garborit et al. have studied the relationship between epicardial fat and visceral fat, and found an association between these two deposits in a population of subjects with severe obesity [127].

Arterial Stiffness

Arterial stiffness, assessed according to pulse wave velocity and to intima-media thickness of the common carotid artery, is a marker of cardiovascular risk. It has been shown that abdominal obesity is a predictor for arterial stiffness in morbidly obese patients [128], and that arterial stiffness is strongly correlated with VAT area measured by CT [129].

CONCLUSION

Substantial evidence highlights the importance of abdominal fat repartition to determine the risk of cardiovascular disease, but this is less clear for extreme obesity. A problem remains for metabolically healthy obese subjects: does morbid obesity carry a different risk of mortality according to the amount of visceral fat?

Although very few specific data exist for this population regarding abdominal obesity, the gold standards for evaluating visceral obesity are still MRI and CT.

If one unique marker is insufficient to predict the abundance of VAT and to more accurately define the phenotype of massive obesity, a combination of several markers (anthropometric, biological, imaging, and histological) could improve our understanding of disease staging. Further investigations are needed to identify a "score" for visceral fat, which would improve the clinical study of these patients who also face various technical difficulties when extreme BMIs are explored.

Acknowledgments

The authors want to thank the funding agencies that support the pathophysiological studies of morbid obesity: the French National Agency of Research (ANR) and the Assistance Publique-Hôpitaux de Paris (Clinical Research Contracts, PHRC, CRCs).

References

[1] Whitlock G, Lewington S, Sherliker P, Clarke R, Emberson J, Halsey J, et al. Body-mass index and cause-specific mortality in 900 000 adults: collaborative analyses of 57 prospective studies Lancet 2009;373(9669):1083–96 [Epub 2009/03/21].

[2] Basdevant A, Charles MA. E. E. OBEPI: enquête épidémiologique nationale sur le surpoids et l'obésité. Paris: Inserm / Kantar Health / Roche; 2012.

[3] Sturm R. Increases in clinically severe obesity in the United States, 1986–2000. Arch Intern Med 2003;163(18):2146–8 [Epub 2003/10/15].

[4] Katzmarzyk PT, Mason C. Prevalence of class I, II and III obesity in Canada. Can Med Asso J (J de l'Assoc Med Can) 2006;174(2):156–7 [Epub 2006/01/18].

[5] Tordjman J, Divoux A, Prifti E, Poitou C, Pelloux V, Hugol D, et al. Structural and inflammatory heterogeneity in subcutaneous adipose tissue: relation with liver histopathology in morbid obesity. J Hepatol 2012;56(5):1152–8 [Epub 2012/01/17].

[6] Smith SR, Lovejoy JC, Greenway F, Ryan D, deJonge L, de la Bretonne J, et al. Contributions of total body fat, abdominal subcutaneous adipose tissue compartments, and visceral adipose tissue to the metabolic complications of obesity. Metab Clin Exp 2001;50(4):425–35 [Epub 2001/04/05].

[7] Kelley DE, Thaete FL, Troost F, Huwe T, Goodpaster BH. Subdivisions of subcutaneous abdominal adipose tissue and insulin resistance. Am J Physiol Endocrinol Metab 2000;278(5):E941–8 [Epub 2000/04/26].

[8] Brochu M, Starling RD, Tchernof A, Matthews DE, Garcia-Rubi E, Poehlman ET. Visceral adipose tissue is an independent correlate of glucose disposal in older obese postmenopausal women. J Clin Endocrinol Metab 2000;85(7):2378–84 [Epub 2000/07/21].

[9] Kuk JL, Katzmarzyk PT, Nichaman MZ, Church TS, Blair SN, Ross R. Visceral fat is an independent predictor of all-cause mortality in men. Obesity (Silver Spring) 2006;14(2):336–41 [Epub 2006/03/31].

[10] Oh TH, Byeon JS, Myung SJ, Yang SK, Choi KS, Chung JW, et al. Visceral obesity as a risk factor for colorectal neoplasm. J Gastroenterol Hepatol 2008;23(3):411–7 [Epub 2007/08/30].

[11] Schapira DV, Clark RA, Wolff PA, Jarrett AR, Kumar NB, Aziz NM. Visceral obesity and breast cancer risk. Cancer 1994;74(2):632–9 [Epub 1994/07/15].

[12] von Hafe P, Pina F, Perez A, Tavares M, Barros H. Visceral fat accumulation as a risk factor for prostate cancer. Obes Res 2004;12(12):1930–5 [Epub 2005/02/03].

[13] Tsujinaka S, Konishi F, Kawamura YJ, Saito M, Tajima N, Tanaka O, et al. Visceral obesity predicts surgical outcomes after laparoscopic colectomy for sigmoid colon cancer. Dis Colon Rectum 2008;51(12):1757–65 [discussion 65-7. Epub 2008/07/05].

[14] Thomas EL, Parkinson JR, Frost GS, Goldstone AP, Dore CJ, McCarthy JP, et al. The missing risk: MRI and MRS phenotyping of abdominal adiposity and ectopic fat. Obesity (Silver Spring) 2012;20(1):76–87 [Epub 2011/06/11].

[15] Muller MJ, Bosy-Westphal A, Krawczak M. Genetic studies of common types of obesity: a critique of the current use of phenotypes. Obesity Rev 2010;11(8):612–8 [Epub 2010/03/30].

[16] Gallagher D, Visser M, Sepulveda D, Pierson RN, Harris T, Heymsfield SB. How useful is body mass index for comparison of body fatness across age, sex, and ethnic groups? Am J Epidemiol 1996;143(3):228–39 [Epub 1996/02/01].

[17] Prentice AM, Jebb SA. Beyond body mass index. Obes Rev 2001;2(3):141–7 [Epub 2002/07/18].

[18] Ashwell M, Cole TJ, Dixon AK. Obesity: new insight into the anthropometric classification of fat distribution shown by computed tomography. Br Med J (Clin Res Ed) 1985;290(6483):1692–4 [Epub 1985/06/08].

[19] Seidell JC, Oosterlee A, Thijssen MA, Burema J, Deurenberg P, Hautvast JG, et al. Assessment of intra-abdominal and subcutaneous abdominal fat: relation between anthropometry and computed tomography. Am J Clin Nutr 1987;45(1):7–13 [Epub 1987/01/01].

[20] Baumgartner RN, Heymsfield SB, Roche AF, Bernardino M. Abdominal composition quantified by computed tomography. Am J Clin Nutr 1988;48(4):936–45 [Epub 1988/10/01].

[21] Kvist H, Chowdhury B, Grangard U, Tylen U, Sjostrom L. Total and visceral adipose-tissue volumes derived from measurements with computed tomography in adult men and women: predictive equations. Am J Clin Nutr 1988;48(6):1351–61 [Epub 1988/12/01].

[22] Seidell JC, Oosterlee A, Deurenberg P, Hautvast JG, Ruijs JH. Abdominal fat depots measured with computed tomography: effects of degree of obesity, sex, and age. Eur J Clin Nutr 1988;42(9):805–15 [Epub 1988/09/01].

[23] Ferland M, Despres JP, Tremblay A, Pinault S, Nadeau A, Moorjani S, et al. Assessment of adipose tissue distribution by computed axial tomography in obese women: association with body density and anthropometric measurements. Br J Nutr 1989;61(2):139–48 [Epub 1989/03/01].

[24] Seidell JC, Bjorntorp P, Sjostrom L, Sannerstedt R, Krotkiewski M, Kvist H. Regional distribution of muscle and fat mass in men—new insight into the risk of abdominal obesity using computed tomography. Int J Obes 1989;13(3):289–303 [Epub 1989/01/01].

[25] Despres JP, Prud'homme D, Pouliot MC, Tremblay A, Bouchard C. Estimation of deep abdominal adipose-tissue accumulation from simple anthropometric measurements in men. Am J Clin Nutr 1991;54(3):471–7 [Epub 1991/09/01].

[26] Ross R, Leger L, Morris D, de Guise J, Guardo R. Quantification of adipose tissue by MRI: relationship with anthropometric variables. J Appl Physiol 1992;72(2):787–95 [Epub 1992/02/01].

[27] Camhi SM, Bray GA, Bouchard C, Greenway FL, Johnson WD, Newton RL, et al. The relationship of waist circumference and BMI to visceral, subcutaneous, and total body fat: sex and race differences. Obesity (Silver Spring) 2011;19(2):402–8 [Epub 2010/10/16].

[28] Kuk JL, Lee S, Heymsfield SB, Ross R. Waist circumference and abdominal adipose tissue distribution: influence of age and sex. Am J Clin Nutr 2005;81(6):1330–4 [Epub 2005/06/09].

[29] Han TS, Sattar N, Lean M. ABC of obesity. Assessment of obesity and its clinical implications. BMJ 2006;333(7570):695–8 [Epub 2006/09/30].

[30] Drapeau V, Lemieux I, Richard D, Bergeron J, Tremblay A, Biron S, et al. Waist circumference is useless to assess the prevalence of metabolic abnormalities in severely obese women. Obes Surg 2007;17(7):905–9 [Epub 2007/09/27].

[31] Kamel EG, McNeill G, Van Wijk MC. Usefulness of anthropometry and DXA in predicting intra-abdominal fat in obese men and women. Obes Res 2000;8(1):36–42 [Epub 2000/03/11].

[32] Ross R, Berentzen T, Bradshaw AJ, Janssen I, Kahn HS, Katzmarzyk PT, et al. Does the relationship between waist circumference, morbidity and mortality depend on measurement protocol for waist circumference? Obesity Rev 2008;9(4):312–25 [Epub 2007/10/25].

[33] Mason C, Katzmarzyk PT. Effect of the site of measurement of waist circumference on the prevalence of the metabolic syndrome. Am J Cardiol 2009;103(12):1716–20 [Epub 2009/06/23].

[34] van der Kooy K, Leenen R, Seidell JC, Deurenberg P, Visser M. Abdominal diameters as indicators of visceral fat: comparison between magnetic resonance imaging and anthropometry. Br J Nutr 1993;70(1):47–58 [Epub 1993/07/01].

[35] Kullberg J, von Below C, Lonn L, Lind L, Ahlstrom H, Johansson L. Practical approach for estimation of subcutaneous and visceral adipose tissue. Clin Physiol Funct Imaging 2007;27(3):148–53 [Epub 2007/04/21].

[36] Yim JY, Kim D, Lim SH, Park MJ, Choi SH, Lee CH, et al. Sagittal abdominal diameter is a strong anthropometric measure of visceral adipose tissue in the Asian general population. Diabetes Care 2010;33(12):2665–70 [Epub 2010/09/17].

[37] Guzzaloni G, Minocci A, Marzullo P, Liuzzi A. Sagittal abdominal diameter is more predictive of cardiovascular risk than abdominal fat compartments in severe obesity. Int J Obes (Lond) 2009;33(2):233–8 [Epub 2009/01/14].

[38] Ben-Noun L, Sohar E, Laor A. Neck circumference as a simple screening measure for identifying overweight and obese patients. Obes Res 2001;9(8):470–7 [Epub 2001/08/14].

[39] Preis SR, Massaro JM, Hoffmann U, D'Agostino Sr RB, Levy D, Robins SJ, et al. Neck circumference as a novel measure of cardiometabolic risk: the Framingham Heart study. J Clin Endocrinol Metab 2010;95(8):3701–10 [Epub 2010/05/21].

[40] Yang L, Samarasinghe YP, Kane P, Amiel SA, Aylwin SJ. Visceral adiposity is closely correlated with neck circumference and represents a significant indicator of insulin resistance in WHO grade III obesity. Clin Endocrinol (Oxf) 2010;73(2):197–200 [Epub 2010/01/07].

[41] Lohman TG, Martorell R. Anthropometric standardization reference manual. Champaign, IL: Human Kinetics Books; 1988. RAF

[42] Seidell JC, Cigolini M, Charzewska J, Ellsinger BM, Deslypere JP, Cruz A. Fat distribution in European men: a comparison of anthropometric measurements in relation to cardiovascular risk factors. Int J Obes Relat Metab Disord 1992;16(1):17–22 [Epub 1992/01/01].

[43] Ribeiro-Filho FF, Faria AN, Azjen S, Zanella MT, Ferreira SR. Methods of estimation of visceral fat: advantages of ultrasonography. Obes Res 2003;11(12):1488–94 [Epub 2003/12/25].

[44] Hayes PA, Sowood PJ, Belyavin A, Cohen JB, Smith FW. Subcutaneous fat thickness measured by magnetic resonance imaging, ultrasound, and calipers. Med Sci Sports Exerc 1988;20(3):303–9 [Epub 1988/06/01].

[45] Peterson MJ, Czerwinski SA, Siervogel RM. Development and validation of skinfold-thickness prediction equations with a

4-compartment model. Am J Clin Nutr 2003;77(5):1186–91 [Epub 2003/04/30].

[46] Huxley R, James WP, Barzi F, Patel JV, Lear SA, Suriyawongpaisal P, et al. Ethnic comparisons of the cross-sectional relationships between measures of body size with diabetes and hypertension. Obes Rev 2008;9(Suppl 1):53–61 [Epub 2008/03/01].

[47] Abate N, Burns D, Peshock RM, Garg A, Grundy SM. Estimation of adipose tissue mass by magnetic resonance imaging: validation against dissection in human cadavers. J Lipid Res 1994;35(8):1490–6 [Epub 1994/08/01].

[48] Rossner S, Bo WJ, Hiltbrandt E, Hinson W, Karstaedt N, Santago P, et al. Adipose tissue determinations in cadavers—a comparison between cross-sectional planimetry and computed tomography. Int J Obes 1990;14(10):893–902 [Epub 1990/10/01].

[49] Kyle UG, Bosaeus I, De Lorenzo AD, Deurenberg P, Elia M, Manuel Gomez J, et al. Bioelectrical impedance analysis-part II: utilization in clinical practice. Clin Nutr 2004;23(6):1430–53 [Epub 2004/11/24].

[50] Gray DS, Bray GA, Gemayel N, Kaplan K. Effect of obesity on bioelectrical impedance. Am J Clin Nutr 1989;50(2):255–60 [Epub 1989/08/01].

[51] Segal KR, Van Loan M, Fitzgerald PI, Hodgdon JA, Van Itallie TB. Lean body mass estimation by bioelectrical impedance analysis: a four-site cross-validation study. Am J Clin Nutr 1988; 47(1):7–14 [Epub 1988/01/01].

[52] Coppini LZ, Waitzberg DL, Campos AC. Limitations and validation of bioelectrical impedance analysis in morbidly obese patients. Curr Opin Clin Nutr Metab Care 2005;8(3):329–32 [Epub 2005/04/06].

[53] Waki M, Kral JG, Mazariegos M, Wang J, Pierson Jr RN, Heymsfield SB. Relative expansion of extracellular fluid in obese vs. nonobese women. Am J Physio 1991;261(2 Pt 1):E199–203 [Epub 1991/08/11].

[54] Nagai M, Komiya H, Mori Y, Ohta T, Kasahara Y, Ikeda Y. Development of a new method for estimating visceral fat area with multi-frequency bioelectrical impedance. Tohoku J Exp Med 2008;214(2):105–12 [Epub 2008/02/21].

[55] Demura S, Sato S. Prediction of visceral fat area at the umbilicus level using fat mass of the trunk: the validity of bioelectrical impedance analysis. J Sports Sci 2007;25(7):823–33 [Epub 2007/04/25].

[56] Treuth MS, Hunter GR, Kekes-Szabo T. Estimating intraabdominal adipose tissue in women by dual-energy X-ray absorptiometry. Am J Clin Nutr 1995;62(3):527–32 [Epub 1995/09/01].

[57] Hill AM, LaForgia J, Coates AM, Buckley JD, Howe PR. Estimating abdominal adipose tissue with DXA and anthropometry. Obesity (Silver Spring) 2007;15(2):504–10 [Epub 2007/02/15].

[58] Park YW, Heymsfield SB, Gallagher D. Are dual-energy X-ray absorptiometry regional estimates associated with visceral adipose tissue mass? Int J Obes Relat Metab Disord 2002;26(7):978–83 [Epub 2002/06/25].

[59] Bredella MA, Ghomi RH, Thomas BJ, Torriani M, Brick DJ, Gerweck AV, et al. Comparison of DXA and CT in the assessment of body composition in premenopausal women with obesity and anorexia nervosa. Obesity (Silver Spring) 2010;18(11):2227–33 [Epub 2010/01/30].

[60] Bertin E, Marcus C, Ruiz JC, Eschard JP, Leutenegger M. Measurement of visceral adipose tissue by DXA combined with anthropometry in obese humans. Int J Obes Relat Metab Disord 2000;24(3):263–70 [Epub 2000/04/11].

[61] Micklesfield LK, Goedecke JH, Punyanitya M, Wilson KE, Kelly TL. Dual-energy X-ray performs as well as clinical computed tomography for the measurement of visceral fat. Obesity (Silver Spring) 2012;20(5):1109–14 [Epub 2012/01/14].

[62] Bredella MA, Gill CM, Keating LK, Torriani M, Anderson EJ, Punyanitya M, et al. Assessment of abdominal fat compartments using DXA in premenopausal women from anorexia nervosa to morbid obesity. Obesity (Silver Spring) 2013 [Epub 2013/03/21].

[63] Armellini F, Zamboni M, Robbi R, Todesco T, Rigo L, Bergamo-Andreis IA, et al. Total and intra-abdominal fat measurements by ultrasound and computerized tomography. Int J Obes Relat Metab Disord 1993;17(4):209–14 [Epub 1993/04/01].

[64] Bellisari A, Roche AF, Siervogel RM. Reliability of B-mode ultrasonic measurements of subcutaneous adipose tissue and intra-abdominal depth: comparisons with skinfold thicknesses. Int J Obes Relat Metab Disord 1993;17(8):475–80 [Epub 1993/08/01].

[65] Cucchi E, Piatti PM, Orena C, Pontiroli AE, Martino E, Paesano PL, et al. L'ecografia e una metodica adeguata per la valutazione dello spessore del grasso intraaddominale? Confronto con la Tomografia Computerizzata. [Is echography an adequate method for assessing the thickness of intra-abdominal fat? A comparison with computed tomography]. Radiol Med 1997;94(4):329–34 [Epub 1998/02/18].

[66] Pontiroli AE, Pizzocri P, Giacomelli M, Marchi M, Vedani P, Cucchi E, et al. Ultrasound measurement of visceral and subcutaneous fat in morbidly obese patients before and after laparoscopic adjustable gastric banding: comparison with computerized tomography and with anthropometric measurements. Obes Surg 2002;12(5):648–51 [Epub 2002/11/27].

[67] Sjostrom L, Kvist H, Cederblad A, Tylen U. Determination of total adipose tissue and body fat in women by computed tomography, 40K, and tritium. Am J Physiol 1986;250(6 Pt 1):E736–45 [Epub 1986/06/01].

[68] Tokunaga K, Matsuzawa Y, Ishikawa K, Tarui S. A novel technique for the determination of body fat by computed tomography. Int J Obes 1983;7(5):437–45 [Epub 1983/01/01].

[69] Lee S, Janssen I, Ross R. Interindividual variation in abdominal subcutaneous and visceral adipose tissue: influence of measurement site. J Appl Physiol 2004;97(3):948–54 [Epub 2004/05/04].

[70] Ross R, Freeman J, Hudson R, Janssen I. Abdominal obesity, muscle composition, and insulin resistance in premenopausal women. J Clin Endocrinol Metab 2002;87(11):5044–51 [Epub 2002/11/05].

[71] Ross R, Aru J, Freeman J, Hudson R, Janssen I. Abdominal adiposity and insulin resistance in obese men. Am J Physiol Endocrinol Metab 2002;282(3):E657–63 [Epub 2002/02/08].

[72] Pare A, Dumont M, Lemieux I, Brochu M, Almeras N, Lemieux S, et al. Is the relationship between adipose tissue and waist girth altered by weight loss in obese men? Obes Res 2001;9(9):526–34 [Epub 2001/09/15].

[73] Thomas EL, Bell JD. Influence of undersampling on magnetic resonance imaging measurements of intra-abdominal adipose tissue. Int J Obes Relat Metab Disord 2003;27(2):211–8 [Epub 2003/02/15].

[74] Rothschild PA, Domesek JM, Eastham ME, Kaufman L. MR imaging of excessively obese patients: the use of an open permanent magnet. Magn Reson Imaging 1991;9(2):151–4 [Epub 1991/01/01].

[75] Busetto L, Perini P, Giantin V, Valente P, Segato G, Belluco C, et al. Relationship between energy expenditure and visceral fat accumulation in obese women submitted to adjustable silicone gastric banding (ASGB). Int J Obes Relat Metab Disord 1995;19(4):227–33 [Epub 1995/04/01].

[76] Seidell JC, Bakker CJ, van der Kooy K. Imaging techniques for measuring adipose-tissue distribution—a comparison between computed tomography and 1.5-T magnetic resonance. Am J Clin Nutr 1990;51(6):953–7 [Epub 1990/06/01].

[77] Heymsfield SB, Wang Z, Baumgartner RN, Ross R. Human body composition: advances in models and methods. Annu Rev Nutr 1997;17:527–58 [Epub 1997/01/01].

[78] Shen W, Wang Z, Punyanita M, Lei J, Sinav A, Kral JG, et al. Adipose tissue quantification by imaging methods: a proposed classification. Obes Res 2003;11(1):5–16 [Epub 2003/01/17].

[79] Han TS, Kelly IE, Walsh K, Greene RM, Lean ME. Relationship between volumes and areas from single transverse scans of intra-abdominal fat measured by magnetic resonance imaging. Int J Obes Relat Metab Disord 1997;21(12):1161–6 [Epub 1998/01/14].

[80] Shen W, Punyanitya M, Wang Z, Gallagher D, St-Onge MP, Albu J, et al. Visceral adipose tissue: relations between single-slice areas and total volume. Am J Clin Nutr 2004;80(2):271–8 [Epub 2004/07/28].

[81] Shen W, Punyanitya M, Wang Z, Gallagher D, St-Onge MP, Albu J, et al. Total body skeletal muscle and adipose tissue volumes: estimation from a single abdominal cross-sectional image. J Appl Physiol 2004;97(6):2333–8 [Epub 2004/08/18].

[82] Despres JP, Lemieux I, Prud'homme D. Treatment of obesity: need to focus on high risk abdominally obese patients. BMJ 2001;322(7288):716–20 [Epub 2001/03/27].

[83] Fujioka S, Matsuzawa Y, Tokunaga K, Tarui S. Contribution of intra-abdominal fat accumulation to the impairment of glucose and lipid metabolism in human obesity. Metab Clin Exp 1987;36(1):54–9 [Epub 1987/01/01].

[84] McNamara JR, Jenner JL, Li Z, Wilson PW, Schaefer EJ. Change in LDL particle size is associated with change in plasma triglyceride concentration. Arterioscler Thromb 1992;12(11):1284–90 [Epub 1992/11/01].

[85] Tchernof A, Lamarche B, Prud'Homme D, Nadeau A, Moorjani S, Labrie F, et al. The dense LDL phenotype. Association with plasma lipoprotein levels, visceral obesity, and hyperinsulinemia in men. Diabetes Care 1996;19(6):629–37 [Epub 1996/06/01].

[86] Bergstrom RW, Newell-Morris LL, Leonetti DL, Shuman WP, Wahl PW, Fujimoto WY. Association of elevated fasting C-peptide level and increased intra-abdominal fat distribution with development of NIDDM in Japanese-American men. Diabetes 1990;39(1):104–11 [Epub 1990/01/01].

[87] Hayashi T, Boyko EJ, Leonetti DL, McNeely MJ, Newell-Morris L, Kahn SE, et al. Visceral adiposity and the risk of impaired glucose tolerance: a prospective study among Japanese Americans. Diabetes Care 2003;26(3):650–5 [Epub 2003/03/01].

[88] Sparrow D, Borkan GA, Gerzof SG, Wisniewski C, Silbert CK. Relationship of fat distribution to glucose tolerance. Results of computed tomography in male participants of the normative aging study. Diabetes 1986;35(4):411–5 [Epub 1986/04/01].

[89] Lemieux S, Prud'homme D, Tremblay A, Bouchard C, Despres JP. Anthropometric correlates to changes in visceral adipose tissue over 7 years in women. Int J Obes Relat Metab Disord 1996;20(7):618–24 [Epub 1996/07/01].

[90] Kissebah AH, Freedman DS, Peiris AN. Health risks of obesity. Med Clin North Am 1989;73(1):111–38 [Epub 1989/01/01].

[91] Pouliot MC, Despres JP, Nadeau A, Moorjani S, Prud'Homme D, Lupien PJ, et al. Visceral obesity in men. Associations with glucose tolerance, plasma insulin, and lipoprotein levels. Diabetes 1992;41(7):826–34 [Epub 1992/07/01].

[92] Whitehead JP, Richards AA, Hickman IJ, Macdonald GA, Prins JB. Adiponectin—a key adipokine in the metabolic syndrome. Diabetes Obes Metab 2006;8(3):264–80 [Epub 2006/04/26].

[93] Arita Y, Kihara S, Ouchi N, Takahashi M, Maeda K, Miyagawa J, et al. Paradoxical decrease of an adipose-specific protein, adiponectin, in obesity. Biochem Biophys Res Commun 1999;257(1):79–83 [Epub 1999/03/27].

[94] Park KG, Park KS, Kim MJ, Kim HS, Suh YS, Ahn JD, et al. Relationship between serum adiponectin and leptin concentrations and body fat distribution. Diabetes Res Clin Pract 2004;63(2):135–42 [Epub 2004/01/24].

[95] Bidulescu A, Liu J, Hickson DA, Hairston KG, Fox ER, Arnett DK, et al. Gender differences in the association of visceral and subcutaneous adiposity with adiponectin in African Americans: the Jackson heart study. BMC Cardiovasc Disord 2013;13:9 [Epub 2013/02/26].

[96] Hanley AJ, Bowden D, Wagenknecht LE, Balasubramanyam A, Langfeld C, Saad MF, et al. Associations of adiponectin with body fat distribution and insulin sensitivity in nondiabetic Hispanics and African-Americans. J Clin Endocrinol Metab 2007;92(7):2665–71 [Epub 2007/04/12].

[97] Nakamura Y, Sekikawa A, Kadowaki T, Kadota A, Kadowaki S, Maegawa H, et al. Visceral and subcutaneous adiposity and adiponectin in middle-aged Japanese men: the ERA JUMP study. Obesity (Silver Spring) 2009;17(6):1269–73 [Epub 2009/07/09].

[98] Yatagai T, Nagasaka S, Taniguchi A, Fukushima M, Nakamura T, Kuroe A, et al. Hypoadiponectinemia is associated with visceral fat accumulation and insulin resistance in Japanese men with type 2 diabetes mellitus. Metab Clin Exp 2003;52(10):1274–8 [Epub 2003/10/18].

[99] Despres JP, Lemieux I. Abdominal obesity and metabolic syndrome. Nature 2006;444(7121):881–7 [Epub 2006/12/15].

[100] van Harmelen V, Dicker A, Ryden M, Hauner H, Lonnqvist F, Naslund E, et al. Increased lipolysis and decreased leptin production by human omental as compared with subcutaneous preadipocytes. Diabetes 2002;51(7):2029–36 [Epub 2002/06/28].

[101] Van Harmelen V, Reynisdottir S, Eriksson P, Thorne A, Hoffstedt J, Lonnqvist F, et al. Leptin secretion from subcutaneous and visceral adipose tissue in women. Diabetes 1998;47(6):913–7 [Epub 1998/05/30].

[102] Masuzaki H, Hosoda K, Ogawa Y, Shigemoto M, Satoh N, Mori K, et al. Augmented expression of obese (ob) gene during the process of obesity in genetically obese-hyperglycemic wistar fatty (fa/fa) rats. FEBS Lett 1996;378(3):267–71 [Epub 1996/01/15].

[103] Vettor R, Vicennati V, Gambineri A, Pagano C, Calzoni F, Pasquali R. Leptin and the hypothalamic-pituitary-adrenal axis activity in women with different obesity phenotypes. Int J Obes Relat Metab Disord 1997;21(8):708–11 [Epub 1997/08/01].

[104] Haffner SM, Gingerich RL, Miettinen H, Stern MP. Leptin concentrations in relation to overall adiposity and regional body fat distribution in Mexican Americans. Int J Obes Relat Metab Disord 1996;20(10):904–8 [Epub 1996/10/01].

[105] Takahashi M, Funahashi T, Shimomura I, Miyaoka K, Matsuzawa Y. Plasma leptin levels and body fat distribution. Horm Metab Res 1996;28(12):751–2 [Epub 1996/12/01].

[106] Minocci A, Savia G, Lucantoni R, Berselli ME, Tagliaferri M, Calo G, et al. Leptin plasma concentrations are dependent on body fat distribution in obese patients. Int J Obes Relat Metab Disord 2000;24(9):1139–44 [Epub 2000/10/18].

[107] Weigle DS, Ganter SL, Kuijper JL, Leonetti DL, Boyko EJ, Fujimoto WY. Effect of regional fat distribution and Prader-Willi syndrome on plasma leptin levels. J Clin Endocrinol Metab 1997;82(2):566–70 [Epub 1997/02/01].

[108] Bertin E, Rich N, Schneider N, Larbre H, Marcus C, Durlach V, et al. Insulin and body fat distribution have no direct effect on plasma leptin levels in obese Caucasian women with and without type 2 diabetes mellitus. Diabetes Metab 1998;24(3):229–34 [Epub 1998/08/05].

[109] Terra X, Auguet T, Quesada I, Aguilar C, Luna AM, Hernandez M, et al. Increased levels and adipose tissue expression of visfatin in morbidly obese women: the relationship with proinflammatory cytokines. Clin Endocrinol (Oxf) 2012;77(5):691–8 [Epub 2011/12/21].

[110] Lim U, Turner SD, Franke AA, Cooney RV, Wilkens LR, Ernst T, et al. Predicting total, abdominal, visceral and hepatic adiposity with circulating biomarkers in Caucasian and Japanese

American women. PLoS One 2012;7(8):e43502 [Epub 2012/08/23].

[111] Cartier A, Cote M, Bergeron J, Almeras N, Tremblay A, Lemieux I, et al. Plasma soluble tumour necrosis factor-alpha receptor 2 is elevated in obesity: specific contribution of visceral adiposity. Clin Endocrinol (Oxf) 2010;72(3):349–57 [Epub 2009/08/05].

[112] Lemieux I, Pascot A, Prud'homme D, Almeras N, Bogaty P, Nadeau A, et al. Elevated C-reactive protein: another component of the atherothrombotic profile of abdominal obesity. Arterioscler Thromb Vasc Biol 2001;21(6):961–7 [Epub 2001/06/09].

[113] Shimomura I, Funahashi T, Takahashi M, Maeda K, Kotani K, Nakamura T, et al. Enhanced expression of PAI-1 in visceral fat: possible contributor to vascular disease in obesity. Nat Med 1996;2(7):800–3 [Epub 1996/07/01].

[114] Markman B, Barton Jr FE. Anatomy of the subcutaneous tissue of the trunk and lower extremity. Plast Reconstr Surg 1987;80(2):248–54 [Epub 1987/08/01].

[115] Hoffstedt J, Arner E, Wahrenberg H, Andersson DP, Qvisth V, Lofgren P, et al. Regional impact of adipose tissue morphology on the metabolic profile in morbid obesity. Diabetologia 2010;53(12):2496–503 [Epub 2010/09/11].

[116] Cancello R, Tordjman J, Poitou C, Guilhem G, Bouillot JL, Hugol D, et al. Increased infiltration of macrophages in omental adipose tissue is associated with marked hepatic lesions in morbid human obesity. Diabetes 2006;55(6):1554–61 [Epub 2006/05/30].

[117] Harman-Boehm I, Bluher M, Redel H, Sion-Vardy N, Ovadia S, Avinoach E, et al. Macrophage infiltration into omental versus subcutaneous fat across different populations: effect of regional adiposity and the comorbidities of obesity. J Clin Endocrinol Metab 2007;92(6):2240–7 [Epub 2007/03/22].

[118] Lafontan M, Girard J. Impact of visceral adipose tissue on liver metabolism. Part I: heterogeneity of adipose tissue and functional properties of visceral adipose tissue. Diabetes Metab 2008;34(4 Pt 1):317–27 [Epub 2008/06/14].

[119] Tordjman J, Poitou C, Hugol D, Bouillot JL, Basdevant A, Bedossa P, et al. Association between omental adipose tissue macrophages and liver histopathology in morbid obesity: influence of glycemic status. J Hepatol 2009;51(2):354–62 [Epub 2009/05/26].

[120] Michaud A, Drolet R, Noel S, Paris G, Tchernof A. Visceral fat accumulation is an indicator of adipose tissue macrophage infiltration in women. Metab Clin Exp 2012;61(5):689–98 [Epub 2011/12/14].

[121] Divoux A, Moutel S, Poitou C, Lacasa D, Veyrie N, Aissat A, et al. Mast cells in human adipose tissue: link with morbid obesity, inflammatory status, and diabetes. J Clin Endocrinol Metab 2012;97(9):E1677–85 [Epub 2012/06/30].

[122] Divoux A, Tordjman J, Lacasa D, Veyrie N, Hugol D, Aissat A, et al. Fibrosis in human adipose tissue: composition, distribution, and link with lipid metabolism and fat mass loss. Diabetes 2010;59(11):2817–25 [Epub 2010/08/18].

[123] Kantartzis K, Machann J, Schick F, Fritsche A, Haring HU, Stefan N. The impact of liver fat vs visceral fat in determining categories of prediabetes. Diabetologia 2010;53(5):882–9 [Epub 2010/01/26].

[124] van der Poorten D, Milner KL, Hui J, Hodge A, Trenell MI, Kench JG, et al. Visceral fat: a key mediator of steatohepatitis in metabolic liver disease. Hepatology 2008;48(2):449–57 [Epub 2008/07/16].

[125] Choudhary NS, Duseja A, Kalra N, Das A, Dhiman RK, Chawla YK. Correlation of adipose tissue with liver histology in Asian Indian patients with nonalcoholic fatty liver disease (NAFLD). Ann Hepatol 2012;11(4):478–86 [Epub 2012/06/16].

[126] Bedossa P, Poitou C, Veyrie N, Bouillot JL, Basdevant A, Paradis V, et al. Histopathological algorithm and scoring system for evaluation of liver lesions in morbidly obese patients. Hepatology 2012;56(5):1751–9 [Epub 2012/06/19].

[127] Gaborit B, Kober F, Jacquier A, Moro PJ, Cuisset T, Boullu S, et al. Assessment of epicardial fat volume and myocardial triglyceride content in severely obese subjects: relationship to metabolic profile, cardiac function and visceral fat. Int J Obes (Lond) 2012;36(3):422–30 [Epub 2011/07/07].

[128] Recio-Rodriguez JI, Gomez-Marcos MA, Patino-Alonso MC, Agudo-Conde C, Rodriguez-Sanchez E, Garcia-Ortiz L. Abdominal obesity vs general obesity for identifying arterial stiffness, subclinical atherosclerosis and wave reflection in healthy, diabetics and hypertensive. BMC Cardiovasc Disord 2012;12:3 [Epub 2012/02/02].

[129] Nordstrand N, Gjevestad E, Dinh KN, Hofso D, Roislien J, Saltvedt E, et al. The relationship between various measures of obesity and arterial stiffness in morbidly obese patients. BMC Cardiovasc Disord 2011;11:7 [Epub 2011/02/03].

CHAPTER

7

Beyond Nutrition Is There Any Role for Physical Activity in Nonalcoholic Fatty Liver Disease Therapy?

Giovanni Tarantino[a] and Carmine Finelli[b]

[a]Department of Clinical Medicine and Surgery, Federico II University Medical School of Naples, Naples, Italy and INT "Fondazione Pascale" - Cancer Research Center of Mercogliano, Mercogliano (AV), Italy; [b]Center of Obesity and Eating Disorders, Stella Maris Mediterraneum Foundation, Chiaromonte, Potenza, Italy

Abbreviations

BMI, body mass index; CT, computed tomography; IAT, intra-abdominal adipose tissue; NAFLD, nonalcoholic fatty liver disease; MFC, muscle fat content; MS, metabolic syndrome; PhA, physical activity; SAT, subcutaneous adipose tissue; VAT, visceral adipose tissue; WC, waist circumference; WHR, waist-hip ratio

INTRODUCTION

Obesity is a widespread and growing problem around the world [1]. Excess adipose tissue, mainly subcutaneous and visceral adipose tissue (SAT and VAT), releases inflammatory cytokines that increase insulin resistance in skeletal muscles [2]. Moreover, central obesity, which is defined as a state of excessive visceral fat accumulation, is associated with a decreased production of adiponectin, an adipose-specific molecule with antidiabetic, anti-atherosclerotic, and anti-inflammatory functions [3]. In recent years, central obesity has been identified as a predominant risk factor for metabolic syndrome (MS) [4,5], a condition in which a cluster of cardiovascular biomarkers correlate with an increased probability of heart disease, stroke, diabetes, and the spectrum of liver abnormalities collectively referred to as nonalcoholic fatty liver disease (NAFLD) [6–13]. These biomarkers include high plasma triacylglycerol, low high-density lipoprotein (LDL) cholesterol, high plasma blood glucose, high blood pressure, and high transaminases.

Numerous studies have investigated the effects of diet, drugs, and physical activity (PhA) on reductions in weight, total fat mass, and/or visceral fat mass [14,15]. Generally, diet therapy is the most effective method for rapidly decreasing weight and total fat mass because it more easily results in a negative energy balance, as compared with PhA or drug therapies [16].

However, it has been suggested that aerobic PhA has specific effects on decreasing visceral fat mass because it may lead to increased sympathetic tonus, thereby increasing lipolysis, especially in abdominal fat [17]. For that reason, PhA therapy is expected to be one of the most effective methods for improving central obesity.

PhA is a critical determinant of visceral fat in adults, even independent of relations between PhA and whole-body fat and between whole-body fat and visceral adiposity [18–20]. For adults with similar body mass index (BMI), those with higher fitness levels have lower abdominal fat than do their less fit counterparts [20,21], even though adults matched only on BMI that differ in fitness are likely to have different whole-body fat levels. PhA interventions, even without concurrent weight loss, lead to visceral fat reductions in adults [22–24].

In this chapter, we systematically reviewed the literature to clarify the role of PhA on the specific body components SAT and VAT, particularly in patients with NAFLD.

THE MEASUREMENT OF SUBCUTANEOUS AND VISCERAL ADIPOSE TISSUE

Reductions in visceral fat have been shown to improve glucose tolerance and insulin sensitivity in nondiabetic [25,26] and noninsulin-dependent diabetes

Nutrition in the Prevention and Treatment of Abdominal Obesity
http://dx.doi.org/10.1016/B978-0-12-407869-7.00007-6

mellitus subjects [27], and changes in trunk fat correlate with improved glycemic control in type 2 diabetics [28].

Studies have demonstrated the predictive relationship of waist circumference (WC) and waist-hip ratio (WHR) with SAT or VAT [25,29] and the associated metabolic risk [30]. The International Diabetes Foundation currently has identified the WC limit as one of the necessary requirements for the diagnosis of MS, as reported by Zimmet et al. [31].

Recommendations for WC upper limits are based on ethnic origin: for men, these are ≥94 cm for Europids, ≥90 cm for South Asians and Chinese, and ≥85 cm for Japanese; for women, these are ≥80 cm for Europids, South Asian, and Chinese, and ≥90 cm for Japanese. The World Health Organization MONICA Project [32] surveyed multiple populations and demonstrated that, for men with a WC ≥94 cm and women with a WC of ≥80 cm, the sensitivity of WC as a screening tool varied between 40% and 80% in men and between 51% and 86% in women when compared with cutoff points based on a BMI (≥25 kg/m^2) and WHR (≥0.95 for men and ≥0.80 for women). Precision was high (≥ 90%) for all populations. At a WC ≥102 cm in men and ≥88 cm in women (BMI ≥30 kg/m^2), sensitivity varied from 22% to 64% in men and from 26% to 67% in women, whereas accuracy was >95% in all populations. In addition, the MONICA project recommended population-specific cutoff points for screening and cautioned against the exclusion of BMI measures.

Many factors should be taken into consideration when predicting the relationship between anthropometry and internal fat topography such as the homogeneity of the population sample [33,34] and the measurement methodologies [35]. For the same WC, men and women may show comparable levels of VAT [30,36]; on the other hand, threshold values of waist girth corresponding to critical amounts of VAT vary with age within genders and are lower in postmenopausal compared with premenopausal women [37]. Studies have shown that increased WC correlates to abdominal fat mass in women and visceral fat mass in both men and women [29,38], while decreased WC is associated with improvements in glucose metabolism [39]. For these reasons, WC and WHR are easy and cost-effective field measures. Nevertheless, they are not without limitations in public health applications [40].

PHYSICAL ACTIVITY

Numerous cross-sectional studies have showed an inverse relationship between PhA and WC [41–43], WHR [42,44,45], abdomen-to-hip ratio [46] and abdominal fat mass measured via DEXA [43,47–49] and computed tomography (CT) scan [50]. The so-called *master athletes*, when measured against age- and BMI-matched controls, have smaller WCs [51]; equally, physically active women have lower WHRs than inactive women. Activity of low intensity is correlated with reduced waist girth [41]; nevertheless, Tremblay and colleagues reported an inverse relationship between both WC and WHR and the intensity of activity independent of energy expenditure for men and women [52]. In a study of monozygotic and dizygotic female twins, after controlling for genetic and environmental factors, the influence of PhA was greater than that of other measured environmental factors, and participants with a genetic predisposition to obesity did not show a reduced effect of PhA on body fat mass [53]. An increasing number of intervention studies have since explored this relationship.

THE INFLUENCE OF PHYSICAL ACTIVITY ON SUBCUTANEOUS AND VISCERAL ADIPOSE TISSUE

SAT and VAT are associated with type 2 diabetes mellitus (T2DM), MS, NAFLD, and metabolic abnormalities [54–59]. SAT, VAT, and liver fat are also independent risk factors for all-cause mortality [22,60]. As previously reported, several studies using novel models of visceral obesity have demonstrated that the relationship between visceral fat and survival is causal, while the accrual of subcutaneous fat does not appear to play an important role in the etiology of disease risk [61]. Although obesity is closely associated with NAFLD, excessive visceral fat storage is reckoned to be just as or even more important [54].

Slentz et al. showed that, for overweight and obese individuals who want to reduce VAT and SAT measures, a moderate amount of aerobic exercise is the most time-efficient and effective exercise mode [62]. Borel et al. examined whether changes in cardiometabolic risk markers after a 1-year lifestyle intervention in viscerally obese men were associated with changes in VAT or with changes in SAT [63]. The reduction in VAT was independently related to the reduction in global adiposity and to the improvement in cardiorespiratory fitness [63].

The degree of fat deposition in muscle and its implications for obesity-related complications in children and adolescents are not well understood [64]. Muscle fat content (MFC) has been measured in the psoas muscle by proton magnetic resonance spectroscopy [64]. Severely obese children and adolescents tend to have a high MFC, which is associated with elevated VAT [64]. An increased MFC may be associated with impaired metabolic processes, which may predispose these young people to obesity-related complications [64].

Body fat and the specific depot in which adipose tissue is stored can contribute to cardiometabolic health risks in children and adolescents [65]. Imaging procedures including magnetic resonance imaging and CT enable the exploration of individual and group differences in pediatric adiposity [65]. Obtaining evidence is difficult because there is no consistent methodology or definition by which to estimate and define depot-specific adiposity, and many analyses have compared SAT and VAT without controlling for total body fat [65]. Future research should include longitudinal examinations of adiposity changes over time in representative samples of young people to enable generalizations to be made regarding the entire pediatric population and to examine variations in organ-specific body fat [65].

Ayabe et al. found that very short bouts of PhA lasting <1 min do not play a significant role in controlling abdominal fat distribution [66]. In addition, Kazlauskaite et al. showed that PhA predicts intra-abdominal adipose tissue (IAT), but has not been established whether energy intake predicts IAT independently of PhA in a community-based, naturalistic environment [67]. Self-reported energy intake was associated with preferential IAT accumulation in middle-aged women, independent of PhA [67]. This association was significantly stronger in Caucasians than in African-American women [67]. Future longitudinal studies are needed to explore lifestyle predictors of IAT accumulation during the menopausal transition [67].

AGE AND GENDER DIFFERENCES IN THE RESPONSE OF SUBCUTANEOUS AND VISCERAL ADIPOSE TISSUE TO PHYSICAL ACTIVITY

It is well-known that middle-aged and older age groups benefit from exercise, even though the number of studies is insufficient to determine whether gender differences exist regarding reductions in abdominal fat. In any case, it is common believed that abdominal adiposity can be reduced in middle-aged and older men and women with exercise. A small number of studies suggest that significant results are less likely in mixed gender and mixed age groups. Gender differences in regional responsiveness of subcutaneous fat, visceral fat, WHR, and WC [68], and in sensitivity to exercise training [69,70], may contribute to this. To determine whether there are gender differences in the response of VAT to PhA would require large samples matched or randomized at baseline for age, different levels of overall obesity, and absolute and relative proportions of subcutaneous and deep abdominal fat. As reported by Ohkawara et al. [71], for both sexes of the same age and BMI, there may be substantial baseline differences in VAT. In addition, it has been calculated that the energy cost of exercise interventions is usually lower for men and women [71], and energy expenditure associated with self-reported sedentary behavior may also differ significantly between genders [72]. Kay suggests that if baseline body composition, sedentary energy expenditure, physiological responsiveness, and the energy cost of exercise interventions all differ according to age and gender, then research design should ensure sufficient power for middle-aged and older men and women to be analyzed independently, thus ensuring that these factors are carefully controlled [73].

PHYSIOLOGICAL EFFECT OF EXERCISE ON OBESITY AND SUBCUTANEOUS AND VISCERAL ADIPOSE TISSUE

Exercise physiology and the salutatory effects on weight loss, fat reduction and insulin sensitivity have been described in great detail. These beneficial effects are at the moment considered to reflect, at least in part, the effect of exercise on the activation of 5′-AMP-activated protein kinase (AMPK). In obese nondiabetics, exercise has been shown to reduce the risk of developing T2DM by up to 46% [74].

Physical exercise, consisting of 20 min of cycling or running, or alternatively of 20 min of swimming below the maximal heart rate, followed by 20 min of warm up and cool down three times per week for 4 weeks, gave rise to a significant weight loss and a decrease in percentage body fat, and this effect was coupled with ameliorated glucose uptake, reduced fasting insulin levels, and higher circulating adiponectin and mRNA expression in muscle. It is important to emphasize that patients suffering from T2DM can reduce fasting plasma glucose by augmenting their amount of exercise [75].

To what extent exercise should be performed to obtain improvements in metabolic profiles has been evaluated by several researchers. O'Donovan and colleagues studies the effects of 24 weeks of moderate-intensity exercise [consisting of cycling three times weekly at 60% peak oxygen consumption (VO_{2max}), to burn 400 kcal] vs. high-intensity exercise (consisting of cycling three times weekly at 80% VO_{2max} to burn 400 kcal) vs.no exercise on insulin sensitivity and other parameters such as serum triglycerides and glucose [76]. Training at 60% $VO_{2\,max}$ gave the same result as training at 80% VO_{2max} when 400 kcal were used at each session. These data provide evidence that moderate exercise, expending 400 kcal per session, at least three times per week ameliorates insulin sensitivity [76]. The total energy expenditure obtained during each work-out session seems to be more useful than the intensity of the exercise. This surprise finding is supported by two recent investigations of obese populations [77,78]. Daily exercise for 3 months, performed for almost an hour per session, at not greater than 70%

VO_{2max} (about 80% maximum heart rate) on a treadmill to achieve 700 kcal energy expenditure gave rise to an 8% body weight reduction. This was followed by a beneficial reduction in abdominal obesity, WC, and insulin resistance [77]. Interestingly, this research emphasized that exercise without weight loss can lead to decreases in both abdominal and visceral fat. Ray et al. [78] made the interesting discovery that daily aerobic exercise for 50–60 min, starting at 60–65% maximum heart rate and increasing to 80–85% maximum heart rate (about 70% VO_{2max}) over 4 weeks reduced the percentage visceral fat content. This effect was related to an overall recovery of glucose metabolism, resulting in improved insulin sensitivity. These surprising results were obtained with a weight reduction of only 3% over this period.

The health effects of aerobic vs. restrictive exercise have given rise to endless debate. A Turkish study evaluated the effects of aerobic exercise, consisting of walking briskly for 15 min and exercising on a stationary bicycle for 12–15 min three times per week during the first month, exercising for 20–30 min four times per week during the second month, and exercising for 30–45 min five times per week during the third month, in a small population of 20 obese women in comparison with restrictive exercise utilizing a stationary exercise unit in a similar group of women over a 3-month period [79]. As reported below [118], despite ameliorated BMI and reduced fasting glucose and postprandial glycemia were obtained in both groups, reduced fat mass (as measured by bioelectric impedance), decreased LDL, and decreased insulin resistance were observed only in the group that underwent aerobic exercise. In another study, well-tolerated resistance exercise reduced intrahepatic lipid, increased insulin sensitivity, and improved metabolic flexibility in NAFLD patients independent of weight loss [80]. The absolute effect of resistance exercise studied in isolation was modest but similar to that of aerobic exercise [80]. The benefits of resistance exercise combined with caloric restriction in the clinical management of NAFLD will depend upon the long-term maintenance and sustainability of exercise—this now needs to be investigated [80].

NONALCOHOLIC FATTY LIVER DISEASE, PHYSICAL ACTIVITY, AND ADIPOSE TISSUE

To date, reducing body weight is the only confirmed therapy for the treatment of NAFLD, and lifestyle interventions remain the cornerstone of management [81,82]. Glucagon-like peptide 1 receptor (GLP-1R) agonists are effective in improving human liver lipid metabolism [83,84], although progressive weight gain, side effects, and cost have prevented the use of these drugs in routine care. Lifestyle interventions have been shown to reduce markers of liver lipid and metabolic control [85–87], in addition to reducing intrahepatic lipid [88–91]. Nevertheless, weight loss is difficult to achieve and sustain. PhA and exercise in NAFLD management may therefore be effective in decreasing intrahepatic lipid levels.

It should be emphasized that the distribution of adiposity (fat storage tissue) may be more important in ectopic fat accumulation into the liver (steatosis) than in determining total adipose mass [13]. Obese persons with excess VAT, or abdominal obesity, are at a higher risk of metabolic syndrome (MS) components than those whose fat is subcutaneous and predominantly in the lower body [9,92]. Furthermore, "lean" nonalcoholic steatohepatitis patients usually have abdominal obesity, or increased VAT [9,13]. WC is highly correlated to VAT and, therefore, should now be used as a surrogate marker for abdominal obesity: this has been recommended in the Asia-Pacific Guidelines on NAFLD [13]. Kim et al. have shown that *ob/ob* mice, which are genetically predisposed to obesity, T2DM, MS, and fatty liver, can be rescued from all of these metabolic complications by expression of an adiponectin transgene [93]. The biological effect of such forced expression of adiponectin was to expand the SAT mass [93]. As reported by Finelli et al. [54], the observation that increasing adiposity in the adiponectin transgenic *ob/ob* mouse protects against fatty liver and MS when fat is distributed into its physiological storage sites (i.e. under the skin) is consistent with the proposal that fat only distributes into the liver and other nonphysiological sites (skeletal and cardiac myocytes and pancreatic beta cells) when access to SAT becomes restricted—that is, when it is full up! [54]. This conclusion is further supported by the observation that persons with severe obesity and a high ratio of central adiposity (VAT) to total body fat have an increased risk of fatty liver and MS than those with lower ratios [94].

Clinical and epidemiological studies using WC to estimate VAT mass have found a direct association between abdominal fat and liver fat content, independent of total adipose mass and BMI [13,94–96]. Furthermore, several recent studies have used imaging methods to demonstrate that VAT, rather than subcutaneous abdominal fat (i.e. SAT), has more influence than BMI in terms of predicting the presence of NAFLD [94–99]. In one such study, obese subjects with hepatic steatosis had higher ratios of truncal:total body fat compared with similarly obese persons without fatty liver [95]. Nevertheless, the sensitivity and specificity of available imaging methods for measuring liver fat content are unsatisfactory compared to proton (^1H) magnetic resonance spectroscopy; the latter modality is usually not available outside a research setting [97–103]. Conflicting results on the accuracy of different modalities have been reported, which may be related both to an inadequate "gold standard" (liver biopsy, also burdened by conspicuous sampling errors, is unusually performed in this experimental context) and to technical factors [99,102,103].

Liver attenuation by CT is a validated quantitative measure that is inversely related to liver fat burden. CT has been used to examine race and sex differences on the distribution of liver attenuation, corresponding to one of the first stages of NAFLD, and the predictors of these mean differences in European American and African-American participants of the Family Heart Study [104]. This study confirmed that there are important sex differences and race-by-sex interaction effects on the distribution of liver attenuation, the prevalence of NAFLD, and the influence of metabolic risk factors on liver attenuation and NAFLD [104].

VAT is a key pathogenic fat depot in MS, but ectopic fat storage into the liver may also play an important role. Associations of VAT and fatty liver with MS in normal weight, overweight, and obese men and women have been evaluated [105]. VAT and fatty liver were associated with MS independently of each other, and these relationships were modified by BMI class such that VAT was the more important depot at lower levels of obesity and fatty liver at higher levels [105]. Importantly, NAFLD is accepted as a metabolic risk factor in overweight and obese individuals.

Kantartzis et al. [106] showed that, in all 50 adults with NAFLD studies, VAT and SAT was decreased and fitness increased by a lifestyle intervention including diet modification and increased PhA. Another study showed that diet with or without exercise results in significant decreases in intrahepatic fat content accompanied by considerable improvements in insulin sensitivity in obese older adults [107]. The addition of exercise to diet therapy improves physical function and other obesity- and aging-related metabolic abnormalities [107]. Hallsworth et al. [108] demonstrated that resistance exercise specifically improves NAFLD independent of any change in body weight. This study demonstrated that resistance exercise may be beneficial in the management of NAFLD; the long-term impact of resistance exercise now requires evaluation [108].

Recently, Lee et al. [109] showed that either aerobic exercise or resistance exercise alone is effective in reducing abdominal fat and intrahepatic lipids in obese adolescent boys. Resistance exercise, but not aerobic exercise, is also associated with significant improvements in insulin sensitivity [109]. Furthermore, De Piano et al. [110] showed that long-term interdisciplinary therapy with an aerobic plus resistance training protocol was more effective in significantly improving noninvasive biomarkers of NAFLD associated with the highest risk of disease progression in the pediatric population.

CONCLUDING REMARKS

The therapeutic role of PhA in the prevention, treatment, and control of cardiovascular and metabolic disease, such as NAFLD, may involve multiple mechanisms. One of these pathways appears to function via effects on abdominal fat [111,112]. Due to technical improvements to imaging, the great contribution of intra-abdominal fat to metabolic abnormalities and coronary risk factors has now been highlighted [112–115]. On the other hand, a major role for subcutaneous abdominal fat and intramuscular fat cannot be excluded [116]. If the positive influence of exercise on metabolic and cardiovascular health is essentially dependent on changes in abdominal fat, then we may now have a specific direction to apply the best interventions and best methods to measure outcomes.

From the perspective of NAFLD patients, weekly or daily walking, swimming, or cycling might seem to be as simple as jumping off a cliff. It seems that in NAFLD patients even small increments in regular PhA can improve liver enzymes; therefore, this encouraging information can be provided to patients.

PhA had an effect on visceral fat reduction that was additive to that of dietary restriction, despite the absence of an additive effect on body weight reduction [117]. Increased total energy expenditure reduced levels of visceral fat, but only moderate-intensity exercise was necessary to improve insulin sensitivity [118]. Thus, recommendations in behavioral targets should lead to an energy deficit and increase and maintain patient motivation [118].

It is necessary to determine how much visceral fat reduction is required to induce favorable metabolic changes in humans; however, early intervention has the greatest potential to decrease visceral fat and reduce the risk of obesity-related metabolic problems [61]. Regular PhA is correlated with low body weight and low body fat mass [119]. The negative fat balance is probably secondary to this negative energy balance [119]. SAT and VAT reduction significantly correlate with weight reduction during aerobic exercise intervention, although a significant SAT and VAT reduction may also occur without significant weight loss. More rigorous, controlled studies of longer duration and with defined histopathological end-points comparing exercise alone and other treatment are needed before better, evidence-based PhA modification guidelines can be established, since several questions remain unanswered. The most intriguing of these arises from recent research showing that the serine/threonine-protein kinase mTOR complex is suppressed by exercise [120]: translating this discovery into a pharmacological approach, it is possible that mTOR inhibitors can slow down MS-related diseases? [121].

References

[1] Affenito SG, Franko DL, Striegel-Moore RH, Thompson D. Behavioral determinants of obesity: research findings and policy implications. J Obes 2012;2012:150732. Epub 2012 Aug 16.

[2] Alam I, Ng TP, Larbi A. Does inflammation determine whether obesity is metabolically healthy or unhealthy? The aging perspective. Mediators Inflamm 2012;2012:456456. Epub 2012 Oct 4.

[3] Chen SJ, Yen CH, Huang YC, Lee BJ, Hsia S, Lin PT. Relationships between inflammation, adiponectin, and oxidative stress in metabolic syndrome. PLoS One 2012;7(9):e45693. Epub 2012 Sep 19.

[4] Carr DB, Utzschneider KM, Hull RL, Kodama K, Retzlaff BM, Brunzell JD, et al. Intra-abdominal fat is a major determinant of the National Cholesterol Education Program Adult Treatment Panel III criteria for the metabolic syndrome. Diabetes 2004;53(8):2087–94.

[5] Ford ES, Giles WH, Dietz WH. Prevalence of the metabolic syndrome among US adults: findings from the third National Health and Nutrition Examination Survey. JAMA 2002;287(3):356–9.

[6] Colicchio P, Tarantino G, del Genio F, Sorrentino P, Saldalamacchia G, Finelli C, et al. Non-alcoholic fatty liver disease in young adult severely obese non-diabetic patients in South Italy. Ann Nutr Metab 2005;49(5):289–95.

[7] Tarantino G, Colicchio P, Conca P, Finelli C, Di Minno MN, Tarantino M, Capone D, Pasanisi F. Young adult obese subjects with and without insulin resistance: what is the role of chronic inflammation and how to weigh it non-invasively? J Inflamm (Lond) 2009;6:6.

[8] Tarantino G, Colao A, Capone D, Conca P, Tarantino M, Grimaldi E, et al. Circulating levels of cytochrome C, gamma-glutamyl transferase, triglycerides and unconjugated bilirubin in overweight/obese patients with non-alcoholic fatty liver disease. J Biol Regul Homeost Agents 2011;25(1):47–56.

[9] Hall AM, Kou K, Chen Z, Pietka TA, Kumar M, Korenblat KM, et al. Evidence for regulated monoacylglycerol acyltransferase expression and activity in human liver. J Lipid Res 2012.

[10] Savastano S, Di Somma C, Pizza G, De Rosa A, Nedi V, Rossi A, et al. Liver-spleen axis, insulin-like growth factor-(IGF)-I axis and fat mass in overweight/obese females. J Transl Med 2011;9:136.

[11] Tarantino G, Caputi A. JNKs, insulin resistance and inflammation: a possible link between NAFLD and coronary artery disease. World J Gastroenterol 2011;17(33):3785–94.

[12] Tarantino G, Finelli C, Colao A, Capone D, Tarantino M, Grimaldi E, et al. Are hepatic steatosis and carotid intima media thickness associated in obese patients with normal or slightly elevated gamma-glutamyl-transferase? J Transl Med 2012;10(1):50.

[13] Farrell GC, Chitturi S, Lau GK, Sollano JD. Asia-Pacific Working Party on NAFLD. Guidelines for the assessment and management of non-alcoholic fatty liver disease in the Asia-Pacific region: executive summary. J Gastroenterol Hepatol 2007;22(6):775–7.

[14] Wu T, Gao X, Chen M, van Dam RM. Long-term effectiveness of diet-plus-exercise interventions vs. diet-only interventions for weight loss: a meta-analysis. Obes Rev 2009;10(3):313–23.

[15] Douketis JD, Macie C, Thabane L, Williamson DF. Systematic review of long-term weight loss studies in obese adults: clinical significance and applicability to clinical practice. Int J Obes (Lond) 2005;29(10):1153–67.

[16] Stiegler P, Cunliffe A. The role of diet and exercise for the maintenance of fat-free mass and resting metabolic rate during weight loss. Sports Med 2006;36(3):239–62.

[17] Manjoo P, Joseph L, Dasgupta K. Abdominal adiposity and daily step counts as determinants of glycemic control in a cohort of patients with type 2 diabetes mellitus. Nutr Diabetes 2012;2:e25.

[18] Green JS, Stanforth PR, Rankinen T, Leon AS, Rao Dc D, Skinner JS, et al. The effects of exercise training on abdominal visceral fat, body composition, and indicators of the metabolic syndrome in postmenopausal women with and without estrogen replacement therapy: the HERITAGE family study. Metabolism 2004;53(9):1192–6.

[19] Saelens BE, Seeley RJ, van Schaick K, Donnelly LF, O'Brien KJ. Visceral abdominal fat is correlated with whole-body fat and physical activity among 8-y-old children at risk of obesity. Am J Clin Nutr 2007;85(1):46–53.

[20] Santos DA, Silva AM, Baptista F, Santos R, Gobbo LA, Mota J, et al. Are cardiorespiratory fitness and moderate-to-vigorous physical activity independently associated to overweight, obesity, and abdominal obesity in elderly? Am J Hum Biol 2012;24(1):28–34.

[21] Ross R, Katzmarzyk PT. Cardiorespiratory fitness is associated with diminished total and abdominal obesity independent of body mass index. Int J Obes Relat Metab Disord 2003;27(2):204–10.

[22] Jung JY, Han KA, Ahn HJ, Kwon HR, Lee JH, Park KS, et al. Effects of aerobic exercise intensity on abdominal and thigh adipose tissue and skeletal muscle attenuation in overweight women with type 2 diabetes mellitus. Diabetes Metab J 2012;36(3):211–21.

[23] Lesser IA, Yew AC, Mackey DC, Lear SA. A cross-sectional analysis of the association between physical activity and visceral adipose tissue accumulation in a multiethnic cohort. J Obes 2012;2012:703941.

[24] Hall CW, Holmstrup ME, Koloseus J, Anderson D, Kanaley JA. Do overweight and obese individuals select a "moderate intensity" workload when asked to do so? J Obes 2012;2012:919051.

[25] Ross R, Dagnone D, Jones PJ, Smith H, Paddags A, Hudson R, et al. Reduction in obesity and related comorbid conditions after diet-induced weight loss or exercise-induced weight loss in men. A randomized, controlled trial. Ann Intern Med 2000;133(2):92–103.

[26] Ross R, Freeman JA, Janssen I. Exercise alone is an effective strategy for reducing obesity and related comorbidities. Exerc Sport Sci Rev 2000;28(4):165–70.

[27] Jung JY, Han KA, Ahn HJ, Kwon HR, Lee JH, Park KS, et al. Effects of aerobic exercise intensity on abdominal and thigh adipose tissue and skeletal muscle attenuation in overweight women with type 2 diabetes mellitus. Diabetes Metab J 2012;36(3):211–21.

[28] Castaneda C, Layne JE, Munoz-Orians L, Gordon PL, Walsmith J, Foldvari M, et al. A randomized controlled trial of resistance exercise training to improve glycemic control in older adults with type 2 diabetes. Diabetes Care 2002;25(12):2335–41.

[29] Kuk JL, Lee S, Heymsfield SB, Ross R. Waist circumference and abdominal adipose tissue distribution: influence of age and sex. Am J Clin Nutr 2005;81(6):1330–4.

[30] Bédard A, Dodin S, Corneau L, Lemieux S. The impact of abdominal obesity status on cardiovascular response to the mediterranean diet. J Obes 2012;2012:969124.

[31] Zimmet P, Magliano D, Matsuzawa Y, Alberti G, Shaw J. The metabolic syndrome: a global public health problem and a new definition. J Atheroscler Thromb 2005;12(6):295–300.

[32] Molarius A, Seidell JC, Sans S, Tuomilehto J, Kuulasmaa K. Varying sensitivity of waist action levels to identify subjects with overweight or obesity in 19 populations of the WHO MONICA project. J Clin Epidemiol 1999;52(12):1213–24.

[33] Ferland M, Després JP, Tremblay A, Pinault S, Nadeau A, Moorjani S, et al. Assessment of adipose tissue distribution by computed axial tomography in obese women: association with body density and anthropometric measurements. Br J Nutr 1989;61(2):139–48.

[34] Saelens BE, Grow HM, Stark LJ, Seeley RJ, Roehrig H. Efficacy of increasing physical activity to reduce children's visceral fat: a pilot randomized controlled trial. Int J Pediatr Obes 2011;6(2):102–12.

[35] Houmard JA, McCulley C, Roy LK, Bruner RK, McCammon MR, Israel RG. Effects of exercise training on absolute and relative measurements of regional adiposity. Int J Obes Relat Metab Disord 1994;18(4):243–8.

[36] Lemieux S, Prud'homme D, Nadeau A, Tremblay A, Bouchard C, Després JP. Seven-year changes in body fat and visceral adipose tissue in women. Association with indexes of plasma glucose-insulin homeostasis. Diabetes Care 1996;19(9):983–91.

[37] Lemieux S, Prud'homme D, Tremblay A, Bouchard C, Tremblay A, Després JP. A single threshold value of waist girth identifies normal-weight and overweight subjects with excess visceral adipose tissue. Am J Clin Nutr 1996;64(5):685–93.

[38] Ross R, Janssen I, Dawson J, Kungl AM, Kuk JL, Wong SL, et al. Exercise-induced reduction in obesity and insulin resistance in women: a randomized controlled trial. Obes Res 2004;12(5):789–98.

[39] Katzel LI, Bleecker ER, Colman EG, Rogus EM, Sorkin JD, Goldberg AP. Effects of weight loss vs aerobic exercise training on risk factors for coronary disease in healthy, obese, middle-aged and older men. A randomized controlled trial. JAMA 1995;274(24):1915–21.

[40] Seidell JC, Kahn HS, Williamson DF, Lissner L, Valdez R. Report from a centers for disease control and prevention workshop on use of adult anthropometry for public health and primary health care. Am J Clin Nutr 2001;73(1):123–6.

[41] Pescatello LS, Murphy D. Lower intensity physical activity is advantageous for fat distribution and blood glucose among viscerally obese older adults. Med Sci Sports Exerc 1998;30(9):1408–13.

[42] Sörensen L, Smolander J, Louhevaara V, Korhonen O, Oja P. Physical activity, fitness and body composition of Finnish police officers: a 15-year follow-up study. Occup Med (Lond) 2000;50(1):3–10.

[43] Van Pelt RE, Davy KP, Stevenson ET, Wilson TM, Jones PP, Desouza CA, et al. Smaller differences in total and regional adiposity with age in women who regularly perform endurance exercise. Am J Physiol 1998;275(4 Pt 1):E626–34.

[44] Hu HH, Li Y, Nagy TR, Goran MI, Nayak KS. Quantification of absolute fat mass by magnetic resonance imaging: a validation study against chemical analysis. Int J Body Compos Res 2011;9(3):111–22.

[45] Slattery ML, McDonald A, Bild DE, Caan BJ, Hilner JE, Jacobs Jr DR, et al. Associations of body fat and its distribution with dietary intake, physical activity, alcohol, and smoking in blacks and whites. Am J Clin Nutr 1992;55(5):943–9.

[46] Troisi RJ, Heinold JW, Vokonas PS, Weiss ST. Cigarette smoking, dietary intake, and physical activity: effects on body fat distribution—the Normative Aging Study. Am J Clin Nutr 1991;53(5):1104–11.

[47] Douchi T, Yamamoto S, Oki T, Maruta K, Kuwahata R, Yamasaki H, et al. The effects of physical exercise on body fat distribution and bone mineral density in postmenopausal women. Maturitas 2000;35(1):25–30.

[48] Fabbri A, Giannini D, Aversa A, De Martino MU, Fabbrini E, Franceschi F, et al. Body-fat distribution and responsiveness of the pituitary-adrenal axis to corticotropin-releasing-hormone stimulation in sedentary and exercising women. J Endocrinol Invest 1999;22(5):377–85.

[49] Horber FF, Kohler SA, Lippuner K, Jaeger P. Effect of regular physical training on age-associated alteration of body composition in men. Eur J Clin Invest 1996;26(4):279–85.

[50] Hunter GR, Kekes-Szabo T, Treuth MS, Williams MJ, Goran M, Pichon C. Intra-abdominal adipose tissue, physical activity and cardiovascular risk in pre- and post-menopausal women. Int J Obes Relat Metab Disord 1996;20(9):860–5.

[51] Pratley RE, Hagberg JM, Rogus EM, Goldberg AP. Enhanced insulin sensitivity and lower waist-to-hip ratio in master athletes. Am J Physiol 1995;268(3 Pt 1):E484–90.

[52] Tremblay A, Després JP, Leblanc C, Craig CL, Ferris B, Stephens T, et al. Effect of intensity of physical activity on body fatness and fat distribution. Am J Clin Nutr 1990;51(2):153–7.

[53] Samaras K, Kelly PJ, Chiano MN, Spector TD, Campbell LV. Genetic and environmental influences on total-body and central abdominal fat: the effect of physical activity in female twins. Ann Intern Med 1999;130(11):873–82.

[54] Finelli C, Tarantino G. Is visceral fat reduction necessary to favour metabolic changes in the liver? J Gastrointestin Liver Dis 2012;21(2):205–8.

[55] Després JP, Couillard C, Gagnon J, Bergeron J, Leon AS, Rao DC, et al. Race, visceral adipose tissue, plasma lipids, and lipoprotein lipase activity in men and women: the Health, Risk Factors, Exercise Training, and Genetics (HERITAGE) family study. Arterioscler Thromb Vasc Biol 2000;20(8):1932–8.

[56] Frayn KN. Visceral fat and insulin resistance—causative or correlative? Br J Nutr 2000;83(Suppl. 1):S71–7.

[57] Liu J, Fox CS, Hickson D, Bidulescu A, Carr JJ, Taylor HA. Fatty liver, abdominal visceral fat, and cardiometabolic risk factors: the Jackson Heart Study. Arterioscler Thromb Vasc Biol 2011;31(11):2715–22.

[58] Slentz CA, Aiken LB, Houmard JA, Bales CW, Johnson JL, Tanner CJ, et al. Inactivity, exercise, and visceral fat. STRRIDE: a randomized, controlled study of exercise intensity and amount. J Appl Physiol 2005;99(4):1613–8.

[59] Kotronen A, Yki-Järvinen H. Fatty liver: a novel component of the metabolic syndrome. Arterioscler Thromb Vasc Biol 2008;28(1):27–38.

[60] Katzmarzyk PT, Mire E, Bouchard C. Abdominal obesity and mortality: the Pennington Center Longitudinal Study. Nutr Diabetes 2012;27(2):e42.

[61] Finelli C, Tarantino G. Should visceral fat, strictly linked to hepatic steatosis, be depleted to improve survival? Hepatol Int 2012;18.

[62] Slentz CA, Bateman LA, Willis LH, Shields AT, Tanner CJ, Piner LW, et al. Effects of aerobic vs. resistance training on visceral and liver fat stores, liver enzymes, and insulin resistance by HOMA in overweight adults from STRRIDE AT/RT. Am J Physiol Endocrinol Metab 2011;301(5):E1033–9.

[63] Borel AL, Nazare JA, Smith J, Alméras N, Tremblay A, Bergeron J, et al. Visceral and not subcutaneous abdominal adiposity reduction drives the benefits of a 1-year lifestyle modification program. Obesity (Silver Spring) 2012;20(6):1223–33.

[64] Fonvig CE, Bille DS, Chabanova E, Nielsen TR, Thomsen HS, Holm JC. Muscle fat content and abdominal adipose tissue distribution investigated by magnetic resonance spectroscopy and imaging in obese children and youths. Pediatr Rep 2012;4(1):e11.

[65] Staiano AE, Katzmarzyk PT. Ethnic and sex differences in body fat and visceral and subcutaneous adiposity in children and adolescents. Int J Obes (Lond) 2012;36(10):1261–9.

[66] Ayabe M, Kumahara H, Morimura K, Sakane N, Ishii K, Tanaka H. Accumulation of short bouts of non-exercise daily physical activity is associated with lower visceral fat in Japanese female adults. Int J Sports Med 2012.

[67] Kazlauskaite R, Karavolos K, Janssen I, Carlson K, Shipp KJ, Dugan SA, et al. The association between self-reported energy intake and intra-abdominal adipose tissue in perimenopausal women. J Obes 2012;2012:567320.

[68] Wilmore JH, Després JP, Stanforth PR, Mandel S, Rice T, et al. Alterations in body weight and composition consequent to 20weeks of endurance training: the HERITAGE Family Study. Am J Clin Nutr 1999;70(3):346–52.
[69] Després JP, Tremblay A, Nadeau A, Bouchard C. Physical training and changes in regional adipose tissue distribution. Acta Med Scand Suppl 1988;723:205–12.
[70] Andersson B, Xu XF, Rebuffé-Scrive M, Terning K, Krotkiewski M, Björntorp P. The effects of exercise, training on body composition and metabolism in men and women. Int J Obes 1991;15(1):75–81.
[71] Ohkawara K, Tanaka S, Miyachi M, Ishikawa-Takata K, Tabata I. A dose-response relation between aerobic exercise and visceral fat reduction: systematic review of clinical trials. Int J Obes (Lond) 2007;31(12):1786–97.
[72] Gal DL, Santos AC, Barros H. Leisure-time versus full-day energy expenditure: a cross-sectional study of sedentarism in a Portuguese urban population. BMC Public Health 2005;5:16.
[73] Kay SJ, Fiatarone Singh MA. The influence of physical activity on abdominal fat: a systematic review of the literature. Obes Rev 2006;7(2):183–200.
[74] Shen J, Goyal A, Sperling L. The emerging epidemic of obesity, diabetes, and the metabolic syndrome in china. Cardiol Res Pract 2012;2012:178675.
[75] Aoi W, Naito Y, Yoshikawa T. Dietary exercise as a novel strategy for the prevention and treatment of metabolic syndrome: effects on skeletal muscle function. J Nutr Metab 2011;2011:676208.
[76] O'Donovan G, Kearney EM, Nevill AM, Woolf-May K, Bird SR, et al. The effect of 24weeks of moderate- or high-intensity exercise on insulin resistance. Eur J Appl Physiol 2005;95:522–8.
[77] Benatti FB, Lira FS, Oyama LM, do Nascimento CM, Lancha Jr AH. Strategies for reducing body fat mass: effects of liposuction and exercise on cardiovascular risk factors and adiposity. Diabetes Metab Syndr Obes 2011;4:141–54.
[78] Ray L, Lipton RB, Zimmerman ME, Katz MJ, Derby CA. Mechanisms of association between obesity and chronic pain in the elderly. Pain 2011;152:53–9.
[79] Fenkci S, Sarsan A, Rota S, Ardic F. Effects of resistance or aerobic exercises on metabolic parameters in obese women who are not on a diet. Adv Ther 2006;23(3):404–13.
[80] Hallsworth K, Fattakhova G, Hollingsworth KG, Thoma C, Moore S, Taylor R, et al. Resistance exercise reduces liver fat and its mediators in non-alcoholic fatty liver disease independent of weight loss. Gut 2011;60:1278–83.
[81] Harrison SA, Day CP. Benefits of lifestyle modification in NAFLD. Gut 2007;56(12):1760–9.
[82] Mark N, de Alwis W, Day CP. Current and future therapeutic strategies in NAFLD. Curr Pharm Des 2010;16(17):1958–62.
[83] Ravikumar B, Gerrard J, Dalla Man C, Firbank MJ, Lane A, English PT, et al. Pioglitazone decreases fasting and postprandial endogenous glucose production in proportion to decrease in hepatic triglyceride content. Diabetes 2008;57(9):2288–95.
[84] Cuthbertson DJ, Irwin A, Gardner CJ, Daousi C, Purewal T, Furlong N, Goenka N, et al. Improved glycaemia correlates with liver fat reduction in obese, type 2 diabetes, patients given glucagon-like peptide-1 (GLP-1) receptor agonists. PLoS One 2012;7(12):e50117.
[85] Bhat G, Baba CS, Pandey A, Kumari N, Choudhuri G. Life style modification improves insulin resistance and liver histology in patients with non-alcoholic fatty liver disease. World J Hepatol 2012;4(7):209–17.
[86] Petta S, Macaluso FS, Barcellona MR, Cammà C, Cabibi D, Di Marco V, et al. Serum -glutamyl transferase levels, insulin resistance and liver fibrosis in patients with chronic liver diseases. PLoS One 2012;7(12):e51165.
[87] Bae JC, Suh S, Park SE, Rhee EJ, Park CY, Oh KW, et al. Regular exercise is associated with a reduction in the risk of NAFLD and decreased liver enzymes in individuals with NAFLD independent of obesity in Korean adults. PLoS One 2012;7(10):e46819.
[88] Finucane FM, Sharp SJ, Purslow LR, Horton K, Horton J, Savage DB, et al. The effects of aerobic exercise on metabolic risk, insulin sensitivity and intrahepatic lipid in healthy older people from the Hertfordshire Cohort Study: a randomised controlled trial. Diabetologia 2010;53(4):624–31.
[89] Solomon TP, Sistrun SN, Krishnan RK, Del Aguila LF, Marchetti CM, O'Carroll SM, et al. Exercise and diet enhance fat oxidation and reduce insulin resistance in older obese adults. J Appl Physiol 2008;104(5):1313–9.
[90] Zelber-Sagi S, Ratziu V, Oren R. Nutrition and physical activity in NAFLD: an overview of the epidemiological evidence. World J Gastroenterol 2011;17(29):3377–89.
[91] Shah K, Stufflebam A, Hilton TN, Sinacore DR, Klein S, Villareal DT. Diet and exercise interventions reduce intrahepatic fat content and improve insulin sensitivity in obese older adults. Obesity (Silver Spring) 2009;17(12):2162–8.
[92] Hamdy O, Porramatikul S, Al-Ozairi E. Metabolic obesity: the paradox between visceral and subcutaneous fat. Curr Diab Rev 2006;2:367–73.
[93] Kim JY, van de Wall E, Laplante M, Azzara A, Trujillo ME, Hofmann SM, et al. Obesity-associated improvements in metabolic profile through expansion of adipose tissue. J Clin Invest 2007;117(9):2621–37.
[94] Vega GL, Chandalia M, Szczepaniak LS, Grundy SM. Metabolic correlates of nonalcoholic fatty liver in women and men. Hepatology 2007;46:716–22.
[95] Jakobsen MU, Berentzen T, Sørensen TI, Overvad K. Abdominal obesity and fatty liver. Epidemiol Rev 2007;29:77–87.
[96] Koda M, Kawakami M, Murawaki Y, Senda M. The impact of visceral fat in nonalcoholic fatty liver disease: cross-sectional and longitudinal studies. J Gastroenterol 2007;42:897–903.
[97] Radetti G, Kleon W, Stuefer J, Pittschieler K. Non-alcoholic fatty liver disease in obese children evaluated by magnetic resonance imaging. Acta Paediatr 2006;95:833–7.
[98] Thamerc C, Machann J, Stefan N, Haap M, Schäfer S, Brenner S, et al. High visceral fat mass and high liver fat are associated with resistance to lifestyle intervention. Obesity 2007;15:531–8.
[99] Décarie PO, Lepanto L, Billiard JS, Olivié D, Murphy-Lavallée J, Kauffmann C, et al. Fatty liver deposition and sparing: a pictorial review. Insights Imaging 2011;2(5):533–8.
[100] Springer F, Machann J, Claussen CD, Schick F, Schwenzer NF. Liver fat content determined by magnetic resonance imaging and spectroscopy. World J Gastroenterol 2010;16(13):1560–6.
[101] Perseghin G, Lattuada G, De Cobelli F, Ragogna F, Ntali G, Esposito A, et al. Habitual physical activity is associated with intrahepatic fat content in humans. Diabetes Care 2007;30:683–8.
[102] Saadeh S, Younossi ZM, Remer EM, Gramlich T, Ong JP, Hurley M, et al. The utility of radiological imaging in nonalcoholic fatty liver disease. Gastroenterology 2002;123:745–50.
[103] Ducluzeau PH, Manchec-Poilblanc P, Roullier V, Cesbron E, Lebigot J, Bertrais S, et al. Distribution of abdominal adipose tissue as a predictor of hepatic steatosis assessed by MRI. Clin Radiol 2010;65(9):695–700.
[104] North KE, Graff M, Franceschini N, Reiner AP, Feitosa MF, Carr JJ, et al. Sex and race differences in the prevalence of fatty liver disease as measured by computed tomography liver attenuation in European American and African American participants of the NHLBI family heart study. Eur J Gastroenterol Hepatol 2011.
[105] Kim LJ, Nalls MA, Eiriksdottir G, Sigurdsson S, Launer LJ, Koster A, et al. AGES-Reykjavik study investigators.

Associations of visceral and liver fat with the metabolic syndrome across the spectrum of obesity: the AGES-Reykjavik study. Obesity (Silver Spring) 2011;19(6):1265–71.

[106] Kantartzis K, Thamer C, Peter A, Machann J, Schick F, Schraml C, et al. High cardiorespiratory fitness is an independent predictor of the reduction in liver fat during a lifestyle intervention in non-alcoholic fatty liver disease. Gut 2009;58(9):1281–8.

[107] Shah K, Stufflebam A, Hilton TN, Sinacore DR, Klein S, Villareal DT. Diet and exercise interventions reduce intrahepatic fat content and improve insulin sensitivity in obese older adults. Obesity (Silver Spring) 2009;17(12):2162–8.

[108] Hallsworth K, Fattakhova G, Hollingsworth KG, Thoma C, Moore S, Taylor R, Day CP, Trenell MI. Resistance exercise reduces liver fat and its mediators in non-alcoholic fatty liver disease independent of weight loss. Gut 2011;60(9):1278–83.

[109] Lee S, Bacha F, Hannon T, Kuk JL, Boesch C, Arslanian S. Effects of aerobic versus resistance exercise without caloric restriction on abdominal fat, intrahepatic lipid, and insulin sensitivity in obese adolescent boys: a randomized, controlled trial. Diabetes 2012;61(11):2787–95.

[110] de Piano A, de Mello MT, Sanches Pde L, da Silva PL, Campos RM, Carnier J, et al. Long-term effects of aerobic plus resistance training on the adipokines and neuropeptides in nonalcoholic fatty liver disease obese adolescents. Eur J Gastroenterol Hepatol 2012;24(11):1313–24.

[111] Fujioka S, Matsuzawa Y, Tokunaga K, Kawamoto T, Kobatake T, Keno Y, et al. Improvement of glucose and lipid metabolism associated with selective reduction of intra-abdominal visceral fat in premenopausal women with visceral fat obesity. Int J Obes 1991;15(12):853–9.

[112] Ross R, Freeman J, Hudson R, Janssen I. Abdominal obesity, muscle composition, and insulin resistance in premenopausal women. J Clin Endocrinol Metab 2002;87(11):5044–51.

[113] Saelens BE, Grow HM, Stark LJ, Seeley RJ, Roehrig H. Efficacy of increasing physical activity to reduce children's visceral fat: a pilot randomized controlled trial. Int J Pediatr Obes 2011;6(2):102–12.

[114] Lee KK, Park HS, Yum KS. Cut-off values of visceral fat area and waist-to-height ratio: diagnostic criteria for obesity-related disorders in Korean children and adolescents. Yonsei Med J 2012;53(1):99–105.

[115] Kaul S, Rothney MP, Peters DM, Wacker WK, Davis CE, Shapiro MD, et al. Dual-energy X-ray absorptiometry for quantification of visceral fat. Obesity (Silver Spring) 2012;20(6):1313–8.

[116] Jung JY, Han KA, Ahn HJ, Kwon HR, Lee JH, Park KS, et al. Effects of aerobic exercise intensity on abdominal and thigh adipose tissue and skeletal muscle attenuation in overweight women with type 2 diabetes mellitus. Diabetes Metab J 2012;36(3):211–21.

[117] Finelli C, Tarantino G. Is there any consensus as to what diet or lifestyle approach is the right one for NAFLD patients? J Gastrointestin Liver Dis 2012;21(3):293–302.

[118] Finelli C, Tarantino G. Have guidelines addressing physical activity been established in nonalcoholic fatty liver disease? World J Gastroenterol 2012;18(46):6790–800.

[119] Finelli C, Gioia S, La Sala N. Physical activity: an important adaptative mechanism for body-weight control. ISRN Obes 2012;2012:675285. http://dx.doi.org/10.5402/2012/675285.

[120] Williamson DL, Kubica N, Kimball SR, Jefferson LS. Exercise-induced alterations in extracellular signal-regulated kinase 1/2 and mammalian target of rapamycin (mTOR) signalling to regulatory mechanisms of mRNA translation in mouse muscle. J Physiol 2006;573(Pt 2):497–510. Epub 2006 Mar 1.6

[121] Tarantino G, Capone D. Inhibition of the mTOR pathway: a possible protective role in coronary artery disease. Ann Med 2013. May 13. [Epub ahead of print].

CHAPTER

8

Abdominal Fat and African-Americans: Incidence and Relationship to Disease

Lyndsey M. Hornbuckle[a] and Gary R. Hunter[b]

[a]Department of Exercise Science & Sport Management, Kennesaw State University, Kennesaw, GA, USA; [b]Department of Human Studies, University of Alabama, Birmingham, AL, USA

INTRODUCTION

The most recent National Health and Nutrition Examination Survey (NHANES) estimates of obesity in the United States show that non-Hispanic black adults (≥20 years) have the highest prevalence of grade 1 [49.6%; body mass index (BMI) ≥ 30 kg/m^2], grade 2 (26.2%; BMI ≥ 35 kg/m^2), and grade 3 obesity (13.3%; BMI ≥ 40 kg/m^2) compared to non-Hispanic whites, Hispanics, and Mexicans [1]. Perhaps even more unsettling are the most recent NHANES data indicating that non-Hispanic black children and adolescents, 2–19 years of age, have the highest prevalence of obesity (24.3%; ≥ 95th percentile for BMI-for-age growth charts) compared to children and adolescents of the same races and ethnicities [2]. As the obesity prevalence in non-Hispanic black adults, adolescents, and children is well above that of the next highest race/ethnicity [1,2], the health implications of these data are a concern. However, not all adipose tissue makes an equal contribution to metabolic disease.

It is well established that abdominal obesity, and more specifically visceral adipose tissue (VAT), is linked to an increased prevalence of multiple biomarkers for cardiometabolic disease compared to subcutaneous fat (SAT), which is more commonly stored in the lower body [3]. Although abdominal obesity is composed of both SAT and VAT, an excess accumulation of VAT plays a more pathogenic role [4,5]. When compared to SAT cells, VAT cells are less sensitive to the antilipolytic and re-esterification effects of insulin, while they are more sensitive to the lipolytic effect of catecholamines, thus encouraging a further increase in free fatty acid (FFA) flux [6]. It has also been suggested that acute increases in plasma FFAs promote hyperinsulinemia, while chronic FFA elevations can lead to lipotoxicity and pancreatic beta cell apoptosis [7]. There is evidence in both mice and humans to support the "portal hypothesis," which suggests that VAT lipolysis releases an excess of FFAs and inflammatory cytokines into the portal vein, directly exposing the liver to these substances [8,9]. Since FFAs come mainly from adipose tissue lipolysis, especially in obesity, these molecules are also considered to be adipokines [7].

Whereas adipose tissue was once considered to function mainly as a passive form of storage for excess energy, there is now evidence that it functions as an endocrine organ, significantly affecting the function of the vascular walls and other body organs through the secretion of bioactive adipokines [10,11]. The accumulation of VAT leads to the dysregulated production of several common adipokines including leptin (which controls satiety, energy expenditure, and neuroendocrine function), adiponectin (which controls glucose and lipid metabolism), interleukin-6 (IL-6; an immune-controlling cytokine and inflammatory mediator), plasminogen activator inhibitor 1 (PAI-1; a fibrinolysis inhibitor), tumor necrosis factor (TNF-α; a proinflammatory mediator), angiotensinogen (a proinflammatory mediator), and C-reactive protein (CRP; a proinflammatory mediator) [7]. Hyposecretion of the defensive adipokines such as adiponectin and hypersecretion of the offending adipokines such as TNF-α, PAI-1, and CRP may make major contributors to the pathogenesis of the obesity-associated components of metabolic syndrome and cardiovascular diseases, including type 2 diabetes mellitus (T2DM), hyperlipidemia, hypertension, and atherosclerosis [11].

Racial differences in the amount of abdominal fat, as well as in VAT stores, have been reported in multiple investigations over the past several years [5]. Despite the statistics showing that African-American (AA) adults have a greater prevalence of obesity [1], studies have

Nutrition in the Prevention and Treatment of Abdominal Obesity
http://dx.doi.org/10.1016/B978-0-12-407869-7.00008-8

consistently shown proportionately lower amounts of metabolically harmful VAT in AAs compared to other races and ethnicities [12–20]. This is the case in both the overweight and obese states [18], as well as after reaching a normal weight after weight loss [21]. AA children have also been shown to distribute less fat in the viscera compared to other races [22,23]. Since AAs appear to have less visceral fat than other races and ethnicities, even when matched for BMI, it may be expected that cardiovascular and metabolic disease risk would also be lower in AAs. However, there is evidence that this speculation does not hold true. Therefore, the purpose of this chapter is to review the incidence of abdominal fat and VAT in AAs compared to other races and ethnicities, and to examine its relationship to chronic disease. Throughout the chapter, specific reference terms for race/ethnicity have been used based on those used by the original authors of the work referenced.

INCIDENCE OF ABDOMINAL OBESITY AND CARDIOMETABOLIC RISK: AFRICAN-AMERICAN ADULTS

Brief Review

As the term *abdominal obesity* can include a variety of adipose tissue, it is important to distinguish exactly which types of fat are included in a given measurement. Anthropometric measurements, such as waist circumference (WC), include all of the mass within the abdomen, which includes all adipose tissue and lean mass. Laboratory methods, such as computed tomography (CT) and magnetic resonance imaging (MRI), allow investigators to separate VAT, SAT, and lean mass. This separation is critical when assessing the link between abdominal obesity and cardiometabolic abnormalities, especially in AAs.

There are data showing higher WC measurements in AAs compared to other races and ethnicities, which may be counterintuitive given the substantial amount of evidence showing smaller amounts of VAT in this population. Okosun et al. [24] used NHANES data from 1988–1994 to examine 8488 black, Hispanic, and white women and found that black women had the highest BMI values, WCs, and prevalence of hypertension compared to both of the other groups. In addition, when analyzed in 10-year increments, black women had the highest WC values for every decade of life from 20 to 79 years of age. Black men in this study had a lower mean WC than white and Hispanic men, which held true at all age groups; however, they had the highest prevalence of hypertension. BMI was different among the three groups of men. Okosun et al. [25] followed this by analyzing NHANES data from 1999–2002 only to discover similar results. Compared to Mexican-American and white women, black women had significantly higher BMI values, abdominal obesity (WC $\geq$ 88 cm in women and $\geq$102 cm in men), truncal obesity (estimated as the ratio of subscapular to triceps skinfold thickness), coexistence of abdominal and truncal obesity, and prevalence of hypertension. Black men had significantly higher BMI values and hypertension prevalence than both of the other groups; however, a significantly higher percentage of black men had abdominal obesity compared to Mexican-American men. Truncal obesity was significantly higher in black men than in white men, but not in Mexican-American men. This analysis also showed that the coexistence of abdominal and truncal obesity greatly increased the likelihood of hypertension in both women and men of all races.

In a different study, Okosun et al. [26] found that WC was positively correlated with plasma glucose, fasting insulin, triglycerides, systolic and diastolic blood pressures, total cholesterol, and total cholesterol:high-density lipoprotein (HDL) cholesterol ratio in black and white women and men. These data also showed that, compared to white women, black women had significantly higher BMI values, serum insulin levels, prevalence of T2DM, and prevalence of hypertension, while black men had a significantly higher prevalence of T2DM and hypertension compared to whites.

Howard et al. [27] examined postmenopausal women and found the greatest mean WC in black women compared to Hispanic/Latino, white, and Asian/Pacific Island women. Black women also had the highest BMI values, insulin resistance, and fasting insulin levels compared to the same three subgroups. Fasting blood glucose was least favorable in Asian/Pacific Island women, followed by Hispanic/Latino, black, and then white women. A study by Matthews et al. [28] found that healthy premenopausal AA women had the highest median WCs and the only values placing any subgroup at risk for cardiometabolic disease, when compared to their Hispanic and white peers. In addition, 48.9% of AA women in this study were obese (BMI $\geq$ 30 kg/m^2), compared to 32.7% of Hispanic, 28.9% of white, 4.5% of Japanese, and 4.4% of Chinese women. There was also a larger percentage of AA women who were on hypertensive medication compared to Hispanic, white, Japanese, and Chinese women.

Barreira et al. [29] took a cross-sectional look at 2037 AA and white adults 18–69 years of age and found that AA men had significantly lower WCs, while AA women had significantly higher WCs compared to whites. When compared to whites, both AA men and women had more favorable HDL cholesterol and triglycerides, and AA women had less favorable hypertension prevalence and glucose. In AA women, CT-measured VAT had a significant positive correlation with total cholesterol, low-density lipoprotein (LDL) cholesterol, glucose, triglycerides, and systolic and diastolic blood pressure, and a significant negative correlation with HDL cholesterol. Correlations between VAT and glucose and between VAT and systolic blood pressure were stronger than the same correlations in white women. In AA men, VAT had a significant positive correlation with LDL cholesterol, glucose, triglycerides, and diastolic blood pressure, and a significant negative correlation with HDL cholesterol. With the exception of triglycerides, correlations between VAT and each biomarker were stronger than the same correlations in white men.

Research using methodologies that enable differentiation between the types of adipose tissue present have consistently shown that AAs distribute a smaller proportion of their body fat as the more harmful VAT. Conway et al. [17] examined a sample of obese black and white women participating in a weight loss study. Data were collected at baseline, after a 12-week very-low-calorie diet, and after a 12-week refeeding period. A lateral view of the lower lumbar spine at the L2-L3 and L4-L5 levels was measured via CT. The areas for VAT, SAT, and total adipose tissue were calculated: all three areas decreased in a similar fashion in both races with weight loss. Black females had significantly less VAT at all three measurement points in the L2-L3 area and there was no significant racial difference in SAT and total adipose tissue in this area. In the L4-L5 region, blacks again had less VAT; however, this difference was not significant. There was also no significant difference between SAT and total adipose tissue between the two groups in the L4-L5 area.

An investigation by Albu et al. [18] showed again that black women had less VAT compared to white women in a sample of nondiabetic, overweight, or obese females aged 26–49 years. VAT and SAT were measured in most participants by MRI, but four subjects were measured via CT scans due to claustrophobia and/or excessive body weight. Measurements were taken at the midpoint between the last rib and the iliac crest, which for most subjects was the L2-L3 level of the lumbar spine. The two groups of women were closely matched for age, body fat, fat-free mass, BMI, and WC. After adjusting for total body fat mass, black women were shown to have significantly less VAT and a lower VAT:SAT ratio compared to the white women. In both groups, WC was significantly correlated to VAT and SAT.

Lovejoy et al. [30] compared fat distribution and health risk factors in middle-aged white and AA women. This investigation did not show as clearly that AA women had less VAT; however, it did show that VAT is the strongest predictor of metabolic and cardiovascular risk factors in both racial groups. Body composition was measured by dual-energy X-ray absorptiometry and abdominal fat distribution was determined using a CT scan at the level between the L4 and L5 vertebrae. After adjustments were made for age and total body fat, results showed that SAT and superficial SAT were significantly higher in AA women, with only a slight and nonsignificant trend for this population to have less VAT than their white counterparts. There were no significant racial differences in total or deep SAT. It was also shown that VAT was the strongest independent predictor of fasting blood glucose, fasting insulin, HDL cholesterol, LDL cholesterol, and total cholesterol in AA women. VAT was also the strongest predictor of most of these factors in white women, with the exception of fasting glucose. These results provide further support that VAT is generally a good predictor of health risk in both populations.

Ardern et al. [31] observed significantly lower VAT in 77 sedentary black men compared to 206 white men at baseline prior to the introduction of a 20-week aerobic exercise training protocol, as measured by CT at the L4-L5 vertebrae. These men were participating in the Health, Risk Factors, Exercise Training, and Genetics (HERITAGE) family study [32], a large, multicenter clinical trial that included participants from a large age range (17–65 years). North et al. [33] also observed lower amounts of VAT and higher amounts of SAT in both AA men and women ($n=506$) compared to European Americans ($n=2221$) who were enrolled in the National Heart, Lung, and Blood Institute (NHLBI) Family Heart Study. Data from this cohort were consistent with those of other studies showing that AA men and women had more favorable HDL cholesterol and triglyceride levels, yet higher BMI values and a greater level of insulin resistance compared to their European American counterparts.

Taken together, these studies show that AAs may be more vulnerable to elevated BMI, but that at similar BMIs, AAs tend to distribute less fat in the viscera than do other racial/ethnic groups. Also, after adjusting for BMI, AAs typically show more favorable triglyceride and HDL cholesterol levels, but higher blood pressure and less insulin sensitivity. These data show that when evaluating abdominal obesity in AAs and other populations, choosing appropriate measurement methods is critical for assessing cardiometabolic risk. When evaluating such risk independent of overall obesity, laboratory methodologies such as CT and MRI should be used over anthropometric measurements in order to closely monitor VAT as a critical marker for health risk.

Visceral Adipose Tissue Thresholds

Research using CT has investigated thresholds for ideal VAT and shown that, compared to white adults, AA adults have a lower threshold for VAT levels that are associated with an increased risk of cardiometabolic disease. Katzmarzyk et al. [34] recently examined a sample of AA and white women and men aged 18–74 years and showed that AA women ($91.0 \pm 49.2\,cm^2$) and men

($90.3 \pm 57.9\,cm^2$) had significantly lower VAT compared to white women ($121.8 \pm 61.2\,cm^2$) and men ($140.9 \pm 70.8\,cm^2$). This study went on to identify lower risk factor thresholds for AA women ($97\,cm^2$) and men ($82\,cm^2$) compared to white women ($141\,cm^2$) and men ($140\,cm^2$). Risk factors included in the threshold analyses were systolic and diastolic blood pressure, glucose, triglycerides, and HDL cholesterol, in addition to the presence of metabolic syndrome.

Additional studies examining VAT thresholds in other ethnicities confirm that Katzmarzyk's suggested thresholds in AAs are much lower than in other races and ethnicities. In a sample of white males aged 30–71 years, Hunter et al. [35] identified both an upper ($>131\,cm^2$) and lower threshold ($<71\,cm^2$) for cardiovascular risk. The upper threshold was associated with an increased risk of abnormal systolic and diastolic blood pressure, HDL cholesterol, and total cholesterol, and the lower threshold was associated with a decreased risk of these markers. Williams et al. [36] identified cutoff points associated with a greater cardiovascular risk in pre- and postmenopausal Caucasian women ages 18–77 years. They concluded that intra-abdominal adipose tissue levels $>110\,cm^2$ were associated with a higher risk of cardiovascular disease, while risk was not affected at levels $<40\,cm^2$. Lim et al. [37] suggested optimal cutoff points for predicting metabolic syndrome in an elderly Korean cohort aged 65 years and older. They found that cutoff points of 100 and $140\,cm^2$ VAT in women and men, respectively, were associated with a greater risk of metabolic syndrome. After adjusting for age, exercise, alcohol consumption, and smoking, the threshold for men decreased to $122\,cm^2$, while the women's threshold did not change. Interestingly, Hayashi et al. [38] showed that Japanese Americans have relatively low VAT thresholds, which appear more similar to those of AAs compared to thresholds shown in the white subjects of previous studies. In Japanese women and men ≤ 57 years of age, they found that the VAT thresholds associated with metabolic syndrome were 51.5 and $88.6\,cm^2$, respectively. In women and men over 57 years of age, the thresholds were 86.3 and $96.1\,cm^2$, respectively.

In summary, the specific thresholds associated with an increased risk of cardiometabolic risk factors vary across studies and populations. However, the lower the VAT threshold, the greater the clinical significance of any accumulation of VAT. The research reviewed in this chapter showing lower thresholds in AAs compared to whites suggests that VAT may have more of an impact on risk factors in AA adults. Further research is needed in AAs to more clearly define a race-specific pattern of VAT thresholds at which cardiometabolic risk is increased. Obtaining a more lucid understanding of VAT- and obesity-related thresholds is highly relevant as future investigators continue to explore and recommend interventions for fat loss as an approach to reduce the prevalence of chronic cardiometabolic diseases.

Hormonal Influence and Variation

Sex steroid hormones have also been linked to abdominal obesity in both men and women. In women, the increase in WC and resulting metabolic disturbances that are common at menopause suggests that estrogen may be a major factor in controlling VAT and metabolism [5,39]. Low total testosterone levels have been linked to abdominal obesity and greater amounts of VAT in men [5]. Hormone replacement therapy has been shown to be a great catalyst in the reduction of central adiposity in both women and men: estrogen and antiandrogens elicited improvements in women, and increases in testosterone levels were successful for the men [40]. Therefore, hormone replacement therapy may be a particularly beneficial addition to obesity interventions in populations that have been afflicted by sex steroid deficiencies and/or those who are specifically looking to reduce VAT in order to improve their cardiometabolic profile. A recent study also showed that lower serum concentrations of sex hormone-binding globulin (SHBG) were associated with an increased risk of several obesity-related diseases in women, including hormone-sensitive cancers, T2DM, metabolic syndrome, and cardiovascular disease, while increased VAT seems to be one of the main factors influencing decreases in SHBG [41]. This study found that, despite lower VAT, AA women did not have increased SHBG, suggesting lower cutoff points for VAT in AA women concerning SHBG.

Elevated adiponectin and decreased leptin values are normally associated with improved metabolic health. Despite a more favorable fat distribution, AA women have shown lower adiponectin and increased leptin compared to Caucasian women [42]. This result again suggests that lower VAT cutoff points are warranted in AA women in order to minimize these particular hormonal disturbances. Interestingly, a large cohort study showed a gender difference in serum adiponectin levels among AAs [43]. This study showed that AA men had significantly higher amounts of VAT and lower levels of both adiponectin and SAT compared to AA women. In addition, VAT was inversely related to adiponectin in only the women of this study, even after adjusting for BMI and WC. However, VAT was not a predictor of adiponectin in the men of this study and SAT in the abdomen seemed to be protective.

INCIDENCE OF ABDOMINAL OBESITY AND CARDIOMETABOLIC RISK: AFRICAN-AMERICAN CHILDREN AND ADOLESCENTS

Brief Review

As obesity in the childhood and adolescent years has also become an epidemic in the United States, it is critical to also assess VAT and its contribution to cardiometabolic risk in young AAs. Morrison et al. [44] provide longitudinal evidence from the NHLBI Growth and Health Study [45] that an increased prevalence of metabolic syndrome in AA women begins as early as adolescence. In this 10-year cohort study of black ($n=584$) and white ($n=608$) girls, they found that only one girl (0.2%) of each race had ≥3 factors related to metabolic syndrome at ages 9 and 10 years. However, by ages 18 and 19 years, 20 out of 567 black girls (3.5%) and 12 out of 511 white girls (2.3%) had metabolic syndrome. At baseline, black girls had significantly higher values for WC, BMI, insulin, glucose, insulin resistance, and systolic blood pressure, while white girls had significantly less favorable levels for HDL cholesterol and triglycerides. There was no difference between the groups for diastolic blood pressure at baseline. After 10 years, diastolic blood pressure became significantly higher in black girls, while all the previous racial differences remained and, in most categories, became even more evident. It was also notable that the 18- and 19-year-old black girls had a mean BMI of 27.5 kg/m^2, categorizing them as overweight at an early age, whereas the white girls at that age had a mean BMI of 23.7 kg/m^2. Additionally, 25.7% of the black vs. 11.8% of the 18- and 19-year-old white girls had WCs >88 cm, placing them at a greater risk of cardiometabolic disorders [46].

Messiah [47] more recently used 1999–2008 NHANES data to examine ethnic group differences in cardiometabolic risk in 3510 8–11-year-old boys and girls. Both before and after adjusting for BMI, they found that WCs differed significantly by ethnic group. Non-Hispanic black children also had more favorable HDL cholesterol levels compared to both Hispanics and non-Hispanic whites. In addition, non-Hispanic blacks were less likely to have high triglycerides levels when compared to non-Hispanic whites. Although racial and ethnic differences in neither systolic nor diastolic blood pressure were shown, the blood lipid data point to racial and ethnic disparities in cardiometabolic risk that are not solely related to BMI.

Herd et al. [22] examined the influence of body fat distribution on serum lipids in AA and Caucasian prepubertal children (mean age of 8.6 years). After adjusting for total fat mass, Caucasian children had significantly greater amounts of abdominal fat, SAT in the abdomen, and VAT compared to the AA children. AA children had more favorable triglycerides and HDL cholesterol levels compared to the Caucasian children, which could be explained by the difference in VAT. These results are consistent with other studies, as shown in a recent review of ethnic differences in body fat in children and adolescents. This review, by Staiano et al. [23], confirms that studies have consistently shown that Hispanic and white children were more likely to have greater amounts of VAT, while AA children most often had higher SAT. However, despite lower amounts of VAT, AA youths have still shown lower insulin sensitivity and greater risk for diabetes when compared to their counterparts of other races/ethnicities.

Collectively, the data described above in children and adolescents are aligned with the body fat distribution and cardiometabolic risk tendencies in adults of their respective races and ethnicities, which were reviewed earlier in this chapter. This congruence between adult and youth patterns supports suggestions of a genetic influence in body fat distribution [5] and should be considered in cardiometabolic disease prevention strategies involving children and adolescents. Initiating methods to minimize abdominal obesity and cardiometabolic risk during the childhood and adolescent years (i.e. encouraging healthy eating, physical activity, and smoking cessation) could be a critical determinant of the long-term health in AAs.

INTERVENTION STRATEGIES

Lifestyle factors can play a crucial role in the effort to prevent and/or treat abdominal obesity and VAT accumulation in AAs. As mentioned previously, these methods should be adopted early and, if possible, should be culturally relevant in order to encourage reinforcement within the community and long-term adherence. As exercise and dietary consumption are lifestyle components that have a well-established influence on body composition and a host of other cardiometabolic health indicators, these modifiable factors are often a topic of focus when researching effective intervention strategies for improving body composition.

A recent systematic review and meta-analysis examining the effect of exercise on VAT showed several different modalities of exercise to be effective in VAT reduction in both men and women [48]. Exercise has even been associated with a disproportionate decrease in VAT in both younger and older women [49,50]. Hunter et al. [49] showed that both resistance and aerobic training prevented VAT gain for 1 year following a 27 lb (12.2 kg) diet-induced weight loss in premenopausal AA ($n=52$) and white ($n=45$) women. Despite modest weight regains, both resistance and aerobic exercise were successful in slowing weight regain and preventing VAT gain. These results strongly suggest that exercise must somehow be involved in fat redistribution away from the viscera and toward the periphery, leading to a more favorable fat distribution for metabolic health. These data did not show any racial differences in the response to exercise, indicating that it is equally beneficial for AA and white women. Treuth et al. [50] observed significant reductions in VAT after only 16 weeks of strength training in 15 postmenopausal women. Race was not specified, but this study further emphasizes the benefit of exercise, even in a population that has negative hormonal influences. In a different study, Treuth et al. [51] showed that 5 months of strength training led to VAT maintenance in 11 prepubertal, obese girls, while both their weight and total body fat mass increased. Race was also not specified in this study. Wilmore et al. [52] examined a sample of 557 black and white men and women participating in the HERITAGE family study [32] and found improvements in VAT after 20 weeks of aerobic exercise training in black men and women. In a different data analysis of this clinical trial, Ardern et al. [31] showed that blood lipids were more closely linked to VAT in blacks compared to whites, both at baseline and after the training. This suggests that exercise for body composition and VAT improvements may be an especially effective way to improve blood lipids in AAs, if needed.

In examining more culturally relevant strategies for health promotion in AA communities, there are data showing success in faith-based diet and physical activity interventions [53–55], as well as in health education dissemination in beauty shops [56]. Since these community-based studies typically do not include laboratory testing, there is little evidence that these types of interventions have improved abdominal obesity. However, the significant health improvements found using these strategies indicate that abdominal obesity could be positively impacted if measured in future studies.

Faith-based interventions launched in the AA community may be more culturally relevant compared to traditional nutrition and exercise interventions, as the church provides a critical foundation for social guidance in AA communities [57]. Yanek et al. [55] examined the effects of a 1-year nutrition and physical activity intervention on cardiovascular disease risk profiles in 529 AA women from 16 churches. When compared to controls, those who participated in either the standard or the spiritual intervention had physiological improvements in body weight, BMI, WC, and systolic blood pressure, in addition to positive dietary changes in total caloric intake, total dietary fat intake, and dietary sodium intake. More recently, Wilcox et al. [53] and Woods et al. [54] both showed health improvements in predominantly AA communities through faith-based interventions. Wilcox and colleagues [53] studied the effects of a 15-month combined physical activity and nutrition faith-based educational intervention in 1257 members from 74 churches. They showed improvements in self-reported leisure-time moderate- to vigorous-intensity physical activity compared to controls, as well as a positive intervention effect on self-reported fruit and vegetable consumption. Woods and colleagues [54] showed improvements in body weight, BMI, total percentage of body fat, and physical fitness compared to controls after an 8-week faith-based intervention in 106 adults from five churches. It is also notable that the intervention group had 97% retention compared to 75% in the control group. Kleindorfer et al. [56] showed improvements in knowledge of the warning signs of a stroke in a group of 318 black women who were educated in the topic by their beauticians during appointments.

While these community-based studies measured neither VAT nor cardiometabolic biomarkers in the blood, their results (improvements in body weight, total body composition, physical activity levels, and physical fitness) suggest that perhaps improvements in VAT could be obtained in such interventions. Measuring VAT in interventions designed to be culturally relevant in the AA community should be a consideration in future research studies.

CONCLUSIONS

There is a vast amount of scientific evidence showing that AAs have less VAT contributing to their abdominal obesity when compared to other races and ethnicities, particularly whites. This pattern of body fat distribution persists in adults, adolescents, and children. However, with the exception of evidence that AAs generally have more favorable blood lipid profiles compared to whites, the lower levels of VAT do not appear to diminish the prevalence of other risk factors for cardiovascular disease in AAs. In addition, the VAT thresholds shown to be associated with an increased risk for cardiometabolic abnormalities are lower in AAs, which may essentially negate any perceived advantage of having less VAT in the abdomen. A common hypothesis of the physiological reason for racial and ethnic differences in VAT is that an individual's fat compartments are genetically predisposed to store a specific type of lipid [5,58].

Further investigations are needed to pinpoint specific VAT thresholds at which AAs experience an increased risk of cardiometabolic disease. In a recent review of the topic, Tchernof and Despres [5] suggest, and the current authors agree, that large epidemiological studies using CT measures of VAT are warranted to identify population-specific thresholds. Population-specific interventions designed to modify lifestyle factors and ultimately reduce VAT and overall body fat should also be an area of focus for future research in order to treat, or preferably prevent, health disparities in this area.

References

[1] Flegal KM, Carroll MD, Kit BK, Ogden CL. Prevalence of obesity and trends in the distribution of body mass index among US adults, 1999–2010. JAMA 2012;307(5):491–7.

[2] Ogden CL, Carroll MD, Kit BK, Flegal KM. Prevalence of obesity trends in body mass index among US children and adolescents, 1999–2010. JAMA 2012;307(5):483–90.

[3] Hamdy O, Porramatikul S, Al-Ozairi E. Metabolic obesity: the paradox between visceral and subcutaneous fat. Curr Diabetes Rev 2006;2(3):367–73.
[4] Freedland ES. Role of critical visceral adipose tissue threshold (CVATT) in metabolic syndrome: implications for controlling dietary carbohydrates: a review. Nutr Metab 2004;1(1):12–35.
[5] Tchernof A, Despres J-P. Pathophysiology of human visceral obesity: an update. Physiol Rev 2013;93(1):359–404.
[6] Lewis GF, Carpentier A, Adeli K, Giacca A. Disordered fat storage and mobilization in the pathogenesis of insulin resistance and type 2 diabetes. Endocr Rev 2002;23(2):201–29.
[7] Hutley L, Prins J. Fat as an endocrine organ: relationship to the metabolic syndrome. Am J Med Sci 2005;330(6):280–9.
[8] Nielsen S, Guo Z, Johnson M, Hensrud DD, Jensen MD. Splanchnic lipolysis in human obesity. J Clin Invest 2004;113(11):1582–8.
[9] Rytka JM, Wueest S, Schoenle EJ, Konrad D. The portal theory supported by venous drainage-selective fat transplantation. Diabetes 2011;60(1):56–63.
[10] Matsuzawa Y. Therapy insight: adipokines in metabolic syndrome and related cardiovascular disease. Nat Clin Pract Cardiovasc Med 2006;3(1):35–42.
[11] Matsuzawa Y. White adipose tissue and cardiovascular disease. Best Pract Res Clin Endocrinol Metab 2005;19(4):637–47.
[12] Hoffman DJ, Wang Z, Gallagher D, Heymsfield SB. Comparison of visceral adipose tissue mass in adult African Americans and whites. Obes Res 2005;13(1):66–74.
[13] Camhi SM, Bray GA, Bouchard C, et al. The relationship of waist circumference and BMI to visceral, subcutaneous, and total body fat: sex and race differences. Obesity 2011;19(2):402–8.
[14] Carroll JF, Chiapa AL, Rodriquez M, et al. Visceral fat, waist circumference, and BMI: impact of race/ethnicity. Obesity 2008;16(3):600–7.
[15] Katzmarzyk PT, Bray GA, Greenway FL, et al. Racial differences in abdominal depot-specific adiposity in white and African American Adults. Am J Clin Nutr 2010;91(1):7–15.
[16] Lovejoy JC, de la Bretonne JA, Klemperer M, Tulley R. Abdominal fat distribution and metabolic risk factors: effects of race. Metabolism 1996;45(9):1119–24.
[17] Conway JM, Yanovski SZ, Avila NA, Hubbard VS. Visceral adipose tissue differences in black and white women. Am J Clin Nutr 1995;61(4):765–71.
[18] Albu JB, Murphy L, Frager DH, Johnson JA, Pi-Sunyer FX. Visceral fat and race-dependent health risks in obese nondiabetic premenopausal women. Diabetes 1997;46(3):456–62.
[19] Hunter GR, Chandler-Laney PC, Brock DW, Lara-Castro C, Fernandez JR, Gower BA. Fat distribution, aerobic fitness, blood lipids, and insulin sensitivity in African-American and European-American women. Obesity 2010;18(2):274–81.
[20] Despres J-P, Couillard C, Gagnon J, et al. Race, visceral adipose tissue, plasma lipids, and lipoprotein lipase activity in men and women: the Health, Risk Factors, Exercise Training, and Genetics (HERITAGE) Family Study. Arterioscler Thromb Vasc Biol 2000;20(8):1932–8.
[21] Weinsier RL, Hunter GR, Gower BA, Schutz Y, Darnell BE, Zuckerman PA. Body fat distribution in white and black women: different patterns of intraabdominal and subcutaneous abdominal adipose tissue utilization with weight loss. Am J Clin Nutr 2001;74(5):631–6.
[22] Herd S, Gower BA, Dashti N, Goran M. Body fat, fat distribution and serum lipids, lipoproteins and apolipoproteins in African-American and Caucasian-American prepubertal children. Int J Obes Relat Metab Disord 2001;25(2):198–204.
[23] Staiano AE, Katzmarzyk PT. Ethnic and sex differences in body fat and visceral and subcutaneous adiposity in children and adolescents. Int J Obes Relat Metab Disord 2012;36(10):1261–9.
[24] Okosun IS, Prewitt TE, Cooper RS. Abdominal obesity in the United States: prevalence and attributable risk of hypertension. J Human Hypertens 1999;13(7):425–30.
[25] Okosun IS, Boltri JM, Hepburn VA, Eriksen MP, Davis-Smith M. Regional fat localizations and racial/ethnic variations in odds of hypertension in at-risk American adults. J Human Hypertens 2006;20(5):362–71.
[26] Okosun IS, Cooper RS, Prewitt E, Rotimi CN. The relation of central adiposity to components of the insulin resistance syndrome in a biracial US population sample. Ethn Dis 1999;9(2):218–29.
[27] Howard BV, Criqui MH, Curb JD, et al. Risk factor clustering in the insulin resistance syndrome and its relationship to cardiovascular disease in postmenopausal white, black, Hispanic, and Asian/Pacific Islander women. Metabolism 2003;52(3):362–71.
[28] Matthews KA, Sowers MF, Derby CA, et al. Ethnic differences in cardiovascular risk factor burden among middle-aged women: Study of Women's Health Across the Nation (SWAN). Am Heart J 2005;149(6):1066–73.
[29] Barreira TV, Staiano AE, Harrington DM, et al. Anthropometric correlates of total body fat, abdominal obesity, and cardiovascular disease risk factors in a biracial sample of men and women. Mayo Clin Proc 2012;87(5):452–60.
[30] Lovejoy JC, Smith SR, Rood JC. Comparison of regional fat distribution and health risk factors in middle-aged white and African American women: the Healthy Transitions Study. Obes Res 2001;9(1):10–16.
[31] Ardern CI, Katzmarzyk PT, Janssen I, et al. Race and sex similarities in exercise-induced changes in blood lipids and fatness. Med Sci Sports Exerc 2004;36(8):1610–5.
[32] Bouchard C, Leon AS, Rao DC, Skinner JS, Wilmore JH, Gagnon J. The HERITAGE family study. Aims, design, and measurement protocol. Med Sci Sports Exerc 1995;27(5):721–5.
[33] North KE, Graff M, Franceschni N, et al. Sex and race differences in the prevalence of fatty liver disease as measured by CT liver attenuation in European American and African American participants of the NHLBI Family Heart Study. Eur J Gastroenterol Hepatol 2012;24(1):9–16.
[34] Katzmarzyk PT, Heymsfield SB, Bouchard C. Clinical utility of visceral adipose tissue for the identification of cardiometabolic risk in white and African American adults. Am J Clin Nutr 2013;97(3):480–6.
[35] Hunter GR, Snyder SW, Kekes-Szabo T, Nicholson C, Berland L. Intra-abdominal adipose tissue values associated with risk of possessing elevated blood lipids and blood pressure. Obes Res 1994;2(6):563–8.
[36] Williams MJ, Hunter GR, Kekes-Szabo T, et al. Intra-abdominal adipose tissue cut-points related to elevated cardiovascular risk in women. Int J Obes Relat Metab Disord 1996;20(7):613–7.
[37] Lim S, Kim JH, Yoon JW, et al. Optimal cut points of waist circumference (WC) and visceral fat area (VFA) predicting for metabolic syndrome (MetS) in elderly population in the Korean Longitudinal Study on Health and Aging (KLoSHA). Arch Gerontol Geriatr 2012;54(2):e29–34.
[38] Hayashi T, Boyko EJ, McNeely MJ, Leonetti DL, Kahn SE, Fujimoto WY. Minimum waist and visceral fat values for identifying Japanese Americans at risk for the metabolic syndrome. Diabetes Care 2007;30(1):120–7.
[39] Bjorntorp P. Visceral obesity: a "civilization syndrome". Obes Res 1993;1(3):206–22.
[40] Mayes JS, Watson GH. Direct effects of sex steroid hormones on adipose tissues and obesity. Obes Rev 2004;5(4):197–216.
[41] Azrad M, Gower BA, Hunter GR, Nagy TR. Intra-abdominal adipose tissue is independently associated with sex-hormone binding globulin in premenopausal women. Obesity 2012;20(5):1012–5.

[42] Azrad M, Gower BA, Hunter GR, Nagy TR. Racial differences in adiponectin and leptin in healthy premenopausal women. Endocrine 2013;43(3):586–92.

[43] Bidulescu A, Liu J, Hickson DA, et al. Gender differences in the association of visceral and subcutaneous adiposity with adiponectin in African Americans: the Jackson Heart Study. BMC Cardiovasc Disord 2013;13(9).

[44] Morrison JA, Friedman LA, Harlan WR, et al. Development of the metabolic syndrome in black and white adolescent girls: a longitudinal assessment. Pediatrics 2005;116(5):1178–82.

[45] The NHLBI Growth and Health Study Research Group . Obesity and cardiovascular disease risk factors in black and white girls: the NHLBI Growth and Health Study. Am J Public Health 1992;82(12):1613–20.

[46] American College of Sports Medicine . Health-related physical fitness testing and interpretation. In: Thompson PD, , Riebe D, Pescatello LS, editors. ACSM's Guidelines for Exercise Testing and Prescription. 9th ed. Baltimore: Lippincott Williams & Wilkins; 2013.

[47] Messiah SE, Arheart KL, Lopez-Mitnik G, Lipshultz SE, Miller TL. Ethnic group differences in cardiometabolic disease risk factors independent of body mass index among American youth. Obesity 2013;21(3):424–8.

[48] Vissers D, Hens W, Taeymans J, Baeyens J-P, Poortmans J, Gaal LV. The effect of exercise on visceral adipose tissue in overweight adults: a systematic review and meta-analysis. PLoS One 2013;8(2):e56415.

[49] Hunter GR, Brock DW, Byrne NM, Chandler-Laney PC, Coral PD, Gower BA. Exercise training prevents regain of visceral fat for 1-year following weight loss. Obesity 2010;18(4):690–5.

[50] Treuth MS, Hunter GR, Kekes-Szabo T, Weinsier RL, Goran M, Berland L. Reduction in intra-abdominal adipose tissue after strength training in older women. J Appl Physiol 1995;78(4):1425–31.

[51] Treuth MS, Hunter GR, Figueroa-Colon R, Goran M. Effects of strength training on intra-abdominal adipose tissue in obese prepubertal girls. Med Sci Sports Exerc 1998;30(12):1738–43.

[52] Wilmore JH, Despres J-P, Stanforth PR, et al. Alterations in body weight and composition consequent to 20 weeks of endurance training: the HERITAGE family study. Am J Clin Nutr 1999;70(3):346–52.

[53] Wilcox S, Parrott A, Baruth M, et al. The faith, activity, and nutrition program: a randomized controlled trial in African-American churches. Am J Prev Med 2013;44(2):122–31.

[54] Woods G, Levinson AH, Jones G, et al. The Living Well by Faith health and wellness program for African Americans: an exemplar of community-based participatory research. Ethn Dis 2013;23(2):223–9.

[55] Yanek LR, Becker DM, Moy T, Gittelson J, Koffman DM. Project Joy: faith based cardiovascular health promotion for African American women. Public Health Rep 2001;116(Suppl. 1):68–81.

[56] Kleindorfer D, Miller R, Sailor-Smith S, Moomaw CJ, Khoury J, Frankel M. The challenges of community-based research: the beauty shop stroke education project. Stroke 2008;39(8):2331–5.

[57] Levin JS. The role of the black church in community medicine. J Natl Med Assoc 1985;76(5):477–83.

[58] Katzmarzyk PT, Perusse L, Bouchard C. Genetics of abdominal visceral fat levels. Am J Hum Biol 1999;11(2):225–35.

PART B

ABDOMINAL OBESITY AND METABOLIC SYNDROME

CHAPTER

9

Visceral Fat and Hypertension: Sex Differences

Zdenka Pausova

The Hospital for Sick Children, University of Toronto, Toronto, Canada

OVERVIEW

Hypertension is a leading cause of death, stroke, cardiovascular disease, and renal disease [1–4]. The prevalence of hypertension is rising worldwide [1,5]. Much of this rise has been attributed to the growing prevalence of obesity. In fact, obesity is a leading risk factor for hypertension [6,7].

The relationship between obesity and hypertension is not simple, however. About 50% of adults classified as being "obese" do not develop hypertension [8] and over 25% of adults classified as being of "normal weight" do develop the disease [9]. To some extent, this may be an artifact of the measurement method. For over 150 years, obesity has been assessed by body mass index (BMI; weight/height^2), which is an imprecise, and possibly misleading [10], metric of body fat. This is because BMI is influenced not only by fat mass but also by muscle mass and bone mass, among others [11]. Moreover, obesity-related risk for hypertension increases not only with the quantity but also with the specific distribution of body fat—individuals who store body fat viscerally rather than elsewhere in the body (mostly subcutaneously) are at a greater risk for hypertension [12–14]. Consistent with these observations, the surgical removal of visceral fat (VF) but not of subcutaneous fat (SF) improves cardiometabolic health in humans and experimental animals [15–17]. Large interindividual differences exist in the quantities of VF and SF and in their proportions (Fig. 9.1).

Why VF is more cardiometabolically dangerous than SF is still unclear. Obesity-related risk for hypertension is mainly the consequence of excess adipose tissue secreting free fatty acids (FFAs) and adipocytokines. Once released within the tissue and into the circulation, these molecules promote the development of hypertension (Fig. 9.2) [18]. Compared with SF, VF exhibits a more *adverse secretory profile* [19–22]. In addition, by virtue of its *anatomical location*, VF (and not SF) drains directly into the portal circulation and liver, where it enhances dyslipidemia and insulin resistance, important mediators of the link between obesity and hypertension [22,23]. Moreover, a growing body of research suggests that SF may even be cardiometabolically protective in overweight and obese individuals [24–26]. This effect has been related to the so-called *expandability of SF,* which is thought to be a biological property of SF that allows excess body fat to accumulate preferentially in this fat depot; through this effect, it protects the body from the cardiometabolically adverse accumulation of VF [27,28]. This biological property of SF is thought to be related to its capacity to form new, insulin-sensitive adipocytes to store excess energy [28]. Perhaps, also through this mechanism, the body can be protected from the cardiometabolically adverse deposition of fat in tissues and organs regulating glucose and lipid metabolism (liver, muscle, and pancreas) and cardiovascular function (heart and kidney) [29].

Finally, marked sex differences exist in the quantities of VF and SF (Fig. 9.3), as well as in their cellular properties. Not surprisingly then, sex differences also exist in the mechanisms of obesity-related hypertension. In this chapter, we will review some of these sex differences and their possible underlying pathways.

SEX DIFFERENCES IN QUANTITY AND DISTRIBUTION OF VISCERAL AND SUBCUTANEOUS FAT

SF and VF are two main components of total body fat. SF, which holds about 90% of total body fat, is defined as the layer of adipose tissue between the skin and muscles;

Nutrition in the Prevention and Treatment of Abdominal Obesity
http://dx.doi.org/10.1016/B978-0-12-407869-7.00009-X

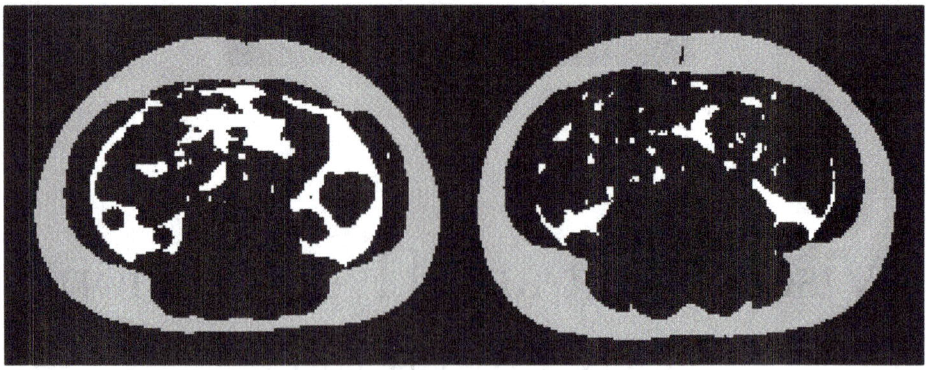

FIGURE 9.1 Interindividual differences in the quantities of visceral fat and subcutaneous fat and in their proportions. Cross-sectional magnetic resonance images of abdomen at the level of the umbilicus in two individuals are shown. Visceral fat is indicated in white and subcutaneous fat is denoted in gray.

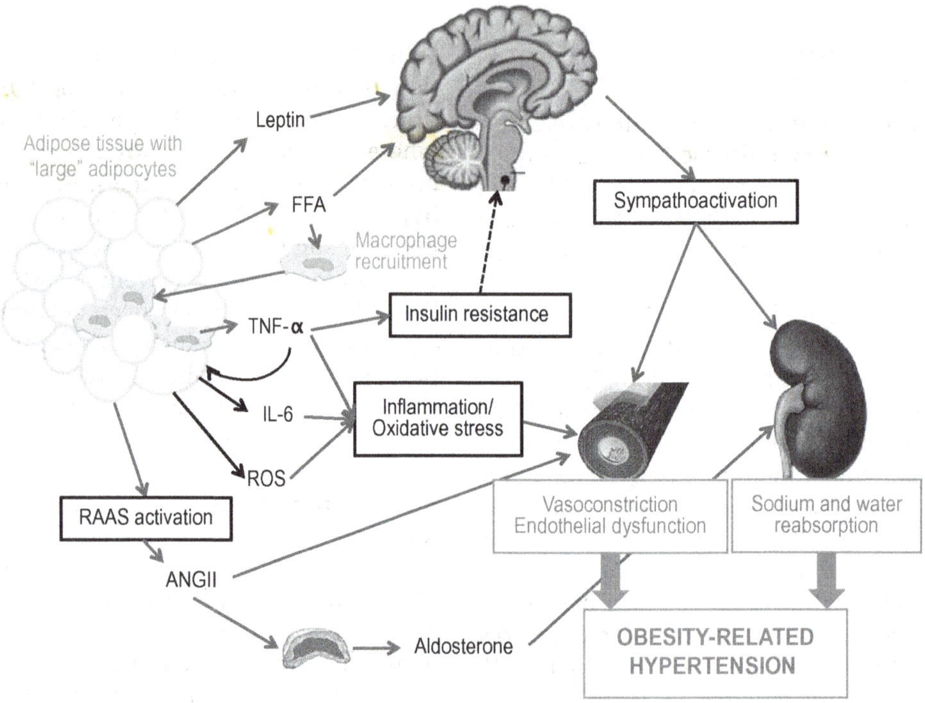

FIGURE 9.2 Simplified scheme of "mechanistic" pathways leading from increased adiposity to elevated blood pressure. ANGII, angiotensin II; FFA, free fatty acids; IL-6, interleukin-6; RAAS, renin-angiotensin-aldosterone system; ROS, reactive oxygen species; TNF-α, tumor necrosis factor (see color plate at the back of the book).

VF, which holds the remaining 10% of total body fat, is broadly defined as adipose tissue lying within the innermost parts of the abdominal cavity and not contained within other abdominal organs or muscles.

Females compared with males have more total body fat [30]. This difference becomes marked during adolescence [31,32] when, on average, fat represents 25% (≈15 kg) of body weight in females but only 15% (≈10 kg) of body weight in males [26]. Most of this extra fat in females is deposited subcutaneously, as females (vs. males) have a substantially higher quantity of SF and a similar or lower quantity of VF [12,26,33–36]. When measured at the level of the umbilicus in 12- to 18-year-old adolescents, for example, females (vs. males) had about 40% more of SF and 10% less of VF [26]. These differences constitute the commonly quoted sexual dimorphism in body-fat distribution—the relative quantity of VF to SF is greater in males than females [12,24,37,38]. Further, there is a sexual dimorphism within SF itself, as most SF is deposited in the gluteofemoral region in females but is deposited in the abdominal region in males. With age, adiposity increases in both males and

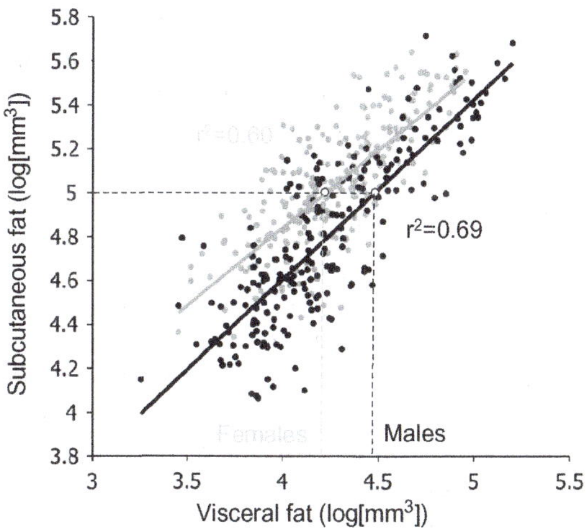

FIGURE 9.3 Sex differences in the relationship between visceral fat and subcutaneous fat. Males are shown in black and females are shown in gray. The graph indicates that, for any given quantity of subcutaneous fat, males tend to have more visceral fat compared with females. Source: reference [135] with permission.

females but, starting in middle age, these increases tend to be greater for VF than SF in both sexes [39]. Consequently, sex differences in body-fat distribution become gradually less pronounced with age [40].

Sex differences in body-fat distribution are determined, to a large degree, by sex hormones. Thus, female-to-male transsexuals treated with the male sex hormone, testosterone, show increases in VF and a disappearance of SF (mainly in the gluteofemoral region), whereas male-to-female transsexuals treated with the female sex hormone, estrogen, demonstrate the opposite pattern [41–43]. These principal effects of sex hormones on body fat distribution may, however, become attenuated with increasing adiposity. In men, excess body fat can produce estrogens through the action of aromatase, an enzyme that converts testosterone to estradiol and is present at higher concentrations in SF than in VF [44]. Consequently, in obese men, excessive SF has been associated with higher serum levels of estrogens [45,46]. In females, on the other hand, excess body-fat can augment the ovarian production of androgens, including testosterone. This is thought to occur through obesity-induced insulin resistance and hyperinsulinemia because insulin has been shown to act as a cogonadotropin with luteinizing hormone and to stimulate ovarian androgen production [47,48]. This pathway may contribute to the development of the polycystic ovary syndrome (PCOS), which is characterized not only by the presence of hyperinsulinemia and hyperandrogenism but also by the enhanced accumulation of VF [49]. In women with PCOS, treatments that reduce hyperinsulinemia (e.g. weight loss and insulin-sensitizing drugs) decrease androgen levels and change body-fat distribution toward less VF [49].

SEX DIFFERENCES IN CELLULARITY AND SECRETORY PROFILES OF VISCERAL AND SUBCUTANEOUS FAT

The human body stores excess energy in the form of lipids (triacylglycerols), which accumulate mostly in adipocytes. This process of energy-to-lipid storage occurs through *adipocyte proliferation*—when the lipids are stored in newly created adipocytes—or *adipocyte differentiation*—when the lipids are stored in preexisting adipocytes. Mature adipocytes develop from precursor cells, i.e. preadipocytes, which reside in the stromal vascular fraction of adipose tissue [50]. Under excess-energy conditions, these cells can *proliferate* and/or *differentiate*. During the latter process, they become larger (up to 10-times) and rounder; their capacity for lipid storage increases and their cytoplasm initially fills with multiple small lipid droplets that ultimately fuse into a single, large lipid droplet that fills almost the entire cell [51]. Alongside these changes, adipocytes increase their production of molecular signals that promote the adverse cardiometabolic consequences of obesity (e.g. FFAs and adipocytokines; Fig. 9.2). This relationship between size and adverse secretory profile means that adipose tissue consisting of *large adipocytes* is cardiometabolically more adverse than the same mass of adipose tissue consisting of *small adipocytes* [18,52].

The potential of adipose tissue to increase the number and/or size of adipocytes during weight gain varies by anatomical location. In most studies, however, this parameter has only been compared between various SF depots (e.g. abdominal vs. gluteofemoral) and not between SF and VF depots; this is most likely due to the fact that SF is relatively easy to access (through a simple needle biopsy) whereas VF is not (accessible only through surgery under general anesthesia). Thus, one such recent study has shown that overfeeding normal-weight adults for 8 weeks enlarged both abdominal SF and gluteofemoral SF, but the enlargement of the abdominal SF was predominantly mediated by adipocyte hypertrophy, whereas the enlargement of the gluteofemoral SF was chiefly through adipocyte proliferation (an estimated 2.6 billion new adipocytes) [53].

The number and size of adipocytes differ between males and females, and the degree of these sex differences varies by anatomical location. Consistent with the overall greater body adiposity of females compared with males, females have a higher number of adipocytes, with this difference being most pronounced in gluteofemoral SF and least pronounced in VF [54]. Regarding the size of adipocytes, gluteofemoral subcutaneous adipocytes are larger in females than males, abdominal subcutaneous adipocytes are of similar sizes in the two sexes, and visceral adipocytes are smaller in females than in males [55]. During weight gain, the expansion of adipose tissues tends to be associated with an increase in adipocyte number in females and an enlargement in adipocyte size in males; this sex difference is again most pronounced in gluteofemoral SF and least pronounced in VF [53,56]. Overall, these regional sex differences in the number and size of adipocytes may in part determine sex differences in the risk of obesity-induced cardiometabolic diseases because the gluteofemoral adipose tissue in women may simply provide a safe lipid reservoir for excess energy [57].

SEX DIFFERENCES IN OBESITY-INDUCED HYPERTENSION

In this section, we will first describe the epidemiology and pathophysiology of obesity-induced hypertension and then explain what is known about the sex differences in these two areas.

Epidemiology

Obesity-induced hypertension is a major public health problem. Hypertension is a leading cause of death, stroke, cardiovascular disease, and renal disease [1–4]. The prevalence of hypertension is on the rise worldwide [1], including in Canada [5]. In Ontario, Canada, for example, the prevalence of hypertension rose almost two-fold between 1995 and 2005, affecting 50% of over 50-year-old and close to 10% of 20–49-year-old individuals in 2005 [5]. Much of this rise has been attributed to the growing prevalence of obesity. Obesity has become highly prevalent in most industrialized countries, spanning all age groups, including adolescents. In Canada and the USA, for example, around 60% of adults and 30% of adolescents are currently overweight or obese [8,58–60]. Over the last 30 years, the proportion of obese adolescents has tripled in both Canada [60] and the USA [61]. These trends are highly alarming because obesity enhances risk for many common disorders, including hypertension [1,2]. The prevalence of hypertension increases with the severity of overweight or obesity: 23% of normal weight individuals and more than 35% and 50% of overweight and obese individuals, respectively, are hypertensive [8].

Pathophysiology

Several mechanisms have been implicated in linking excess body fat to blood pressure (BP) elevation. Most of these are related to molecular signals, such as various lipids and adipocytokines, that are produced by adipose tissue and that, once released into the circulation, increase BP through their actions on the vessels, brain, and kidneys, leading to vasoconstriction, fluid retention (increased circulating volume), endothelial dysfunction (impaired vasodilation), and vascular remodeling (increased vessel stiffness) [18,62,63]. These effects are mediated by (1) *enhanced sympathetic outflow from the central nervous system (CNS)*; (2) *activation of the renin-angiotensin-aldosterone system*; and (3) *induction of low-grade inflammation and oxidative stress* (Fig. 9.2).

Obesity-Induced Sympathoactivation

Obesity-induced sympathoactivation (i.e. *enhanced sympathetic outflow from the* CNS) is considered to be a key mechanism of obesity-induced hypertension. Sympathoactivation may increase BP through the augmentation of vascular tone (vasoconstriction) and stimulation of renal sodium and water reabsorption (fluid retention) [62–64]. Obese (vs. lean) individuals demonstrate higher sympathetic activity [65], and a combined α- and β-sympathetic blockade decreases BP more effectively in obese vs. lean individuals [66]. Moreover, obese individuals who are hypertensive show a higher sympathetic activity than obese individuals who are not [67].

Adipose tissue-released molecular signals that can increase sympathetic activity include, for example, FFAs. FFAs are released from adipocytes through lipolysis of stored triacylglycerols during fasting conditions. In human studies, fasting plasma FFAs are elevated in obesity and predict hypertension [68]. FFA plasma levels in obese hypertensive individuals are approximately double those in lean normotensive individuals [69] and correlate directly with BP [69]. Moreover, acute administration of fatty acids (either free or bound in triacylglycerols) into the circulation increases not only BP but also sympathetic activity [70–74]. Although it is not known exactly how circulating FFAs stimulate sympathetic activity, some evidence suggests that they may do so via the vagal afferents from the vasculature to the brain or via direct FFA detection in the hypothalamus (FFAs can easily cross the blood-brain barrier) [75].

Visceral Fat Plays a Unique Role in Obesity-Induced Hypertension

Population-based studies measuring VF and SF directly with magnetic resonance imaging or computed tomography have shown that VF but not SF is associated with hypertension (and BP) above and beyond routine clinical measures of obesity, i.e. BMI and waist circumference (WC) [12,76]. This may be related to the differences between VF and SF in anatomical location (i.e., relative position to the liver), cellularity, and secretory profile.

Visceral Fat but not Subcutaneous Fat is Associated with Sympathoactivation

Human studies show that the quantity of VF but not that of SF correlates with sympathetic activity [77,78]. Certain biological properties of VF may promote sympathoactivation in obesity and these may be related to a greater flux of lipids from VF than from other fat depots. Thus, VF compared with SF exhibits greater lipid turnover. Under postprandial conditions (after a high-fat test meal), VF shows a higher fat uptake compared with SF and, under fasting conditions, visceral adipocytes are more lipolytically active compared with subcutaneous adipocytes: they are more sensitive to sympathetic lipolytic effects (they show higher sensitivity and expression of β3-adrenoreceptors) and are more resistant to insulin antilipolytic effects [reviewed in 79]. As a result of these metabolic differences, VF can contribute relatively more to elevated plasma lipids in obesity than SF can. It has been estimated that, under overnight fasting conditions, only 6–17% of systemic FFAs come from the visceral area in lean normoinsulinemic individuals, whereas the figure is >40% in obese hyperinsulinemic individuals [79]. Moreover, VF drains directly into the portal circulation and the liver, where excess FFAs from enlarged VF in obesity can contribute to the enhanced de novo synthesis of triacylglycerols, which are released into the circulation bound to very-low-density lipoproteins [79].

Specific Plasma Lipid Species May Link Visceral Obesity to Sympathoactivation and Blood Pressure Elevation

Obesity and obesity-induced hypertension are associated with increased plasma FFAs and triacylglycerols [68,69] and, as indicated above, acute systemic administration of FFAs and triacylglycerols have been shown to increase sympathetic activity and BP in animals and humans [70–74]. However, the novel application of mass spectrometry profiling to the identification of lipid species at the molecular level (i.e., *lipidomics*) is beginning to show that the lipid perturbations in obesity and related cardiometabolic abnormalities may be more complex: rather than involving whole groups of lipids (i.e., FFAs and triacylglycerols), they may be restricted to specific pathogenic molecular species and additional, previously unsuspected, classes of lipids, namely phospholipids and their metabolites. For example, it has been shown that plasma triacylglycerols are a heterogeneous moiety, consisting of subfractions with distinct functionalities [80,81], and that triacylglycerols containing saturated and monounsaturated fatty acids are positively correlated with insulin resistance, whereas triacylglycerols containing the essential linoleic acid are negatively correlated with insulin resistance [80]. Consistent with these data, a higher proportion of saturated fatty acids in plasma has been prospectively and positively associated with an increased risk of cardiovascular disease [82] and type 2 diabetes mellitus [83]. With respect to additional novel classes of lipids, it has been shown that obesity is associated with increases in lysophosphatidylcholine (LPC) species, found mainly in proinflammatory and proatherogenic conditions [84]. LPC species are immediate precursors and metabolites of phospholipids, which are components of cellular membranes and plasma lipoproteins [chylomicrons and both high-density lipoprotein (HDL) and low-density lipoprotein (LDL)]. It has also been demonstrated that hypertension is associated with lower plasma concentrations of "good" antiatherogenic alkylacylphosphorylcholines (i.e., alkylacylphosphorylethanolamines) and ether-linked glycerophosphocholines) [85].

Visceral Fat and Subcutaneous Fat May Make Different Contributions to Plasma Lipid Profiles

It has been reported that BMI, total body fat, and SF inversely correlate with specific phospholipids, while VF does not; VF, on the other hand, correlates positively with medium-chain sphingomyelin (SM) species, and this relationship is not seen with any other fat depot [84]. Perhaps related to the VF-SM specific relationship, it has also been demonstrated that VF compared with SF contains more ceramides [86], which are not only the most basic SM species but also bioactive products of SM species, generated through their metabolism by sphingomyelinases. In fact, both long-chain glycerophospholipid (GP) and SM species may impact cardiometabolic health through either direct effects or the effects of their catabolic products (i.e. lyso-GP or ceramide second messengers and FFAs). Arachidonic acid, for example, is further metabolized to prostaglandins and eicosanoids that modulate activity of sympathetic neurons in vitro [87]. VF may also contribute to an abnormal lipid profile through the release of specific lipid metabolism-related enzymes. Visceral adipocytes secrete markedly high levels of secretory type II phospholipase A_2 ($sPLA_2$-II) [88], which may enhance the production of FFAs in the circulation through phospholipase remodeling (hydrolysis) of GPs contained in HDLs and LDLs. $sPLA_2$ displays a high affinity for ether-linked 1-*O*-alkyl-phosphorylcholines [89,90]. As such, it augments the metabolism of ether-linked glycerophosphocholines contained in HDL and LDL particles, and can (1) decrease the circulating levels of these antiatherogenic ether-linked GPs and (2) increase the circulating levels of FFAs and atherogenic phospholipid second messengers (i.e. lysophospholipids and alkyl-lysophospholipids). Notably, the latter changes have recently been linked to hypertension [85] and obesity [84], as described above.

Obesity-Induced Activation of the Renin-Angiotensin-Aldosterone System

Obesity-induced activation of the renin-angiotensin-aldosterone system (RAAS) is an additional potential mechanism of obesity-induced BP elevation. The RAAS is a key system for BP regulation and its components [such as angiotensinogen (AGT)] are produced in adipose tissue (in addition to their primary production sites: liver, lung, and kidneys) [91]. Adipose tissue RAAS production may also contribute to higher circulating levels of RAAS components seen in obese vs. lean individuals and may thus contribute to elevating BP in obesity [91]. Consistent with this possibility, targeted AGT overexpression in adipocytes increased circulating AGT levels and BP in both wild-type and AGT knockout mice [92], whereas targeted AGT deficiency in adipocytes prevented obesity-induced elevations in plasma angiotensin II (the primary BP-elevating component of the RAAS) and BP [93]. RAAS activation in obesity may also contribute to obesity-induced sympathoactivation, insulin resistance, and oxidative stress [94]. Most of these deleterious actions of the RAAS appear to be mediated via activation of the type-1 angiotensin II receptor (AT1R) and increased production of aldosterone [reviewed in 95]. Some components of the adipose tissue RAAS, namely AGT and AT1R are expressed at higher levels in VF than SF in humans [96].

Obesity-Induced Low-Grade Inflammation and Oxidative Stress

Obesity-induced low-grade inflammation and oxidative stress are additional potential mechanisms for obesity-induced BP elevation. Thus, in obese individuals, adipose tissue becomes infiltrated with immune cells (macrophages), and the degree of this infiltration increases with whole-body adiposity [97]. FFA released from adipocytes may promote this process. FFA overflow from enlarged adipocytes enhances adipose tissue recruitment of macrophages and stimulates their production of tumor necrosis factor (TNF-α); this, in turn, stimulates neighboring adipocytes to secrete other inflammatory cytokines, such as inteleukin-1 (IL-1) and IL-6 [97], some of which are then released into the systemic circulation and stimulate the liver production of C-reactive protein (CRP) [98], an established marker of systemic inflammation and atherosclerosis. Circulating levels of CRP are higher in both obesity and hypertension [99–101], but their causal relationship to BP elevation is controversial [102] and the role of obesity (and body-fat distribution) in this relationship has not been sufficiently studied.

Proinflammatory changes in adipose tissue may increase BP indirectly through the production of reactive oxygen species (ROS) and subsequent systemic *oxidative stress*. Oxidative stress, defined as a redox state in which prooxidant capacity overwhelms antioxidant capacity, may augment BP through the modulation of endothelial function and vascular remodeling [103]. In humans and animal models of obesity, the degree of adiposity closely correlates with markers of systemic oxidative stress [104]. In animal models of obesity, ROS production is increased in adipose tissue but not in the liver, skeletal muscle, or aorta [104]. In addition, ROS production from 3T3-L1 adipocytes increases in parallel with adipocyte size [104]. Besides adipocytes, adipose tissue macrophages may contribute to local ROS production [reviewed in 105]. Human obesity is associated with endothelial dysfunction [106–108], which in turn is associated with hypertension [109–111]; the latter relationship, however, may not be causal [112]. Similar to CRP, the role of obesity (and body-fat distribution) in the relationship endothelial dysfunction-hypertension of endothelial dysfunction to hypertension has not been sufficiently studied.

Further, proinflammatory changes in adipose tissue enhance the adipocyte production of *leptin* [113], which (based on animal studies) may also stimulate sympathetic activity and elevate BP via its action in the hypothalamus [114–117]. Leptin is an adipocytokine produced mainly by adipocytes (in proportion to body adiposity) [118]. Obese individuals exhibit high circulating levels of leptin, but they are leptin resistant. This leptin resistance may be selective, with only the metabolic effects of leptin on appetite and energy expenditure being diminished and the sympathomimetic effects of leptin on vasculature and kidneys (and hence BP) being preserved [116]. Consistent with this possibility, circulating leptin levels have been associated with hypertension and elevated BP [119,120] and, as expected [118], these associations become diminished when adjusted for a measure of total body adiposity [119–121]. In rats, systemic administration of leptin activates the sympathetic nervous system and increases BP [114,117], further supporting a possible role for leptin in BP elevation.

Finally, some adipose tissue-produced cytokines, such as TNF-α [122], contribute to the development of systemic *insulin resistance* and compensatory hyperinsulinemia [123]—two conditions that are almost invariably present in obese individuals with hypertension [124]. However, studies demonstrating that chronic infusion of insulin increases BP in rats [125], but not in dogs [126] and humans [127], make the primary role of hyperinsulinemia in elevating BP controversial.

In obesity, VF and SF may contribute differently to obesity-associated low-grade inflammation and oxidative stress. VF exhibits a higher degree of macrophage infiltration compared with SF [19]. Consistent with this observation, population-based studies show that only VF (and not SF) remains positively associated with circulating markers of low-grade inflammation (such as CRP and IL-6) above and beyond their associations with BMI and WC [128]. They also show that VF but not SF remains associated with endothelial dysfunction (which is promoted by low-grade inflammation and excess ROS) above and beyond its association with BMI and WC [108]. In contrast, obesity-induced hyperleptinemia is linked more closely with SF than with VF, as leptin production is higher in SF than VF adipocytes [129].

Sex Differences

The prevalence of both hypertension and BP are higher in males than females from adolescence until middle age, when they become first similar and then higher in females than in males [130–132]. In contrast, both the prevalence obesity and adiposity are higher in females than males [133]: females have higher quantities of SF (which forms the majority body fat) and lower (or similar) quantities of VF (which forms the minority of body fat) [12,26,33–36]. The greater degree of adiposity in females than males holds throughout life, but the sex differences in body-fat distribution, similarly to the sex difference in BP, become less pronounced beginning in middle age [40].

Sex differences in obesity-induced hypertension are still not fully understood. Obesity is a risk factor for hypertension in both males and females [134], but the relationships of individual fat depots with BP differ between the two sexes, with the degree of these sex differences varying by developmental stage. In adolescence, VF (adjusted for SF) is associated with higher BP in males but not in females (Fig. 9.4) [26,37]. During middle and old age, this association is present in both sexes but is stronger in males than females [12]. On the other hand, SF (adjusted for VF) is associated with higher BP in females but not males [24,26]. During adolescence, this relationship in females is only apparent during and immediately after mental stress (Fig. 9.4) [26], but during middle age it is also present at rest [24]. In males, SF may

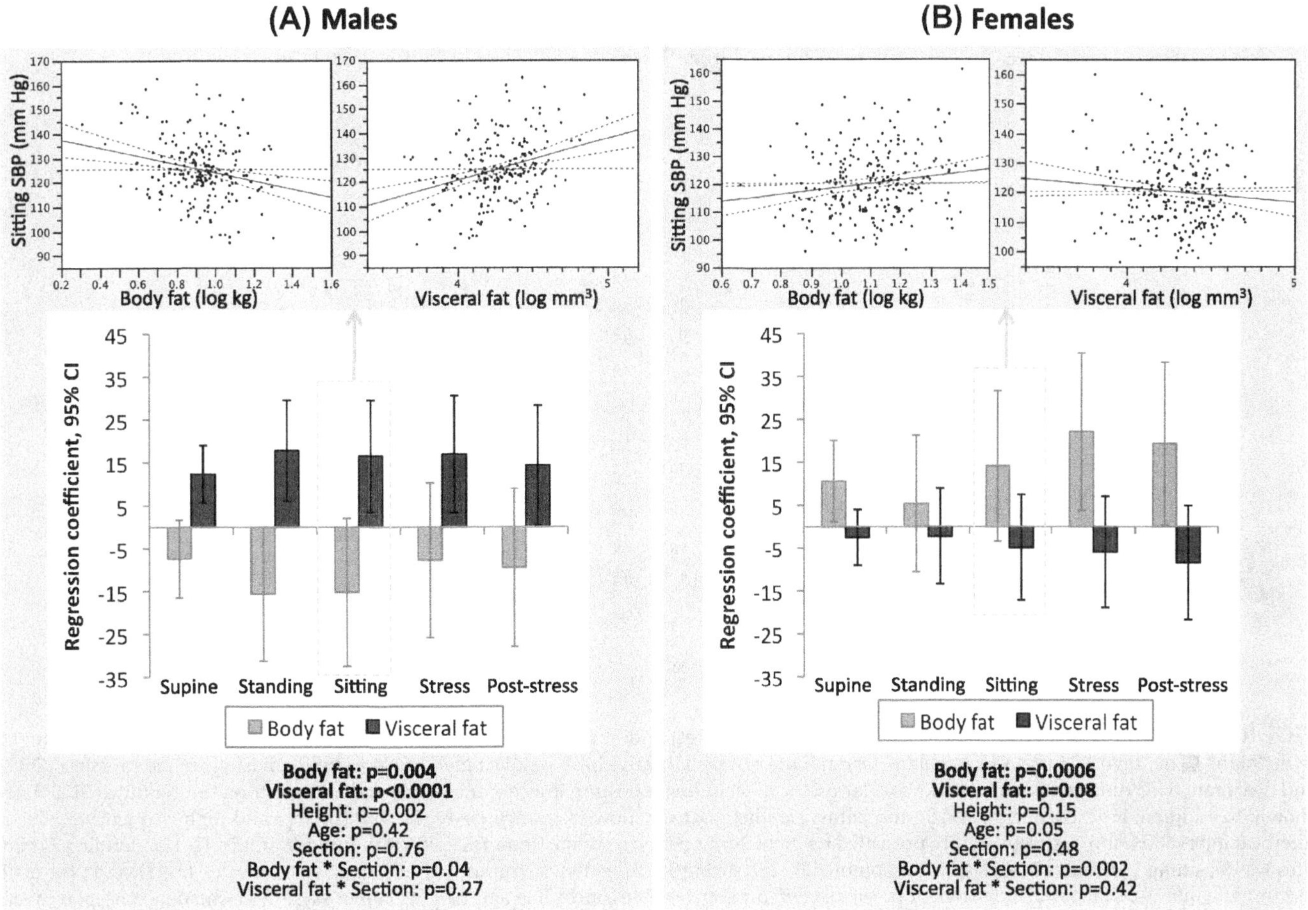

FIGURE 9.4 Multivariable relationships of systolic blood pressure with total body fat and visceral fat in males and females. A multivariable mixed linear model was used to estimate the relative contribution (model coefficient with 95% confidence interval) of each total body fat and visceral fat to systolic blood pressure (SBP) in males (*A*) and females (*B*), while adjusting for interindividual differences in height. SBP means of five consecutive sections of a 52-min cardiovascular protocol (i.e. supine, standing, sitting, stress, and poststress) were included in these analyses as repeated measures. Representative scatter plots of the multivariate associations of SBP with visceral fat and total body fat are also shown; for this purpose, the sitting section of the protocol was chosen (see color plate at the back of the book). Source: reference [26] with permission.

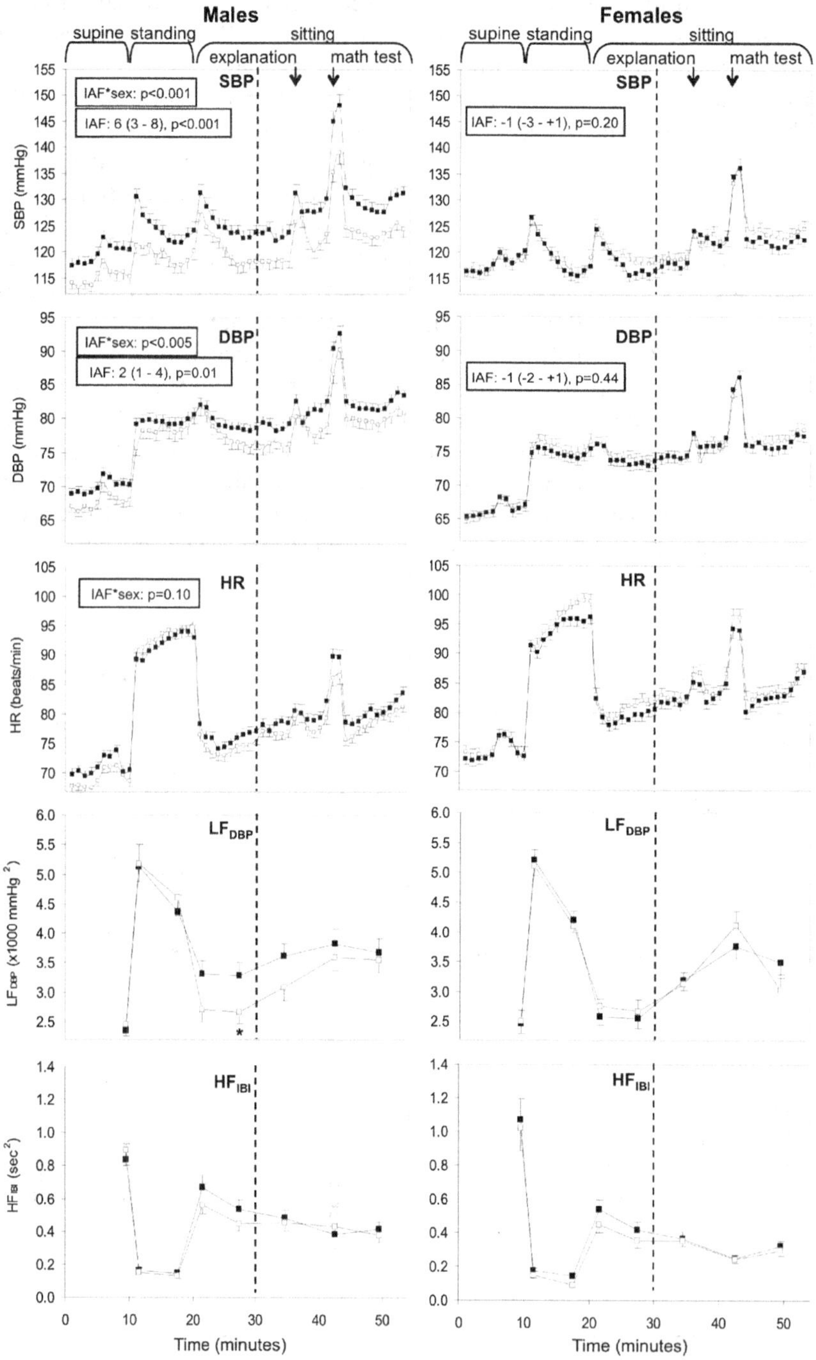

FIGURE 9.5 Cardiovascular and autonomic nervous system at rest and in response to postural and mental challenges in males and females with "high" ■ or "low" □ intra-abdominal fat. One-minute means of beat-to-beat systolic blood pressure (SBP), diastolic blood pressure (DBP), and heart rate (HR) during a 53-min cardiovascular protocol, including a posture test (minutes 1–30) and a math stress test (minutes 31–53), are shown. In addition, indexes of sympathetic and parasympathetic activity [low-frequency power of DBP (LFdbp) and high-frequency power of interbeat interval (HFibi), respectively] are presented for eight 2-min periods: supine (minutes 9–10), standing 1 (minutes 11–12), standing 2 (minutes 17–18), sitting 1 (minutes 21–22), sitting 2 (minutes 27–28), sitting 3 (pre-math test, minutes 34–35), math test (minutes 42–43), and post-math test (minutes 49–50). Data are all adjusted for potential confounding variables, including age, height, Tanner stage, household income, and prenatal exposure to maternal cigarette smoking. They are presented as the means (SEM); solid squares indicate the mean for individuals with high intra-abdominal fat (IAF; =visceral fat) and open squares show the mean for individuals with low IAF. The dashed vertical line indicates the end of the posture test. The 53 1-min means of SBP, DBP, and HR were analyzed with mixed-model regression analyses. Statistics show the *P* value of the IAF-sex interaction and the estimated difference (95% confidence interval) and *P* value for high vs. low IAF in males and females. The eight estimates of sympathetic (LFdbp) and parasympathetic (HFibi) nervous system functions, calculated for specific 2-min periods, were analyzed using multiple linear regression analysis. *, statistical significance for a difference between males with high and low IAF ($P=0.04$). Source: reprinted from reference [37] with permission.

even have BP-lowering effects: in adolescent males, SF (adjusted for VF) is associated with lower BP (particularly during standing; Fig. 9.4) [26]. The underlying mechanisms of these sex differences in fat depot-specific relationships with BP are not very clear. They may be related to sex differences in obesity-induced (1) sympathoactivation associated with VF (and VF-released lipids) and with SF (and SF-released leptin); (2) induction of low-grade inflammation; and (3) conversion of testosterone to estradiol by excessive SF.

Obesity-Induced Sympathoactivation Associated with Visceral Fat

Obesity-induced sympathoactivation associated with VF (and released lipids) may be greater in males than in females (at least during adolescence; Fig. 9.5) [37,77,78] and, as such, it may contribute to the positive association between VF and BP seen in males only during adolescence [26,37] and being stronger in males (vs. females) during adulthood [12]. This sex difference may in part be the result of testosterone effects—a functional variant in the androgen receptor gene, which mediates the androgenic effects of testosterone, is associated with higher VF, sympathetic vasomotor tone, and BP in adolescent males but not in females (Fig. 9.6) [135]. On the other hand, *obesity-induced sympathoactivation associated with SF* (and released leptin) may be greater in females than males. Leptin, which may elevate BP via its action on sympathetic outflow from the hypothalamus to the kidneys [115,116], is secreted by adipocytes, with its production being higher in SF than in VF [129] and its circulating

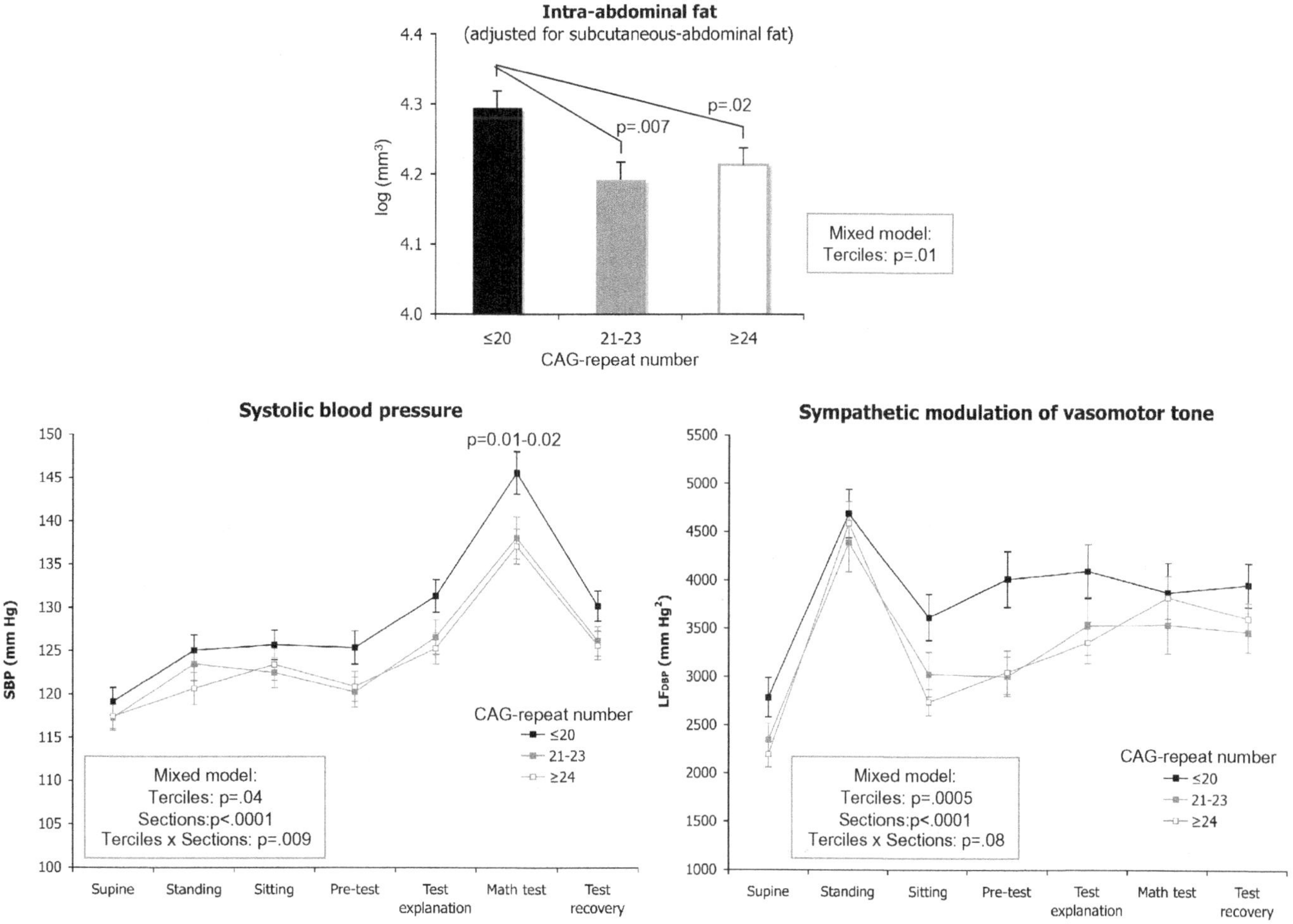

FIGURE 9.6 CAG-repeat tertiles in the androgen receptor gene and intra-abdominal fat, blood pressure, and an index of sympathetic modulation of vasomotor tone. Mean ± SE of (top) intra-abdominal fat (IAF), (lower left) systolic blood pressure (SBP), and (lower right) an index of sympathetic modulation of vasomotor tone (LFdbp) are presented for groups of males with low, intermediate, and high CAG-repeat number. SBP and LFdbp are shown for seven periods of an hour-long protocol, defined by various experimental conditions (i.e. supine, standing, sitting, pre-test, test explanation, math test, and test recovery). All of the variables shown were adjusted for five potential confounders (age, height, puberty stage, family income, and prenatal exposure to maternal cigarette smoking). IAF was additionally adjusted for subcutaneous abdominal fat. Male-specific tertile differences in IAF, SBP, and LFdbp were assessed with a mixed-model analysis, adjusting for the specified potential confounders. Source: reprinted from reference [135] with permission.

levels being higher in females than in males [136]. As such, this relationship may contribute to the positive association between SF and BP seen in females but not in males (Fig. 9.4) [26]. Of note, sympathetic nerve activity (assessed as muscle sympathetic nerve activity) shows a similar developmental trend as BP: it is higher in males than in females from adolescence until middle age, when it first becomes similar and then becomes higher in females than in males [130,137]. It is unclear whether these changes are related, at least in part, to the changes in body-fat distribution that occur with age in females (i.e. the central redistribution of body fat).

Obesity-Induced Low-Grade Inflammation

Obesity-induced low-grade inflammation may also contribute to the positive association between SF and BP seen in females (Fig. 9.4). Females (vs. males) demonstrate a stronger relationship between adiposity and low-grade inflammation [30]. Although both SF and VF are positively associated with circulating markers of low-grade inflammation, the latter relationships are generally stronger in females than in males [128].

Adipose Tissue Conversion of Testosterone to Estradiol

The adipose tissue conversion of testosterone to estradiol seen in obese males may contribute to the inverse relationship between SF and BP in adolescent males (Fig. 9.4) [26]. This observation is consistent with a previous study demonstrating that elevated SF reduces risk for the metabolic syndrome, which includes hypertension, in adult men with high VF [36]. Excess SF has been associated with higher serum estrogens in obese adult men [45,46], and estrogens have BP-lowering effects [138]. In men, adipose tissue can produce estrogens by the conversion of testosterone to estradiol by aromatase, an enzyme found at higher concentrations in SF than in VF [44].

CONCLUSION

Obesity is a major risk factor for hypertension, and VF appears to be more dangerous than SF in this respect, particularly in males. Marked sex differences exist in the quantities of VF and SF, as well as in their cellular properties. Sex differences also exist in the mechanisms of obesity-related hypertension. Our understanding of these mechanisms is critical for appropriate sex-specific prevention and treatment strategies for this disease.

References

[1] Kearney PM, Whelton M, Reynolds K, Muntner P, Whelton PK, He J. Global burden of hypertension: analysis of worldwide data. Lancet 2005;365(9455):217–23.

[2] MacMahon S, Peto R, Cutler J, et al. Blood pressure, stroke, and coronary heart disease. Part 1, Prolonged differences in blood pressure: prospective observational studies corrected for the regression dilution bias. Lancet 1990;335(8692):765–74.

[3] Stamler J, Stamler R, Neaton JD. Blood pressure, systolic and diastolic, and cardiovascular risks. US population data. Arch Intern Med 1993;153(5):598–615.

[4] Tunstall-Pedoe H, Kuulasmaa K, Amouyel P, Arveiler D, Rajakangas AM, Pajak A. Myocardial infarction and coronary deaths in the World Health Organization MONICA Project. Registration procedures, event rates, and case-fatality rates in 38 populations from 21 countries in four continents. Circulation 1994;90(1):583–612.

[5] Tu K, Chen Z, Lipscombe LL. Prevalence and incidence of hypertension from 1995 to 2005: a population-based study. CMAJ 2008;178(11):1429–35.

[6] Whyte HM. Blood pressure and obesity. Circulation 1959;19(4):511–6.

[7] Kannel WB, Brand N, Skinner Jr JJ, Dawber TR, McNamara PM. The relation of adiposity to blood pressure and development of hypertension. The Framingham study. Ann Intern Med 1967;67(1):48–59.

[8] Must A, Spadano J, Coakley EH, Field AE, Colditz G, Dietz WH. The disease burden associated with overweight and obesity. Jama 1999;282(16):1523–9.

[9] Wildman RP, Muntner P, Reynolds K, et al. The obese without cardiometabolic risk factor clustering and the normal weight with cardiometabolic risk factor clustering: prevalence and correlates of 2 phenotypes among the us population (NHANES 1999–2004). Arch Intern Med 2008;168(15):1617–24.

[10] Pou KM, Massaro JM, Hoffmann U, et al. Patterns of abdominal fat distribution: the Framingham Heart Study. Diabetes Care 2009;32(3):481–5.

[11] Muller MJ, Lagerpusch M, Enderle J, Schautz B, Heller M, Bosy-Westphal A. Beyond the body mass index: tracking body composition in the pathogenesis of obesity and the metabolic syndrome. Obes Rev 2012;13(Suppl. 2):6–13.

[12] Fox CS, Massaro JM, Hoffmann U, et al. Abdominal visceral and subcutaneous adipose tissue compartments: association with metabolic risk factors in the Framingham Heart Study. Circulation 2007;116(1):39–48.

[13] Demerath EW, Reed D, Rogers N, et al. Visceral adiposity and its anatomical distribution as predictors of the metabolic syndrome and cardiometabolic risk factor levels. Am J Clin Nutr 2008;88(5):1263–71.

[14] Smith JD, Borel AL, Nazare JA, et al. Visceral adipose tissue indicates the severity of cardiometabolic risk in patients with and without type 2 diabetes: results from the INSPIRE ME IAA study. J Clin Endocrinol Metab 2012;97(5):1517–25.

[15] Gabriely I, Ma XH, Yang XM, et al. Removal of visceral fat prevents insulin resistance and glucose intolerance of aging: an adipokine-mediated process? Diabetes 2002;51(10):2951–8.

[16] Thorne A, Lonnqvist F, Apelman J, Hellers G, Arner P. A pilot study of long-term effects of a novel obesity treatment: omentectomy in connection with adjustable gastric banding. Int J Obes Relat Metab Disord 2002;26(2):193–9.

[17] Klein S, Fontana L, Young VL, et al. Absence of an effect of liposuction on insulin action and risk factors for coronary heart disease. N Engl J Med 2004;350(25):2549–57.

[18] Pausova Z. From big fat cells to high blood pressure: a pathway to obesity-associated hypertension. Curr Opin Nephrol Hypertens 2006;15(2):173–8.

[19] Harman-Boehm I, Bluher M, Redel H, et al. Macrophage infiltration into omental versus subcutaneous fat across different populations: effect of regional adiposity and the comorbidities of obesity. J Clin Endocrinol Metab 2007;92(6):2240–7.

[20] Liu A, McLaughlin T, Liu T, et al. Differential intra-abdominal adipose tissue profiling in obese, insulin-resistant women. Obes Surg 2009;19(11):1564–73.

[21] Bolinder J, Kager L, Ostman J, Arner P. Differences at the receptor and postreceptor levels between human omental and subcutaneous adipose tissue in the action of insulin on lipolysis. Diabetes 1983;32(2):117–23.

[22] Hocking S, Samocha-Bonet D, Milner KL, Greenfield JR, Chisholm DJ. Adiposity and Insulin Resistance in Humans: The Role of the Different Tissue and Cellular Lipid Depots. Endocr Rev 2013;34(4):463–500.

[23] Bjorntorp P. "Portal" adipose tissue as a generator of risk factors for cardiovascular disease and diabetes. Arteriosclerosis 1990;10(4):493–6.

[24] Porter SA, Massaro JM, Hoffmann U, Vasan RS, O'Donnel CJ, Fox CS. Abdominal subcutaneous adipose tissue: a protective fat depot? Diabetes Care 2009;32(6):1068–75.

[25] Tran TT, Yamamoto Y, Gesta S, Kahn CR. Beneficial effects of subcutaneous fat transplantation on metabolism. Cell Metab 2008;7(5):410–20.

[26] Pausova Z, Mahboubi A, Abrahamowicz M, et al. Sex differences in the contributions of visceral and total body fat to blood pressure in adolescence. Hypertension 2012;59(3):572–9.

[27] Alligier M, Gabert L, Meugnier E, et al. Visceral fat accumulation during lipid overfeeding is related to subcutaneous adipose tissue characteristics in healthy men. J Clin Endocrinol Metab 2013;98(2):802–10.

[28] McLaughlin T, Lamendola C, Liu A, Abbasi F. Preferential fat deposition in subcutaneous versus visceral depots is associated with insulin sensitivity. J Clin Endocrinol Metab 2011;96(11):E1756–60.

[29] Virtue S, Vidal-Puig A. Adipose tissue expandability, lipotoxicity and the Metabolic Syndrome—an allostatic perspective. Biochim Biophys Acta 2010;1801(3):338–49.

[30] Khera A, Vega GL, Das SR, et al. Sex differences in the relationship between C-reactive protein and body fat. J Clin Endocrinol Metab 2009;94(9):3251–8.

[31] Veldhuis JD, Roemmich JN, Richmond EJ, et al. Endocrine control of body composition in infancy, childhood, and puberty. Endocr Rev 2005;26(1):114–46.

[32] Blouin K, Boivin A, Tchernof A. Androgens and body fat distribution. J Steroid Biochem Mol Biol 2008;108(3–5):272–80.

[33] Westerbacka J, Corner A, Tiikkainen M, et al. Women and men have similar amounts of liver and intra-abdominal fat, despite more subcutaneous fat in women: implications for sex differences in markers of cardiovascular risk. Diabetologia 2004;47(8):1360–9.

[34] Chung SA, Dorey F, Mittelman S, Gilsanz V. Effect of gender on intra-abdominal fat in teenagers and young adults. Pediatr Radiol 2011;41(4):469–75.

[35] Vega GL, Adams-Huet B, Peshock R, Willett D, Shah B, Grundy SM. Influence of body fat content and distribution on variation in metabolic risk. J Clin Endocrinol Metab 2006;91(11):4459–66.

[36] Demerath EW, Reed D, Rogers N, et al. Visceral adiposity and its anatomical distribution as predictors of the metabolic syndrome and cardiometabolic risk factor levels. Am J Clin Nutr 2008;88(5):1263–71.

[37] Syme C, Abrahamowicz M, Leonard GT, et al. Intra-abdominal adiposity and individual components of the metabolic syndrome in adolescence: sex differences and underlying mechanisms. Arch Pediatr Adolesc Med 2008;162(5):453–61.

[38] Gutin B, Johnson MH, Humphries MC, et al. Relationship of visceral adiposity to cardiovascular disease risk factors in black and white teens. Obesity (Silver Spring) 2007;15(4):1029–35.

[39] Toth MJ, Tchernof A, Sites CK, Poehlman ET. Menopause-related changes in body fat distribution. Ann N Y Acad Sci 2000;904:502–6.

[40] Tchernof A, Despres JP. Sex steroid hormones, sex hormone-binding globulin, and obesity in men and women. Horm Metab Res 2000;32(11–12):526–36.

[41] Elbers JM, Asscheman H, Seidell JC, Gooren LJ. Effects of sex steroid hormones on regional fat depots as assessed by magnetic resonance imaging in transsexuals. Am J Physiol 1999;276(2 Pt 1):E317–325.

[42] Elbers JM, Asscheman H, Seidell JC, Megens JA, Gooren LJ. Long-term testosterone administration increases visceral fat in female to male transsexuals. J Clin Endocrinol Metab 1997;82(7):2044–7.

[43] Elbers JM, Giltay EJ, Teerlink T, et al. Effects of sex steroids on components of the insulin resistance syndrome in transsexual subjects. Clin Endocrinol (Oxf) 2003;58(5):562–71.

[44] Wajchenberg BL. Subcutaneous and visceral adipose tissue: their relation to the metabolic syndrome. Endocr Rev 2000;21(6):697–738.

[45] Schneider G, Kirschner MA, Berkowitz R, Ertel NH. Increased estrogen production in obese men. J Clin Endocrinol Metab 1979;48(4):633–8.

[46] Tajar A, Forti G, O'Neill TW, et al. Characteristics of secondary, primary, and compensated hypogonadism in aging men: evidence from the European Male Ageing Study. J Clin Endocrinol Metab 2010;95(4):1810–8.

[47] Dunaif A. Insulin resistance and the polycystic ovary syndrome: mechanism and implications for pathogenesis. Endocr Rev 1997;18(6):774–800.

[48] Poretsky L, Cataldo NA, Rosenwaks Z, Giudice LC. The insulin-related ovarian regulatory system in health and disease. Endocr Rev 1999;20(4):535–82.

[49] Burt Solorzano CM, Beller JP, Abshire MY, Collins JS, McCartney CR, Marshall JC. Neuroendocrine dysfunction in polycystic ovary syndrome. Steroids 2012;77(4):332–7.

[50] Spalding KL, Arner E, Westermark PO, et al. Dynamics of fat cell turnover in humans. Nature 2008;453(7196):783–7.

[51] Liu J, DeYoung SM, Zhang M, Zhang M, Cheng A, Saltiel AR. Changes in integrin expression during adipocyte differentiation. Cell Metab 2005;2(3):165–77.

[52] Arner E, Westermark PO, Spalding KL, et al. Adipocyte turnover: relevance to human adipose tissue morphology. Diabetes 2010;59(1):105–9.

[53] Tchoukalova YD, Votruba SB, Tchkonia T, Giorgadze N, Kirkland JL, Jensen MD. Regional differences in cellular mechanisms of adipose tissue gain with overfeeding. Proc Natl Acad Sci USA 2010;107(42):18226–31.

[54] Krotkiewski M, Bjorntorp P, Sjostrom L, Smith U. Impact of obesity on metabolism in men and women. Importance of regional adipose tissue distribution. J Clin Invest 1983;72(3):1150–62.

[55] Fried SK, Kral JG. Sex differences in regional distribution of fat cell size and lipoprotein lipase activity in morbidly obese patients. Int J Obes 1987;11(2):129–40.

[56] Tchoukalova YD, Koutsari C, Karpyak MV, Votruba SB, Wendland E, Jensen MD. Subcutaneous adipocyte size and body fat distribution. Am J Clin Nutr 2008;87(1):56–63.

[57] Karastergiou K, Smith SR, Greenberg AS, Fried SK. Sex differences in human adipose tissues—the biology of pear shape. Biol Sex Differ 2012;3(1):13.

[58] Anis AH, Zhang W, Bansback N, Guh DP, Amarsi Z, Birmingham CL. Obesity and overweight in Canada: an updated cost-of-illness study. Obes Rev 2009;1(1):31–40.

[59] Ogden CL, Carroll MD, Flegal KM. High body mass index for age among US children and adolescents, 2003–2006. Jama 2008;299(20):2401–5.
[60] Survey CCH. Prevalence of adolescent overweight and obesity in Canada in 1978/79 and 2004, <www.geog.ubc.ca/courses/geob370/students/class10/ddchan/www/images/docs/Shields.pdf>; 2004 [accessed 25.09.13].
[61] Ogden CL, Flegal KM, Carroll MD, Johnson CL. Prevalence and trends in overweight among US children and adolescents, 1999–2000. Jama 2002;288(14):1728–32.
[62] Esler M, Straznicky N, Eikelis N, Masuo K, Lambert G, Lambert E. Mechanisms of sympathetic activation in obesity-related hypertension. Hypertension 2006;48(5):787–96.
[63] Biaggioni I. Should we target the sympathetic nervous system in the treatment of obesity-associated hypertension? Hypertension 2008;51(2):168–71.
[64] da Silva AA, do Carmo J, Dubinion J, Hall JE. The role of the sympathetic nervous system in obesity-related hypertension. Curr Hypertens Rep 2009;11(3):206–11.
[65] Grassi G, Seravalle G, Cattaneo BM, et al. Sympathetic activation in obese normotensive subjects. Hypertension 1995;25(4 Pt 1):560–3.
[66] Wofford MR, Anderson Jr DC, Brown CA, Jones DW, Miller ME, Hall JE. Antihypertensive effect of alpha- and beta-adrenergic blockade in obese and lean hypertensive subjects. Am J Hypertens 2001;14(7 Pt 1):694–8.
[67] Grassi G, Seravalle G, Dell'Oro R, Turri C, Bolla GB, Mancia G. Adrenergic and reflex abnormalities in obesity-related hypertension. Hypertension 2000;36(4):538–42.
[68] Fagot-Campagna A, Balkau B, Simon D, et al. High free fatty acid concentration: an independent risk factor for hypertension in the Paris Prospective Study. Int J Epidemiol 1998;27(5):808–13.
[69] Egan BM, Hennes MM, Stepniakowski KT, O'Shaughnessy IM, Kissebah AH, Goodfriend TL. Obesity hypertension is related more to insulin's fatty acid than glucose action. Hypertension 1996;27(3 Pt 2):723–8.
[70] Haastrup AT, Stepniakowski KT, Goodfriend TL, Egan BM. Intralipid enhances alpha1-adrenergic receptor mediated pressor sensitivity. Hypertension 1998;32(4):693–8.
[71] Florian JP, Pawelczyk JA. Non-esterified fatty acids increase arterial pressure via central sympathetic activation in humans. Clin Sci (Lond) 2010;118(1):61–9.
[72] Florian JP, Pawelczyk JA. Sympathetic and haemodynamic responses to lipids in healthy human ageing. Exp Physiol 2010;95(4):486–97.
[73] Stojiljkovic MP, Zhang D, Lopes HF, Lee CG, Goodfriend TL, Egan BM. Hemodynamic effects of lipids in humans. Am J Physiol Regul Integr Comp Physiol 2001;280(6):R1674–1679.
[74] Grekin RJ, Vollmer AP, Sider RS. Pressor effects of portal venous oleate infusion. A proposed mechanism for obesity hypertension. Hypertension 1995;26(1):193–8.
[75] Katagiri H, Yamada T, Oka Y. Adiposity and cardiovascular disorders: disturbance of the regulatory system consisting of humoral and neuronal signals. Circ Res 2007;101(1):27–39.
[76] Hayashi T, Boyko EJ, Leonetti DL, et al. Visceral adiposity and the prevalence of hypertension in Japanese Americans. Circulation 2003;108(14):1718–23.
[77] Alvarez GE, Beske SD, Ballard TP, Davy KP. Sympathetic neural activation in visceral obesity. Circulation 2002;106(20):2533–6.
[78] Alvarez GE, Ballard TP, Beske SD, Davy KP. Subcutaneous obesity is not associated with sympathetic neural activation. Am J Physiol Heart Circ Physiol 2004;287(1):H414–418.
[79] Votruba SB, Jensen MD. Regional fat deposition as a factor in FFA metabolism. Annu Rev Nutr 2007;27:149–63.
[80] Kotronen A, Velagapudi VR, Yetukuri L, et al. Serum saturated fatty acids containing triacylglycerols are better markers of insulin resistance than total serum triacylglycerol concentrations. Diabetologia 2009;52(4):684–90.
[81] Kontush A, Chapman MJ. Lipidomics as a tool for the study of lipoprotein metabolism. Curr Atheroscler Rep 2010;12(3):194–201.
[82] Wang L, Folsom AR, Eckfeldt JH. Plasma fatty acid composition and incidence of coronary heart disease in middle aged adults: the Atherosclerosis Risk in Communities (ARIC) Study. Nutr Metab Cardiovasc Dis 2003;13(5):256–66.
[83] Wang L, Folsom AR, Zheng ZJ, Pankow JS, Eckfeldt JH. Plasma fatty acid composition and incidence of diabetes in middle-aged adults: the Atherosclerosis Risk in Communities (ARIC) Study. Am J Clin Nutr 2003;78(1):91–8.
[84] Pietilainen KH, Sysi-Aho M, Rissanen A, et al. Acquired obesity is associated with changes in the serum lipidomic profile independent of genetic effects—a monozygotic twin study. PLoS One 2007;2(2):e218.
[85] Graessler J, Schwudke D, Schwarz PE, Herzog R, Shevchenko A, Bornstein SR. Top-down lipidomics reveals ether lipid deficiency in blood plasma of hypertensive patients. PLoS One 2009;4(7):e6261.
[86] Kotronen A, Seppanen-Laakso T, Westerbacka J, et al. Comparison of lipid and fatty acid composition of the liver, subcutaneous and intra-abdominal adipose tissue, and serum. Obesity (Silver Spring) 2010;18(5):937–44.
[87] Liu L, Rittenhouse AR. Arachidonic acid mediates muscarinic inhibition and enhancement of N-type Ca2+ current in sympathetic neurons. Proc Natl Acad Sci U S A 2003;100(1):295–300.
[88] Dutour A, Achard V, Sell H, et al. Secretory type II phospholipase A2 is produced and secreted by epicardial adipose tissue and overexpressed in patients with coronary artery disease. J Clin Endocrinol Metab 2010;95(2):963–7.
[89] Pruzanski W, Stefanski E, de Beer FC, et al. Lipoproteins are substrates for human secretory group IIA phospholipase A2: preferential hydrolysis of acute phase HDL. J Lipid Res 1998;39(11):2150–60.
[90] Ramadan E, Rosa AO, Chang L, Chen M, Rapoport SI, Basselin M. Extracellular-derived calcium does not initiate in vivo neurotransmission involving docosahexaenoic acid. J Lipid Res 2010;51(8):2334–40.
[91] Engeli S, Negrel R, Sharma AM. Physiology and pathophysiology of the adipose tissue renin-angiotensin system. Hypertension 2000;35(6):1270–7.
[92] Massiera F, Bloch-Faure M, Ceiler D, et al. Adipose angiotensinogen is involved in adipose tissue growth and blood pressure regulation. Faseb J 2001;15(14):2727–9.
[93] Yiannikouris F, Gupte M, Putnam K, et al. Adipocyte deficiency of angiotensinogen prevents obesity-induced hypertension in male mice. Hypertension 2012;60(6):1524–30.
[94] Grassi G, Seravalle G, Dell'Oro R, et al. Comparative effects of candesartan and hydrochlorothiazide on blood pressure, insulin sensitivity, and sympathetic drive in obese hypertensive individuals: results of the CROSS study. J Hypertens 2003;21(9):1761–9.
[95] Lastra-Lastra G, Sowers JR, Restrepo-Erazo K, Manrique-Acevedo C, Lastra-Gonzalez G. Role of aldosterone and angiotensin II in insulin resistance: an update. Clin Endocrinol (Oxf) 2009;71(1):1–6.
[96] Giacchetti G, Faloia E, Mariniello B, et al. Overexpression of the renin-angiotensin system in human visceral adipose tissue in normal and overweight subjects. Am J Hypertens 2002;15(5):381–8.
[97] Weisberg SP, McCann D, Desai M, Rosenbaum M, Leibel RL, Ferrante Jr AW. Obesity is associated with macrophage accumulation in adipose tissue. J Clin Invest 2003;112(12):1796–808.
[98] Zhang S, Liu Q, Wang J, Harnish DC. Suppression of interleukin-6-induced C-reactive protein expression by FXR agonists. Biochem Biophys Res Commun 2009;379(2):476–9.

[99] Sesso HD, Buring JE, Rifai N, Blake GJ, Gaziano JM, Ridker PM. C-reactive protein and the risk of developing hypertension. JAMA 2003;290(22):2945–51.
[100] Lakoski SG, Cushman M, Criqui M, et al. Gender and C-reactive protein: data from the Multiethnic Study of Atherosclerosis (MESA) cohort. Am Heart J 2006;152(3):593–8.
[101] Lakoski SG, Herrington DM, Siscovick DM, Hulley SB. C-reactive protein concentration and incident hypertension in young adults: the CARDIA study. Arch Intern Med 2006;166(3):345–9.
[102] Smith G, Lawlor DA, Harbord R, et al. Association of C-reactive protein with blood pressure and hypertension: life course confounding and mendelian randomization tests of causality. Arterioscler Thromb Vasc Biol 2005;25(5):1051–6.
[103] Touyz RM. Reactive oxygen species, vascular oxidative stress, and redox signaling in hypertension: what is the clinical significance? Hypertension 2004;44(3):248–52.
[104] Furukawa S, Fujita T, Shimabukuro M, et al. Increased oxidative stress in obesity and its impact on metabolic syndrome. J Clin Invest 2004;114(12):1752–61.
[105] Bouloumie A, Curat CA, Sengenes C, Lolmede K, Miranville A, Busse R. Role of macrophage tissue infiltration in metabolic diseases. Curr Opin Clin Nutr Metab Care 2005;8(4):347–54.
[106] Steinberg HO, Chaker H, Leaming R, Johnson A, Brechtel G, Baron AD. Obesity/insulin resistance is associated with endothelial dysfunction. Implications for the syndrome of insulin resistance. J Clin Invest 1996;97(11):2601–10.
[107] Brook RD, Bard RL, Rubenfire M, Ridker PM, Rajagopalan S. Usefulness of visceral obesity (waist/hip ratio) in predicting vascular endothelial function in healthy overweight adults. Am J Cardiol 2001;88(11):1264–9.
[108] Parikh NI, Keyes MJ, Larson MG, et al. Visceral and subcutaneous adiposity and brachial artery vasodilator function. Obesity (Silver Spring) 2009;17(11):2054–9.
[109] Benjamin EJ, Larson MG, Keyes MJ, et al. Clinical correlates and heritability of flow-mediated dilation in the community: the Framingham Heart Study. Circulation 2004;109(5):613–9.
[110] Panza JA, Quyyumi AA, Brush Jr JE, Epstein SE. Abnormal endothelium-dependent vascular relaxation in patients with essential hypertension. N Engl J Med 1990;323(1):22–7.
[111] Wallace SM, Yasmin McEniery CM, et al. Isolated systolic hypertension is characterized by increased aortic stiffness and endothelial dysfunction. Hypertension 2007;50(1):228–33.
[112] Shimbo D, Muntner P, Mann D, et al. Endothelial dysfunction and the risk of hypertension: the multi-ethnic study of atherosclerosis. Hypertension 2010;55(5):1210–6.
[113] Grunfeld C, Zhao C, Fuller J, et al. Endotoxin and cytokines induce expression of leptin, the ob gene product, in hamsters. J Clin Invest 1996;97(9):2152–7.
[114] Shek EW, Brands MW, Hall JE. Chronic leptin infusion increases arterial pressure. Hypertension 1998;31(1 Pt 2):409–14.
[115] Mark AL, Correia M, Morgan DA, Shaffer RA, Haynes WG. State-of-the-art-lecture: obesity-induced hypertension: new concepts from the emerging biology of obesity. Hypertension 1999;33(1 Pt 2):537–41.
[116] Rahmouni K, Morgan DA, Morgan GM, Mark AL, Haynes WG. Role of selective leptin resistance in diet-induced obesity hypertension. Diabetes 2005;54(7):2012–8.
[117] Carlyle M, Jones OB, Kuo JJ, Hall JE. Chronic cardiovascular and renal actions of leptin: role of adrenergic activity. Hypertension 2002;39(2 Pt 2):496–501.
[118] Considine RV, Sinha MK, Heiman ML, et al. Serum immunoreactive-leptin concentrations in normal-weight and obese humans. N Engl J Med 1996;334(5):292–5.
[119] Ma D, Feitosa MF, Wilk JB, et al. Leptin is associated with blood pressure and hypertension in women from the National Heart, Lung, and Blood Institute Family Heart Study. Hypertension 2009;53(3):473–9.
[120] Shankar A, Xiao J. Positive relationship between plasma leptin level and hypertension. Hypertension 2010;56(4):623–8.
[121] Wannamethee SG, Tchernova J, Whincup P, et al. Plasma leptin: associations with metabolic, inflammatory and haemostatic risk factors for cardiovascular disease. Atherosclerosis 2007;191(2):418–26.
[122] Hotamisligil GS, Shargill NS, Spiegelman BM. Adipose expression of tumor necrosis factor-alpha: direct role in obesity-linked insulin resistance. Science 1993;259(5091):87–91.
[123] Pradhan AD, Manson JE, Rifai N, Buring JE, Ridker PM. C-reactive protein, interleukin 6, and risk of developing type 2 diabetes mellitus. JAMA 2001;286(3):327–34.
[124] Kaplan NM. The deadly quartet. Upper-body obesity, glucose intolerance, hypertriglyceridemia, and hypertension. Arch Intern Med 1989;149(7):1514–20.
[125] Brands MW, Harrison DL, Keen HL, Gardner A, Shek EW, Hall JE. Insulin-induced hypertension in rats depends on an intact renin-angiotensin system. Hypertension 1997;29(4):1014–9.
[126] Brands MW, Mizelle HL, Gaillard CA, Hildebrandt DA, Hall JE. The hemodynamic response to chronic hyperinsulinemia in conscious dogs. Am J Hypertens 1991;4(2 Pt 1):164–8.
[127] Anderson EA, Hoffman RP, Balon TW, Sinkey CA, Mark AL. Hyperinsulinemia produces both sympathetic neural activation and vasodilation in normal humans. J Clin Invest 1991;87(6):2246–52.
[128] Pou KM, Massaro JM, Hoffmann U, et al. Visceral and subcutaneous adipose tissue volumes are cross-sectionally related to markers of inflammation and oxidative stress: the Framingham Heart Study. Circulation 2007;116(11):1234–41.
[129] van Harmelen V, Dicker A, Ryden M, et al. Increased lipolysis and decreased leptin production by human omental as compared with subcutaneous preadipocytes. Diabetes 2002;51(7):2029–36.
[130] Narkiewicz K, Phillips BG, Kato M, Hering D, Bieniaszewski L, Somers VK. Gender-selective interaction between aging, blood pressure, and sympathetic nerve activity. Hypertension 2005;45(4):522–5.
[131] Wolf-Maier K, Cooper RS, Banegas JR, et al. Hypertension prevalence and blood pressure levels in 6 European countries, Canada, and the United States. Jama 2003;289(18):2363–9.
[132] Meigs JB, Wilson PW, Nathan DM, D'Agostino Sr RB, Williams K, Haffner SM. Prevalence and characteristics of the metabolic syndrome in the San Antonio Heart and Framingham Offspring Studies. Diabetes 2003;52(8):2160–7.
[133] Lovejoy JC, Sainsbury A. Sex differences in obesity and the regulation of energy homeostasis. Obes Rev 2009;10(2):154–67.
[134] Hall JE. Pathophysiology of obesity hypertension. Curr Hypertens Rep 2000;2(2):139–47.
[135] Pausova Z, Abrahamowicz M, Mahboubi A, et al. Functional variation in the androgen-receptor gene is associated with visceral adiposity and blood pressure in male adolescents. Hypertension 2010;55(3):706–14.
[136] Nedungadi TP, Clegg DJ. Sexual dimorphism in body fat distribution and risk for cardiovascular diseases. J Cardiovasc Transl Res 2009;2(3):321–7.
[137] Ng AV, Callister R, Johnson DG, Seals DR. Age and gender influence muscle sympathetic nerve activity at rest in healthy humans. Hypertension 1993;21(4):498–503.
[138] Reckelhoff JF. Sex steroids, cardiovascular disease, and hypertension: unanswered questions and some speculations. Hypertension 2005;45(2):170–4.

CHAPTER

10

Remission of Metabolic Syndrome After Sleeve Gastrectomy

Jaime Ruiz-Tovar and Rafael Calpena

Department of Surgery, Bariatric Surgery Unit, General University Hospital Elche, Alicante, Spain

Impaired glucose tolerance, hypertension, and dyslipidemia have been described as metabolic syndrome (MS). MS is associated with an increased cardiovascular risk [1], and a close association between morbid obesity and MS has been highlighted in several clinical studies. Disease risk increases with increasing body mass index (BMI) [2,3]. Bariatric surgery has been shown to be effective in achieving and maintaining weight change and reducing obesity related comorbidities [4].

Laparoscopic sleeve gastrectomy (LSG) is a restrictive bariatric procedure that involves subtotal gastric resection of the fundus and body to create a long, tubular gastric conduit constructed along the lesser curvature of the stomach. There is little long-term information available because this procedure has only recently been used as a primary weight loss surgery procedure. It was originally described as a first-stage bariatric procedure followed by Roux-en-Y gastric bypass or duodenal switch in high-risk patients. However, with the benefit of low risk due to less invasiveness, ease of surgery, and success in terms of sustained weight loss, surgeons have accepted LSG as a primary bariatric procedure. Most bariatric surgeons calibrate the sleeve with 32-40F bougies, and the use of smaller diameter bougies is associated with higher weight loss rates [5–7].

LSG not only reduces the volume of the stomach, which makes it a restrictive procedure, but also changes gastrointestinal hormone levels such as serum ghrelin, peptide YY (PYY) and glucagon-like peptide 1 (GLP-1). Recent reports have shown that LSG may have similar resolution rates of the MS and a weight loss curve similar to that of the Roux-en-Y bypass [8–10]. However, there is still little mid- and long-term information available about the metabolic effects of LSG.

EFFECT OF LAPAROSCOPIC SLEEVE GASTRECTOMY ON TYPE 2 DIABETES MELLITUS

The mechanisms underlying type 2 diabetes mellitus (T2DM) remission following LSG have yet to be fully determined, but some studies have reported favorable changes in insulin sensitivity [11]. Abbatini et al. [12] have demonstrated a near-normalization of insulin resistance in patients treated with LSG. The improvement in insulin sensitivity is thought to be primarily due to weight loss, reduction in inflammatory mediators, and decreased caloric intake, although the contribution of weight-independent mechanisms seems very likely. In our recently published study, we could not demonstrate a correlation between weight loss and reduction in glucose levels [13]. It has been established that diabetes improvement appears before a significant weight loss occurs [14]. Despite a progressive reduction of glucose levels in our case series, this did not achieve statistically significance up to 3 months after surgery; however, it was associated with a loss of excessive BMI by 45.6%. Some authors have reported glycemic control in >80% of patients after 1 month. In our series, including diabetic and euglycemic patients, significant differences from preoperative glucose values could only be observed after 3 months. However, 83.3% of our diabetic patients discontinued their hypoglycemic medication after 1 month, similar to other reported findings [13,14].

The exclusion of the proximal small intestine was initially thought to play a major role in the rapid improvement in the metabolic control of diabetes. Therefore, malabsorptive or mixed bariatric procedures were considered to be much more effective than purely restrictive ones. In this way, additional mechanisms, such as ileal interposition, have been added to sleeve gastrectomy with the aim of achieving better metabolic results [15].

Nutrition in the Prevention and Treatment of Abdominal Obesity
http://dx.doi.org/10.1016/B978-0-12-407869-7.00010-6

However, diverse studies have demonstrated that LSG as a unique bariatric procedure, compared with Roux-en-Y gastric bypass, achieves similar improvements in the glucose homeostasis [9,16,17]. Some studies have shown that LSG is associated with a marked reduction in the secretion of ghrelin, an orexigenic peptide produced by the gastric fundus and involved in mealtime hunger regulation. Ghrelin also exerts several diabetogenic effects (increases in somatotropin/growth hormone, cortisol, and epinephrine); therefore, its suppression could contribute to improve glucose homeostasis [18,19].

Previous studies have shown diabetes resolution occurring in 66–80% of patients undergoing LSG, and the maintenance of reduced plasma levels after 15 months follow-up. In our series, the short-term results are in line with those described in the literature, and good glycemic control persisted after a minimum follow-up of 24 months [13], thus confirming the midterm effectiveness of glycemic control described by other groups [10,19].

EFFECT OF LAPAROSCOPIC SLEEVE GASTRECTOMY ON LIPID PROFILE

Diverse studies have shown a significant reduction in cardiovascular risk, with increased high-density lipoprotein (HDL) cholesterol and decreased triglycerides after 1 year [7,20]. As with glucose homeostasis, there is also a lack of long-term results describing changes in the lipid profile. One year after surgery, increases in HDL of 12% and reductions in triglycerides of up to 23% have been described. We have observed an increase of 30% in HDL levels and a reduction of >60% in triglyceride levels, and these levels were maintained after a minimum follow-up of 24 months; however, total cholesterol and low-density lipoprotein cholesterol levels were not significantly changed. A relationship between lipid profile changes and weight loss or BMI changes during follow-up could not be demonstrated [13].

Low serum lipid profiles in morbidly obese patients may be affected by alterations in the expression of a recently described receptor that mediates the absorption of dietary cholesterol in the intestine; abnormal intestinal flora; or serum leptin levels [7,21,22]. Our data highlight this paradox, with LSG achieving an excess BMI loss of 76.9% in 1 year and no change in total cholesterol values [13]. Increases in serum cholesterol have even been noted during the weight loss period, with cholesterol being mobilized from adipose tissue as it is metabolized [7].

It has been known for more than 40 years that some extremely obese subjects have normal serum cholesterol, although they still have a high cardiovascular risk [23]. On the other hand, weight loss is associated with a lower cardiovascular risk. This means that other cardiovascular risk factors must improve after weight loss. The triglyceride:HDL ratio has been described as one of the strongest predictor of a heart attack and of other cardiovascular complications [24]. Ratio levels >4 are associated with a high cardiovascular risk. In our patients, we observed a significant reduction in this ratio from 4.2 to 3.5 after 1 year, which was maintained at 3.4 2 years after surgery [13]. The triglyceride:HDL ratio has been proposed as an early marker of insulin resistance, which improves with LSG. The improvement in diabetes could be one of the factors contributing to decreased cardiovascular risk. Vila et al. [25] recently reviewed published studies about lipid changes after different types of weight loss surgery, but there were no data on sleeve gastrectomies. In general, malabsorptive procedures improved all variables of the lipid profile, while the restrictive procedures tended to primarily increase HDL and reduce triglycerides, as we observed for LSG. However, decreased global cardiovascular risk was similarly observed following both restrictive and malabsorptive procedures.

EFFECT OF LAPAROSCOPIC SLEEVE GASTRECTOMY ON HYPERTENSION

Obesity surgery also improves hypertension. Slight weight loss is associated with a significant reduction in blood pressure values. Following Buchwald classification, an excess weight loss of 1% correlates with a reduction of 2 mmHg in diastolic blood pressure [26]. Different studies have demonstrated that bariatric surgery globally reduces hypertension rate to 50%, represented as treatment discontinuation and a 25% reduction in the amount of antihypertensive drugs needed [27]. In contrast to effects on T2DM, improvements in blood pressure values are achieved several months postoperatively.

Moreover, the improvement in hypertension seems to be independent of the bariatric technique performed, although a greater reduction is obtained in those patients with greater weight loss [28]. Resolution of hypertension has been described in 43% of cases following adjustable gastric banding, in 69% after gastric bypass, and in 83% after biliopancreatic diversion. Surprisingly, in our series of morbidly obese patients undergoing LSG with a hypertension rate of 30%, this comorbidity showed complete resolution in all patients (100%), allowing discontinuation of all antihypertensive treatment 6 months after surgery. We observed a mean reduction of 37 mmHg in systolic blood pressure and of 19 mmHg in diastolic blood pressure; however, this reduction did not show any correlation with weight loss. We cannot currently explain these extraordinary results in our patients.

EFFECT OF LAPAROSCOPIC SLEEVE GASTRECTOMY ON CORTISOL LEVELS

Increased cortisol levels have been proposed to contribute to the pathogenesis of MS, although only mild hypercortisolism occurs in MS and morbid obesity, in contrast to Cushing syndrome [29,30]. Furthermore, it has been demonstrated that weight loss normalizes cortisol levels and improves insulin resistance [31].

Because the diagnostic features of MS are partially shared with Cushing syndrome, which results from endogenous or exogenous hypercortisolism, it has been proposed that cortisol contributes to the pathogenesis of both disease states, although only mild hypercortisolism occurs in MS [32]. Central obesity is one of the main components of MS. Cortisol appears to play a role in adiposity in MS: circulating cortisol concentrations are higher in patients with MS and in obese patients than in healthy subjects [33]; our results are consistent with this, showing increased median preoperative cortisol levels. However, we observed no significant difference between morbidly obese patients with and without MS [34].

It is also well documented that cortisol promotes the differentiation and proliferation of human adipocytes, and that cortisol receptors are more abundant in visceral than in subcutaneous adipose tissue. Cortisol also redistributes adiposity from peripheral to central depots, which is metabolically more active, thus activating lipolysis and the release of free fatty acids into the circulation, leading to an increased risk of atheromatosis and finally to an increased cardiovascular risk [32,35]. Although an association between higher cortisol levels and both high triglyceride and low HDL cholesterol levels has been described, we could not demonstrate this in our patients. However, during postoperative follow-up, a significant association was observed between cortisol levels and a cardiovascular risk predictor (triglyceride:HDL cholesterol ratio) from the sixth month onward [34]. It is widely accepted that weight loss reduces cardiovascular risk in obese patients. In the same way, weight loss tends to normalize cortisol levels [36], but our study is the first one in which all patients displayed the normal range after 1 year [34]. According to this data, decreased cortisol levels may reflect reduced cardiovascular risk during the weight loss following sleeve gastrectomy. In our field, two predictors of cardiovascular risk are widely employed: the triglyceride:HDL cholesterol ratio and the Framingham Risk Score, which analyzes age, gender, total cholesterol, HDL cholesterol, tobacco habit, and systolic blood pressure. The Framingham Risk Score appears to be a more recent and sophisticated method of determining longitudinal cardiac risk.

References

[1] Bray GA. Medical consequences of obesity. J Clin Endocrinol Metab 2004;89:2583–9.

[2] Sullivan PW, Ghushchyan VH, Ben-Joseph R. The impact of obesity on diabetes, hyperlipidemia and hypertension in the United States. Qual Life Res 2008;17:1063–71.

[3] Nguyen NT, Magno CP, Lane KT, Hinojosa MW, Lane JS, Association of hypertension, diabetes, dyslipidemia and metabolic syndrome with obesity:findings from the National Health and Nutrition Examination Survey 1999 to 2004. J Am Coll Surg 2008;207:928–34.

[4] Buchwald H, Avidor Y, Braunwald E, et al. Bariatric surgery: a systematic review and meta-analysis. JAMA 2004;292:1724–37.

[5] Cottam D, Qureshi FG, Mattar SG, et al. Laparoscopic sleeve gastrectomy as an initial weight-loss procedure for high-risk patients with morbid obesity. Surg Endosc 2006;20:859–63.

[6] Melissas J, Daskalakis M, Koukouraki S, et al. Sleeve gastrectomy—a "food limiting" operation. Obes Surg 2008;18:1251–6.

[7] Zhang F, Strain GW, Lei W, et al. Changes in lipid profiles in morbidly obese patients after laparoscopic sleeve gastrectomy. Obes Surg 2011;21:305–9.

[8] Langer FB, Reza Hoda MA, et al. Sleeve gastrectomy and gastric banding: effects on plasma ghrelin levels. Obes Surg 2005;15:1024–9.

[9] Peterli R, Wolnerhanssen B, Peters T, et al. Improvement in glucose metabolism after bariatric surgery: comparison of laparoscopic Roux-en-Y gastric bypass and laparoscopic sleeve gastrectomy: a prospective randomized trial. Ann Surg 2009;250:234–41.

[10] Vidal J, Ibarzabal A, Romero F, et al. Type 2 diabetes mellitus and the metabolic syndrome following sleeve gastrectomy in severely obese patients. Obes Surg 2008;18:1077–82.

[11] Rizzello M, Abbatini F, Casella G, et al. Early postoperative insulin-resistance changes alter sleeve gastrectomy. Obes Surg 2010;20:50–5.

[12] Abbatini F, Rizzello M, Casella G, et al. Long-term effects of sleeve gastrectomy, gastric bypass and adjustable gastric banding on type 2 diabetes. Surg Endosc 2010;24:1005–10.

[13] Ruiz-Tovar J, Oller I, Tomas A, et al. Midterm impact of sleeve gastrectomy, calibrated with a 50-Fr bougie, on weight loss, glucose hemostasis, lipid profiles and comorbidities in morbidly obese patients. Am Surg 2012;78:969–74.

[14] Shah PS, Todkar JS, Shah SS. Effectiveness of laparoscopic sleeve gastrectomy on glycemic control in obese Indians with type 2 diabetes mellitus. Surg Obes Relat Dis 2010;6:138–41.

[15] DePaula AL, Macedo AL, Mota BR, Schraibman V. Laparoscopic ileal interposition associated to a diverted sleeve gastrectomy is an effective operation for the treatment of type 2 diabetes mellitus patients with BMI 21–29. Surg Endosc 2009;23:1313–20.

[16] Woelnerhanssen B, Peterli R, Steinert RE, et al. Effects of postbariatric surgery weight loss on adipokines and metabolic parameters: comparison of laparoscopic Roux-en-Y gastric bypass and laparoscopic sleeve gastrectomy-a prospective randomized trial. Surg Obes Relat Dis 2011;7:561–8.

[17] Chambers AP, Stefater MA, Wilson-Perez HE, et al. Similar effects of Roux-en-Y gastric bypass and vertical sleeve gastrectomy on glucose regulation in rats. Physiol Behav 2011;105:120–3.

[18] Li F, Zhang G, Liang J, et al. Sleeve gastrectomy provides a better control of diabetes by decreasing ghrelin in the diabetic Goto-Kakizaki rats. J Gastrointest Surg 2009;13:2302–8.

[19] Nosso G, Angrisani L, Saldalamacchia G, et al. Impact of sleeve gastrectomy on weight loss, glucose homeostasis, and comorbidities in severly obese type 2 diabetic subjects. J Obes 2011;2011:340867.

[20] Marantos G, Daskalakis M, Karkavitsas N, et al. Changes in metabolic profile and adipoinsular axis in morbidly obese premenopauseal females treated with restrictive bariatric surgery. World J Surg 2011;35:2022–30.

[21] Hauser H, Dyer JH, Nandy A, et al. Identification of a receptor mediating absorption of dietary cholesterol in the intestine. Biochemistry 1998;37:17843–50.

[22] Vierhapper H, Heinze G, Nowotny P, Bieglmayer C. Serum concentrations of dehydroepiandrosterone sulphate and leptin in obese patients with normal serum cholesterol. Metabolism 2003;52:379–81.

[23] Vierhapper H, Nardi A, Grosser P. Prevalence of paradoxically normal serum cholesterol in morbidly obese women. Metabolism 2000;49:607–10.

[24] Gaziano JM, Hennekens CH, O'Donnell CJ, et al. Fasting triglycerides, high-density lipoprotein, and risk of myocardial infarction. Circulation 1997;96:2520–5.

[25] Vila M, Ruiz O, Belmonte M, et al. Changes in lipid profile and insulin resistance in obese patients after Scopinaro biliopancreatic diversion. Obes Surg 2009;19:299–306.

[26] Buchwald H, Estok R, Fahrbach K, et al. Weight and type 2 diabetes after bariatric surgery: systematic review and meta-analysis. Am J Med 2009;122:248–56.

[27] Sjöström L, Lindroos AK, Peltonen M, et al. Swedish Obese Subjects Study Scientific Group. Lifestyle, diabetes, and cardiovascular risk factors 10 years after bariatric surgery. N Engl J Med 2004;351:2683–93.

[28] Sjöström CD, Peltonen M, Wedel H, et al. Differentiated long-term effects of intentional weight loss on diabetes and hypertension. Hypertension 2000;36:20–5.

[29] Pasquali R, Vicennati V, Cacciari M, et al. The hypothalamic-pituitary-adrenal axis activity in obesity and the metabolic syndrome. Ann NY Acad Sci 2006;1083:111–28.

[30] Walker BR. Cortisol—cause and cure for metabolic syndrome? Diabet Med 2006;23:1281–8.

[31] Reinher T, Andler W. Cortisol and its relation to insulin resistance before and after weight loss in obese children. Horm Res 2004;62:107–12.

[32] Anagnostis P, Athyros VG, Tzionalos K, et al. The pathogenetic role of cortisol in the metabolic syndrome: a hypothesis. J Clin Endocrinol Metab 2009;94:2692–701.

[33] Third report of the National Cholesterol Education Program . (NCEP) Expert panel on detection, evaluation and treatment of high blood cholesterol in adults (Adult treatment panel III) final report 2002. Circulation 2002;106:3143–421.

[34] Ruiz-Tovar J, Oller I, Galindo I, et al. Change in levels of C-reactive protein (CRP) and serum cortisol in morbidly obese patients after laparoscopic sleeve gastrectomy. Obes Surg 2013;23(6):764–9.

[35] Rao SR. Inflammatory markers and bariatric surgery. Inflamm Res 2012;61:789–807.

[36] Reinher T, Andler W. Cortisol and its relation to insulin resistance before and after weight loss in obese children. Horm Res 2004;62:107–12.

CHAPTER

11

Serum Magnesium and Abdominal Obesity and its Consequences

Teresa Kokot, Małgorzata Muc-Wierzgoń, Ewa Nowakowska-Zajdel, and Sylwia Dzięgielewska-Gęsiak

Department of Internal Diseases, Silesian Medical University, Katowice, Poland

INTRODUCTION

Magnesium is an essential mineral, with several dietary sources including whole grains, green leafy vegetables, legumes, and nuts. As a macroelement, it is one of the four most important cations (sodium, potassium, calcium, and magnesium) and the second—after potassium—most important intracellular element necessary for life. The adult human organism contains approximately 24–30 g (1000 mM) of magnesium, roughly 60% of which is contained in bones and 39% in soft tissues (brain, heart, liver, kidneys, and skeletal muscles), and with only 1% present in intercellular fluids, including plasma. The intracellular magnesium level is several times higher than the extracellular level. Approximately 16% of systemic magnesium is exchangeable. The normal magnesium range is 0.8–1.0 mM, which corresponds to only 1% of systemic resources, and approximately 70% occurs in a bound form. The total magnesium level in blood serum is divided into three fractions: protein associated (mainly albumin), 19%; anions (citrate, lactate, and hydrocarbonate) and phospholipid associated, 14%; and ionized calcium-associated, 67%. Considering that most magnesium is intracellular, its serum level does not provide an accurate measure of total magnesium. Free magnesium levels range between 0.5 and 0.6 mM, and only 2–3% of magnesium occurs in a free form [1,2].

Magnesium as a critical cofactor for hundreds of enzymes and a direct antagonist of intracellular calcium [3]. Is necessary for glucose transportation, glucose oxidation, reactions involving phosphorylation, and energy exchange. It is also important for the action of insulin [4].

Magnesium regulation mechanisms are based on its ability to bind to other ligands (e.g. adenosine triphosphate (ATP)-dependent enzymes), to enzymatic active sites (e.g. pyruvate kinase and pyrophosphatase), to cause structural changes in proteins during catalytic processes (e.g. ATPases), and also to initiate protein aggregation during the formation of multienzyme complexes (e.g. aldehyde dehydrogenase). Magnesium is an activator of the sodium-potassium ATPase, which is present in the cellular membrane and maintains the transmembrane potential by exchanging three intracellular sodium ions for two extracellular potassium ions. The transmembrane calcium ion concentration gradient is also maintained by the magnesium-dependent calcium ATPase. Several other enzymes whose activity depends on the level of magnesium ions are phosphofructokinase, creatine kinase, adenylate and guanylate cyclase, and phosphoribosyl pyrophosphate synthetase. It is believed that cellular magnesium levels provide a measure of its metabolic activity [5,6].

MAGNESIUM DEFICIENCY AND ITS HEALTH-ASSOCIATED CONSEQUENCES

Nutritional norms indicate the average daily magnesium demand of an adult human to be 300–350 mg, and a traditional diet satisfies approximately two-thirds of that demand.

Disturbance of magnesium homeostasis is a relatively common phenomenon: although hypermagnesemia is rather rare, mostly as an effect of excessive dietary magnesium supply or a consequence of impaired elimination of the element, magnesium deficiencies (usually chronic) are relatively common. Hypomagnesemia is a common (occurring in roughly 60% of adults) and underestimated phenomenon. There may be various reasons for this condition, including:

Nutrition in the Prevention and Treatment of Abdominal Obesity
http://dx.doi.org/10.1016/B978-0-12-407869-7.00011-8

- gastrointestinal losses, e.g. acute or chronic diarrhea, malabsorption and steatorrhea, small bowel bypass surgery, primary intestinal hypomagnesemia, or acute pancreatitis;
- renal losses, e.g. use of loop and thiazide-type diuretics, and many nephrotoxic drugs;
- volume expansion, e.g. primary hyperaldosteronism;
- alcohol abuse;
- hypercalcemia;
- dietary errors, e.g. phosphate, phytic compounds, and a fiber-rich diet.

Magnesium deficiency causes cardiovascular disorders and menstruation disorders, and favors spontaneous abortions, premature births, and puerperal eclampsia. It is associated with a higher susceptibility to infections and allergic reactions, including urticaria and bronchial asthma.

Muscular and neuropsychiatric symptoms are the earliest clinical signs of magnesium deficiency. Hyperexcitability symptoms, including Chvostek and Trousseau sign, tremors, muscular fasciculations, and tetani, are the most common. Those abnormalities are caused by a reduction in the axon excitability threshold and the acceleration of nervous conduction.

Daily demand for magnesium increases with increased gastrointestinal passage, with excessive alcohol consumption, in stressful situations, and following excessive physical strain. Decreased tissue magnesium levels are accompanied by reduced potassium and increased sodium levels, and also often by increased calcium levels. This causes further homeostatic disorder and causes tissue- and organ-associated disturbances [2,7]. The exact mechanism for hypopotassemia is not fully understood; however, it may be associated with the activity of Na+/K+-ATPase, Na+ and KCl transporters, and potassium channels and mechanisms for magnesium transmembrane transport. On the other hand, hypocalcemia, a phenomenon secondary to hypomagnesemia, is associated with reduced secretion of parathyroid hormone (PTH), cellular resistance to PTH, reduced production of active form of vitamin D3 and the associated reduction in intestinal calcium absorption, and cellular resistance to vitamin D3.

Red blood cell magnesium seems to be a better indicator of magnesium status than serum levels [8–10].

ABDOMINAL OBESITY

Abdominal obesity is a recognized risk factor for metabolic syndrome. The incidence of this syndrome is steadily increasing [7,9].

At present, the most commonly used measure of overweight and obesity is the body weight index (BMI). A diagnosis of abdominal obesity (android or visceral) is made if the waist-hip ratio (WHR) is equal to or higher than 0.8 in females, and equal to or higher than 1.0 in males.

Many researchers claim that waist circumference (WC) is a better predictor than BMI of diabetes. Although obesity is commonly associated with diabetes, WC measurement may be useful for individuals who are not obese but are nevertheless at risk of diabetes because of an increased volume of abdominal fat. Whereas the fat on hips, thighs, and other body areas is relatively harmless (i.e. passive and serving as insulation protecting against heat loss and injuries), abdominal fat accumulates not only subcutaneously but also in internal organs such as the heart, pancreas, and liver, and in skeletal muscles (i.e. visceral fat), thus affecting their function. Visceral fat is metabolically different from subcutaneous fat. Whereas abdominal adipose tissue is an active organ of internal secretion, subcutaneous fat releases active, hormone-like chemicals into the circulation. The majority of these are carried to the liver [11].

The chain of biochemical reactions that may cause insulin resistance—the cause of type 2 diabetes, coronary disease, cerebral stroke, and breast and prostate cancer, as well as renal failure and Alzheimer disease—originates in the abdominal fat [12].

Abdominal adipocytes are characterized by their significant lipolytic activity, which leads to an excess of free fatty acids in the liver and portal circulation. Moreover, increased blood serum triglyceride levels [very-low-density lipoprotein (VLDL) fraction], reduced high-density lipoprotein (HDL) cholesterol levels, the occurrence of small, dense low-density lipoproteins (LDLs) of high atherogenicity, and the retention of postprandial lipoproteins (triglyceride-rich lipoprotein remnants) is observed [9,13]. Abdominal obesity increases the risk of thrombus formation because it favors the rise in certain postthrombotic factors, including fibrinogen, factor VII, and plasminogen activator inhibitor 1 (PAI-1).

It was demonstrated that chronic stress causes the release of a large volume of neuropeptide Y (NPY; a hormone responsible for the accumulation of fat in cells) [14]. Together with cortisone, this hormone triggers abdominal obesity through mechanisms that include increased appetite. Adipose tissue in the abdominal area is equipped with the highest number of cortisone-sensitive receptors, causing the "opening" of adipocytes and thus increasing their storage capacity. Abdominal fat also releases many other substances, including hormones responsible for appetite regulation and compounds that influence the immune system. Stressful situations cause also increased production of leptin (a hormone produced in adipose tissue), with an effect similar to that of NPY. Stressful situations are accompanied by the increased production of noradrenalin—a hormone responsible for uncontrolled appetite for carbohydrates. The consumption of high amounts of carbohydrates favors the production of serotonin, a substance that cheers us up.

Pasaric et al. evaluated the effect of growth hormone on reducing the amount of visceral fat. Numerous studies have demonstrated that growth hormone reduces the amount of adipose tissue, and particularly of visceral fat [11,14,15].

MECHANISM OF MAGNESIUM DEFICIENCY IN OBESITY

Human studies also indicate that a low magnesium status is strongly correlated with increased inflammatory and oxidative stress [16–19]. Lower serum magnesium levels are associated with insulin resistance and with elevated serum concentrations of tumor necrosis factor (TNF-α), interleukin-6 (IL-6) [18], and C-reactive protein (CRP) [17]. Low serum magnesium occurs much more commonly in obese individuals (than in individuals of normal weight) and may be one of the stress-inducing factors leading to the activation of inflammatory pathways.

The following pathways should be considered [20]:

- Cellular entry of calcium and priming of phagocytic cells;
- Opening of calcium channels and activation of specific receptors;
- Release of neurotransmitters, e.g. substance P; and
- Membrane oxidation and activation of nuclear factor-kappa-B (NF-κB).

Not all obese people have increased inflammatory indexes. Therefore, other factors, including nutrients, may also participate in its development. A lack of magnesium is associated with a rapid drop in the extracellular magnesium level, which initiates an inflammatory reaction [14,21]. An increase in intracellular calcium levels activates cellular phagocytes (i.e. priming), leading to the release of proinflammatory cytokines.

A significant dietary magnesium deficiency causes a drop in extracellular magnesium levels within a few days.

MAGNESIUM AND ABDOMINAL OBESITY

Numerous recent epidemiological studies have demonstrated a correlation between both low magnesium levels and low magnesium consumption and an increased risk of some diseases, including arterial hypertension, asthma, atheromatosis, diabetes, metabolic syndrome, and osteoporosis [1]. Numerous reports [22] indicate that the appropriate systemic magnesium level and dietary uptake of the element play a significant role in reducing the risk of obesity.

The relation between obesity and magnesium is also unclear [23]. Many studies show that abdominal obesity is associated with low levels of magnesium, zinc, and vitamins C and E. However, increased visceral adiposity is known to predispose to reduced insulin sensitivity, which in turn may worsen magnesium status. Thus, a greater resistance to insulin activity could explain the strong association between WC and hypomagnesemia. Laires et al. [24], in the group of 136 postmenopausal women, observed a direct correlation in both groups (obese BMI $\geq$ 25 kg/m^2 and nonobese BMI < 25 kg/m^2) of women between magnesium values in red blood cells (RBC-Mg) and insulin. Paolisso et al. [5] reported an increase in intracellular magnesium upon insulin modulation. Insulin may therefore be responsible for shifting magnesium from the extracellular to intracellular space [5,25].

The observed correlation between RBC-Mg and the homeostasis model assessment index is independent of obesity, but the correlation is weaker in obese women [24]: this phenomenon may be explained by the significantly higher incidence of glucose levels exceeding 100 mg/dL in that group of subjects. Insulin is involved in erythrocyte magnesium transport, especially in the presence of normal glucose levels [8]. However, the higher value of RBC-Mg in the obese can be linked to higher insulin levels and normoglycemic status [12].

Metabolic syndrome is a disease of modern times [1]. The first studies on serum magnesium levels in young individuals with metabolic syndrome were initiated in 1985. In 2002, following 15 years of observation, metabolic syndrome was confirmed in 74% of the study participants, and a correlation was demonstrated between magnesium level and metabolic syndrome. A low magnesium level (<0.74 mM or 1.8 mg/dL) was observed in 66% of patients with metabolic syndrome, but in only 4.9% of healthy individuals (control) [1]. Another cross-sectional study, the Women's Health Study, on young individuals (aged 18–30 years) indicated the existence of a correlation between magnesium consumption and metabolic syndrome. Young people who consumed more magnesium were at a lower risk of developing metabolic syndrome (including abdominal obesity), and the risk was dose dependent [7].

Corica et al. found a significant negative correlation between WHR and plasma magnesium in obese subjects [18].

There are no accurate data indicating that magnesium participation in maintaining homeostasis may facilitate the maintenance of normal body weight [2]. It is suggested that magnesium in the form of insoluble soaps in the small intestine may prevent the absorption of dietary fat. Another study indicated that magnesium deficiency in obese adults and children may explain their observed insulin resistance [26].

Cross-sectional studies (in various populations) have measured the bioelectric impedance of adipose tissue and noted that people with a higher fatty tissue content have lower serum magnesium and are more exposed to the oxidative stress. Apparently, magnesium modulates adipocyte function by stimulating adenylate cyclase activity and increasing the production of cyclic AMP. Importantly, such changes in adipocyte function may be involved in energy metabolism, energy storage, and control of glucose [2].

Further studies are needed to tease out the specific molecular and cellular mechanisms through which magnesium modulates adipocyte biochemistry and physiology, and to discover how such events may potentiate fat storage in those with or at risk of metabolic syndrome [2].

CONCLUSION

Studies indicate a correlation between chronic magnesium deficiency and obesity. Hypomagnesemia is a proven risk factor for metabolic syndrome and type 2 diabetes—both of which are commonly associated with obesity, and particularly with abdominal obesity. Correct magnesium supplementation improves insulin sensitivity even in normomagnesemic, overweight, nondiabetic subjects, thus emphasizing the need for an early optimization of magnesium status to prevent insulin resistance and subsequent type 2 diabetes [27,28,29].

It is unclear whether hypomagnesemia is a separate risk factor for obesity, independent of the other risk factors described in literature, or whether its presence adds an additional risk to the global calculated risk. Even if that doubt is justified, there is agreement that body weight reduction is one of the basic principles of primary and secondary prophylaxis in overweight and obese patients.

References

[1] Geiger H, Wanner Ch. Magnesium in disease. Clin Kidney J 2012(Suppl. 1):25–38.

[2] Belin RJ, He K. Magnesium physiology and pathogenic mechanisms that contribute to the development of the metabolic syndrome. Magnes Res 2007;20(2):107–29.

[3] Elin RJ. Magnesium metabolism in health and disease. Dis Mon 1998 on Niedworok E, Muc-Wierzgoñ M, Nowakowska-Zajdel E. Influence of magnesium on fatty acids and Their esters in isolated rat hepatocytes. J Biol Regul Homeost Agents 2010.

[4] Paolisso G, Scheen A, D'Onofrio F, Lefebvre P. Magnesium and glucose homeostasis. Diabetologia 1990;33:511–4.

[5] Paolisso G, Barbagallo M. Hypertension, diabetes mellitus, and insulin resistance. The role of intracellular magnesium. Am J Hypertens 1997;10:346–55.

[6] Barbagallo M, Dominguez LJ. Magnesium intake in the pathophysiology and treatment of the cardiometaboliic syndrome: where are we in 2006? JCMS 2006;6104:356–7.

[7] Simmons D, Joshi S, Shaw J. Hypomagnesaemia is associated with diabetes: not pre-diabetes, obesity or the metabolic syndrome. Diab Res Clin Pract 2010;87:261–6.

[8] Delva P, Pellegrini P, Degan M, Pastori C, Lecchi A. Na+ K- Cl co-transport mediates insulin in vitro effects on celluar ionised magnesium. Eleventh European Meeting on Hypertension (abstract) 2001;S43-P1:88.

[9] Randell EW, Mathews M, Gadag V, Zhang H, Sun G. Relationship between serum magnesium values, lipids and anthropometric risk factor. Atherosclerosis 2008;196:413–9.

[10] Ghaasemi A, Zahediasl S, Syedmoradi L, Azizi F. Low serum magnesium levels in elderly subjects with metabolic syndrome. Biol Trace Elem Res 2001;136:18–25.

[11] Pasarica M, Zachwieja JJ, et al. Effect of growth hormone on body composition and visceral adiposity in middle-aged men with visceral obesity. J Clin Endocrinol Metab 2007;92:4265–70.

[12] Ishizuka J, Bold RJ, Towsend Jr CM, Thompson JC. In vitro relationship between magnesium and insulin secretion. Magnes Res 1994;7:17–22.

[13] He K, Song Y, Belin RJ, Chen Y. Magnesium intake and the metabolic syndrome: epidemilogic evidence to date. JCMS 2006;I:351–5.

[14] Nielsen FH. Magnesium, inflammation, and obesity in chronic disease. Nutr Rev 2010;68(6):333–40.

[15] Evangelopoulos AA, Vallianou NG, Panagiotakos DB, Georgiou AG, Zacharias GA, Alevra AN, et al. An inverse relationship between cumulating components of the metabolic syndrome and serum magnesium levels. Nutr Res 2008;28:659–63.

[16] Guerrero-Romero F, Rodriguez-Moran M. Low serum magnesium levels and metabolic syndrome. Acta Diabetol 2002;39:209–13.

[17] King DE, Mainous AG, Geesey ME, Woolson RF. Dietary magnesium and C-reactive protein levels. J Am Coll Nutr 2005;24:166–71.

[18] Rodriguez-Hemandez H, Gonzalez IL, Rodriguez-Moran M, Guerrero-Romero F. Hypomagnesemia, insulin resistance, and non-alcoholic steatohepatis in obese subjects. Arch Med Res 2005;36:362–6.

[19] He K, Liu K, Daviglus ML, Morris SJ, Loria CM, Van Horn L. Magnesium intake and incidence of metabolic syndrome among young adults. Circulation 2006;113:1675–82.

[20] Liana A, Miu RM, Andreica M. Obesity and magnesium deficiency: is oxidative stress involved? Clu Jul Medical 2010;83(4):581–3.

[21] Chacko SA, Sul J, Song Y, Li X, LeBlanc J, You Y. Magnesium supplementation, metabolic and inflammatoty markers, and global genomic and proteomic profiling: a randomized, double-blind, controlled, crossover trial in overweight individuals. Am J Clin Nutr 2011;93:463–73.

[22] Johansson HE, Zethelius B, Öhrvall M, Sundbom M, Haenni A. Serum magnesium ststus after gastric bypass surgery in obesity. Obes Surg 2009;19:1250–5.

[23] Kurpad AV, Aeberli I. Low serum magnesium and obesity—causal role or diet biomarker? Indian Pediatr 2012;49(16):100–1.

[24] Laire MJ, Moreira H, Monteiro CP, Sardinha L, Limao F, Veiga L, et al. Magnesium, Insulin resistance and Body Composition in Healthy Postmenopausal Women. J Am Coll Nutr 2004;23(5):510S–3S.

[25] Barbagallo M, Gupta RK, Bardicef M, Resnick LM. Altered ionic effect of insulin in hypertension: role of basal ion levels in determining cellular responsiveness. J Clin Endocrinol Metab 1997;82:1761–5.

[26] Takaya J, Higashino H, Kotera F, Kobayashi Y. Intracellular magnesium of platelets in children with diabetes and obesity. Metabolism 2003;52(4):468–71.
[27] Mooren FC, Krüger K, Völker K, Golf SW, Wadepuhl M, Kraus A. Oral magnesium supplementation reduces insulin resistance in non-diabetic subjects—a double-blind, placebo-controlled, randomized trial. Diabetes Obes Metab 2011 Mar;13(3):281–4.
[28] Hadjistavri LS, Sarafidis PA, Georglanos PI, Tziolas IM, Arodltis CP, Hltoglou-Makedou A, et al. Beneficial effects of oral magnesium supplementation on insulin sensitivity and serum lipid profile. Med Sci Monit 2010;16(6):CR307–12.
[29] Watson RR, Preedy VR, Zibadi S. Magnesium in human health and disease. New York: Humana Press; 2013.

PART C

NUTRITION, ABDOMINAL OBESITY, AND TYPE 2 DIABETES

CHAPTER

12

Abdominal Adipose Tissue and Insulin Resistance: The Role of Ethnicity

Danijela Gasevic[a], Simi Kohli[a], Nadia Khan[b], and Scott A. Lear[c]

[a]Department of Biomedical Physiology and Kinesiology, Simon Fraser University, Burnaby, British Columbia, Canada; [b]Department of Medicine, University of British Columbia, Vancouver, British Columbia, Canada; [c]Faculty of Health Sciences, Simon Fraser University, Vancouver, British Columbia, Canada

INTRODUCTION

Obesity is a chronic and debilitating condition, and its prevalence in the world is rising rapidly [1]. Currently, obesity is defined in clinical and research practice as a body mass index (BMI) of 30 kg/m^2 or greater [2,3]. The BMI is a simple, inexpensive, and noninvasive clinical tool to identify and measure obesity; however, its use is limited as it is a measure of excess weight rather than excess body fat because the BMI cannot delineate between excessive weight due to bone, lean muscle, or fat mass. For example, BMI measures may mistakenly place muscular individuals in an overweight or obesity category. Furthermore, there is also an assumption that weight is evenly distributed throughout the body [4], thereby disregarding the heterogeneity that exists within body fat distribution. It is this regional distribution that has been found to play an integral role in obesity-related health risk [5,6].

French physician Jean Vague was the first to report that the health complications associated with obesity are related to regional distribution of body fat rather than to overall obesity [7]. He also observed sex differences in body fat distribution, whereby men tend to accumulate adipose tissue in the trunk area (termed *android obesity*), whereas premenopausal women are prone to accumulate adipose tissue in the thighs and hips (*gynoid obesity*). However, it took the medical community several decades to confirm Dr Vague's observations. The results of several prospective studies indicate that abdominal adipose tissue deposition, or central obesity, measured predominantly using anthropometrics such as waist-hip ratio (WHR) and skinfolds, is associated with an increased risk of myocardial infarction, stroke, and mortality [8]; the occurrence of ischemic heart disease and stroke [9]; and the development of coronary heart disease [10,11] and diabetes [12]. These findings were independent of overall obesity measured by BMI. The use of anthropometric measurements as surrogates for abdominal adiposity, although relatively simple and inexpensive, is limited in the information it can provide; thus, the use of advanced imaging techniques such as computed tomography (CT) and magnetic resonance imaging (MRI) not only enable the objective measurement of abdominal adipose tissue but also distinguishes adipose tissue from muscle, bone, and other tissues in the abdominal cavity. Furthermore, these imaging methods assisted in identifying distinct abdominal adipose tissue compartments such as subcutaneous (SAT) and intra-abdominal adipose tissue [visceral adipose tissue (VAT) in particular] that exhibit different anatomical and physiological characteristics [13–15]. This chapter focuses on these distinct abdominal adipose tissue compartments and their relationship with insulin resistance in ethnic groups.

Insulin resistance syndrome, also known as *Syndrome X*, was first described by Dr Gerald Reaven in 1988. He observed metabolic and hemodynamic abnormalities such as glucose intolerance, dyslipidemia, and elevated blood pressure to be clustered in similar individuals, thereby increasing their risk of type 2 diabetes mellitus (T2DM) and cardiovascular disease (CVD) [16,17]. Given that techniques for assessing insulin sensitivity, such as the hyperinsulinemic-euglycemic clamp, are invasive, time consuming, labor intensive, and expensive, measuring insulin sensitivity in a clinical setting is not feasible [18]. For this reason, major health organizations such as the World Health Organization [19], National Cholesterol Education Program Adult Treatment Panel III (NCEP-ATP III) [20], and the International Diabetes Federation

Nutrition in the Prevention and Treatment of Abdominal Obesity
http://dx.doi.org/10.1016/B978-0-12-407869-7.00012-X

[21] proposed the use of parameters that are now regularly measured in clinical practice and that would, taken together, most probably identify insulin-resistant individuals at increased risk of T2DM and CVD. A proposed cluster of clinical parameters with their respective cutoff values was termed *metabolic syndrome*. Given that the definition of metabolic syndrome slightly differs across health organizational bodies and this can largely influence the risk assessment [22–27], the definition has recently been harmonized to enable a common approach to identifying individuals with metabolic syndrome and, therefore, permit international comparisons [28]. According to the harmonized definition, common criteria for the clinical diagnosis of metabolic syndrome include elevated waist circumference (WC); elevated triglycerides $\geq$150 mg/dL (1.7 mM) or drug treatment for elevated triglycerides; reduced high-density lipoprotein cholesterol [HDL-C; <40 mg/dL (1.0 mM) in males or <50 mg/dL (1.3 mM) in females] or drug treatment for reduced HDL-C; elevated blood pressure (systolic $\geq$130 mmHg and/or diastolic $\geq$85 mmHg) or antihypertensive medication treatment with a history of hypertension; and elevated fasting blood glucose [$\geq$100 mg/dL (5.6 mM)] or drug treatment for elevated glucose. The presence of three out of five clinical criteria constitutes the diagnosis of metabolic syndrome. In addition, the harmonized definition of metabolic syndrome recognizes that cardiovascular risk associated with certain WC measurement will vary among different ethnic groups [29]. This is important, as it has been shown that various ethnic groups accumulate abdominal adipose tissue differently, which affects their risk of CVD and T2DM [28,30].

Regardless of the criteria used for metabolic syndrome, multiple research groups have described a significant association between metabolic syndrome and T2DM [31–34], CVD morbidity and mortality [27,33,35–40], and all-cause mortality [35,36,39,41]. In the prospective Kuopio Ischaemic Heart Disease Risk Factor study, which recruited men between ages 42 and 60 years without CVD, cancer, or diabetes, even after adjustment for conventional cardiovascular risk factors, the risk of all-cause mortality was two-fold higher while the risk of cardiovascular mortality was two- to three-fold higher among men with the metabolic syndrome compared to their counterparts without the syndrome [42]. Given the debilitating consequences of metabolic syndrome, it is alarming that the prevalence of metabolic syndrome is high and rising in both developed [43–47] and developing countries [48–52]. Multiple factors contribute to metabolic syndrome such as genetic predisposition, age, sex, ethnicity, physical inactivity, increased consumption of energy dense diet, smoking, alcohol consumption, obesity, neuroendocrine abnormalities, stress, chronic inflammation, and drugs [53,54]; however, mounting evidence shows that increased abdominal adipose tissue is predictive for the presence of individual or clustered cardiometabolic abnormalities, which are components of metabolic syndrome [55–61]. Abdominal adipose tissue, its association with insulin resistance, and the role of ethnicity are discussed below.

ABDOMINAL ADIPOSE TISSUE

Abdominal adipose tissue can be divided anatomically into two main compartments: the SAT compartment and the intra-abdominal adipose tissue compartment. In clinical and research practice, anthropometric indexes such as WHR, WC, and abdominal sagittal diameter provide an estimate of the amount of abdominal adipose tissue and thus an associated health risk level; however, imaging techniques such as CT, MRI, and ultrasound permit a more accurate assessment of subcompartments of abdominal adipose tissue [13]. The most superficial layer, SAT, is located beneath the skin and above the abdominal musculature. This layer can also be further subdivided by the *fascia superficialis*, which is visible by imaging techniques [62,63], into superficial subcutaneous adipose tissue (SSAT) and deep subcutaneous adipose tissue (DSAT). SSAT is located immediately beneath the skin and overlaying the abdominal wall fascia, while DSAT is located between the abdominal wall fascia and the parietal peritoneum. Intra-abdominal adipose tissue is located in the abdominal cavity and is composed of intraperitoneal or VAT and retroperitoneal adipose tissue. The VAT depot is located between the layers of visceral peritoneum (omental and mesenteric adipose tissue), while retroperitoneal adipose tissue includes peripancreatic, periaortic, pararenal, and perirenal adipose tissue.

Significant anatomical and physiological differences have been observed between subcompartments of abdominal adipose tissue [13–15]. While SAT venous blood is drained through systemic veins and thus proceeds directly to the systemic circulation, the VAT venous blood is initially drained to the liver through the portal vein. According to the "portal vein theory," insulin resistance and related cardiometabolic complications arise from a VAT-generated high flux of free fatty acids in the portal vein that further stimulates gluconeogenesis, increases triglyceride rich lipoprotein synthesis in the liver, and decreases hepatic clearance of insulin [64,65]. Although it is often widely stated that, compared to SAT, VAT adipocytes are larger and exhibit higher lipolytic activity [15], evidence for this is not conclusive. That is, while some evidence indicates that, compared to SAT, VAT adipocytes are more sensitive to catecholamine-induced lipolysis [66–69] and have a decreased response to insulin's antilipolytic effect [70], other research demonstrates a larger adipocyte size [71–73] and higher basal lipolytic activity for SAT [73–75] than that for VAT adipocytes. Similarly, while the majority of evidence illustrates a strong relationship between VAT and insulin resistance and associated cardiometabolic complications [55,56,76–85], there is also some evidence demonstrating a significant relationship between SAT and cardiometabolic abnormalities [86,87], even independent of VAT [88,89]. With that said, it is important to note that when the relationship between weight loss-induced change in regional body fat distribution and insulin sensitivity was examined in adults with obesity, it was found that the reduction in VAT was the only regional adipose tissue depot that predicted improvement in insulin sensitivity [90]. This was confirmed in animal studies demonstrating that surgical removal of visceral fat reduces insulin resistance and the development of diabetes [91,92], and was further confirmed in patients with severe obesity in whom surgical removal of VAT, through omentectomy, resulted in significant improvements in insulin sensitivity [93]. In contrast, surgical removal of abdominal SAT (i.e. liposuction) in obese women had no significant effect on insulin resistance or other obesity-associated metabolic abnormalities, thereby suggesting that decreasing SAT alone does not lead to improvements in the metabolic profile of patients [94]. Although both SAT and VAT have been shown to be associated with insulin resistance, VAT appears to be of greater clinical importance in regulating insulin resistance [95].

The role of SAT and whether it has a detrimental effect on cardiovascular risk or a cardioprotective role remains unclear [96]. While evidence has shown that both SAT and VAT contribute to cardiovascular risk [95,97–100], studies that investigated the interaction between SAT and VAT and its association with insulin resistance demonstrated a distinct contribution of SAT to cardiometabolic risk at different levels of VAT [95,96,98]. Demerath et al. [98] explored associations among SAT, VAT, and their interaction with metabolic syndrome among non-Hispanic white adults. They found a significant association between both SAT and VAT and metabolic syndrome, and reported a significant SAT × VAT interaction in men but not in women. This interaction is consistent with the notion that at lower levels of VAT individuals in the top tertile of SAT were at greater risk for metabolic syndrome compared to their counterparts with lower levels of SAT; however, among individuals with higher levels of VAT, having more SAT was associated with lower cardiometabolic risk [98]. Other studies have also shown that an increase in SAT lessens the adverse effects of VAT among African-American but not white women [96] and among individuals without obesity but not among obese individuals [95]. In a study conducted by Porter et al. [101], participants from the Framingham Heart Study were stratified into VAT tertiles, within which the relationship of SAT tertiles with cardiometabolic risk factors was explored. Similar to the aforementioned studies, an increase in SAT was associated with increases in risk factor prevalence among individuals with less VAT (the bottom two VAT tertiles). However, among people with most VAT (the top VAT tertile), an increase in SAT exhibited a beneficial effect on triglycerides but not on other risk factors, the prevalence of which increased with increases in SAT [101].

In an attempt to explain the contribution of SAT to insulin resistance, Freedland [14] recently proposed a new critical VAT threshold (CVATT) hypothesis. Being unique for each individual, CVATT "represents a range for the accumulation of a critical mass of VAT that when achieved, leads to the development of metabolic syndrome" [14]. According to this theory, once VAT expands and reaches CVATT, thereby initiating metabolic syndrome, adipose tissue in the VAT depot may influence the central SAT depot adipocytes so that they become more lipolytic and less sensitive to insulin action [14]. Studies researching subcompartments of SAT indeed showed significant functional and morphological differences between SSAT and DSAT [102], demonstrating a higher lipolytic activity of adipocytes in the DSAT depot [69] and a stronger association between DSAT and insulin resistance when compared to SSAT [103–105]. Furthermore, it has been shown that there is a general trend toward increased adipocyte irregularity and vascularization from the outermost compartment toward the inner most compartment, i.e. from the SSAT to DSAT and finally to the VAT depot [106]. Consequently, in order to gain an adequate understanding of the relationship between body composition and insulin resistance, the SSAT and DSAT depots should not be regarded as a single adipose tissue depot but rather as two anatomically and physiologically distinct compartments [104].

DEFINING ETHNICITY

Ethnicity is a strong predictor of health and health-related behaviors [107]. The term *ethnicity* is believed to originate from the Greek term *ethnos* used in reference to band, tribe, race, and people [108]; however, there is no single definition or theory to describe ethnic groups [109]. Hutchinson and Smith [108] defined an ethnic group or *ethnie* as consisting of six characteristics including a name for the group, common ancestry, historical memories, elements of common culture, and a link with a homeland; however, they did note that the presence of all six features is not critical for an ethnic group to exist. In medical research and practice, the term *ethnicity* is commonly used together with *race* such that researchers often combine the two categories to form a single dimension, *race/ethnicity* [30,110–113]. This approach is justified only if it is generally believed that the terms *ethnicity* and *race* are synonymous [114]; however, while *ethnicity*, as regarded by social scientists, emphasizes cultural differences, *race* pertains to common physical characteristics [115].

Although ethnicity/race research may help us to understand the differences in disease risk factors and symptoms among different ethnic/racial groups, elucidate disease etiology, or explore equity in access to health care, researching ethnic/racial differences in disease risk does not come without its challenges. One of the main challenges stems from categorizing ethnicity/race. There is still no standardized scientific classification for ethnicity/race, thus making these terms challenging to measure [116,117]. Approaches used for assessing ethnicity/race are inconsistent and can include self-reporting, assessment by another by observation (i.e. observer-coded) [118], or the use of computer programs [119] or surname lists [120] for defining ethnicity. Although race and ethnicity are commonly lumped together to form a single race/ethnicity dimension [30,110–113], the two terms represent two distinct concepts [121]. This is especially emphasized in the heterogeneity within ethnic/racial groups. For example, within a "white" race group, there are multiple groups that differ according to lifestyle and cultural practices. Similarly, the South Asian ethnic group includes individuals from Bangladesh, India, Pakistan, and Sri Lanka and the religious, behavioral, and cultural practices differ significantly not only between the aforementioned countries but also within the countries. Furthermore, while an individual's race is biologically static, their ethnicity can be fluid [121]. For example, which ethnicity a person will self-categorize into may depend on their personal, social, and political environment; the way the ethnicity question is phrased within a survey; or the way people consider their answers may be used [121]. Another challenge lies in the observation that people often identify themselves as belonging to multiple races and multiple ethnic groups. Indeed, according to data from the 2000 U.S. Census, nearly 7 million people identified themselves as members of more than one race [122]. Given that *race* and *ethnicity* are commonly presented as a single dimension, in this chapter the term *ethnicity* is used to denote any racial/ethnic differences in adipose tissue accumulation or clinical outcomes.

ETHNICITY AND INSULIN RESISTANCE

A growing body of research has explored ethnic differences in insulin resistance syndrome, and significant differences were found in both developed and developing countries. In Canada, in a cross-sectional study conducted by Anand et al. [123], who randomly selected 1276 adults of Chinese, European, Native American, and South Asian origin from three large Canadian cities (Hamilton, Toronto, and Edmonton) and the Six Nations reserve (Ohsweken, Ontario), the prevalence of metabolic syndrome, as defined by the NCEP-ATP III guidelines [20], was highest among Aboriginals (41.6%) followed by South Asians (25.9%), Europeans (22.0%), and Chinese (11.0%). Additionally, among 797 apparently healthy adults between ages of 30 to 65 years of Native Americans, Chinese, European, and South Asian origin from Vancouver, Canada, participants of the Multicultural Community Health Assessment Trial (M-CHAT), the prevalence of metabolic syndrome, as defined using a harmonized [29] definition, was highest among South Asians (37%), followed by Aboriginals and Europeans (26% for both), while the lowest prevalence of metabolic syndrome was observed among Chinese individuals (23%) [124].

In the United Kingdom, data collected in Southall [125] and Brent [126] using identical protocols were pooled by Tillin et al. [127], who found significant ethnic differences in the age-standardized metabolic syndrome prevalence, irrespective of the criteria used to define metabolic syndrome. Using World Health Organization (WHO) [128]/NCEP-ATP III criteria [20], metabolic syndrome was more prevalent among both South Asian men (46.3%/28.8%) and women (30.8%/31.8%) than among African Caribbean men (26.7%/15.5%) and women (26.4%/23.4%) or among European men (18.8%/18.4%) and women (9.1%/14.4%) [127]. Furthermore, in the Wandsworth Heart and Stroke Study conducted in South London (1994–1996), the prevalence of metabolic syndrome (NCEP-ATP III [20]) was again highest among South Asians (26.7%), followed by that of white participants and those of African origin (16.4% and 16.1%, respectively) [129]. Similarly, the Newcastle Heart Project, which collected prevalence data on three ethnic groups between 1991 and 1997, demonstrated that regardless of the metabolic syndrome definition used (WHO 1999 [128], NCEP-ATP III 2001 [20] and 2005 [130], or International Diabetes Federation 2005 [21] criteria), the South Asian population (men, 23.9–49.3%; women, 24.1–38.0%) consistently had a higher prevalence of metabolic syndrome when compared to European men (22.3–30.7%) and women (14.9–23.3%); the lowest prevalence of metabolic syndrome was observed among Chinese men (3.6–12.3%) and women (8.8–16.5%) [131]. However, according to the Leicester Ethnic Atherosclerosis and Diabetes Risk study, which assessed 3099 participants (71.4% white Europeans and the remainder of South Asian origin), the gender-adjusted prevalence of metabolic syndrome as defined by the NCEP-ATP III [20] criteria did not statistically differ between South Asians (30.6%) and white Europeans (29.3%) [132].

In the United States, the analysis of data regarding 8814 adults aged 20 years or older from the third National Health and Nutrition Examination Survey (NHANES;

1988–1984) revealed highest metabolic syndrome prevalence (NCEP-ATP III criteria [20]) among the Mexican Americans (31.9%) followed by white (23.8%) and African-Americans (21.6%) [133]. Using the same population, but focusing solely on normal weight Americans, ethnic-specific differences were apparent across all BMI categories. Both men and women of Hispanic and white origins had a higher prevalence of metabolic syndrome compared to black individuals in the BMI categories 23.0–24.9 kg/m^2 and 25.0–26.9 kg/m^2; however, in the BMI range of 18.5–22.9 kg/m^2, the prevalence of metabolic syndrome was higher in white men and women than in their Hispanic and black counterparts [134]. Using the same criteria for metabolic syndrome, a more recent NHANES 2003–2006 demonstrated an overall higher prevalence of metabolic syndrome in the American population compared to that reported by the NHANES 1988–1984. The highest prevalence of metabolic syndrome persisted among Mexican American men (33.2%) and women (40.6%); the prevalence of metabolic syndrome among black women (38.8%) was greater than among white women (31.5%), while the opposite was noted for black men (25.3%) and white men (37.2%) [44]. Moreover, among 5810 participants of the Multi-Ethnic Study of Atherosclerosis aged 45–84 years with no evidence of clinical CVD before recruitment, the prevalence of metabolic syndrome was highest among Hispanic (33.4%) and lowest among Chinese (20.5%) participants [112]. In the same study, metabolic syndrome prevalence among black and white participants was similar, reaching 25.6% and 27.5%, respectively [112]. However, in the Coronary Artery Risk Development in Young Adults study, there was a significant difference in the rates of metabolic syndrome between black and white young adults aged between 18 and 30 years: after an average of 13.6 years of follow-up, black women had the highest rate of metabolic syndrome followed by white men, black men, and white women [135]. Furthermore, metabolic syndrome, as defined by NCEP-ATP III [20] criteria, was found to be more prevalent among women of Filipino origin (32.6%) than in white women (13.8%) [136].

According to data from the 1998 Singapore National Health Survey involving 4724 adults aged 18–69 years, South Asians had the highest prevalence of metabolic syndrome (28.8%), followed by Malays (24.2%) and Chinese (14.8%) [137]. Similarly, using a harmonized [29] definition, the highest prevalence of metabolic syndrome in Malaysia was again observed among South Asians (35.6%), while the lowest prevalence was observed among Chinese (26.2%) [138]. In the same study, the prevalence of metabolic syndrome was higher in indigenous Sarawakians (30.5%) than in Malays (26.4%) [138]. According to data from India, the prevalence of metabolic syndrome ranges from 9.8% to 36.4% in Indian men and from 10.5% to 47.8% in Indian women [139–145]. Moreover, in studies researching metabolic syndrome in Chinese population, the metabolic syndrome prevalence ranged from 7.3% to 23.3% [51,146–149]: the prevalence in Chinese men ranged from 9.8% to 22.9%, while that of Chinese women was between 17.8% and 29.1% [148,150,151]. Furthermore, according to the results of the Korean National Health and Nutrition Examination Surveys, the metabolic syndrome prevalence among Korean adults increased from 24.9% in 1998 to 31.3% in 2007 [47]. In Mexico, the results of the Mexican National Survey of Chronic Diseases [11] showed an overall metabolic syndrome prevalence of 26.6% when using NCEP-ATP III [20] criteria. This percentage has increased substantially over the years; according to the National Health and Nutrition Survey from 2006, the prevalence of metabolic syndrome (NCEP-ATP III [20] criteria) among Mexican adults aged 20 years or older was 41.6% [152]. In addition, in a more recent study, the prevalence of metabolic syndrome among the urban Mexican population greatly exceeded 50% [153].

Thus, evidence indicates a high prevalence of metabolic syndrome in both developed and developing countries. Furthermore, it can be seen that not all ethnic groups are equally affected by metabolic syndrome and consequently by cardiovascular risk. It is believed that these differences across ethnic groups are attributable to genetic factors and the interplay between ethnicity and an individual's environment [154]. Given the strong association between abdominal adipose tissue and metabolic syndrome, ethnic disparities in metabolic syndrome prevalence and individual cardiometabolic risk factors may be attributed to ethnic differences in the accumulation of abdominal adipose tissue. This evidence is reviewed in the next section.

ETHNICITY AND ABDOMINAL ADIPOSITY

Many studies have demonstrated ethnic-specific differences in the regional distribution of body fat. The M-CHAT study, conducted in Canada, measured and compared body fat distribution in a European population (continental Europe, Ireland, and the United Kingdom) to that of an Aboriginal, Chinese (China, Hong Kong, and Taiwan), and South Asian (Bangladesh, India, Nepal, Pakistan and Sri Lanka) population [155]. The M-CHAT study illustrated that abdominal adipose tissue, assessed via CT, significantly differed among ethnic groups (Fig. 12.1); at the same BMI, and after adjusting for age and sex, SAT of Aboriginals and South Asians was significantly higher than that of Europeans [28]. Furthermore, the regression analyses controlled for age, sex, household income, maximum level of education,

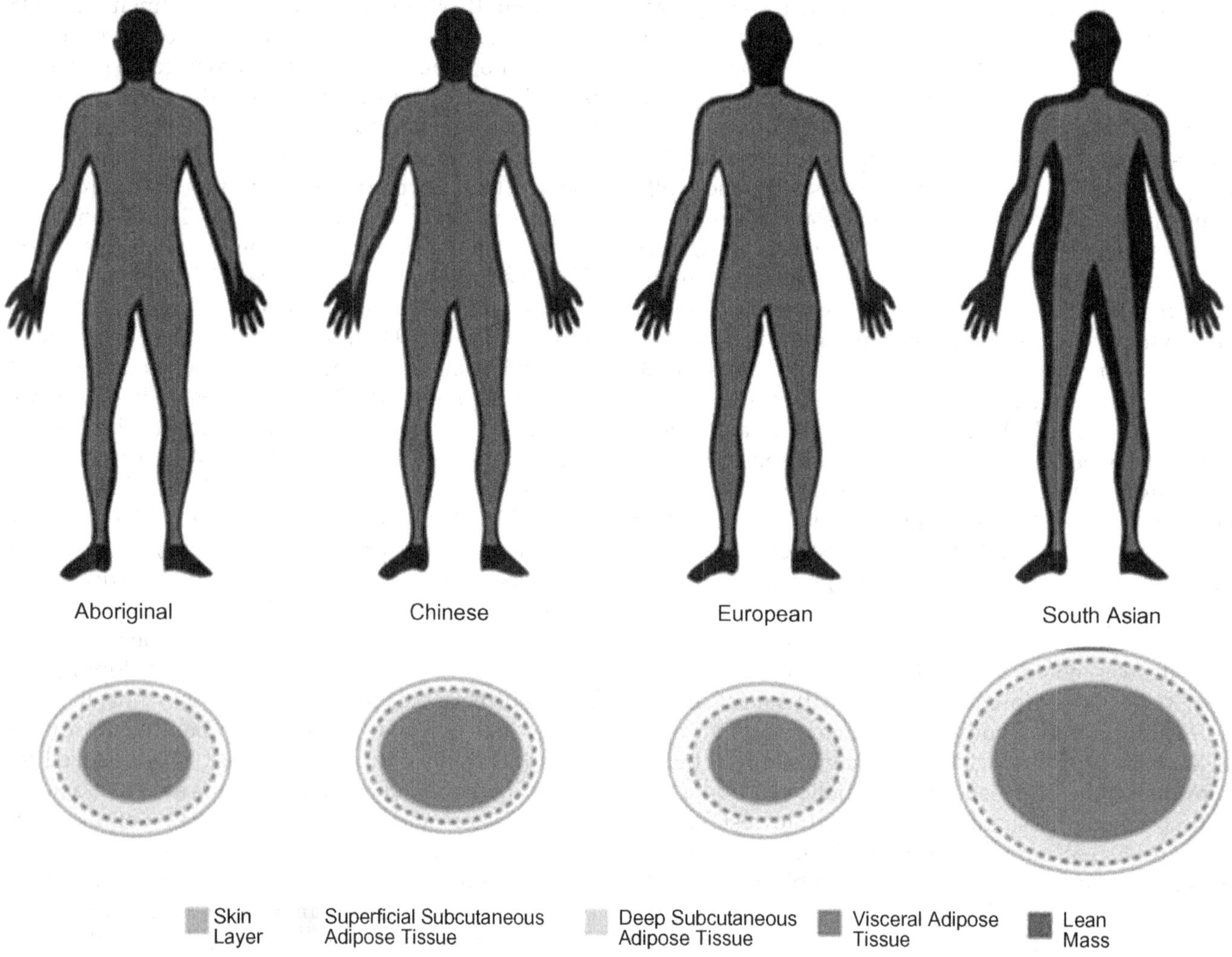

FIGURE 12.1 Ethnic differences in abdominal adipose tissue distribution. Schematic representation of adipose tissue and lean tissue mass (upper part) and cross-sectional area of abdominal adipose tissue (lower part) in individuals of Aboriginal, Chinese, European, and South Asian origin.

humerus breadth, smoking status, and physical activity revealed higher VAT among Chinese and South Asians than among Europeans [28]. Ethnic differences in abdominal adipose tissue corresponded to ethnic differences in cardiometabolic risk factors: after adjusting for age and sex, fasting insulin and homeostasis model assessment of insulin resistance (HOMA-IR) were higher among Aboriginals and South Asians compared to Europeans and Chinese [156]. Additionally, South Asians exhibited the lowest levels of HDL-C and the highest levels of triglycerides, triglyceride:HDL-C ratio, low-density lipoprotein cholesterol (LDL-C), and non-HDL-C [156].

The results of a substudy performed on the M-CHAT population, which focused exclusively on European and South Asian populations and their differences in abdominal SAT compartments, indicate that the amount of DSAT was significantly higher among South Asians compared to their European counterparts (Fig. 12.1), while no significant ethnic difference was observed for SSAT [63]. A more recent Canadian study, the Molecular Study of Health and Risk in Ethnic Groups, explored differences in abdominal fat distribution, as determined by MRI, between South Asians and white Caucasians [157]. The results of the study indicated that South Asians had less SSAT (as a percentage of their total abdominal fat) and more DSAT and VAT when compared to white Caucasians. Furthermore, South Asians had a greater maximum adipocyte diameter and area of adipocytes than did white Caucasians; they further exhibited greater cardiometabolic risk by having higher insulin concentrations, lower HDL-C, and lower adiponectin (adjusted for age, sex, and BMI) [157].

In a study from the United States that explored differences in body fat distribution and insulin resistance between healthy South Asians and Caucasian aged 20–65 years, of similar age and BMI, South Asians had more total abdominal fat and VAT than did Caucasians, while no statistically significant ethnic difference was observed for SAT [158]. Additionally, compared to Caucasians, South Asians had lower glucose disposal rates, measured by the euglycemic hyperinsulinemic clamp technique; higher levels of insulin, triglycerides, LDL-C, and plasminogen activator inhibitor 1 (PAI-1); and lower levels of HDL-C [158]. It has been demonstrated that increases in cardiometabolic risk factors among South Asians, compared to Europeans, are predominantly mediated by VAT, which is greater in South Asians [159]. Conversely, a study from Dallas, Texas, concluded that, compared to Caucasian men, South Asian men were more insulin resistant, with lower plasma adiponectin and higher plasma leptin levels, yet no significant ethnic difference in intraperitoneal fat was observed; interestingly, South Asians also had greater amounts of SAT than Caucasians at a similar BMI and a lower intraperitoneal fat-to-subcutaneous abdominal fat ratio [160]. Furthermore, the results of abdominal subcutaneous area adipose tissue biopsy revealed greater adipocyte cell size in the South Asian population compared to their Caucasian counterparts [160]. Consequently, the authors concluded that it is less likely that the increased insulin resistance among South Asians could be explained by the preferential accumulation of VAT [160].

A recently conducted large multicenter trial, the International Study of Prediction of Intra-Abdominal Adiposity and its Relationship with Cardiometabolic Risk/Intra-Abdominal Adiposity (INSPIRE ME IAA), recruited 4097 patients between 2006 and 2008 by 297 physicians in 29 countries within Asia, Europe, Latin America, and North America. The participants were classified into five ethnic groups [whites, African Caribbean blacks (non-Hispanic blacks), Hispanics (non-black North and Latin American Hispanics), East Asians (mainly from China, Japan, and Korea), and Southeast Asians (mainly from Malaysia and Vietnam)] and assessed for body composition (SAT, SSAT, DSAT, and VAT), using CT, and cardiometabolic risk [30]. In both men and women, the largest VAT area was observed among white patients, while the smallest VAT area was among East Asians. Similarly, East Asian men and women had lowest SAT, SSAT, and DSAT. The DSAT: SSAT ratio was highest among white and Hispanic male patients and lowest among East Asian men and Southeast Asian women; however, the VAT:SAT ratio was highest in East Asians compared to patients from other ethnic groups [30]. Furthermore, with respect to cardiometabolic risk factors, while no ethnic difference was observed for triglycerides, East Asians had the highest concentrations of HDL-C and the lowest HOMA-IR levels and high-sensitivity C-reactive protein (hs-CRP) concentrations [30].

Many investigators have reported lower VAT among African-American men [30,161–167] and women [30,163, 165,166,168–172] compared to their white counterparts. A higher accumulation of VAT among whites was observed for any level of total body fat, supporting the notion that whites are more prone to VAT accumulation than are African-Americans [162]. These results are also supported by several additional studies observing lower VAT among African-American women compared to white women; however, the ethnic differences in these studies did not reach statistical significance [162,173–178]. In contrast, there are two studies in which VAT among African-American women was higher on average than that of white women; however, in these studies, African-American women had significantly higher BMIs than did white women [161,164]. Moreover, many investigators have observed higher amounts of SAT among African-American men [179,180] and women [161–165,167,171,176–178] compared to that of white men and women. Among women, both SSAT and DSAT were significantly higher in African-Americans than in whites [176]. However, among obese individuals, women of African ancestry, compared to white women, had on average higher SAT, higher SSAT, and lower VAT, while no difference was observed for DSAT [181,182]. Lower VAT and higher SAT in African-American men and women, compared to their white counterparts, persisted even after adjusting for age and total adipose tissue [179,180]. Conversely, several groups did not find ethnic differences in SAT between African-American and white men [30,161–167] and women [30,166,168–170,173–175]. Additionally, compared to whites, while a lower VAT:SAT ratio was observed among African-American men [30,179] and women [30,161,165,170,177], no such ethnic difference in VAT:SAT ratio was noted for either men [161,165,166] or women [166,174,178]. Despite their lower levels of VAT, African-American women are characterized by a more favorable cardiometabolic risk profile than are white women; African-American women were observed to have higher HDL-C [168,174], lower levels of triglycerides [162,163,168,172–174,177], apolipoprotein B (ApoB) [162], blood glucose [168,169,174,175], and insulin [176]. Similarly, a more favorable cardiometabolic profile was noted in African-American men than in white men [162]. Thus, this more favorable cardiometabolic profile among African-Americans may be explained by their lower VAT and their higher postheparin lipoprotein lipase (LPL) and lower postheparin hepatic lipase activity [162]. However, some research groups have not detected an ethnic difference in glucose, insulin, and HOMA-IR [171,178] or in lipids [169,176] between African-American and white women, and no difference in glucose, insulin, and HOMA-IR between African-American and white men [163]. In contrast, a very few investigators had observed higher levels of fasting insulin [163,177] and HOMA-IR [163] in African-American compared to white women. African-American women were more insulin resistant than their white counterparts even when matched for age, degree of obesity, and WHR [173]. Similarly, in the Insulin Resistance Atherosclerosis Study, African-Americans were more insulin resistant compared to whites after adjusting for obesity, body fat distribution, and behavioral factors [183]. In addition, African-American men and women were found to be more insulin resistant than their Hispanic and white counterparts for any level of intraperitoneal adiposity [167]. Furthermore, studies that explored differences in abdominal adipose tissue between African-Americans and Hispanics reported lower VAT [95,166,167] and VAT:SAT ratios [95,166] among African-American men and women compared to their Hispanic counterparts. Despite their higher levels of VAT, Hispanics were observed to be more insulin sensitive than African-Americans [95]; however, some studies found no significant ethnic difference in insulin [167] and HOMA-IR [30,167] between Hispanics and African-Americans.

Ethnic differences in abdominal adipose tissue and cardiometabolic risk may lead to differences in the association between abdominal adipose tissue and insulin resistance among different ethnicities; this topic is discussed next.

ETHNIC DIFFERENCES IN THE ASSOCIATION BETWEEN ABDOMINAL ADIPOSE TISSUE AND INSULIN RESISTANCE

Evidence indicates that there are significant ethnic differences in the association between abdominal adipose tissue and insulin resistance. In the INSPIRE ME IAA study [30], increases in DSAT and VAT were associated with a greater odds ratio of metabolic syndrome in both men and women; however, while no ethnic difference in these associations was observed for women, there were significant ethnic differences in the association between DSAT and metabolic syndrome for men. In particular, for one standard deviation increase in DSAT, the odds of meeting the criteria for metabolic syndrome among East Asian male patients were 6%, 48%, 60%, and 70% higher than those of their Southeast Asian, white, Hispanic, and African Caribbean black counterparts, respectively [30]. Similarly, although not reaching statistical significance for ethnic differences, increases in VAT resulted in a higher odds ratio of metabolic syndrome among East Asian men and women compared to their Hispanic and white counterparts. These findings are interesting, given the fact that patients of East Asian origin are observed to have lowest levels of DSAT and VAT compared to African Caribbean black, Hispanic, Southeast Asian, and white patients [30]. These findings suggest that ethnic differences in cardiometabolic risk may not necessarily stem from the ethnic differences in the amount of abdominal fat tissue within the depots; rather, they may originate from ethnic differences in the susceptibility to DSAT and VAT deposition for a given amount of total or abdominal body fat. Indeed, despite having the lowest levels of DSAT and VAT, East Asians showed the largest increase in VAT per 1 kg/m^2 increase in BMI compared to African Caribbean blacks, Hispanics, and Southeast Asians [30]. Furthermore, in the substudy of the Multiethnic Cohort Study that recruited equal numbers of Japanese and white women (aged 60–65 years) across all ranges of BMI, greater VAT adiposity was observed among Japanese than among white women with similar levels of overall adiposity [184]. Moreover, in a study that looked at differences in abdominal fat distribution between Japanese and Caucasian American men aged 40–49 years, Japanese men had less VAT on average compared to their Caucasian counterparts; however, once VAT was compared at similar levels of WC (i.e. WC quartiles), at each WC level, VAT amount in Japanese subjects was greater than in Caucasian Americans [185].

In a study from Chennai, India, VAT, but not SAT, was associated with metabolic syndrome in South Indians without T2DM after adjusting for age, sex, and BMI [186]. This is consistent with an earlier published study by Banerji et al. [187], who found a significant association between VAT and insulin resistance, while no such association reached significance for SAT. In contrast, in another recent study from India in which 100 healthy adults without known heart disease or diabetes were recruited and assessed for abdominal adipose tissue (using MRI) and metabolic syndrome, SAT was found to be a more significant predictor of metabolic syndrome, compared to VAT [89]. Although this study showed that both SAT and VAT were significantly associated with metabolic syndrome, once both were inserted into the same model, VAT no longer showed a significant association with metabolic syndrome [89]. Similarly, among participants of the M-CHAT study, after adjusting for confounders, the association between VAT and metabolic syndrome was stronger than that between SAT and metabolic syndrome among Aboriginals, Chinese, and Europeans; however, SAT showed a stronger association with metabolic syndrome than did VAT among South Asians [124].

From the aforementioned studies investigating ethnic-specific differences in body fat distribution and cardiometabolic risk, it can be seen that South Asians have a greater susceptibility toward central obesity and have more SAT and VAT compared to their ethnic counterparts. South Asians tend to have higher levels of cardiometabolic risk factors, and the prevalence of metabolic syndrome in this group is higher than in other ethnic groups. Furthermore, insulin resistance has been observed among South Asians at BMI levels considered to be "healthy" (i.e. <25 kg/m^2) [188]. Thus, we are left asking the question: What can explain these ethnic differences in body fat distribution and cardiometabolic risk? It is thought that such clinical and biochemical characteristics commonly found among South Asians are attributable to the "Asian Indian phenotype" or the "thin-fat phenotype" [189,190]. The "thin-fat phenotype" refers to a relatively low BMI, but with increased total, subcutaneous, and central (truncal and abdominal) body fat [191]. There is evidence that the "thin-fat phenotype" of South Asians is present from birth, is more prevalent among South Asian than Caucasian babies, and continues to persist into childhood [192–194]. Furthermore, this phenotype has been shown to be preserved in South Asian newborns of the fourth to fifth generation after migration from India to another country [195]. According to results of the M-CHAT study, at any given body fat mass, South Asian adults have less lean mass than their Aboriginal, Chinese, and European counterparts (Fig. 12.1); additionally, after adjusting for age, South Asian men and women have significantly higher fat to lean mass ratio (F:LM) than do men and women of Aboriginal, Chinese, and European origins [196]. Moreover, the higher levels of insulin and HOMA-IR observed among South Asians, compared to Chinese and Europeans, persisted after adjusting for age, height, humerus breadth (a proxy for frame size), diet, and physical activity; however, the additional adjustment for F:LM resulted in differences in insulin and HOME-IR among South Asian, Chinese, and European men and women being no longer significant, suggesting that greater insulin resistance among South Asians may be largely attributed to their higher F:LM compared to other ethnic groups [196]. Also of interest, Sniderman et al. [197] put forward "the adipose tissue overflow hypothesis," which states that differences in cardiometabolic risk between South Asians and whites are founded in ethnic differences in the primary adipose tissue compartment, the SSAT compartment, which is present throughout the body and constitutes the majority of adipose tissue in the lower limb. According to the adipose tissue overflow hypothesis, the SSAT compartment is better developed and larger in whites than in South Asians, who consequently have a reduced capacity to store fatty acids in the SSAT. As obesity develops, South Asians fill up SSAT with fatty acids quicker than do whites, and fatty acids start to "overflow" into the DSAT and VAT secondary compartments, which are not meant to withstand larger amounts of adipose tissue. This results in the development of cardiometabolic complications at lower absolute masses of adipose tissue in South Asians compared to whites [197]. In addition, Wells suggests that the ethnic differences in adipose tissue biology originate in evolutionary interactions between diverse agricultural practices and local climate conditions [198]. For instance, individuals originally from tropical areas tend to have less developed adipose tissue compartments; thus, the overflow of adipose tissue upon accumulation spills into less well-developed compartments (DSAT and VAT) [197].

With respect to African-American populations, in the Jackson Heart Study elevated VAT levels were significantly associated with metabolic syndrome in black adults aged 21–94 years [199]. Similarly, in the Framingham Heart Study elevated VAT was associated with an adverse metabolic risk profile and metabolic syndrome among the white population [97]. That said, significant differences in abdominal adipose tissue depots and insulin resistance were observed among African-Americans and whites: as discussed earlier, on average, African-Americans had lower VAT, higher SAT, and were more insulin resistant than their white counterparts. Insulin sensitivity in blacks is lower than in whites for all levels of body fat and abdominal fat area [200]. Furthermore, higher insulin resistance was noted among both lean and obese women of African ancestry [182,200]. In both African-American and white women, higher VAT was found to be associated with lower insulin action, lower glucose disposal, and higher levels of fasting insulin [173]. Other reports also indicate no ethnic differences in the association between VAT with insulin action [95,174] and insulin and HOMA [96,171]. In spite of this, there is no evidence of an association between VAT and insulin, the insulin:glucose ratio [169], or insulin sensitivity [182,200] among black women, while such relationships were seen among white women. Furthermore, other reports indicate that in African-Americans, but not in whites, SAT has a negative correlation with insulin action [173]. Among African-American and white women aged 42–52 years, participants of the Study of Women's Health Across the Nation Heart study, both SAT and VAT were found to be positively associated with insulin resistance; however, in African-American, but not in white women, at the highest amounts of VAT, higher amounts of SAT were associated with lower insulin resistance [96]. With regards to the subcompartments of SAT, both SSAT and DSAT correlate with insulin sensitivity in both black and white populations [182,200].

Low VAT but higher insulin resistance among black individuals of African ancestry seems to contradict the established positive association between VAT and insulin resistance. Despite previous hypothesis that the increased prevalence of insulin resistance in blacks may be due to higher adipose tissue lipolysis rates, there is no strong evidence to suggest that differences in insulin resistance between whites and blacks can be explained by ethnic differences in adipose tissue lipolysis [201]. Although it has been shown within the group of black individuals that those with higher VAT are more insulin resistant, a link between high levels of insulin resistance and low VAT observed in blacks and not in whites suggests that factors other than excess VAT may play a significant role in driving insulin resistance among black populations [173]. It has recently been shown that gluteal adipose tissue may play a vital role in the development of insulin resistance among blacks: that is, higher gluteal fat mass associated with lower insulin sensitivity in black individuals, while no such association was observed in white individuals [182]. Furthermore, gluteal adipocyte size was found to be larger in black than in white women [201], and was positively associated with insulin resistance in black but not in white women [172]. Moreover, it has recently been shown that in black individuals more than in white, obesity impairs gluteal SAT adipogenesis and storage, potentially leading to insulin resistance and an increased risk of T2DM in blacks [181]. Consequently, although gluteofemoral SAT was shown to be associated with lower cardiometabolic risk [202], this protective role of gluteal SAT may not hold for black individuals.

CONCLUSIONS

We have presented evidence for substantial ethnic and racial differences in abdominal adipose tissue distribution, the prevalence of insulin resistance, and the association between abdominal adipose tissue and insulin resistance. Some challenges in ethnicity research have also been identified, such as the lack of standardized scientific classification of ethnicity, inconsistent approaches for assessing ethnicity, and the lumping together of ethnicity and race, despite these terms representing two distinct concepts. Additionally, a major challenge in clinical research is the lack of normal values and measurement instruments for specific ethnic groups, given that the ones in current use are predominantly derived from research on white/European populations [154]. Specifically, with regards to metabolic syndrome, current standard WC cutoffs may not be appropriate for all ethnic groups worldwide [203]. Moreover, ethnic-specific WC cutoff values that have already been proposed have not always been validated against direct imaging data of visceral fat and clinical outcomes, indicating that further work on defining high-risk abdominal obesity in various ethnicities is warranted [53].

Given the increasing ethnic/racial diversity worldwide, and especially in high-income countries such as Australia, Canada, the United Kingdom, and the United States, standardized and consistent methods for assessing ethnicity/race would enable the collection of higher quality data and allow direct comparisons to be made among research studies [117]. Furthermore, specific biological, behavioral, social, and cultural factors should also be assessed in order to capture multiple dimensions of ethnicity/race [121]. This comprehensive assessment of ethnicity/race may shed more light on the mechanisms underlying the ethnic/racial differences in disease risk factors and diseases, and guide the development and implementation of targeted disease prevention and treatment strategies.

References

[1] World Health Organization. Obesity and overweight. Fact sheet no. 311. <http://www.who.int/mediacentre/factsheets/fs311/en/>; 2013 [accessed 11.04.13].

[2] National Institutes of Health. Clinical guidelines on the identification, evaluation, and treatment of overweight and obesity in adults. The evidence, report No. 98-4083; September 1998.

[3] Lau DCW, Douketis JD, Morrison KM, Hramiak IM, Sharma AM, Ur E. Obesity Canada Practice Guidelines Expert Panel. 2006 Canadian clinical practice guidelines on the management and prevention of obesity in adults and children (summary). CMAJ 2007;176(8 Suppl.):S1–S13.

[4] Bray GA, Bouchard C, James WPT, editors. Handbook of obesity. New York: Marcel Dekker; 1988.

[5] Despres JP, Lemieux I, Prud'homme D. Treatment of obesity: need to focus on high risk abdominally obese patients. BMJ 2001;322:716–20.

[6] Jensen MD. Role of body fat distribution and the metabolic complication of obesity. J Clin Endocrinol Metab 2008;93(11 Suppl.):S57–63.

[7] Vague J. La Differenciation sexuelle, facteur determinant des forms de l'obesite. Presse Med 1947;55:339–40.

[8] Lapidus L, Bengtsson C, Larsson B, Pennert K, Rybo K, Sjostrom L. Distribution of adipose tissue and risk of cardiovascular disease and death: a 12 year follow up of participants in the population study of women in Gothenburg, Sweden. BMJ 1984;289(6454):1257–61.

[9] Larsson B, Svardsudd K, Welin L, Wilhelmsen L, Bjorntrop P, Tibblin G. Abdominal adipose tissue distribution, obesity, and risk of cardiovascular disease and death: 13 year follow up of participants in the study of men born in 1913. BMJ 1984;288(6428):1401–4.

[10] Donahue RP, Bloom E, Abbott R, Reed D, Yano K. Central obesity and coronary heart disease in men. Lancet 1987;329(8537):821–4.

[11] Ducimetiere P, Richard J, Cambien F. The pattern of subcutaneous fat distribution in middle-aged men and the risk of coronary heart disease: the Paris Prospective Study. Int J Obes 1986;10(3):229–40.

[12] Ohlson LO, Larsson B, Svardsudd K, Welin L, Eriksson L, Wilhelmsen L, et al. The influence of body fat distribution on the incidence of diabetes mellitus. 13.5 years of follow-up of the participants in the study of men born in 1913. Diabetes 1985;34(10):1055–8.

[13] Wajchenberg BE. Subcutaneous and visceral adipose tissue: their relation to metabolic syndrome. Endocr Rev 2000;21(6):697–738.

[14] Freedland ES. Role of critical visceral adipose tissue thresholds (CVATT) in metabolic syndrome: implications for controlling for dietary carbohydrates: a review. Nutr Metab 2004;1:12.

[15] Ibrahim MM. Subcutaneous and visceral adipose tissue: structural and functional differences. Obes Rev 2010;11:11–18.

[16] Reaven GM. Bunting lecture 1988. Role of insulin resistance in human disease. Diabetes 1988;1988(37):1595–607.

[17] Reaven GM. Role of insulin resistance in human disease (syndrome X): an expanded definition. Annu Rev Med 1993; 44:121–31.

[18] Ferranini E, Mari A. How to measure insulin sensitivity. J Hypertens 1998;16(7):895–906.

[19] Alberti KG, Zimmet PA. Definition, diagnosis and classification of diabetes mellitus and its complications. Part 1: Diagnosis and classification of diabetes mellitus provisional report of a WHO consultation. Diabet Med 1998;15:539–53.

[20] Adult Treatment Panel III. Executive summary of The Third Report of The National Cholesterol Education Program (NCEP) Expert Panel on detection, evaluation, and treatment of high blood cholesterol in adults (Adult Treatment Panel III). JAMA 2001;285:2486–97.

[21] Alberti KG, Zimmet P, Shaw J. The metabolic syndrome—a new worldwide definition. Lancet 2005;366:1059–62.

[22] De Simone G, Devereux RB, Chinali M, Best LG, Lee ET, Galloway JM, et al. for the Strong Heart Study Investigators. Prognostic impact of metabolic syndrome by different definitions in a population with high prevalence of obesity and diabetes. Diabetes Care 2007;30(7):1851–6.

[23] Aguilar-Salinas CA, Rojas R, Gomez-Perez FJ, Valles V, Rios-Torres JM, Franco A, et al. High prevalence of metabolic syndrome in Mexico. Arch Med Res 2004;35(1):76–81.

[24] Moebus S, Hanisch JU, Aidelsburger P, Bramlage P, Wasem J, Jockel K-H. Impact of 4 different definitions used for the assessment of the prevalence of the metabolic syndrome in primary health care: The German Metabolic and Cardiovascular Risk Project (GEMCAS). Cardiovasc Diabetol 2007;6:22.

[25] Cameron AJ, Magliano DJ, Zimmet PZ, Welborn T, Shaw JE. The metabolic syndrome in Australia: prevalence using four definitions. Diabetes Res Clin Pract 2007;77(3):471–8.

[26] Lioudaki E, Vrentzos GE, Mavrogeni H, Zeniodi M-H, Ganotakis ES, Mikhailidis DP, et al. Prevalence of metabolic syndrome according to different definitions in a hypertensive population. Angiology 2012;63:39–47.

[27] Vinluan CM, Zreikat HH, Levy JR, Cheang KI. Comparison of different metabolic syndrome definitions and risks of incident cardiovascular events in elderly. Metabolism 2012;61(3):302–9.

[28] Lear SA, Humphries KH, Kohli S, Chockalingam A, Frohlich JJ, Birmingham CL. Visceral adipose tissue accumulation differs according to ethnic background: results of the Multicultural Community Health Assessment Trial (M-CHAT). Am J Clin Nutr 2007;86(2):353–9.

[29] Alberti KGMM, Eckel RH, Grundy SM, Zimmet PZ, Cleeman JI, Donato KA, et al. Harmonizing the metabolic syndrome. A joint interim statement of the International Diabetes Federation Task Force on Epidemiology and Prevention; National Heart, Lung and Blood Institute; American Heart Association; World Heart Federation; International Atherosclerosis Society; and International Association for the Study of Obesity. Circulation 2009;120:1640–5.

[30] Nazare JA, Smith JD, Borel AL, Haffner SM, Balkau B, Ross R, et al. Ethnic influences on the relations between abdominal subcutaneous and visceral adiposity, liver fat, and cardiometabolic risk profile: the International Study of Prediction of Intra-Abdominal Adiposity and Its Relationship With Cardiometabolic Risk/Intra-Abdominal Adiposity. Am J Clin Nutr 2012; 96:714–26.

[31] Ford ES, Li C, Sattar N. Metabolic syndrome and incident diabetes: current state of evidence. Diabetes Care 2008;31(9):1898–904.

[32] Gupta AK, Prieto-Merino D, Dahloft B, Sever PS, Roulter NRon behalf of the ASCOT investigators. Metabolic syndrome, impaired fasting glucose and obesity, as predictors of incident diabetes in 14120 hypertensive patients of ASCOT-BPLA: comparison of their relative predictability using a novel approach. Diabet Med 2011;28:941–7.

[33] Hivert MF, Dusseault-Belanger F, Cohen A, Courteau J, Vanasse A. Modified metabolic syndrome criteria for identification of patients at risk of developing diabetes and coronary heart diseases: longitudinal assessment via electronic health records. Can J Cardiol 2012;28(6):744–9.

[34] Salminen M, Kuoppamaki M, Vahlberg T, Raiha I, Irjala K, Kivela SL. Metabolic syndrome defined by modified International Diabetes Federation criteria and type 2 diabetes mellitus risk: a 9-year follow-up among the aged in Finland. Diab Vasc Dis Res 2013;10(1):11–16.

[35] Ford ES. Risk of all-cause mortality, cardiovascular disease, and diabetes associated with the metabolic syndrome: a summary of the evidence. Diabetes Care 2005;28(7):1769–78.

[36] Galassi A, Reynolds K, He J. Metabolic syndrome and risk of cardiovascular disease: a meta-analysis. Am J Med 2006; 119(10):812–9.

[37] Gami AS, Witt BJ, Howard DE, Erwin PJ, Gami LA, Somers VK, et al. Metabolic syndrome and risk of incident cardiovqascular events and death: a systematic review and meta-analysis of longitudinal studies. JACC 2007;49(4):403–14.

[38] Li W, Ma D, Liu M, Liu H, Feng S, Hao Z, et al. Association between metabolic syndrome and risk of stroke: a meta-analysis of cohort studies. Cerebrovasc Dis 2008;25(6):539–47.

[39] Motillo S, Filion KB, Genest J, Joseph L, Pilote L, Poirier P, et al. The metabolic syndrome and cardiovascular risk: a systematic review and meta-analysis. JACC 2010;56(14):1113–32.

[40] Schmidt C, Bergstrom GM. The metabolic syndrome predicts cardiovascular events: results of a 13-year follow-up in initially healthy 58-year old men. Metab Syndr Relat Disord 2012;10(6):394–9.

[41] Wu SH, Liu Z, Ho SC. Metabolic syndrome and all-cause mortality: a meta-analysis of prospective cohort studies. Eur J Epidemiol 2010;25(6):375–84.

[42] Lakka HM, Laaksonen DE, Lakka TA, Niskanen LK, Kumpusalo E, Tuomilehto J, et al. The metabolic syndrome and total and cardiovascular disease mortality in middle-aged men. JAMA 2002;288(21):2709–16.

[43] Ford ES, Giles WH, Mokdad AH. Increasing prevalence of the metabolic syndrome among U.S. adults. Diabetes Care 2004;27(10):2444–9.

[44] Ervin RB. Prevalence of metabolic syndrome among adults 20 years of age and over, by sex, age, race and ethnicity, and body mass index: United States 2003-2006. National Health Statistics Reports, Number 13, <http://www.cdc.gov/nchs/data/nhsr/nhsr013.pdf>; May 2009 [accessed 19.06.13].

[45] Ford ES, Li C, Zhao G. Prevalence and correlates of metabolic syndrome based on a harmonious definition among adults in the US. J Diab 2010;2:180–93.

[46] Riediger ND, Clara I. Prevalence of metabolic syndrome in the Canadian adult population. CMAJ 2011;183(15):E1127–34.

[47] Lim S, Shin H, Song JH, Kwak SH, Kang SM, Won Yoon J, et al. Increasing prevalence of metabolic syndrome in Korea: the Korean National Health and Nutrition Examination Survey for 1998-2007. Diabetes Care 2011;34(6):1323–8.

[48] Mohan V, Deepa M. The metabolic syndrome in developing countries. Diabetes Voice 2006;51:15–17.

[49] Misra A, Misra R, Wijesuriya M, Banerjee D. The metabolic syndrome in South Asians: continuing escalation and possible solutions. Indian J Med Res 2007;125:345–54.

[50] Misra A, Khurana L. Obesity and metabolic syndrome in developing countries. J Clin Endocrinol Metab 2008;93(11suppl1):S9–S30.

[51] Lao XQ, Zhang YH, Wong MCS, Xu YJ, Xu HF, Nie SP, et al. The prevalence of metabolic syndrome and cardiovascular risk factors in adults in southern China. BMC Public Health 2012;12:64.

[52] Shen J, Goyal A, Sperling L. The emerging epidemic of obesity, diabetes, and the metabolic syndrome in China. Cardiology Research and Practice 2012;2012:178675. http://dx.doi.org/10.1155/2012/178675.

[53] Despres JP, Lemieux I, Bergeron J, Pibarot P, Mathieu P, Larose E, et al. Abdominal obesity and the metabolic syndrome: contribution to global cardiometabolic risk. Arterioscl Thromb Vasc Biol 2008;28(6):1039–49.

[54] Wild SH, Byrne CD. The epidemiology of the metabolic syndrome and its association with diabetes, cardiovascular disease and other conditions. In: Byrne CD, Wild SH, editors. The metabolic syndrome. 2nd ed.. Oxford, UK: Wiley-Blackwell; 2011.

[55] Despres JP, Moorjani S, Lupien PJ, Tremblay A, Nadeau A, Bouchard C. Regional distribution of body fat, plasma lipoproteins, and cardiovascular disease. Arteriosclerosis 1990; 10:497–511.

[56] Ross R, Aru J, Freeman J, Hudson R, Janssen I. Abdominal adiposity and insulin resistance in obese men. Am J Physiol, Endocrinol Metab 2002;282:E657–63.

[57] Nieves DJ, Cnop M, Retzlaff B, Walden CE, Brunzell JD, Knopp RH, et al. The atherogenic lipoprotein profile associated with obesity and insulin resistance is largely attributable to intra-abdominal fat. Diabetes 2003;52:172–9.

[58] Carr DB, Utzschneider KM, Hull RL, Kodama K, Retzlaff BM, Brunzell JD, et al. Intra-abdominal fat is a major determinant of the National Cholesterol Education Program Adult Treatment Panel III Criteria for the metabolic syndrome. Diabetes 2004;53(8):2087–94.

[59] Lebovitz HE, Banerji MA. Point: visceral adiposity is causally related to insulin resistance. Diabetes Care 2005;28:2322–5.

[60] Tong J, Boyko EJ, Utschneider KM, McNeely MJ, Hayashi T, Carr DB, et al. Intra-abdominal fat accumulation predicts the development of the metabolic syndrome in non-diabetic Japanese-Americans. Diabetologia 2007;50(6):1156–60.

[61] Nakao YM, Miyawaki T, Yasuno S, Nakao K, Tanaka S, Ida M, Hirata M, et al. Intra-abdominal fat area is a predictor for new onset of individual components of metabolic syndrome: Metabolic syndrome and abdominal ObesiTy (MERLOT study). Proc Jpn Acad Ser B Phys Biol Sci 2012;88(8):454–61.

[62] Johnson D, Dixon AK, Abrahams PH. The abdominal subcutaneous tissue: computed tomographic, magnetic resonance, and anatomical observations. Clin Anat 1996;9:19–24.

[63] Kohli S, Sniderman AD, Tchernof A, Lear SA. Ethnic-specific differences in abdominal subcutaneous adipose tissue compartments. Obesity 2010;18(11):2177–83.

[64] Bjorntrop P. "Portal" adipose tissue as a generator of risk factors for cardiovascular disease and diabetes. Arterioscler Thromb Vasc Biol 1990;10:493–6.

[65] Bergman RN, Van Citters GW, Mittelman SD, Dea MK, Hamilton-Wessler M, Kin SP, Ellmerer M. Central role of the adipocyte in the metabolic syndrome. J Invest Med 2001;49(1):119–26.

[66] Hellmer J, Marcus C, Sonnefeld T, Arner P. Mechanisms for differences in lipolysis between human subcutaneous and omental fat cells. J Clin Endocrinol Metab 1992;75(1):15–20.

[67] Marin P, Andersson B, Ottoson M, Olbe L, Chowdhury B, Kvist H, Holm G, Sjostrom L, et al. The morphology and metabolism of intraabdominal adipose tissue in men. Metabolism 1992;41(11):1242–8.

[68] Arner P. Differences in lipolysis between human subcutaneous and omental adipose tissues. Ann Med 1995;27(4):435–8.

[69] Monzon JR, Basile R, Heneghan S, Udupi V, Green A. Lipolysis in adipocytes isolated from deep and superficial subcutaneous adipose tissue. Obes Res 2002;10(4):266–9.

[70] Zierath JR, Livingston JN, Thorne A, Bolinder J, Reynisdottir S, Lonnqvist F, et al. Regional difference in insulin inhibition of non-esterified fatty acid release from human adipocytes: relation to insulin receptor phosphorylation and intracellular signaling through the insulin receptor substrate-1 pathway. Diabetologia 1998;41(11):1343–54.

[71] Revnisdottir S, Dauzats M, Thorne A, Langin D. Comparison of hormone-sensitive lipase activity in visceral and subcutaneous human adipose tissue. J Clin Endocrinol Metab 1997;82 (12):4162–6.

[72] Garaulet M, Perex-Llamas F, Fuente T, Zamora S, Tebar FJ. Anthropometric, computed tomography and fat cell data in an obese population: relationship with insulin, leptin, tumor necrosis factor-alpha, sex hormone-binding globulin and sex hormones. Eur J Endocrinol 2000;143(5):657–66.

[73] Tchernof A, Belanger C, Morisset AS, Richard C, Mailloux J, Laberge P, et al. Regional differences in adipose tissue metabolism in women: minor effect of obesity and body fat distribution. Diabetes 2006;55(5):1353–60.

[74] Edens NK, Fried SK, Kral JG, Hirsch J, Leibel RL. In vitro lipid synthesis in human adipose tissue from three abdominal sites. Am J Physiol 1993;265(3Pt1):E374–9.

[75] Fried SK, Leibel RL, Edens NK, Kral JG. Lypolisis in intraabdominal adipose tissues of obese women and men. Obes Res 1993;1(6):443–8.

[76] Fujioka S, Matsuzawa Y, Tokunaga K, Tarui S. Contribution of intra-abdominal fat accumulation to the impairment of glucose and lipid metabolism in human obesity. Metabolism 1987;36 (1):54–9.

[77] Pouliot MC, Despres JP, Nadeau A, Moorjani S, Prud'Homme D, Lupien PJ, et al. Visceral obesity in men: associations with glucose tolerance, plasma insulin, and lipoprotein levels. Diabetes 1992;41(7):826–34.

[78] Fujimoto WY, Bergstrom RW, Boyko EJ, Chen KW, Leonetti DL, Newell-Morris L, et al. Visceral adiposity and incident coronary heart disease in Japanese-American men. The 10-year follow-up results of the Seattle Japanese-American Community Diabetes Study. Diabetes Care 1999;22(11):1808–12.

[79] Boyko EJ, Fujimoto WY, Leonetti DL, Newell-Morris L. Visceral adiposity and risk of type 2 diabetes: a prospective study among Japanese Americans. Diabetes Care 2000;23(4):465–71.

[80] Brochu M, Starling RD, Tchernof A, Matthewes DE, Garcia-Rubi E, Poehlman ET. Visceral adipose tissue is an independent correlate of glucose disposal in older obese postmenopausal women. J Clin Endocrinol Metab 2000;85(7):2378–84.

[81] Ross R, Freeman J, Hudson R, Janssen I. Abdominal obesity, muscle composition, and insulin resistance in premenopausal women. J Clin Endocrinol Metab 2002;87(11):5044–51.

[82] Gastaldelli A, Sironi AM, Ciociaro D, Positano V, Buzzigoli E, Giannessi D, et al. Visceral fat and beta cell function in non-diabetic humans. Diabetologia 2005;48:2090–6.

[83] Despres JP. Is visceral obesity the cause of the metabolic syndrome? Ann Med 2006;38(1):52–63.

[84] Hayashi T, Boyko E, McNeely MJ, Leonetti DL, Kahn SE, Fujimoto WY. Visceral adiposity, not abdominal subcutaneous fat area, is associated with an increase in future insulin resistance in Japanese Americans. Diabetes 2008;57:1269–75.

[85] Neeland IJ, Turer AT, Ayers CR, Powell-Wiley TM, Vega GL, Farzaneh-Far R, et al. Dysfunctional adiposity and the risk of prediabetes and type 2 diabetes in obese adults. JAMA 2012;308(11):1150–9.

[86] Abate N, Garg A, Peshock RM, Stray-Gundersen J, Grundy SM. Relationships of generalized and regional adiposity to insulin sensitivity in men. J Clin Invest 1995;96(1):88–98.

[87] Abate N, Garg A, Peshock RM, Stray-Gundersen J, Adams-Huet B, Grundy SM. Relationship of generalized and regional adiposity to insulin sensitivity in men with NIDDM. Diabetes 1996;45(12):1684–93.

[88] Goodpaster BH, Thaete FL, Simoneau JA, Kelley DE. Subcutaneous abdominal fat and thigh muscle composition predict insulin sensitivity independently of visceral fat. Diabetes 1997;46(10):1579–85.

[89] Goel K, Misra A, Vikram NK, Poddar P, Gupta N. Subcutaneous abdominal adipose tissue is associated with the metabolic syndrome in Asian Indians independent of intra-abdominal and total body fat. Heart 2010;96:579–83.

[90] Goodpaster BH, Kelley DE, Wing RR, Meier A, Thaete FL. Effects of weight loss on regional fat distribution and insulin sensitivity in obesity. Diabetes 1999;48(4):839–47.

[91] Barzilai N, She L, Liu B-Q, Vuguin P, Cohen P, Wang J, et al. Surgical removal of visceral fat reverses hepatic insulin resistance. Diabetes 1999;48:94–8.

[92] Gabriely I, Ma XH, Yang XM, Atzmon G, Rajala MW, Berg AH, et al. Removal of visceral fat prevents insulin resistance and glucose intolerance of aging: an adipokine-mediated process? Diabetes 2002;51(10):2951–8.

[93] Thorne A, Lonngvist F, Apelman J, Hellers G, Arner P. A pilot study of long-term effects of a novel obesity treatment: omentectomy in connection with adjustable gastric banding. Int J Obes Relat Metab Disord 2002;26(2):193–9.

[94] Klein S, Fontana L, Young VL, Coggan AR, Kilo C, Patterson BW, et al. Absence of an effect of liposuction on insulin action and risk factors for coronary heart disease. NEJM 2004;350:2549–57.

[95] Wagenknecht LE, Langefeld CD, Scherzinger AL, Norris JM, Haffner SM, Saad MF, et al. Insulin sensitivity, insulin secretion, and abdominal fat. The Insulin Resistance Atherosclerosis Study (IRAS) Family Study. Diabetes 2003;52:2490–6.

[96] Wildman RP, Janssen I, Khan UI, Thurston R, Barinas-Mitchell E, El Khoudary SR, et al. Subcutaneous adipose tissue in relation to subclinical atherosclerosis and cardiometabolic risk factors in midlife women. Am J Clin Nutr 2011;93:719–26.

[97] Fox CS, Massaro JM, Hoffmann U, Pou KM, Maurovich-Horvat P, Liu C-Y, et al. Abdominal visceral and subcutaneous adipose tissue compartments: association with metabolic risk factors in the Framingham Heart Study. Circulation 2007;116:39–48.

[98] Demerath EW, Reed D, Rogers N, Sun SS, Lee M, Choh AC, et al. Visceral adiposity and its anatomical distribution as predictors of the metabolic syndrome and cardiometabolic risk factor levels. Am J Clin Nutr 2008;88(5):1263–71.

[99] Tulloch-Reid MK, Hanson RL, Sebring NG, Reynolds JC, Premkumar A, Genovese DJ, et al. Both subcutaneous and visceral adipose tissue correlate highly with insulin resistance in African Americans. Obes Res 2004;12(8):1352–9.

[100] Preis SR, Massaro JM, Robins SJ, Hoffman U, Vasan RS, Irlbeck T, et al. Abdominal subcutaneous and visceral adipose tissue and insulin resistance in the Framingham Heart Study. Obesity 2010;18(11):2191–8.

[101] Porter SA, Massaro JM, Hoffmann U, Vasan RS, O'Donnel CJ, Fox CS. Abdominal subcutaneous adipose tissue: a protective fat depot? Diabetes Care 2009;32(6):1068–75.

[102] Cancello R, Zulian A, Gentilini D, Maestrini S, Barba AD, Invitti C, et al. Molecular and morphologic characterization of superficial and deep-subcutaneous adipose tissue subdivisions in human obesity. Obesity 2013. http://dx.doi.org/10.1002/oby.20417. [Epub ahead of print]

[103] Misra A, Garg A, Abate N, Peshock R, Stray-Gunderson J, Grundy S. Relationship of anterior and posterior subcutaneous abdominal fat to insulin sensitivity in nondiabetic men. Obes Res 1997;5:93–9.

[104] Kelley DE, Thate FL, Troost F, Huwe T, Goodpaster BH. Subdivisions of subcutaneous abdominal adipose tissue and insulin resistance. Am J Physiol Endocrinol Metab 2000;278:E941–8.

[105] Smith SR, Lovejoy JC, Greenway F, Ryan D, deJonge L, de la Bretonne J, et al. Contributions of total body fat, abdominal subcutaneous adipose tissue compartments, and visceral adipose tissue to the metabolic complications of obesity. Metabolism 2001;50(4):425–35.

[106] Markman B, Barton Jr FE. Anatomy of the subcutaneous tissue of the trunk and lower extremity. Plast Reconstr Surg 1987;80(2):248–54.

[107] Cruickshank JK, Beevers DG, editors. Ethnic factors in health and disease. Boston, MA: Wright; 1989.

[108] Hutchinson J, Smith AD. Introduction. In: Hutchinson J, Smith AD, editors. Ethnicity. Oxford and New York: Oxford University Press; 1996. p. 1–14.

[109] Baumann T. Defining ethnicity. The SAA Archeological Record, <http://gbl.indiana.edu/baumann/Baumann%202004%20-%20Defining%20Ethnicity.pdf>; September 2004 [accessed 19.06.13].

[110] Williams DR. Race/ethnicity and socioeconomic status: measurement and methodological issues. Int J Health Serv Plann Adm Eval 1996;26(3):483–505.

[111] Zhu S, Heymsfield SB, Toyoshima H, Wang Z, Pietrobelli A, Heshka S. Race-ethnicity-specific waist circumference cutoffs for identifying cardiovascular disease risk factors. Am J Clin Nutr 2005;81(2):409–15.

[112] Bertoni AG, Wong ND, Shea S, Ma S, Liu K, Preethi S, et al. Insulin resistance, metabolic syndrome, and subclinical atherosclerosis. The Multi-Ethnic Study of Atherosclerosis. Diabetes Care 2007;30(11):2951–6.

[113] Giardina EG, Sciacca RR, Akabas S, Flink LE, Moise N, Paul TK, et al. Relationship between cardiovascular disease knowledge and race/ethnicity, education and weight status. Clin Cardiol 2012;35(1):43–8.

[114] McKenney NR, Bennett CE. Issues regarding data on race and ethnicity: the Census Bureau experience. Public Health Rep 1994;109:16–25.

[115] Berreman GD. Race, caste, and other invidious distinctions in social stratification. Race Class 1972;13:385–414.

[116] Bhopal R. Glossary of terms relating to ethnicity and race: for reflection and debate. J Epidemiol Community Health 2004;58(6):441–5.

[117] Kaneshiro B, Geling O, Gellert K, Limmar L. The challenges of collecting data on race and ethnicity in a diverse multiethnic state. Hawaii Med J 2011;70(8):168–71.

[118] Jones CP. Race, racism, and the practice of epidemiology. Am J Epidemiol 2001;154(4):299–304.

[119] Cummins C, Winter H, Cheng K, Maric R, Silcocks P, Varghese C. An assessment of the Nam Pehchan computer program for the identification of names of South Asian ethnic origin. J Public Health Med 1999;21:401–6.

[120] Quan H, Wang F, Schopflocher D, Norris C, Galbraith D, Faris P, et al. Development and validation of a surname list to define Chinese ethnicity. Med Care 2006;44:328–33.

[121] Lin SS, Kelsey JL. Use of race and ethnicity in epidemiologic research: concepts, methodological issues, and suggestions for research. Epidemiol Rev 2000;22(2):187–202.

[122] Schmitt E. For 7 million people in census, one race category isn't enough. New York times, <http://www.nytimes.com/2001/03/13/us/for-7-million-people-in-census-one-race-category-isn-t-enough.html>; March 13, 2001 [accessed 19.06.13].

[123] Anand SS, Yi Q, Gerstain H, Lonn E, Jacobs R, Vuksan V, et al. Relationship of metabolic syndrome and fibrinolytic dysfunction to cardiovascular disease. Circulation 2003;108:420–5.

[124] Gasevic D, Kohli S, Lear SA. Visceral and subcutaneous abdominal adipose tissue and their association with metabolic syndrome in four ethnic groups. Can J Cardiol 2012;28(5 Suppl.):S172–3 abstract.

[125] McKeigue PM, Shah B, Marmot MG. Relation of central obesity and insulin resistance with high diabetes prevalence and cardiovascular risk in South Asians. Lancet 1991;337(8738):382–6.

[126] Chaturvedi N, McKeigue PM, Marmot MG. Resting and ambulatory blood pressure differences in Afro-Caribbeans and Europeans. Hypertension 1993;22:90–6.
[127] Tillin T, Forouhi N, Johnston DG, McKeigue PM, Chaturvedi N, Godsland IF. Metabolic syndrome and coronary heart disease in South Asians, African-Caribbeans and white Europeans: a UK population-based cross-sectional study. Diabetologia 2005;48:649–56.
[128] World Health Organization. Definition, diagnosis, and classification of diabetes mellitus and its complications. Report of a WHO consultation. Part 1: Diagnosis and classification of diabetes mellitus. Geneva: WHO; 1999.
[129] Barbato A, Cappuccio FP, Folkerd EJ, Strazzullo P, Sampson B, Cook DG, et al. Metabolic syndrome and renal sodium handling in three ethnic groups living in England. Diabetologia 2004;47:40–6.
[130] Grundy SM, Cleeman JI, Daniels SR, Donato KA, Eckel RH, Franklin BA, et al. Diagnosis and management of metabolic syndrome: an American Heart Association/National Heart, Lung, and Blood Institute scientific statement. Circulation 2005;112:2735–52.
[131] Unwin N, Bhopal R, Hayes L, White M, Patel S, Ragoobirsingh D, et al. A comparison of the new International Diabetes Federation of metabolic syndrome to WHO and NCEP definitions in Chinese, European and South Asian origin adults. Ethn Dis 2007;17:522–8.
[132] Khunti K, Taub N, Tringham J, Jarvis J, Farooqi A, Skinner TC, et al. Screening for the metabolic syndrome using simple anthropometric measurements in south Asian and white Europeans: A population-based screening study. The Leicester Ethnic Atherosclerosis and Diabetes Risk (LEADER) study. Prim Care Diabetes 2010;4(1):25–32.
[133] Ford ES, Giles WH, Dietz WH. Prevalence of the metabolic syndrome among US adults. Findings from the third National Health and Nutrition Examination Survey. JAMA 2002;287:356–9.
[134] St-Onge M-P, Janssen I, Heymsfield SB. Metabolic syndrome in normal-weight Americans. Diabetes Care 2004;27:2222–8.
[135] Carnethon MR, Loria CM, Hill JO, Sidney S, Savage PJ, Liu K. Risk factors for the metabolic syndrome. The Coronary Artery Risk Development in Young Adults (CARDIA) study, 1985–2001. Diabetes Care 2004;27(11):2707–15.
[136] Araneta MRG, Barrett-Connor E. Subclinical coronary atherosclerosis in asymptomatic Filipino and White women. Circulation 2004;110:2817–23.
[137] Tan CE, Ma S, Wai D, Chew SK, Tai ES. Can we apply the National Cholesterol Education Program Adult Treatment Panel definition of the metabolic syndrome to Asians? Diabetes Care 2004;27(5):1182–6.
[138] Rampal S, Mahadeva S, Guallar E, Bulgiba A, Mohamed R, Rahmat R, et al. Ethnic differences in the prevalence of metabolic syndrome: results from a Multi-ethnic Population-Based Survey in Malaysia. PLoS One 2012;7(9):e46365.
[139] Gupta A, Gupta R, Sarna M, Rastogi S, Gupta VP, Kothari K. Prevalence of diabetes, impaired fasting glucose and insulin resistance syndrome in an urban Indian population. Diabetes Res Clin Pract 2003;61(1):69–76.
[140] Gupta R, Sarna M, Thanvi J, Rastogi P, Kaul V, Gupta VP. High prevalence of multiple coronary risk factors in Punjabi Bhatia community: Jaipur Heart Watch-3. Indian Heart J 2004;56(6):646–52.
[141] Gupta R, Deedwania PC, Gupta A, Rastogi S, Panwar RB, Kothari K. Prevalence of metabolic syndrome in an Indian urban population. Int J Cardiol 2004;97(2):257–61.
[142] Gupta R, Sarna M, Thanvi J, Sharma V, Gupta VP. Fasting glucose and cardiovascular risk factors in an urban population. J Assoc Physicians India 2007;55:705–9.
[143] Chow CK, Naidu S, Raju K, Joshi R, Sullivan D, Celermajer DS, Neal BC. Significant lipid, adiposity and metabolic abnormalities amongst 4535 Indians from a developing region of rural Andhra Pradesh. Atherosclerosis 2008;196(2):943–52.
[144] Misra A, Wasir JS, Pandey RM. An evaluation of candidate definitions of the metabolic syndrome in adult Asian Indians. Diabetes Care 2005;28(2):398–403.
[145] Ramachandran A, Snehalatha C, Satyavani K, Sivasankari S, Vijay V. Metabolic syndrome in urban Asian Indian adults—a population study using modified ATP III criteria. Diabetes Res Clin Pract 2003;60(3):199–204.
[146] Yi Z, Jing J, Xiu-ying L, Hongxia X, Jianjung Y, Yuhong Z. Prevalence of the metabolic syndrome among rural original adults in NingXia, China. BMC Public Health 2010;10:140.
[147] Further Study of Risk Factors for Stroke and Coronary Heart Disease group. The prevalence of metabolic syndrome in a 11 provinces cohort in China. Zhonghua Yu Fang Yi Xue Za Zhi 2002;36(5):298–300.
[148] Yang W, Reynolds K, Gu D, Chen J, He J. A comparison of two proposed definitions for metabolic syndrome in the Chinese adult population. Am J Med Sci 2007;334(3):184–9.
[149] Fan JG, Cai XB, Li L, Li XJ, Dai F, Zhu J. Alcohol consumption and metabolic syndrome among Shanghai adults: a randomized multistage stratified cluster sampling investigation. World J Gastroenterol 2008;14(15):2418–24.
[150] Gu D, Reynolds K, Wu X, Chen J, Duan X, Reynolds RF, et alInterASIA Collaborative Group. Prevalence of the metabolic syndrome and overweight among adults in China. Lancet 2005;365(9468):1398–405.
[151] Fan JG, Zhu J, Li XJ, Chen L, Lu YS, Li L, et al. Fatty liver and the metabolic syndrome among Shanghai adults. J Gastroenterol Hepatol 2005;20(12):1825–32.
[152] Rojas R, Aguilar-Salinas CA, Jimenez-Corona A, Shamah-Levy T, Rauda J, Avila-Burgos L, et al. Metabolic syndrome in Mexican adults. Results from the National Health and Nutrition Survey 2006. Salud Publica Mex 2010;52(Suppl. 11):S11–8.
[153] Isordia-Salas I, Santiago-German D, Rodriguez-Navarro H, Almaraz-Delgado M, Leanos-Miranda A, Anaya-Gomez F, et al. Prevalence of metabolic syndrome components in an urban Mexican sample: comparisons between two classifications. Exp Diabetes Res 2012;2012:202540. http://dx.doi.org/10.1155/2012/202540.
[154] Tillin T, Forouhi NG. Metabolic syndrome and ethnicity. In: Byrne CD, Wild SH, editors. The metabolic syndrome. 2nd ed. Oxford, UK: Blackwell Publishing Ltd.; 2011.
[155] Lear SA, Birmingham CL, Chockalingam A, Humphries KH. Study design of the Multicultural Community Health Assessment Trial (M-CHAT): a comparison of body fat distribution in four distinct populations. Ethn Dis 2006;16(1):96–100.
[156] Gasevic D, Frohlich J, Mancini GBJ, Lear SA. The association between triglyceride to high-density-lipoprotein cholesterol ratio and insulin resistance in a multiethnic primary prevention cohort. Metabolism 2012;61(4):583–9.
[157] Anand SS, Tarnopolsky MA, Rashid S, Schulze KM, Desai D, Mente A, et al. Adipocyte hypertrophy, fatty liver and metabolic risk factors in south Asians: The Molecular Study of Health and Risk in Ethnic Groups (mol-SHARE). PLoS One 2011;6(7):e22112.
[158] Raji A, Seely EW, Arky RA, Simonson DC. Body fat distribution and insulin resistance in healthy Asian Indians and Caucasians. J Clin Endocrinol Metab 2001;86:5366–71.
[159] Lear SA, Chockalingam A, Kohli S, Richardson CG, Humphries KH. Elevation in cardiovascular disease risk in South Asians is mediated by differences in visceral adipose tissue. Obesity 2012;20:1293–300.
[160] Chandalia M, Lin P, Seenivasan T, Livingston EH, Snell PG, Grundy SM, et al. Insulin resistance and body fat distribution in

South Asian men compared to Caucasian men. PLoS one 2007;2(8):e812.
[161] Hill JO, Sidney S, Lewes CE, tolan K, Scherzinger AL, Stamm ER. Racial differences in amounts of visceral adipose tissue in young adults: the CARDIA (Coronary artery Risk Development in young Adults) study. Am J Clin Nutr 1999;69:381–7.
[162] Despres JP, Couillard C, Gagnon J, Bergeron J, Leon AS, Rao DC, Skinner JS, et al. Race, visceral adipose tissue, plasma lipids, and lipoprotein lipase activity in men and women: the Health, Risk Factors, Exercise Training, and Genetics (HERITAGE) Family Study. Arterioscler Thromb Vasc Biol 2000;20:1932–8.
[163] Vega GL, Adams-Huet B, Peshock R, Willett D, Shah B, Grundy SM. Influence of body fat content and distribution on variation in metabolic risk. J Clin Endocrinol Metab 2006;91:4459–66.
[164] Demerath EW, Sun SS, Rogers N, Lee M, Reed D, Choh AC, et al. Anatomical patterning of visceral adipose tissue: race, sex, and age variation. Obesity 2007;15(12):2984–93.
[165] Bray GA, Jablonski KA, fujimoto WY, Barrett-Connor E, Haffner S, Hanson RL, et al. Diabetes Prevention Program Research Group. Relation of central adiposity and body mass index to the development of diabetes in the Diabetes Prevention Program. Am J Clin Nutr 2008;87(5):1212–8.
[166] Carroll JF, Fulda KG, Chiapa AL, Rodriguez M, Phelps DR, Cardarelli KM, et al. Impact of race/ethnicity on the relationship between visceral fat and inflammatory biomarkers. Obesity 2009;17:1420–7.
[167] Guerrero R, Vega GL, Grundy SM, Browning JD. Ethnic differences in hepatic steatosis: an insulin resistance paradox. Hepatology 2009;49(3):791–801.
[168] Conway JM, Yanovski SZ, Avila NA, Hubbard VS. Visceral adipose tissue differences in black and white women. Am J Clin Nutr 1995;61:765–71.
[169] Perry AC, Applegate EB, Jackson ML, Deprima S, Goldberg RB, Ross R, et al. Racial differences in visceral adipose tissue but not anthropometric markers of health-related variables. J Appl Physiol 2000;89:636–43.
[170] Weinsier RL, Hunter GR, Gower BA, Schutz Y, Darnell BE, Zukerman PA. Body fat distribution in white and black women: different patterns of intraabdominal and subcutaneous abdominal adipose tissue utilization with weight loss. Am J Clin Nutr 2001;74:631–6.
[171] Kanaley JA, Giannopoulou I, Tillapaugh-Fay G, Nappi JS, Ploutz-Snyder LL. Racial differences in subcutaneous and visceral fat distribution in postmenopausal black and white women. Metabolism 2003;52(2):186–91.
[172] Tittlebach TJ, Berman DM, Nicklas BJ, Ryan AS, Goldberg AP. Racial differences in adipocyte size and relationship to the metabolic syndrome in obese women. Obes Res 2004;12(6):990–8.
[173] Lovejoy JC, de la Bretonne JA, Klemperer M, Tulley R. Abdominal fat distribution and metabolic risk factors: effect of race. Metabolism 1996;45(9):1119–24.
[174] Albu JB, Murphy L, Frager DH, Johnson JA, Pi-Sunyer FX. Visceral fat and race-dependent health risks in obese nondiabetic premenopausal women. Diabetes 1997;46:456–62.
[175] Marcus MA, Murphy L, Pi-Sunyer FX, Albu JB. Insulin sensitivity and serum triglyceride level in obese white and black women: relationship to visceral and truncal subcutaneous fat. Metabolism 1999;48(2):194–9.
[176] Lovejoy JC, Smith SR, Rood JC. Comparison of regional fat distribution and health risk factors in middle-aged white and African American women: The Healthy Transition study. Obes Res 2001;9(1):10–16.
[177] Berman DM, Rodrigues LM, Nicklas BJ, Ryan AS, Dennis KE, Goldberg AP. Racial disparities in metabolism, central obesity, and sex hormone-binding globulin in postmenopausal women. J Clin Endocrinol Metab 2001;86:97–103.
[178] Araneta MR, Barrett-Connor E. Ethnic differences in visceral adipose tissue and type 2 diabates: Filipino, African-American, and white women. Obes Res 2005;13(8):1458–65.
[179] Hoffman DJ, Wang Z, Gallagher D, Heymsfield SB. Comparison of visceral adipose tissue mass in adult African Americans and Whites. Obes Res 2005;13(1):66–74.
[180] Katzmarzyk PT, Bray GA, Greenway FL, Johnson WD, Newton Jr RL, Ravussin E, et al. Racial differences in abdominal depot-specific adiposity in white and African American adults. Am J Clin Nutr 2010;91:7–15.
[181] Goedecke JH, Evans J, Keswell D, Stimson RH, Livingstone DEW, Hayes P, et al. Reduced gluteal expression of adipogenic and lipogenic genes in black South African women is associated with obesity-related insulin resistance. J Clin Endocrinol Metab 2011;96(12):E2029–33.
[182] Hayes P, Adams K, Dave JA, Goedecke JH. Ethnic-specific associations between abdominal and gluteal fat distribution and the metabolic complications of obesity: implications for the use of liposuction. PlasticSurgIntJ2013(2013).http://dx.doi.org/10.5171/2013.796359.
[183] Haffner SM, D'Agostino R, Saad MF, Rewers M, Mykkanen L, Selby J, et al. Increased insulin resistance and insulin secretion in nondiabetic African-Americans and Hispanics compared with Non-Hispanic Whites. Diabetes 1996;45:742–8.
[184] Lim U, Ernst T, Buchtal SD, Latch M, Albright CL, Wilkens LR, et al. Asian women have greater abdominal and visceral adiposity than Caucasian women with similar body mass index. Nutr Diab 2011;1(5):e6.
[185] Kadowaki T, Sekikawa A, Murata K, Maegawa H, Takamiya T, Okamura T, et al. Japanese men have larger areas of visceral adipose tissue than Caucasian men in the same levels of waist circumference in a population-based study. Int J Obes 2006;30:1163–5.
[186] Sandeep S, Gokulakrishnan K, Velmurugan K, Deepa M, Mohan V. Visceral and subcutaneous abdominal fat in relation to insulin resistance and metabolic syndrome in non-diabetic south Indians. Indian J Med Res 2010;131:629–35.
[187] Banerji MA, Faridi N, Atluri R, Chaiken RL, Lebovitz HE. Body composition, visceral fat, leptin, and insulin resistance in Asian Indian men. J Clin Endocrinol Metab 1999;84:137–44.
[188] Snehalatha C, Viswanathan V, Ramachandran A. Cutoff values for normal anthropometric variables in Asian Indian adults. Diabetes Care 2003;26(5):1380–4.
[189] Deepa R, Sandeep S, Mohan V. Abdominal obesity, visceral fat and type 2 diabetes—"Asian Indian Phenotype". In: Mohan V, Gundu R, editors. Type 2 diabetes in South Asians; Epidemiology, risk factors and prevention. New Delhi: Jaypee Medical Publishers; 2006. p. 138–52.
[190] Gupta M, Singh N, Verma S. South Asians and cardiovascular risk: what clinicians should know. Circulation 2006;113:e924–9.
[191] Prasad DS, Kabir Z, Dash AK, Das BC. Abdominal obesity, and independent cardiovascular risk factor in Indian subcontinent: a clinic epidemiological evidence summary. J Cardiovasc Dis Res 2011;2(4):199–205.
[192] Yajnik CS, Fall CH, Coyaji KJ, Hirve SS, Rao S, Barker DJ, et al. Neonatal anthopometry: the thin-fat Indian baby. The Pune Maternal Nutrition Study. Int J Obes Relat Metab Disord 2003;27(2):173–80.
[193] Krishnaveni GV, Hill JC, Veena SR, Leary SD, Saperia J, Chachyamma KJ, et al. Truncal adiposity is present at birth and in early childhood in South Indian children. Indian Pediatr 2005;42(6):527–38.
[194] Kulkarni ML, Mythri HP, Kulkarni AM. 'Thinfat' phenotype in newborns. Indian J Pediatr 2009;76(4):369–73.
[195] Van Steijn L, Karamali NS, Kanhai HH, Ariëns GA, Fall CH, Yajnik CS, et al. Neonatal anthropometry: thin-fat phenotype in fourth to fifth generation South Asian neonates in Surinam. Int J Obes 2009;33(11):1326–9.

[196] Lear SA, Kohli S, Bondy GP, Tchernof A, Sniderman AD. Ethnic variation in fat and lean body mass and the association with insulin resistance. J Clin Endocrinol Metab 2009;94(12):4696–702.
[197] Sniderman AD, Bhopal R, Prabhakaran D, Sarrafzadegan N, Tchernof A. Why might South Asians be so susceptible to central obesity and its atherogenic consequences? The adipose tissue overflow hypothesis. Int J Epidemiol 2007;36:220–5.
[198] Wells JCK. Commentary: Why are South Asians susceptible to central obesity?—the El Nino hypothesis. Int J Epidemiol 2007; 36:226–7.
[199] Liu J, Fox CS, Hickson D, Bidulescu A, Carr JJ, Taylor HA. Fatty liver, abdominal visceral fat, and cardiometabolic risk factors. The Jackson Heart Study. Arterioscler Thromb Vasc Biol 2011;31:2715–22.
[200] Goedecke JH, Levitt NS, Lambert EV, Utzschneider KM, Faulenbach MV, Dave JA, West S, et al. Differential effects of abdominal adipose tissue distribution on insulin sensitivity in black and white South African women. Obesity 2009;17: 1506–12.
[201] Goedecke JH, Levitt NS, Evans J, Ellman N, Hume DJ, Kotze L, Tootla M, et al. The role of adipose tissue in insulin resistance in women of African ancestry. J Obes 2013;2013:952916.
[202] Monolopoulos KN, Karpe F, Frayn KN. Gluteofemoral body fat as a determinant of metabolic health. Int J Obes 2010;34:949–59.
[203] Crowther NJ, Norris SA. The current waist circumference cut points used for the diagnosis of metabolic syndrome in Sub-Saharan African Women is not appropriate. PLoS One 2012;7(11):e48883.

CHAPTER

13

Visceral Fat Predicts Ectopic Fat Accumulation Mechanisms and Health Consequences

Andrea P. Rossi, Francesco Fantin, Paolo Bertassello, Valeria Zanandrea, E. Sartori, and Mauro Zamboni

Division of Geriatric Medicine, University of Verona, Ospedale Maggiore, Verona, Italy

INTRODUCTION

Ultimately, interactions between many environmental factors, including an excess caloric balance due to increased food intake or a reduction in physical activity, within a predisposing genetic background lead to a particular type of obesity characterized by increased visceral adipose tissue. This type of obesity is associated with insulin resistance, atherogenic dyslipidemia, and metabolic syndrome. The chronic inflammatory state associated with predominantly central fat deposition associated with the production of metabolically active cytokines, the release of circulating free fatty acids (FFAs), the state of leptin resistance, and the reduction of adiponectin levels leads to increased lipolysis and the increased release of FFAs to tissues other than adipose (particularly the liver, pancreas, and muscles) and to a reduction in their oxidation and clearance capacity, and the consequent deposition of ectopic fat in these organs [1]. Organ dysfunction caused by lipotoxicity and lipoapoptosis, and the different mechanisms for altering insulin signaling lead, in the end, to the major manifestations of metabolic syndrome [2].

PREDICTORS OF ECTOPIC FAT DEPOSITION

In adulthood, fat tissue becomes increasingly dysfunctional. Fat cell size and body fat distribution change, insulin sensitivity decreases, the response to lipolytic agents declines, and inflammatory cytokine production by adipose tissue increases [3–5]. Since the late twentieth century, it has been reported that these changes are accompanied by the increased prevalence of diabetes, dyslipidemia, hypertension, and atherosclerosis, accompanied by lipid deposition and lipotoxicity in nonadipose tissues compartments [6].

In normal conditions, preadipocytes, which comprise 15–50% of cells within fat tissue, defend against lipotoxicity by sequestering circulating FFAs [5]. Preadipocytes, from which new fat cells develop throughout the life span and which reside in a high fatty acid microenvironment, are themselves increasingly subject to lipotoxicity. Decreased adipogenesis in response to fatty acids may contribute to this [7]. Preadipocyte aging results in lowered defenses against lipotoxicity related to inherent cellular aging processes such as DNA damage, the effects of reactive oxygen species, mitochondrial dysfunction, and cellular stress response pathway activation [7]. Preadipocyte susceptibility to lipotoxicity may directly contribute to fat tissue dysfunction, by impairing the capacity of fat tissue to protect nonadipose tissues from ectopic fat deposition, thus leading to lipotoxicity in the liver, pancreas, muscle, heart, and other organs.

During our life span, we observe a progressive increase in fat mass, which normally peaks at approximately 65 years of age in men and later in women [8]. This increase in total adiposity is independent of changes in body weight caused by concomitant decreases in muscle mass observed with aging, the so-called *sarcopenia* [9,10].

Body fat distribution also changes with age: visceral abdominal fat increases and decreased subcutaneous abdominal fat [9–11] is related to a reduced capacity of subcutaneous adipose tissue to act as a lipid store that can provide adequate circulating FFA uptake [12].

It has been proposed that dysregulation of lipid metabolism in subcutaneous adipocytes may partly

Nutrition in the Prevention and Treatment of Abdominal Obesity
http://dx.doi.org/10.1016/B978-0-12-407869-7.00013-1

explain not only the increase in visceral adiposity but also ectopic fat deposition within nonadipose tissue such as skeletal and cardiac muscle, liver, and pancreas (Fig. 13.1) [13–16]. Studies performed in mice confirm impaired lipid mobilization related to abnormalities in apolipoprotein gene expression [17]. Adipogenesis and impaired hydrolysis of triglycerides by intracellular adipocytes cause an imbalance in intracellular FFA esterification that results in a net release of FFAs into the systemic circulation [18].

Increased FFA delivery to other organs, especially when combined with defective FFA oxidation, leads to ectopic triglyceride storage in these organs, thus contributing to lipotoxicity and systemic dysfunction [19].

Ectopic Fat Deposition in Liver

It has been shown that aging is associated with lipid accumulation within the hepatocytes [20], although a stronger independent association has been particularly observed between obesity and visceral fat accumulation [14,15]. Recent findings have shown that central obesity, particularly visceral adipose tissue accumulation [21–23], can be more strongly related to hepatic steatosis than body mass index (BMI), but all of the factors influencing ectopic lipid accumulation in the liver have not yet been identified.

Abdominal adipose tissue includes different anatomical depots, i.e. the subcutaneous fat depot and the visceral fat depot, which can be subclassified as intraperitoneal or retroperitoneal [24]. Subcutaneous fat differs from visceral fat in that venous drainage from subcutaneous fat is directed into the systemic circulation, whereas venous drainage from visceral fat is directed into the portal vein. Visceral fat directly releases FFAs and adipokines, thereby exposing the liver to fat accumulation [25].

Using methods involving tracers, Nielsen et al. found a direct association between the amount of visceral fat and the release of FFAs to the liver [26].

In a recent study, an association between ectopic deposition of fat in the liver and deep subcutaneous adipose tissue, but not with superficial subcutaneous adipose tissue, was observed [14]. Some studies involving imaging techniques to determine the abdominal fat mass have reported a significant association between nonalcoholic fatty liver disease and subcutaneous adipose tissue [21,27,28], while others found no relationship [22,29,30]. Different metabolic roles for deep subcutaneous adipose tissue and superficial adipose tissue have previously been demonstrated [31,32] For example, Kelley et al. [31] observed that deep subcutaneous adipose tissue, but not superficial subcutaneous adipose tissue, is strongly associated with peripheral insulin resistance and features of insulin resistance in nondiabetic subjects. Myazaki et al. [32] showed an association between deep subcutaneous adipose tissue and indexes of hepatic insulin resistance in males but not in females. Rossi et al. observed a significant association between lipid infiltration of the liver and deep subcutaneous adipose tissue, but not superficial subcutaneous adipose tissue, regardless of gender [14]. Adipocytes present in deep subcutaneous adipose tissue have increased lipolytic activity compared to those in superficial subcutaneous adipose tissue [33], which could partly explain the relationship among insulin resistance, hepatic fat depots, and deep subcutaneous adipose tissue [32].

An association has been shown between dietary fat and ectopic fat deposition in the liver and pancreas. These results are in line with previous studies demonstrating that the exposure of the liver to FFAs due to lipid intake in the diet is a determining factor in increased lipid content in the liver. The exposure to fatty acids may be due to the contribution of dietary fat and the release of FFAs from abdominal fat, especially from visceral adipose tissue [34], resulting in the deposition of ectopic fat in the liver and pancreas. This hypothesis was recently confirmed by Fraulob et al. in a murine model in which obesity is induced by excess caloric intake. In this study, they demonstrate that mice fed high-fat meals have increased deposition of ectopic fat in both the liver and pancreas [35]. Gender differences have been observed in the degree of lipid infiltration into the liver. In fact, men usually present with higher postprandial levels of plasma triglycerides and FFAs compared to women [36].

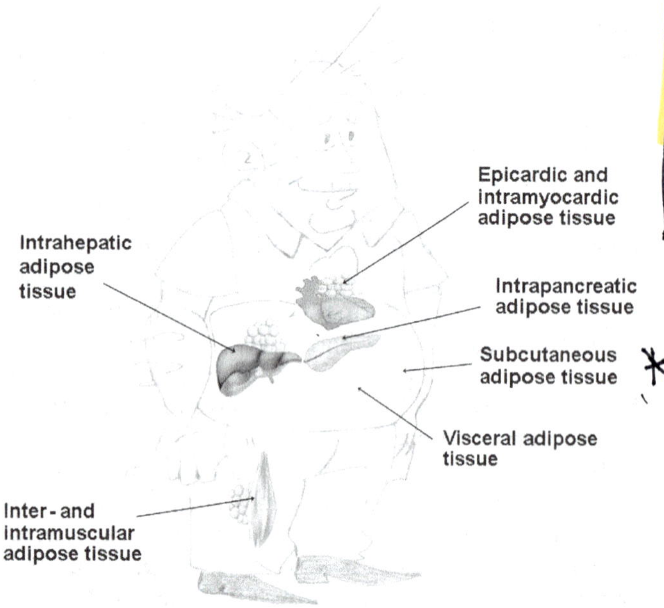

FIGURE 13.1 Ectopic fat deposition in obese subject. Different sites of ectopic fat deposition shown in an obese subject.

Ectopic Fat Deposition in Muscle

In muscle, we can distinct between two different lipid depots: intermuscular adipose tissue, which is mainly composed of triglycerides interspersed with adipocytes and located between muscle fibers (these are also known as *extramyocellular lipids*); and intramyocellular lipids, which are located within muscle fibers in the form of cytosolic triacylglycerols [37,38]. The size of both depots increases with age [39] and is associated with decreased muscle strength and mobility limitations in elderly men and women independent of age, race, and obesity [40–42]. Elderly adults show altered mitochondrial activity along with increased adiposity, oxidative stress, and insulin resistance independent of obesity [43]. In an animal model, Korach-André et al. showed that the high-fat diet-induced increase in intramyocellular lipid was strongly related to fat accumulation in the abdominal area and increased insulin resistance [44], although a causal relationship has not yet been established. However, this finding is unsurprising considering recent reports that intramyocellular lipids and visceral adipose tissue accumulation are both present at an early stage in the development of peripheral insulin resistance in obese young subjects [45].

Lipid Deposition in the Pancreas

In recent years, great attention has been devoted to lipid infiltration of the pancreas; it has been suggested that fat deposition in and around beta cells is involved in altering pancreatic function [46] and in the development of type 2 diabetes mellitus (T2DM) [47,48].

In a study using computed tomography (CT) in more than 2000 subjects of wide age range, Saisho et al. showed that after 60 years of age, both total and parenchymal pancreas volumes gradually decline, while pancreatic fat volume increases linearly with aging, leading to an increase in the fat:functional parenchyma ratio in both genders [49]. In the same study, the authors examined the effect of BMI on pancreas volume and confirmed that the pancreas parenchymal volume increases in line with obesity, with a concomitant accumulation of fat that is greater (by nearly 70%) in overweight and obese compared with lean subjects.

Previously studies only partly addressed the relationship between the release of FFAs from adipose tissue and visceral lipid accumulation in the pancreas. However, recent studies showed that body fat distribution, in particular visceral fat deposition, is the main predictor of ectopic fat deposition in the pancreas [14,50]. In a recent study analyzing the accumulation of fatty acids and their composition in mice fed with a high-fat diet (and a control group), it was discovered that the triglycerides present in the pancreas were composed of fatty acids of a similar profile to that of visceral adipose tissue [51].

An association between pancreatic lipid content, evaluated using a chemical shift technique, and visceral adipose tissue, evaluated by magnetic resonance imaging, has been observed [14]. A previously reported strong association between pancreatic lipid content, evaluated using an ultrasound method, and visceral adipose tissue has been observed in a cross-sectional study [50]. Associations between pancreatic fat accumulation and liver fat content, quantified by an opposed-phase magnetic resonance imaging technique, have been observed in a population of obese, but otherwise healthy, individuals. However, after adjusting for potential confounding variables, these associations were found to be largely mediated by the amount of visceral adipose tissue [52].

A negative correlation between adiponectin and hepatic lipid content and pancreatic fat has been shown [53,54]. Adiponectin is believed to protect hepatocytes from the accumulation of triglycerides, probably by increasing the beta-oxidation of FFAs and/or reducing the de novo production of FFAs in hepatocytes [55]. In a relatively large study, involving 80 patients with nonalcoholic fatty liver disease, lower levels of adiponectin were independently associated with nonalcoholic steatohepatitis (NASH) [54]. In another study, adiponectin levels were lower in the 174 patients with nonalcoholic fatty liver disease compared to 42 controls, and correlated inversely with steatosis in 116 patients undergoing liver biopsy [56]. These data could explain the lower degree of lipid infiltration in the liver in female subjects, who usually show higher levels of adiponectin, even after adjustment for BMI [57].

Cardiac Fat Deposition

More recently, great interest has been also focused on fat depots in and around the heart, i.e. intramyocardial and epicardial fat, respectively.

Despite a relation between age and intramyocardial lipid levels, i.e. the storage of triglyceride droplet within cardiomyocytes, it is unclear whether a relation also exists with obesity [58,59]. This fat depot has important health consequences: it has been shown to be associated with left ventricular thickness and heart failure [58]. In fact, it has been hypothesized that increased lipid content cause increased production of reactive oxygen species and ceramides, which leads to cardiac remodeling and cardiomyocytes apoptosis, and a consequent reduction in contractility [58,59]. Epicardial adipose tissue, i.e. fat located between the myocardium and pericardium, is reported to be strongly associated with abdominal adiposity and, from an anatomical point of view, is considered as visceral fat inside the thoracic region. In studies of middle-aged and older groups, no relation between this depot and aging was generally observed [60,61]. Conversely, studies with a wide range of age groups reported a positive association [62].

Human studies have shown that epicardial fat is positively associated with left ventricular hypertrophy and with coronary artery disease [61–63–70].

WEIGHT LOSS, VISCERAL FAT, AND ECTOPIC FAT DEPOSITION

Several studies showed that even moderate weight loss improves metabolic complications of obesity [63,64]. This may be due to the preferential loss of visceral compared to subcutaneous fat [9,65], or to a reduction in ectopic fat content [66–68]. In fact, it has been demonstrated that ectopic fat deposition (i.e. liver, pancreas, and muscle fat infiltration) significantly contributes to the insulin resistance and metabolic alterations observed in obese subjects [66].

It was recently shown in a murine model that impaired glucose homeostasis and insulin resistance are associated with hepatosteatosis [68] and triglyceride hyperaccumulation in the pancreas [10] consequent to long-term high-fat feeding. Using CT at the midthigh level, Mazzali et al. observed a significant decrease in muscle lipid content after moderate weight loss in obese sedentary subjects [66,67]. Using magnetic resonance, Colles et al. [69] observed a significant decline in liver volume (a proxy of liver fat infiltration) after a mean weight loss of 10% in obese subjects. In eight obese subjects with T2DM, Petersen et al. [70] observed that a weight loss of 8 kg normalized fasting glucose; this improvement was associated with an 81% decline in intrahepatic lipid content.

There is a general lack of reported studies evaluating the effect of weight loss on multiple organ ectopic fat depots. In a weight loss intervention study on a population of 24 obese subjects, variations in liver lipid infiltration was shown to be positively correlated with variations in visceral adipose tissue, deep subcutaneous adipose tissue, and high-sensitivity C-reactive protein (CRP), while lipid infiltration into the pancreas was found to be positively related to changes in visceral adipose tissue. In the same population, a positive association between changes in liver and pancreatic lipid content was observed [71]. Using multiple regression models in which pancreatic and hepatic lipid content were considered as dependent variables and related variables considered as independent variables, altered visceral adipose tissue was the main predictor of changes in ectopic deposition in both organs, explaining 43.1% and 30.7%, respectively, of the variance [71].

Changes in liver fat content in a population of obese females following laparoscopic gastric banding surgery was evaluated by Philips and colleagues, who observed a significant decline in liver lipid infiltration after 3 months [72]. Similar results were observed by Hearth and colleagues in a population of 18 female obese subjects who underwent laparoscopic adjustable gastric banding surgery: they used magnetic resonance imaging (MRI) and magnetic resonance spectroscopy (MRS) to quantify abdominal subcutaneous and visceral adipose tissue areas and liver fat content before and 3 and 12 months after surgery [73].

HEALTH CONSEQUENCES OF VISCERAL ADIPOSE TISSUE AND ECTOPIC FAT DEPOSITION

Total body fat, and adipose tissue distribution in particular, has been shown to be strictly related to the pathogenesis of insulin resistance and T2DM. In epidemiological studies, visceral adipose tissue is considered a major risk factor for cardiovascular disease, stroke, metabolic syndrome, and death [74]. The mechanism linking visceral fat with the metabolic syndrome is not completely clear, but it has been shown that its anatomical location plays a role, leading to the so-called *portal effect*, consisting of increased FFA release directly into the portal vein [25]. Studies have shown that subcutaneous and visceral abdominal fat have biologically distinct roles, with visceral fat demonstrating greater proinflammatory characteristics compared to subcutaneous fat.

Adipose tissue is an active endocrine organ per se, secreting a wide variety of cytokines (referred to as adipokines) involved in inflammation and the dysregulation of insulin action [2]. Growing evidence supports the notion that high amounts of visceral fat are predictive of insulin resistance, and the presence of related metabolic abnormalities is commonly referred to as *metabolic syndrome* [75]. First, visceral adipose tissue shows resistance to the action of insulin and contributes, via portal circulation, to exposure of the liver to high concentrations of FFAs; this has several metabolic consequences, such as hyperinsulinemia, glucose intolerance, and hypertriglyceridemia.

Adipose tissue is a source of proinflammatory adipokines, which contribute both directly and indirectly to insulin resistance and a thrombotic and hypertensive state, which forms a characteristic feature of visceral obesity. Excess visceral fat is considered a marker of the relative incapacity of subcutaneous adipose tissue to act as a protective metabolic sink because of its inability to expand (lipodystrophy) or because it has become dysfunctional and insulin resistant, with consequent ectopic fat deposition [76].

Since the late twentieth century, in addition to regional adipose tissue distribution and the causative role of adipokines in metabolic abnormalities in obese subjects, attention has also focused on the infiltration of ectopic lipids. Ectopic fat usually increases in obese and diabetic subjects, and may itself be responsible for relevant clinical consequences. Ectopic fat is defined as the storage of triglycerides within cells outside of adipose tissue as a result of excess food intake and a sedentary lifestyle [77]. This infiltration is caused by a failure of the homeostatic system of lipid metabolism inside white adipocytes, which in normal conditions should prevent lipotoxicity in the organs [78]. The mechanisms that lead to homeostatic failure are multiple and probably act in a synergistic way and include increased caloric intake in the diet, a reduction in lipid oxidation, and alterations to the adipogenesis processes [78]. The deposition of ectopic fat is therefore an important pathophysiological process that is associated with cell dysfunction and death in the tissues in which it is present. This phenomenon is defined as lipotoxicity and lipoapoptosis [79].

Ectopic fat deposition has often been shown to be simultaneous with and to contribute to a worsening glycometabolic profile. Liver fat is elevated in insulin-resistant subjects [80]; furthermore, it is strongly correlated with the amount of visceral fat in the prediabetic population [81]. In addition, intramuscular adipose tissue is a well-known marker of insulin resistance [82]. Therefore, the determination of visceral fat and ectopic fat depots at the liver and muscle level is thought to be a predictor for cardiovascular disease, T2DM, and insulin resistance.

Recently, Taira et al. [83] showed that lipid deposition in various sites within skeletal muscle and the liver shows a correlation with visceral fat accumulation in a population of middle-aged Japanese men affected by metabolic syndrome. In the same population, they also showed that antidiabetic medication has various effects on fat deposition in the different ectopic sites. In fact, after weight loss visceral fat and liver ectopic fat was mobilized faster compared to other depots, such as intra- and intermuscular fat, suggesting that they are controlled by different regulatory mechanisms.

Lipid Infiltration of the Liver

Ectopic lipid deposition in the liver leads to the commonly observed hepatic steatosis, also known as nonalcoholic fatty liver disease (NAFLD), a clinical condition predisposing to cirrhosis and liver failure [84]. Visceral obesity and insulin resistance represent the most important risk factors for the development of NAFLD [85]. NAFLD is associated with increased hepatic insulin resistance and is very common in patients with metabolic syndrome [86]. NAFLD can thus be considered an early predictor of metabolic disorders, even in the normal weight population [87], and early detection of NAFLD could have benefits in clinical practice.

The prevalence of NAFLD increases by 74% in obese and 90% in obese subjects with metabolic morbidity [88]. Recent studies have shown that visceral adipose tissue is the most important factor in the genesis of hepatic steatosis, compared to BMI [21,22]. The causes of NAFLD have not yet been fully elucidated, but it is well known that the intake of dietary fat, the release of FFAs from adipose tissue, and de novo lipogenesis in the liver cells are involved in this process. The mechanism by which the fatty liver leads to insulin resistance has not been clarified, but lipid intermediate products seem to play a major role. The increase in diacylglycerol activates serine protein kinase F, which blocks the activation of insulin receptor substrate 1 (IRS-1) and IRS-2, and in turn reduces the activation of phosphoinositide 3-kinase (PI3K) and Akt [79]. Therefore, glycogen accumulation is reduced and endogenous glucose production is increased, contributing to the development of impaired glucose tolerance and T2DM. Hepatic insulin resistance is also associated with raised serum insulin levels, which stimulate de novo lipogenesis and in turn contribute to a further increase in hepatic steatosis. In some studies performed in animal models, it was observed that insulin can increase the expression of sterol regulatory element-binding protein 1c (SREB-1c), which activates the transcription of many genes involved in lipogenesis [89]. Lipid infiltration of the liver, as well as insulin resistance, is implicated in the development of inflammatory lesions of the liver.

It is well known, in fact, that NAFLD can develop from NASH and hepatitis. Although the pathogenesis of the latter is not yet fully elucidated, it has been suggested that, following the accumulation of fatty acids, oxidative stress plays an important role. An imbalance between oxidants (reactive oxygen intermediates) and antioxidant agents has been observed in NAFLD patients, and this can lead to lipid peroxidation [90]. It follows, therefore, that direct cellular damage with a subsequent amplified response of the immune system leads to inflammation and collagen hyper production and results in progressive fibrosis [91]. Excessive oxidation of FFAs in hepatocytes causes oxidative damage to these cells through mitochondrial dysfunction and induction of hepatic cytochrome P450 2E1 (CYP2E1) [92]. CYP2E1is therefore increased in the hepatocytes of patients with NASH; as ketones and FFAs are substrates of this cytochrome, this would result in their increased expression. Cell damage in turn induces the production of tumor necrosis factor (TNF-α), which has a central role in the development of the inflammatory response [93], thus transforming a reversible metabolic event, such as hepatic steatosis, into a condition of permanent damage.

Lipid Infiltration of the Pancreas

In the study of metabolic abnormalities related with obesity, ectopic fat deposition in the pancreas, also known as *fatty pancreas* or *nonalcoholic fatty pancreas disease* [94], has gained much attention since the early 2000s. It has been observed that obese and/or elderly subjects show a higher prevalence of nonalcoholic fatty pancreas compared to young nonobese subjects. From a histological point of view, such infiltration is both interlobular and intralobular, with the presence of perilipin-positive adipocytes within the pancreatic tissue. Immunohistochemical studies have demonstrated that lipid deposits primarily accumulate in adipocytes that are present among exocrine cells [95], but also take the form of triglyceride droplets within the pancreatic cells. In obese subjects, increased lipolysis causes high levels of circulating FFAs, and hepatic insulin resistance also causes the release of triglyceride-rich particles from the liver; in association with the altered production of adipokines, these particles seem to participate to lipid infiltration of the pancreas. Studies in humans have confirmed, through evaluation with MRI, the presence of fat in the pancreatic parenchyma, and a correlation between visceral obesity and lipid infiltration of the pancreas, as well as between lipid infiltration of the pancreas and insulin resistance [50]. In fact, numerous studies have identified a relationship between high levels of FFAs and pancreatic beta cell dysfunction [46]. Several mechanisms have been proposed to explain this dysfunction, including FFAs reducing insulin production by altering the expression of the proinsulin gene, and the possibility that long-chain fatty acyl-CoA may mediate the harmful effects of FFAs on beta cells. Long-chain fatty acyl-CoA can activate adenosine triphosphate (ATP)-sensitive potassium channels and hyperpolarize beta cells, thus making glucose-mediated depolarization more difficult by reducing glucose-mediated insulin secretion. Reserves of long-chain fatty acyl-CoA may cause a reduction in the activity of specific isoforms of protein kinase F, thus suppressing the incretin effect on insulin secretion [86]. In addition, it seems that palmitate induces apoptosis of beta cells, with a consequent reduction of their proliferative capacity: high levels of palmitate correlate with the de novo synthesis of ceramides, which are implicated in the apoptotic pathways of many cells, including pancreas beta cells [96].

In summary, therefore, lipid infiltration of pancreatic islets causes a reduction in insulin secretion and a progressive reduction in beta cells mass and increased susceptibility to the development of T2DM. It has been observed in fact that in T2DM patients, the percentage of pancreatic fat is almost twice that of nondiabetic subjects (20.4% vs 9.7%) [46].

It has been shown that fatty pancreas may promote the development of chronic pancreatitis [97,98] and pancreatic cancer [94] and exacerbate the severity of acute pancreatitis [97,98]. Moreover, fatty pancreas facilitates the dissemination and lethality of pancreatic cancer [99], and the formation of pancreatic fistulas after pancreatic surgery [100,101]. Pancreatic fat replacement associated with acinar cell death and pancreatic fat infiltration due to obesity both contribute to pancreatic steatosis [97]. In addition, it has been suggested that fatty pancreas could play a role in T2DM. In rats, chronic exposure to a high-fat diet induces both interlobular and intralobular fat accumulation, inflammatory cell infiltration, and fibrosis in the pancreas, thus causing damage to the normal pancreatic architecture and islets [102]. Likewise, C57BL/6 mice fed a high-fat diet develop insulin resistance and features of both NAFLD and fatty pancreas [35–103]. In human studies, pancreatic fat content is closely associated with BMI [104], insulin resistance [21,50], metabolic syndrome [50,104], and hepatic fat content [104–107]. However, only a few studies have evaluated the relationship between fatty pancreas and beta cell function, and these show conflicting results: some indicate that pancreatic lipid content is negatively associated with insulin secretion in nondiabetic subjects [46] or individuals with prediabetes [108], while others suggest that there is no relationship between beta cell function and pancreatic fat in prediabetic or type 2 diabetic subjects [46].

Recently, in a large-scale study of Chinese subjects, Ou and colleagues confirmed that both NAFLD and fatty pancreas are associated with diabetes independent of age, gender, adiposity, and other cardiometabolic risk factors. Moreover, they observed a relationship between prediabetes status and both pancreatic fat infiltration and glycometabolic profile [109].

Intramyocardial and Epicardial Lipid Infiltration

The mechanisms by which abdominal obesity, and in particular visceral fat deposition, can negatively influence cardiac function are not completely understood, but it has been proposed that ectopic fat deposition in and around the heart can lead to so-called *cardiac lipotoxicity* [110]. This phenomenon is caused by different pathological mechanisms that directly and indirectly affect cardiac muscle function.

Intra- and extramyocellular fat in the heart are closely related with visceral fat deposition in both animals [111] and humans [58]. Fat accumulation in the myocardium is associated with left ventricle hypertrophy and dysfunction. In fact, the contractile function of myocardium seems to be negatively influenced by lipid infiltration, as evaluated with magnetic resonance spectroscopy [58]. Fat deposition inside the myocardium is also related with heart anatomical remodeling and, in particular, with left ventricle concentric hypertrophy. Excess pericardial fat is also associated with cardiac remodeling and is considered to be a novel indicator of cardiovascular risk [112]. This fat depot shares with visceral fat the capacity to secrete cytokines, with the amount being related to intra-abdominal adipose tissue quantity.

Recent evidence supports the finding that the amount of epicardial adipose tissue, measured by multidetector computer tomography, is strongly associated with the incidence of atrial fibrillation, independent of traditional risk factors including left atrial enlargement [113]. This result has been confirmed in a large population from the Framingham Heart Study: pericardial fat volume was associated with atrial fibrillation even after adjusting for BMI and others risk factors [114]. In particular, it has been shown that the amount of periatrial fat is a better prognostic predictor of future atrial fibrillation episodes compared with the amount of whole epicardial adipose tissue [115].

Lipid Infiltration of Skeletal Muscle

Lipid accumulation in human skeletal muscle was described for the first time in 1976 by Dagenais et al. through their analysis of forearm muscle biopsy samples

[116]. Subsequently, microscopic methods were developed that used specific dyes for quantifying fat located within the cell in the form of intramyocellular lipids. It has been shown that fat can be stored at the ectopic level not only in tissues such as skeletal muscle but also in organs such as the liver and pancreas [117]. However, until the advent of magnetic resonance spectroscopy, studies into the effects of lipid infiltration on muscle biochemistry were limited to an analysis of skeletal muscle biopsy specimens.

It has been demonstrated that the lipid infiltration of muscle is associated with negative effects on metabolism and function. The first to propose a correlation between lipid infiltration and muscle insulin resistance was Falholt et al. in 1985, who conducted a study in hyperinsulinemic dogs, which showed an increased triglyceride content in muscle compared to levels in normoglycemic controls [117]. A possible relation between insulin resistance and muscle lipid infiltration was proposed by Falholt and colleagues for the first time in 1988 that measured a significantly higher triglyceride content within the rectus abdominis muscle of patients with T2DM compared to a healthy control group [117]. Subsequent studies have confirmed significant association between insulin resistance and the accumulation of intracellular muscular adipose tissue, in both animal models and humans [118]. Kelley and colleagues [119] showed in obese patients that muscle lipid infiltration, as assessed by CT scans measured at the midthigh was a better predictor of insulin resistance than was visceral adiposity or subcutaneous fat.

The existence of a close relationship between insulin resistance and lipid infiltration of the muscle seems to contradict the "metabolic athlete's paradox" [120]. In fact, higher lipid content has been demonstrated in the muscles of highly trained athletes, despite good peripheral insulin sensitivity [120]. This physiological phenomenon, referred to as the *metabolic paradox* may be due to the balance between the availability of fatty acids into the circulation and their cellular uptake and oxidation [120]. Intracellular muscular fat is in fact a readily available source of energy during exercise and its reduction during prolonged and intense muscle activity; it is stored in the more oxidative type I muscle fibers [121].

In 2001, Goodpaster et al. demonstrated that the association between the intramuscular lipid content and insulin sensitivity in athletes was influenced by the oxidative capacity of skeletal muscle itself. It has been hypothesized that the increased capacity of glucose transport in the skeletal muscle of trained subjects may facilitate the synthesis of intracellular triglycerides and at the same time increase the sensitivity to insulin. The increase in muscle intracellular fat observed in sedentary individuals is caused by an increased caloric intake, especially of the fat component, and a sedentary lifestyle, and is not due to muscle training [120].

Lipid infiltration adversely affects not only the muscle metabolic profile but also muscle function, and has been implicated in the onset of disability in the elderly. A reduction in muscle strength represents an important risk factor for a decline in physical performance and the appearance of genuine disability. With aging has been documented a progressive loss of strength and muscle mass [122], along with a reduction in type II muscle fibers and a decrease in contractile force [123]. In addition to these phenomena, muscle lipid infiltration is also associated with aging, and this is considered to be a causative factor in the age-related loss of muscle mass and strength, known as *sarcopenia* [40]. Such lipid infiltration may lead to changes in contractility, muscle fiber recruitment, and muscle metabolism. However, the exact mechanism through which the lipid infiltration affects muscle strength and function remains largely unknown.

References

[1] Deprés JP, Lemieux I, Bergeron J, Pibarot P, Mathieu P, Larose E. Abdominal obesity and the metabolic syndrome: contribution to global cardiometabolic risk. Arterioscler Thromb Vasc Biol 2008;28:1039–49.

[2] Unger RH. Lipotoxic diseases. Annu Rev Med 2002;53:319–36.

[3] Dax EM, Partilla JS, Gregerman RI. Mechanism of the age-related decrease of epinephrine stimulated lipolysis in isolated rat adipocytes: β-adrenergic receptor binding, adenylate cyclase activity, and cyclic AMP accumulation. J Lipid Res 1981;22:934–43.

[4] Kirkland JL, Dobson DE. Preadipocyte function and aging: links between age-related changes in cell dynamics and altered fat cell function. J Amer Geriatr Soc 1997;45:959–67.

[5] Kirkland JL, Tchkonia T, Pirtskhalava T, Han J, Karagiannides I. Adipogenesis and aging: Does aging make fat go MAD? Exp Gerontol 2002;37:757–67.

[6] Unger RH. Lipid overload and overflow: metabolic trauma and the metabolic syndrome. Trends Endocrinol Metab 2003;14:398–403.

[7] Guo W, Pirtskhalava T, Tchkonia T, et al. Aging results in paradoxical susceptibility of fat cell progenitors to lipotoxicity. Am J Physiol Endocrinol Metab 2007;292:E1041–51.

[8] Prentice AM, Jebb SA. Beyond body mass index. Obes Rev 2001;2:141–7.

[9] Zamboni M, Armellini F, Harris T, et al. Effects of age on body fat distribution and cardiovascular risk factors in women. Am J Clin Nutr 1997;66:111–5.

[10] Gallagher D, Ruts E, Visser M, et al. Weight stability masks sarcopenia in elderly men and women. Am J Physiol Endocrinol Metab 2000;279:E366–75.

[11] Enzi G, Gasparo M, Biondetti PR, Fiore D, Semisa M, Zurlo F. Subcutaneous and visceral fat distribution according to sex, age, and overweight, evaluated by computed tomography. Am J Clin Nutr 1986;44:739–46.

[12] Uranga AP, Levine J, Jensen M. Isotope tracer measures of meal fatty acid metabolism: reproducibility and effects of the menstrual cycle. Am J Physiol Endocrinol Metab 2005;288:E547–55.

[13] Despres JP, Lemieux I. Abdominal obesity and metabolic syndrome. Nature 2006;444:881–7.

[14] Rossi AP, Fantin F, Zamboni GA, Mazzali G, Rinaldi CA, Del Giglio M, et al. Predictors of ectopic fat deposition in liver and pancreas in obese men and women. Obesity 2011;19:1747–54.

[15] Machann J, Thamer C, Schnoedt B, Stefan N, Stumvoll M, Haring HU, et al. Age and gender related effects on adipose

tissue compartments of subjects with increased risk for type 2 diabetes: a whole body MRI/MRS study. MAGMA 2005;18:128–37.

[16] Rabkin SW. Epicardial fat: properties, function and relationship to obesity. Obes Rev 2007;8:253–61.

[17] Sepe A, Tchkonia T, Thomou T, Zamboni M, Kirkland JL. Aging and regional differences in fat cell progenitors—a mini-review. Gerontology 2011;57:66–75.

[18] Araki S, Okazaki M, Goto S. Impaired lipid metabolism in aged mice as revealed by fasting-induced expression of apolipoprotein mRNAs in the liver and changes in serum lipids. Gerontology 2004;50:206–15.

[19] Tchkonia T, Corkey BE, Kirkland JL. Current views of the fat cell as an endocrine cell: lipotoxicity. Endocrine Update 2003;26:105–18.

[20] Cree MG, Newcomer BR, Katsanos CS, Sheffield-Moore M, Chinkes D, Aarsland A, et al. Intramuscular and liver triglycerides are increased in the elderly. J Clin Endocrinol Metab 2004;89:3864–71.

[21] Cree MG, Newcomer BR, Katsanos CS, Sheffield-Moore M, Chinkes D, Aarsland A, et al. Hepatic triglyceride content and its relation to body adiposity: a magnetic resonance imaging and proton spectroscopy study. Gut 2005;54:122–7.

[22] Eguchi Y, Eguchi T, Mizuta T, Ide Y, Yasutake T, Iwakiri R, et al. Visceral fat accumulation and insulin resistance are important risk factors in nonalcoholic fatty liver disease. J Gastroenterol 2006;41:462–9.

[23] Jakobsen MU, Berentzen T, Sorensen TIA, Overvad K. Abdominal Obesity and fatty liver. Epidemiol Rev 2007;29:77–87.

[24] Frayn KN. Visceral fat and insulin resistance-causative or correlative? Br J Nutr 2000;83(suppl 1):S71–7.

[25] Bjorntorp P. "Portal" adipose tissue as a generator of risk factors for cardiovascular disease and diabetes. Arteriosclerosis 1990;10:493–6.

[26] Nielsen S, Guo Z, Johnson CM, Hensrud DD, Jensen MD. Splanchnic lipolysis in human obesity. J Clin Invest 2004;113:1582–8.

[27] Sabir N, Sermez Y, Kazil S, Zencir M. Correlation of abdominal fat distribution and liver steatosis: importance of ultrasonographic and anthropometric measurement. Eur J Ultrasound 2001;14:121–8.

[28] Church TS, Kuk JL, Ross R, Priest EL, Biltoft E, Blair SN. Association of cardiorespiratory fitness, body mass index, and waist circumference to non-alcoholic fatty liver disease. Gastroenterology 2006;130:2023–30.

[29] Targher G, Bertolini L, Scala L, Zoppini G, Zenari L, Falezza G. Non-alcoholic hepatic steatosis and its relation to increased plasma biomarkers of inflammation and endothelial dysfunction in non-diabetic men. Role of visceral adipose tissue. Diabet Med 2005;22:1354–8.

[30] Chalasani N, Deeg MA, Persohn S, Crabb DW. Metabolic and anthropometric evaluation of insulin resistance in nondiabetic patients with non-alcoholic steatohepatitis. Am J Gastroenterol 2003;98:1849–55.

[31] Kelley DE, Thaete FL, Troost F, Huwe T, Goodpaster BH. Subdivision of subcutaneous abdominal adipose tissue and insulin resistance. Am J Physiol Endocrinol Metab 2000;278:E941–8.

[32] Miyazaki Y, Glass L, Triplitt C, Wajcberg E, Mandarino LJ, DeFronzo RA. Abdominal fat distribution and peripheral and hepatic insulin resistance in type 2 diabetes mellitus. Am J Physiol Endocrinol Metab 2002;283:E1135–43.

[33] Monzon JR, Basile R, Henegan S, Udupi V, Green A. Lipolysis in adipocytes isolated from deep and superficial subcutaneous adipose tissue. Obes Res 2002;10:266–9.

[34] Westerbacka J, Lammi K, Hakkinen AM, Rissanen A, Salminen I, Aro A, et al. Dietary fat content modifies liver fat in overweight nondiabetic subjects. J Clin Endocrinol Metab 2005;90:2804–9.

[35] Fraulob JC, Ogg-Diamantino R, Fernandes-Santos C, Aguila MB, Mandarim-de-Lacerda CA. A mouse model of metabolic syndrome: insulin resistance, fatty liver and non-alcoholic fatty pancreas disease (NAFPD) in C57BL/6 mice fed a high fat diet. J Clin Biochem Nutr 2010;46:212–23.

[36] Couillard C, Bergeron N, Prud'homme D, Bergeron J, Tremblay A, Bouchard C, et al. Gender difference in postprandial lipemia: importance of visceral adipose tissue accumulation. Aterioscler Tromb Vasc Biol 1999;19:2448–55.

[37] Gallagher D, Kuznia P, Heshka S, Albu J, Heymsfield SB, Goodpaster B, et al. Adipose tissue in muscle: a novel depot similar in size to visceral adipose tissue. Am J Clin Nutr 2005;81:903–10.

[38] Rossi A, Zoico E, Goodpaster BH, Sepe A, Di Francesco V, Fantin F, et al. Quantification of intermuscular adipose tissue in the erector spinae muscle by MRI: agreement with histological evaluation. Obesity 2010;18:2379–84.

[39] Ryan AS, Nicklas BJ. Age-related changes in fat deposition in mid-thigh muscle in women: relationships with metabolic cardiovascular disease risk factors. Int J Obes Relat Metab Disord 1999;23:126–32.

[40] Visser M, Kritchevsky SB, Goodpaster BH, Newman AB, Nevitt M, Stamm E, et al. Leg muscle mass and composition in relation to lower extremity performance in men and women aged 70 to 79: the health, aging and body composition study. J Am Geriatr Soc 2002;50:897–904.

[41] Goodpaster BH, Carlson CL, Visser M, Kelley DE, Scherzinger A, Harris TB, et al. Attenuation of skeletal muscle and strength in the elderly: the health ABC study. J Appl Physiol 2001;90:2157–65.

[42] Katsiaras A, Newman AB, Kriska A, Brach J, Krishnaswami S, Feingold E, et al. Skeletal muscle fatigue, strength, and quality in the elderly: the health ABC study. J Appl Physiol 2005;99:210–6.

[43] Johannsen DL, Conley KE, Bajpeyi S, Punyanitya M, Gallagher D, Zhang Z, et al. Ectopic lipid accumulation and reduced glucose tolerance in elderly adults are accompanied by altered skeletal muscle mitochondrial activity. J Clin Endocrinol Metab 2012;97:242–50.

[44] Korach-André M, Gao J, Gounarides JS, Deacon R, Islam A, Laurent D. Relationship between visceral adiposity and intramyocellular lipid content in two rat models of insulin resistance. Am J Physiol Endocrinol Metab 2005;288:E106–16.

[45] Weiss R, Dufour S, Taksali SF, Tamborlane WV, Petersen KF, Bonadonna RC, et al. Prediabetes in obese youth: a syndrome of impaired glucose tolerance, severe insulin resistance, and altered myocellular and abdominal fat partitioning. Lancet 2003;362:951–7.

[46] Tushuizen ME, Bunck MC, Pouwels PJ, Bontemps S, van Waesberghe JH, Schindhelm RK, et al. Pancreatic fat content and beta-cell function in men with and without type 2 diabetes. Diabetes Care 2007;30:2916–21.

[47] Lee Y, Hirose H, Ohneda M, Johnson JH, McGarry JD, Unger RH. Beta-cell lipotoxicity in the pathogenesis of non- insulin-dependent diabetes mellitus of obese rats: impairment in adipocyte-beta call relationships. Proc Natl Acad Sci USA 1994;91:10878–82.

[48] Nolan CJ, Madiraju MS, Delghingaro-Augusto V, Peyot ML. Fatty acid signalling in the beta-cell and insulin secretion. Diabetes 2006;55(Suppl2):S16–23.

[49] Saisho Y, Butler AE, Meier JJ, Monchamp T, Allen-Auerbach M, Rizza RA, et al. Pancreas volumes in humans from birth to age

on hundred taking into account sex, obesity, and presence of type 2 diabetes. Clin Anat 2007;20:933–42.
[50] Lee SL, Kim SH, Jun DW, Han JH, Jang EC, Park JY, et al. Clinical implications of fatty pancreas: correlations between fatty pancreas and metabolic syndrome. World J Gastroenterol 2009;15:1869–75.
[51] Pinnick KE, Collins SC, Londos C, Gauguier D, Clark A, Fielding BA. Pancreatic ectopic fat is characterized by adipocyte infiltration and altered lipid composition. Obesity 2008;16:522–9.
[52] Targher G, Rossi AP, Zamboni GA, Fantin F, Antonioli A, Corzato F, et al. Pancreatic fat accumulation and its relationship with liver fat content and other fat depots in obese individuals. J Endocrinol Invest 2012;35:748–53.
[53] You M, Considine RV, Leone TC, Kelly DP, Crabb DW. Role of adiponectin in the protective action of dietary saturated fat against alcoholic fatty liver in mice. Hepatology 2005;42:568–77.
[54] Hui JM, Hodge A, Farrel GC, Kench JG, Kriketos A, George J. Beyond insulin resistance in NASH: TNF-alpha or adiponectin? Hepatology 2004;40:46–54.
[55] Musso G, Gambino R, Biroli G, Carello M, Fagà E, Pacini G, et al. Hypoadiponectinemia predicts the severity of hepatic fibrosis and pancreatic Beta-cell dysfunction in nondiabetic nonobese patients with nonalcoholic steatohepatitis. Am J Gastroenterol 2005;100:2438–46.
[56] Bugianesi E, Pagotto U, Manini R, Vanni E, Gastaldelli A, de Iasio R, et al. Plasma adiponectin in non-alcoholic fatty liver is related to hepatic insulin resistance and hepatic fat content, not to liver disease severity. J Clin Endocrinol Metab 2005;90:3498–504.
[57] Cnop M, Havel PJ, Utzschneider KM, Carr DB, Sinha MK, Boyko EJ, et al. Relationship of adiponectin to body fat distribution, insulin sensitivity and plasma lipoproteins: Evidence for independent roles of age and sex. Diabetologia 2003;46:459–69.
[58] Szczepaniak LS, Babcock EE, Schick F, Dobbins RL, Garg A, Burns DK, et al. Measurement of intracellular triglyceride stores by H spectroscopy. Am J Physiol 1999;276:E977–89.
[59] Sharma S, Adrogue JV, Golfman L, Uray I, Lemm J, Youker K, et al. Intramyocellular lipid accumulation in the failing human heart resembles the lipotoxic rat heart. FASEB J 2004;18:1692–700.
[60] Iacobellis G, Assael F, Ribaudo MC, Zappaterreno A, Alessi G, Di Mario U, et al. Epicardial fat from echography: a new method to for viscerla adipose tissue prediction. Obes Res 2003;11:304–10.
[61] Iacobellis G, Ribaudo MC, Assael F, Vecci E, Tiberti C, Zappaterreno A, et al. Echocardiographic epicardial adipose tissue is related to anthropometric and clinical parameters of metabolixc syndrome: a new indicator cardiovascular risk. J Clin Endocrinol Metab 2003;88:5163–8.
[62] Silaghi A, Piercecchi-Marti MD, Grino M, Leonetti G, Alessi MC, Clement K, et al. Epicardial adipose tissue e xtent: relationship with age, body fat distribution, and coronaropathy. Obesity 2008;16:2424–30.
[63] Tuomilehto J, Lindstrom J, Eriksson JG, Valle TT, Hämäläinen H, Ilanne-Parikka P, et al. Prevention of type 2 diabetes mellitus by changes in lifestyle among subjects with impaired glucose tolerance. N Engl J Med 2001;344:1343–50.
[64] Knowler WC, Barrett-Connor E, Fowler SE, Hamman RF, Lachin JM, Walker EA, et al. Diabetes Prevention Program Research Group. Reduction in the incidence of type 2 diabetes with lifestyle intervention or metformin. N Engl J Med 2002;346:393–403.
[65] Goodpaster BH, Kelley DE, Wing RR, Meier A, Thaete FL. Effects of weight loss on regional fat distribution and insulin sensitivity in obesity. Diabetes 1999;48:839–47.
[66] Mazzali G, Di Francesco V, Zoico E, Fantin F, Zamboni G, Benati C, et al. Interrelations between fat distribution, muscle lipid content, adipocytokines, and insulin resistance: effect of moderate weight loss in older women. Am J Clin Nutr 2006;84:1193–9.
[67] Goodpaster BH, Delany JP, Otto AD, Kuller L, Vockley J, South-Paul JE, et al. Effects of diet and physical activity interventions on weight loss and cardiometabolic risk factors in severely obese adults: a randomized trial. JAMA 2010;304:1795–802.
[68] Medrikova D, Jilkova ZM, Bardava K, Janovska P, Rossmeisl M, Kopecky J. Sex differences during the course of diet-induced obesity in mice: adipose tissue expandability and glycemic control. Int J Obes 2011;36(2):262–72.
[69] Colles SL, Dixon JB, Marks P, Strauss BJ, O'Brien PE. Preoperative weight loss with a very low energy diet: quantitation of changes in liver and abdominal fat by serial imaging. Am J Clin Nutr 2006;84:304–11.
[70] Petersen KF, Dufour S, Befroy D, Lehrke M, Hendler RE, Shulman GI. Reversal nonalcoholic hepatic steatosis, hepatic insuline resistance and hyperglycemia by moderate weight reduction in patients with type 2 of diabetes. Diabetes 2005;54:603–8.
[71] Rossi AP, Fantin F, Zamboni GA, Mazzali G, Zoico E, Bambace C, et al. Effect of moderate weight loss on hepatic, pancreatic and visceral lipids in obese subjects. Nutr Diabetes 2012;2:e32.
[72] Phillips ML, Boase S, Wahlroos S, Dugar M, Kow L, Stahl J, et al. Associates of change in liver fat content in the morbidly obese after laparoscopic gastric banding surgery. Diabetes Obes Metab 2008;10:661–7.
[73] Heath ML, Kow L, Slavotinek JP, Valentine R, Toouli J, Thompson CH. Abdominal adiposity and liver fat content 3 and 12 months after gastric banding surgery. Metabolism 2009;58:753–8.
[74] Deprés JP, Lemieux I. Abdominal obesity and metabolic syndrome. Nature 2006;444:881–7.
[75] Pouliot MC, Deprés JP, Nadeau A, Moorjani S, Prud'Homme D, Lupien PJ, et al. Visceral obesity in men. Association with glucose tolerance, plasma insulin, and lipoproteins level. Diabetes 1992;41:826–34.
[76] Brunzell JD, Hokanson JE. Dyslipidemia of central obesity and insulin resistance. Diabetes Care 1999;22(Suppl 3):C10–3.
[77] Rasuoli N, Molavi B, Elbein SC, Kern PA. Ectopic fat accumulation and metabolic syndrome. Diab Obes Metab 2007;9:1–10.
[78] Heilbronn L, Smith SR, Ravussin E. Failure of fat cell proliferation, mitochondrial function and fat oxidation results in ectopic fat storage, insulin resistance and type II diabetes mellitus. Int J Obes 2004;28:S12–21.
[79] van Herpen NA, Schrauwen-Hinderling VB. Lipid accumulation in non-adipose tissue and lipotoxicity. Physiol Behav 2008;94:231–41.
[80] Thamer C, Machann J, Stefan N, Haap M, Schäfer S, Brenner S, et al. High visceral fat mass and high liver fat are associated with resistance to lifestyle intervention. Obesity 2007;15:531–8.
[81] Thamer C, Machann J, Haap M, Stefan N, Heller E, Schnödt B, et al. Intrahepatic lipids are predicted by visceral adipose tissue mass in healthy subjects. Diabetes Care 2004:2726–9.
[82] Kelley DE, Goodpaster BH, Storlien S. Muscle triglyceride and insulin resistance. Ann Rev Nutr 2002;22:325–46.
[83] Taira S, Shimabukuro M, Higa C, Yabiku K, Kozuka C, Ueda R, et al. Lipid deposition in various sites of skeletal muscle and liver shows correlation with visceral fat accumulation in male patients with metabolic syndrome. J Med Invest 2013;60:1–14.
[84] Angulo P. Nonhalcoholic fatty liver disease. New Eng J Med 2002;346:1221–31.
[85] Stranges S, Dorn JM, Muti P, Freudenheim JL, Farinaro E, Russell M, et al. Body composition, relative weigh, and liver enzyme levels: a population-based study. Hepatology 2004;39:754–63.

[86] Marchesini G, Bugianesi E, Forlani G, Cerrelli F, Lenzi M, Manini R, et al. Nonalcoholic fatty liver, steatohepatitis, and the metabolic syndrome. Hepatology 2003;37:917–23.
[87] Kim HJ, Kim HJ, Lee KE, Kim DJ, Kim SK, Ahn CW, et al. Metabolic significance of nonalcoholic fatty liver disease in nonobese, nondiabetic adults. Arch Intern Med 2004;164:2169–75.
[88] Angulo P. Treatment of nonalcoholic fatty liver disease. Ann Hepatol 2002;1:12–19.
[89] Shimomura I, Bashmakov Y, Horton JD. Increased levels of nuclear SREBP-1c associated with fatty livers in two mouse models of diabetes mellitus. J Biol Chem 1999;274:30028–32.
[90] McCullogh AJ. Pathophysiology of nonalcoholic steatohepatitis. J Clin Gastroenterol 2006;40:S17–29.
[91] Aronis A, Madar Z, Tirosh O. Mechanism underlying oxidative stress-mediated lipotoxicity: exposure of J774.2 macrophages to triacylglyceroles facielities mithochondrial reactive oxygen species production and cellular necrosis. Free Radic Biol Med 2005;38:1221–30.
[92] Lieber CS. Cytochrome P-4502E1: its physiological and pathological role. Physiol Rev 1997;77:517–44.
[93] Diehl AM. Tumor necrosis factor and its potential role in insuline resistence and nonalcoholic fatty liver didease. Clin Liver Dis 2004;8:619–38.
[94] Mathur A, Marine M, Lu D, Swartz-Basile DA, Saxena R, Zyromski NJ, et al. Nonalcoholic fatty pancreas disease. HPB 2007;9:312–8.
[95] Pinnick KE, Collins SC, Londos C, Gauguier D, Clark A, Fielding BA. Pancreatic ectopic fat in characterized by adipocyte infiltration and altered lipid composition. Obesity 2008;16:522–30.
[96] Newshalme P, Keane D, Welters HJ, Morgan NG. Life and death decision of the pancreatic β-cell: the role of fatty acid. Clin Sci 2007;112:27–42.
[97] Smits M, van Geenen E. The clinical significance of pancreatic steatosis. Nat Rev Gastroenterol Hepatol 2011;8:169–77.
[98] Pitt H. Hepato-pancreato-biliary fat: the good, the bad and the ugly. HPB 2007;9:92–7.
[99] Mathur A, Zyromski N, Pitt H, Al-Azzawi H, Walker JJ, Saxena R, et al. Pancreatic steatosis promotes dissemination and lethality of pancreatic cancer. J Am Coll Surg 2009;208:989.
[100] Mathur A, Pitt HA, Marine M, Saxena R, Schmidt CM, Howard TJ, et al. Fatty pancreas: a factor in postoperative pancreatic fistula. Ann Surg 2007;246:1058–64.
[101] Gaujoux S, Cortes A, Couvelard A, Noullet S, Clavel L, Rebours V, et al. Fatty pancreas and increased body mass index are risk factors of pancreatic fistula after pancreaticoduodenectomy. Surgery 2010;148:15–23.
[102] Zhang X, Cui Y, Fang L, Li F. Chronic high-fat diets induce oxide injuries and fibrogenesis of pancreatic cells in rats. Pancreas 2008;37:e31–8.
[103] Fernandes-Santos C, Evangelista Carneiro R, de Souza Mendonca L, Barbosa Aguila M, Mandarim-de-Lacerda CA. Rosiglitazone aggravates nonalcoholic fatty pancreatic disease in C57BL/6 mice fed high-fat and high-sucrose diet. Pancreas 2009;38:e80–6.
[104] Sepe PS, Ohri A, Sanaka S, Berzin TM, Sekhon S, Bennett G, et al. A prospective evaluation of fatty pancreas by using EUS. Gastrointest Endosc 2011;73:987–93.
[105] Hannukainen JC, Borra R, Linderborg K, Kallio H, Kiss J, Lepomäki V, et al. Liver and pancreatic fat content and metabolism in healthy monozygotic twins with discordant physical activity. J Hepatol 2011;54:545–52.
[106] van Geenen EJ, Smits MM, Schreuder TC, van der Peet DL, Bloemena E, Mulder CJ. Nonalcoholic fatty liver disease is related to nonalcoholic fatty pancreas disease. Pancreas 2010;39:1185–90.
[107] Al-Haddad M, Khashab M, Zyromski N, et al. Risk factors for hyperechogenic pancreas on endoscopic ultrasound: a case-control study. Pancreas 2009;38:672–5.
[108] Heni M, Machann J, Staiger H, Schwenzer NF, Peter A, Schick F, et al. Pancreatic fat is negatively associated with insulin secretion in individuals with impaired fasting glucose and/or impaired glucose tolerance: a nuclear magnetic resonance study. Diabetes Metab Res Rev 2010;26:200–5.
[109] Ou H-Y, Wang C-Y, Yang Y-C, Chen M-F, Chang C-J. The association between nonalcoholic fatty pancreas disease and diabetes. PLoS ONE 2013;8:e62561.
[110] Shimabukuro M, Kozuka C, Taira S, Yabiku K, Dagvasumberel M, Ishida M, et al. Ectopic fat deposition and global cardiometabolic risk: new paradigm in cardiovascular medicine. J Med Invest 2013;60:1–14.
[111] Shimabukuro M, Meng F, Zhou YT, Grayburn PA, Karim MA. Increased extracellular matrix remodeling during the development of a specific diabetic cardiomyopathy in the Zucker fatty rats. Circulation 1998;98(Suppl):180. (Meeting Abstract)
[112] Ding J, Hsu FC, Harris TB, Liu Y, Kritchevsky SB, Szklo M, et al. The association of pericardial fat with incident coronary heart disease. The Multi-Ethnic Study of Atherosclerosis (MESA). Am J Clin Nutr 2009;90:499–504.
[113] Al Chekakie MO, Welles CC, Metoyer R, Ibrahim A, Shapira AR, Cytron J, et al. Perivascular fat is independently associated with human atrial fibrillation. J Am Coll Cardiol 2010;56:784–8.
[114] Thanassoulis G, Massaro JM, O'Donnell CJ, Hoffmann U, Levy D, Ellinor PT, et al. Pericardial fat is associated with prevalent atrial fibrillation: the Framingham Heart Study. Circ Arrhythm Electrophysiol 2010;3:345–50.
[115] Nakanishi K, Fukuda S, Tanaka A, Otsuka K, Sakamoto M, Taguchi H, et al. Peri-atrial epicardial adipose tissue is associated with newonset nonvalvular atrial fibrillation. Circ J 2012;76:2748–54.
[116] Dagenais GR, Tancredi RG, Zierler KL. Free fatty acid oxidation by forearm muscle at rest, and evidence for an intramuscolar lipid pool in the human forearm. J Clin Invest 1976;58:421–31.
[117] Falholt K, Jensen I, Lindkaer Jensen S, Mortensen H, Vølund A, Heding LG, et al. Carbohydrate and lipid metabolism of skeletal muscle in type 2 diabetic patients. Diabet Med 1988;5:27–31.
[118] Corcoran MP, Lamon-Fava S, Fielding RA. Skeletal muscle lipid deposition and insulin resistance: effect of dietary fatty acids and exercise. Am J Clin Nutr 2007;85:662–77.
[119] Kelley DE, Slasky BS, Janosky J. Skeletal muscle density: effects of obesity and non-insulin-dependent diabetes mellitus. Am J Clin Nutr 1991;54:509–15.
[120] Goodpaster BH, He J, Watkins S, Kelley DE. Skeletal muscle lipid content and insulin resistance: evidence for a paradox in endurance trained athletes. J Clin Endocrinol Metab 2001;86:5755–61.
[121] Schrauwen-Hinderling VB, Hesselink MKC, Schrauwen P, Kooi ME. Intramyocellular lipid content in human skeletal muscle. Obesity 2006;14:357–67.
[122] Roubenoff R, Hughes VA. Sarcopenia: current concepts. J Gerontol 2000;55:M716–24. 26
[123] Larsson L, Li X, Frontera WR. Effects of aging on shortening velocity and myosin isoform composition in single human skeletal muscle cells. Am J Physiol Cell Physiol 1997;272:C638–49.

CHAPTER

14

Blood Pressure Regulation in Abdominal Obesity

Marie-Ève Leblanc and Paul Poirier

Université Laval and Institut Universitaire de Cardiologie et de Pneumologie de Québec, Quebec City, Quebec, Canada

INTRODUCTION

Obesity and hypertension commonly coexist. Abdominal obesity is undoubtedly linked with high blood pressure as a consequence of multiple mechanisms that are enhanced by visceral fat. The objective of this chapter is to discuss how blood pressure regulation is influenced by abdominal obesity. Health-care professionals should be aware of the risks encountered by fat accumulation and of their ability to correctly estimate abdominal obesity. Useful clinical tools will be presented including waist circumference (WC) and the waist-hip ratio (WHR), which are the most popular adiposity indexes. Some mechanisms explaining the role of two types of adipokines, namely apelin and leptin, in hypertension will be presented. Complex pathways stimulated by visceral fat will be highlighted: activation of the sympathetic nervous and the renin-angiotensin system, structural dysfunction of the kidneys, and exercise-induced hypertension. When health-care professionals meet abdominally obese patients, one priority should be to encourage and motivate them to improve their lifestyle behavior, since exercise and dietetic recommendations have been proven to be efficient ways to improve weight management and blood pressure regulation.

OBESITY: A DEFINITION

Since the 1990s, a drastic increase in the prevalence and incidence of obesity has been observed in both developed and developing countries. According to the National Health and Nutrition Examination Survey (NHANES), which measured the prevalence of obesity in the United States from 2009 to 2010, 35.7% of American adults are obese [1]. According to the Canadian Health Measures Survey (2007–2009), 24.1% of Canadian adults are obese [2].

Obesity is defined using the body mass index (BMI), calculated as weight in kilograms divided by height in meters squared (kg/m^2). For adults aged 18 years or older, overweight is defined as a BMI of 25.0–29.9 kg/m^2 and obesity is defined as a BMI of 30.0 kg/m^2 or higher [3,4]. Obesity may be divided into several grades: grade 1 (BMI of 30.0–34.9 kg/m^2), grade 2 (BMI of 35–39.9 kg/m^2), grade 3 (BMI of 40 kg/m^2 or higher), grade 4 (BMI of 50.0 kg/m^2 or higher), and grade 5 (BMI 60.0 kg/m^2 or higher) [5,6]. In addition, obesity guidelines [4,7] recommend the assessment of abdominal obesity using WC when BMI is 25–34.9 kg/m^2, whereas obesity experts also recommend measuring WC even if BMI is normal [8–11] because *metabolically obese, normal weight* individuals have been described.

Excess adiposity should be considered a chronic health disease associated with serious health consequences. Systemic hypertension and obesity are chronic diseases that are frequently linked, as reported in the United States [12–14] and Canada [15–17], including Inuit [18] and Indian populations [19].

SYSTEMIC HYPERTENSION: A DEFINITION

Approximately 20% of adults in Canada [20] and 30% of adults in the United States [21–23] have blood pressure ≥140/90 mmHg. Systemic hypertension has been recognized as the primary cause of major cardiovascular diseases worldwide, including stroke [24,25]. Hypertension guidelines recommend aggressive blood pressure control by maintaining blood

Nutrition in the Prevention and Treatment of Abdominal Obesity
http://dx.doi.org/10.1016/B978-0-12-407869-7.00014-3

TABLE 14.1 Tools Available for Body Composition Assessments in Research and the Clinic

Method		Used in Research	Used in the Clinic
Hydrodensitometry		X	–
Dual-energy X-ray absorptiometry		X	–
Computed tomography		X	–
Magnetic resonance imaging		X	–
Bioelectrical impedance		X	X
Body mass index		X	X
Skinfold thickness		↓	↓
Waist circumference		X	X
Ratios	WHR	X	X
	WHtR	X	–

Source: adapted from reference [9]. WHR, waist-hip ratio; WHtR, waist-height ratio; X, actually used; –, not recommended for clinical use; ↓, used in the past but now rarely used.

pressure ≤130/80 mmHg among patients at risk for coronary artery disease, including individuals with diabetes mellitus, chronic kidney, or coronary artery risk equivalent, or with a 10-year Framingham risk score equivalent to or over 10% [22]. NHANES survey reported in 1999 that the estimated prevalence ratio of systemic hypertension was 4.6 and 5.5 times more elevated in men and women, respectively, aged <55 years with a BMI ≥40 kg/m^2 [14].

Recommendations for obese individuals are not covered in depth in the Canadian hypertension guidelines [20], whereas specific precautions regarding obese patients can be found in the American guidelines [23]. The difficulty of properly managing blood pressure in an obese patient is that an accurate measurement of blood pressure may be difficult to obtain, especially when a patient's arm circumference is >52 cm, since an appropriate cuff may not be readily available. An alternative may be to substitute a forearm blood pressure measurement for the standard upper-arm blood pressure measurement [23,26].

Moreover, individuals with elevated blood pressure are two and a half times more likely to develop diabetes within 5 years [27], largely because metabolic abnormalities like insulin resistance may be exacerbated by some antihypertensive medications [28]. Lifestyle interventions are always preferred as the initial approach to treat most patients with uncomplicated high blood pressure. Indeed, lifestyle interventions should be initiated aggressively as soon as possible when health-care professionals are facing patients at a high risk of developing abnormal or impaired glucose metabolism [29].

WHICH ADIPOSITY INDEX IS THE BEST FOR EXPLAINING THE LINK BETWEEN SYSTEMIC HYPERTENSION RISK AND OBESITY?

There are many methods and clinical body assessments tools available to measure body composition (Table 14.1). Clinically, the most useful adiposity indexes to assess body fat distribution are WC and WHR.

Waist Circumference

WC is an easy method for assessing central obesity, which has an excellent correlation with abdominal imaging and a high correlation with systemic hypertension risk [30,31], blood pressure level [31–34], cardiovascular risk [35,36], and mortality [37]. In a cohort of 1847 individuals, WC showed a better correlation with blood pressure than with BMI and insulin sensitivity [33]. In a large international, noninterventional, cross-sectional study called the International Day for the Evaluation of Abdominal Obesity (IDEA), carried out in 63 countries among 168,000 patients, Balkau et al. reported a stronger relationship between cardiovascular disease, including stroke, and WC than with BMI [38]. In a cross-sectional descriptive study in 305 individuals (33% diabetics, 37% hypertensive subjects, and 30% healthy controls), for every centimeter WC increment, arterial stiffness (measured by pulse wave velocity) increased [39]. A recent literature review reported that WC methods using different location points [40] have no substantial influence on the association between WC, cardiovascular disease, diabetes, and all-cause and cardiovascular disease mortality [40]. The National Institutes of Health and the National Heart, Lung and Blood Institute recommend that WC should be taken at the level of the iliac crest [9]. This appears to be the simplest method, since bony structures are stable over time and easy to locate in the majority of patients. It is most important to standardize the procedure over time by using the same approach for each patient WC during the follow-up [41].

Waist-Hip and Waist-Height Ratios

The most popular ratios for characterizing obesity are the WHR (i.e. WC in meters divided by hip circumference in meters) and the waist-height ratio (WHtR; WC in meters divided by height in meters). These measurements are easy to calculate and numerous studies have reported their association with cardiovascular disease [37,42–45]. In the Asian population, WHtR appears one of the best adiposity measurements for assessing metabolic and cardiovascular risk [42,46,47]. A recent systematic review and meta-analysis involving 300,000 adults, including several different ethnic groups, showed the superiority of WHtR over WC and BMI for the detection of cardiometabolic risk factors in both genders [48]. The WHtR also appears to correlate better with pulse wave velocity: for every 0.1 point WHtR increment, the pulse wave velocity increased by 0.0029 m/s [39]. WHR and WHtR are associated with systemic hypertension and/or the level of blood pressure in many studies [46,49–51]. Therefore, there seems to be a potential clinical utility and add-on value for assessing WHR and WHtR in an evaluation of the hypertension risk for a given individual.

ABDOMINAL OBESITY AND ITS IMPACT ON BLOOD PRESSURE

Adipose tissue is not simply a fat storage organ but is now considered to be a complex organ that interacts with the inflammatory system and the vascular wall [52]. Several potential mechanisms have been proposed to explain the interplay between adipocytes and hypertension development. First, the hemodynamic pattern of obesity-related hypertension is probably related to multiple mechanisms: (1) volume expansion [53]; (2) increased cardiac output [54]; (3) increased systemic vascular resistance that fails to decrease sufficiently to counteract the higher cardiac output [55]; and (4) activation of the sympathetic nervous and the renin-angiotensin-aldosterone systems [56]. Second, important consideration should also be given to fat cells. Fat cells produce a large number of biologically active molecules called *adipokines*, which may be partly responsible for the relationship between obesity and hypertension [57].

HEMODYNAMIC PATTERN: MECHANISMS

Volume Expansion, Increased Cardiac Output, and Systemic Vascular Resistance

Obese hypertensive individuals usually present with elevated cardiac output due to excessive intravascular volume [53]. The increment in systemic blood flow encountered in obesity cannot be solely explained by increased requirements caused by adipose tissue perfusion because the enlarged vascular bed of adipose tissue is less vascularized than is other tissue [58]. Indeed, it was reported in 2744 participants that stroke volume and cardiac output are more strongly related to fat free mass than to other variables such as adipose mass, age, sex, diabetes, blood pressure, or cardioactive medications [54].

Sympathetic Nervous Activation

Sympathetic overactivity is one of the most important mechanisms linking obesity with systemic hypertension [56,57,59]. It is possible that weight gain stimulates the sympathetic nervous system to compensate in order to burn excessive fat. This situation, however, is detrimental for the kidney and for vascular smooth muscle [57]. Experimental studies support a role for renal sympathetic nerves in the development of hypertension in obesity [60]. The blockade of adrenergic activity lowers blood pressure to a greater extent in obese individuals than in hypertensive lean individuals [61]. Sympathetic activation of the kidney is probably another important modulatory factor [62]. This phenomenon was explored using a norepinephrine kinetic design study, which revealed that neural activity to skeletal muscle is more closely related to abdominal visceral fat than to total fat mass or abdominal subcutaneous fat [63]. However, neural activity to the kidney and to skeletal muscle is elevated in obese normotensive as well as in obese hypertensive individuals [63]. This raises the possibility that blood pressure associated in obesity-related neural activity is strongly influenced by environmental factors. As an example, Pima Indians are mostly obese but their prevalence of hypertension is low, as shown in a study that reported low muscle sympathetic nerve activity in this population [64]. In response to environmental factors and psychological "stress," physiological mechanisms are triggered, particularly those associated with activation of the adrenomedullary and adrenocortical system [61]. It is possible that different sympathetic responses occur in different environments or in different genetic backgrounds in the presence of similar levels of adiposity.

Renin-Angiotensin-Aldosterone System Activation

Obesity and metabolic syndrome (MetS) can enhance salt sensitivity and, consequently, aggravate renal sodium retention and impair natriuresis pressure [62]. The renin-angiotensin system plays a central role in salt and water homeostasis, as well as in the maintenance of vascular tone. Modulation of the renin-angiotensin system raises or lowers blood pressure [65,66]. Abnormal renin-angiotensin system regulation in obesity can result in a primary increase in the production of renin-angiotensin pathway components like angiotensinogen, angiotensin II, and aldosterone. It is important to emphasize that most components of the renin-angiotensin system [e.g. angiotensinogen, aldosterone, and angiotensin-converting enzyme (ACE)] are found in the adipose tissue [67]. To some degree, this may explain the pathophysiology of hypertension in obesity [66]. Animal studies have also demonstrated that modifying the amount of angiotensin directly influences body weight and adiposity [68]. It was shown in 30 menopausal women that a reduction in body weight by 5% leads to a meaningful reduction in renin-angiotensin-aldosterone levels in both plasma and adipose tissue [69]. The plasma angiotensin decrement was highly correlated with a WC reduction ($r=0.74$, $P<0.001$), and reductions in both weight and renin-angiotensin-aldosterone levels was accompanied by a 7mmHg reduction in ambulatory blood pressure [69].

Structural Alteration to the Kidneys

An association between renal sinus fat, hypertension, and kidney disease has been proposed [70]. Enhanced renal norepinephrine spillover in obesity may have implications for the development of hypertension because enhanced visceral oxygen consumption in the kidneys has been reported [71]. Investigators suggested that compression of the renal vasculature, particularly affecting renal veins, may increase renal venous pressure, causing sodium retention and hypertension [71]. Foster et al. [72], using a subset of the Framingham Heart Study cohort, quantified renal sinus fat and abdominal adipose tissue using computed tomography. The authors observed that fatty kidney was present in almost one-third of the subjects and was associated with a higher odds ratio of hypertension and chronic kidney disease, even after adjusting for BMI or abdominal visceral adipose tissue [72].

ABDOMINAL OBESITY AND EXERCISED-INDUCED HYPERTENSION

Exercise-induced hypertension has been defined as systolic blood pressure ≥220mmHg and diastolic blood pressure ≥110mmHg at the end of exercise [73]. This phenomenon has been studied to determine the factors that may contribute to elevated blood pressure. In a study including 179 abdominally obese men with MetS without type 2 diabetes mellitus (T2DM), the most important predictor of exercised-induced hypertension was WC [74]. WC was higher in the group with exercised-induced hypertension than in the group without (111 ± 8cm vs. 106 ± 4cm, respectively, $P<0.001$). Other findings showed that individuals with exercise-induced hypertension presented a worse anthropometric profile than did abdominally obese men with normal exercise blood pressure and higher weight, systolic blood pressure, high-density lipoprotein cholesterol, and apolipoprotein B (ApoB) at baseline [74].

ADIPOKINES

Adipocytes are recognized as an endocrine organ with many secretory products: over 50 different adipocyte-derived substances (called *adipokines*) have been identified and studied with regard to their potential contribution to blood pressure control [62]. Currently, two promising adipokines (leptin and apelin) link adiposity and high blood pressure.

Apelin

Apelin is a protein secreted in adipocytes that shows predominant vascular effects in vivo in both animals [75,76] and humans [77]. Apelin exerts multiple physiological functions, including effects on (1) fluid homeostasis, (2) food intake, (3) cell proliferation, (4) blood pressure regulation, (5) angiogenesis, and (6) glucose utilization [78]. From a renal perspective, apelin plays a counter-regulatory role against the pressor action of angiotensin II [76]. Vascular effects of apelin were assessed in 24 healthy volunteers: forearm blood flow was measured by venous occlusion plethysmography with or without intrabrachial nitric oxide (NO) infusion [77]. Although having no apparent effect on venous tone, apelin causes NO-dependent arterial vasodilatation in the forearm vascular bed during NO infusion [77]. Therefore, apelin appears to be a beneficial adipokine with hypotensive effects [76] and antiobesity properties. Although this may be a promising therapeutic target in metabolic disorders, further research is needed to demonstrate the clinical utility of apelin [79].

Leptin

Leptin is a well-studied protein [62] secreted by adipocytes; it acts on the hypothalamus, which regulates energy metabolism by helping to create a satiety sensation and, consequently, reducing food ingestion [57]. The effects of leptin are primarily mediated by receptors

TABLE 14.2 Metabolic Syndrome Definitions from Two Different Organizations

	National Cholesterol Education Program Adult Treatment Panel III report [85]	International Diabetes Federation [84]
Diagnostic criteria	≥3 criteria	Abdominal obesity and ≥2 other criteria
Fasting plasma glucose	≥5.6 mM	≥5.6 mM (or a previous diagnosis type 2 diabetes)
Blood pressure	≥130/85 mmHg	≥130/85 mmHg (or being treated with specific medication)
TG level	≥1.7 mM	≥1.7 mM (or being treated with specific medication)
HDL-C	Men: <1.0 mM Women: <1.3 mM	Men: <1.03 mM Women: <1.29 mM
Abdominal obesity defined by WC	Men: ≥102 cm Women: ≥88 cm	Americans: Men: >102 cm Women: >88 cm Europoids, Sub-Saharan Africans, Eastern Mediterranean and Middle East populations: Men: >94 cm Women: >88 cm South Asians, Chinese, Japanese, Ethnic South and Central Americans Men: ≥88 cm Women: ≥80 cm

Source: adapted from references [84,85]. HDL-C, high-density lipoprotein cholesterol; TG, triglycerides; WC, waist circumference.

located in the central nervous system [62]. Serum leptin levels are elevated in hypertensive compared with normotensive individuals, independent of BMI and body fat distribution. Leptin is recognized as being associated with reduced food intake and increased energy expenditure [80], and also facilitates physical activity and reduced insulin resistance [81]. Despite high leptin levels in obese individuals, adiposity and weight gain increases are encountered in most cases of obesity, as a result of so-called *leptin resistance* [82]. Interestingly, in a small study involving 10 hypertensive, severely obese patients, indexes of abdominal obesity (i.e. WC and WHR) showed a better correlation than BMI with leptin levels [83].

METABOLIC SYNDROME: A COMBINATION OF CARDIOVASCULAR RISK FACTORS INCLUDING HIGH BLOOD PRESSURE

MetS is defined as a condition in which an individual has at least three out of the five cardiovascular disease risk factors: (1) abdominal obesity assessed by WC; (2) reduced high-density lipoprotein (HDL) cholesterol; (3) high triglycerides levels; (4) high blood pressure; and (5) elevated fasting glucose. The National Cholesterol Education Program Adult Treatment Panel III (NCEP-ATP III) report [84] and the International Diabetes Federation [85] define MetS slightly differently (Table 14.2). The rationale for not having WC as a mandatory criterion was that some individuals can be characterized as having MetS even if they are lean or with normal blood pressure [8]. Experts recommend that a distinction must clearly be made between MetS as a concept and the criteria used in clinical practice to identify individuals with features of MetS. We should keep in mind that initial indicators of high-risk abdominal obesity are an increased WC combined with raised fasting glucose and high blood pressure [86].

MANAGEMENT OF SYSTEMIC HYPERTENSION IN OBESITY; BENEFITS FROM WEIGHT REDUCTION

Regulation of blood pressure in obesity can be managed by weight reduction [87–90]. Weight loss is considered to be a difficult and time-consuming process that includes many lifestyle interventions [91]. The adoption of healthy eating habits, moderation of alcohol

TABLE 14.3 Lifestyle Modifications to Prevent and Manage Hypertension

Modifications	Recommendations
Weight reduction	Maintain a normal body mass index[a] and a healthy waist circumference Example: for Americans, <102 cm for men and <88 cm for women[b]
Eating plan	Adopt healthy eating pattern: diet rich in fruits products and vegetables, low-fat dairy with a reduced content of saturated and total fat Example: the DASH diet
Dietary sodium reduction	Reduce dietary sodium intake to ≤100 mmol/day (or 2.4 g) sodium, or 6 g sodium chloride, or one "full" tablespoon
Physical activity	Engage in regular aerobic physical activity such as brisk walking for at least 30 min/day, 5 days/week
Moderation of alcohol consumption	≤2 drinks[c]/day or ≤14 drinks/week for men and ≤1 drink/day or a maximum of 9 drinks/week for women

Source: adapted from [103].
[a]*Normal body mass index: 18.5–24.9 kg/m². [b]Adjust waist circumference limits for each ethnic group. [c]One drink is the equivalent of 24 fl oz (≈700 mL) beer, 10 fl oz (≈300 mL) wine, or 3 fl oz (≈90 mL) 80-proof whiskey.*

consumption, and the adoption of physical activities should always be included in a comprehensive weight loss program [92]. When abdominal obesity is linked with hypertension, dietary sodium reduction is critical [53,93]. The influence of weight reduction on blood pressure has been reported in many studies [94–96]. In a recent meta-analysis of randomized controlled trials including 4874 participants, the blood pressure reduction was significantly larger in populations with an average weight loss of >5 kg than in populations with smaller weight loss, for both systolic [−6.63 mmHg (95% CI, −8.43 to −4.82) vs. −2.70 mmHg (95% CI, −4.59 to −0.81)] and diastolic [−5.12 mmHg (95% CI, −6.48 to −3.75) vs. −2.01 mmHg (95% CI, −3.47 to −0.54)] blood pressure [88]. Lifestyle interventions are summarized in Table 14.3.

A DISCOVERY EMERGING FROM AGGRESSIVE DIET AND EXERCISE THERAPY IN ABDOMINAL OBESITY

Studies aimed at achieving a better understanding of the efficacy of diet and exercise in the management of cardiovascular risk factors in patients with obesity and T2DM have been undertaken. As recommended for hypertensive obese individuals, these study designs could probably be applied to similar populations with hypertension and overweight or obesity. Indeed, the SYNERGIE lifestyle intervention study, which included 144 men with MetS, identified which components of a 1-year lifestyle intervention program (physical activity, energy and macronutrient intake, and diet quality) had the most influence on visceral adipose tissue loss [97]. The results highlight a strong contribution of dietary quality beyond macronutrient and energy content to changes in body composition and suggest that synergistic changes in both dietary quality and physical activity levels optimally reduce the amount of visceral adipose tissue in men [97] leading to improvements in cardiometabolic risk [98].

A summary of those studies in which lifestyle interventions were the central approaches to improve dyslipidemia, blood pressure, impaired fasting glucose, or glycemic control in obese patients with impaired tolerance or T2DM is provided in Table 14.4.

The Finnish Diabetes Prevention Study

The Finnish Diabetes Prevention Study (DPS) included 522 overweight Finnish adults with impaired glucose tolerance, who were divided into two groups: these were given (1) standard intervention or (2) intensive therapy. The median follow-up for participants was 7 years [99]. In the intensive therapy group, the strategy consisted of weight reduction, limited total and saturated fat intake, and the consumption of fiber, whole-grain products, vegetables, fruit, low-fat milk, soft margarines, and vegetable oils rich in monounsaturated fat, combined with an increase in exercise [100]. After 3.2 years of follow-up, WC was reduced by 4.4 cm in the intensive therapy group compared to 1.3 cm in the control group, and blood pressure was reduced by 5/5 mmHg in the intensive group compared to 1/3 mmHg in the intervention group for systolic/diastolic blood pressure [100].

Look AHEAD

The Look AHEAD study involved 5145 obese patients with T2DM, with inclusion criteria being glycated hemoglobin [hemoglobin A1c (HbA1c)] of <11%, blood pressure <160/100 mmHg, and triglycerides <6.84 mM. Follow-up lasted a maximum of 13.5 years [91]. The cohort was divided into two treatment groups and given (1) lifestyle intervention with an intensive program designed to reduce initial weight by >7% and increase physical activity with a physical activity goal of ≥175 min/week of moderate intensity activity to be achieved by the sixth month, in which participants were

TABLE 14.4 Interventions and Main Results of the Diabetes Prevention Study and Look AHEAD

			Main Result			
Study	**Group**	**Intervention**	**Hypertension: Blood Pressure Control**	**Type 2 Diabetes (HbA1c Level)**	**Dyslipidemia**	**Weight Loss, Organ Damage, Cardiovascular Events**
Diabetes Prevention Study [100,102]	1	Oral and written information about diet and exercise without individualized programs	G2: lower blood pressure	G2: onset and prevalence of type 2 diabetes ↓ by 58%	G2: best improvement in triglyceride levels	G2: better weight loss and improvement in waist circumference
	2	Detailed advice about how to achieve a reduction in weight of >5% Daily energy intake: <30% fat, <10% saturated fat, ≥15 g fiber intake/day, frequent ingestion of whole grains, vegetables, fruits, low-fat milk and meat products, soft margarines, and vegetable oils rich in monounsaturated fat				
Look AHEAD [101]	1	Usual medical care and an intensive program designed to increase physical activity and reduce initial weight by >7%	G1: lower blood pressure	G1: better HbA1c level	G1: best improvement in triglyceride, LDL, and HDL levels	G1: better % initial weight loss
	2	Usual medical care and three educational sessions/year				

Source: adapted from [103]. HbA1c, glycated hemoglobin; HDL, high-density lipoprotein; LDL, low-density lipoprotein.

instructed to engage in brisk walking or a similar aerobic activity; or (2) standard care, including diabetes support and educational group sessions. After 4 years, there was a significant improvement in the lifestyle intervention group compared with the standard care group in terms of initial weight loss (−6.15 vs. −0.88%, $P<0.001$), systolic blood pressure (−5.3 vs. −2.9 mmHg), and diastolic blood pressure (−2.9 vs. −2.5 mmHg; $P<0.001$) [101]. However, lifestyle interventions did not reduce the rate of cardiovascular events in overweight or obese adults with T2DM [91].

Findings

As reported in the DPS and the Look AHEAD study, aggressive lifestyle interventions are efficient in achieving goals related to weigh loss and on improving chronic condition such as hypertension. Commonalities in the studies are related to the intensity of the interventions, including moderate exercise and healthy eating patterns, as well as the inclusion of health-care professionals, such as nutritionists and kinesiologists, in order to provide regular support to the participants during their follow-up.

CONCLUSION

Many factors can promote hypertension development in abdominal obesity. Most important factors seem to be related to the deleterious effects of adipocyte overactivity at a molecular level and also to overstimulation of the sympathetic nervous system, which controls the mechanisms responsible for blood pressure regulation. Abdominal obesity assessed by WC is frequently associated with blood pressure dysregulation, as well as with other metabolic abnormalities like high fasting plasma glucose levels and dyslipidemia, which can lead to MetS. Promising intensive interventions centered on increasing physical activity and recommending specific dietary patterns, as reported by the Diabetes Prevention Program, Look AHEAD and SYNERGIE studies, should be replicated by health-care professionals in the promotion of aggressive nonpharmacological approaches for treating high blood pressure in patients with abdominal obesity.

References

[1] Ogden CL, Carroll MD, Kit BK, Flegal KM. Prevalence of obesity in the united states, 2009–2010. Cent Dis Control Prev Natl Cent Health Stat Data Brief 2012;82:1–8.

[2] Shields M, Carroll MD, Ogden CL. Adult obesity prevalence in Canada and the United States. Natl Cent Health Stat Data Brief 2011;56:1–8.

[3] World Health Organization expert committee on physical status. Physical status: the use and interpretation of anthropometry. Geneva, Switzerland: World Health Organization; 1995.

[4] National Institutes for Health and Clinical Excellence. Obesity guidance on the prevention, identification, assessment and management of overweight and obesity in adults and children. London: National Institute for Health and Clinical Excellence; 2006.

[5] Poirier P, Cornier M-A, Mazzone T, Stiles S, Cummings S, Klein S, et al. Bariatric surgery and cardiovascular risk factors: A scientific statement from the American Heart Association. Circulation 2011;123(15):1683–701.

[6] Poirier P, Alpert MA, Fleisher LA, Thompson PD, Sugerman HJ, Burke LE, et al. Cardiovascular evaluation and management of severely obese patients undergoing surgery: a science advisory from the American Heart Association. Circulation 2009;120: 86–95.

[7] Lau DC, Douketis JD, Morrison KM, Hramiak IM, Sharma AM, Ur E, et al. Canadian clinical practice guidelines on the management and prevention of obesity in adultss and children. CMAJ 2007;176:S1–S13.

[8] Tchernof A, Després J-P. Pathophysiology of human visceral obesity: an update. Physiol Rev 2013;93:359–404.

[9] Cornier MA, Després JP, Davis N, Grossniklaus DA, Klein S, Lamarche B, et al. American Heart Association Obesity Committee of the Council on Nutrition; Physical Activity and Metabolism; Council on Arteriosclerosis; Thrombosis and Vascular Biology; Council on Cardiovascular Disease in the Young; Council on Cardiovascular Radiology and Intervention; Council on Cardiovascular Nursing, Council on Epidemiology and Prevention; Council on the Kidney in Cardiovascular Disease, and Stroke Council. Assessing adiposity: a scientific statement from the American Heart Association. Circulation 2011;124(18):1996–2019. Nov 1.

[10] Ruderman NB, Berchtold P, Schneider S. Obesity-associated disorders in normal-weight individuals: some speculations. Int J Obes 1982;6(Suppl, 1):151–7.

[11] Ruderman NB, Schneider SH, Berchtold P. The "metabolically -obese", normal-weight individual. Am J Clin Nutr 1981;34: 1617–21.

[12] Okosun IS, Chandra KMD, Choi S, Christman J, Dever GEA, Prewitt TE. Hypertension and type 2 diabetes comorbidity in adults in the United States: Risk of Overall and Regional Adiposity. Obes Res 2001;9:1–9.

[13] Okosun IS, Prewitt TE, Cooper RS. Abdominal obesity in the United States: prevalence and attributable risk of hypertension. J Hum Hypertens 1999;13:425–30.

[14] Must A, Spadano J, Coakley EH, Field AE, Colditz G, Dietz WH. The disease burden associated with overweight and obesity. JAMA 1999;282:1523–9.

[15] Salvadori M, Sontrop JM, Garg AX, Truong J, Suri RS, Mahmud FH, et al. Elevated blood pressure in relation to overweight and obesity among children in a rural Canadian community. Pediatrics 2008;122:e821–7.

[16] Reeder BA, Angel A, Ledoux M, Rabkin SW, Young K, Lamont SE, et al. Obesity and its relation to cardiovascular disease risk factors in Canadian adults. Can Med Assoc J 1992;146:2009–19.

[17] Leenen FHH, McInnis NH, Fodor G. Obesity and the prevalence and management of hypertension in Ontario, Canada. Am J Hypertens 2010;23:1000–6.

[18] Chateau-Degat M-L, Dewailly E, Noël M, Valera B, Ferland A, Counil E, et al. Hypertension among the Inuit from Nunavik: should we expect an increased because of obesity? Int J Circumpolar Health 2010;69:361–72.

[19] Young TK, Sevenhuysen G. Obesity in northern Canadian Indians: patterns, determinants, and consequences. Am J Clin Nutr 1989;49:786–93.

[20] Hackam DG, Quinn RR, Ravani P, Rabi DM, Dasgupta K, Daskalopoulou SS, et al. The 2013 Canadian hypertension education program recommendations for blood pressure measurement, diagnosis, assessment of risk, prevention, and treatment of hypertension. Can J Cardiol 2013;29:528–42.

[21] Rosendorff C, Black HR, Cannon CP, Gersh BJ, Gore J, Izzo JL, et al. Treatment of hypertension in the prevention and management of ischemic heart disease: a scientific statement from the American Heart Association Council for high blood pressure research and the councils on Clinical Cardiology and Epidemiology and Prevention. Circulation 2007;115:2761–88.

[22] Bertoia ML, Waring ME, Gupta PS, Roberts MB, Eaton CB. Implications of new hypertension guidelines in the United States. Hypertension 2012;60:639–44.

[23] Pickering TG, Hall JE, Appel LJ, Falkner BE, Graves J, Hill MN, et al. Recommendations for blood pressure measurement in humans and experimental animals: Part 1: Blood pressure measurement in humans: a statement for professionals from the subcommittee of professional and public education of the American Heart Association Council on high blood pressure research. Circulation 2005;111:697–716.

[24] 'INTERSTROKE Study' top 10 stroke risk factors. *AACN Bold Voices* 2010; 2: 13.

[25] Goldstein LB, Bushnell CD, Adams RJ, Appel LJ, Braun LT, Chaturvedi S, et al. Guidelines for the primary prevention of stroke: a guideline for healthcare professionals from the American Heart Association/American Stroke Association. Stroke 2011;42:517–84.

[26] Leblanc ME, Croteau S, Ferland A, Bussières J, Cloutier L, Hould FS, et al. Blood pressure assessment in severe obesity; validation of a forearm approach. Obesity 2013. [Epub ahead of print].

[27] Gress TW, Nieto FJ, Shahar E, Wofford MR, Brancati FL. Hypertension and antihypertensive therapy as risk factors for type 2 diabetes mellitus. N Engl J Med 2000;342:905–12.

[28] Hinderliter AL, Babyak MA, Sherwood A, Blumenthal JA. The DASH diet and insulin sensitivity. Curr Hypertens Rep 2011;13:67–73.

[29] American Diabetes Association . Standards of medical care in diabetes—2011. Diabetes Care 2011;34(Suppl. 1):S11–61.

[30] Gus M, Fuchs SC, Moreira LB, Moraes RS, Wiehe M, Silva AF, et al. Association between different measurements of obesity and the incidence of hypertension. Am J Hypertens 2004;17:50–3.

[31] Chuang S-Y, Chou P, Hsu P-F, Cheng H-M, Tsai S-T, Lin IF, et al. Presence and progression of abdominal obesity are predictors of future high blood pressure and hypertension. Am J Hypertens 2006;19:788–95.
[32] Siani A, Cappuccio FP, Barba G, Trevisan M, Farinaro E, Iacone R, et al. The relationship of waist circumference to blood pressure: The Olivetti Heart Study. Am J Hypertens 2002;15:780–6.
[33] Poirier P, Lemieux I, Mauriege P, Dewailly E, Blanchet C, Bergeron J, et al. Impact of waist circumference on the relationship between blood pressure and insulin: The Quebec Health Survey. Hypertension 2005;45:363–7.
[34] Zhou Z, Hu D, Chen J. Association between obesity indices and blood pressure or hypertension: which index is the best? Public Health Nutr 2009;12:1061–71.
[35] Christian AH, Mochari H, Mosca LJ. Waist circumference, body mass index, and their association with cardiometabolic and global risk. J Cardiometab Syndr 2009;4:12–19.
[36] Brenner DR, Tepylo K, Eny KM, Cahill LE, El-Sohemy A. Comparison of body mass index and waist circumference as predictors of cardiometabolic health in a population of young Canadian adults. Diabetol Metab Syndr 2010;2:28.
[37] Taylor AE, Ebrahim S, Ben-Shlomo Y, Martin RM, Whincup PH, Yarnell JW, et al. Comparison of the associations of body mass index and measures of central adiposity and fat mass with coronary heart disease, diabetes, and all-cause mortality: a study using data from 4 UK cohorts. Am J Clin Nutr 2010;91:547–56.
[38] Balkau B, Deanfield JE, Després J-P, Bassand J-P, Fox KAA, Smith SC, et al. International Day for the Evaluation of Abdominal Obesity (IDEA): A study of waist circumference, cardiovascular disease, and diabetes mellitus in 168 000 primary care patients in 63 countries. Circulation 2007;116:1942–51.
[39] Recio-Rodriguez JI, Gomez-Marcos MA, Patino-Alonso MC, Agudo-Conde C, Rodriguez-Sanchez E, Garcia-Ortiz L. Abdominal obesity vs general obesity for identifying arterial stiffness, subclinical atherosclerosis and wave reflection in healthy, diabetics and hypertensive. BMC Cardiovasc Disord 2012;12:1–8.
[40] Ross R, Berentzen T, Bradshaw AJ, Janssen I, Kahn HS, Katzmarzyk PT, et al. Does the relationship between waist circumference, morbidity and mortality depend on measurement protocol for waist circumference? Obes Rev 2008;9:312–25.
[41] Cloutier L, Grenier-Michaud S, Houle J. Le tour de taille: une mesure qui en dit long. Perspect Infirmière 2010;7:32–4.
[42] Lin WY, Lee LT, Chen CY, Lo H, Hsia HH, Liu IL, et al. Optimal cut-off values for obesity: using simple anthropometric indices to predict cardiovascular risk factors in Taiwan. Int J Obes Relat Metab Disord 2002;26:1232–8.
[43] Huang KC, Lin WY, Lee LT, Chen CY, Lo H, Hsia HH, et al. Four anthropometric indices and cardiovascular risk factors in Taiwan. Int J Obes Relat Metab Disord 2002;26:1060–8.
[44] Bodenant M, Kuulasmaa K, Wagner A, Kee F, Palmieri L, Ferrario MM, et al. Measures of abdominal adiposity and the risk of stroke: the MOnica Risk, Genetics, Archiving and Monograph (MORGAM) study. Stroke 2011;42:2872–7.
[45] Hsieh SD, Ashwell M, Muto T, Tsuji H, Arase Y, Murase T. Urgency of reassessment of role of obesity indices for metabolic risks. Metab Clin Exp 2010;59:834–40.
[46] Jayawardana R, Ranasinghe P, Sheriff MHR, Matthews DR, Katulanda P. Waist to height ratio: a better anthropometric marker of diabetes and cardio-metabolic risks in South Asian adults. Diabetes Res Clin Pract 2013;99:292–9.
[47] Li W-C, Chen IC, Chang Y-C, Loke S-S, Wang S-H, Hsiao K-Y. Waist-to-height ratio, waist circumference, and body mass index as indices of cardiometabolic risk among 36,642 Taiwanese adults. Eur J Nutr 2013;52:57–65.
[48] Ashwell M, Gunn P, Gibson S. Waist-to-height ratio is a better screening tool than waist circumference and BMI for adult cardiometabolic risk factors: systematic review and meta-analysis. Obes Rev 2012;13:275–86.
[49] Syed S, Hingorjo MR, Charania A, Qureshi MA. Anthropometric and metabolic indicators in hypertensive patients. J Coll Physic Surg Pak 2009;19:421–7.
[50] Doll S, Paccaud F, Bovet P, Burnier M, Wietlisbach V. Body mass index, abdominal adiposity and blood pressure: consistency of their association across developing and developed countries. Int J Obes Relat Metab Disord 2002;26:48–57.
[51] Hartz A, He T, Rimm A. Comparison of adiposity measures as risk factors in postmenopausal women. J Clin Endocrinol Metab 2012;97:227–33.
[52] Mathieu P, Poirier P, Pibarot P, Lemieux I, Després J-P. Visceral obesity: the link among inflammation, hypertension, and cardiovascular disease. Hypertension 2009;53:577–84.
[53] Díaz ME. Hypertension and obesity. J Hum Hypertens 2002;16(Suppl 1):S18–22.
[54] Collis T, Devereux RB, Roman MJ, de Simone G, Yeh J-L, Howard BV, et al. Relations of stroke volume and cardiac output to body composition: The Strong Heart Study. Circulation 2001;103:820–5.
[55] Esler M, Straznicky N, Eikelis N, Masuo K, Lambert G, Lambert E. Mechanisms of sympathetic activation in obesity-related hypertension. Hypertension 2006;48:787–96.
[56] Rahmouni K. Obesity, sympathetic overdrive, and hypertension: the leptin connection. Hypertension 2010;55:844–5.
[57] Kaplan NM, Victor RG. Chapter 3: Primary hypertension: pathogenesis. In: Kaplan NM, Victor RG, editors. Kaplan's clinical hypertension. Philadelphia: Lippincott Williams & Wilkins; 2010.
[58] Poirier P, Giles TD, Bray GA, Hong Y, Stern JS, Pi-Sunyer FX, et al. Obesity and cardiovascular disease: pathophysiology, evaluation, and effect of weight loss: an update of the 1997 American Heart Association Scientific Statement on Obesity and Heart Disease from the Obesity Committee of the Council on Nutrition, Physical Activity, and Metabolism. Circulation 2006;113:898–918.
[59] Kurukulasuriya LR, Stas S, Lastra G, Manrique C, Sowers JR. Hypertension in obesity. Endocrinol Metab Clin North Am 2008;37:647–62.
[60] Hall JE. The kidney, hypertension, and obesity. Hypertension 2003;41:625–33.
[61] Lambert EA, Straznicky NE, Lambert GW. A sympathetic view of human obesity. Clin Auton Res 2013;23:9–14.
[62] Kotchen TA. Obesity-related hypertension: epidemiology, pathophysiology, and clinical Management. Am J Hypertens 2010;23:1170–8.
[63] Alvarez GE, Beske SD, Ballard TP, Davy KP. Sympathetic Neural Activation in Visceral Obesity. Circulation 2002;106:2533–6.
[64] Weyer C, Pratley RE, Snitker S, Spraul M, Ravussin E, Tataranni PA. Ethnic differences in insulinemia and sympathetic tone as links between obesity and blood pressure. Hypertension 2000;36:531–7.
[65] Sarzani R, Salvi F, Dessì-Fulgheri P, Rappelli A. Renin-angiotensin system, natriuretic peptides, obesity, metabolic syndrome, and hypertension: an integrated view in humans. J Hypertens 2008;26:831–43.
[66] Jeunemaitre X, Soubrier F, Kotelevtsev YV, Lifton RP, Williams CS, Charru A, et al. Molecular basis of human hypertension: Role of angiotensinogen. Cell 1992;71:169–80.
[67] Giacchetti G, Faloia E, Mariniello B, Sardu C, Gatti C, Camilloni MA, et al. Overexpression of the renin-angiotensin system in human visceral adipose tissue in normal and overweight subjects. Am J Hyperten 2002;15:381–8.

[68] Thethi T, Kamiyama M, Kobori H. The link between the renin-angiotensin-aldosterone system and renal injury in obesity and the metabolic syndrome. Curr Hypertens Rep 2012;14:160–9.
[69] Engeli S, Böhnke J, Gorzelniak K, Janke J, Schling P, Bader M, et al. Weight loss and the renin-angiotensin-aldosterone system. Hypertension 2005;45:356–62.
[70] Hamm LL, Chen J. Fat chance for hypertension and chronic kidney disease. Hypertension 2011;58:756–7.
[71] Vaz M, Jennings G, Turner A, Cox H, Lambert G, Esler M. Regional sympathetic nervous activity and oxygen consumption in obese normotensive human subjects. Circulation 1997;96:3423–9.
[72] Foster MC, Hwang S-J, Porter SA, Massaro JM, Hoffmann U, Fox CS. Fatty kidney, hypertension, and chronic kidney disease: The Framingham Heart Study. Hypertension 2011;58:784–90.
[73] Pescatello L, Franklin B, Fagard R, Farquhar W, Kelley G, Ray C, et al. Position stand: exercise and hypertension. Med Sci Sports Exerc 2004;36:533–53.
[74] Gaudreault V, Després J-P, Rhéaume C, Alméras N, Bergeron J, Tremblay A, et al. Exercise-induced hypertension in men with metabolic syndrome: anthropometric, metabolic, and hemodynamic features. Metab Syndr Relat Disord 2013;11:7–14.
[75] Lee DK, Cheng R, Nguyen T, Fan T, Kariyawasam AP, Liu Y, et al. Characterization of Apelin, the Ligand for the APJ Receptor. J Neurochem 2000;74:34–41.
[76] Ishida J, Hashimoto T, Hashimoto Y, Nishiwaki S, Iguchi T, Harada S, et al. Regulatory roles for APJ, a seven-transmembrane receptor related to angiotensin-type 1 receptor in blood pressure in vivo. J Biol Chem 2004;279:26274–9.
[77] Japp AG, Cruden NL, Amer DAB, Li VKY, Goudie EB, Johnston NR, et al. Vascular effects of apelin in vivo in man. J Am Coll Cardiol 2008;52:908–13.
[78] Falcão-Pires I, Castro-Chaves P, Miranda-Silva D, Lourenço AP, Leite-Moreira AF. Physiological, pathological and potential therapeutic roles of adipokines. Drug Discovery Today 2012;17:880–9.
[79] Castan-Laurell I, Dray C, Attané C, Duparc T, Knauf C, Valet P. Apelin, diabetes, and obesity. Endocrine 2011;40:1–9.
[80] Webber J. Energy balance in obesity. Proc Nutr Soc 2003;62:539–43.
[81] Al-Daghri N, Bartlett WA, Jones AF, Kumar S. Role of leptin in glucose metabolism in type 2 diabetes. Diabetes Obes Metab 2002;4:147–55.
[82] Considine RV, Sinha MK, Heiman ML, Kriauciunas A, Stephens TW, Nyce MR, et al. Serum immunoreactive-leptin concentrations in normal-weight and obese humans. N Engl J Med 1996;334:292–5.
[83] Stępień M, Wlazeł RN, Paradowski M, Banach M, Rysz M, Misztal M, et al. Serum concentrations of adiponectin, leptin, resistin, ghrelin and insulin and their association with obesity indices in obese normo- and hypertensive patients—pilot study. Arch Med Sc 2012;8:431–6.
[84] Grundy SM, Hansen B, Smith SC, Cleeman JI, Kahn RA. Clinical management of metabolic syndrome: report of the American Heart Association/National Heart, Lung, and Blood Institute/American Diabetes Association conference on scientific issues related to management. Arterioscler Thromb Vasc Biol 2004;24:e19–24.
[85] Alberti KGMM, Zimmet P, Shaw J. Metabolic syndrome—a new world-wide definition. A Consensus Statement from the International Diabetes Federation. J Br Diab Assoc 2006;23:469–80.
[86] Despres J-P, Lemieux I. Abdominal obesity and metabolic syndrome. Nature 2006;444:881–7.
[87] Mulrow C, Chiquette E, Angel L, Cornell J, Summerbell C, Anagnostelis B, et al. Dieting to reduce body weight for controlling hypertension in adults (Review). *The Cochrane, Library* 2008:1–44.
[88] Neter JE, Stam BE, Kok FJ, Grobbee DE, Geleijnse JM. Influence of weight reduction on blood pressure: a meta-Analysis of randomized controlled trials. Hypertension 2003;42:878–84.
[89] Mertens IL, Van Gaal LF. Overweight, obesity, and blood pressure: the effects of modest weight reduction. Obes Res 2000;8:270–8.
[90] Aucott L, Poobalan A, Smith WCS, Avenell A, Jung R, Broom J. Effects of weight loss in overweight/obese individuals and long-term hypertension outcomes: a systematic review. Hypertension 2005;45:1035–41.
[91] Look AHEAD Research Group, Wing RR, Bolin P, Brancati FL, Bray GA, Clark JM, Coday M, et al. Cardiovascular effects of intensive lifestyle intervention in type 2 diabetes. N Engl J Med 2013;369:145–54.
[92] Pi-Sunyer FX, Kokkoris P, Szeto IMY. Obesity in Hypertension. In: Black HR, Elliott WJ, editors. Hypertension: a companion to Braunwald's Heart Disease. 2nd ed. Philadelphia: Elsevier Saunders; 2012.
[93] Poirier P. The obesity epidemic and the cardiovascular risk. In: Eckel RH, editor. Metabolic risk for cardiovascular disease. United Kingdom: Wiley-Blackwell; 2010.
[94] Pasanisi F, Contaldo F, de Simone G, Mancini M. Benefits of sustained moderate weight loss in obesity. Nutr Metab Cardiovasc Dis 2001;11:401–6.
[95] Davis BR, Blaufox MD, Oberman A, Wassertheil-Smoller S, Zimbaldi N, Cutler JA, et al. Reduction in long-term antihypertensive medication requirements. Effects of weight reduction by dietary intervention in overweight persons with mild hypertension. Arch Int Med 1993;153:1773–82.
[96] Sartorio A, Lafortuna CL, Vangeli V, Tavani A, Bosetti C, La Vecchia C. Short-term changes of cardiovascular risk factors after a non-pharmacological body weight reduction program. Eur J Clin Nutr 2001;55:865–9.
[97] Nazare J-A, Smith J, Borel A-L, Alméras N, Tremblay A, Bergeron J, et al. Changes in both global diet quality and physical activity level synergistically reduce visceral adiposity in men with features of metabolic syndrome. J Nutr 2013;143:1074–83.
[98] Borel A-L, Nazare J-A, Smith J, Alméras N, Tremblay A, Bergeron J, et al. Visceral and not subcutaneous abdominal adiposity reduction drives the benefits of a 1-year lifestyle modification mrogram. Obesity 2012;20:1223–33.
[99] Lindström J, Ilanne-Parikka P, Peltonen M, Aunola S, Eriksson JG, Hemiö K, et al. Sustained reduction in the incidence of type 2 diabetes by lifestyle intervention: follow-up of the Finnish Diabetes Prevention Study. Lancet 2006;368:1673–9.
[100] Tuomilehto J, Lindström J, Eriksson JG, Valle TT, Hämäläinen H, Ilanne-Parikka P, et al. Prevention of type 2 diabetes mellitus by changes in lifestyle among subjects with impaired glucose tolerance. N Engl J Med 2001;344:1343–50.
[101] The Look AHEAD Research Group. Long-term effects of a lifestyle intervention on weight and cardiovascular risk factors in individuals with type 2 diabetes mellitus: four-year

results of the Look AHEAD trial. Arch Intern Med 2010;170: 1566–75.

[102] Lindström J, Peltonen M, Tuomilehto J. Lifestyle strategies for weight control: experience from the Finnish Diabetes Prevention Study. Proc Nutr Soc 2005;64:81–8.

[103] Leblanc M-E, Rhéaume C, Cloutier L, Lefebvre J, Poirier P. Nonpharmacological management of hypertension in diabetes. In Management of Hypertension in Diabetes: Future Medicine Ltd 2011; 16-29.

SECTION 2

DIET, SUPPLEMENTS AND FOODS IN THE MANAGEMENT OF VISCERAL OBESITY

PART D

MECHANISMS OF ALTERING ABDOMINAL OBESITY

CHAPTER

15

Effect of Glucagon-Like Peptide 1 Receptor Agonists on Visceral Fat Adiposity, Appetite, and Food Preference

Yuya Fujishima and Norikazu Maeda

Department of Metabolic Medicine, Graduate School of Medicine, Osaka University, Osaka, Japan

INTRODUCTION

Obesity, defined as a body mass index (BMI) of $\geq 30\,kg/m^2$, has reached epidemic proportions worldwide. The World Health Organization (WHO) estimates that 2.30 billion adults will be overweight and >700 million will be obese by 2015 [1]. Obesity increases the risk of type 2 diabetes mellitus (T2DM), hypertension, dyslipidemia, and death from cardiovascular diseases [2].

Metabolic parameters such as blood pressure, lipid metabolism, and glucose tolerance are improved by a 5–10% weight reduction [3]. A meta-analysis indicates that a maximum 8.5 kg weight reduction is obtained only by lifestyle modification such as diet and exercise, but it is very difficult to maintain for a long period (over 6 months) [4]. Many types of drugs appeared on the market for the treatment of obesity, but most were withdrawn due to serious adverse events. In the United States, orlistat is the only drug that is currently available for use over a long period. Another drug, phentermine, is also approved, but is restricted for short-term use only (up to 12 weeks). Therefore, a new pharmacological agent that is well tolerated and will decrease the risk of obesity-related comorbidities is desired as an alternative approach for treating obesity.

Glucagon-like peptide 1 (GLP-1) is a naturally occurring incretin hormone and is characterized as having antidiabetic effects by inducing insulin secretion and reducing glucagon secretion only under conditions of hyperglycemia [5]. GLP-1 is a 30-amino-acid peptide hormone that is secreted from L cells in the small intestine following differential processing of proglucagon [6]. Native GLP-1, which is degraded by dipeptidyl peptidase 4 (DPP-IV) to GLP-1(9-36)amide [7,8], has a short elimination half-life of about 1–2 min [9]. Exenatide, a synthetic version of exendin-4, is the first GLP-1 receptor (GLP-1R) agonist to be approved by the Food and Drug Administration (FDA) and has 53% sequence identity to native human GLP-1; therefore, exenatide is partially resistant to DPP-IV degradation, resulting in a half-life extension to 2.4 h [10]. Liraglutide, another novel GLP-1R agonist, has 97% structural homology to human GLP-1. Subcutaneously injected liraglutide reaches a maximal concentration at around 13 h and has a long half-life; thus, liraglutide can be administered once a day [11]. Both GLP-1R agonists are generally well tolerated and almost free from the risk of hypoglycemia. These drugs therefore have become rapidly available worldwide as new therapeutic alternatives for T2DM subjects.

In addition, GLP-1 delays gastric emptying and induces satiety, leading to a decreased energy intake and consequent weight reduction. The underlying mechanisms of weight loss are thought to be the combined effects of GLP-1 on the gastrointestinal tract and the brain [12]. GLP-1 also has various extrapancreatic effects such as a protective role for cardiovascular system [1]. Hence, GLP-1R agonists are now considered to be promising new agents for the treatment of obesity and obesity-related comorbidities. In this chapter, we summarize and discuss the effects of GLP-1 on body weight, body fat composition, and food preference.

CENTRAL AND PERIPHERAL ACTIONS OF GLP-1 ON APPETITE AND FOOD INTAKE

The glucagon-containing peptides are reported to be present in the brain and are speculated to have effects on food intake [13]. Since GLP-1 was discovered in the

Nutrition in the Prevention and Treatment of Abdominal Obesity
http://dx.doi.org/10.1016/B978-0-12-407869-7.00015-5

brain [14], a central role for GLP-1 in appetite regulation has been investigated by many researchers. In the central nervous system (CNS), the caudal part of the nucleus of the solitary tract is confirmed to be the sole region of GLP-1 synthesis, occurring through a similar process to its synthesis in intestinal L cells [15]. Additionally, all GLP-1-containing neural fibers are thought to arise from the solitary tract nucleus; these neural fibers are specifically projected into the hypothalamus, which is involved in appetite control [16]. In contrast, GLP-1Rs are expressed in many regions of the brain, especially the arcuate nucleus and other hypothalamic regions [17]. Taken together, GLP-1 has a role in appetite control as a neurotransmitter substance in the CNS. Actually, intracerebroventricular GLP-1 administration inhibits food intake in rats in a dose-dependent manner [18–20]. A similar result is observed following exendin-4 administration, and is inhibited by concomitant administration of the GLP-1 antagonist, GLP-1(9-36). Activation of the paraventricular nucleus, supraoptic nucleus, and arcuate nucleus of the hypothalamus are observed after intracerebroventricular administration of GLP-1 (shown by *Fos* expression) [18,19]. As perinatal monosodium glutamate-mediated destruction of the arcuate nucleus blocks the inhibitory effects on food intake by intracerebroventricular GLP-1 administration [21], the arcuate nucleus may be essential for the GLP-1 response. GLP-1-dependent inhibition of food intake was originally considered to be a short-term effect, but later studies indicated that the appetite suppression was sustained and that continuous body weight reduction was induced by prolonged intracerebroventricular GLP-1 administration [22,23]. In addition, intracerebroventricular GLP-1 treatment completely suppressed the increase in food intake induced by melanin-concentrating hormone (MCH) and neuropeptide Y (NPY) [24].

Several studies using animal models and human subjects have shown that systemic administration of GLP-1 also reduces food intake [25,26]. However, the precise mechanism for appetite inhibition by peripheral GLP-1 administration is not yet fully understood. GLP-1 is reported to pass through the blood-brain barrier [27] or to access the brain via breaks in the blood-brain barrier such as the subfornical organ and the area postrema [28], suggesting that GLP-1 acts directly on the CNS. DPP-IV is present throughout the body, including the circulatory system, and can rapidly inactivate GLP-1; therefore, >70% of endogenous GLP-1 secreted from intestine may be inactivated before passing through the liver. Small amounts of active GLP-1 reach the systemic circulation; thus, crossing the blood-brain barrier may be an extremely inefficient route to reaching the target CNS area. However, higher molecular weight GLP-1R agonists, such as the albumin-bound GLP-1 agonist, also induce satiety and restrict food consumption although they cannot cross the blood-brain barrier [29]. Another possibility is that GLP-1 acts on the CNS via the peripheral sensory nervous system. GLP-1R is expressed in nodose ganglion cells distributed in the intestinal tract and hepatoportal bed, from which the vagal afferent fibers arise before passing through the nucleus of the solitary tract and onwards to hypothalamus [30]. Abdominal vagal nerves may be observed in localized areas of GLP-1-secreting cells or in the portal tract before GLP-1 passes through the liver, and GLP-1 may elicit its effects via central nerves through this mechanism [31]. Gastric distension elevates the *Fos* expression in brainstem neurons that produce GLP-1 [32] and deafferentation of the vagal afferent fibers abolishes the suppressive effects of GLP-1 on food intake and appetite [33,34]. These results suggest that the vagal afferent pathway also plays an essential role in mediating the effects of GLP-1 on appetite.

Importantly, GLP-1 inhibits gastrointestinal motility. If unabsorbed carbohydrate and fat flow into the ileum after a meal, gastric emptying is inhibited. Since L cells secreting GLP-1 are generally distributed within the distal ileum, it is speculated that GLP-1 inhibits gastrointestinal motility in a negative-feedback manner [35]. Intravenous or subcutaneous administration of GLP-1 inhibits gastric emptying and duodenal motility in healthy volunteers in a dose-dependent manner at physiological and supraphysiological concentrations [36,37]. An elevation in circulating GLP-1 levels within a physiological range also inhibits gastrin-induced acid secretion and pancreatic secretion [38,39]. These GLP-1 actions on the gastrointestinal tract are dependent on the vagal efferent pathway [40]. Peripherally circulating GLP-1 may exert its inhibitory effects on the gastrointestinal tract via the neural reflex, consisting of the vagal afferent fibers as inputs and the vagal efferent fibers as outputs. GLP-1R is also expressed in gastric parietal cells; thus, GLP-1 may exhibit direct actions such as delaying gastric emptying and regulating gastric acid secretion [41].

As mentioned above, GLP-1-induced suppression of food intake is thought to be mediated by inhibition of gastric motility and emptying. However, GLP-1-induced appetite reduction can be observed in subjects under fasting conditions [42]. Taken together, these findings indicate that GLP-1 synergistically acts on the hypothalamic appetite center and the gastrointestinal tract to decrease food intake.

EFFECTS ON BODY WEIGHT

Continuous GLP-1 infusion for 6 weeks not only improves glycemic control, insulin sensitivity, and beta cell function but also results in weight loss, suggesting that GLP-1 may be an effective treatment for T2DM and obesity [43]. However, native GLP-1 is rapidly degraded by DPP-IV, which limits its clinical use. Therefore, DPP-IV-resistant GLP-1 analogs with a longer half-life have been developed.

Liraglutide, a long-acting GLP-1R agonist, was originally developed to treat T2DM subjects. Further studies showed that subcutaneous injection of a maximum dose of 1.8 mg once per day improved not only glycemic control [44] but also beta cell function [45,46] and hypertension [47]. The Liraglutide Effect and Action in Diabetes (LEAD) studies, which are multicenter randomized double-blind, parallel-group trials, showed dose-dependent weight loss in addition to reduced glycated hemoglobin (HbA1c) levels [48]. Hence, liraglutide is expected to be not only an antidiabetic drug but also an antiobesity agent. An effective therapeutic strategy for obese T2DM patients should be developed without delay, but maintaining body weight in this patient group is often difficult. Early intensive therapy for T2DM subjects resulted in fine glycemic control and the prevention of microvascular and macrovascular complications over a long period [49], while intensive insulin therapy tended to increase body weight [50,51]. In addition, oral glucose-lowering agents, such as sulfonylurea and thiazolidinedione, also increase body weight by enhancing glucose uptake into adipocytes. In treating T2DM, it should be noted that weight gain and obesity develop into significant risk factors for cardiovascular events. In T2DM patients, every 5 kg/m^2 increase in BMI leads to a 30% increase in the risk of cardiovascular death [52]. Therefore, liraglutide is expected to be an effective drug producing unprecedented benefits in both improving glycemic control and reducing body weight.

In LEAD trials, substantial weight reductions were obtained in liraglutide-treated patient groups. The LEAD-3 study showed that liraglutide monotherapy at 1.2 mg/day and 1.8 mg/day significantly altered body weight by −2.1 kg and −2.5 kg, respectively, while glimepiride, a trial comparator, increased body weight by 1.1 kg (Fig. 15.1). Liraglutide monotherapy resulted in weight loss primarily in the first 16 weeks, but this effect was maintained throughout the entire 52 weeks of the study. In addition, reductions in HbA1c from baseline levels were significantly greater with both liraglutide doses than with glimepiride [53]. Furthermore, the follow-up study revealed that body weight loss by liraglutide was sustained for 2 years (1.2 mg/day liraglutide, −2.3 kg; 1.8 mg/day liraglutide, −2.8 kg; glimepiride, +1.0 kg) [54]. The LEAD-1 study was performed to evaluate the efficacy of combined liraglutide-glimepiride therapy. Over a 26-week period, 1.8 mg/day liraglutide resulted in a 0.2 kg weight reduction, which was significantly different from the 2.1 kg weight gain observed with rosiglitazone [55]. A comparative study of liraglutide with insulin therapy was performed in the LEAD-5 study, in which subjects treated with metformin and glimepiride were randomized to liraglutide or the ultra-long-acting insulin, glargine [56]. This study demonstrated that 1.8 mg/day liraglutide led to a body weight reduction of 1.8 kg from baseline; in contrast, treatment with glargine caused a significant weight gain of 1.6 kg from baseline.

Another GLP-1R agonist, exenatide, is also reported to induce clear weight reductions [57]. Exenatide was directly compared with liraglutide in the LEAD-6 study (Fig. 15.1). Over the 26-week observation period, both drugs exerted similar effects on weight reduction

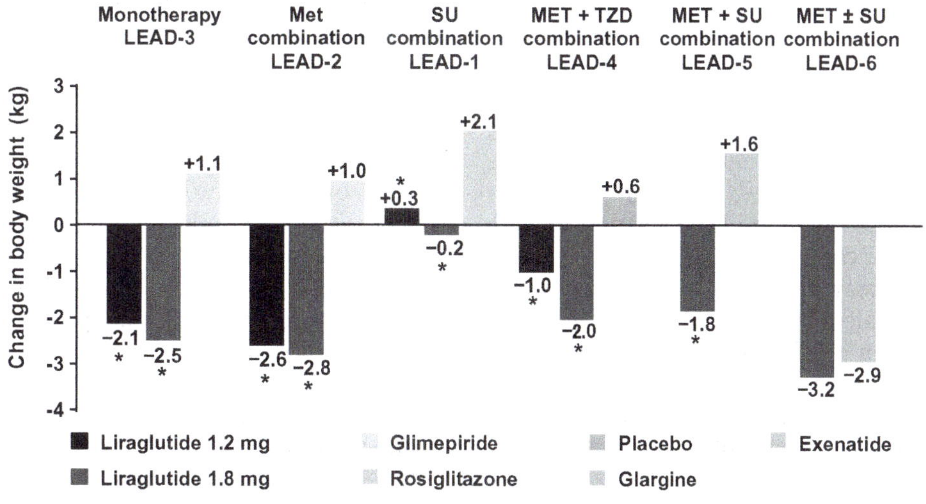

FIGURE 15.1 Changes in body weight from baseline observed in the LEAD trials [55,56,58]. *, statistical significance compared to a trial comparator. LEAD, Liraglutide Effect and Action in Diabetes; Met, metformin; SU, sulfonylurea; TZD, thiazolidinediones. (See color plate at the back of the book.)

(1.8 mg/day liraglutide, −3.2 kg; 10 μg/day exenatide, −2.9 kg), although the reduction in HbA1c was greater with liraglutide than with exenatide [58]. However, the other head-to-head study, comparing liraglutide with once-weekly slow-releasing exenatide for 26 weeks, showed that weight loss in the liraglutide group was significantly greater than in the exenatide group (liraglutide, −3.9 kg; exenatide, −2.7 kg) and glycemic control in the liraglutide group was also better than in the exenatide group [59]. Although adverse events were mild or moderate with both drugs, gastrointestinal side effects and withdrawals due to adverse events were more frequent in the liraglutide group in this study, indicating that liraglutide may have a greater effect on weight loss.

We recently reported the long-term effects of liraglutide in Japanese obese T2DM subjects (BMI > 25 kg/m^2) [60]. In this study, liraglutide was introduced during hospitalization for the medical treatment of diabetes and its effect was compared with insulin therapy. Liraglutide treatment significantly decreased body weight, even 6 months after discharge, compared to at admission (at discharge, −6.3%; at 6 months after discharge, −9.8%), even though the maximum dose permitted in Japan is 0.9 mg/day. In contrast, in the insulin group (most of the patients received insulin administration more than three times per day), body weight was significantly reduced from admission to discharge, which may have been due to the special educational program for diet therapy during hospitalization, while there were no changes in body weight from discharge to 6 months (at discharge, −4.5%; at 6 months after discharge, −3.8%). Moreover, the reduction in HbA1c levels was not different between the liraglutide and insulin groups.

As mentioned above, most clinical trials of GLP-1R agonists, as represented by the LEAD studies, were designed for T2DM subjects who are obese or overweight, but there are few trials evaluating body weight changes as a primary end point in obese subjects without diabetes. In the phase II study for obesity (BMI, 30–40 kg/m^2), up to 3.0 mg/day liraglutide for 20 weeks resulted in a dose-dependent weight reduction even in nondiabetic obese subjects (1.2 mg/day, −4.8 kg; 1.8 mg/day, −5.5 kg; 2.4 mg/day, −6.3 kg; 3.0 mg/day, −7.2 kg) [61]. Particularly in the high-dose groups (>2.4 mg/day), weight loss with liraglutide was significantly larger than the −4.1 kg obtained in subjects treated with orlistat. In addition, a follow-up study revealed that the differences in body weight change between liraglutide and orlistat were sustained over the following 2 years (2.4/3.0 mg/day liraglutide, −5.3 kg; orlistat, −2.3 kg) and the proportion of prediabetic subjects was significantly decreased in the liraglutide treatment groups [62]. Likewise, another study evaluating the efficacy of exenatide in obese subjects without diabetes (mean BMI of 39.6 kg/m^2) showed that exenatide treatment also resulted in a significant weight reduction of 5.1 kg compared to placebo at 24 weeks [63]. Although other studies are ongoing, further evidence is needed to fully elucidate the effects of GLP-1R agonists for the treatment of obesity.

EFFECTS ON BODY FAT COMPOSITION

Abdominal obesity caused by visceral fat accumulation strongly correlates with insulin resistance [64] and a high risk for T2DM [65,66]. Several studies have demonstrated that atherosclerosis proceeds through the inflammatory process: visceral fat accumulation causes dysfunction of adipocytes, which results in dysregulation of adipocytokines, such as tumor necrosis factor (TNF-α), plasminogen activator inhibitor 1 (PAI-1), and adiponectin, which then accelerates the development of atherosclerotic cardiovascular diseases [67–69]. Therefore, reducing visceral fat should be an essential therapeutic strategy for abdominal obesity, since reducing the visceral fat area decreases the risk of cardiovascular events [70].

As discussed in Chapter 3, there is increasing evidence to demonstrate that GLP-1R agonists effectively reduce body weight. A recent meta-analysis of GLP-1R agonist-dependent weight reduction showed that administration of these agents resulted in around 3% weight reduction at 6 months [71]. However, very few studies have examined changes in body fat composition caused by GLP-1R agonists. In animal models, administration of exendin (1–30) and exendin-4 significantly reduced visceral fat mass [72,73]. In human studies, the LEAD-2 and LEAD-3 trials evaluated body composition using dual-energy X-ray absorptiometry (DEXA) [74]. These studies indicated that liraglutide-induced weight reduction was mainly dependent on fat tissue rather than on lean tissue. Furthermore, in the LEAD-2 trial, abdominal fat composition was measured by single-slice abdominal computed tomography (CT) at both the time of entry and the time of completion (26 weeks). Both 1.2 mg/day and 1.8 mg/day liraglutide significantly reduced visceral fat area compared to glimepiride. Visceral fat area was eventually decreased by 30.4 cm^2 (−16%) in the 1.8 mg/day liraglutide group [74]. The other study that enrolled nondiabetic obese subjects also demonstrated that body weight reduction by liraglutide was primarily a result of decreased fat tissue [62].

In a pilot study involving Japanese T2DM inpatients, we previously reported that the estimated visceral fat area, as measured by abdominal bioelectrical impedance analysis [75], was significantly reduced by liraglutide treatment for 20 days [76]. In addition, short-term liraglutide treatment decreased the levels of biomarkers related to atherosclerosis, such as high-sensitivity C-reactive protein (hs-CRP) and soluble intercellular adhesion molecule 1 (sICAM-1), while significant changes were not observed with other glucose-lowering agents. Previous studies showed a lack of GLP-1R expression in adipocytes [77], but recent work has demonstrated that GLP-1R is expressed in adipocytes [78]. These studies suggest that liraglutide reduces visceral fat adiposity either directly or indirectly, although GLP-1 activity and GLP-1R signaling in adipocytes have not yet been fully elucidated.

Adiponectin, which is specifically secreted from adipocytes, possesses multiple effects on organ protection, including antiarteriosclerotic, antidiabetic, and anti-inflammatory effects [69]. Adiponectin is characterized by a decreased serum level in obesity, despite its restricted expression in adipocytes. Importantly, hypoadiponectinemia is closely associated with diabetes and atherosclerosis [79]. Exenatide treatment for 3 months increased adiponectin serum levels, along with a significant reduction in body weight and waist circumference [80]. In vitro experiments showed that exendin-4 has direct effects on adipocytes and induces adiponectin expression [78], suggesting that GLP-1R agonist-dependent elevation of circulating adiponectin levels is independent of weight reduction. However, further evidence for an effect of GLP-1 on adiponectin expression is required.

It is well known that long-term excessive caloric intake and/or physical inactivity cause extra fat accumulation in organs other than adipose tissue. Nonalcoholic fatty liver disease (NAFLD), a condition of excess fat deposition within the liver, is a disease with a poor prognosis that is associated with inflammation, fibrosis, and cell death, ultimately progressing to cirrhosis [81]. NAFLD frequently coexists with T2DM and abdominal obesity, but the current therapeutic strategy for NAFLD is limited to weight reduction by lifestyle modifications involving diet and exercise [82,83] because there is no approved pharmacological therapy of proven benefit for NAFLD [84]. In in vitro studies, GLP-1R agonists exhibited direct actions on hepatocytes and enhanced hepatic fatty acid oxidation via the 5′-AMP-activated protein kinase (AMPK) pathway and insulin signaling pathway [85,86]. Recent clinical research demonstrated the expression of GLP-1Rs in the liver, indicating the possibility that GLP-1R agonists can be applied clinically for the treatment of NAFLD [87]. In LEAD trials, treatment with 1.8 mg/day liraglutide for 26 weeks significantly reduced alanine transaminase (ALT) levels, especially in patients with elevated ALT at baseline, but this effect was lost after adjusting for weight loss by liraglutide [88]. Subanalysis of the LEAD-2 trial showed that liraglutide tends to improve hepatic steatosis [88]. In a small population, liraglutide treatment was reported to significantly reduce intrahepatic lipid levels (quantified by liver proton magnetic resonance spectroscopy) by 42% from baseline, which correlated with improvements in HbA1c [89].

In conclusion, long-term prospective studies are needed to determine whether GLP-1R agonists improve various metabolic parameters and reduce the risk of cardiovascular events.

EFFECTS ON FOOD PREFERENCE AND EATING BEHAVIOR

The peripheral infusion of native GLP-1 enhanced satiety and reduced food intake in healthy subjects in a dose-dependent manner [25,26]. The effect of GLP-1 on satiety and food intake is also seen in individuals with T2DM and obesity [90,91]. Although very few effects on food intake have been shown (plasma levels of GLP-1 are comparable to those seen in the physiological state after meals [92,93]), GLP-1 itself may have therapeutic potential in obesity as well as being a physiological regulator of appetite.

Reductions in body weight and fat mass by GLP-1R agonists should result from a decreased total caloric intake. First, it is speculated that appetite-suppressive effects are associated with inhibition of gastric emptying. In fact, gastrointestinal events, such as nausea and vomiting, were the most frequently reported adverse events for GLP-1R agonists. Although the frequency of these gastrointestinal side effects gradually decreases over time and decline to <10% by 4 weeks [47], GLP-1R agonist-dependent weight reduction is known to be sustained for long periods, indicating the possibility that GLP-1 may also influence eating behavior and food preference.

Liraglutide reduces both dietary intake and body weight in rats. More interestingly, liraglutide treatment influenced food choice, which shifted in favor of normal chow rather than candy consumption. Conversely, these effects were not observed with a DPP-IV inhibitor, vildagliptin, suggesting that GLP-1R agonists may be able to reduce sugar and fat intake [94]. Similarly, meal size and feeding frequency were decreased with liraglutide treatment in minipig obesity model [95]. Furthermore, a recent study of obese T2DM subjects revealed that a once-daily injection of liraglutide, compared to placebo and glimepiride, induced less fasting hunger and a shorter meal duration and suppressed gastric emptying, leading to decreased energy intake [96]. There was no significant effect of liraglutide on resting energy expenditure. Another randomized placebo-controlled, double-blind crossover study also showed that both postprandial hunger and energy intake during the subsequent ad libitum lunch were reduced after 3 weeks of liraglutide treatment [97].

It is generally difficult to intervene in eating behavior in obese human subjects, although abnormal eating behavior may form a background to obesity [98]. The effect of GLP-1R agonists on eating behavior has not been fully examined in human subjects; we therefore recently investigated the effect of liraglutide on eating behavior in Japanese obese patients (BMI > 25 kg/m^2) with T2DM [60]. In this study, liraglutide was introduced to patients during their hospitalization for the medical treatment for diabetes, and eating behavior was assessed by using the Guideline for Obesity questionnaire issued by the Japan Society for the Study of Obesity. This questionnaire consists of 55-item questions of seven major scales as follows: (1) recognition of weight and constitution (e.g. "Do you think it is easier for you to gain weight than others?"); (2) external eating behavior (e.g. "If food smells and looks good, do you eat more than usual?"); (3) emotional eating behavior (e.g. "Do you have the desire to eat when you are irritated?"); (4) sense of hunger (e.g. "Do you become irritated when you feel hungry?"); (5) eating style (e.g. "Do you eat fast?"); (6) food preference (e.g. "Do you like meat?"); and (7) regularity of eating habits (e.g. "Is your dinner time too late at night?"). Interestingly, the scores for obese T2DM patients at admission were higher in all major scales than in nonobese subjects. Liraglutide administration decreased these scores and maintained improvements in all scales (except for the emotional eating behavior scale) until 6 months after discharge. The total score for eating behavior in liraglutide-treated patients eventually showed a significant decreased to match the score in nonobese healthy subjects. Further, the extent of weight reduction at 6 months after discharge significantly correlated with the reduction in scores for the sense of hunger and for eating style (a more significant improvement was observed for the response to the question about eating quickly), suggesting that liraglutide-induced weight reduction is partly mediated through improvements in eating behavior (Fig. 15.2). The intake of animal fat, especially of saturated fat, is considered to be associated with T2DM and cardiovascular diseases [99]. Liraglutide treatment significantly decreased the score for fat requirement. Actually, liraglutide significantly reduced high-density lipoprotein cholesterol levels 6 months after discharge. These results indicate that liraglutide effectively improves eating behavior in obese T2DM subjects.

CONCLUSIONS

Many studies since the mid-1990s have demonstrated that GLP-1 has direct effects on appetite and food intake, in addition to its actions on pancreatic islet cells. There is

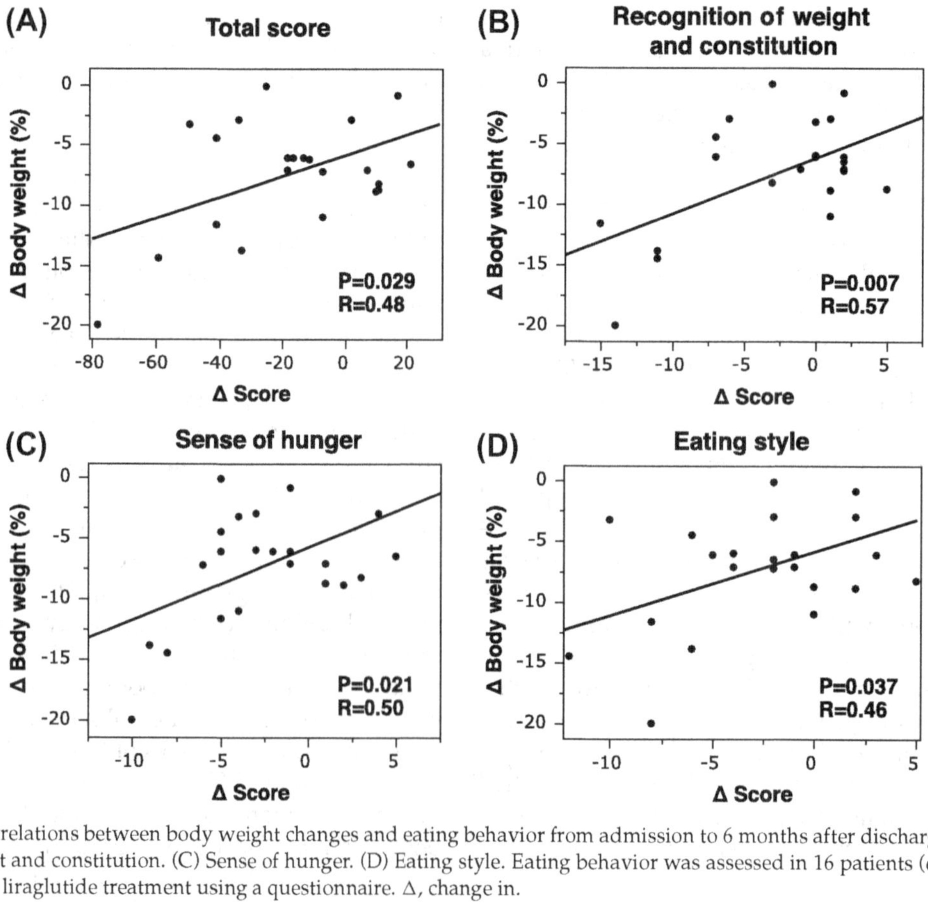

FIGURE 15.2 Correlations between body weight changes and eating behavior from admission to 6 months after discharge.(A) Total score. (B) Recognition of weight and constitution. (C) Sense of hunger. (D) Eating style. Eating behavior was assessed in 16 patients (eight males and eight females) treated with liraglutide treatment using a questionnaire. Δ, change in.

increasing evidence that GLP-1R agonists not only ameliorate hyperglycemia in diabetic subjects but also reduce body weight and alter food preference. GLP-1R agonists are expected to form a new class of antiobesity drugs. However, the effect of weight reduction and improvements in eating behavior should be further examined in the future as part of a double-blind, placebo-controlled clinical trial.

References

[1] Chilton R, Wyatt J, Nandish S, Oliveros R, Lujan M. Cardiovascular comorbidities of type 2 diabetes mellitus: defining the potential of glucagonlike peptide-1-based therapies. Am J Med 2011;124: S35–53.

[2] Van Gaal LF, Mertens IL, De Block CE. Mechanisms linking obesity with cardiovascular disease. Nature 2006;444:875–80.

[3] Wing RR, Lang W, Wadden TA, Safford M, Knowler WC, Bertoni AG, Hill JO, Brancati FL, Peters A, Wagenknecht L. Look AHEAD Research Group. Benefits of modest weight loss in improving cardiovascular risk factors in overweight and obese individuals with type 2 diabetes. Diabetes Care 2011;34:1481–6.

[4] Franz MJ, VanWormer JJ, Crain AL, Boucher JL, Histon T, Caplan W, Bowman JD, Pronk NP. Weight-loss outcomes: a systematic review and meta-analysis of weight-loss clinical trials with a minimum 1-year follow-up. J Am Diet Assoc 2007;107:1755–67.

[5] Holst JJ, Orskov C. The incretin approach for diabetes treatment: modulation of islet hormone release by GLP-1 agonism. Diabetes 2004;53:S197–204.

[6] Frezza EE, Wachtel MS, Chiriva-Internati M. The multiple faces of glucagon-like peptide-1—obesity, appetite, and stress: what is next? A Review Dig Dis Sci 2007;52:643–9.

[7] Deacon CF, Johnsen AH, Holst JJ. Degradation of glucagon-like peptide-1 by human plasma in vitro yields an N-terminally truncated peptide that is a major endogenous metabolite in vivo. J Clin Endocrinol Metab 1995;80:952–7.

[8] Kieffer TJ, McIntosh CH, Pederson RA. Degradation of glucose-dependent insulinotropic polypeptide and truncated glucagon-like peptide 1 in vitro and in vivo by dipeptidyl peptidase IV. Endocrinology 1995;136:3585–96.

[9] Drucker DJ, Nauck MA. The incretin system: glucagon-like peptide-1 receptor agonists and dipeptidyl peptidase-4 inhibitors in type 2 diabetes. Lancet 2006;368:1696–705.

[10] Byetta Package Insert, <http://pi.lilly.com/us/byetta-pi.pdf>; 2009 [accessed 6.04.09].

[11] Agersø H, Jensen LB, Elbrønd B, Rolan P, Zdravkovic M. The pharmacokinetics, pharmacodynamics, safety and tolerability of NN2211, a new long-acting GLP-1 derivative, in healthy men. Diabetologia 2002;45:195–202.

[12] Abu-Hamdah R, Rabiee A, Meneilly GS, Shannon RP, Andersen DK, Elahi D. Clinical review: the extrapancreatic effects of glucagon-like peptide-1 and related peptides. J Clin Endocrinol Metab 2009;94:1843–52.

[13] Tager H, Hohenboken M, Markese J, Dinerstein RJ. Identification and localization of glucagon-related peptides in rat brain. Proc Natl Acad Sci USA 1980;77:6229–33.

[14] Jin SL, Han VK, Simmons JG, Towle AC, Lauder JM, Lund PK. Distribution of glucagonlike peptide I (GLP-I), glucagon, and glicentin in the rat brain: an immunocytochemical study. J Comp Neurol 1988;271:519–32.

[15] Larsen PJ, Tang-Christensen M, Holst JJ, Orskov C. Distribution of glucagon-like peptide-1 and other preproglucagon-derived peptides in the rat hypothalamus and brainstem. Neuroscience 1997;77:257–70.

[16] Larsen PJ, Holst JJ. Glucagon-related peptide 1 (GLP-1): hormone and neurotransmitter. Regul Pept 2005;128:97–107.

[17] Göke R, Larsen PJ, Mikkelsen JD, Sheikh SP. Distribution of GLP-1 binding sites in the rat brain: evidence that exendin-4 is a ligand of brain GLP-1 binding sites. Eur J Neurosci 1995;7:2294–300.

[18] Turton MD, O'Shea D, Gunn I, Beak SA, Edwards CM, Meeran K, Choi SJ, Taylor GM, Heath MM, Lambert PD, Wilding JP, Smith DM, Ghatei MA, Herbert J, Bloom SR. A role for glucagon-like peptide-1 in the central regulation of feeding. Nature 1996;4(379):69–72.

[19] Tang-Christensen M, Larsen PJ, Göke R, Fink-Jensen A, Jessop DS, Møller M, Sheikh SP. Central administration of GLP-1-(7–36) amide inhibits food and water intake in rats. Am J Physiol 1996;271:R848–56.

[20] Navarro M, Rodriquez de Fonseca F, Alvarez E, Chowen JA, Zueco JA, Gomez R, Eng J, Blázquez E. Colocalization of glucagon-like peptide-1 (GLP-1) receptors, glucose transporter GLUT-2, and glucokinase mRNAs in rat hypothalamic cells: evidence for a role of GLP-1 receptor agonists as an inhibitory signal for food and water intake. J Neurochem 1996;67:1982–91.

[21] Tang-Christensen M, Vrang N, Larsen PJ. Glucagon-like peptide 1(7–36) amide's central inhibition of feeding and peripheral inhibition of drinking are abolished by neonatal monosodium glutamate treatment. Diabetes 1998;47:530–7.

[22] Davis Jr HR, Mullins DE, Pines JM, Hoos LM, France CF, Compton DS, Graziano MP, Sybertz EJ, Strader CD, Van Heek M. Effect of chronic central administration of glucagon-like peptide-1 (7–36) amide on food consumption and body weight in normal and obese rats. Obes Res 1998;6:147–56.

[23] Meeran K, O'Shea D, Edwards CM, Turton MD, Heath MM, Gunn I, Abusnana S, Rossi M, Small CJ, Goldstone AP, Taylor GM, Sunter D, Steere J, Choi SJ, Ghatei MA, Bloom SR. Repeated intracerebroventricular administration of glucagon-like peptide-1-(7–36) amide or exendin-(9–39) alters body weight in the rat. Endocrinology 1999;140:244–50.

[24] Tritos NA, Vicent D, Gillette J, Ludwig DS, Flier ES, Maratos-Flier E. Functional interactions between melanin-concentrating hormone, neuropeptide Y, and anorectic neuropeptides in the rat hypothalamus. Diabetes 1998;47:1687–92.

[25] Flint A, Raben A, Astrup A, Holst JJ. Glucagon-like peptide 1 promotes satiety and suppresses energy intake in humans. J Clin Invest 1998;101:515–20.

[26] Verdich C, Flint A, Gutzwiller JP, Näslund E, Beglinger C, Hellström PM, Long SJ, Morgan LM, Holst JJ, Astrup A. A meta-analysis of the effect of glucagon-like peptide-1 (7–36) amide on ad libitum energy intake in humans. J Clin Endocrinol Metab 2001;86:4382–9.

[27] Kastin AJ, Akerstrom V, Pan W. Interactions of glucagon-like peptide-1 (GLP-1) with the blood-brain barrier. J Mol Neurosci. 2002;18:7–14.

[28] Orskov C, Poulsen SS, Møller M, Holst JJ. Glucagon-like peptide I receptors in the subfornical organ and the area postrema are accessible to circulating glucagon-like peptide I. Diabetes 1996;45:832–5.

[29] Baggio LL, Huang Q, Brown TJ, Drucker DJ. A recombinant human glucagon-like peptide (GLP)-1-albumin protein (albugon) mimics peptidergic activation of GLP-1 receptor-dependent pathways coupled with satiety, gastrointestinal motility, and glucose homeostasis. Diabetes 2004;53:2492–500.

[30] Nakagawa A, Satake H, Nakabayashi H, Nishizawa M, Furuya K, Nakano S, Kigoshi T, Nakayama K, Uchida K. Receptor gene expression of glucagon-like peptide-1, but not glucose-dependent insulinotropic polypeptide, in rat nodose ganglion cells. Auton Neurosci 2004;110:36–43.

[31] Vahl TP, Tauchi M, Durler TS, Elfers EE, Fernandes TM, Bitner RD, Ellis KS, Woods SC, Seeley RJ, Herman JP, D'Alessio DA. Glucagon-like peptide-1 (GLP-1) receptors expressed on nerve terminals in the portal vein mediate the effects of endogenous GLP-1 on glucose tolerance in rats. Endocrinology 2007:4965–73.

[32] Vrang N, Phifer CB, Corkern MM, Berthoud HR. Gastric distension induces c-Fos in medullary GLP-1/2-containing neurons. Am J Physiol Regul Integr Comp Physiol 2003;285:R470–8.

[33] Talsania T, Anini Y, Siu S, Drucker DJ, Brubaker PL. Peripheral exendin-4 and peptide YY(3–36) synergistically reduce food intake through different mechanisms in mice. Endocrinology 2005;146:3748–56.

[34] Rüttimann EB, Arnold M, Hillebrand JJ, Geary N, Langhans W. Intrameal hepatic portal and intraperitoneal infusions of glucagon-like peptide-1 reduce spontaneous meal size in the rat via different mechanisms. Endocrinology 2009;150:1174–81.

[35] Ahrén B. GLP-1 and extra-islet effects. Horm Metab Res 2004;36:842–5.

[36] Nauck MA, Niedereichholz U, Ettler R, Holst JJ, Orskov C, Ritzel R, Schmiegel WH. Glucagon-like peptide 1 inhibition of gastric emptying outweighs its insulinotropic effects in healthy humans. Am J Physiol 1997;273:E981–8.

[37] Schirra J, Kuwert P, Wank U, Leicht P, Arnold R, Göke B, Katschinski M. Differential effects of subcutaneous GLP-1 on gastric emptying, antroduodenal motility, and pancreatic function in men. Proc Assoc Am Phys 1997;109:84–97.

[38] Schjoldager BT, Mortensen PE, Christiansen J, Orskov C, Holst JJ. GLP-1 (glucagon-like peptide 1) and truncated GLP-1, fragments of human proglucagon, inhibit gastric acid secretion in humans. Dig Dis Sci 1989;34:703–8.

[39] Wettergren A, Schjoldager B, Mortensen PE, Myhre J, Christiansen J, Holst JJ. Truncated GLP-1 (proglucagon 78–107-amide) inhibits gastric and pancreatic functions in man. Dig Dis Sci 1993;38:665–73.

[40] Wettergren A, Wøjdemann M, Holst JJ. Glucagon-like peptide-1 inhibits gastropancreatic function by inhibiting central parasympathetic outflow. Am J Physiol 1998;275:G984–92.

[41] Schmidtler J, Dehne K, Allescher HD, Schusdziarra V, Classen M, Holst JJ, Polack A, Schepp W. Rat parietal cell receptors for GLP-1-(7–36) amide: northern blot, cross-linking, and radioligand binding. Am J Physiol 1994;267:G423–32.

[42] Gutzwiller JP, Göke B, Drewe J, Hildebrand P, Ketterer S, Handschin D, Winterhalder R, Conen D, Beglinger C. Glucagon-like peptide-1: a potent regulator of food intake in humans. Gut 1999;44:81–6.

[43] Zander M, Madsbad S, Madsen JL, Holst JJ. Effect of 6-week course of glucagon-like peptide 1 on glycaemic control, insulin sensitivity, and beta-cell function in type 2 diabetes: a parallel-group study. Lancet 2002;359:824–30.

[44] Garber AJ. Long-acting glucagon-like peptide 1 receptor agonists: a review of their efficacy and tolerability. Diabetes Care 2011;34:S279–84.

[45] Vilsbøll T, Brock B, Perrild H, Levin K, Lervang HH, Kølendorf K, Krarup T, Schmitz O, Zdravkovic M, Le-Thi T, Madsbad S. Liraglutide, a once-daily human GLP-1 analogue, improves pancreatic B-cell function and arginine-stimulated insulin secretion during hyperglycaemia in patients with Type 2 diabetes mellitus. Diabet Med 2008;25:152–6.

[46] Mari A, Degn K, Brock B, Rungby J, Ferrannini E, Schmitz O. Effects of the long-acting human glucagon-like peptide-1 analog liraglutide on beta-cell function in normal living conditions. Diabetes Care 2007;30:2032–3.

[47] Nauck M, Frid A, Hermansen K, Shah NS, Tankova T, Mitha IH, Zdravkovic M, Düring M. Matthews DR; LEAD-2 Study Group. Efficacy and safety comparison of liraglutide, glimepiride, and placebo, all in combination with metformin, in type 2 diabetes: the LEAD (liraglutide effect and action in diabetes)-2 study. Diabetes Care 2009;32:84–90.

[48] Blonde L, Russell-Jones D. The safety and efficacy of liraglutide with or without oral antidiabetic drug therapy in type 2 diabetes: an overview of the LEAD 1–5 studies. Diabetes Obes Metab 2009(Suppl. 3):26–34.

[49] Holman RR, Paul SK, Bethel MA, Matthews DR, Neil HA. 10-year follow-up of intensive glucose control in type 2 diabetes. N Engl J Med 2008;359:1577–89.

[50] UK Prospective Diabetes Study (UKPDS) Group . Intensive blood-glucose control with sulphonylureas or insulin compared with conventional treatment and risk of complications in patients with type 2 diabetes (UKPDS 33). Lancet 1998;352:837–53.

[51] Russell-Jones D, Khan R. Insulin-associated weight gain in diabetes—causes, effects and coping strategies. Diabetes Obes Metab 2007;9:799–812.

[52] Inzucchi SE. Oral antihyperglycemic therapy for type 2 diabetes: scientific review. JAMA 2002;287:360–72.

[53] Vilsbøll T, Zdravkovic M, Le-Thi T, Krarup T, Schmitz O, Courrèges JP, Verhoeven R, Bugánová I, Madsbad S. Liraglutide, a long-acting human glucagon-like peptide-1 analog, given as monotherapy significantly improves glycemic control and lowers body weight without risk of hypoglycemia in patients with type 2 diabetes. Diabetes Care 2007;30:1608–10.

[54] Garber A, Henry RR, Ratner R, Hale P, Chang CT, Bode B. LEAD-3 (Mono) Study Group. Liraglutide, a once-daily human glucagon-like peptide 1 analogue, provides sustained improvements in glycaemic control and weight for 2 years as monotherapy compared with glimepiride in patients with type 2 diabetes. Diabetes Obes Metab 2011;13:348–56.

[55] Marre M, Shaw J, Brändle M, Bebakar WM, Kamaruddin NA, Strand J, Zdravkovic M, Le Thi TD, Colagiuri S. LEAD-1 SU study group. Liraglutide, a once-daily human GLP-1 analogue, added to a sulphonylurea over 26 weeks produces greater improvements in glycaemic and weight control compared with adding rosiglitazone or placebo in subjects with Type 2 diabetes (LEAD-1 SU). Diabet Med 2009;26:268–78.

[56] Russell-Jones D, Vaag A, Schmitz O, Sethi BK, Lalic N, Antic S, Zdravkovic M, Ravn GM, Simó R. Liraglutide Effect and Action in Diabetes 5 (LEAD-5) met+SU Study Group. Liraglutide vs insulin glargine and placebo in combination with metformin and sulfonylurea therapy in type 2 diabetes mellitus (LEAD-5 met+SU): a randomised controlled trial. Diabetologia 2009;52:2046–55.

[57] Klonoff DC, Buse JB, Nielsen LL, Guan X, Bowlus CL, Holcombe JH, Wintle ME, Maggs DG. Exenatide effects on diabetes, obesity, cardiovascular risk factors and hepatic biomarkers in patients with type 2 diabetes treated for at least 3 years. Curr Med Res Opin 2008;24:275–86.

[58] Buse JB, Rosenstock J, Sesti G, Schmidt WE, Montanya E, Brett JH, Zychma M, Blonde L. LEAD-6 Study Group. Liraglutide once a day versus exenatide twice a day for type 2 diabetes: a 26-week randomised, parallel-group, multinational, open-label trial (LEAD-6). Lancet 2009;374:39–47.

[59] Buse JB, Nauck M, Forst T, Sheu WH, Shenouda SK, Heilmann CR, Hoogwerf BJ, Gao A, Boardman MK, Fineman M, Porter L, Schernthaner G. Exenatide once weekly versus liraglutide once daily in patients with type 2 diabetes (DURATION-6): a randomised, open-label study. Lancet 2013;381:117–24.

[60] Fujishima Y, Maeda N, Inoue K, Kashine S, Nishizawa H, Hirata A, Kozawa J, Yasuda T, Okita K, Imagawa A, Funahashi T, Shimomura I. Efficacy of liraglutide, a glucagon-like peptide-1 (GLP-1) analogue, on body weight, eating behavior, and glycemic control, in Japanese obese type 2 diabetes. Cardiovasc Diabetol 2012;11:107.

[61] Astrup A, Rössner S, Van Gaal L, Rissanen A, Niskanen L, Al Hakim M, Madsen J, Rasmussen MF, Lean ME. NN8022-1807 Study Group. Effects of liraglutide in the treatment of obesity: a randomised, double-blind, placebo-controlled study. Lancet 2009;374:1606–16.

[62] Astrup A, Carraro R, Finer N, Harper A, Kunesova M, Lean ME, Niskanen L, Rasmussen MF, Rissanen A, Rössner S, Savolainen MJ, Van Gaal L. NN8022-1807 Investigators. Safety, tolerability

and sustained weight loss over 2 years with the once-daily human GLP-1 analog, liraglutide. Int J Obes (Lond) 2012;36:843–54.
[63] Rosenstock J, Klaff LJ, Schwartz S, Northrup J, Holcombe JH, Wilhelm K, Trautmann M. Effects of exenatide and lifestyle modification on body weight and glucose tolerance in obese subjects with and without pre-diabetes. Diabetes Care 2010;33:1173–5.
[64] Hansen E, Hajri T, Abumrad NN. Is all fat the same? The role of fat in the pathogenesis of the metabolic syndrome and type 2 diabetes mellitus. Surgery 2006;139:711–6.
[65] Freemantle N, Holmes J, Hockey A, Kumar S. How strong is the association between abdominal obesity and the incidence of type 2 diabetes? Int J Clin Pract 2008;62:1391–6.
[66] DeFronzo RA. Insulin resistance, lipotoxicity, type 2 diabetes and atherosclerosis: the missing links. The Claude Bernard Lecture 2009. Diabetologia 2010;53:1270–87.
[67] Hotamisligil GS, Shargill NS, Spiegelman BM. Adipose expression of tumor necrosis factor-alpha: direct role in obesity-linked insulin resistance. Science 1993;259:87–91.
[68] Shimomura I, Funahashi T, Takahashi M, Maeda K, Kotani K, Nakamura T, Yamashita S, Miura M, Fukuda Y, Takemura K, Tokunaga K, Matsuzawa Y. Enhanced expression of PAI-1 in visceral fat: possible contributor to vascular disease in obesity. Nat Med 1996;2:800–3.
[69] Matsuzawa Y, Funahashi T, Kihara S, Shimomura I. Adiponectin and metabolic syndrome. Arterioscler Thromb Vasc Biol Jan 2004;24(1):29–33.
[70] Okauchi Y, Kishida K, Funahashi T, Noguchi M, Morita S, Ogawa T, Imagawa A, Nakamura T, Matsuzawa Y, Shimomura I. 4-year follow-up of cardiovascular events and changes in visceral fat accumulation after health promotion program in the Amagasaki Visceral Fat Study. Atherosclerosis 2010;212:698–700.
[71] Monami M, Dicembrini I, Marchionni N, Rotella CM, Mannucci E. Effects of glucagon-like peptide-1 receptor agonists on body weight: a meta-analysis. Exp Diabetes Res 2012;2012:672658.
[72] Doyle ME, McConville P, Theodorakis MJ, Goetschkes MM, Bernier M, Spencer RG, Holloway HW, Greig NH, Egan JM. In vivo biological activity of exendin (1–30). Endocrine 2005;27:1–9.
[73] Mack CM, Moore CX, Jodka CM, Bhavsar S, Wilson JK, Hoyt JA, Roan JL, Vu C, Laugero KD, Parkes DG, Young AA. Antiobesity action of peripheral exenatide (exendin-4) in rodents: effects on food intake, body weight, metabolic status and side-effect measures. Int J Obes (Lond) 2006;30:1332–40.
[74] Jendle J, Nauck MA, Matthews DR, Frid A, Hermansen K, Düring M, Zdravkovic M, Strauss BJ, Garber AJ. LEAD-2 and LEAD-3 Study Groups. Weight loss with liraglutide, a once-daily human glucagon-like peptide-1 analogue for type 2 diabetes treatment as monotherapy or added to metformin, is primarily as a result of a reduction in fat tissue. Diabetes Obes Metab 2009;11:1163–72.
[75] Ryo M, Maeda K, Onda T, Katashima M, Okumiya A, Nishida M, Yamaguchi T, Funahashi T, Matsuzawa Y, Nakamura T, Shimomura I. A new simple method for the measurement of visceral fat accumulation by bioelectrical impedance. Diabetes Care 2005;28:451–3.
[76] Inoue K, Maeda N, Kashine S, Fujishima Y, Kozawa J, Hiuge-Shimizu A, Okita K, Imagawa A, Funahashi T, Shimomura I. Short-term effects of liraglutide on visceral fat adiposity, appetite, and food preference: a pilot study of obese Japanese patients with type 2 diabetes. Cardiovasc Diabetol 2011;10:109.
[77] Hansotia T, Maida A, Flock G, Yamada Y, Tsukiyama K, Seino Y, Drucker DJ. Extrapancreatic incretin receptors modulate glucose homeostasis, body weight, and energy expenditure. J Clin Invest 2007;117:143–52.
[78] Kim Chung le T, Hosaka T, Yoshida M, Harada N, Sakaue H, Sakai T, Nakaya Y. Exendin-4, a GLP-1 receptor agonist, directly induces adiponectin expression through protein kinase A pathway and prevents inflammatory adipokine expression. Biochem Biophys Res Commun 2009;390:613–8.
[79] Funahashi T, Matsuzawa Y. Metabolic syndrome: clinical concept and molecular basis. Ann Med 2007;39(7):482–94.
[80] Bunck MC, Diamant M, Eliasson B, Cornér A, Shaginian RM, Heine RJ, Taskinen MR, Yki-Järvinen H, Smith U. Exenatide affects circulating cardiovascular risk biomarkers independently of changes in body composition. Diabetes Care 2010;33:1734–7.
[81] Cohen JC, Horton JD, Hobbs HH. Human fatty liver disease: old questions and new insights. Science 2011;332:1519–23.
[82] Harrison SA, Day CP. Benefits of lifestyle modification in NAFLD. Gut 2007;56:1760–9.
[83] Lazo M, Solga SF, Horska A, Bonekamp S, Diehl AM, Brancati FL, Wagenknecht LE, Pi-Sunyer FX, Kahn SE, Clark JM. Fatty Liver Subgroup of the Look AHEAD Research Group. Effect of a 12-month intensive lifestyle intervention on hepatic steatosis in adults with type 2 diabetes. Diabetes Care 2010;33:2156–63.
[84] Sanyal AJ, Brunt EM, Kleiner DE, Kowdley KV, Chalasani N, Lavine JE, Ratziu V, McCullough A. Endpoints and clinical trial design for nonalcoholic steatohepatitis. Hepatology 2011;54:344–53.
[85] Ben-Shlomo S, Zvibel I, Shnell M, Shlomai A, Chepurko E, Halpern Z, Barzilai N, Oren R, Fishman S. Glucagon-like peptide-1 reduces hepatic lipogenesis via activation of AMP-activated protein kinase. J Hepatol 2011;54:1214–23.
[86] Svegliati-Baroni G, Saccomanno S, Rychlicki C, Agostinelli L, De Minicis S, Candelaresi C, Faraci G, Pacetti D, Vivarelli M, Nicolini D, Garelli P, Casini A, Manco M, Mingrone G, Risaliti A, Frega GN, Benedetti A, Gastaldelli A. Glucagon-like peptide-1 receptor activation stimulates hepatic lipid oxidation and restores hepatic signalling alteration induced by a high-fat diet in nonalcoholic steatohepatitis. Liver Int 2011;31:1285–97.
[87] Gupta NA, Mells J, Dunham RM, Grakoui A, Handy J, Saxena NK, Anania FA. Glucagon-like peptide-1 receptor is present on human hepatocytes and has a direct role in decreasing hepatic steatosis in vitro by modulating elements of the insulin signaling pathway. Hepatology 2010;51:1584–92.
[88] Armstrong MJ, Houlihan DD, Rowe IA, Clausen WH, Elbrønd B, Gough SC, Tomlinson JW, Newsome PN. Safety and efficacy of liraglutide in patients with type 2 diabetes and elevated liver enzymes: individual patient data meta-analysis of the LEAD program. Aliment Pharmacol Ther 2013;37:234–42.
[89] Cuthbertson DJ, Irwin A, Gardner CJ, Daousi C, Purewal T, Furlong N, Goenka N, Thomas EL, Adams VL, Pushpakom SP, Pirmohamed M, Kemp GJ. Improved glycaemia correlates with liver fat reduction in obese, type 2 diabetes, patients given glucagon-like peptide-1 (GLP-1) receptor agonists. PLoS One 2012;7:e50117.
[90] Gutzwiller JP, Drewe J, Göke B, Schmidt H, Rohrer B, Lareida J, Beglinger C. Glucagon-like peptide-1 promotes satiety and reduces food intake in patients with diabetes mellitus type 2. Am J Physiol 1999;276:R1541–4.
[91] Näslund E, Barkeling B, King N, Gutniak M, Blundell JE, Holst JJ, Rössner S, Hellström PM. Energy intake and appetite are suppressed by glucagon-like peptide-1 (GLP-1) in obese men. Int J Obes Relat Metab Disord 1999;23:304–11.
[92] Verdich C, Toubro S, Buemann B, Lysgård Madsen J, Juul Holst J, Astrup A. The role of postprandial releases of insulin and incretin hormones in meal-induced satiety—effect of obesity and weight reduction. Int J Obes Relat Metab Disord 2001;25:1206–14.
[93] Flint A, Raben A, Ersbøll AK, Holst JJ, Astrup A. The effect of physiological levels of glucagon-like peptide-1 on appetite, gastric emptying, energy and substrate metabolism in obesity. Int J Obes Relat Metab Disord 2001;25:781–92.
[94] Raun K, von Voss P, Gotfredsen CF, Golozoubova V, Rolin B, Knudsen LB. Liraglutide, a long-acting glucagon-like peptide-1 analog, reduces body weight and food intake in obese candy-fed rats, whereas a dipeptidyl peptidase-IV inhibitor, vildagliptin, does not. Diabetes 2007;56:8–15.

[95] Raun K, von Voss P, Knudsen LB. Liraglutide, a once-daily human glucagon-like peptide-1 analog, minimizes food intake in severely obese minipigs. Obesity 2007;15:1710–6.

[96] Horowitz M, Flint A, Jones KL, Hindsberger C, Rasmussen MF, Kapitza C, Doran S, Jax T, Zdravkovic M, Chapman IM. Effect of the once-daily human GLP-1 analogue liraglutide on appetite, energy intake, energy expenditure and gastric emptying in type 2 diabetes. Diabetes Res Clin Pract 2012;97:258–66.

[97] Flint A, Kapitza C, Zdravkovic M. The once-daily human GLP-1 analogue liraglutide impacts appetite and energy intake in patients with type 2 diabetes after short-term treatment. Diabetes Obes Metab 2013;15(10):958–62. http://dx.doi.org/10.1111/dom.12108.

[98] Torres SJ, Nowson CA. Relationship between stress, eating behavior, and obesity. Nutrition 2007;23:887–94.

[99] Thanopoulou AC, Karamanos BG, Angelico FV, Assaad-Khalil SH, Barbato AF, Del Ben MP, Djordjevic PB, Dimitrijevic-Sreckovic VS, Gallotti CA, Katsilambros NL, Migdalis IN, Mrabet MM, Petkova MK, Roussi DP, Tenconi MT. Dietary fat intake as risk factor for the development of diabetes: multinational, multicenter study of the Mediterranean Group for the Study of Diabetes (MGSD). Diabetes Care 2003;26:302–7.

CHAPTER

16

Effects of Sleeve Gastrectomy on Calcium Metabolism

Jaime Ruiz-Tovar and Rafael Calpena

Department of Surgery, Bariatric Surgery Unit, General University Hospital of Elche, Alicante, Spain

There has been a progressive increase in obesity in recent years in developed countries, reaching a prevalence of about 30% in the USA and 17.1% in Spain in 2009 [1–3]. In a large number of obese patients, lifestyle modifications and pharmacotherapy fail to result in significant weight loss. Actually, bariatric surgery is the most effective treatment for achieving significant weight loss and improving quality of life and morbidity and mortality rates among obese subjects [4]. Moreover, there is a significant reduction in the prevalence of weight-related morbid conditions after bariatric surgery [5].

Despite the routine supplementation of vitamins and minerals after bariatric surgery, a large number of patients suffer from nutrient deficiencies [6–10]: this is related to the reduction in food intake as well as the physiological impact of surgically-induced anatomical changes on the gastrointestinal tract [10]. Bariatric procedures with malabsorptive effects may lead to an increased risk of postoperative nutrient deficiencies, while restrictive operations tend to cause fewer problems [11]. However, little is still known about the novel restrictive procedure, sleeve gastrectomy, in which food passes faster through the upper gastrointestinal tract, but still contacts the antrum, duodenum, and proximal jejunum.

Initially, laparoscopic sleeve gastrectomy (LSG) was performed as the first part of a staged treatment of super-obese, high-risk patients, and was followed by duodenal switch [12]. However, some studies have shown LSG to be as successful as a single-step operation in many patients [13]. Long-term studies are not yet available for this technique as a single-step procedure. LSG is effective in terms of weight loss as a consequence of simple restriction in combination with accelerating gastric emptying of solids. In contrast, malabsorptive procedures may lead to more deficiencies by bypassing the stomach, duodenum, and proximal jejunum, which are the sites of maximal absorption of several micronutrients such as iron and calcium.

CHANGES IN NUTRITIONAL STATUS

Although some patients present with nutrient deficiencies before surgery, as a consequence of alimentary disorders, the prevalence of abnormalities 1 year after surgery is usually higher [14]. After bariatric surgery, patients mainly suffer from folate, iron, zinc, protein, vitamin B12, and vitamin D deficiencies, as well as secondary hyperparathyroidism [15]. In our experience, patients mainly suffer preoperatively from vitamin D deficiency (96.7%) and have elevated parathyroid hormone (PTH; 20%), although hypoalbuminemia and folic acid deficiencies are also present in isolated cases. Postoperatively, only 6% of patients present with iron deficiency, which can be relieved by oral administration of iron(II) glycine sulfate [16]. Other possible vitamin or mineral deficiencies can be avoided with the routine multivitamin supplementation. Apart from iron, vitamin B12 is the most frequent deficiency after bariatric surgery, despite the use of multivitamin supplements, and requires additional oral or intramuscular cyanocobalamin supplementation [17]. However, vitamin B12 deficiency is much more frequent after malabsorptive procedures rather than after purely restrictive ones, such as LSG. Therefore, it is not surprising that vitamin B12 levels remain in the normal range in all postoperative determinations of our patients.

EFFECTS ON CALCIUM LEVELS

Calcium values are usually normal after bariatric surgery. Johnson et al. [18] reported nonsignificant decreases in serum calcium levels from 9.8 to 9.2 mg/dL during the first year and to 8.8 mg/dL by the second year after bypass procedures. In contrast, we found postoperative calcium levels to show a nonsignificant increase from 9.3

Nutrition in the Prevention and Treatment of Abdominal Obesity
http://dx.doi.org/10.1016/B978-0-12-407869-7.00016-7

to 9.8 mg/dL during the first year, maintaining a level of 9.7 mg/dL by the second year. The duodenum is the main location of calcium absorption. In LSG, the duodenum is not bypassed, which explains the maintenance of calcium levels. Bypassing the duodenum leads to calcium malabsorption and secondary hyperparathyroidism.

EFFECTS ON VITAMIN D LEVELS

Vitamin D deficiency, caused by a reduced intake of food containing vitamin D and less sunlight exposure, may aggravate secondary hyperparathyroidism, causing bone disease [19]. The prevalence of vitamin D deficiency in morbidly obese patients ranges from 33% to 80% [20,21]. Secondary hyperparathyroidism was described preoperatively in up to 48% of patients [21,22]. This is substantially higher than the rate observed in the normal population of same age and may be caused by malnutrition as a consequence of dietary restraints and/or by lower sunlight exposure because of reduced physical performance and increased time spent indoors for psychological reasons [19]. Vitamin D obtained from the diet or cutaneous synthesis is taken up by adipose tissue, which stores vitamin D for subsequent release and metabolism at times when production is reduced, such as during the winter months [23,24]. Levels of adipose tissue appear to inversely correlate with vitamin D status. Several studies have shown that obese individuals tend to have lower serum concentrations of vitamin D than do those of normal weight. This is probably secondary to the sequestration of vitamin D into a larger pool of adipose tissue [23,25]. In a study performed by our group [16], we failed to demonstrate a significant correlation between preoperative vitamin D levels and preoperative body mass index (BMI). However, a significant inverse correlation could be demonstrated between weight loss and increased vitamin D at the third month after surgery, reinforcing the hypothesis of vitamin D sequestration into a larger pool of adipose tissue. Nevertheless, our study was the first to report increased vitamin D levels after bariatric surgery. It is certain that reports describing malabsorptive procedures present higher incidences of vitamin D deficiency than do pure restrictive ones, but even in LSG groups the reported postoperative vitamin D deficiency was higher than the preoperative one [19,26]. A possible factor that may explain these differences is that our study was conducted in Spain, a region with high sunlight exposure, while most other reports describe studies conducted in Northern Europe or North America, i.e. regions with lower sunlight exposure. Moreover, our patients were stimulated to improve their physical performance by participating mainly in outdoor sports and activities, even in the winter months. Most patients preoperatively reported spending more time indoors because they were ashamed of their physical appearance, indicating that their sunlight exposure before surgery was minimal [16].

It has been reported that vitamin D deficiency may even increase cardiovascular risk in this high-risk group of morbidly obese patients. epidemiological evidence supports an association between hypovitaminosis D and increased risk of mortality due to cardiovascular disease, hypertension, stroke, metabolic syndrome, and diabetes [27]. In a previous study [16], we demonstrated a significant inverse correlation between postoperative weight loss and vitamin D increase. It has been widely demonstrated that weight loss after bariatric surgery leads to a reduction in comorbidities in most morbid obese patients [7–9]. In our series, we observed a significant improvement in the control of diabetes mellitus, hypertension, and hypertriglyceridemia. We do not know whether postoperative vitamin D improvement is an independent protective factor for cardiovascular diseases or whether it is associated with weight loss [16].

EFFECTS ON PARATHYROID HORMONE LEVELS

In response to reduced calcium absorption, organisms start bone resorption to maintain serum calcium within the normal range. Such bone resorption is mediated by PTH; thus, PTH levels increase over the postoperative course [28]. In a previous study, we reported a prevalence of preoperative deficiencies of vitamin D of 95%, and 43% of patients with elevated PTH levels. After surgery, vitamin D and PTH levels normalized in all but one case [16]. A progressive decrease in PTH levels parallels the progressive increase in vitamin D. Secondary parathyroidism is normal in patients with vitamin D deficiency. Due to decreased vitamin D-mediated calcium absorption, maintenance of calcium levels occurs mainly from bone resorption. Secondary parathyroidism causes muscle weakness, bone disease, and various other health problems associated with vitamin D deficiency [28].

EFFECTS ON BONE MINERAL DENSITY

Several studies have reported a reduction in bone mineral density (BMD), but most relate to malabsorptive procedures, such as Roux-en-Y gastric bypass (RYGBP) [29–31] and biliopancreatic diversion [31,32].

To our knowledge, only three studies have investigated BMD in patients after LSG. The study conducted by our group had the largest sample size [33]; the two other reports involved a small study also conducted in Spain, including 15 women, and a Czech report including 29 patients. The first Spanish series analyzed 15 women, comparing the results of eight patients who underwent LSG versus seven undergoing RYGBP. They observe a significant BMD decrease in both groups, with no difference between them [34]. The Czech study included 29 patients, who all underwent LSG. They also report a decline in BMD that paralleled body weight reduction [34]. In contrast to these studies, our patients showed a significant increase in BMD. One of the main differences between our series and the other two is that BMD measurement was done in the lumbar spine (L1-L4) in our series, while the measurement was performed in the spine and proximal femur in the others. Both reports describe a more pronounced decrease in BMD in the femur than in the spine, revealing that the femur seems to be more sensitive to BMD changes. Several studies analyzing BMD changes after RYGBP confirmed that the average decrease in BMD is significantly higher in lumbar spine determinations than in those in the proximal femur [35]. Fleischer et al. [36] even reported a decrease of 9.2% in the femoral neck, but did not observe any changes in the lumbar spine. A potential explanation for the detection of different BMDs in the lumbar spine and the proximal femur is that densitometers are unable to accurately measure changes in adipose tissue density and distribution following bariatric surgery [37]. Although the lack of BMD measurements in the proximal femur in our patients was a limitation of the study, we were the first group to describe an increase in BMD in the lumbar spine of up to 7.9% 2 years after surgery.

Most studies have reported an association between weight loss and decreased BMD, showing a more pronounced BMD reduction in those patients with greater weight loss [34,36]. However, some authors have reported that this association is only valid for proximal femur measurements, and not for values obtained from the lumbar spine [38]. We cannot reject this possibility because we could not demonstrate this association in our series, but our measurements were performed in lumbar spine [33].

However, we could demonstrate a direct correlation between BMD and increased vitamin D and an inverse correlation between increased BMD and reduced PTH. It is likely that preoperatively low vitamin D levels led to secondary hyperparathyroidism, which started bone resorption. With weight loss, vitamin D sequestrated within adipose tissue is freed and enters the bloodstream, thus increasing serum levels. Increased serum vitamin D increases the intestinal absorption of calcium, thus stopping bone resorption as source of calcium. Moreover, with sufficient serum calcium and vitamin D availability, calcium can be targeted to the bone to restore the original BMD. We observed a significant increase in vitamin D and decrease in PTH levels to occur after 1 year, and these levels were maintained after 2 years. However, BMD showed a significant but mild increase after 1 year, but a higher increase after 2 years. This suggests that during the first postoperative year, the main goal of the organism is to normalize serum vitamin D values. Once the normal range is attained, the goal is then to restore BMD and preventing bone resorption.

References

[1] Rockholm B, Baker JL, Sorensen TI. The leveling off of the obesity epidemic since the year 1999—a review of evidence and perspectives. Obes Rev 2010;11:835–46.

[2] Flegal KM, Carroll MD, Ogden CL, Curtin LR. Prevalence and trends in obesity among US adults, 1999–2008. JAMA 2010;11: 835–46.

[3] Encuesta Europea de Salud en España. Instituto Nacional de Estadística. INEbase. <http://www.ine.es/jaxi/menu.do?type=pcaxis&path=/t15/p420&file=inebase&L=0>; 2009 [accessed 20.09.13].

[4] Colquitt JL, Picot J, Loveman E, Clegg AJ. Surgery for obesity. Cochrane Database Syst Rev 2009. [CD 003641]

[5] Ruiz-Tovar J, Oller I, Tomas A, Llavero C, Arroyo A, Calero A, et al. Midterm impact of sleeve gastrectomy, calibrated with a 50-Fr bougie, on weight loss, glucose hemostasis, lipid profiles and comorbidities in morbidly obese patients. Am Surg 2012;78:969–74.

[6] Sjostrom L, Lindroos AK, Peltonen M, Torgerson J, Bouchard C, Carlsson B, et al. Lifestyle, diabetes and cardiovascular risk factors 10 years after bariatric surgery. N Engl J Med 2004;351: 2683–93.

[7] Buchwald H, Williams SE. Bariatric surgery worldwide 2003. Obes Surg 2004;14:1157–64.

[8] Maggard MA, Shugarman LR, Suttorp M, Maglione M, Sugerman HJ, Livingston EH, et al. Meta-analysis: surgical treatment of obesity. Ann Intern Med 2005;142:547–59.

[9] Buchwald H, Avidor Y, Braunwald E, Jensen MD, Pories W, Fahrbach K, et al. Bariatric surgery: a systematic review and meta-analysis. JAMA 2004;292:1724–37.

[10] Davies DJ, Baxter JM, Baxter JN. Nutritional deficiencies after bariatric surgery. Obes Surg 2007;17:1150–8.

[11] Giusti V, Suter M, Héraïef E, Gaillard RC, Burckhardt P. Effects of laparoscopic gastric banding on body composition, metabolic profile and nutritional status of obese women: 12-months follow-up. Obes Surg 2004;14:239–45.

[12] Cottam D, Qureshi FG, Mattar SG, Sharma S, Holover S, Bonanomi G, et al. Laparoscopic sleeve gastrectomy as an initial weight-loss procedure for high-risk patients with morbid obesity. Surg Endosc 2006;20:859–63.

[13] Melissas J, Daskalakis M, Koukouraki S, Askoxylakis I, Metaxari M, Dimitriadis E, et al. Sleeve gastrectomy—a "food limiting" operation. Obes Surg 2008;18:1251–6.

[14] Toh SY, Zarshenas N, Jorgensen J. Prevalence of nutrient deficiencies in bariatric patients. Nutrition 2009;25:1150–6.

[15] Vargas-Ruiz AG, Hernandez-Rivera G, Herrera MF. Prevalence of iron, folate and vitamin B12 deficiency anemia after laparoscopic Roux-en-Y gastric bypass. Obes Surg 2008;18:288–93.

[16] Ruiz-Tovar J, Oller I, Tomás A, Llavero C, Arroyo A, Calero A, et al. Mid-term effects of sleeve gastrectomy on calcium metabolism parameters, vitamin D and parathormone (PTH) in morbid obese women. Obes Surg 2012;22:797–801.

[17] Brolin RE, Leung M. Survey of vitamin and mineral supplementation after gastric bypass and biliopancreatic diversion for morbid obesity. Obes Surg 1999;9:150–4.

[18] Johnson JM, Maher JW, Samuel I, Heitshusen D, Doherty C, Downs RW. Effects of gastric bypass procedures on bone mineral

density, calcium, para thyroid hormone and vitamin D. J Gastrointest Surg 2005;9:1106–10.
[19] Gehrer S, Kern B, Peters T, Christoffel-Courtin C, Peterli R. Fewer nutrient deficiencies after laparoscopic sleeve gastrectomy than after laparoscopic Roux-Y-Gastric bypass—a prospective study. Obes Surg 2010;20:447–53.
[20] Ybarra J, Sánchez-Hernández J, Gich I, De Leiva A, Rius X, Rodríguez-Espinosa J, et al. Unchanged hypovitaminosis D and secondary hyperparathyroidism in morbid obesity after bariatric surgery. Obes Surg 2005;15:330–5.
[21] Carlin AM, Rao DS, Yager KM, Genaw JA, Parikh NJ, Szymanski W. Effect of gastric bypass surgery on vitamin D nutritional status. Surg Obes Relat Dis 2006;2:638–42.
[22] Carlin AM, Rao DS, Meslemani AM, Genaw JA, Parikh NJ, Levy S, et al. Prevalence of vitamin D depletion among morbidly obese patients seeking gastric bypass surgery. Surg Obes Relat Dis 2006;2:98–103.
[23] Tsiaras WG, Weinstock MA. Factors influencing vitamin D status. Acta Derm Venereol 2011;91:115–24.
[24] Blum M, Dolnikowski G, Seyoum E, Harris SS, Booth SL, Peterson J, et al. Vitamin D(3) in fat tissue. Endocrine 2008;33:90–4.
[25] Holick MF. Vitamin D deficiency. N Engl J Med 2007;357:266–81.
[26] Johnson JM, Maher JW, DeMaria EJ, Downs RW, Wolfe LG, Kellum JM. The long-term effects of gastric bypass on vitamin D metabolism. Ann Surg 2006;243:701–4.
[27] Maxwell CS, Wood RJ. Update on vitamin D and type 2 diabetes. Nutr Rev 2011;69:291–5.
[28] Schaan Casagrande D, Repetto G, Cora Mottin C, Shah J, Pietrobon R, Worni M, et al. Changes in bone mineral density in women following 1-year gastric bypass surgery. Obes Surg 2012;22:1287–92.
[29] Vilarrasa N, San Jose P, Garcia I, Gómez-Vaquero C, Miras PM, de Gordejuela AG, et al. Evaluation of bone mineral density loss in morbidly obese women after gastric bypass: 3-year follow-up. Obes Surg 2011;21:465–72.
[30] Mahdy T, Atia S, Farid M, Adulatif A. Effect of Roux-en-Y gastric bypass on bone metabolism in patients with morbid obesity: Mansoura experiences. Obes Surg 2008;18:1526–31.
[31] Balsa JA, Botella-Carretero JI, Peromingo R, Caballero C, Muñoz-Malo T, Villafruela JJ, et al. Chronic increase of bone turnover markers after biliopancreatic diversion is related to secondary hyperparathyroidism and weight loss. Relation with bone mineral density. Obes Surg 2010;20:468–73.
[32] Tsiftsis DD, Mylonas P, Mead N, Kalfarentzos F, Alexandrides TK. Bone mass decreases in morbidly obese women after long limb-biliopancreatic diversion and marked weight loss without secondary hyperparathyroidism. A physiological adaptation to weight loss? Obes Surg 2009;19:1497–503.
[33] Ruiz-Tovar J, Oller I, Priego P, Arroyo A, Calero A, Diez M, et al. Short and mid-term changes in body mineral density alter laparoscopic sleeve gastrectomy. Obes Surg 2013. [PMID: 23315187]
[34] Nogués X, Goday A, Peña MJ, Benaiges D, de Ramón M, Crous X, et al. Pérdida de masa ósea tras gastrectomía tubular: Estudio prospectivo comparativo con el bypass gástrico. Cir Esp 2010;88:103–9.
[35] Vilarrasa N, Gómez JM, Elio I, Gómez-Vaquero C, Masdevall C, Pujol J, et al. Evaluation of bone disease in morbidly obese women after gastric bypass and risk factors implicated in bone loss. Obes Surg 2009;19:860–6.
[36] Fleischer J, Stein EM, Bessler M, Della Badia M, Restuccia N, et al. The decline in hip bone density after gastric bypass surgery is associated with extent of weight loss. J Clin Endocrinol Metab 2008;93:3735–40.
[37] Tothill P. Dual-energy X-ray absorptiometry measurements of total body bone mineral during weight change. J Clin Densitom 2005;8:31–8.
[38] Pluskiewicz W, Buzga M, Holeczy P, Bortlik L, Smajstrla V, Adamczyk P. Bone mineral changes in spine and proximal femur in individual obese women after laparoscopic sleeve gastrectomy: a short-term study. Obes Surg 2012;22:1068–76.

CHAPTER

17

Intermittent Versus Daily Calorie Restriction in Visceral Fat Loss

John F. Trepanowski and Krista A. Varady

Department of Kinesiology and Nutrition, University of Illinois, Chicago, IL, USA

INTRODUCTION

Visceral adiposity is associated with a number of metabolic abnormalities, including insulin resistance [1], high triglyceride concentrations [2], low high-density lipoprotein (HDL) concentrations [2], and small, dense low-density lipoprotein (LDL) and HDL particles [3]. It is also related to several disease states, including hypertension [4] and other forms of cardiovascular disease [5]; several forms of cancer, such as colorectal, breast, prostate, and esophageal [6–9]; and obstructive sleep apnea [10]. Visceral adiposity also strongly and independently predicts all-cause mortality in men [11].

Diet-induced weight loss has been demonstrated to reduce visceral fat and improve many of its associated metabolic abnormalities [12]. The most popular weight loss diet is daily calorie restriction (DCR), in which energy intake is reduced below energy expenditure (typically by 15–40%) every day. An alternative to DCR that has grown in recognition since the early 2000s is intermittent calorie restriction (ICR) [13]. ICR regimens alternate between "fast periods" of greatly reduced energy intake (e.g. 75%) and "feast periods" of unrestricted intake, leading to approximately the same average reduction in daily energy intake as DCR.

Several reasons suggest that ICR may be a more effective diet regimen for reducing visceral fat compared to DCR. First, dietary adherence may be greater for ICR than DCR. Adherence to DCR begins to decline at 6–8 weeks and progressively worsens thereafter [14], which may be due to chronic feelings of deprivation caused by restricting energy intake every single day. In contrast, ICR incorporates feast periods designed to attenuate feelings of deprivation and might therefore improve dietary adherence, ultimately resulting in greater weight loss and reductions in visceral fat. Second, the percentage of weight lost as visceral fat may be greater for ICR than for DCR. A meta-analysis of weight loss trials found that the ratio of visceral fat reduction to subcutaneous fat reduction correlated positively with the degree of energy restriction independently of weight loss during the first 12 weeks of treatment [15]. As the fast periods of ICR involve approximately double the degree of energy restriction as compared to DCR, they may promote greater utilization of visceral fat to meet energy needs.

Therefore, this chapter will review human weight loss studies involving DCR or ICR to determine whether the latter is indeed a superior method for reducing visceral fat. Additionally, this chapter will examine whether dietary adherence is greater for ICR than for DCR, and also whether the percentage of weight lost as visceral fat is greater for ICR than for DCR.

METHODS

For a study to have been included in this chapter, all of the following criteria must have been satisfied: (1) randomized controlled trial; (2) primary endpoint of weight loss or change in body composition; (3) DCR or ICR as the primary intervention; (4) study duration of 8–30 weeks; (5) study population consisting entirely of adult, overweight or obese, nondiabetics; (6) publication date of year 2000 or later; and (7) total fat mass measured via dual-energy X-ray absorptiometry (DEXA), hydrodensitometry, air displacement plethysmography, computed tomography (CT), or magnetic resonance imaging (MRI). Due to the small number of ICR studies that met these inclusion criteria, the criteria were amended for this group to allow for the measurement of total fat mass via bioelectrical impedance analysis (BIA); this yielded three additional eligible studies [16–18]. Investigations including

Nutrition in the Prevention and Treatment of Abdominal Obesity
http://dx.doi.org/10.1016/B978-0-12-407869-7.00017-9

a cointervention that probably affected body composition (e.g. exercise) were included in this review only if the study featured a diet-only arm or were otherwise able to isolate the effects of the dietary intervention on visceral fat reduction.

On 1 February 2013, a PubMed search was conducted using the following input: ("calorie restriction" or "intermittent calorie restriction" or "alternate-day fasting" or "caloric restriction") and ("body weight" or "weight loss" or "body composition") and ("visceral fat" or "waist circumference"). Additional trials were identified using the references listed in these manuscripts. After applying the aforementioned inclusion criteria, this yielded 11 DCR studies (Table 17.1) and 5 ICR studies (Table 17.2) that were eligible for review. Investigations were grouped by trial duration and classified as short term (8–12 weeks) or moderate term (13–30 weeks).

We used two separate methodologies for estimating dietary adherence. First, we defined percentage adherence as (percent energy restriction achieved/percent energy restriction prescribed) × 100. We allowed for values >100%, as this would indicate that a weight loss diet was so effective that participants reduced energy intake even more than the prescribed reduction (which, in an overweight and obese population, should be viewed positively). A limitation of this approach is that most of the data pertaining to the percentage energy restriction achieved was derived from food records, which tend to underestimate food intake (especially in an overweight and obese population) [19]. We therefore used percentage

TABLE 17.1 Daily Calorie Restriction: Effects on Body Weight and Body Composition

Reference	Subjects	Trial Length	Prescribed CR Regimen	Estimated Daily CR Achieved	Body Weight Change (%)	Total Fat Mass Change (%)	WC Change (%)	WC Change/ Total Fat Mass Change
[20]	n=13; F,M	8 weeks	60% CR daily (food provided)	–	−9%	−13%	−6%	0.46
	Age, 50±3 years							
	BMI, 36±1							
[21]	n=11; F,M	8 weeks	25% CR daily (food provided)	29% (food records)	−12%	−20%	–	–
	Age, 50±3 years							
	BMI, 34±2							
[22]	n=22; F,M	11 weeks	50% CR daily +LC diet (food provided)	–	−7%	−11%	–	–
	Age, 43±4 years		50% CR daily +HC diet (food provided)	–	−8%	−11%	–	–
	BMI, 37±1							
[23]	n=9; F,M	12 weeks	15% CR daily (food provided)	16% (unspecified)	−6%	−13%	–	–
	Age, 58±2 years							
	BMI, 30±0							
[24]	n=26; F,M	12 weeks	Unspecified (food provided initially, then self-selected)	33% (food records)	−11%	−19%	−7%	0.37
	Age, 50±3 years							
	BMI, 29±1							
[25]	n=12; F,M	12 weeks	25% CR daily (food provided)	18% (DLW)	−7%	−16%	–	–
	Age, 39±5 years							
	BMI, 28±1							

(Continued)

TABLE 17.1 Continued

Reference	Subjects	Trial Length	Prescribed CR Regimen	Estimated Daily CR Achieved	Body Weight Change (%)	Total Fat Mass Change (%)	WC Change (%)	WC Change/ Total Fat Mass Change
[28]	$n=15$; F	14 weeks	25% CR daily (food not provided)	19% (food records)	−8%	−10%	−4%	0.40
	Age, 44 ± 5 years							
	BMI, 32 ± 3							
[29]	$n=10$, F	15 weeks	Unspecified (food not provided)	21% (food records)	−12%	−24%	−10%	0.42
	Age, 61 ± 7 years							
	Body weight, 78 ± 10 kg							
[30]	$n=29$; F	20 weeks	25% CR daily (food provided)	23% (self-reported)	−13%	−19%	−9%	0.47
	Age, 58 ± 6 years							
	BMI, 34 ± 4							
[31]	$n=71$; F	24 weeks	34% CR daily (food not provided)	–	−6%	−11%	−4%	0.36
	Age, 58 ± 5 years							
	BMI, 32 ± 5							
[18]	$n=47$; F	24 weeks	25% CR daily (food not provided)	20% (food records)	−5%	−10%	−4%	0.40
	Age, 40 ± 4 years							
	BMI, 31 ± 5							
				Mean change	−9%	−15%	−6%	0.42

BMI, body mass index (in kg/m²); CR, calorie restriction; DLW, doubly labeled water; F, female; HC, high-carbohydrate; LC, low-carbohydrate; M, male; WC, waist circumference.

TABLE 17.2 Intermittent Calorie Restriction: Effects on Body Weight and Body Composition

Reference	Subjects	Trial Length	Prescribed CR Regimen	Estimated Daily CR Achieved	Body Weight Change (%)	Total Fat Mass Change (%)	WC Change (%)	WC Change/ Total Fat Mass Change
[27]	$n=32$; F	8 weeks	HF diet: fast day, 75% CR; feed day, 125% energy needs (food provided)	–	−5%	−12%	−7%	0.58
	Age, 43 ± 3 years		LF diet: fast day, 75% CR; feed day, 125% energy needs (food provided)	–	−4%	−10%	−8%	0.80
	BMI, 35 ± 1							
[16]	$n=16$; F,M	8 weeks	Fast day: 75% CR	37% (food records)	−6%	−11%	−4%	0.36
	Age, 46 ± 2 years		Feed day: *ad libitum* fed					
	BMI, 34 ± 1		(food provided on fast day initially, then self-selected)					

(*Continued*)

TABLE 17.2 Continued

Reference	Subjects	Trial Length	Prescribed CR Regimen	Estimated Daily CR Achieved	Body Weight Change (%)	Total Fat Mass Change (%)	WC Change (%)	WC Change/ Total Fat Mass Change
[17]	$n=16$; F,M	12 weeks	Fast day: 75% CR	–	−3%	−5%	−5%	1.00
	Age, 42±2 years		Feed day: *ad libitum* fed					
	BMI, 35±1		(food provided on fast day initially, then self-selected)					
[18]	$n=42$; F	24 weeks	2 fast days (75% CR) alternated with 5 ad libitum feed days (food not provided)	30% (food records)	−7%	−13%	−6%	0.46
	Age, 40±4 years							
	BMI, 31±5							
[29]	$n=12$; F	30 weeks	5-week period of unspecified energy restriction alternated with 5-week period of 100% energy needs	23% (food records)	−13%	−23%	−10%	0.43
	Age, 61±7 years		(food not provided)					
	Body weight 81±11 kg							
				Mean change	−7%	−13%	−7%	0.52

BMI, body mass index (in kg/m^2); CR, calorie restriction, F, female; HF, high-fat; LF, low-fat; M, male; WC, waist circumference.

change in total fat mass as a second indicator of dietary adherence. For this analysis, a diet regimen was regarded as having greater adherence if it reduced total fat by ≥2.0% more (absolute difference) than its competitor.

Each of the ICR trials used waist circumference as an estimate for visceral fat, and none of them measured subcutaneous fat. Consequently, while it would have been preferable to compare the ratio of visceral fat reduction to subcutaneous fat reduction between DCR and ICR studies, instead we compared the ratio of waist circumference reduction to total fat mass reduction.

RESULTS

Description of Weight Loss Interventions: Short Term (8–12 weeks)

Six short-term DCR studies were included in this chapter [20–25]. One trial [24] provided food initially and then allowed participants to self-select their diet, while the other investigations provided food to the participants throughout the intervention. The degree of prescribed energy restriction in these trials ranged from 15% to 60%. Three studies measured or estimated the degree of energy restriction that was actually achieved by the participants. Luscombe et al. [21] and Pierce et al. [24] estimated (via food records) the degree of energy restriction achieved to be 29% and 33%, respectively, while Redman et al. [25] calculated this number (via doubly labeled water) to be 18%. Kirk and colleagues [22] compared a high-carbohydrate diet (65% carbohydrate, 20% fat, 15% protein) to a low-carbohydrate diet (10% carbohydrate, 75% fat, 15% protein) and found that they equally reduced body weight, total fat mass, and visceral fat mass. One trial [24] examined a high-fat diet (30% carbohydrate, 60% fat, 10% protein). One study [25] investigated a diet that complied with the American Heart Association dietary guidelines (55% carbohydrate, 30% fat, 15% protein) [26], while another [23] examined a similar diet that was slightly lower in carbohydrate (45%) and higher in both fat (35%) and protein (20%). Two investigations [20,21] examined high-protein formula diets (approximately 40% carbohydrate, 10% fat, 50% protein). All six short-term DCR studies measured total fat mass via DEXA.

Three short-term ICR trials were included in this chapter [16,17,27]. One study [27] provided food to the participants throughout the intervention, while the other two [16,17] provided food initially and then allowed the participants to self-select their diet at around the midpoint of the intervention. Each of the trials utilized alternate-day modified fasting [13], a form of ICR that alternates between a "fast day" (75% energy restriction) and a "feast day" (ad libitum intake, or in the case of one study [27], consumption of 125% of energy needs). Only one study [16] determined the degree of average daily energy restriction that was actually achieved by the participants (37%, estimated via food records). Klempel and colleagues [27] compared a high-fat diet (40% carbohydrate, 45% fat, 15% protein) to a low-fat diet (60% carbohydrate, 25% fat, 15% protein) and found that they equally reduced body weight, total fat mass, and waist circumference. The other two investigations also examined low-fat diets (55% carbohydrate, 25% fat, 20% protein for Bhutani et al. [16]; and 52% carbohydrate, 24% fat, 24% protein for Bhutani et al. [17]). Two trials measured total fat mass via BIA [16,17], while Klempel et al. [27] used DEXA.

Description of Weight Loss Interventions: Moderate Term (13–30 weeks)

Five moderate-term DCR studies were included in this review [18,28–31]. Only one trial [30] provided food to the participants. The degree of prescribed energy restriction in these studies ranged from 25% to 34%, while the degree of energy restriction that was actually achieved by the participants (estimated via food records or self-reporting) ranged from 19% to 23%. Four investigations [28–31] examined diets that complied with the American Heart Association dietary guidelines (50–60% carbohydrate, 25–30% fat, 15–20% protein) [26], and a fifth study [18] examined a low-glycemic index, Mediterranean diet (45% carbohydrate, 30% fat, 25% protein). Three trials measured total fat mass via DEXA [29–31], one trial utilized MRI [28], while a fifth study utilized BIA [18].

Two moderate-term ICR trials [18,29] were included in this chapter. Coincidentally, these were the only two studies featured in this review (short term or moderate term) that directly compared an ICR regimen to a DCR one. Neither trial provided food to the participants. The ICR regimen in the Harvie et al. study [18] alternated between a 2-day period of 75% energy restriction and a 5-day period of intake equal to 100% of energy needs. The ICR regimen in the Arguin et al. investigation [29] alternated between 5-week periods of weight loss (unspecified energy restriction prescription) or weight maintenance. Both investigations used food records to estimate the average daily energy restriction actually achieved by the participants: this was 30% for the Harvie et al. study [18] and 23% for the weight loss periods of the Arguin et al. study [29]. Information pertaining to diet macronutrient distributions as well as the measurements of total fat mass in the Arguin et al. [29] and Harvie et al. [18] studies can be found in the previous section.

Effects of Average Daily Energy Reduction

The average daily energy reduction was 24% in short-term DCR studies, which represented 97% of the prescribed energy reduction. In moderate-term DCR investigations, the average daily energy reduction was 21%, representing only 83% of the prescribed energy reduction. Only one short-term ICR study [16] and one moderate-term ICR study [18] compared actual versus prescribed energy intake. Bhutani and colleagues [16] reported a 37% reduction in actual intake, representing 99% of the prescribed energy reduction. Harvie and colleagues [18] reported a 30% reduction in actual intake, which represented 120% of the prescribed energy reduction. Thus, the percentage of prescribed energy reduction that was actually achieved appears to be similar between DCR and ICR in the short term. However, this percentage decreases considerably in moderate-duration DCR studies, suggesting that patients adhere less to this diet regimen over time. There is currently not enough information available to determine whether a similar phenomenon occurs for ICR, but results from Harvie et al. [18] suggest that this may not be the case.

Effects on Body Weight and Total Fat Mass

In short-term studies, DCR was more effective at reducing body weight (8.8%) and total fat mass (15.3%) than was ICR (4.5% and 9.0%, respectively). However, these trends were not observed in studies of moderate duration. In these latter studies, weight loss was similar between DCR (8.8%) and ICR (10.0%), and ICR was more effective at reducing total fat mass (18.0%) than was DCR (14.8%). The two studies that directly compared DCR and ICR regimens [18,29] observed no between-group differences in weight loss or total fat mass reduction.

There were some methodological differences between the short-term DCR and ICR studies that could have affected changes in body composition. The participants in the short-term ICR trials were younger (44 years vs. 49 years), were comprised of more women (90% vs. 59%), and were probably comprised of more African-Americans (58% in the ICR studies, whereas all but one DCR study [23] did not report on ethnicity) compared to the participants in the short-term DCR trials; each of these factors is associated with less weight loss in randomized controlled trials [32,33]. On the other hand, the participants in the short-term ICR studies were also heavier at baseline [body mass index (BMI) of 35 vs. 32], which is associated with greater weight loss in randomized controlled trials [32,33]. Another methodological difference that may have affected the results was the instrument used to measure total fat mass. Two of the three short-duration ICR studies [16,17] measured total fat mass via BIA, while all the short-duration DCR studies used the more accurate DEXA. However, BIA appears to be reasonably accurate compared to DEXA at measuring body composition changes during weight loss [34,35]. In contrast to the short-term studies, the moderate-term ICR and DCR studies were similar to each other regarding the age, ethnicity, gender, and baseline BMI of the participants. The moderate-duration DCR and ICR studies also measured total fat mass in a similar way. Other potential confounding variables that were examined in this review include sample size and whether food was provided to the subjects; however, these variables were similar between DCR and ICR studies of comparable duration.

Effects on Percentage of Weight Lost as Visceral Fat

In short-term studies, the ratio of waist circumference reduction to total fat mass reduction was greater for ICR (0.68) than for DCR (0.42). This effect was not observed in moderate-term studies, in which the respective ratios for ICR (0.45) and DCR (0.41) were similar.

As mentioned in the previous section, the short-term DCR and ICR investigations differed from one another regarding the baseline BMI, gender, ethnicity, and age of participants; these differences may have affected the percentage of weight lost as visceral fat. A meta-analysis found that the percentage of weight lost as visceral fat is unaffected by baseline BMI and gender [15]. Whether ethnicity affects this variable is less straightforward: two studies reported that Caucasian women lost a greater percentage of weight as visceral fat compared to African-American women [36,37], while a third study reported no ethnicity-related difference in this variable [38]. Whether age affects the percentage of weight lost as visceral fat is an important question that has not been fully answered to date.

Effects on Visceral Fat

Waist circumference reduction was comparable between short-term ICR (5.5%) and DCR trials (6.5%). However, ICR was more effective at reducing waist circumference (8.0%) than was DCR (6.2%) in moderate-term trials. The two studies that directly compared DCR and ICR regimens [18,29] observed no between-group differences in waist circumference reduction.

The total amount of visceral fat reduction is affected by the amount of total fat that is reduced, as well as by the percentage of weight lost as visceral fat. Consequently, methodological differences between the short-term DCR and ICR studies that may have affected total fat mass reduction and the percentage of weight lost as visceral fat (see sections entitled "Effects on Body Weight and Total Fat Mass" and "Effects on Percentage of Weight Lost as Visceral Fat") may have also affected the total amount of visceral fat that was reduced.

DISCUSSION

The key finding from this chapter is that ICR appears to reduce visceral fat (estimated via waist circumference) more effectively than DCR in moderate-duration (13–30 weeks) trials. This contrasts with short-duration trials, for which the reduction in visceral fat is similar between DCR and ICR.

ICR also reduced total fat mass (and possibly also body weight) more effectively than did DCR in moderate-duration studies. Thus, the greater reduction in visceral fat for ICR compared to DCR appears to be due to better dietary adherence. To date, no trial has directly examined whether individuals are less prone to "cheat" (i.e. consume more energy than prescribed) on an ICR diet than on a DCR one. Such a phenomenon seems plausible, as ICR includes feast periods that are designed to restore satiety and satisfaction, thus reducing the urge to cheat. There was initial concern that individuals on ICR would binge (consume well above 100% of energy needs) during the feast periods but, at least in alternate-day modified fasting models, this does not appear to be the case [39].

In short-term studies, ICR reduces visceral fat as effectively as does DCR despite producing less weight loss and total fat reduction. This occurs because the percentage of weight lost as visceral fat (ratio of waist circumference reduction to total fat mass reduction) is greater for ICR than for DCR. Interestingly, this result is consistent with the finding from a recent meta-analysis that the ratio of visceral fat reduction to subcutaneous fat reduction correlates positively with the degree of energy restriction independently of weight loss during the first 12 weeks of treatment [15]. Visceral adipocytes are more responsive to lipolytic stimuli than their subcutaneous counterparts [40]. Thus, if intense, intermittent energy restriction produces a greater lipolytic stimulus compared to moderate, continuous energy restriction, then the former may be better suited for reducing visceral fat, at least during the first 12 weeks of dieting.

This chapter has some limitations that are worth mentioning. Only five ICR investigations met the inclusion criteria, highlighting the need for additional research in this area. Long-duration ICR studies are particularly needed, as no published work to date has examined ICR beyond 30 weeks. We are currently awaiting the results of a year-long trial (6-month weight loss period followed by a 6-month weight-maintenance period) comparing alternate-day modified fasting to DCR. Defining visceral fat change as change in waist circumference was another limitation of this chapter; this was necessitated by the lack of more robust techniques for measuring visceral fat in the ICR studies. There were also some methodological differences between the short-term DCR and ICR investigations, such as differences in the age, ethnicity, baseline BMI, and gender of subjects, as well as differences in how total fat mass was measured, that may have affected the findings generated in this review. Finally, unlike in a meta-analysis, the comparisons in this chapter do not include measures of statistical significance.

In conclusion, ICR may be more effective than DCR for visceral fat reduction at 13–30 weeks of treatment. This may be due to greater dietary adherence to ICR, as suggested by a greater reduction in total fat (and possibly also body weight). Additional research is needed to confirm these findings, and also to examine whether the greater reduction in visceral fat for ICR continues past 30 weeks of treatment.

CONFLICTS OF INTEREST

The authors have no conflicts of interest to declare.

Acknowledgments

Funding: Departmental grant from Kinesiology and Nutrition, University of Illinois, Chicago.

References

[1] Despres J. Abdominal obesity as important component of insulin-resistance syndrome. Nutrition 1993;9(5):452–9.

[2] Després J, Moorjani S, Lupien PJ, Tremblay A, Nadeau A, Bouchard C. Regional distribution of body fat, plasma lipoproteins, and cardiovascular disease. Arterioscler Thromb Vasc Biol 1990;10(4):497–511.

[3] Pascot A, Lemieux I, Prud'homme D, et al. Reduced HDL particle size as an additional feature of the atherogenic dyslipidemia of abdominal obesity. J Lipid Res 2001;42(12):2007–14.

[4] Hayashi T, Boyko EJ, Leonetti DL, McNeely MJ, Newell-Morris L, Kahn SE, et al. Visceral adiposity and the prevalence of hypertension in Japanese Americans. Circulation 2003;108(14):1718–23.

[5] Dagenais GR, Yi Q, Mann JF, Bosch J, Pogue J, Yusuf S. Prognostic impact of body weight and abdominal obesity in women and men with cardiovascular disease. Am Heart J 2005;149(1):54–60.

[6] Larsson SC, Wolk A. Obesity and colon and rectal cancer risk: a meta-analysis of prospective studies. Am J Clin Nutr 2007;86(3): 556–65.

[7] Rose DP, Haffner SM, Baillargeon J. Adiposity, the metabolic syndrome, and breast cancer in African-American and white American women. Endocr Rev 2007;28(7):763–77.

[8] von Hafe P, Pina F, Pérez A, Tavares M, Barros H. Visceral fat accumulation as a risk factor for prostate cancer. Obes Res 2004;12(12):1930–5.

[9] Ryan AM, Duong M, Healy L, Ryan SA, Parekh N, Reynolds JV, et al. Obesity, metabolic syndrome and esophageal adenocarcinoma: Epidemiology, etiology and new targets. Cancer epidemiology 2011;35(4):309–19.

[10] Malhotra A, White DP. Obstructive sleep apnoea. Lancet 2002;360(9328):237–45.

[11] Kuk JL, Katzmarzyk PT, Nichaman MZ, Church TS, Blair SN, Ross R. Visceral fat Is an independent predictor of all-cause mortality in men. Obesity 2006;14(2):336–41.

[12] Goodpaster BH, DeLany JP, Otto AD, et al. Effects of diet and physical activity interventions on weight loss and cardiometabolic risk factors in severely obese adults. JAMA 2010;304(16): 1795–802.

[13] Varady KA, Hellerstein MK. Alternate-day fasting and chronic disease prevention: a review of human and animal trials. Am J Clin Nutr 2007;86(1):7–13.

[14] Hall KD. Predicting metabolic adaptation, body weight change, and energy intake in humans. Am J Physiol Endocrinol Metab 2010;298(3):E449–66.

[15] Chaston T, Dixon J. Factors associated with percent change in visceral versus subcutaneous abdominal fat during weight loss: findings from a systematic review. Int J Obes 2008;32(4):619–28.

[16] Bhutani S, Klempel MC, Berger RA, Varady KA. Improvements in coronary heart disease risk indicators by alternate-day fasting involve adipose tissue modulations. Obesity 2010;18(11):2152–9.

[17] Bhutani S, Klempel Mc, Kroeger C, Trepanowski JF, Varady KA. Alternate day fasting and endurance exercise combine to reduce body weight and favorably alter plasma lipids in obese humans. Obesity 2013;21(7):1370–9.

[18] Harvie MN, Pegington M, Mattson MP, et al. The effects of intermittent or continuous energy restriction on weight loss and metabolic disease risk markers: a randomized trial in young overweight women. Int J Obes 2010;35(5):714–27.

[19] Winkler J. The fundamental flaw in obesity research. Obes Rev 2005;6(3):199–202.

[20] Haugaard SB, Vaag A, Høy C, Madsbad S. Desaturation of skeletal muscle structural and depot lipids in obese individuals during a very-low-calorie diet intervention. Obesity 2007;15(1):117–25.

[21] Luscombe ND, Tsopelas C, Bellon M, Clifton PM, Kirkwood I, Wittert GA. Use of [14C]-sodium bicarbonate/urea to measure total energy expenditure in overweight men and women before and after low calorie diet induced weight loss. Asia Pac J ClinNutr 2006;15(3):307–16.

[22] Kirk E, Reeds DN, Finck BN, Mayurranjan MS, Patterson BW, Klein S. Dietary fat and carbohydrates differentially alter insulin sensitivity during caloric restriction. Gastroenterology 2009;136(5): 1552–60.

[23] Coker RH, Williams RH, Yeo SE, Kortebein PM, Bodenner DL, Kern PA, et al. The impact of exercise training compared to caloric restriction on hepatic and peripheral insulin resistance in obesity. J Clin Endocrinol Metab 2009;94(11):4258–66.

[24] Pierce GL, Beske SD, Lawson BR, Southall KL, Benay FJ, Donato AJ, et al. Weight loss alone improves conduit and resistance artery endothelial function in young and older overweight/obese adults. Hypertension 2008;52(1):72–9.

[25] Redman LM, Heilbronn LK, Martin CK, Alfonso A, Smith SR, Ravussin E. Effect of calorie restriction with or without exercise on body composition and fat distribution. J Clin Endocrinol Metab 2007;92(3):865–72.

[26] National Cholesterol Education Program (NCEP). Expert Panel on Detection, Evaluation, and Treatment of High Blood Cholesterol in Adults (Adult Treatment Panel III). Third report of the National Cholesterol Education Program (NCEP) expert panel

on detection, evaluation, and treatment of high blood cholesterol in adults (Adult Treatment Panel III) final report. Circulation 2002;106(25):3143–421.

[27] Klempel MC, Kroeger CM, Varady KA. Alternate day fasting (ADF) with a high-fat diet produces similar weight loss and cardio-protection as ADF with a low-fat diet. Metabolism 2013;62(1):137–43.

[28] Ross R, Janssen I, Dawson J, et al. Exercise-induced reduction in obesity and insulin resistance in women: a randomized controlled trial. Obes Res 2004;12(5):789–98.

[29] Arguin H, Dionne IJ, Sénéchal M, et al. Short-and long-term effects of continuous versus intermittent restrictive diet approaches on body composition and the metabolic profile in overweight and obese postmenopausal women: a pilot study. Menopause 2012;19(8):870–6.

[30] Nicklas BJ, Wang X, You T, et al. Effect of exercise intensity on abdominal fat loss during calorie restriction in overweight and obese postmenopausal women: a randomized, controlled trial. Am J Clin Nutr 2009;89(4):1043–52.

[31] Brochu M, Malita MF, Messier V, et al. Resistance training does not contribute to improving the metabolic profile after a 6-month weight loss program in overweight and obese postmenopausal women. J Clin Endocrinol Metab 2009;94(9):3226–33.

[32] Finkler E, Heymsfield SB, St-Onge M. Rate of weight loss can be predicted by patient characteristics and intervention strategies. J Acad Nutr Diet 2012;112(1):75–80.

[33] Stubbs J, Whybrow S, Teixeira P, et al. Problems in identifying predictors and correlates of weight loss and maintenance: implications for weight control therapies based on behaviour change. Obes Rev 2011;12(9):688–708.

[34] Frisard MI, Greenway FL, DeLany JP. Comparison of methods to assess body composition changes during a period of weight loss. Obes Res 2005;13(5):845–54.

[35] Thomson R, Brinkworth GD, Buckley JD, Noakes M, Clifton PM. Good agreement between bioelectrical impedance and dual-energy X-ray absorptiometry for estimating changes in body composition during weight loss in overweight young women. Clin Nutr 2007;26(6):771–7.

[36] Gower BA, Weinsier RL, Jordan JM, Hunter GR, Desmond R. Effects of weight loss on changes in insulin sensitivity and lipid concentrations in premenopausal African American and white women. Am J Clin Nutr 2002;76(5):923–7.

[37] Weinsier RL, Hunter GR, Gower BA, Schutz Y, Darnell BE, Zuckerman PA. Body fat distribution in white and black women: different patterns of intraabdominal and subcutaneous abdominal adipose tissue utilization with weight loss. Am J Clin Nutr 2001;74(5):631–6.

[38] Nicklas BJ, Dennis KE, Berman DM, Sorkin J, Ryan AS, Goldberg AP. Lifestyle intervention of hypocaloric dieting and walking reduces abdominal obesity and improves coronary heart disease risk factors in obese, postmenopausal, African-American and Caucasian women. J Gerontol A Biol Sci Med Sci 2003;58(2): M181–9.

[39] Klempel M, Bhutani S, Fitzgibbon M, Freels S, Varady K. Dietary and physical activity adaptations to alternate day modified fasting: implications for optimal weight loss. Nutr J 2010;9(1):35.

[40] Arner P. Differences in lipolysis between human subcutaneous and omental adipose tissues. Ann Med 1995;27(4):435–8.

CHAPTER

18

Stress-Induced Eating Dampens Physiological and Behavioral Stress Responses

Laura E. Finch and A. Janet Tomiyama

Department of Psychology, University of California, Los Angeles, CA, USA

INTRODUCTION

Perceived stress influences health behaviors across multiple domains, with high stress levels associated with a high-fat diet, less frequent exercise, and cigarette smoking [1]. A recent national survey found that 44% of adults report feeling greater stress now than they did 5 years ago, and 39% report eating too much or eating unhealthy foods due to feelings of stress in the past month [2]. Chronic life stress is associated with increased consumption of energy- and nutrient-dense "comfort foods," particularly high-fat and high-sugar foods [3]. This altered eating behavior in times of stress is referred to as *stress-induced eating*, *emotional eating*, or *comfort eating*. While the first term refers to eating behavior being specifically altered in response to feelings of stress, the latter two terms may be used to describe altered eating in response to a range of emotional states (e.g. stress, sadness, anger, or boredom). Here we primarily focus on stress-induced eating because it is clearly operationally defined across species and is most commonly examined in existing research.

Acute psychological stress in humans is associated with increased food intake even in the absence of hunger [4]. For example, in student populations, exams or high workload have been associated with higher energy and fat intake [5] or a decreased quality of dietary nutrition [6]. Furthermore, chronic stress exposure also promotes stress-induced eating behavior. Psychological stress due to interpersonal and work-related daily hassles is associated with an increased consumption of high-fat and high-sugar between-meal snacks and with decreased consumption of main meals and vegetables [7].

Not all individuals increase their food intake in response to stress; in studies of self-reported stress and food intake, approximately 40–70% of humans report increasing and 30–60% report decreasing their food intake under stress [8,9]. Researchers have yet to fully identify which factors account for these individual differences, but body mass index (BMI) may matter. Data from the Whitehall II study indicated that under stress conditions, individuals with higher initial BMI tend to gain weight and vice versa [10]. Twin studies indicate that stress-induced eating may also be partially heritable [11]. Some researchers have also observed gender [12] and racial/ethnic differences [13] in the levels of stress-induced eating, with females and black individuals engaging in more emotional eating, and others not [14]. Individuals characterized by restrained eating and sensitivity to chronic stress may also be particularly susceptible to stress-induced eating [4]. Regardless of whether the overall *amount* of food consumption changes under stress, all individuals (including nonhuman animals) alter their eating habits to consume palatable foods characterized by high-calorie, high-sugar, and high-fat content [15].

Persistent stress-induced eating behavior over time results in intra-abdominal obesity [16], which is strongly associated with metabolic syndrome, hypertension, type 2 diabetes mellitus, cardiovascular disease, morbidity, and mortality [17,18]. The association of stress-induced eating with increased visceral fat accumulation has motivated the development of stress-induced eating interventions on the premise that stress eating is unequivocally harmful [19]. However, there is a growing literature demonstrating the potentially salutary role of stress-induced eating behavior in dampening both physiological and behavioral stress responses.

Nutrition in the Prevention and Treatment of Abdominal Obesity
http://dx.doi.org/10.1016/B978-0-12-407869-7.00018-0

In this chapter, we review cross-species literatures describing how experiences of stress affect eating behavior and fat distribution, and vice versa. First, we review research demonstrating the effects of both acute and chronic stressors in promoting stress-induced eating. Next, we discuss how repeated engagement in stress-induced eating under chronic stress conditions leads to the accumulation of visceral fat, as evidenced primarily in studies of nonhuman animals. We then review the burgeoning literature supporting the joint role of stress-induced eating and abdominal fat in attenuating stress responses, focusing on glucocorticoids and insulin as endocrine promoters of these processes. We go on to describe potential affective and neural mechanisms for perpetuating the cycle of stress-induced eating. The vast majority of data regarding the physiological and behavioral effects of stress-induced eating comes from studies of nonhuman animals. However, to the extent that these effects have been tested in humans, consistent results have been observed. We conclude our discussion with a summary of the remaining gaps in the literature and suggestions for future research.

GLUCOCORTICOIDS AND INSULIN PROMOTE STRESS-INDUCED EATING

Both physical and psychological stressors are known to stimulate the hypothalamic-pituitary-adrenal (HPA) axis. Stress-induced activation of the HPA axis begins with the release of corticoliberin [corticotropin-releasing factor (CRH), encoded by the *CRH* gene] from the hypothalamus, which stimulates the release of adrenocorticotropic hormone (ACTH) from the anterior pituitary gland. ACTH then circulates through the bloodstream to the adrenal cortex, where it stimulates glucocorticoid secretion [20].

Increased glucocorticoid secretion following HPA axis activation appears to be a central pathway through which stress promotes the consumption of palatable foods. In a sample of healthy premenopausal women, individuals who exhibited a higher total cortisol output in response to a laboratory stressor consumed more calories that day compared to those with a lower total cortisol response [21]. Furthermore, oral administration of glucocorticoids in healthy white males has been shown to increase their intake of total energy, carbohydrate, and protein, but not of fat [22]. Dose-response effects of glucocorticoid concentrations on eating behavior may be robustly tested through the study of adrenalectomized organisms, as they lack the capability to naturally produce glucocorticoids via the adrenal glands. In adrenalectomized rats, the administration of corticosterone directly affects the consumption of both saccharin and sucrose in a dose-response manner, with larger corticosterone doses resulting in a greater proportional intake of these substances [23,24].

Importantly, increased glucocorticoid concentrations stimulate insulin secretion [25]. In a series of experiments in rats, La Fleur and colleagues identified complex interactions between corticosterone and insulin in the regulation of food intake, finding that glucocorticoids elicit dose-related increases in total caloric intake, and that increased insulin concentrations stimulated by glucocorticoids specifically regulate the amount of fat consumed [26]. These effects are evidenced in studies of adrenalectomized, diabetic rats, in which concurrent glucocorticoids and insulin promote a shift in intake toward fat and sugar, whereas glucocorticoids in the absence of insulin promote the consumption of bland rat chow. Therefore, it seems that glucocorticoids function to increase general food-associated drives, while insulin influences preferences for which types of foods are consumed.

GLUCOCORTICOIDS AND INSULIN PROMOTE VISCERAL FAT ACCUMULATION

Insulin and glucocorticoids also have complex interactions in fat accumulation. These hormones have acutely antagonistic effects, with glucocorticoids inhibiting energy storage and insulin promoting energy storage [27]. However, in the location of fat stores, insulin and high glucocorticoids act synergistically to promote visceral fat accumulation, especially under chronically stressful conditions [28,29]. Cortisol binds to glucocorticoid receptors and activates lipoprotein lipase (LPL), thus increasing triglyceride accumulation in adipocytes. In the presence of insulin, cortisol also inhibits the lipid-mobilizing system, resulting in triglyceride retention [28]. Concurrent cortisol and insulin also promote visceral fat accumulation indirectly by inhibiting the activity of somatotropin/growth hormone, which otherwise exerts lipolytic effects [30]. These processes are amplified in intra-abdominal adipose tissue, where there is a particularly high density of glucocorticoid receptors compared to other fat depots [28]. Visceral fat accumulation further perpetuates this cycle by providing increased intracellular glucocorticoids [31]. These effects are particularly apparent in patients with Cushing syndrome, who are both hypercortisolemic and hyperinsulinemic and have high levels of intra-abdominal obesity [32].

These processes have been demonstrated experimentally. In rats, the administration of high glucocorticoid concentrations in the presence of insulin increases fat stores [26,33]. Although no experimental studies are known to have been conducted in humans, preliminary evidence suggests that some of the same processes are at work. For example, the synergistic role of these hormones in promoting stress-induced eating and weight gain is supported in a sample of healthy medical students who categorized themselves as consistently eating either more or less during stress [34]. Students that characterized themselves as normatively eating more during stress tended to gain more weight and also demonstrated increases in urinary cortisol and insulin levels during exam periods, controlling for baseline. Although this study did not test for expected increases in fat and sugar consumption related to increased insulin, the increase in total food intake self-reported by the "eat-more" group is consistent with their corresponding elevated cortisol concentrations.

STRESS-INDUCED EATING DAMPENS PHYSIOLOGICAL AND BEHAVIORAL STRESS RESPONSES

There is increasing evidence from animal models supporting an important therapeutic role of comfort eating in inhibiting the HPA axis response to both acute and chronic stressors. Studies in nonhuman animals have demonstrated what Dallman and colleagues have termed a *chronic stress response network* model, that is, a process through which stress-induced eating decreases neuroendocrine activity associated with the physiological stress response [33]. For example, in rats exposed to chronic restraint stress, the provision of palatable lard or sucrose has been shown to dampen stress responses compared to a diet of less palatable chow [35]. In particular, there is an attenuated physiological stress response in the form of reduced ACTH secretion. The consumption of palatable food may reduce HPA outflows even in the absence of stress; nonstressed rats given the palatable diet showed reduced *Crh* expression compared to nonstressed rats given chow. Similarly, in rats exposed to chronic unpredictable physical stress, the provision of daily limited access to sucrose or saccharin solutions decreased *Crh* mRNA expression in the paraventricular nucleus of the hypothalamus [36]. Furthermore, sucrose ingestion reduced the plasma corticosterone response to restraint in these chronically stressed rats. Additional research suggests that a palatable diet is also effective in dampening physiological responses to acute stressors. A study in rats tested the effects of prior access (7 days) to chow versus palatable foods on HPA axis activation following 4 h of acute restraint stress [37]. Rats with prior access to palatable foods showed inhibited ACTH and corticosterone responses, as well as reduced *Crh* mRNA in the hypothalamus and oval nucleus of the bed nuclei of the stria terminalis. In summary, these studies suggest that the consumption of palatable foods decreases endocrine responses to both acute and chronic physical stressors.

In addition to attenuating physiological stress responses, the consumption of palatable food has also been shown to ameliorate behavioral responses to stressors. In rats, the ingestion of palatable food reduces the effects of chronic maternal separation stress, decreasing anxiety and depressive-like behaviors [38]. Likewise, in mice exposed to chronic unpredictable social defeat and overcrowding stress, concurrent subjection to a high-fat diet decreased the expression of anxiety and depressive-like behaviors, compared to mice on a concurrent low-fat diet. However, a high-fat diet appears to protect from some but not other behavioral effects of chronic social stress; for example, social avoidance and anhedonic behavior were not affected [39]. Finally, in male rats, the short-term (7 days) intake of a high-fat diet reduced acute behavioral anxiety response to an elevated plus maze stressor. This effect appears to be highly dependent upon macronutrient content, as comparison high-carbohydrate and high-protein diets did not decrease anxiety behaviors [40]. These results consistently support the protective role of a palatable diet in reducing anxiety and depressive behaviors in response to both acute and chronic psychosocial stressors. While no known studies to date have experimentally tested these behavioral effects in humans, these findings in rodent models may be particularly relevant to human populations; compared to the administration of physical stressors, the psychosocial stress paradigms employed in these behavioral studies bear a closer resemblance to the types of stressors naturally experienced by some humans.

REINFORCEMENT OF STRESS-INDUCED EATING VIA AFFECTIVE RESPONSES, THE REWARD SYSTEM, AND ENHANCED MEMORY

Stress and food intake interact in a bidirectional manner. Just as stress and mood can alter eating behavior, food choice can conversely impact stress and mood, whether deliberate or unintended. As reviewed by Gibson [41], choosing to eat particular foods can alter mood via sensory or hedonic effects, associated social context, cognitive expectations, psychological distraction, changes in appetite, or nutritional modulation of brain function. For example, high-sugar, high-fat foods low in protein may ameliorate stress via enhanced functioning of the serotonergic system. Laboratory experiments have also demonstrated that sweet-tasting substances may provide analgesic effects during acute stressors, e.g. increasing pain threshold latency and pain tolerance during cold-pressor tasks [42,43]. Taken together, these findings suggest a general capability of comfort foods to elicit desirable affective or sensory responses in humans, which may function to reinforce stress-induced eating behavior.

The experience of eating can be both pleasurable and rewarding. Indeed, the addiction literature suggests that repeated activation of neural reward circuitry may also drive stress-induced eating. Food intake stimulates the release of endogenous opiates and activates neural substrates such as dopamine in a similar manner to drugs of abuse, albeit with differences in intensity [44]. Consequently, opiate release may serve to protect an organism from the detrimental effects of stress by decreasing HPA axis activity and dampening the stress response. In a reward-based stress eating model, repeated stimulation of reward pathways coinciding with stress-induced eating may result in neurobiological adaptations that promote the compulsive nature of overeating [31]. Reward-related consumption can result in caloric intake exceeding requirements, and may be a critical etiological pathway in the development of obesity, in particular abdominal obesity [45].

In addition, the cycle of stress-induced eating may also be perpetuated by learning and memory via the action of glucocorticoids. Considerable evidence has accumulated indicating that glucocorticoids are crucially involved in the regulation of memory, specifically enhancing memory consolidation of emotionally arousing experiences [46]. Thus, when stress promotes glucocorticoid-induced palatable food intake, glucocorticoids also facilitate the formation of cognitive associations between comfort food indulgence and subsequent positive affect.

ROLE OF GLUCOCORTICOIDS AND VISCERAL FAT IN DAMPENING STRESS RESPONSES

In addition to their role in promoting stress-induced eating and memory formation, glucocorticoids are also crucial in the development of visceral fat accumulation [28], which in turn attenuates stress responses [33]. The effect of stress-induced glucocorticoid secretion on subsequent ACTH secretion is dependent upon the chronicity of stressors. Within hours of acute stressors, glucocorticoids directly inhibit further activity in the HPA axis [47], but across the course of days the chronic actions of glucocorticoids on the brain are directly excitatory [33]. As summarized by Dallman and colleagues [33], chronically high glucocorticoid concentrations act in three functionally congruent ways: (1) increasing the expression of *Crh* mRNA in the amygdala; (2) increasing the salience of pleasurable or compulsive activities, including the motivation to consume "comfort food"; and (3) systematically increasing visceral fat stores. These visceral stores then send a negative feedback signal to inhibit both catecholamines in the brainstem and CRH expression in hypothalamic neurons that regulate ACTH. Indeed, studies in chronically stressed rats have consistently demonstrated a strong negative correlation between intra-abdominal fat stores and hypothalamic CRH expression [16,48]. Therefore, it seems that under chronic stress conditions, abdominal fat serves as a surrogate for the negative feedback signal of glucocorticoids that is normally present under acute stress conditions, thus inhibiting further HPA activation. Although the particular signal to the brain that represents increased abdominal fat stores remains unidentified, it is apparent that this signal does indeed act in the brain to decrease the adverse effects of the chronic stress response, plausibly promoting feelings of well-being [16].

While stress-induced palatable eating and greater abdominal fat stores have consistently been shown to reduce signs of stress in rodent models, there is a dearth of research examining these processes in other organisms. However, preliminary evidence suggests that these processes are indeed conserved across species.

In a study by our group [50], women with high chronic perceived stress reported more emotional eating and had significantly greater BMI and sagittal diameter in comparison to low-stress women. Emotional eating behavior was measured using the Dutch Eating Behavior Questionnaire (DEBQ) [51], a well-validated measure of eating behavior. In addition to these cross-sectional results, a laboratory component of the study also measured HPA axis activation in response to an acute laboratory stressor, the Trier Social Stress Test (TSST) [52]. This is a procedure designed to induce psychological and physiological stress responses via the performance of both a speech task and mental arithmetic task in front of an evaluative audience. Following the TSST, the chronic high-stress women showed a blunted cortisol response and lower diurnal cortisol levels compared to low-stress women. While these findings are consistent with rodent models, this study is limited by its lack of direct measurement of eating behavior following stressor exposure.

Two additional studies in humans expand upon previous findings by directly measuring food intake after exposure to an acute laboratory stressor. The first study compared female students with extremely high or low scores on emotional eating, as measured by the DEBQ [53]. The study exposed participants to a modified TSST, subsequently assessing total cortisol response to the stressor, as well as their food intake. Results revealed emotional eating to be a significant moderator of the relationship between cortisol stress reactivity and food intake. High emotional eaters with a blunted cortisol response consumed more food after stress than those with an elevated cortisol response, whereas no relationship was found in low emotional eaters. Thus, these results are consistent with previous studies demonstrating a relationship between blunted cortisol stress response and increased stress-induced eating in high emotional eaters.

Using a similar experimental design, Tryon et al. assessed both food intake and total cortisol response following administration of the TSST [54]. In this sample of healthy, perimenopausal women, responses to the stressor were compared on the basis of high vs. low self-reported chronic stress levels, as measured by the Wheaton Social Stress Index [55]. Women with high chronic stress and low cortisol reactivity consumed more calories from chocolate cake in response to the stressor. Moreover, the combination of high chronic stress and low cortisol reactivity was positively associated with total fat mass and regional fat percentage. This finding supports the previously discussed concept of a metabolic feedback pathway, in which a signal sent from adipose tissue inhibits activation of the HPA axis. In conclusion, early studies in humans repeatedly show correlations between high chronic stress, high emotional eating, greater abdominal fat, and decreased cortisol responses to acute laboratory stressors. Future studies should expand upon this work by investigating how stress-induced eating and abdominal fat stores affect responses to naturalistic stressors in humans.

Additional evidence from an epidemiological study supports the chronic stress response network model. In black individuals, the relationship between stressors and meeting major-depression criteria was buffered in obese individuals, compared to nonobese individuals [13]. Although this study was limited by its lack of a direct measurement of eating behavior, it suggests a significant paradox in which obesity (a proxy for overeating) serves a protective role for mental health outcomes, while simultaneously contributing to negative physical health outcomes in the form of higher rates of chronic conditions, morbidity, and mortality. Further research is needed to test the potential protective role of obesity and stress-induced eating behavior for mental health by specifically exploring its capacity for dampening psychological stress responses.

While stress-induced eating has been shown to reliably attenuate stress responses in rodents, and preliminarily in humans, these effects may be variable in other species. For example, in a study of 10 adult female rhesus monkeys, stress-induced eating was shown to decrease behavioral, but not physiological stress responses [56]. For a period of 3 weeks of social subordination stress exposure, the females were assigned to either a low-calorie diet or to a choice condition with the provision of both a low- and high-calorie diet. Food intake, cortisol secretion, and socioemotional behavior were assessed over time in both subordinate females and nonstressed dominant females. Of the females in the diet-choice condition, subordinate females consumed more calories from the high-calorie diet and gained more weight compared to dominant females. However, the provision of a high-calorie diet was associated with a flattening of the diurnal cortisol rhythm and did not decrease the cortisol response to acute social separation. Although these physiological findings are inconsistent with previous work in other species, diet condition did indeed influence behavioral stress responses over time. While females in the low-calorie diet condition exhibited increasing rates of anxiety-like behaviors, females in the diet-choice condition showed decreasing rates of these behaviors. Interestingly, rates of aggressive behavior directed at other females were significantly higher for females in the no-choice condition with only the low-calorie diet available. In summary, stress-induced eating may decrease physiological stress responses in some, but not all, species. Nevertheless, cross-species data consistently show decreased behavioral stress responses with the provision of a palatable diet.

CONCLUSION AND FUTURE DIRECTIONS

There is strong evidence across species that both acute and chronic stressors promote increased consumption of palatable comfort foods. Furthermore, studies in rodents have consistently shown that chronic persistence in stress-induced eating behavior results in increased visceral fat accumulation, which functions to attenuate HPA axis activation in response to stressors. These effects have only just begun to be tested in humans; however, preliminary evidence is consistent with the dampened stress responses demonstrated in rodents. Of the few studies that have investigated these processes in humans, the outcome measures of stress have been responses to acute social evaluative stressors administered in the laboratory setting. Additional research is needed to explore how stress-induced eating might reduce experiences of stress related to more heterogeneous and naturally occurring stressors outside the laboratory.

In addition to exploring how the chronic stress response network functions in humans, future studies should also include experimental designs aimed to investigate multiple stress systems. Previous research has primarily focused on HPA axis activation as the principal outcome measure of dampened stress responsivity. However, autonomic and immune system activity is also heavily influenced by exposure to stressors. Therefore, future work should evaluate the potential role of stress-induced eating in similarly attenuating responses to stress across these additional physiological systems.

Furthermore, little is known about how stress dampening may be particularly dependent upon the macronutrient content of palatable foods. Are characteristically high-sugar, high-fat foods necessary for decreasing stress responsivity or can high-protein, or simply high-calorie, foods also elicit these responses?

Future research should also carefully delineate which specific types of circumstances or emotional exposures are most responsible for triggering the stress-induced eating process. For example, is general stress driving this behavior, or do certain characteristic types of stress, such as uncontrollable or unpredictable stress experiences, have the same effect? Alternatively, are experiences with other types of negative emotion (e.g. anger, sadness, or worry), or even positive emotion, also effective in eliciting stress-induced eating and its corresponding attenuated stress response?

Similarly, researchers should investigate which individuals are particularly (1) susceptible to stress-induced eating and (2) effective in dampening stress responses via stress-induced eating. Some evidence supports genetics, BMI, and demographic characteristics such as gender and race/ethnicity as potential candidates for the former; virtually no research exists on the latter.

Finally, existing research has yet to conclusively identify the peripheral negative feedback signal to the brain that promotes the inhibition of further HPA axis activation during chronic stress exposure [for a review, see 56]. Potential signal mechanisms and structures include insulin activity, vagus nerve stimulation, and neural alterations in the activity of the prefrontal cortex.

Although obesity is known to develop from myriad genetic and environmental factors, the growing literature on stress-induced eating will elucidate the complex relationships between stress, eating, and obesity. If stress-induced eating leads to the consumption of food in excess of nutritive requirements, then this behavior may culminate in abdominal weight gain and obesity. However, the dampened physiological and behavioral stress responses demonstrated in numerous studies suggest that stress-induced eating provides short-term amelioration of stress. This ostensible benefit of stress-induced eating has important implications for evaluating whether attempts at stress-induced eating intervention are an appropriate response to the behavior. Further research evaluating the causes and effects of stress-induced eating will improve our understanding of why individuals engage in this behavior and how it functions as a contributing factor in the etiology of obesity.

References

[1] Ng DM, Jeffery RW. Relationships between perceived stress and health behaviors in a sample of working adults. Health Psychol 2003;22:638–42.

[2] American Psychological Association Press Release. Stress in America: Our health at risk. <http://www.apa.org/news/press/releases/stress/2011/final-2011.pdf> [accessed 02.04.13].

[3] Torres SJ, Nowson CA. Relationship between stress, eating behavior, and obesity. Nutrition 2007;23:887–94.

[4] Rutters F, Nieuwenhuizen AG, Lemmens SG, Born JM, Westerterp-Plantenga MS. Acute stress-related changes in eating in the absence of hunger. Obesity 2008;17:72–7.

[5] Michaud C, Kahn JP, Musse N, Burlet C, Nicolas JP, Mejean L. Relationships between a critical life event and eating behaviour in high-school students. Stress Med 1990;6:57–64.

[6] Weidner G, Kohlmann CW, Dotzauer E, Burns LR. The effects of academic stress on health behaviors in young adults. Anxiety Stress Copin 1996;9:123–33.

[7] O'Connor DB, Jones F, Conner M, McMillan B, Ferguson E. Effects of daily hassles and eating style on eating behavior. Health Psychol 2008;27:S20–31.

[8] Oliver G, Wardle J. Perceived effects of stress on food choice. Physiol Behav 1999;66:511–5.

[9] Kandiah J, Yake M, Willett H. Effects of stress on eating practices among adults. Fam Consum Sci Res J 2008;37:27–38.

[10] Kivimaki M, Head J, Ferrie JE, et al. Work stress, weight gain and weight loss: evidence for bidirectional effects of job strain on body mass index in the Whitehall II study. Int J Obes 2006;30:982–7.

[11] Sung J, Lee K, Song YM, Lee MK, Lee DH. Heritability of eating behavior assessed using the DEBQ (Dutch Eating Behavior Questionnaire) and weight-related traits: the healthy twin study. Obesity 2010;18:1000–5.

[12] Snoek HM, Van Strien T, Janssens JM, Engels RC. Emotional, external, restrained eating and overweight in Dutch adolescents. Scand J Psychol 2007;48:23–32.

[13] Jackson JS, Knight KM, Rafferty JA. Race and unhealthy behaviors: chronic stress, the HPA axis, and physical and mental health disparities over the life course. Am J Public Health 2010;100:933–9.

[14] Ledoux T, Watson K, Baranowski J, Tepper BJ, Baranowski T. Overeating styles and adiposity among multiethnic youth. Appetite 2011;56:71–7.

[15] Dallman MF. Stress-induced obesity and the emotional nervous system. Trends Endocrinol Metab 2010;21:159–65.

[16] Dallman MF, Pecoraro NC, la Fleur SE. Chronic stress and comfort foods: self-medication and abdominal obesity. Brain Behav Immun 2005;19:275–80.

[17] Wajchenberg BL. Subcutaneous and visceral adipose tissue: their relation to the metabolic syndrome. Endocr Rev 2000;21:697–738.

[18] Björntorp P. " Portal" adipose tissue as a generator of risk factors for cardiovascular disease and diabetes. Arteriosclerosis 1990;10:493–6.

[19] Daubenmier J, Kristeller J, Hecht FM, Maninger N, Kuwata M, Jhaveri K, et al. Mindfulness intervention for stress eating to reduce cortisol and abdominal fat among overweight and obese women: an exploratory randomized controlled study. J Obes 2011;2011:651936.. http://dx.doi.org/10.1155/2011/651936.

[20] Lovallo WR, Thomas TL. Stress hormones in psychophysiological research: emotional, behavioral, and cognitive implications. In: Cacioppo JT, , Tassinary LG, Berntson GG, editors. Handbook of psychophysiology. 2nd ed.. New York: Cambridge University Press; 2000. p. 342–67.

[21] Epel E, Lapidus R, McEwen B, Brownell K. Stress may add bite to appetite in women: a laboratory study of stress-induced cortisol and eating behavior. Psychoneuroendocrinology 2001;26:37–49.

[22] Tataranni P, Larson D. Effects of glucocorticoids on energy metabolism and food intake in humans. Am J Physiol 1996;271: E317–25.

[23] Bhatnagar S, Bell ME, Liang J, Soriano L, Nagy TR, Dallman MF. Corticosterone facilitates saccharin intake in adrenalectomized rats: does corticosterone increase stimulus salience? J Neuroendocrinol 2000;12:453–60.

[24] Bell ME, Bhatnagar S, Liang J, Soriano L, Nagy TR, Dallman MF. Voluntary sucrose ingestion, like corticosterone replacement, prevents the metabolic deficits of adrenalectomy. J Neuroendocrinol 2001;12:461–70.

[25] Miller WL, Tyrrell JB. The adrenal cortex. In: Felig P, , Baxter JD, Frohman LA, editors. Endocrinology and metabolism. 3rd ed.. New York: McGraw-Hill; 1995. p. 555–711.

[26] La Fleur SE, Akana SF, Manalo SL, Dallman MF. Interaction between corticosterone and insulin in obesity: regulation of lard intake and fat stores. Endocrinology 2004;145:2174–85.

[27] Strack AM, Sebastian RJ, Schwartz MW, Dallman MF. Glucocorticoids and insulin: reciprocal signals for energy balance. Am J Physiol 1995;268:R142–9.

[28] Björntorp P. Do stress reactions cause abdominal obesity and comorbidities? Obes Rev 2001;2:73–86.

[29] Hauner H, Schmid P, Pfeiffer EF. Glucocorticoids and insulin promote the differentiation of human adipocyte precursor cells into fat cells. J Clin Endocrinol Metab 1987;64:832–5.

[30] Ottosson M, Lönnroth P, Björntorp P, Edén S. Effects of cortisol and growth hormone on lipolysis in human adipose tissue. J Clin Endocrinol Metab 2000;85:799–803.

[31] Adam TC, Epel ES. Stress, eating and the reward system. Physiol Behav 2007;91:449–58.

[32] Rebuffé-Scrive M, Krotkiewski M, Elfverson J, Björntorp P. Muscle and adipose tissue morphology and metabolism in Cushing's syndrome. J Clin Endocrinol Metab 1988;67:1122–8.

[33] Dallman MF, Pecoraro N, Akana SF, et al. Chronic stress and obesity: a new view of "comfort food". Proc Natl Acad Sci USA 2003;100:11696–701.

[34] Epel E, Jimenez S, Brownell K, Stroud L, Stoney C, Niaura R. Are stress eaters at risk for the metabolic syndrome? Ann NY Acad Sci 2004;1032:208–10.

[35] Pecoraro N, Reyes F, Gomez F, Bhargava A, Dallman MF. Chronic stress promotes palatable feeding, which reduces signs of stress: feedforward and feedback effects of chronic stress. Endocrinology 2004;145:3754–62.

[36] Ulrich-Lai YM, Ostrander MM, Thomas IM, et al. Daily limited access to sweetened drink attenuates hypothalamic-pituitary-adrenocortical axis stress responses. Endocrinology 2007;148:1823–34.

[37] Foster MT, Warne JP, Ginsberg AB, et al. Palatable foods, stress, and energy stores sculpt corticotropin-releasing factor, adrenocorticotropin, and corticosterone concentrations after restraint. Endocrinology 2009;150:2325–33.

[38] Maniam J, Morris MJ. Palatable cafeteria diet ameliorates anxiety and depression-like symptoms following an adverse early environment. Psychoneuroendocrinology 2010;35:717–28.

[39] Finger BC, Dinan TG, Cryan JF. High-fat diet selectively protects against the effects of chronic social stress in the mouse. Neuroscience 2011;192:351–60.

[40] Prasad A, Prasad C. Short-term consumption of a diet rich in fat decreases anxiety response in adult male rats. Physiol Behav 1996;60:1039–42.

[41] Gibson EL. Emotional influences on food choice: sensory, physiological and psychological pathways. Physiol Behav 2006;89:53–61.

[42] Miller A, Barr RG, Young SN. The cold pressor test in children: methodological aspects and the analgesic effect of intraoral sucrose. Pain 1994;56:175–83.

[43] Leweekowski MD, Ditto B, Roussos M, Young SN. Sweet taste and blood pressure-related analgesia. Pain 2003;106:181–6.

[44] Grigson PS. Like drugs for chocolate: separate rewards modulated by common mechanisms? Physiol Behav 2002;76:389–95.

[45] Kuo LE, Kitlinska JB, Tilan JU, et al. Neuropeptide Y acts directly in the periphery on fat tissue and mediates stress-induced obesity and metabolic syndrome. Nat Med 2007;13:803–11.

[46] de Quervain DJ, Aerni A, Schelling G, Roozendaal B. Glucocorticoids and the regulation of memory in health and disease. Front Neuroendocrinol 2009;30:358–70.

[47] Keller-Wood ME, Dallman MF. Corticosteroid inhibition of ACTH secretion. Endocr Rev 1984;5:1–24.

[48] Houshyar H, Manalo S, Dallman MF. Time-dependent alterations in mRNA expression of brain neuropeptides regulating energy balance and hypothalamo-pituitary-adrenal activity after withdrawal from intermittent morphine treatment. J Neurosci 2004;24:9414–24.

[49] Tomiyama AJ, Dallman MF, Epel ES. Comfort food is comforting to those most stressed: evidence of the chronic stress response network in high stress women. Psychoneuroendocrinology 2011;36:1513–9.

[50] van Strien T, Frijters JE, Bergers G, Defares PB. The Dutch Eating Behavior Questionnaire (DEBQ) for assessment of restrained, emotional, and external eating behavior. Int J Eat Disord 1986;5:295–315.

[51] Kirschbaum C, Pirke KM, Hellhammer DH. The 'Trier Social Stress Test'—a tool for investigating psychobiological stress responses in a laboratory setting. Neuropsychobiology 2008;28:76–81.

[52] van Strien T, Roelofs K, de Weerth C. Cortisol reactivity and distress-induced emotional eating. Psychoneuroendocrinology 2013;38:677–84.

[53] Tryon MS, DeCant R, Laugero KD. Having your cake and eating it too: A habit of comfort food may link chronic social stress exposure and acute stress-induced cortisol hyporesponsiveness. Physiol Behav 2013;114–115:32–7.

[54] Turner RJ, Wheaton B, Lloyd DA. The epidemiology of social stress. Am Sociol Rev 1995;60:104–25.

[55] Arce M, Michopoulos V, Shepard KN, Ha QC, Wilson ME. Diet choice, cortisol reactivity, and emotional feeding in socially housed rhesus monkeys. Physiol Behav 2010;101:446–55.

[56] Warne JP. Shaping the stress response: interplay of palatable food choices, glucocorticoids, insulin and abdominal obesity. Mol Cell Endocrinol 2009;300(1–2):137–46.

CHAPTER

19

Fructose-Induced Hypertriglyceridemia: A Review

Eric Campbell, Anna Schlappal, Eliana Geller and Thomas W. Castonguay

Department of Nutrition and Food Science, University of Maryland, College Park, MD, USA

INTRODUCTION

Nikkila and Ojala [1] were among the first to report that fructose consumption leads to a dramatic increase in circulating triglycerides. Since that time, fructose-induced hypertriglyceridemia (FIH) has been reported by dozens of investigators [2–4], many of whom have proposed mechanisms to explain how fructose is uniquely and quickly converted from sugar to circulating fat. This chapter attempts to summarize the major factors involved in FIH. However, it is by no means comprehensive, and we apologize if we have inadvertently omitted someone's contribution to the literature. On the other hand, we hope that this introduction to the phenomenon contributes to a deeper understanding of how fructose can be added to the long list of factors promoting obesity, and particularly abdominal obesity.

The obesity epidemic that we are experiencing in the USA is a national concern that affects all Americans. It does not discriminate among age, race, class, or gender. In 1985, the rate of obesity across our country was under 14%, but by 2010 the rate exceeded 30% [5]. Furthermore, obesity is quickly becoming a leading cause of major health problems and death [6]. The research community, along with policy makers and health-care officials are grappling to find the causes of this relatively sudden increase in American's girth. Several researchers have targeted high-fructose corn syrup (HFCS) as a potential factor contributing to the obesity epidemic [7–10]. They and their supporters have pointed out that fructose has become more prevalent in our diets over the past century. In 1900, the average fructose intake was 15 g/day, and fructose was consumed mainly through eating fruits and vegetables, which have the added benefit of fiber [11]. However, as of 2010, fructose consumption had risen to 73 g/day and was being consumed in highly processed forms [11]. One particularly attractive hypothesis linking obesity and fructose consumption is that increased fructose intake can disrupt normal hepatic metabolism, leading to increased hepatic lipogenesis [12]. The purpose of this review is to summarize the evidence supporting this hypothesis while focusing on one manifestation of this disruption, that of FIH.

Fructose and Appetite

It is currently believed that normal hunger and satiety signals operate to alert the body when to initiate or end eating. One of these protein signals, leptin, decreases food intake when in excess and is therefore said to have anorexigenic effects [12,13]. Leptin is produced within adipose cells at levels related to the amount of adipose in the body, and travels to the arcuate nucleus. When excess adipose tissue exists, the excess leptin produced signals the body to stop eating. Another signal, ghrelin, is produced in the absence of food in the stomach and stimulates food intake [14,15]. Ghrelin is said to have orexigenic effects, and travels through the blood system to the hypothalamus to signal hunger [15]. Recently, we have reported that overnight access to sucrose or fructose solutions can dramatically increase liver corticosteroid 11-beta-dehydrogenase isozyme 1 [11β-hydroxysteroiddehydrogenase1(11β-HSD1)], an enzyme linked to omental obesity [16,17]. Further, we have demonstrated that both fructose and sucrose can have significant effects on hypothalamic leptin, ghrelin, and several other factors that help to control appetite [18,19]. We believe that dietary obesity arises when normal hunger and satiety signals are disrupted, causing food intake dysregulation in the form of overeating. While fructose has become a

http://dx.doi.org/10.1016/B978-0-12-407869-7.00019-2

target of many research topics surrounding obesity, it is important to remember that sucrose (i.e. table sugar) is comprised of two molecules, one of glucose and one of fructose. Not surprisingly, sucrose and fructose have been shown to have similar effects on weight gain.

Fructose can increase the palatability of some foods and as a result can cause normal signals for fullness to be ignored, thereby causing increased intake and subsequent weight gain [20,21]. Others have confirmed this effect with other sugars by showing that sugary foods motivate intake despite satiety [22]. Rats fed high-fructose diets had increased body adiposity after 3-6 weeks [23–25]. Furthermore, rats continuously fed fructose develop leptin resistance, which in turn accelerates high-fat-induced obesity [26]. Additionally, diet-induced obesity causes leptin resistance by inhibiting both leptin transport across the blood-brain barrier and central leptin signaling in mice [27]. Thus, the long-term consequences of fructose consumption and weight gain may override normal satiety signals.

Fructose and Reward

In addition to the effect of fructose on satiety signals, sucrose can induce addiction-like behaviors such as bingeing and dependence [28–30]. Hoebel and his associates have shown that underweight rats release more dopamine in the nucleus accumbens during a sucrose binge, indicating a potential mechanism for the induction of addiction-like behaviors by sucrose [31]. Additionally, intermittent sucrose bingeing decreased D2 receptors and μ-opioid receptors in rats; this effect is similar to that seen with morphine, thus indicating a role for sucrose in reward via its dopamine pathway [32]. These data make it clear that sugar (either sucrose or fructose) can have a major impact on reward and possibly addiction, as both phenomena are mediated by dopaminergic pathways. Additionally this research may shed light on how sugary foods override satiety and result in overeating through mechanisms other than direct effects on satiety signals of the hypothalamus.

Fructose and Liver

Sugar also has effects on peripheral metabolic mechanisms that influence intake. For example, fructose may increase lipogenesis in the liver, beginning at the molecular level. Miyazaki [33] reported that sterol regulatory element-binding protein 1 (SREBP-1), an integral part of hepatic lipogenesis, was increased in the livers of rats receiving high-fructose diets. This enzyme is a critical factor that transforms excess energy into triglycerides. Thus, excess SREBP-1 will increase triglyceride formation. Additionally, elevated levels of glucocorticoids have been linked to visceral obesity and metabolic complications [34]. In a recent study, 11β-HSD1 (a regulator of intracellular glucocorticoids) was increased in the livers of rats after 24-h of fructose access [17]. Additionally, sucrose increases 11β-HSD1 in adipose tissue, which is a characteristic of human and animal models of obesity [15]. In a study that assessed the effect of fructose and glucose in humans, overweight and obese subjects consuming 25% of their energy (for 10 weeks) as either glucose- or fructose-sweetened beverages gained weight regardless of the type of sugar used [34]. Interestingly, in subjects consuming fructose the visceral adipose volume was significantly higher than in both control and glucose groups [34]. Rats fed high-fructose diets (for 6 weeks) displayed hypertriglyceridemia and hyperinsulinemia, and became glucose intolerant [35]. Oxysterols receptor LXR beta and alpha (or liver X receptors β and α) are nuclear receptors that help regulate carbohydrate and lipid metabolism, which decrease and increase, respectively, in response to chronic fructose consumption [35]. Taken together, these results indicate a potential connection between liver metabolism dysfunction, fructose, and increased visceral obesity.

All of the data described above show that sugars, and particularly fructose, have the potential to be major contributors in supporting at least part of the obesity epidemic. However, not all authorities agree that sugar consumption is solely responsible for this. For example, the American Heart Association concluded that cardiovascular disease (CVD) and sugar consumption are not linked and that the effect on triglycerides seen with a high-sugar, high-carbohydrate diet can be reduced through exercise. Fried has proposed that long-term, randomized clinical studies are needed to assess whether there is a threshold at which fructose and sucrose content in diets can cause abnormalities in triacylglycerol metabolism.

The work summarized above reviews how sugars enter our diets and our bodies, and how they bypass some of the controls of intake and metabolism. The following section attempts to outline how fructose is metabolized and how it uniquely contributes to adiposity via hypertriglyceridemia.

Fructose Metabolism: An Overview

Before attempting to explain how fructose causes hypertriglyceridemia, a short review of how it is absorbed and metabolized may be of help.

Absorption

Glucose is readily absorbed through the intestinal lumen via the diffusive solute carrier family 2, facilitated glucose transporter member 2 (GLUT-2) protein and an active sodium/glucose cotransporter (SGLT) pump in humans [36–39]. GLUT-2 is found on the basolateral membrane of epithelial cells and functions to transport glucose into circulation [37]. GLUT-2 exhibits a low affinity for fructose and is responsible for only a fraction of the total fructose absorption [37]. In contrast, many investigators reported that intestinal fructose absorption is incomplete in humans [40–42]. Fructose is predominantly taken into the intestinal epithelial cells from the intestinal lumen passively via the GLUT-5 protein transporter in humans [42]. GLUT-5 is also expressed on the basolateral side of intestinal epithelial cells, which allows fructose to exit the epithelial cell and enter into circulation [43]. Some evidence suggests that fructose can exit epithelial cells via GLUT-2 as well as GLUT-5 [44].

The liver can extract 40–70% of dietary fructose in both rats and humans [45–48]. The high efficiency of fructose extraction by the liver is due to the fact that the liver is the main source of GLUT-5 [42]. Anatomically, the liver is the first organ to receive absorbed nutrients via the portal vein; in that way, it contributes to fructose extraction. In contrast, the liver accounts for a smaller percentage of glucose extraction for glycogen restoration [49].

Fructose Metabolism

Fructose metabolism is best understood by considering three enzymes: fructokinase, fructose-bisphosphate aldolase B, and adenosine triphosphate (ATP)-dependent dihydroxyacetone kinase (or triokinase). All three of these are only found in the liver and kidneys of rats and humans. In the liver, fructose is rapidly converted to fructose 1-phosphate via fructokinase. Fructose 1-phosphate is then converted into the trioses dihydroxyacetone phosphate and glyceraldehyde via aldolase B. Aldolase B also functions in the liver for normal glycolysis (glucose metabolism). Glyceraldehyde is then converted to glyceraldehyde-3-phosphate via triokinase. Up until this point in fructose metabolism, there have been no rate-limiting steps and, as a result, there is an increased amount of substrate leading to metabolic pathways from triose phosphate (i.e. glycolysis, glycogenesis, glyconeogenesis, lipogenesis, and fatty acid esterification). Glyceraldehyde-3-phosphate is next metabolized to pyruvate via the rate-limiting enzyme, pyruvate kinase. Fructose enhances the activation of pyruvate kinase and thus leads to an increased flux of pyruvate into the Krebs's cycle. It should be noted that fructose metabolism does not promote an insulin response (Fig. 19.1).

Glucose Metabolism

Glucose typically enters liver cells and is phosphorylated via glucokinase to form glucose-6-phosphate. Glucose-6-phosphate has two fates: conversion to fructose-6-phosphate via phosphoglucoseisomerase; or storage in the form of glycogen. Fructose-6-phosphate is further phosphorylated by phosphofructokinase to produce fructose-1,6-bisphosphate. Phosphofructokinase is the main rate-limiting step in glycolysis. Aldolase, as seen in fructose metabolism, next converts fructose-1,6-bisphosphate into dihydroxyacetone phosphate and glyceraldehyde-3-phosphate. Dihydroxyacetone phosphate lies at the crossroads between glucose and fructose metabolism [12,51]. The metabolic fate of glucose relies heavily on the body's energy needs at the time. The integrated pathways of glucose metabolism include glycogenesis, glycogenolysis, glycolysis, the pentose phosphate pathway, lipogenesis, and the tricarboxylic acid cycle (Fig. 19.2).

Theories on Fructose-Induced Hypertriglyceridemia

A diet high in fructose can produce adverse metabolic changes such as increased plasma triglycerides, hepatic insulin resistance, and hepatic steatosis [52]. These changes usually occur in people consuming large amounts of fructose and under hypercaloric conditions [52]. Tappy has suggested that sugar calories should be limited to 140 kcal/day for men and 100 kcal/day for women [52]. Fructose can alter normal lipid metabolism in the liver by generating unregulated surges of pyruvate. Pyruvate enters the mitochondria via pyruvate dehydrogenase and forms acetyl coenzyme A (acetyl-CoA). Acetyl-CoA acts as a carbon source for three different pathways: the citric acid cycle, lipogenesis, and the formation of ketone bodies. In the lipogenic pathways, acetyl-CoA is shuttled across the mitochondrial membrane as citrate and is restored to acetyl-CoA in the mitochondrial cytosol by ATP citrate lyase. Here, acetyl-CoA acts as a substrate for the production of long-chain fatty acids. Fatty acid synthase is a multienzyme complex that helps facilitate the conversion of acetyl-CoA to long-chain fatty acids. Rats fed 63% fructose for 24-48 h and then fasted developed liver steatosis because fructose is highly lipogenic [53,54].

Most of the information presented above focuses on the potential effects of fructose consumption. We should point out that not only *can* these shifts in metabolism take place, but there is growing evidence that they *are* taking place in the population. For example, the amount of added sugars in the average American diet is currently 477 kcal/day [10]. This contrasts with the recommendation from the World Health Organization that only 10% of the total daily energy intake should come from added sugars [55]. Stanhope and her associates have shown that leptin production drops by 20–30% when subjects consumed fructose-sweetened beverages (30% of caloric intake) compared to glucose-sweetened beverages [56,57]. They hypothesize that the leptin reduction observed during prolonged consumption of diets high in fructose may

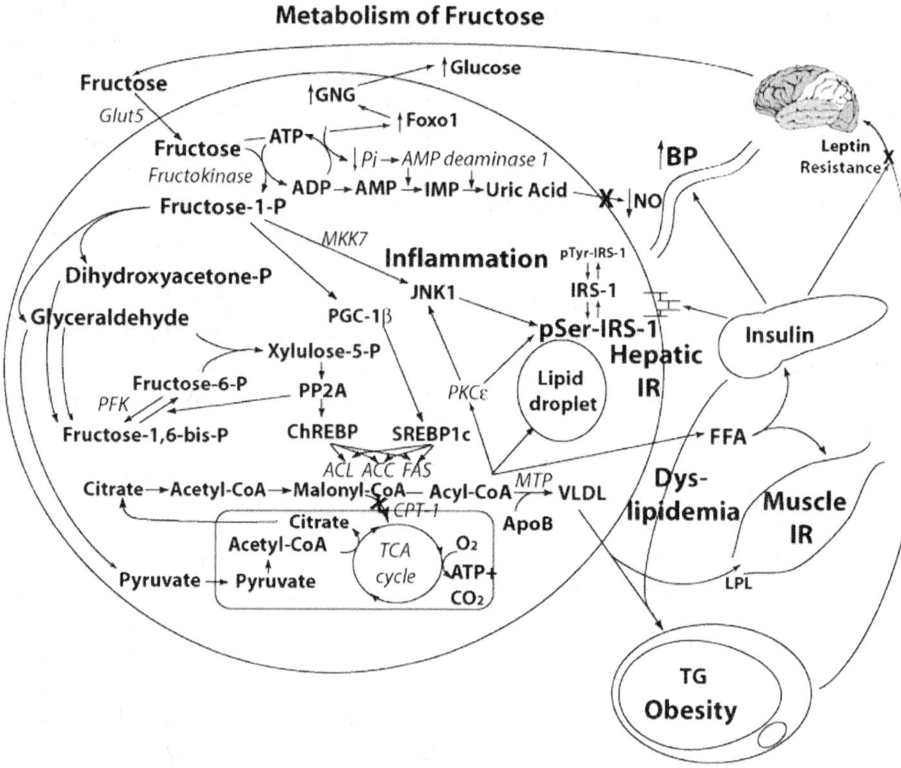

FIGURE 19.1 Hepatic Metabolism of Fructose. Outlined is the metabolism of a 20% fructose load as it passes through the liver. Fructose induces substrate-dependent phosphate depletion, thereby increasing uric acid. Fructose metabolism contributes to hypertension by inhibiting endothelial nitric oxide synthase and reducing nitric oxide (NO). Fructose also contributes to de novo lipogenesis (DNL), dyslipidemia, hepatic lipid droplet formation, and steatosis due to inadequate clearance of lipid produced during fructose metabolism. Fructose also contributes to muscle insulin resistance and activates mitogen-activated protein kinase/c-Jun N-terminal kinase (JNK-1), both of which are linked to hepatic insulin resistance. Hepatic insulin resistance promotes hyperinsulinemia and encourages metabolites to deposit into fat. Fructose increases forkhead box protein O1 (FOXO1), leading to gluconeogenesis and hyperglycemia and central nervous system (CNS) hyperinsulinemia. CNS hyperinsulinemia results in central leptin signaling upregulation and, in that way, stimulates continued energy intake. ACC, acetyl-CoA carboxylase; AMP, adenosine monophosphate; ApoB, apolipoprotein B; ChREBP, carbohydrate response element-binding protein; FFA, free fatty acid; Glut5, solute carrier family 2, facilitated glucose transporter member 5; Glut2, solute carrier family 2, facilitated glucose transporter member 2; Glut4, solute carrier family 2, facilitated glucose transporter member 4; LPL, lipoprotein lipase; PFK, phosphofructokinase; SREBP-1c, sterol regulatory element-binding protein 1c; VLDL, very-low-density lipoprotein. *Source: Adapted from* [50].

lead to increased energy intake and/or decreased energy expenditure and weight gain. In fact, in subjects consuming fructose there is a decrease in energy expenditure and fat oxidation when compared to subjects consuming glucose. In rhesus monkeys, the consumption of fructose over 3- and 6-month periods resulted in significant weight gain and decreased energy expenditure [10]. In a steady state fructose feeding study, postprandial levels of very-low-density lipoprotein (VLDL) triglycerides increased in parallel with total triglycerides, and it is likely that delayed triglyceride clearance also contributes to this rise [10]. Rebollo [55] reported that sucrose-sweetened beverages significantly increase triglyceride deposition in the liver, skeletal muscle, and visceral adipose tissue. Additionally, fructose consumption can increase triglycerides over a 24-h period, as well as the apolipoprotein B (ApoB) concentration [56]. In a study comparing the effects of consuming glucose, fructose, or HFCS (25% energy), triglycerides increased during HFCS and fructose consumption over a 24-h period [57]. Fasting low-density lipoprotein and ApoB concentrations were also increased as a result of fructose and HFCS consumption [57]. In an earlier study assessing the effects of fructose and glucose in humans, Stanhope [34] reported that overweight and obese subjects consuming 25% of their energy over 10weeks as either glucose- or fructose-sweetened beverages gained weight regardless of the type of sugar used. Interestingly, in subjects consuming fructose, the visceral adipose volume was significantly higher than in both control and glucose groups.

Additional Factors Contributing to Fructose-Induced Hypertriglyceridemia

Recently, it has been discovered that hepatic lipogenesis is regulated by several transcription factors, most

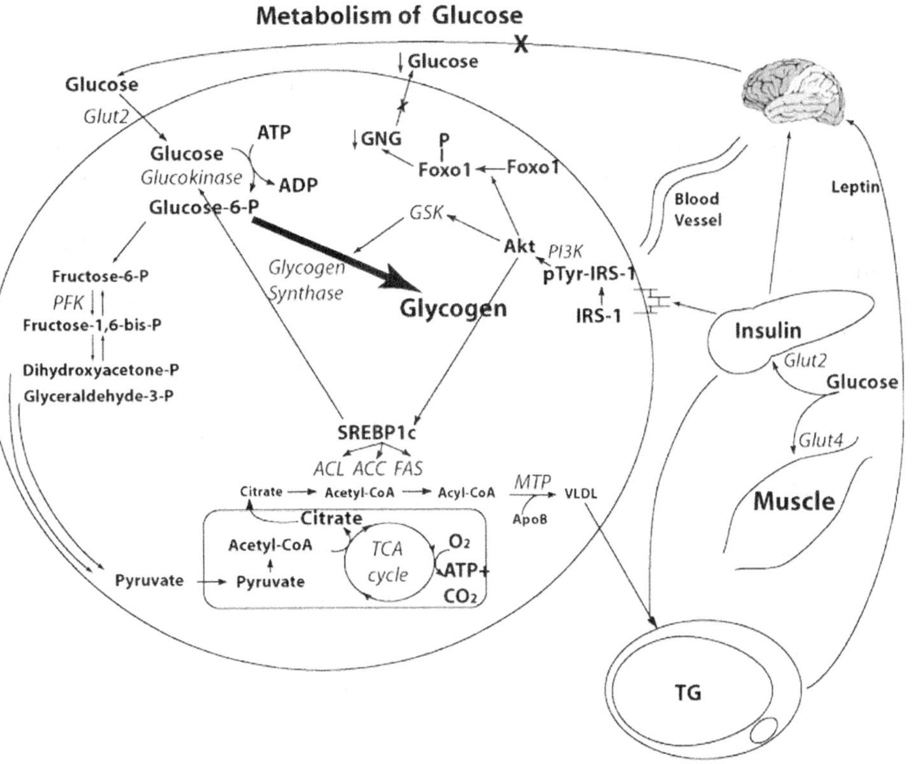

FIGURE 19.2 Hepatic Metabolism of Glucose. Illustrated in the figure is the fate of a 20% glucose load as it is metabolized through the liver. With insulin activation, glycogen synthase is released and most of the glucose being metabolized is turned into glycogen, the storage form of glucose. Insulin activates sterol response element-binding protein 1c (SREBP-1c), which then activates the lipogenic pathway. Insulin activation also results in phosphorylation of the forkhead box protein O1 (FOXO1), keeping FOXO1 from entering the nucleus and thus suppressing activation of the enzymes involved in gluconeogenesis. ADP, adenosine diphosphate; ATP, adenosine triphosphate; TG, triglyceride. *Source: Adapted from* [48].

notably the SREBP-1c and the carbohydrate-responsive element-binding protein (ChREBP) [58,59]. SREBP-1c can induce expression of the fatty acid synthase complex, which leads to increased triglyceride production and secretion [60]. Fructose increases hepatic expression of SREBP-1 and ChREBP family proteins; thus, the lipogenic enzymes responsible for triglyceride synthesis [59,61].

Additional discoveries involving peroxisome proliferator-activated receptors alpha and beta (PPAR-α and PPAR-β) provide additional insights into the regulation of fatty acids in the liver [62]. PPAR-γ coactivator-1-beta (PGC-1β) mediates SREBP-1c regulation of lipogenesis [63]: PGC-1β is a direct coactivator of the transcription factor for SREBP-1c. Interestingly, Nagai showed that PGC-1β knockout protects rats from fructose-induced hyperlipidemia [61].

PPAR-α is a liver transcription factor that enhances fatty acid beta-oxidation. Fructose directly suppresses PPAR-α, which leads to less fatty acid oxidation and thus promotes hypertriglyceridemia. In rats fed 10% fructose solutions, PPAR-α was reduced; these changes were not observed in glucose fed rats [64]. Additionally, fructose reduced levels of hepatic fatty oxidation and increased levels of the proinflammatory transcription factor, nuclear factor-kappa-B (NF-κB) [64]. Many compounds, such as fibrates and some fatty acids, successfully enhance PPAR-α activity and remedy FIH [61].

No list of the factors promoting FIH would be complete without including forkhead box protein O1 (FOXO1), which is involved in carbohydrate and lipid metabolism. FOXO1 is required for the activation of gluconeogenic gene expression in hepatic cells [65]. Fructose can stimulate FOXO1 expression, which favors a gluconeogenic state [66]. Additionally, it has been suggested that FOXO1 increases hepatic expression of a potent lipoprotein lipase (LPL) inhibitor, ApoC-III [67]. ApoC-III is produced in the liver and released into circulation attached to VLDLs [68]. In the presence of insulin, LPL plays a pivotal role in the clearance of plasma triglycerides [69]. Thus, it seems that fructose is a dual threat to plasma triglyceride clearance through its ability to activate ApoC-III and its inability to produce significant insulin release.

Lastly, protein-tyrosine phosphatase 1B (PTP-1B) is a receptor localized on the cytoplasmic side of endoplasmic reticulum. It negatively regulates insulin signaling in vivo [70,71]. Normally, PTP-1B will regulate insulin signaling to match the body's demand. The greatest expression of PTP-1B occurs in the absence of insulin and in insulin-resistant states. Overexpression of PTP-1B leads to the dephosphorylation of insulin receptors and downregulation of insulin signaling molecules [72]. Chronic fructose feeding causes PTP-1B overexpression in hamsters [73] and mice [74]. PTP-1B overexpression shifts hepatic lipid metabolism to favor an increase in lipoprotein secretion by increasing ApoB-100, a substrate required for lipoprotein production [74]. In that way, fructose promotes increased VLDL synthesis and release, and contributes to FIH.

THERAPEUTICS

Recently, some researchers have focused on finding therapeutic drugs to ameliorate FIH. Several exogenous compounds have been tested for their ability to interfere at different steps in the fructose metabolism pathway. Some of these findings are discussed below.

Insulin requires nitric oxide to stimulate glucose uptake. Fructose raises uric acid levels, and uric acid inhibits nitric oxide bioavailability. Allopurinol is a xanthene oxidase inhibitor, and thus interferes with uric acid synthesis. Nakagawa reported that allopurinol effectively reduced uric acid even in combination with a HFCS diet [75]. Additionally, it inhibited hyperinsulinemia, hypertriglyceridemia, and hyperuricemia seen in rats fed only HFCS diets without the drug. These data provide evidence that uric acid may be an important link between fructose consumption and metabolic syndrome development.

Vila reported that atorvastatin can inhibit triglycerides in plasma, and is effective in preventing increased plasma and liver triglyceride accumulation in rats fed a high-fructose diet [76]. Atorvastatin also reduced fatty acid beta-oxidation. It also increased expression of several genes that control fatty acid catabolism, prevented activation of ChREBP transcriptional activity, blunted liver incorporation of fructokinase, and prevented histological damage by fructose-induced liver inflammation. Rasineni [77] showed that *Catharanthus roseus* (a subshrub, also known as Lochnerarosea) can prevent FIH and lower hepatic fructokinase activity. Another therapeutic, *Enicostemma littorale* Blume extract (EL), successfully lowered triglyceride levels by ameliorating glucose tolerance [78]. EL has 3-hydroxy-3-methylglutaryl-coenzyme A reductase (HMG-CoA reductase) activity that allows it to have a hypolipidemic effect, as well as beneficial effects on platelet aggregation and blood coagulation [78].

Finally, an antisense oligonucleotide against ChREBP (ChREBP ASO; a therapeutic aimed at reducing triglycerides) successfully decreased plasma triglyceride concentrations compared with control ASO treatments in rats fed high-fat and high-fructose diets [79]. Additionally, fructose-fed rats treated with ChREBP ASO had increased plasma uric acid, alanine transaminase, and aspartate aminotransferase concentrations due to decreased fructose aldose and fructokinase expression [79].

Fibrates are a class of plasma triglyceride-lowering drugs that are routinely used in clinical practice [80]. The fibrates act as ligands for PPAR-α and induce expression of their associated fatty acid beta-oxidation genes. Additionally, fibrates also act to increase the sensitivity of LPL by reducing expression of the LPL inhibitor, ApoC-III [81]. These three actions by fibrates can lower plasma triglycerides by increasing fatty acid beta-oxidation, by interfering with lipolysis, and by increasing LPL sensitivity, respectively. Several investigators have reported that fibrates can ameliorate FIH in animal models [61,66,82,83].

Thiazolidinediones (TZD) are a class of antidiabetic drugs that target PPAR-γ in adipocytes to improve insulin sensitivity. TZDs can reverse and/or prevent FIH is animal models [84–87].

SUMMARY

Long-term exposure to dietary fructose (as opposed to glucose) results in marked increases in several enzymes that lead to metabolic dysfunction in rats and humans. The increases in gene expression such as those described above, as well as a lack of key regulatory steps in initial fructose metabolism favors de novo lipogenesis (synthesis of triglycerides) in the liver. As a consequence, there is overproduction of VLDL and triglycerides that are released into circulation, leading to hypertriglyceridemia [10,55,56]. In contrast, glucose does not increase gene expression that facilitates de novo lipogenesis, and thus spares a massive unregulated surge of metabolites favoring lipid production. One of the questions for future research deals with the safety of the USA's continued use of fructose as a principal sweetening agent in our food supply. As attributed to Paracelsus "The dose makes the poison." Is there a safe level of exposure? If so, how does it vary across the life span? Also, there are financial implications to altering a major component of the country's diet that need to be factored into making such a decision. We look forward to several years of scientific debate.

The review of fructose intake and metabolism presented above is intended to facilitate a thorough examination of FIH. Presented below is a list of the work that has been reviewed. The reference list is by no means exhaustive, but is offered to the reader as an initial guide into an important body of literature as we continue to

TABLE 19.1 Relevant References Sorted by Principle Contribution

Topic	References
Obesity epidemic	BRFSS CDC; Cawley and Meherhoefer 2012; Stanhope 2012; Rebollo 2012
Food intake	Havel 2005; Farooqi 2005; Wren 200; Wren 2001
Fructose and food intake	Pelchat 2002; Erlanson-Albertsson 2005; Zheng 2009
Fructose and obesity	Glickman 2012; Bocarsly 2010; Malik and Hu 2012; Stanhope 2012; Vos 2008; London and Castonguay 2007; London 2011; Colley 2011; Colley and Castonguay 2013; Rizkalla 1990, 1992, and 1993; Shapiro 2008; El-Haschimi 2000; Stanhope 2009; Tappy 2010; Stanhope 2012; Rebollo 2012
Fructose digestion	Ravich 1983; Kneepkens 1984; Truswell 1988; Burant 1992; Angelpoulos 2009; Lanaspa 2012
Hepatic metabolism	Lin 2005; Braissant 1996; Motsumoto 2006; Kellet 2005; Elchelby 1999; Haj 2002; Qiu 2004
Fructose hepatic metabolism	Havel 2005; Miyazaki 2004; London 2010; London 2007; Kruse 2012; Topping1976; Mendeloff 1953; Topping 2008; Burant 1992; Tappy 2010; Castro 2013; Rebollo 2012; Stanhope 2011; Lanaspa 2012; Nagai 2009; Lizuka 2004; Roglans 2007; Qu 2007; Altomonte 2004; Taghibiglou 2002; Qiu 2004; Faeh 2007
Glucose metabolism	Groen 1937; Kellet 2000, 2005; Semenza 1984; Kruse 2012
Glucose hepatic metabolism	Radziuk 1978; Blakemore 1995
Fructose and triglycerides	Rebollo 2012; Stanhope 2011; Tappy 2010; Moon 2001; Nagai 2009; Lizuka 2004; Eckel 1989; Storlien 1993; Stanhope 2012
Dopamine pathway	Spangler 2004
Therapeutic interventions	Nakagawa 2006; Lee 1994; Collino 2010; Saltiel 1996
Sugar addiction	Avena 2006; Avean 2008; Colanutoni 2002; Grim 2005; Wideman 2005

grapple with developing a thorough assessment of the effects of our use of sugars in our diets. These summaries are divided into three types of FIH papers: reviews (like this one); papers that focus on some component of the pathway (from fructose intake to circulating triglycerides); and papers that focus on assessing the efficacy of exogenous compounds that suppress circulating triglycerides. We have organized the references into a table (Table 19.1), which groups references cited within this review based on the major topic to which it contributes.

Acknowledgments

This work was supported in part by grants from the Maryland Agricultural Experiment Station, the Vice President for Research at the University of Maryland, and the USDA Cooperative Agreement 58-1235-2-112 to TWC.

References

[1] Nikkilä EA, Ojala K. Acute effects of fructose and glucose on the concentration and removal rate of plasma triglyceride. Life Sci 1966;5:89–94.

[2] Storlein LH, Oakes ND, Pan DA, Kusunoki M, Jenkins AB. Syndromes of insulin resistance in the rat. Inducement by diet and amelioration with benfluorex. Diabetes 1993;42:457–62.

[3] Kanarek RB, Orthen-Gambill N. Differential effects of sucrose, fructose, and glucose on carbohydrate-induced obesity in rats. J Nutr 1982;112:1546–54.

[4] Bar-On H, Stein Y. Effect of glucose and fructose administrations on lipid metabolism in the rat. J Nutr 1967;94:95–105.

[5] State Obesity Prevalence. CDC, Published May 2011, <http://www.cdc.gov/obesity/data/adult.html>; 2013 [accessed 22.05.13].

[6] Cawley John, Meyerhoefer Chad. The medical care costs of obesity: an instrumental variables approach. J Health Econ 2012;31:219–30.

[7] Institute of Medicine (US). Committee on Accelerating Progress in Obesity Prevention,Glickman D. Accelerating Progress in Obesity Prevention: Solving the Weight of the Nation. National Academies Press; 2012.

[8] Bocarsly ME, Powell ES, Avena NM, Hoebel BG. High-fructose corn syrup causes characteristics of obesity in rats: increased body weight, body fat and triglyceride levels. Pharmacol Biochem Behavior 2010;97:101–6.

[9] Malik VS, Hu FB. Sweeteners and risk of obesity and type 2 diabetes: the role of sugar-sweetened beverages. Curr Diab Rep 2012;12:195–203.

[10] Stanhope KL. Role of fructose-containing sugars in the epidemics of obesity and metabolic syndrome. Annu Rev Med 2012;63: 329–43.

[11] Vos MB, Kimmons JE, Gillespie C, Welsh J, Blanck HM. Dietary fructose consumption among US children and adults: the Third National Health and Nutrition Examination Survey. The Medscape Journal of Medicine 2008;10:160.

[12] Havel PJ. Dietary fructose: implications for dysregulation of energy homeostasis and lipid/carbohydrate metabolism. Nutr Rev 2005;63:133–57.

[13] Farooqi IS, Bullmore E, Keogh J, Gillard J, O'Rahilly S, Fletcher PC. Leptin regulates striatal regions and human eating behavior. Science 2007;317:1355.

[14] Wren AM, Small CJ, Ward HL, Murphy KG, Dakin CL, Taheri S, et al. The novel hypothalamic peptide ghrelin stimulates food intake and growth hormone secretion. Endocrinology 2000;141:4325–8.

[15] Wren AM, Small CJ, Abbott CR, Dhillo WS, Seal LJ, Cohen MA, et al. Ghrelin causes hyperphagia and obesity in rats. Diabetes 2001;50:2540–7.

[16] London E, Lala G, Berger R, Panzenbeck A, Kohli AA, Renner M, et al. Sucrose access differentially modifies 11-hydroxysteroid dehydrogenase-1 and hexose-6-phosphate dehydrogenase message in liver and adipose tissue in rats. J Nutr 2007;137:2616–21.

[17] London E, Castonguay T. High fructose diets increase 11β-hydroxysteroid dehydrogenase type 1 in liver and visceral adipose in rats within 24-h exposure. Obesity 2010;19:925–32.

[18] Colley D, London E, Jiang B, Khural J, Castonguay TW. Fructose and the control of food intake. In: Johnston BM, Collins AB, editors. Fructose and the synthesis, functions and health implications. Hauppage, NY: Nova Science Publishers; 2012. p. 129–43.

[19] Colley D, Castonguay TW. The effects of sugar solutions on hypothalamuc appetite regulation. J Nutr 2013. (submitted)

[20] Pelchant ML. Of human bondage: food craving, obsession, compulsion, and addiction. Physiol Behav 2002;76:347–52.

[21] Erlanson-Albertson C. How palatable food disrupts appetite regulation. Basic Clin Pharmacol Toxicol 2004;97:61–73.

[22] Zheng H, Shin AC, Lenard NR, Townsend RL, Patterson LM, Sigalet DL, et al. Meal patterns, satiety, and food choice in a rat model of Roux-en-Y gastric bypass surgery. American Journal of Physiology-Regulatory, Integrative and Comparative Physiology 2009;297:R1273–82.

[23] Rizkalla SR, Hellal I, Boillot J. Comparative metabolic effects of 10 week starch, glucose, fructose in normal rats. Insulin Cell Memb 1990:443–50.

[24] Rizkalla SW et al. Comparative effects of 6 week fructose, dextrose and starch feeding on fat-cell lipolysis in normal rats: effects of isoproterenol, theophylline and insulin. Mol Cell Biochem 1992;109:127–32.

[25] Rizkalla SW, Boillot J, Tricottet V, Fontvieille AM, Luo J, Salzman JL, et al. Effects of chronic dietary fructose with and without copper supplementation on glycaemic control, adiposity, insulin binding to adipocytes and glomerular basement membrane thickness in normal rats. British Journal of Nutrition 1993;70:199–209.

[26] Shapiro A, Mu W, Roncol C, Cheng K, Johnson RJ, Scarpace PJ. Fructose-induced leptin resistance exacerbates weight gain in response to subsequent high-fat feeding. Am J Physiol Regul Integr Comp Physiol 2008;295:R1370–5.

[27] El-Haschimi K, Pierroz DD, Hileman SM, Bjorbaek C, Flier JS. Two defects contribute to hypothalamic leptin resistance in mice with diet-induced obesity. J Clin Invest 2000;105:1827–32.

[28] Avena Nicole M. Examining the addictive-like properties of binge eating using an animal model of sugar dependence. Exp Clin Psychopharmacol 2007;15:481–91.

[29] Grimm Jeffrey W, Fyall Amber M, Osincup Dan P. Incubation of sucrose craving: effects of reduced training and sucrose pre-loading. Physiol Behav 2005;84:73–9.

[30] Wideman CH, Nadzam GR, Murphy HM. Implications of an animal model of sugar addiction, withdrawal and relapse for human health. Nutr Neurosci 2005;8:5–6.

[31] Avena NM, Rada P, Hoebel BG. Underweight rats have enhanced dopamine release and blunted acetylcholine response in the nucleus accumbens while bingeing on sucrose. Neuroscience 2008;156:865–71.

[32] Spangler R, Wittkowski KM, Goddard NL, Avena NM, Hoebel BG, Leibowitz SF. Opiate-like effects of sugar on gene expression in reward areas of the rat brain. Brain Res Mol Brain Res 2004;124:134–42.

[33] Miyazaki M, Dobrzyn A, Man WC, Chu K, Sampath H, Kim HJ, et al. Stearoyl-CoA desaturase 1 gene expression is necessary for fructose-mediated introduction of lipogenic gene expression by sterol regulatory element-binding protein-1c-dependent and – independent mechanisms. J Biol Chem 2004;279:25164–71.

[34] Björntorp P. The regulation of adipose tissue distribution in humans. Int J Obes Relat Metab Disord 1996;20:291–302.

[35] Stanhope KL, Schwarz JM, Keim NL, Griffen SC, Bremer AA, Graham JL, et al. Consuming fructose-sweetened, not glucose-sweetened, beverages increases visceral adiposity and lipids and decreases insulin sensitivity in overweight/obese humans. J Clin Invest 2009;119:1322–34.

[36] Kruse MS, Rey M, Vega MC, Coirini H. Alterations of LXRα and LXRβ expression in the hypothalamus of glucose-intolerant rats. J Endocrinol 2012;215:51–8.

[37] Rasineni K, Bellamkonda R, Singareddy SR, Desireddy S. Abnormalities in carbohydrates and lipid metabolism in high-fructose dietfed insulin-resistant rats: amelioration by Catharanthusroseus treatments. J Physiol Biochem 2013;69: 459–66.

[38] Kellett GL, Helliwell PA. The diffusive component of intestinal glucose absorption is mediated by the glucose-induced recruitment of GLUT2 to the brush-border membrane. Biochem J 2000;350:155.

[39] Semenza G, Kessler M, Hosang M, Weber J, Schmidt U. Biochemistry of the Na+, D-glucose cotransporter of the small-intestinal brush-border membrane. The state of the art in 1984. Biochim Biophys Acta 1984;779:343.

[40] Ravich WJ, Bayless TM, Thomas M. Fructose: incomplete intestinal absorption in humans. Gastroenterology 1983;84:26.

[41] Kneepkens CM, Vonk RJ, Fernandes J. Incomplete intestinal absorption of fructose. Arch Dis Child 1984;59:735–8.

[42] Truswell AS, Seach JM, Thorburn AW. Incomplete absorption of pure fructose in healthy subjects and the facilitating effect of glucose. Am J Clin Nutr 1988;48:1424–30.

[43] Burant CF, Takeda J, Brot-Laroche E, Bell GI, Davidson NO. Fructose transporter in human spermatozoa and small intestine is GLUT5. J Biol Chem 1992;267:14523–6.

[44] Blakemore SJ, Aledo JC, James J, Campbell FC, Lucocq JM, Hunda HS. The GLUT5 hexose transporter is also localized to the basolateral membrane of the human jejunum. Biochem J 1995;309:7.

[45] Kellett GL, Brot-Laroche E. Apical GLUT2 a major pathway of intestinal sugar absorption. Diabetes 2005;54:3056–62.

[46] Topping DL, Mayes PA. Comparative effects of fructose and glucose on the lipid and carbohydrate metabolism of perfused rat liver. Br J Nutr 1976;36:113–26.

[47] Topping DL, Mayes PA. The concentrations of fructose, glucose and lactate in the splanchnic blood vessels of rats absorbing fructose. Nutr Metab 2008;13:331–8.

[48] Mendeloff AI, Weichselbaum TE. Role of the human liver in the assimilation of intravenously administered fructose. Metabolism 1953;2:450.

[49] Radziuk J, McDonald TJ, Rubenstein D, Dupre J. Initial splanchnic extraction of ingested glucose in normal man. Metabolism 1978;27:657–69.

[50] Lustig Robert H. Fructose: metabolic, hedonic, and societal parallels with ethanol. J Am Diet Assoc 2010;110:1307–21.

[51] Mayes PA. Intermediary metabolism of fructose. Am J Clin Nutr 1993;58:754S–65S.

[52] Tappy L, Le KA, Tran C, Paquot N. Fructose and metabolic diseases: new findings, new questions. Nutrition 2010;26:1044–9.

[53] Castro GSF, Cardoso JFR, Vannucchi H, Zucoloto S, Jordao AA. Fructose and NAFLD: metabolic implications and models of induction in rats. Acta Cir Bras 2011;26:45–50.

[54] Castro MC, Massa ML, Schinella G, Gagliardino JJ, Francini F. Lipoic acid prevents liver metabolic changes induced by administration of a fructose-rich diet. Biochim Biophys Acta 2013;1830: 2226–32.

[55] Rebollo A, Roglans N, Alegret M, Laguna JC. Way back for fructose and liver metabolism: bench side to molecular insights. World J Gastroenterol 2012;7:6552–9.

[56] Teff KL, Elliott SS, Tschop M, Kieffer TJ, Rader D, Heiman M, et al. Dietary fructose reduces circulating insulin and leptin, attenuates postprandial suppression of ghrelin, and increases triglycerides in women. J Clin Endocrin Metab 2004;89:2963–72.

[57] Teff KL, Grudziak J, Townsend RR, Dunn TN, Grant RW, Adams SH, et al. Endocrine and metabolic effects of consuming fructose- and glucose-sweetened beverages with meals in obese men and women: influence of insulin resistance on plasma triglyceride responses. J Clin Endocrinol Metab 2009;94:1562–9.

[58] Horton JD, Goldstein JL, Brown MS. SREBPs: activators of the complete program of cholesterol and fatty acid synthesis in the liver. J Clin Invest 2002;109:1125–31.

[59] Lizuka K, Bruick RK, Liang G, et al. Deficiency of carbohydrate response element-binding protein (ChREBP) reduces lipogenesis as well as glycolysis. Proc Natl Acad Sci USA 2004;101:7281–6.

[60] Moon YA, Shah NA, Mohapatra S, Warrington JA, Horton JD. Identification of a mammalian long chain fatty acyl elongase regulated by sterol regulatory element-binding proteins. J Biol Chem 2001;276:45358–66.

[61] Nagai Y, Nishio Y, Nakamura T, Maegawa H, Kikkawa R, Kashiwagi A. Amelioration of high fructose-induced metabolic derangements by activation of PPARα. Am J Physiol Endocrinol Metab 2002;282:E1180–90.

[62] Braissant O, Foufelle F, Scotto C, Dauca M, Wahli W. Differential expression of peroxisome proliferator-activated receptors (PPARs): tissue distribution of PPAR-alpha, -beta, and -gamma in the adult rat. Endocrinology 1996;137:354–66.

[63] Lin J, Yang R, Tarr PT, Wu PH, Handschin C, Li S, et al. Hyperlipidemic effects of dietary saturated fats mediated through PGC-1β coactivation of SREBP. Cell 2005;120:261–73.

[64] Roglans N, Vila L, Farre M, Alegret M, Sanchez RM, Vazquez-Carrerra M, et al. Impairment of hepatic Stat-3 activation and reduction of PPARalpha activity in fructose fed rats. Hepatology 2007;45:778–88.

[65] Matsumoto M, Han S, Kitamura T, Accili D. Dual role of transcription factor Fox01 in controlling hepatic insulin sensitivity and lipid metabolism. J Clin Invest 2006;116:2464–72.

[66] Qu S, Su D, Altomonte J, Kamagate A, He J, Perdomo G, et al. PPARα mediates the hypolipidemic action of fibrates by antagonizing Fox01. Am J Physiol Endocrinol Metab 2007;292: E421–34.

[67] Altomonte J, Cong L, Harbaran S, Richter A, Xu J, Meseck M, Dong HH. Fox01 mediates insulin action on apoC-III and triglyceride metabolism. J Clin Invest 2004;114:1493–503.

[68] Jong MC, Hofker MH, Havekes LM. Role of ApoCs in lipoprotein metabolism functional differences between ApoC1, apoC2, and ApoC3. Arterioscler Thromb Vasc Biol 1999;19:472–84.

[69] Eckel RH. Lipoprotein lipase. a multifunctional enzyme relevant to common metabolic diseases. N Engl J Med 1989;320:1060.

[70] Elchebly M, Payette P, Michaliszyn E, Cromlish . Increased insulin sensitivity and obesity resistance in mice lacking the protein tyrosine phosphatase-1B gene. Science 1999;283:1544–8.

[71] Haj FG, Verveer PJ, Squire A, Neel BG, Bastiaens PI. Imaging sites of receptor dephosphorylation by PTP1B on the surface of the endoplasmic reticulum. Sci Signal 2002;295:1708.

[72] Cheng A, Dube N, Gu F. Coordinated action of protein tyrosine phosphatases in insulin signal transduction. FEBS J 2002;262:1050–9.

[73] Taghibiglou C, Rashid-Kolvear F, Van Iderstine SC, et al. Hepatic very low density lipoprotein-ApoB overproduction is associated with attenuated hepatic insulin signaling and overexpression of protein-tyrosine phosphatase 1B in a fructose-fed hamster model of insulin resistance. J Biol Chem 2002;277:793–803.

[74] Qiu W, Avramoglu RK, Dubé N, Chong TM, Naples M, Au C, et al. Hepatic PTP-1B Expression Regulates the Assembly and Secretion of Apolipoprotein B-Containing Lipoproteins Evidence From Protein Tyrosine Phosphatase-1B Overexpression, knock-out, and RNAiStudies. Diabetes 2004;53:3057–66.

[75] Nakagawa T, Hu H, Zharikov S, Tuttle KR, Short RA, Glushakova O, et al. A casual role for uric acid in fructose-induced metabolic syndrome. Am J Phyisol Renal Physiol 2006;290:F625–31.

[76] Vila L, Rebollo A, Adalsteisson GS, Alegret M, Merlos M, Roglans N, et al. Reduction of liver fructokinase expression and improved hepatic inflammation and metabolism in liquid fructose-fed rats after atorvastatin treatment. Toxicol Appl Pharmacol 2011;15: 32–40.

[77] Rasineni K, Bellamkonda R, Singareddy SR, Desireddy S. Abnormalities in carbohydrates and lipid metabolism in high-fructose dietfed insulin-resistant rats: amelioration by Catharanthus-roseus treatments. J Physiol Biochem 2013;69:459–66.

[78] Bhatt NM, Chavda M, Desai D, Zalawadia R, Patel VB, Burade V, et al. Cardioprotective and antihypertensive effects of EnicostemmalittoraleBlume extract in fructose-fed rats. Can J Physiol Pharmacol 2012;90:1065–73.

[79] Erion DM, Popov V, Hsiao . The role of the carbohydrate response element-binding protein in male fructose-fed rats. Endocrinology 2013;154:36–44.

[80] Staels B, Schoonjans K, Fruchart JC, Auwerx J. The effects of fibrates and thiazolidinesdiones on plasma triglyceride metabolism are mediated by distinct peroxisome proliferator activated receptors (PPARs). Biochimie 1997;79:95–9.

[81] Malmendier CL, Lontie JF, Delcroix C, Dubois DY, Magot T, De Roy L. Apolipoproteins C-II and C-III metabolism in hypertriglyceridemic patients Effect of a drastic triglyceride reduction by combined diet restriction and fenofibrate administration. Atherosclerosis 1989;77:139–49.

[82] Ackerman Z, Oron-Herman M, Rosenthal T, Pappo O, Link G, Sela BA, Grozovski M. Effects of amlodipine, captopril, and bezafibrate on oxidative milieu in rats with fatty liver. Dig Dis Sci 2008;53:777–84.

[83] Bastow MD, Durrington PN, Ishola M. Hypertriglyceridemia and hyperuricemia: effects of two fibric acid derivatives (bezafibrate and fenofibrate) in a double-blind, placebo-controlled trial. Metabolism 1988;37:217–20.

[84] Sharabi Y, Oron-Herman M, Kamari Y, Avni I, Peleg E, Shabtay Z, et al. P-543: Effect of PPAR-γ agonist-rosiglitazone-on adiponectin level in the metabolic syndrome. Am J Hypertens 2005;18: 204A.

[85] Collino M, Aragno M, Castiglia S, Miglio G, Tomasinelli C, Boccuzzi G, et al. Pioglitazone improves lipid and insulin levels in overweight rats on a high cholesterol and fructose diet by decreasing hepatic inflammation. Br J Pharmacol 2010;160:1892–902.

[86] Saltiel AR, Olefsky JM. Thiazolidinediones in the treatment of insulin resistance and type II diabetes. Diabetes 1996;45:1661–9.

[87] Lee MK, Miles PD, Khoursheed M, Gao KM, Moossa AR, Olefsky JM, et al. Metabolic effects of troglitazone on fructose-induced insulin resistance in the rat. Diabetes 1994;43:1435–9.

CHAPTER

20

Impact of Sex and Lifestyle of Adolescents and Their Parents on Obesity

Masao Yoshinaga[a], *Ayumi Miyazaki*[b], *Masaki Shinomiya*[c], *Machiko Aoki*[d], *Takashi Hamajima*[e], *and Masami Nagashima*[f]

[a]Department of Pediatrics, National Hospital Organization Kagoshima Medical Center, Kagoshima, Japan; [b]Department of Pediatrics, Japan Community Health Care Organization Takaoka-Fushiki Hospital, Takaoka, Toyama, Japan; [c]Department of Internal Medicine, Nishifuna Naika, Funabashi, Chiba, Japan; [d]Department of Pediatrics, Aoki Clinic of Internal Medicine, Cardiovascular Medicine & Pediatrics, Fukuoka, Japan; [e]Department of Endocrinology and Metabolism, Aichi Children's Health and Medical Center, Motiokamachi, Obu, Aichi, Japan; [f]Department of Rehabilitation, Aichi Saiseikai Rehabilitation Hospital, Nishi-ku, Nagoya, Japan

INTRODUCTION

The prevalence of overweight or obese children has increased since the late twentieth century in most industrialized countries [1]. This prevalence doubled or trebled between the early 1970s and late 1990s in Australia, Brazil, Canada, Chile, Finland, France, Greece, Japan, the UK, and the USA [2]. However, recent data have shown that this increase in childhood obesity might be declining [1].

Cross-sectional analysis has shown that the prevalence of obesity has gradually decreased since the early 2000s, with the highest prevalence in the late 1990s to early 2000s in Japan [3]. Longitudinal studies have shown that the critical periods for developing obesity are in late infancy (between 5 and 6 years of age) and during the high school period in boys, and is mainly in late infancy in girls [3]. Another issue to be solved in Japan is the rapid increase in severe obesity in senior high school adolescents [4].

The development of cardiovascular disease (CVD) risk factors, including obesity, is associated with adverse behavioral patterns, such as decreased physical activity [5,6,8,9]; increased sedentary lifestyle, in particular television watching [5–10]; and unhealthy dietary habits [5,6,9]. Parental obesity is also strongly associated with CVD risk factors in children and adolescents [5,6,9].

Therefore, the present chapter aims to evaluate the effect of lifestyles of adolescents and their parents on the levels of CVD risk factors in adolescents based on data obtained from adolescent volunteers.

METHODS

Subjects

Two studies have been conducted in Japan. The first study was conducted from 2006 to 2008 and was announced through the local boards of education in three areas: Toyama, Chiba, and Kagoshima prefectures. The background of the first study has been described in detail elsewhere [9]. The study included 1358 healthy adolescent volunteers (587 males and 771 females), comprising senior high school students aged 15 to 18 years. All of the subjects gave written informed consent. The study consisted of a medical examination and a questionnaire. Volunteers were asked to complete the questionnaires before their medical examination. The questionnaire collected data on the lifestyles of both the subjects and their parents. Of the 1358 subjects, 54 participated in the study twice, and only data from the first visit were used. Of the remaining 1304 subjects, 549 did not complete the questionnaire and were excluded. Therefore, a total of 755 volunteers were included in the study (331 males and

Nutrition in the Prevention and Treatment of Abdominal Obesity
http://dx.doi.org/10.1016/B978-0-12-407869-7.00020-9

424 females). Subjects of both sexes included in the study had lower mean levels of several CVD risk factors than those who were excluded (data not shown), suggesting that adolescent volunteers with more healthy lifestyles were more likely to completely answer the questionnaire. We obtained permission from the ethics committee of the National Hospital Organization Kagoshima Medical Center to use and analyze the data under the condition that the confidentiality would be maintained for all subjects.

The second study was conducted from 2012 onwards. The subjects in this study were children and adolescents in kindergartens, elementary schools, and junior high schools in Japan. This ongoing study was conducted in Kagoshima, Toyama, Fukuoka, and Aichi areas, and a total of 954 children and adolescents participated during 2012. Of these, 200 adolescents aged 12–15 years in junior high schools were the final subjects of the study. All subjects in the second study also gave written informed consent. The second study was done using the same methods as the first study. Volunteers were asked to complete questionnaires before their medical examination. All subjects in the second study completed the questionnaires.

Physical and Blood Biochemistry Parameters

Height was measured to the nearest 0.1 cm and weight was measured to the nearest 0.1 kg. Body mass index (BMI) was calculated as (weight in kg)/(height in m)^2. Blood pressure was measured three times using a TM-2571 automated oscillatory system (A&D Co. Ltd, Tokyo, Japan) after subjects had rested for 10 min in a seated position, and the mean value of the second and third measurements was used. Waist circumference was measured at the umbilical level to the nearest 0.1 cm.

Blood samples were collected the morning after an overnight fast. Levels of high-density lipoprotein (HDL) cholesterol were determined using a direct quantitative assay. Triglyceride and fasting plasma glucose (FPG) levels were measured using enzymatic assays and analyzed using a JCA-BM9030 automated analyzer (JEOL Ltd, Tokyo, Japan). Insulin levels were measured using a chemiluminescence immunologic assay and an automated Lumipulse PrestoII analyzer (Fujirebio Inc., Tokyo, Japan). All assays were performed by SRL Inc, Tokyo, Japan). The homeostasis model assessment of insulin resistance (HOMA-IR) was used as a surrogate marker for insulin resistance [11], and calculated as fasting insulin (in μU/mL) × fasting glucose (in mg/dL)/405.

Levels of adiponectin, leptin, and high-sensitivity C-reactive protein (hs-CRP) were measured at the same laboratory (SRL Inc). These adipocytokines and/or inflammatory markers are hereafter collectively referred to as biomarkers. Adiponectin was measured using the Human Adiponectin ELISA kit (Otsuka Pharmaceutical Inc, Tokyo, Japan), leptin measurement was done using the Human Leptin RIA KIT (Linco Research Inc, St. Charles, MO, USA), and hs-CRP was measured using the N-Latex CRP II (Dade Behring Inc, Marburg, Germany).

Definition of Cardiovascular Disease Risk Factors, Metabolic Syndrome, and Obesity

Abdominal obesity, hypertension, elevated triglyceride levels, decreased HDL cholesterol levels, and hyperglycemia were used as CVD risk factors in the present study. The definition of CVD risk factors was based on that of the International Diabetes Federation for the ages of 10–16 years as follows [12]: triglycerides, ≥150 mg/dL; HDL cholesterol, <40 mg/dL; blood pressure, ≥130 mmHg systolic or ≥85 mmHg diastolic; and FPG, ≥100 mg/dL. Preliminary 90th percentile values in male and female junior high school adolescents for waist circumference were ≥80 cm and ≥75 cm, respectively, based on data from the participants of the present study. The definition of CVD risk factors for ages >16 years was based on that for adults as follows [13]: triglycerides, ≥150 mg/dL; HDL cholesterol, <40 mg/dL in males and <50 mg/dL in females; blood pressure, ≥130 mmHg systolic or ≥85 mmHg diastolic; and FPG, ≥100 mg/dL. Preliminary 90th percentile values in male and female high school adolescents for waist circumference were ≥80 cm based on data from the participants of the present study. The definition of metabolic syndrome was based on that of the International Diabetes Federation [12,13].

The Examination Committee of Criteria for Obesity Disease in Japan recommended a BMI ≥25 kg/m^2 as the definition of obesity in the adult Japanese population [14]. Therefore, adolescent obesity in the present study was defined using the age- and sex-specific International Obesity Task Force standard corresponding to a BMI cutoff of 25 kg/m^2 at the age of 18 years [15].

Assessment of the Lifestyles of Adolescents and Their Parents

Self-reported lifestyle parameters for all subjects included regular times of going to bed and waking up; participation in school-based extracurricular (EC) physical activities; time spent in exercise, including walking, jogging, cycling, and EC physical activities on weekdays and holidays; time spent watching a screen, including watching television, non-school-related computer use, and games on weekdays and holidays; and score for eating breakfast (1, seldom; 2, occasional; 3, regular). Age, height, weight, and the following lifestyle information for both parents were also recorded: regular times for going to bed and waking up; time spent taking exercise,

TABLE 20.1 Characteristics of Adolescents[a,b]

Characteristic	Junior High School Adolescents			Senior High School Adolescents		
	Males	Females	*P* value	Males	Females	*P* value
Number	99	101	–	337	442	–
Age (years)	14.0 (0.9)	14.0 (1.0)	0.88	16.5 (0.8)***	16.7 (0.9)***	0.01
Height (cm)	162.5 (8.4)	155.7 (5.5)	<0.001	170.5 (6.1)***	158.3 (5.3)***	<0.001
Weight (kg)	50.9 (10.7)	47.4 (6.7)	0.006	60.8 (10.3)***	51.1 (6.5)***	<0.001
Body mass index (kg/m^2)	19.1 (2.8)	19.5 (2.4)	0.32	20.9 (3.1)***	20.4 (2.3)***	0.01
Waist circumference (cm)	68.0 (8.1)	68.1 (6.5)	0.89	72.3 (8.2)***	71.2 (5.9)***	0.03
Systolic BP (mmHg)	106 (9)	100 (9)	<0.001	116 (10)***	106 (10)***	<0.001
Diastolic BP (mmHg)	58 (8)	56 (7)	0.02	63 (9)***	62 (9)***	0.02
Total cholesterol (mg/dL)	161 (23)	170 (30)	0.03	161 (28)	174 (27)	<0.001
LDL cholesterol (mg/dL)	89 (20)	97 (26)	0.02	89 (24)	96 (23)	<0.001
HDL cholesterol (mg/dL)	61 (12)	61 (11)	0.95	59 (12)	65 (13)**	<0.001
Triglycerides (mg/dL)	54 (39, 79)	63 (46, 84)	0.13	53 (41, 74)	52 (39, 69)***	0.23
FPG (mg/dL)	87 (6)	85 (5)	0.004	88 (7)	86 (6)	<0.001
Insulin (μU/mL)	7.2 (5.3, 10.7)	87 (5.7, 11.2)	0.07	6.4 (4.3, 9.1)*	7.0 (5.1, 9.5)**	0.07
HOMA-IR	1.6 (1.1, 2.3)	1.8 (1.2, 2.5)	0.16	1.4 (0.9, 2.0)	1.5 (1.1, 2.1)**	0.26
No of CV risks	0.2 (0.4)	0.2 (0.4)	0.65	0.7 (0.9)**	0.6 (0.8)	0.11
Adiponectin (μg/mL)	10.0 (4.1)	9.9 (4.6)	0.89	10.5 (4.0)	12.0 (4.6)***	<0.001
Leptin (ng/mL)	2.3 (1.8, 4.3)	7.9 (5.7, 12.8)	<0.001	1.1 (0.8, 2.2)***	6.2 (4.2, 8.6)***	<0.001
Hs-CRP (ng/mL)	82 (52, 177)	69 (25, 147)	0.053	111 (152, 268)*	58 (50, 137)*	<0.001
Birth weight (g)	3036 (533)	3014 (401)	0.74	3154 (425)*	3053 (407)	<0.001
Breast feeding (mo)	10.3 (4.3)	8.3 (4.9)	–	7.3 (5.5)***	7.8 (5.2)	0.29
Lifestyle factor						
EC activities (%)	73	47	<0.001	62	35	<0.001
Exercise (w, m)	90 (58, 120)	60 (30, 120)	0.16	120 (35, 150)	40 (10, 120)	<0.001
Exercise (h, m)	120 (30, 218)	60 (0, 180)	0.006	120 (30, 210)	30 (0, 120)	<0.001
Exercise (av, m)	90 (51, 150)	73 (25, 137)	0.04	120 (39, 167)	40 (13, 129)	<0.001
Screen (w, m)	90 (60, 150)	90 (60, 120)	0.46	120 (60, 180)	90 (60, 150)	0.70
Screen (h, m)	180 (120, 278)	180 (120, 240)	0.48	180 (120, 240)	180 (120, 240)	0.10
Screen (av, m)	118 (77, 177)	120 (77, 171)	0.92	120 (77, 184)	120 (69, 180)	0.21
Regular breakfast (%)	96%	93%	0.54	96%	92%	0.05

[a]*Data are expressed as the mean (standard deviation).* [b]*Statistical analysis was performed for each sex between junior and high school adolescents; significance levels are shown as:*$^*P<0.05$. $^{**}P<0.01$. $^{***}P<0.001$.

Variables with highly skewed distribution (triglycerides, insulin, HOMA-IR, leptin, high-sensitive CRP, exercise time, and screen time) are expressed as the mean (95% confidence interval).BP, blood pressure; CVD, cardiovascular; EC activities, extracurricular physical activities; exercise, exercise time; FPG, fasting plasma glucose; HOMA-IR, homeostasis assessment of insulin resistance; hs-CRP, high-sensitivity C-reactive protein; LDL, low-density lipoprotein; screen, screen time; (w, m), (weekday, minutes); (h, m), (holiday, minutes); (av, m), (average value per day, minutes).

TABLE 20.2 Characteristics of Parents[a]

Characteristics	Junior High School Adolescents		Senior High School Adolescents	
	Males	Females	Males	Females
Characteristics and lifestyle of fathers				
Age (years)	44.1 (5.4)	45.3 (6.7)	47.5 (4.6)	48.1 (5.2)
Body mass index (kg/m^2)	24.0 (3.4)	23.8 (3.2)	23.7 (3.2)	23.5 (2.6)
Exercise (av, m)	14 (0, 43)	17 (0, 51)	10 (0, 39)	17 (0, 43)
Screen (av, m)	150 (93, 197)	150 (77, 214)	129 (77, 180)	137 (94, 206)
Having a regular breakfast (%)	76	69	80	81
Smoking rate (%)	39	40	42	42
Characteristics and lifestyle of mothers				
Age (years)	44.1 (5.4)	43.5 (5.2)	44.8 (3.7)	45.4 (4.1)
Body mass index (kg/m^2)	24.0 (3.4)	22.3 (4.2)	21.7 (2.8)	21.7 (3.0)
Exercise (av, m)	0 (0, 21)	0 (0, 21)	9 (0, 30)*	15 (0, 30)[b]
Screen (av, m)	124 (75, 180)	120 (60, 184)	120 (77, 180)	137 (77, 194)
Having a regular breakfast (%)	90	89	89	89
Smoking rate (%)	6	8	11	8

[a]*Data are expressed as the mean (standard deviation).* [b]*Mothers of male and female senior high school adolescents had a longer exercise time than those of junior high school adolescents.*
Highly skewed variables in distribution (exercise time and television-watching time) were log-transformed before analysis to yield unimodal symmetry. These data are expressed as the median (interquartile ranges).Exercise (av, m), exercise time (average value per day, minute); screen (av, m), screen time (average value per day).

including walking, jogging, and cycling on weekdays and holidays; time spent watching a screen, including watching television and playing television- and/or computer-based games on weekdays and holidays; score for eating breakfast (1, seldom; 2, occasional; 3, regular); and history of smoking. Information on birth weight of the adolescents and duration of breastfeeding during infancy was obtained from the mothers.

Statistical Analysis

Data are expressed as the mean and standard deviation. Data for highly skewed variables in distribution are expressed as the median and interquartile range. Differences in mean values were examined using unpaired Student's t-tests. To determine the effect of lifestyles of adolescents and their parents on the levels of adolescent CVD risk factors, multivariate regression analyses were performed using each CVD risk level as a dependent variable, and the significant variables (P value <0.05) in previous simple regression analyses as independent variables. Highly skewed variables were log-transformed to yield unimodal symmetry, and these are indicated by ln(variable) hereafter to indicate the transformation. In regression analysis, dependent variables included BMI, waist circumference, systolic blood pressure, HDL cholesterol, ln(triglycerides), ln(insulin), ln(HOMA-IR), the number of CVD risk factors, adiponectin, ln(leptin), and ln(hs-CRP). Independent variables include age, presence or absence of participation in EC physical activities, ln(exercise time), ln(screen time), presence or absence of a regular breakfast for adolescent volunteers, age, BMI, ln(exercise time), ln(screen time), and the presence or absence of smoking habits of parents. Statistical analysis was performed using IBM SPSS Statistics version 21.0 (Tokyo, Japan). Results with a two-sided P value <0.05 were considered to be significant.

RESULTS

Characteristics of Subjects

Sex differences were present in junior and senior high school adolescent volunteers. Sex differences in height, weight, systolic and diastolic blood pressure, total cholesterol, FPG, and leptin were found in junior high school adolescents. Sex differences in age, height, weight, BMI, waist circumference, systolic and diastolic blood pressures, total cholesterol, and HDL cholesterol, FPG, insulin, adiponectin, leptin, hs-CRP, and birth weight were

TABLE 20.3 Effect of Lifestyle on Cardiovascular Risk Factors in Junior High School Adolescents by Simple Regression Analysis

	BMI	WC	SBP	HDLc	ln(TG)[a]	FPG	ln (insulin)[a]	ln (HOMA-IR)[a]	No of risk factors	AN	ln(leptin)[a]	ln (hs-CRP)[a]
Males ($n=99$)												
Age	3.66***	3.99***	2.44*	−2.36*	2.09*	–	2.18*	2.15*	–	–	–	–
EC activities[b]	−4.34***	−4.69***	−3.14**	3.73***	−2.81**	–	−2.30*	−2.16*	−2.86**	–	−4.08***	–
ln(screen time)[a]	–	–	–	–	–	–	2.63*	2.46*	–	–	–	–
ln(paternal exercise time)[a]	–	–	–	–	–	–	–	–	–	2.31*	–	–
Maternal BMI	3.19**	3.89**	–	–	–	–	–	–	–	–	3.52***	–
Females ($n=101$)												
Age	2.09*	–	–	–	–	–	–	–	–	–	–	–
EC activities[b]	−2.86**	−2.95**	–	3.60***	−2.24*	–	–	–	–	–	−5.30***	–
ln(exercise time)[a]	−3.66***	−3.49***	−2.85**	3.16**	–	–	–	–	–	–	−3.80***	–
Paternal BMI	3.21**	3.27**	–	−2.26*	–	–	–	–	2.39*	–	2.40*	–
Maternal BMI	3.10**	4.04***	–	−2.07*	–	2.08*	–	–	3.33**	–	2.42*	–

*$P<0.05$. **$P<0.01$. ***$P<0.001$. [a]*Highly skewed variables in distribution (levels of triglycerides, insulin, HOMA-IR, leptin, hs-CRP, exercise time, and screen time) were log-transformed before analysis to yield unimodal symmetry, which are indicated by ln(variable) to indicate the transformation.* [b]*Adolescents were asked whether they participated in EC activities (1, participated; 0, did not participate).*

Values are expressed as t-values obtained by simple regression analysis. Data without significance were not included in the table. –, Variables that were not significant in simple or multivariate regression analyses. AN, adiponectin (in μg/mL); BMI, body mass index (in kg/m^2); EC activities, extracurricular physical activities; exercise or screen time, average time spent (in min) per day for exercise or watching a screen; FPG, fasting plasma glucose (in mg/dL); HDLc, high-density lipoprotein cholesterol (in mg/dL); HOMA-IR, homeostasis model assessment of insulin resistance; hs-CRP, high-sensitivity C-reactive protein (in ng/mL); regular breakfast, regular breakfast consumption; SBP, systolic blood pressure (in mmHg); TG, triglycerides; WC, waist circumference.

found in senior high school adolescents (Table 20.1). Female adolescents showed a significantly lower rate of participation in EC physical activities and spent significantly less time on exercise than did male adolescents in junior and senior high school. In contrast, the amount of screen time was similar for both sexes (Table 20.1). No junior high school volunteers fulfilled the criteria of metabolic syndrome; four senior high school volunteers fulfilled the criteria.

Parental BMIs and time spent watching a screen were similar for both sexes (Table 20.2). Mothers of male and female senior high school adolescents participated in more exercise than did those of junior high school adolescents.

Effect of Lifestyle on Cardiovascular Disease Risk Factor Levels in Junior High School Adolescents

The effect of lifestyle on CVD risk factor levels determined by simple and multivariate regression analysis is shown in Tables 20.3 and 20.4. Multivariate regression analysis showed that the effect of adolescent lifestyle on BMI or waist circumference was different between sexes. In male adolescents, BMI and waist circumference were associated with maternal BMI, but not with paternal BMI. Participation in EC physical activity greatly decreased with worsening BMI and waist circumference. In female adolescents, BMI and waist circumference were associated with paternal and maternal BMI. Participation in EC physical activity was widely associated with improved CVD risk factors, except for obesity, including lowering systolic blood pressure, increasing HDL cholesterol levels, decreasing the level of ln(triglycerides), and decreasing the accumulation of CVD risk factors.

Effect of Lifestyle on Cardiovascular Disease Risk Factor Levels in Senior High School Adolescents

The effect of lifestyle on CVD risk factor levels determined by simple and multivariate regression analysis is shown in Tables 20.5 and 20.6. Multivariate regression analysis showed that the effect of adolescent lifestyle on BMI or waist circumference was sex dependent and was different between junior and senior high school adolescents. In male adolescents, higher paternal and maternal BMI were independently associated with a high BMI and

TABLE 20.4 Effect of Lifestyle on Cardiovascular Risk Factors in Junior High School Adolescents by Multivariate Regression Analysis

	BMI	WC	SBP	HDLc	ln(TG)[a]	ln(insulin)[a]	ln (HOMA-IR)[a]	No of risks	AN	ln(leptin)[a]
Males ($n=99$)										
EC activities[b]	−3.09**	−3.40**	−2.4*	2.99**	−2.14*	–	–	−2.86**	–	−3.74***
ln(screen time)[a]	–	–	–	–	–	2.68**	2.51*	–	–	–
ln(paternal exercise time)[a]	–	–	–	–	–	–	–	–	2.31*	–
Maternal BMI	2.87**	3.64***	–	–	–	–	–	–	–	3.43***
Females ($n=101$)										
EC activities	–	–	–	–	−2.24*	–	–	–	–	−3.18**
ln(exercise time)[a]	–	–	−2.85**	–	–	–	–	–	–	–
Paternal BMI	3.08**	3.03**	–	–	–	–	–	2.48*	–	–
Maternal BMI	2.65**	3.92***	–	–	–	–	–	3.17**	–	2.29*

*$P<0.05$. **$P<0.01$. ***$P<0.001$. [a]*Highly skewed variables in distribution (levels of triglycerides, insulin, HOMA-IR, leptin, hs-CRP, exercise time, and screen time) were log-transformed before analysis to yield unimodal symmetry, which are indicated by ln(variable) to indicate the transformation.* [b]*Adolescents were asked whether they participated in EC activities (1, participated; 0, did not participate).*
Values in the table are expressed as the t-value by multivariate regression analysis. Data without significance were not included in the table.

greater waist circumference. Paternal BMI had a stronger effect on male adolescent BMI and waist circumference than did maternal BMI. Having a regular breakfast was associated with a lower BMI and smaller waist circumference. Conversely, higher maternal BMI, but not higher paternal BMI, was associated with a high BMI and greater waist circumference in female adolescents.

Participation in EC physical activity had a large effect on the following risk factors in male and female senior high school adolescents: levels of HDL cholesterol, ln(triglycerides), ln(insulin), ln(HOMA-IR), adiponectin, and ln(leptin) in both sexes; and systolic blood pressure and the total number of CVD risk factors in male senior high school adolescents. Time spent watching a screen was negatively associated with HDL cholesterol levels for both sexes. Additionally, a longer time spent watching a screen was associated with high levels of ln(triglycerides) and ln(leptin) and low levels of adiponectin in female senior high school adolescents.

Concerning the association between ln(screen time) and obesity in junior and senior high school adolescents, ln(screen time) was weakly associated with a higher waist circumference (abdominal obesity) only in female senior high school adolescents. Screen time of >120 min/day was not associated with the presence of obesity, as defined by international cut offs, or with the presence of abdominal obesity defined by increased waist circumference (data not shown).

Birth weight and duration of breastfeeding were not significant for either sex (data not shown).

DISCUSSION

The present study shows that participation in school-based EC physical activities and parental BMI are strongly associated with the levels of one or more CVD risk factors in adolescents. We also show sex differences and age-specific effects on adolescent BMI and waist circumference, indicating that strategies to prevent the development of CVD risk factors in adolescents should account for sex and age.

Physical activity, especially moderate-to-vigorous physical activity, is associated with beneficial metabolic profiles [8,16]. Participating in EC activities to experience sports or liberal arts are encouraged in junior and senior high schools in Japan. In the present study, multivariate regression analysis showed that participation in EC physical activities is highly associated with improving levels of CVD risk factors in male and female adolescents. Especially in male adolescents, participating in EC physical activities is associated with improvements in many CVD risk factors, such as abdominal obesity, hypertension, low HDL cholesterol levels, and high triglyceride levels in the junior high school period, and hypertension, low HDL cholesterol levels, high triglyceride levels, and insulin resistance in the senior high school period. In female senior high school adolescents, participating in EC activities is associated with improvements in levels of CVD risk factors. The United States Department of Health and Human Services has called for an expansion of school-based EC sports

TABLE 20.5 Effect of Lifestyle on Cardiovascular Risk Factors in Senior High School Adolescents by Simple Regression Analysis

	BMI	WC	SBP	HDLc	ln(TG)[a]	FPG	ln (insulin)[a]	ln (HOMA-IR)[a]	No of risks	AN	ln (leptin)[a]	ln (hs-CRP)[a]
Males ($n=337$)												
Age	–	2.66**	–	–	–	–	–	–	–	−2.10*	–	–
EC activities[b]	–	–	−2.03*	5.29***	−4.49***	–	−3.61***	−4.50***	−4.51***	2.36*	−4.73***	–
ln(exercise time)[a]	–	–	–	3.66***	−3.67***	–	–	−3.34**	–	–	−2.68**	–
ln(screen time)[a]	–	–	2.80**	2.55**	–	–	2.27*	–	2.70**	–	2.13*	–
Regular breakfast[¶]	−2.70**	−3.07**	–	–	–	–	–	−2.21*	–	–	2.88**	–
Paternal BMI	**5.32*** **	4.95***	–	–	–	–	2.55*	2.34*	–	–	3.29**	2.52*
ln(paternal exercise time)[a]	–	–	–	–	−2.16*	–	–	–	–	–	–	–
Maternal BMI	**3.81*** **	3.29***	2.14*	–	–	–	–	–	2.18*	–	–	–
ln(maternal exercise time)[a]	–	–	2.41*	–	–	–	–	–	–	–	–	–
Females ($n=442$)												
Age	–	–	−3.25**	–	–	–	–	–	–	–	–	–
EC activities	–	–	–	6.23***	−3.58***	–	−4.25***	−4.17***	–	2.63**	−6.09***	2.48*
ln(exercise time)[a]	–	–	–	3.58***	−2.35*	–	−4.22***	−4.19***	–	–	−5.10***	2.28*
ln(screen time)[a]	2.33*	2.26*	–	−2.46*	2.11*	–	–	–	–	−2.55*	2.96**	–
Regular breakfast[¶]	–	–	–	–	–	–	–	–	–	–	–	–
Paternal BMI	2.08*	–	–	–	–	–	–	–	–	–	–	–
Maternal BMI	4.38***	3.03**	–	–	–	–	0.49	–	2.33*	–	–	–

*$P<0.05$. **$P<0.01$. ***$P<0.001$. [a]*Highly skewed variables in distribution (levels of triglycerides, insulin, HOMA-IR, leptin, hs-CRP, exercise time, and screen time) were log-transformed before analysis to yield unimodal symmetry, which are indicated by ln(variable) to indicate the transformation.* [b]*Adolescents were asked whether they participated in EC activities (1, participated; 0, did not participate).*[¶]*Adolescents were asked whether they ate breakfast (1: seldom, 2: occasionally, or 3: regularly).*

programs to address the obesity epidemic [16,17]. The present study reinforces the premise that participation in school-based EC physical activities has a considerable impact on the levels of multiple CVD risk factors in adolescents.

Concerning the effect of parental BMI on CVD risk factors in children and adolescents, previous studies have shown a greater influence of maternal BMI than paternal BMI on childhood adiposity [18–20]. Sun et al. reported that, based on data obtained in 2002, maternal obesity was more strongly associated with adolescent obesity than was paternal obesity in 2842 males and 2911 females aged 12–13 years in Japan [21]. From data obtained in 2001, Kazumi et al. reported that adolescent BMI was associated with maternal BMI, but not with paternal BMI, in 148 male adolescents aged 18 years in Japan [22]. The present data shows sex and age differences. In junior high school, BMI in male and female adolescents was associated with maternal BMI, but paternal BMI was not associated with BMI in male adolescents. In senior high school, BMI in male adolescents was associated with paternal or maternal BMI. Importantly, paternal BMI was more strongly associated with BMI in male adolescents than was maternal BMI. BMI in female adolescents was associated with maternal BMI but not with paternal BMI. The reason for sex and age differences between adolescent and parental BMI should be further investigated to determine whether adolescent and/or parental attitudes have been changing. Nevertheless, these data suggest that approaches for adolescent obesity that focus on parents should consider the sex of the parent.

Screen time is well known as being associated with unfavorable body composition and CVD risk factors. In the present study, a longer screen time was not strongly associated with obesity. One reason for this low level of

TABLE 20.6 Effect of Lifestyle on Cardiovascular Risk Factors in Senior High School Adolescents by Multivariate Regression Analysis

	BMI	WC	SBP	HDLc	ln(TG)[a]	FPG	ln (insulin)[a]	ln (HOMA-IR)[a]	No of risks	AN	ln(leptin)	ln (hs-CRP)[a]
Males ($n = 337$)												
Age	–	2.82**	–	–	–	–	–	–	–	–	–	–
EC activities[b]	–	–	–2.40*	3.64***	–2.67**	–	–4.58***	–2.95**	–	2.36*	–3.75***	–
ln(screen time)[a]	–	–	2.58*	–2.02*	–	–	–	–		–	–	–
Regular breakfast[¶]	–2.70**	–2.93**	–	–	–	–	–	–	–	–	2.03*	–
Paternal BMI	5.01***	4.62***	–	–	–	–	2.57*	2.14*	–	–	3.10**	2.47*
Maternal BMI	3.58***	2.61**	–	–	–	–	–	–	2.24*	–	–	–
ln(maternal exercise time)[a]	–	–	2.44*	–	–	–	–	–	–	–	–	–
Females ($n = 442$)												
Age	–	–	–3.25**	–	–	–	–	–	–	–	–	–
EC activities	–	–	–	4.66***	–2.55**	–	–2.27*	–2.20*	–	2.60**	–3.53***	–
ln(exercise time)[a]	–	–	–	–	–	–	–	–	–	–	–2.06*	–
ln(screen time)[a]	–	1.98*	–	–2.59*	2.09*	–	–	–	–	–2.52*	3.14**	–
Maternal BMI	3.95***	2.83**	–	–	–	–	–	–	2.33*	–	–	–

*$P < 0.05$. **$P < 0.01$. ***$P < 0.001$. [a]*Highly skewed variables in distribution (levels of triglycerides, insulin, HOMA-IR, leptin, hs-CRP, exercise time, and screen time) were log-transformed before analysis to yield unimodal symmetry, which are indicated by ln(variable) to indicate the transformation.* [b]*Adolescents were asked whether they participated in EC activities (1, participated; 0, did not participate).* [¶] *Adolescents were asked whether they ate breakfast (1: seldom, 2: occasionally, or 3: regularly).*

association may be that the present data were obtained from volunteer adolescents. However, this issue needs to be further investigated.

The present study was limited by the fact that the present data were obtained from two studies. Data were obtained from senior high school students between 2006 and 2008 and from junior high school between 2012 and 2013. Therefore, the time periods were different in each study. Another major limitation is the cross-sectional nature of the present study. Noninterventional studies on family and physical environmental factors related to health behavior (i.e. diet, physical activity, and sedentary behavior) in adolescents concluded that favorable lifestyles were associated with improved levels of CVD risk factors [6,10]. However, this may be because cross-sectional studies have commonly obtained data form adolescents and their families with favorable lifestyles for prolonged periods. Interventional studies have shown limited effectiveness in reducing the risk of obesity, particularly in the long term, or in increasing positive health behavior despite using a variety of strategies (e.g. reduction in television viewing, increasing physical activities, improving dietary choices, changing health behavior social climates, and providing recreational after school programs) [6]. For adolescents, families, and social groups, the available evidence needs to be used to determine minimal and optimal thresholds for daily sedentary time; daily exercise time by sex, age, and ethnicity; and, when possible, how thresholds differ across health outcomes or demographic status (i.e. age, gender, and ethnicity). Interventional studies are required to test the effect of improved adolescent and/or parental lifestyles on the levels of adolescent CVD risk factors. This could provide strategies for adolescents at a high risk for CVD diseases who may be resistant to ordinary procedures.

CONCLUSION

The present study shows that participation in school-based EC physical activities and parental BMI are associated with the levels of one or more CVD risk factors in adolescents. Among these, participation in EC physical activities has a profound effect on several CVD risk factors, especially for male adolescents. The influence of paternal or maternal obesity on adolescent obesity differs according to sex and age in Japan. Therefore, approaches focusing on the parents should take into account the sex of the adolescents.

Acknowledgments

This study was supported by a Health and Labor Sciences Research Grant (Comprehensive Research on Cardiovascular and Lifestyle Related Diseases [H18-049 and H24-014] of the Ministry of Health, Labour and Welfare in Japan.

References

[1] Han JC, Lawlor DA, Kimm SY. Childhood obesity. Lancet 2010;375:1737–48.

[2] Wang Y, Lobstein T. Worldwide trends in childhood overweight and obesity. Int J Pediatr Obes 2006;1:11–25.

[3] Yoshinaga M, Ichiki T, Tanaka Y, Hazeki D, Horigome H, Takahashi H, et al. Prevalence of childhood obesity from 1978 to 2007 in Japan. Pediatr Int 2010;52:213–7.

[4] Sakimukai S, Yoshinaga M. Cross-sectional and longitudinal studies on the prevalence of obesity in children and adolescents in Japan. Himan Kenkyu 2013;19:101–10. [in Japanese]

[5] Reinehr T, Kleber M, Toschke AM. Lifestyle intervention in obese children is associated with a decrease of the metabolic syndrome prevalence. Atherosclerosis 2009;207:174–80.

[6] Lawman HG, Wilson DK. A review of family and environmental correlates of health behaviors in high-risk youth. Obesity 2010;20:1142–57.

[7] Kang HT, Lee HR, Shim JY, Shin YH, Park BJ, Lee YJ. Association between screen time and metabolic syndrome in children and adolescents in Korea: the 2005 Korean National Health and Nutrition Examination Survey. Diabetes Res Clin Pract 2010;89:72–8.

[8] Carlson SA, Fulton JE, Lee SM, Foley JT, Heitzler C, Huhman M. Influence of limit-setting and participation in physical activity on youth screen time. Pediatrics 2010;126:e89–96.

[9] Yoshinaga M, Hatake S, Tachikawa T, Shinomiya M, Miyazaki A, Takahashi H. Impact of lifestyles of adolescents and their parents on cardiovascular risk factors in the adolescents. J Atheroscler Thromb 2011;18:981–90.

[10] Tremblay MS, LeBlanc AG, Kho ME, Saunders TJ, Larouche R, Colley RC, et al. Systematic review of sedentary behaviour and health indicators in school-aged children and youth. Int J Behav Nutr Phys Act 2011;8:98.

[11] Matthews DR, Hosker JP, Rudenski AS, Naylor BA, Treacher DF, Turner RC. Homeostasis model assessment: insulin resistance and beta-cell function from fasting plasma glucose and insulin concentrations in man. Diabetologia 1985;28:412–9.

[12] Zimmet P, Alberti G, Kaufman F, Tajima N, Silink M, Arslanian S, et al. The metabolic syndrome in children and adolescents. Lancet 2007;369:2059–61.

[13] Alberti KG, Zimmet P, Shaw J. Metabolic syndrome - a new world-wide definition. A Consensus Statement from the International Diabetes Federation. Diabet Med 2006;23:469–80.

[14] Examination Committee of Criteria for 'Obesity Disease' in Japan; Japan Society for the Study of Obesity. New criteria for 'obesity disease' in Japan. Circ J 2002;66:987–92.

[15] Cole TJ, Bellizzi MC, Flegal KM, Dietz WH. Establishing a standard definition for child overweight and obesity worldwide: international survey. BMJ 2000;320(7244):1240–3.

[16] Cohen DA, Taylor SL, Zonta M, Vestal KD, Schuster MA. Availability of high school extracurricular sports programs and high-risk behaviors. J Sch Health 2007;77:80–6.

[17] Keeton VF, Kennedy C. Update on physical activity including special needs populations. Curr Opin Pediatr 2009;21:262–8.

[18] Lawlor DA, Smith GD, O'Callaghan M, Alati R, Mamun AA, Williams GM, et al. Epidemiologic evidence for the fetal overnutrition hypothesis: findings from the mater-university study of pregnancy and its outcomes. Am J Epidemiol 2007;165:418–24.

[19] Harvey NC, Poole JR, Javaid MK, Dennison EM, Robinson S, Inskip HM, et al. Parental determinants of neonatal body composition. J Clin Endocrinol Metab 2007;92:523–6.

[20] Tanaka S, Bin W, Honda M, Nanbu S, Suzuki K, Fukuo K, et al. Associations of 18-year-old daughters' and mothers' serum leptin, body mass index and DXA-derived fat mass. J Atheroscler Thromb 2010;17:1077–81.

[21] Sun Y, Sekine M, Kagamimori S. Lifestyle and overweight among Japanese adolescents: the Toyama Birth Cohort Study. J Epidemiol 2009;19:303–10.

[22] Kazumi T, Kawaguchi A, Yoshino G. Associations of middle-aged mother's but not father's body mass index with 18-year-old son's waist circumferences, birth weight, and serum hepatic enzyme levels. Metabolism 2005;54:466–70.

CHAPTER

21

Physical Activity, Inflammatory Cytokines, Endothelial Dysfunction, and Risk of Coronary Artery Diseases in Visceral Obesity

Pascal Laurant, Catherine Riva, and Agnes Vinet

Laboratoire Pharm-Ecologie Cardiovasculaire, UFRip Sciences Technologies Santé, Université d'Avignon et des Pays du Vaucluse, Avignon, France

INTRODUCTION

Since at least the 1980s, people in developed and developing countries have been becoming more obese and less physically active. Obesity, in particular visceral obesity, is associated with an increased risk of coronary heart disease and stroke, and elevated cardiovascular mortality and morbidity. Metabolic syndrome often accompanies visceral obesity and contributes to the elevated atherothrombotic risk associated with obesity. Visceral obesity is also characterized by local and systemic chronic inflammation. It seems well established that elevation of proinflammatory cytokines may be a link between enlarged adipose tissue reserves and increased risk of coronary diseases. The vascular endothelium plays a major role in the prevention of inflammation and atherogenesis. When it is damaged, endothelial dysfunction becomes a coronary risk factor and is an early step in the pathogenesis of the atherosclerotic cascade. Endothelial dysfunction has been reported in obese patients. Present in all risk factors (type 2 diabetes, hypertension, and dyslipidemia), inflammation promotes atherosclerosis by its deleterious effects on vascular endothelium.

As obesity is considered to be the major public health problem in Westernized and developing societies, it is urgent to find new methods to prevent and treat afflicted patients. Evidence shows that exercise training prevents the progression of vascular diseases and reduces cardiovascular mortality and morbidity. Exercise is known to reduce chronic inflammation and to preserve vascular endothelial function. The purpose of this chapter is to understand the potential mechanisms by which exercise affects obesity-related chronic inflammation and endothelial dysfunction.

DISTURBANCES TO ENDOTHELIAL FUNCTION AND CARDIOVASCULAR INFLAMMATORY PATHWAYS IN VISCERAL OBESITY

Obesity and Endothelial Dysfunction

Endothelial dysfunction is a term that refers to an impairment of endothelium-dependent vasorelaxation caused by a loss of nitric oxide (NO) bioactivity in the vessel wall. Endothelial dysfunction appears to be an early event in the pathogenesis of atherosclerosis, and has profound prognostic implications for adverse cardiovascular events and clinical outcomes [1].

Although some clinical studies reported the absence of endothelial dysfunction or even, paradoxically, improved endothelial function in severe obesity [2,3], numerous research groups have reported impaired endothelium-dependent vasodilation in the obese that is detectable even in prepubertal children with mild-to-moderate obesity [4] and worsens with puberty [5]. Not only the degree but also the duration of obesity is

Nutrition in the Prevention and Treatment of Abdominal Obesity
http://dx.doi.org/10.1016/B978-0-12-407869-7.00021-0

likely to play a significant role in this type of endothelial dysfunction, which is proportional to body mass index (BMI) [6]. The distribution of fat, rather than obesity per se, negatively affects endothelial function. Visceral obesity is associated with endothelial dysfunction [7]. Furthermore, the severity of endothelial dysfunction is correlated with the degree of visceral obesity [6,8]. In fact, in the healthy obese, an increased waist-hip ratio is a powerful predictor of vascular endothelial dysfunction, independent of other cardiovascular risk factors [9]. The more inflammatory fat phenotype is also associated with higher levels of endothelium impairment [10]. The level of impairment in endothelium-dependent vasodilation is proportional to the level of insulin resistance in the obese [11,12]. However, some studies have reported that diabetes and obesity affect endothelial function equally, while smooth muscle cell function is only affected in diabetes [13,14]. In obese patients, elevated free fatty acid levels can impair the function of small forearm vessels, where coupling between blood flow and metabolism takes place [15]. The release of endothelial tissue-type plasminogen activator (t-PA), a key enzyme in initiating an endogenous fibrinolytic response, is blunted in the obese [16], in whom higher plasma levels of t-PA and plasminogen activator inhibitor 1 (PAI-1) antigens correlate with the increased BMI [17].

Several mechanisms are implicated in the pathogenesis of endothelial dysfunction. NO is thought to have a pivotal role in cardiovascular health; its deficiency affects the oxidation of low-density lipoprotein (LDL) cholesterol, which is associated with the initiation and progression of atherosclerosis [1]. Endothelial dysfunction is characterized by the decreased bioavailability of NO. Loss of NO results from decreased expression of endothelial NO synthase (eNOS), loss of eNOS activity, and accelerated NO degradation by radical oxygen species (ROS). Inactivation of NO by excessive ROS production has been reported in patients with cardiovascular risk factors such as obesity and coronary artery diseases [18–21]. Among the many enzymatic systems that are capable of producing ROS, NADPH oxidase appears to play an important pathological role in cardiometabolic diseases. In obese patients, increased NADPH oxidase activity, along with the expression of specific subunits such as neutrophil cytosol factor 1 (NCF-1; or p47-phox) leads to the excessive production of superoxide anions (O_2^-) and rapid inactivation of NO by ROS, thereby causing endothelial oxidative stress and endothelial dysfunction [22]. In obese rats, aortic upregulation of the vascular subunits of NADPH oxidase, increased NADPH oxidase activity, and overproduction of O_2^- generated in response to NADPH [23] have been shown.

The renin-angiotensin system (RAS) is also implicated in the pathogenesis of endothelial dysfunction, oxidative stress, and inflammation [24,25]. Activation of type-1 angiotensin II receptors (AT1Rs) on endothelial cells by angiotensin II promotes oxidative stress through the activation of membrane-bound NADPH oxidase and, thus, the generation of ROS [26]. RAS is hyperactivated in obesity, and evidence suggests a link between insulin resistance, inflammation, endothelial dysfunction, and obesity [27]. In obese Zucker rats, vascular AT1R is overexpressed, suggesting that AT1R activation may be involved in vascular dysfunction and inflammation in obesity [23,28].

Obesity as a State of Chronic Inflammation

Hotamisligil et al. [29] were the first to report a direct link between obesity and inflammation by demonstrating that the proinflammatory cytokine tumor necrosis factor (TNF-α) was expressed in adipose tissue of obese mice and linked to insulin resistance. Substantial evidence now indicates that obesity is associated with a state of chronic low-grade inflammation in metabolically active tissues such adipose tissue, liver, and muscle, as well as in the pancreas and brain [30,31]. Adipose tissue, particularly visceral adiposity, plays a major role in the regulation of inflammation. Adipose tissue expresses and secretes proinflammatory cytokines such as TNF-α and interleukin-6 (IL-6) [32,33]. Systemic concentrations of these cytokines increase with adiposity, and large circulating concentrations of IL-6 and TNF-α originate from adipose tissue. Furthermore, systemic concentrations of these cytokines correlate with the BMI [8,34].

Adipose tissue is a heterogeneous mix of adipocytes, stromal preadipocytes, several types of immune cells (most prominently macrophages and subpopulations of T lymphocytes), and endothelium, which can respond rapidly and dynamically to nutrient excess through adipocyte hypertrophy and hyperplasia [35–37]. In obesity, adipose tissue dysfunction is caused by the interaction of genetic, behavioral, and environmental factors that leads to adipocyte hypertrophy, ectopic fat accumulation, hypoxia, impaired adipose tissue mitochondrial function, and inflammatory processes within adipose tissue. Furthermore, because progressive adipocyte enlargement occurs in obesity, the blood supply to adipocytes may be reduced, with consequent hypoxia [38]. Hypoxia is reported to be associated with increased macrophage infiltration into adipose tissue, which leads to the increased production of proinflammatory cytokines [39–41]. This results in localized inflammation of adipose tissues, which then propagate an overall systemic inflammation associated with the development of obesity-related cardiovascular pathologies [42–44].

Peripheral blood mononuclear cells are known to migrate into adipose tissue, where they become macrophages and release proinflammatory cytokines. In particular, proinflammatory M1-type macrophages expressing proinflammatory cytokines, such as IL-6 and TNF-α, contribute to the increased levels of inflammation in the circulation of obese individuals [45,46]. Furthermore, within the immune cells, regulatory T (Treg) cells are a population of lymphocytes with potent immunosuppressive and anti-inflammatory activities. Whereas adipose tissue of lean individuals is enriched with Tregs, a significant decline was observed in obese mice and humans [47,48] and was correlated with adiposity, inflammation, and glucose intolerance [49,50].

Recent clinical studies in humans have shown that adipose tissue is poorly oxygenated in the obese state [39,40,51–54]. These reports suggest that many adipokines that are related to inflammation, such as angiopoietin-related protein 4 (Angplt4), leptin, macrophage migration inhibitory factor (MIF), matrix metalloproteinases 2 and 9 (MMP-2 and MMP-9), IL-6, PAI-1, and vascular endothelial growth factor (VEGF) are all upregulated by hypoxia. Tissue inflammation was inversely related to tissue oxygenation, which suggests that adipose tissue hypoxia might be a mechanism causing adipose tissue inflammation in humans [55]. The master regulator of hypoxia, oxygen homeostasis, and angiogenesis is the transcription factor hypoxia-inducible factor 1 (HIF1) [56]. In fact, several important hypoxia-associated genes, such as leptin and VEGF, are directly regulated by HIF1 [54]. It has been reported that when adipose tissue VEGF gene and protein expression is altered, adipose tissue capillary density is lowered in obesity [55]. On the other hand, overexpression of VEGF and increased angiogenesis protect against obesity-related hypoxia and insulin resistance [57].

Adipose tissue vasoconstriction is elevated in obesity [13]. Circulating levels of angiotensinogen and angiotensin II proteins have been found to play an important role in vasoconstriction [58], and are elevated in adipose tissue in obesity [59]. On the other hand, blood flow to adipose tissue is substantially reduced in both subcutaneous and visceral adipose tissue in obesity [60].

In summary, visceral adiposity is a crucial key regulator of inflammation, coagulation, and fibrinolysis. Proinflammatory cytokines (particularly IL-6 and TNF-α) secreted and released by adipose tissue seem to play a major role because they can influence endothelial function. In fact, endothelial dysfunction was reported in obesity and resulted in vascular wall damage, accumulation of phagocytes in the subintimal space, and the subsequent release of inflammatory cytokines [43,61–63], and is thus associated with the initiation and development of atherosclerosis and cardiovascular complications, such as the metabolic syndrome.

Increased Proinflammatory State is Linked to Endothelial Damage in Obesity

Obesity with or without other components of the metabolic syndrome (insulin resistance, hypercholesterolemia, elevated free fatty acids, and hypertension), contributes to endothelial activation and dysfunction associated with inflammation in the arterial wall [61,62].

In obese women (in particular, in women with visceral obesity), a close positive correlation has been shown between circulating levels of IL-6 and TNF-α and circulating levels of adhesion molecules [intercellular adhesion molecule (ICAM), P-selectin, and vascular cell adhesion molecule (VCAM)], suggesting that these cytokines are partly responsible for the endothelial activation observed in visceral obesity [8]. Experimental studies have effectively shown that these cytokines can directly influence endothelial function and induce the endothelial expression of chemokines and adhesion molecules [64], which play key roles in the early stage of the atherogenic process [62]. A number of proinflammatory cytokines, such as TNF-α and interferon gamma (IFN-γ), have also been shown to alter endothelial permeability and facilitate leukocytes transmigration [65,66]. TNF-α secreted from endothelial cells, smooth muscle cells, macrophages, and adipose cells enhances monocyte recruitment into developing atherosclerosis lesions, indicating an important role for this cytokine in inflammation at an early stage of atherosclerosis [67]. IL-6, another cytokine secreted by adipose cells, skeletal muscle cells, macrophages, and lymphocytes in response to TNF-α has been linked to all-cause and cardiovascular morbidity. IL-6 stimulates the production of proinflammatory cytokines from monocytes and macrophages, and upregulates C-reactive protein (CRP) production by the liver. However, IL-6 originating from skeletal muscle exerts anti-inflammatory effects by stimulating anti-inflammatory cytokines such as interleukin-1 receptor antagonist (IL-1ra) and IL-10 [68].

Although the role of inflammation in obesity-associated cardiovascular risk is well established, it is less clear how the endothelium is affected by obesity. Obesity is associated with endothelial dysfunction in various vascular beds such as skeletal muscle, mesenteric, visceral adipose tissue, and coronary arteries [69–72]. One aspect of the dysfunction, at least, has been attributed to the effect of factors released from adipose tissue [71,73], such as TNF-α and IL-1β, that are capable of impairing endothelial function [72,74]. One recent study demonstrated that the incubation of resistance arteries taken from diet-induced obese mice with a neutralizing antibody against TNF-α restores endothelial-dependent dilation and NO bioavailability [72]. Therefore, cytokines such as TNF-α seem to be critical mediators of impaired endothelial function in obesity. The mechanisms through which they induce endothelial dysfunction involve reduced NO activation and/or increased oxidative stress [75,76]. Other mechanisms have also been described such as endothelium apoptosis and vascular remodeling [76].

Endothelial dysfunction enhances the synthesis and release of proinflammatory cytokines [63]. In the context of insulin-resistant states such as obesity, endothelial dysfunction is partly caused by the activation of innate immune inflammatory pathways, in which nuclear factor-kappa-B (NF-κB) seems to play a pivotal role [43].

PHYSICAL ACTIVITY PRESERVES ENDOTHELIAL DYSFUNCTION AND EXERTS ANTI-INFLAMMATORY EFFECTS

Physical inactivity is reported to be a leading cause of death in industrialized countries. In obese individuals, a low level of physical activity was shown to be a better predictor of all-cause mortality compared to cholesterol levels, smoking status, and blood pressure [77]. Moreover, evidence from numerous epidemiological studies indicates that national recommendations for physical activity, diet, and combined diet and exercise interventions prevent the progression of cardiovascular diseases and associated risk factors [78]. Numerous clinical and experimental studies have demonstrated that exercise training is an effective strategy to correct all atherosclerotic risk factors associated with obesity, such as endothelial dysfunction and proinflammatory status.

Physical Activity is Linked to Endothelial Protection

Only a few studies have analyzed the effect of exercise training alone on endothelial dysfunction in obese subjects. Exercise improved and even restored endothelial function in adults, as well as in obese children and adolescents [12,79,80]. This improvement was often independent of weight loss [12,81]; it probably occurs through shear stress-related improvements in NO availability, as well as changes in fibrinolytic processes with reduced PAI-1 antigen [82] and increased t-PA release capacity [83] after exercise training, and possibly also changes in free radical degradation of NO, oxidative stress, and inflammation status. Unfortunately, no clinical study has reported relationships between changes in endothelial function and changes in oxidative stress and inflammatory markers after exercise training in obese subjects. Moreover, the extent of improvements in endothelial vasodilation and the increase in insulin sensitivity were not correlated [84].

Exercise training alone improved endothelial function in whichever vascular bed was assessed, i.e. the large conduit artery and resistance vessels [12,79,83–85]. However, when both artery types were explored in the same trained obese subjects, exercise training produced distinctive vascular functional effects that underlie different regulatory mechanisms along the artery tree [12].

Regular aerobic training even with low-intensity exercise, targeted for lipid oxidation, improved endothelial vasodilation in obese adults [12]. All types of exercise training were efficient in increasing endothelial function in obese adults [86]. However, the greatest amelioration was observed after high-intensity interval aerobic training; similar improvements were observed after continuous moderate-intensity aerobic training and strength training [84].

In obese animals, exercise training prevents or restores endothelium- and NO-dependent vascular relaxation [87]. This beneficial effect on the endothelium can be explain by increased expression and activity of eNOS, thus generating NO and modulating ROS production, and leading to the reversal of arterial hypertension and risk factors for metabolic syndrome [87,88]. One possible mechanism may be a powerful stimulus to increase blood flow and shear stress in vascular beds, which, in turn, increases Akt and eNOS expression and/or activity, leading to increased vascular NO production and/or NO bioavailability [89,90]. According to clinical studies [90], training increases vascular Akt phosphorylation at serine-473 and eNOS phosphorylation at serine-1177 in high-fat diet-induced obese rats [87], thus confirming a stimulatory effect of exercise training on Akt-eNOS pathway activation, leading to improve endothelial-dependent vasodilatation. Exercise training could also downregulate vascular AT1Rs and modulate the activity of membrane-bound NADPH oxidase in several experimental models of metabolic disorders [91,92]. These findings also indicate the existence of a distinct signal derived from endothelial cells. Through laminar shear stress activation, exercise training downregulates AT1R expression [93], leading to decreased NADPH oxidase activity and O_2^- production, which in turn decreases ROS generation and preserves endothelial NO bioavailability, which has protective antiatherogenic and anti-inflammatory effects [94]. However, it is unclear whether exercise influences NADPH oxidase activity and NADPH oxidase subunit expression, as well as AT1R expression, in obesity.

Physical Activity has Anti-inflammatory Effects

Human studies examining the effects of chronic exercise on circulating levels of cytokines are contradictory. Cross-sectional studies indicate moderated reductions in the concentration of IL-6 and TNF-α, along with increased levels of anti-inflammatory IL-10. However, other studies report no such beneficial effects [95].

The anti-inflammatory effects of exercise may be mediated via a reduction in visceral fat mass with a subsequent decrease in adipokine release. In obese rodents, exercise training decreased expression of the proinflammatory cytokines TNF-α, IL-1β, and IL-12, and increased expression of anti-inflammatory cytokines, such as IL-10, in visceral adipose tissue [96–99]. Several human studies have shown that chronic exercise reduces proinflammatory cytokine expression in subcutaneous adipose tissue [100,101]. However, it is unknown whether visceral adipose tissue is more important than subcutaneous adipose tissue in chronic inflammation. In healthy obese women, lifestyle modifications, including exercise, lead to decreased cytokine and adhesin serum levels. Furthermore, the improvement in endothelial functions after weight loss is reported to be more marked in obese women who lose more visceral fat and to be strictly associated with decreased cytokine concentrations [8]. These findings strongly suggest that a link exists between the modifiable risk factor, inflammation (especially in visceral fat), and cardiovascular risk is mediated by changes in endothelial function, which can be corrected by lifestyle modifications.

The anti-inflammatory effect of exercise may be also mediated via cells and tissues other than adipose tissue (e.g. endothelial cells, innate immune cells, regulatory T cells, and skeletal muscle tissue). Exercise training reduces endothelial expression and release of adhesion molecules [102–104]. These beneficial effects contribute to reduced leukocyte migration into the vessel wall. Indeed, experimental studies suggest that exercise training contributes to reduced macrophage infiltration in adipose and vascular tissues [91,105]. In patients at cardiovascular risk, exercise training can also reduce the release of proinflammatory cytokines from peripheral mononuclear cells, reduce the number and size of circulating proinflammatory monocytes, and increase the numbers of circulating Treg cells, as well as increasing the circulating level of anti-inflammatory cytokines [106]. In obese mice, exercise training decreases the expression of cell-surface toll-like receptors (TLRs), resulting in a lower production of proinflammatory cytokines [105]. Exercise training is also reported to attenuate inflammation in obese mice by inducing a phenotypic switch from proinflammatory M1 macrophages to anti-inflammatory M2 macrophages [105].

Skeletal muscle fiber contraction is thought to induce the expression and release of myokines, which exert endocrine and paracrine effects that partly explain the anti-inflammatory properties of exercise. Of the myokines, IL-6, appears to play a central role [107]: once released by skeletal muscle, IL-6 exerts a specific endocrine effect on visceral fat, macrophages, and other organs such as liver that opposes the deleterious effects of inflammation. IL-6 increases fat oxidation and lipolysis in adipose tissue and helps ameliorate insulin sensitivity in skeletal muscle. In addition, IL-6 induces the production and release of anti-inflammatory cytokines such IL-10 and IL-1ra, and inhibits production of TNF-α in adipose tissue and infiltrated macrophages [68,94,108].

CONCLUSION

There is increasing evidence to support a relationship between endothelial dysfunction and chronic inflammation in obesity, and especially in visceral obesity. Exercise training is known to improve endothelial function in the obese, but more studies are needed to demonstrate whether exercise influence NADPH oxidase activity and NADPH oxidase subunit expression, as well AT1R expression, in obesity. In animal studies, exercise training is efficient in reducing the expression of proinflammatory cytokines and increasing the expression of anti-inflammatory cytokines. Future clinical studies are needed to clarify the effect of exercise training alone on inflammation status and the link with changes in endothelial function.

References

[1] Davignon J, Ganz P. Role of endothelial dysfunction in atherosclerosis. Circulation 2004;109(suppl. III):27–32.

[2] Biasucci LM, Graziani F, Rizzello V, Liuzzo G, Guidone C, De Caterina AR, et al. Paradoxical preservation of vascular function in severe obesity. Am J Med 2010;123:727–34.

[3] Grassi G, Seravalle G, Scopelliti F, Dell'Oro R, Fattori L, Quarti-Trevano F, et al. Structural and functional alterations of subcutaneous small resistance arteries in severe human obesity. Obesity (Silver Spring) 2010;18:92–8.

[4] Karpoff L, Vinet A, Schuster I, Oudot C, Goret L, Dauzat M, et al. Abnormal vascular reactivity at rest and exercise in obese boys. Eur J Clin Invest 2009;39:94–102.

[5] Montero D, Walther G, Perez-Martin A, Roche E, Vinet A. Endothelial dysfunction, inflammation, and oxidative stress in obese children and adolescents: markers and effect of lifestyle intervention. Obes Rev 2012;13:441–55.

[6] Arkin JM, Alsdorf R, Bigornia S, Palmisano J, Beal R, Istfan N, et al. Relation of cumulative weight burden to vascular endothelial dysfunction in obesity. Am J Cardiol 2008;101:98–101.

[7] Perticone F, Ceravolo R, Candigliota M, Ventura G, Lacopino S, Sinopoli F, et al. Obesity and body fat distribution induce endothelial dysfunction by oxidative stress: protective effect of vitamin C. Diabetes 2001;50:159–65.

[8] Ziccardi P, Nappo F, Guigliano G, Esposito K, Marfella R, Cioffi M, D'Andrea F, et al. Reduction of inflammatory cytokine concentrations and improvement of endothelial function in obese women after weight loss over one year. Circulation 2002;105:804–9.

[9] Brook RD, Bard RL, Rubenfire M, Ridker PM, Rajagopalan S. Usefulness of visceral obesity (waist/hip ratio) in predicting vascular endothelial function in healthy overweight adults. Am J Cardiol 2001;88:1264–9.

[10] Apovian CM, Bigornia S, Mott M, Meyers MR, Ulloor J, Gagua M, et al. Adipose macrophage infiltration is associated with insulin resistance and vascular endothelial dysfunction in obese subjects. Arterioscler Thromb Vasc Biol 2008;28:1654–9.

[11] Pasimeni G, Ribaudo MC, Capoccia D, Rossi F, Bertone C, Leonetti F, Santiemma V. Non-invasive evaluation of endothelial dysfunction in uncomplicated obesity: relationship with insulin resistance. Microvasc Res 2006;71:115–20.
[12] Vinet A, Karpoff L, Walther G, Startun A, Obert P, Goret L, et al. Vascular reactivity at rest and during exercise in middle-aged obese men: effects of short-term, low-intensity, exercise training. Int J Obes 2011;35:820–8.
[13] Sivitz WI, Wayson SM, Bayless ML, Sinkey CA, Haynes WG. Obesity impairs vascular relaxation in human subjects: hyperglycemia exaggerates adrenergic vasoconstriction arterial dysfunction in obesity and diabetes. J Diabetes Comp 2007;21:149–57.
[14] Doupis J, Rahangdale S, Gnardellis C, Pena SE, Malhotra A, Veves A. Effects of diabetes and obesity on vascular reactivity, inflammatory cytokines, and growth factors. Obesity 2011;19:729–35.
[15] Vigili de Kreutzenberg S, Kiwanuka E, Tiengo A, Avogaro A. Visceral obesity is characterized by impaired nitric oxide-independent vasodilation. Eur Heart J 2003;24:1210–5.
[16] Van Guilder GP, Hoetzer GL, Smith DT, Irmiger HM, Greiner JJ, Stauffer BL, et al. Endothelial t-PA release is impaired in overweight and obese adults but can be improved with regular aerobic exercise. Am J Physiol 2005;289:E807–13.
[17] Rosita GA, D'Agostino RB, Massaro J, Lipinska I, Mittleman MA, Sutherland P, et al. Association between obesity and a prothrombotic state: the Framingham offspring study. Thromb Haemost 2004;91:683–9.
[18] Cai H, Harrison DG. Endothelial dysfunction in cardiovascular diseases: the role of oxidant stress. Circ Res 2000;87:840–4.
[19] Fearon IM, Faux SP. Oxidative stress and cardiovascular diseases: novel tools give (free) radical insight. J Mol Cell Cardiol 2009;47:372–81.
[20] Harrison DG, Griendling KK, Landmesser U, Hornig B, Drexler H. Role of oxidative stress in atherosclerosis. Am J Cardiol 2003;91:7A–11A.
[21] Spiekermann S, Landmesser U, Dikalov S, Bredt M, Gamez G, Tatge H, et al. Electron spin resonance characterization of vascular xanthine and NADP(H) oxidase activity in patient with coronary artery disease: relation to endothelium-dependent vasodilation. Circulation 2003;107:1383–9.
[22] Silver AE, Beske SD, Christou DD, Donato AJ, Moreau KL, Eskurza I, et al. Overweight and obese human demonstrate increase vascular endothelial NAD(P)H oxydase-p47phox expression and evidence of endothelial oxidative stress. Circulation 2007;115:627–37.
[23] Shinozaki Z, Nishio Y, Ayajiki K, Yoshida Y, Masada M, Kashiwagi A, et al. Pitavastatin restores vascular dysfunction in insulin-resistant state by inhibiting NAD(P)H oxidase activity and uncoupled endothelial nitric oxide synthase-dependent superoxide production. J Cardiovasc Pharmacol 2007;49:122–30.
[24] Schmidt-Ott KM, Kagiyama S, Phillips MI. The multiple actions of angiotensin II in atherosclerosis. Regul Pept 2000;93:65–77.
[25] Brillante DG, O'Sullivan AJ, Howes LG. Arterial stiffness in insulin resistance: the role of nitric oxide and angiotensin II receptors. Vasc Health Risk Manag 2009;5:73–8.
[26] Bendall JK, Rinze R, Adlam D, Tatham AL, De Bono J, Wilson N, et al. Endothelial Nox2 overexpression potentiates vascular oxidative stress and hemodynamic response to angiotensin II: studies in endothelial targeted Nox2 transgenic mice. Circ Res 2007;100:1016–25.
[27] Kalupahana NS, Moustaid-Moussa N. The renin-angiotensin system: a link between obesity, inflammation and insulin resistance. Obesity Rev 2011;13:136–49.
[28] Vaziri ND, Xu ZG, Shahkarami A, Huang KT, Rodriguez-Iturbe B, Natarajan R. Role of AT-1 receptor in regulation of vascular MCP-1, IL-6, PAI-1, MAP-kinase, and matrix expression in obesity. Kidney Int 2005;68:2787–93.
[29] Hotamisligil GS, Shargill NS, Spiegelman BM. Adipose expression of tumor necrosis factor-alpha: direct role in obesity-linked insulin resistance. Science 1993;259:87–91.
[30] Tanti JF, Ceppo F, Jager J, Berthou F. Implication of inflammatory signaling pathways in obesity-induced insulin resistance. Front Endocrinol 2012;3:181.
[31] Emanuela F, Grazia M, Marco de R, Maria Paola L, Giorgio F, Marco B. Inflammation as a link between obesity and metabolic syndrome. J Nutr Metab 2012;2012:476380.
[32] Kern PA, Saghizadeh M, Ong JM, Bosch RJ, Deem R, Simsolo RB. The expression of tumor necrosis factor in human adipose tissue: regulation by obesity, weight loss, and relationship to lipoprotein lipase. J Clin Invest 1995;95:2111–9.
[33] Mohamed-Ali V, Goodrick S, Rawesh A, Katz DR, Miles JM, Yudkin JS, et al. Human subcutaneous adipose tissue releases IL-6 but not TNF-a in vivo. J Clin Endocrinol Metab 1997;82:4196–200.
[34] Mendall MA, Patel P, Asante M, Ballam L, Morris J, Strachan DP, et al. Relation of serum cytokine concentrations to cardiovascular risk factors and coronary heart disease. Heart 1997;78:273–7.
[35] Halberg N, Wernstedt-Asterholm I, Scherer PE. The adipocyte as an endocrine cell. Endocrinol Metab Clin North Am 2008;37:753–68.
[36] Vielma SA, Klein RL, Levingston CA, Young MR. Adipocytes as immune regulatory cells. Int Immunopharmacol 2013;16:224–31.
[37] Tan CY, Vidal-Puig A. Adipose tissue expandability: the metabolic problems of obesity may arise from the inability to become more obese. Biochem Soc Trans 2008;36:935–40.
[38] Trayhurn P. Hypoxia and adipose tissue function and dysfunction in obesity. Physiol Rev 2013;93:1–21.
[39] Hosogai N, Fukuhara A, Oshima K, Miyata Y, Tanaka S, Segawa K, et al. Adipose tissue hypoxia in obesity and its impact on adipocytokine dysregulation. Diabetes 2007;56:901–11.
[40] Ye J, Gao Z, Yin J, He Q. Hypoxia is a potential risk factor for chronic inflammation and adiponectin reduction in adipose tissue of *ob/ob* and dietary obese mice. Am J Physiol Endocrinol Metab 2007;293:E1118–28.
[41] Rausch ME, Weisberg S, Vardhana P, Tortoriello DV. Obesity in C57BL/6J mice is characterized by adipose tissue hypoxia and cytotoxic T-cell infiltration. Int J Obes 2008;32:451–63.
[42] Trayhurn P, Wood IS. Adipokines: inflammation and the pleiotropic role of white adipose tissue. Br J Nutr 2004;92:347–55.
[43] Bachmayer C, Kemmer A, Ehrmann N, Hasenberg T, Lammert A, Hammes HP. Adipokines and endothelial dysfunction in obesity WHO°III. Microvasc Res 2013;89:129–33.
[44] Van Gaal LF, Mertens IL, De Block CE. Mechanisms linking obesity with cardiovascular disease. Nature 2006;444:875–80.
[45] Ghanim H, Aljada A, Hofmeyer D, et al. Circulating mononuclear cells in the obese are in a proinflammatory state. Circulation 2004;110:1564–71.
[46] Cancello R, Clement K. Is obesity an inflammatory illness? Role of low-grade inflammation and macrophage infiltration in human white adipose tissue. BJOG 2006;113:1141–7.
[47] Deiuliis J, Shah Z, Shah N, Needleman B, Mikami D, Narula V, et al. Visceral adipose inflammation in obesity is associated with critical alterations in T-regulatory cell numbers. PLoS ONE 2011;6:e16376.
[48] Feuerer M, Herrero L, Cipolletta D, Naaz A, Wong J, Nayer A, et al. Lean, but not obese, fat is enriched for a unique population of regulatory T cells that affect metabolic parameters. Nat Med 2009;15:930–9.
[49] Wagner NM, Brandhorst G, Czepluch F, Lankeit M, Eberle C, Herzberg S, et al. Circulating regulatory T cells are reduced in

obesity and may identify subjects at increased metabolic and cardiovascular risk. Obesity (Silver Spring) 2013;21:461–8.
[50] Hamaguchi M, Sakaguchi S. Regulatory T cells expressing PPAR-γ control inflammation in obesity. Cell Metab 2012;16:4–6.
[51] Kabon B, Nagele A, Reddy D, Eagon C, Fleshman JW, Sessler DI, et al. Obesity decreases perioperative tissue oxygenation. Anesthesiology 2004;100:274–80.
[52] Virtanen KA, Lönnroth P, Parkkola R, Peltoniemi P, Asola M, Viljanen T, Tolvanen T, et al. Glucose uptake and perfusion in subcutaneous and visceral adipose tissue during insulin stimulation in nonobese and obese humans. J Clin Endocrinol Metab 2002;87:3902–10.
[53] Chen B, Lam KS, Wang Y, Wu D, Lam MC, Shen J, et al. Hypoxia dysregulates the production of adiponectin and plasminogen activator inhibitor-1 independent of reactive oxygen species in adipocytes. Biochem Biophys Res Commun 2006;341:549–56.
[54] Lolmede K, Durand de Saint Front V, Galitzky J, Lafontan M, Bouloumie A. Effects of hypoxia on the expression of proangiogenic factors in differentiated 3T3-F442A adipocytes. Int J Obes Relat Metab Disord 2003;27:1187–95.
[55] Pasarica M, Sereda OR, Redman LM, Albarado DC, Hymel DT, Roan LE, Smith SR. Reduced adipose tissue oxygenation in human obesity: evidence for rarefaction, macrophage chemotaxis, and inflammation without an angiogenic response. Diabetes 2009;58:718–25.
[56] Koh MY, Powis G. Passing the baton: the HIF switch. Trends Biochem Sci 2012;37:364–72.
[57] Sung HK, Doh KO, Son JE, Park JG, Bae Y, Choi S, et al. Adipose vascular endothelial growth factor regulates metabolic homeostasis through angiogenesis. Cell Metab 2013;17:61–72.
[58] Paul M, Poyan Mehr A, Kreutz R. Physiology of local renin-angiotensin systems. Phys Rev 2006;86:747–803.
[59] Boustany CM, Bharadwaj K, Daugherty A, Brown DR, Randall DC, Cassis LA. Activation of the systemic and adipose renin-angiotensin system in rats with diet-induced obesity and hypertension. Am J Physiol Regul Int Comp Physiol 2004;287:R943–9.
[60] West DB, Prinz WA, Francendese AA, Greenwood MR. Adipocyte blood flow is decreased in obese Zucker rats. Am J Physiol 1987;253:R228–33.
[61] Drexler H. Endothelial dysfunction: clinical implications. Prog Cardiovasc Dis 1997;39:287–324.
[62] Ross R. Atherosclerosis—an inflammatory disease. N Engl J Med 1999;340:115–26.
[63] Libby P. Inflammation in atherosclerosis. Nature 2002;420:868–74.
[64] Romano M, Sironi M, Toniatti C, Polentarutti N, Fruscella P, Ghezzi P, et al. Role of IL-6 and its soluble receptor in induction of chemokines and leukocytes recruitment. Immunity 1997;6:315–25.
[65] Edens HA, Parkos CA. Modulation of epithelial and endothelial paracellular permeability by leukocytes. Adv Drug Deliv Rev 2000;41:315–28.
[66] Wojciak-Stothard B, Entwistle A, Garg R, Ridley AJ. Regulation of TNF-alpha-induced reorganization of the actin cytoskeleleton and cell-cell junctions by Rho, rac, and Cdc42 in human endothelial cells. J Cell Physiol 1998;176:150–65.
[67] Koh KK, Han SH, Quon MJ. Inflammatory markers and the metabolic syndrome. J Am Coll Cardiol 2005;46:1978–85.
[68] Petersen AMW, Pedersen BK. The role of IL-6 in mediating the anti-inflammatory effects of exercise. J Physiol Pharmacol 2006;57(suppl. 10):43–51.
[69] Bouvet C, Belin de Chantemele E, Guilhot AL, Vessiere E, Bocquet A, Dumont O, Jardel A, et al. Flow-induced remodeling in resistance arteries from obese Zucker rats is associated with endothelial dysfunction. Hypertension 2007;50:248–54.
[70] Erdei N, Toth A, Pasztor ET, Papp Z, Edes I, Koller A, et al. High-fat diet-iduced reduction in nitric oxide-dependent arteriolar dilation in rats: role of xanthine oxidase-derived superoxide anion. Am J Physiol 2006;291:H2107–15.
[71] Payne GA, Borbouse L, Kumar S, Neeb Z, Alloosh M, Sturek M, et al. Epicardial perivascular adipose-derived leptin exacerbates coronary endothelial dysfunction in metabolic syndrome via e protein kinase C-beta pathway. Arterioscler Thromb Vasc Biol 2010;30:1711–7.
[72] Donato AJ, Henson GD, Morgan RG, Ene RA, Walker AE, Lesniewski LA. TNF-α impairs endothelial function in adipose tissue resistance arteries of mice with diet-induced obesity. Am J Physiol 2012;303:H672–9.
[73] Farb MG, Ganley-Leal L, Mott M, Liang Y, Ercan B, Widlansky ME, et al. Arteriolar function in visceral adipose tissue is impaired in human obesity. Arterioscler Thromb Vasc Biol 2012;32:467–73.
[74] Vila E, Salaices M. Cytokines and vascular reactivity in resistance arteries. Am J Physiol 2005;288:H1016–21.
[75] Kim F, Gallis B, Corson MA. TNF-α inhibits flow and insulin signaling leading to NO production in aortic endothelial cells. Am J Physiol 2001;280:C1057–65.
[76] Zhang H, Park Y, Wu J, Chen X, Lee S, Yang J, et al. Role of TNF-alpha in vascular dysfunction. Clin Sci (London) 2009;116:219–30.
[77] Wei M, Kampert JB, Barlow CE, Nichaman MZ, Gibbons LW, Paffenbarger RS, et al. Relationship between low cardiorespiratory fitness and Akt in normal-weight, overweight, and obese men. JAMA 1999;282:1547–53.
[78] Roberts CK, Barnard RJ. Effects of exercise and diet on chronic diseases. J Appl Physiol 2005;98:3–30.
[79] Lavrencic A, Salobir BG, Keber I. Physical training improves flow-mediated dilation in patients with the polymetabolic syndrome. Arterioscler Thromb Vasc Biol 2000;20:551–5.
[80] Watts K, Beye P, Siafarikas A, Davis EA, Jones TW, O'Driscoll G, et al. Exercise training normalizes vascular dysfunction and improves central adiposity in obese adolescents. J Am Coll Cardiol 2004;43:1823–7.
[81] Mestek ML, Westby CM, Van Guilder GP, Greiner JJ, Stauffer BL, DeSouza CA. Regular aerobic exercise, without weight loss, improves endothelium-dependent vasodilation in overweight and obese adults. Obesity (Silver Spring) 2010;18:1667–9.
[82] Hamdy O, Ledbury S, Mullooly C, Jarema C, Porter S, Ovalle K, et al. Lifestyle modification improves endothelial function in obese subjects with the insulin resistance syndrome. Diabetes Care 2003;26:2119–25.
[83] De Filippis E, Cusi K, Ocampo G, Berria R, Buck S, Consoli A, et al. Exercise-induced improvement in vasodilatory function accompanies increased insulin sensitivity in obesity and type 2 diabetes mellitus. J Clin Endocrinol Metab 2006;91:4903–10.
[84] Schjerve IE, Tyldum GA, Tjonna AE, Stolen T, Loennechen JP, Hansen HE, et al. Both aerobic endurance and strength training programmes improve cardiovascular health in obese adults. Clin Sci (Lond) 2008;115:283–93.
[85] Pasqualini L, Schillaci G, Innocente S, Pucci G, Coscia F, Siepi D, et al. Lifestyle intervention improves microvascular reactivity and increases serum adiponectin in overweight hypertensive patients. Nutr Metab Cardiovasc Dis 2010;20:87–92.
[86] Stensvold D, Tjønna AE, Skaug EA, Aspenes S, Stølen T, Wisløff U, et al. Strength training versus aerobic interval training to modify risk factors of metabolic syndrome. J Appl Physiol 2010;108:804–10.
[87] Touati S, Meziri F, Devaux S, Berthelot A, Touyz RM, Laurant P. Exercise reverses metabolic syndrome in high-fat diet-induced obese rats. Med Sci Sports Exerc 2011;43:398–407.
[88] Pinheiro AR, Cunha AR, Aguila MB, Mandarin-de-Lacerba CA. Beneficial effects of physical exercise on hypertension and

cardiovascular adverse remodeling of diet-induced obese rats. Nutr Metab Cardiovasc Dis 2007;17:365–75.

[89] Franzoni F, Ghiadoni L, Galetta F, Plantinga Y, Lubrano V, Huang Y, et al. Physical activity, plasma antioxidant capacity, and endothelium-dependent vasodilation in young and older men. Am J Hypertens 2005;18:510–6.

[90] Hambrecht R, Adams V, Erbs S, Linke A, Kränkel N, Shu Y, et al. Regular physical activity improve endothelial function in patients with coronary artery disease by increasing phosphorylation on endothelial nitric oxide synthase. Circulation 2003;107:3152–8.

[91] Pellegrin M, Alonso F, Aubert JF, Bouzourene K, Braunersreuther V, Mach F, et al. Swimming prevents vulnerable atherosclerotic plaque development in hypertensive 2-kidney, 1-clip mice by modulating angiotensin II type 1 receptor expression independently from hemodynamic changes. Hypertension 2009;53:782–9.

[92] Agarwal D, Haque M, Sriramula S, Mariappan N, Pariaut R, Francis J. Role of proinflammatory cytokines and redox homeostasis in exercise-induced delayed progression of hypertension in spontaneously hypertensive rats. Hypertension 2009;54:1393–400.

[93] Ramkhelawon B, Vilar J, Rivas D, Mees D, De Crom R, Tedgui A, et al. Shear stress regulates angiotensin type 1 receptor expression in endothelial cells. Circ Res 2009;105:869–75.

[94] Szostak J, Laurant P. The forgotten face of regular physical exercise: a natural anti-atherogenic activity. Clin Sci (London) 2011;121:91–106.

[95] Brrunsgaard H. Physical activity and modulation of systemic low-level inflammation. J Leukocyte Biol 2005;78:819–35.

[96] Gomez-Merino D, Drogou C, Guezennec CY, Chennaoui M. Effect of chronic exercise on cytokine production in white adipose tissue and skeletal muscle of rats. Cytokine 2007;40:23–9.

[97] Lira FS, Rosa JC, Yamashita AS, Koyama CH, Batista ML, Seelaender M. Endurance training induces depot-specific changes in IL-10/TNF-alpha ratio in rays adipose tissue. Cytokine 2009;45:80–5.

[98] Bradley RL, Jeon JY, Liu FF, Maratos-Flier E. Voluntary exercise improves insulin sensitivity and adipose tissue inflammation in diet-induced obese mice. Am J Physiol 2008;295:E586–94.

[99] Viera VJ, Valentine RJ, Wilund KR, Antao N, Baynard T, Woods JA. Effect of exercise and low-fat diet on adipose tissue inflammation and metabolic complications in obese mice. Am J Physiol 2009;296:E1164–71.

[100] Leick L, Lindegaard B, Stensvold D, Plomgaard P, Saltin B, Pilegaard H. Adipose tissue interleukin-18 mRNA and plasma interleukin-18/ effect of obesity and exercise. Obesity 2007;15:356–63.

[101] Chrstiansen T, Paulsen SK, Bruun JM, Pedersen SB, Richelsen B. Exercise training versus diet-induced weight-loss on metabolic risk factor and inflammatory markers in obese subjects: a 12-week randomized intervention study. Am J Physiol 2010;298:E824–31.

[102] Di Franscicomarino S, Sciartilli A, Di Valerio V, Di Baldassarre A, Gallina S. The effect of physical exercise on endothelial function. Sport Med 2009;39:797–812.

[103] Rector RS, Turk JR, Sun GY, Guilford BL, Toedebusch BW, McClanahan MW, et al. Short-term lifestyle modification alters circulating biomarkers of endothelial health in sedentary, overweight adults. Appl Physiol Nutr Metab 2006;31:512–7.

[104] Yang AL, Chen HI. Chronic exercise reduces adhesion molecules/iNOS expression and partially reverses vascular responsiveness in hypercholesterolemic rabbit aortae. Atherosclerosis 2003;169:11–17.

[105] Kawanishi N, Yano H, Yokogawa Y, Suzuki K. Exercise training inhibits inflammation in adipose tissue via both suppression of macrophage infiltration and acceleration of phenotypic swithching from M1 to M2 macrophages in high-fat-diet-induced obese mice. Exerc Immunol Rev 2010;16:105–18.

[106] You T, Arsenis NC, Disanzo BL, LaMonte MJ. Effects of exercise training on chronic inflammation in obesity. Current evidence and potential mechanisms. Sports Med 2013;43:243–56.

[107] Pedersen BK. The diseasome of physical inactivity and the role of myokines in muscle-fat cross talk. J Physiol 2009;587:5559–68.

[108] Steenberg A, Fischer CP, Keller C, Moller K, Pedersen BK. IL-6 enhances plasma IL-1Ra and IL-10, and cortisol in humans. Am J Physiol Endocrinol Metab 2003;285:E433–7.

PARTE

DIETARY FOODS AND VISCERAL FAT ACCUMULATION AND REMOVAL

CHAPTER

22

Fermented Soypastes, *Doenjang* and *Cheonggukjang*, and Obesity

Myoungsook Lee[a] *and Yongsoon Park*[b]

[a]Department of Food and Nutrition, and Research Institute of Obesity Sciences, Sungshin Women's University, Seoul, Korea; [b]Department of Food and Nutrition, Hanyang University, Seoul, Korea

SOYBEAN AND FERMENTED SOYPASTE

Soybean, a legume species native to East Asia, has been consumed for the past 5000 years in Asia. Soybean contains complex carbohydrates, unsaturated fatty acids, vegetable protein, soluble fiber, oligosaccharides, vitamins, minerals, inositol-derived substances (such as lipintol and pinitol), and phytoestrogens, particularly the isoflavones genistein, daidzein, and glycitein [1,2]. The isoflavones in soybeans have been shown to correlate with their antioxidative, antitumor, antihypertensive, antiosteoporotic, and antiobesity functions [3–7].

Soybeans contain 0.1–5 mg/g of total isoflavones, primarily daidzein, genistein, and glycitein in their biologically inactive glucosidic forms [8]. Once ingested, isoflavone glycosides are readily digested into the biologically active aglycone forms in the intestinal tract [9]. In fact, daidzein, equol, genistein, and *O*-demethyangolensin are the major isoflavones detected in the blood and urine of humans and animals [10].

In contrast, the process of fermentation converts the soybean polyphenols, isoflavones, into the more active compounds, daidzein and genistein [11,12]. Various types of fermented soybean foods are consumed in Asian countries, including China, Indonesia, Japan, Korea, and Vietnam. The most common Korean fermented soybean foods are *Cheonggukjang*, *Doenjang*, *Kochujang*, and soy sauce. *Natto* and *Miso* are the Japanese equivalents of *Cheonggukjang* and *Doenjang*, respectively. China also has various fermented soybean products such as *Dajiang*, *Doubanjiang*, *Douchi*, sweet noodle sauce, *Tauchu*, and yellow soybean paste.

Doenjang has been traditionally manufactured from fermented *meju* formed into regular shapes molded from crushed cooked soybeans. The main microorganisms involved in the fermentation of *meju* are *Bacillus subtilis* and molds such as *Aspergillus*, *Mucor*, and *Rhizopus* spp. [11,12]. When the *meju*-brine mixture is fully fermented, it is separated into liquid and solid parts [11]. The liquid is filtered, boiled, and used as soy sauce; the crushed solids are further ripened in a separated pottery container for 2–6 months, and become *Doenjang*.

The longer the fermentation process, the less acetyl, glycosidyl, malonyl isoflavonoids are present and the more isoflavonoid aglycones, daidzein and genistein, are formed (by 10- to 100-fold) [13]. In fact, *Doenjang* supplementation provides approximately 20–30 mg of isoflavones daily, increasing their plasma concentration up to 300 nM, the typical amount present in oral ingested therapeutics [14].

Another form of traditional Korean fermented soybean food, *Cheonggukjang*, is made from rice straw and boiled soybean using bacterial inoculums. *Cheonggukjang* is predominantly fermented with *B. subtilis* for short periods (approximately 2 days) without salt or other seasoning [15], and has distinct characteristics when compared to *Doenjang*. In addition to the preexisting compounds in soybean, metabolites produced during *Cheonggukjang* fermentation are responsible for its characteristic fragrance and taste [16]. During the fermentation of *Cheonggukjang*, soybean isoflavones are converted from glycosides into their corresponding aglycones, of which most are degraded into small peptides and amino acids [17,18]. *Cheonggukjang* and *Doenjang* were registered on Codex on 4 July 2009 and have since become increasingly present on the world market.

Nutrition in the Prevention and Treatment of Abdominal Obesity
http://dx.doi.org/10.1016/B978-0-12-407869-7.00022-2

ANTIOBESITY EFFECTS OF ISOFLAVONES

The low frequency of obesity and related metabolic disorders in Asian populations has drawn attention to soy, a characteristic component of Asian diets. The antiobesity effect of genistein, the principal soy isoflavone, has been reported in experimental animals fed with diets containing the isoflavone [19]. Although controversy surrounds their efficacy in promoting weight loss, soy products have been shown to increase energy expenditure relative to carbohydrates in overweight men [20].

Several studies have also reported that isoflavone consumption by postmenopausal women correlate with lower body mass index (BMI) and higher high-density lipoprotein (HDL) cholesterol levels [21–23]. Wu et al. [23] observed that postmenopausal Japanese women treated for 24 weeks with isoflavones exhibited a lower fat mass, and Allison et al. [24] also reported that obese patients treated with soy protein isolates for 12 weeks had lower body weight and BMI with decreased serum levels of cholesterol and low-density lipoprotein (LDL) cholesterol.

In contrast, a significant number of studies have reported an absence of beneficial effects of soybean on body weight [25–27]. These may be explained by differences in ethnic background, baseline BMI, gender distribution, and previous weight loss in study populations, as well as differences in experimental design. Additionally, inconsistent results may partly be due to the type of soy or soy product used, such as the type of isoflavones, soybeans, or fermented soypaste. Previous studies suggested that the fermented soypastes, *Cheonggukjang* and *Doenjang*, contain greater amounts of bioactive isoflavones than soybean and bioinactive isoflavones and have a greater effect on obesity in animal models [11,12]. Although it is difficult to draw any conclusions regarding the effect of fermented soypaste on obesity, the underlying cause of the conflicting results may be related to the fermentation process.

MECHANISMS INVOLVED IN FERMENTED SOYPASTE ANTIOBESITY ACTIVITY

The mechanisms by which soy isoflavones reduce adiposity are unclear. However, isoflavones may provide health benefits through their selective estrogen receptor (ER) modulatory activities [28]. By specifically binding to ERs, isoflavones can elicit both estrogenic and antiestrogenic effects depending on the type of tissue, as well as on isoflavone and endogenous estradiol levels. For instance, in various cell lines treated with physiological levels (1 nM) of estradiol, genistein acted as an antiestrogen, whereas at levels of estradiol found in postmenopausal women (0.01 nM), genistein showed additive agonistic effects [29].

Estrogen is reported to affect adiposity either directly by modulating lipogenesis, lipolysis, or adipogenesis or indirectly by modulating appetite or energy expenditure [30]. The idea that estrogen modulates metabolic features was originally derived from the observation that postmenopausal women develop visceral obesity and insulin resistance as a result of low levels of estrogens, whereas hormone replacement therapy normalized these symptoms [31,32]. Estrogen also plays an important role in glucose homeostasis, and is known to modulate insulin sensitivity [33]. Variations in human glucose homeostasis are observed during the menstrual cycle, and diabetes becomes more resistant to treatment during the luteal phase [34]. Individuals with mutations in genes encoding aromatases, enzymes that convert androgens to estrogens, also display truncal obesity, insulin resistance, and hyperlipidemia [35]. In addition, mice lacking genes encoding either ERα or aromatase have increased adiposity and fatty liver [35]. Genistein and daidzein prevent hyperglycemia via reducing hepatic gluconeogenesis and lipogenesis [36]. An in vitro study also showed that daidzein exerts its insulin-sensitizing actions in 3T3-L1 adipocytes by activating peroxisome proliferator-activated receptor gamma (PPAR-γ), the central regulator of insulin and glucose metabolism [37].

An in vitro study using isolated rat adipocytes showed that genistein stimulates lipolysis through the inhibition of cyclic AMP (cAMP) phosphodiesterases; it has a greater inhibitory effect than estrogen [38]. Fats in adipocytes are broken down by hormone-sensitive lipase; the activation of this enzyme is stimulated by protein kinase A and is preceded by elevated cAMP. In vitro studies also reported that genistein enhances the expression of genes involved in fatty acid catabolism by activating PPAR-α [39,40]. In Sprague-Dawley rats fed a high-fat diet, *Doenjang* prevented diet-induced visceral fat accumulation due to increased carnitine *O*-palmitoyltransferase 1 (CPT-1) and decreased fatty acid synthase (FAS) activity. CPT-1 is a rate-limiting enzyme in the beta-oxidation pathway, where its lipogenic capacities in both liver and adipose tissue are controlled by FAS, a multiunit enzyme complex that catalyzes the synthesis of long-chain fatty acids from acetyl coenzyme A (acetyl-CoA) and malonyl-CoA. Suh et al. [41] also observed that expression of *S1c27a2* and *S1c27a5* [encoding the fatty acid transport proteins (FATPs; solute carrier family 27 proteins), very long-chain acyl-CoA synthetase and bile acyl-CoA synthetase, respectively] is also dysregulated by *Cheonggukjang* consumption in mice with diet-induced obesity.

Estrogens have been shown to modulate energy homeostasis indirectly through the central nervous system (CNS) and the hypothalamus. Although how soy-derived compounds modulate energy expenditure via the CNS is unclear, recent data suggest that some effects may be centrally mediated. Recently, it was found that increased energy expenditure and locomotor activity, coupled with a shift toward the use of lipids as a fuel source, were important contributory factors for the leanness observed in mice exposed to dietary phytoestrogens [42]. In mice or rats fed soy-rich diets, the feeding behavior and locomotor activity were significantly affected, suggesting that the central regulation of energy balance in the hypothalamus may be modulated by soy or phytoestrogens [42,43]. For example, in mice exposed to dietary soy, the increased locomotor activity and preferential use of lipids as a fuel source is associated with a 40% decrease in the levels of *Agrp* mRNA [encoding agouti-related protein (AgRP)] in the hypothalamus [42]. AgRP is a key neuropeptide that regulates energy expenditure in the arcuate nucleus of the hypothalamus [44]. Mice lacking AgRP or with a 50% reduction in AgRP levels in the hypothalamus display an increased metabolic rate, lipid utilization, and locomotor activity [45,46]. In a similar study, rats exposed to the same soy-based diet exhibited an approximately 40% higher expression of *Npy* transcripts [encoding neuropeptide Y (NPY)] in the arcuate and paraventricular nuclei of the hypothalamus. NPY is an orexigenic neuropeptide known to stimulate food intake in both rodents and humans [47].

The decrease in fat abundance correlated with increased activation of both 5′-AMP-activated protein kinase (AMPK) and its downstream target acetyl-CoA carboxylase (ACC), two regulator enzymes of fatty acid oxidation, in peripheral tissues. In these mice, two targets of AMPK, PPAR-γ coactivator-1-alpha (PGC-1α) and PPAR-α, which regulate mitochondrial and peroxisomal metabolism respectively, were preferentially upregulated in adipose tissue [48]. In fact, glyceollin-containing fermented soybeans [49] and *Cheonggukjang* [50] increased AMPK and acetyl-CoA in the liver of diabetic mice, and improved both insulin sensitivity and glucose metabolism. The effect of fermented soypastes on obesity mediated by estrogen mimics remains controversial.

In the case of obesity-induced inflammatory responses, adipocyte cell division is associated with the increased presence of intrinsic fat globules due to inflammatory responses or macrophage infiltration. In the initial phase of adipocytic division, tumor necrosis factor (TNF-α) stimulates preadipocyte and endothelial cells to secrete C-C motif chemokine 2 [monocyte chemoattractant protein 1 (MCP-1)], thus inducing the recruitment and accumulation of macrophages in the adipocyte. During this process, body weight is increased due to the increased presence of adipocytes. As a result of the increase in cytokines such as interleukin-6 (IL-6), IL-1β, and TNF-α, insulin resistance also develops [51]. It is known that isoflavones and phytochemicals suppress the secretion of inflammatory cytokines that results from the interaction between adipocytes and macrophages [52–54]. *Doenjang*, derived from black soybeans, modulated the production of cytokines, including IL-2, IL-6, and TNF-α, and showed an anticancer effect. This effect was increased with a longer duration of fermentation. [55]

ANTIOBESITY EFFECTS OF FERMENTED SOYPASTES IN RODENTS

Most of the previous studies have evaluated the effect of soy or isoflavones on adiposity in rodents and suggested that a soy-rich diet or supplementation with genistein can reduce both weight and adipose tissue deposition [28,56–58]. Penza et al. [58] reported that fat mass was increased in mice given daily oral doses of genistein of up to 50 mg/kg/day, but was decreased at doses of 200 mg/kg/day, suggesting that high pharmacological doses of soy-derived phytoestrogens in the micromolar range inhibit adipose tissue deposition. The high pharmacological doses of isoflavones can easily be obtained from fermented soypastes, but only a limited number of studies have evaluated the effect of fermented soypastes on obesity.

Current evidence concerning the role of fermented soy in rodents is based on studies in which animals have been exposed to fermented soy supplemented in the diet itself (Table 22.1). Diets containing 5–40% fermented soypastes, in the form of *Cheonggukjang*, *Doenjang*, and *meju*, decreased body weight or adiposity in high-fat diet-induced obese or diabetic rodents [41,50,59–62]. Body weight was significantly lower in Sprague-Dawley rats and C57BL/6J mice fed with 5% [61] and 40% *Cheonggukjang* [41] in a high-fat diet than in those fed a high-fat diet without *Cheonggukjang*. In addition, the presence of 10% and 20% *Doenjang* in a high-fat diet significantly decreased body weight in C57BL/6J mice [60] and Sprague-Dawley rats [59], compared with controls fed a high-fat diet without *Doenjang*. Kwak et al. [59] reported that *Doenjang* reduced not only body weight gain but also liver weight and hepatic triglyceride and cholesterol content. There was a greater significant reduction of fat depots and adipocyte size in the *Doenjang*-supplemented group than in the soybean group, with no significant differences on body weight gain. The stronger effect of *Doenjang* than of soybean may be associated with increased CPT-1 activity and decreases FAS activity in liver caused by the increased level of aglycone isoflavones synthesized during fermentation [59].

However, feeding Sprague-Dawley rats a high-fat diet containing 5% *Doenjang* [61] and streptozotocin-induced diabetic C57BL/6J mice a diet containing 10% fermented soybean powder in [49] had no significant effect on body

TABLE 22.1 Animal Studies Using Dietary Supplementation with Fermented Soy

Species	Duration	Dose	Compound	Weight	Reference
Sprague-Dawley rats	6 weeks	5%, in high-fat diet	*Doenjang*	No effect	Choi et al. [61]
			Cheonggukjang	Lower body weight	
Sprague-Dawley rats	8 weeks	20%, in high-fat diet	*Doenjang*	Lower body weight	Kwak et al. [59]
C57BL/6J mice	8 weeks	10%, in high-fat diet	*Doenjang*	Lower body weight	Park et al. [60]
C57BL/6J mice	9 weeks	40%, in high-fat diet	*Cheonggukjang*	Lower body weight	Soh et al. [41]
Streptozotocin-induced diabetic C57BL/6J mice	8 weeks	10%, in normal diet	Fermented soybean powder (0.009% isoflavonoid aglycones; 0.0014% glyceollins; 0.012% total isoflavone)	No effect	Park et al. [49]
Pancreatectomized C57BL/6J mice	8 weeks	10%, in normal diet	*Meju* (0.005 and 0.01% isoflavonoid aglycones; 0.011 and 0.014% total isoflavone)	No effect on body weight, but reduced epididymal fat pads	Yang et al. [62]
Pancreatectomized Sprague-Dawley rats	8 weeks	10%, in normal diet	*Cheonggukjang* (0.014% isoflavonoid aglycones; 0.026% total isoflavone)	No effect on body weight, but reduced epididymal fat pads	Yang et al. [50]
Pancreatectomized Sprague-Dawley rats	8 weeks	50%, in high-fat diet	*Cheonggukjang* (0.015% isoflavonoid aglycones; 0.027% total isoflavone)	No effect	Kwon et al. [65]

weight. Choi et al. [61] suggested that 5% *Cheonggukjang* but not *Doenjang* led to decreased body weight in Sprague-Dawley rats because of the higher isoflavone aglycone levels present in *Cheonggukjang* compared with *Doenjang*. Lee at al. [63] reported that isoflavone aglycone levels in soybean were increased in both *Cheonggukjang* and *Doenjang*, with the highest levels being present in *Cheonggukjang*. During fermentation, soybean glycosides are hydrolyzed by beta-glucosidase secreted by microorganisms, resulting in the formation of active aglycones and the promotion of intestinal absorption [11,12]. In addition, a diet containing 10% *Cheonggukjang* and *meju* had no effect on body weight but significantly reduced epididymal fat pads in pancreatectomized C57BL/6J mice [64] and Sprague-Dawley rats [50].

Some traditionally made *Cheonggukjang* lacks consistent efficacy as a functional food because its activity varies according to conditions under which it is prepared such as regional differences in the prevalent microorganisms. In traditionally made *Cheonggukjang*, *B. subtilis* is the major microorganism, but *B. amylofenices* and *B. lichemiformis* may also be present. *Cheonggukjang* fermented with *B. subtilis* and *B. amylofenices* had no effect on body weight or adiposity [64], but *Cheonggukjang* fermented with *B. lichemiformis* reduced body fat [50]. *Cheonggukjang* fermented with *B. lichemiformis* was more effective in increasing insulin-stimulated glucose uptake in 3T3-L1 adipocytes and glucose-stimulated insulin secretion in insulinoma cell than that made with *B. subtilis* [64]. Yang et al. [50] also observed that *Cheonggukjang* fermented with *B. subtilis* and *B. amylofenices* had less antidiabetic activity than *Cheonggukjang* fermented with *B. lichemiformis*. These differences may be related to changes in isoflavonoids and peptides in different *Cheonggukjang* preparations, since the isoflavonoid and peptide patterns of *Cheonggukjang* fermented with *B. subtilis* are similar to those of *Cheonggukjang* fermented with *B. lichemiformis* [50]. Total amounts of isoflavonoid aglycones were higher in all *Cheonggukjang* preparations compared to in unfermented soybeans, but their bioavailability and bioactivity are expected to be increased in *Cheonggukjang* fermented with *B. lichemiformis* [50]. In addition, 1–1.5kDa peptide profiles of *Cheonggukjang* fermented with *B. lichemiformis*, but not with *B. subtilis* or *B. amylofenices*, appears to be associated with improved insulin sensitivity [50]. Kwon et al. [65] previously showed that 3kDa peptides do not contribute to the antidiabetic activity of fermented soybeans. Thus, it is reasonable to conclude that *B. lichemiformis* may be one of the major microorganisms responsible for the functional benefits of *Cheonggukjang* fermented soybeans.

Data on isoflavone levels and bioactive composition are incomplete, but Yang et al. [50,62] reported that 0.005–0.014% bioactive isoflavonoid aglycones were included in their experimental diet. Thus, the questions of (1) which compound is responsible for the observed effects and (2) whether the relative benefits of fermented soy are in fact due to the relatively poor performance of casein, which is usually used as a control, are yet to be answered.

Yang et al. [50] investigated whether there was a dose-dependent effect of fermented soy on adiposity and did not observe any significant differences between 0.005% and 0.01% isoflavonoid aglycones in diet. Pyo and Seong [66] also reported that oral administration of fermented soybean extracts at 200 or 400 mg/kg decreased body weight in a dose-independent manner in rats. Although further research is needed to confirm the dose-dependent effect of fermented soy on adiposity, beneficial effects of the fermented soypastes, *Cheonggukjang* and *Doenjang*, on adiposity in rodents are caused by fermentation enhancing soy bioactivity.

ANTIOBESITY EFFECTS OF FERMENTED SOYPASTES IN HUMANS

Many clinical studies of soybean products in obese population have focused on the use of soy protein or soy protein isolates (SPIs) as calorie replacements in antiobesity treatments (Table 22.2). For instance, a meta-analysis of 38 trials as well as more recent reports demonstrated a significant reduction in plasma total cholesterol (TC) and LDL cholesterol in individuals exposed to soy proteins [67,68]. Obese patients fed with SPIs for 12 weeks had a lower body weight and BMI, with decreased TC and LDL cholesterol [24]. An SPI diet decreased body weight, serum TC, LDL cholesterol, very-low-density lipoprotein cholesterol, and triacylglycerol (TG), compared with a casein diet, in both obese and normal subjects [69]. Soy protein may have a greater benefit than casein for patients who need to take a hypocaloric diet for long periods. As a consequence of the low energy values and the high quantity of essential amino acids in soybeans, obese subjects who consumed soy protein had a greater weight loss rather than who consumed a meat-protein diet [20,70]. However, a significant number of studies have reported an absence of beneficial effects of soy on classical obese parameters [71–73].

Beneficial effects on obese metabolic parameters were shown not only for soy protein but also for the isoflavones present in soy products and their aglycones such as cyanidin, daidzein, genistein, and glycitein [37]. Postmenopausal Japanese women treated for 24 weeks with isoflavones exhibited a lower body fat mass [23]. In a 6-month clinical trial among postmenopausal Taiwanese women, glucose and insulin levels were significantly reduced by soy isoflavones (100 mg/day) and conjugated estrogens (0.625 mg/day) [74]. Daidzein and genistein may enhance insulin sensitivity and plasma HDL cholesterol and decrease BMI [22,27]. However, many studies in postmenopausal women showed no significant changes in lipid profiles and the reduction in body fat in those who consumed 50-150 mg/day isoflavones for up to 6 months [75–77]. These contradictory results may be explained by two recent meta-analyses [78,79]. Eleven randomized controlled trials showed that soy isoflavones significantly lowered lipid profiles without changing HDL cholesterol levels [78]. Another meta-analysis of eight randomized controlled trials has shown that the beneficial effects of isoflavones on hyperinsulinemia and hyperlipidemia were greater when these compounds ingested along with soybean protein [79]. Based on these meta-analyses, clinical trials now should be conducted to demonstrate the dose-dependent or interaction effects of soybean components. Furthermore, equol was produced following daidzein ingestion in at least 30–40% of the study population; it was readily absorbed and had strong estrogenic activity. Asians produced more equol than Westerners, which may contribute to the lower incidences of obesity and related diseases in the Asian population [80].

In many studies, the antiobesigenic and antiatherogenic properties of soybean products or extracts have been demonstrated; however, only a few human studies of fermented soybean products have been conducted. In a 12-week randomized double-blind, placebo-controlled study, *Doenjang* (9.9 g dry weight/day) reduced fat mass and, in particular, visceral fat area ($-8.6\,cm^2$), as measured by CT, compared to control ($-0.6\,cm^2$) in overweight and obese Koreans (BMI ≥ 23, waist-hip ratio ≥ 0.9), but subcutaneous fat mass was not changed [81]. Although *Doenjang* was used as a whole food in this study, the high level of isoflavones in *Doenjang* may be the determining factor in decreasing visceral fat. Unfortunately, the concentration of serum isoflavone, in particular genistein, was not measured. However, the 9.9 g dry weight used in this study is equivalent to 40 g wet weight, which is roughly equivalent to three bowls of *Doenjang* soup containing approximately 20–30 mg of isoflavones (containing 8.57 mg aglycones) per day [13]. This amount produces plasma isoflavone concentrations of around 200–300 nM, which is typical of many orally ingested therapeutics [14]. Moreover, both cholesterol-lowering [by inhibition of 3-hydroxy-3-methylglutaryl-coenzyme A reductase (HMG-CoA reductase)] and TG-lowering substances isolated from *Doenjang* were identified as aglycones [82]. Since the aglycone forms of isoflavones are more effectively absorbed than the glycoside forms, research into the bioavailability of aglycones whether consumed as pure compounds or as whole foods will be necessary in the future. Another possibility

TABLE 22.2 Beneficial Effects of Soybean Products on Obesity: Intervention Studies

Sources	Subjects	Dose and Duration	Effects	References
Soy protein or SPI	Obese men and women	SPI vs. control	Lower body weight, BMI, TC, LDL	Allison et al. [24]
	Overweight/obese men and women	SPI vs. milk	No effects on body weight, FBS, TC, LDL, HDL, TG	Anderson [67]
	Obese men and women	SPI vs. meat	No effects on weight, fat, BMI, FBS, TC, LDL, HDL, TG	Yamashita et al. [71]
	Obese men and women	SPI vs. individual diets	Lower body weight, fat, BMI, FBS No effects on insulin, TC, LDL, HDL, TG.	Li et al. [73]
	Obese men and women	Soy protein vs. casein (375–425 kcal/day, 60–70 days)	Lower body weight, greater reduction in TC and TG	Bosello et al. [69]
	Randomized	Soy protein vs. animal protein (28–29%, 4 days)	Lower 24-h energy expenditure	Mikkelsen et al. [20]
Phytochemicals	Postmenopausal women	Soy protein (15 g with 150 mg/day isoflavones) vs. casein (15 g with 10 mg/day isoflavones)	No effects on body weight, fat, BMI, FBS, insulin, TC, LDL, HDL, TG	Anderson et al. [27]
	Postmenopausal women	Isoflavones, 75 mg/day, 6 months	Lower BMI, body fat, HDLc	Wu et al. [23]
	Postmenopausal women	Isoflavones 150 mg/day, 6 months	No effects on body fat and HDLc	Hsu et al. [75]
	Postmenopausal women	Genistein, >1 mg/day	Lower body fat, WC, HDLc	Goodman-Gruen et al. [22]
	Postmenopausal women	Genistein, 0.001-0.999 mg/day	Lower HDLc and FBS	Anderson et al. [27]
	Obese	Pregnane, 1 g/day, 60 days	2.5% reduction in food intake	
	Obese	Phytosterol, 257 mg/day, 8 weeks	23% reduction in body weight	Kuriyan [95], Oben [96]
Fermented soybean paste	Overweight and obese men/women	*Doenjang*, 9.9 g/day, 12 weeks	Lower body weight, fat, visceral fat (CT); no effects on lipid profiles and subcutaneous fat	Cha et al. [81]
	Overweight and obese men/women with UCP 1 (wild A; 39.2/mutant T; 60.8%)	*Doenjang* 9.9 g/day, 12 weeks	Lower visceral fat and higher FFA in mutant G allele	Lee et al. [88]
	Overweight and obese men/women with PPAR-r (wild C; 81.6/mutant T; 18.4%)	*Doenjang*, 9.9 g/day, 12 weeks	Lower visceral fat and higher FFA levels in mutant T allele; activated radical clearance capacity	Cha et al. [89]
	Overweight and obese men/women	*Cheonggukjang*, 26 g/day, 12 weeks	Lower ApoB and visceral fat (CT)	Back et al. [83]

BMI, body mass index; CT, computed tomography; FBS, fasting blood sugar; FFA, free fatty acid; LDL, low-density lipoprotein; HDL, high-density lipoprotein; HDLc, HDL cholesterol; TC, total cholesterol; TG, triglycerides; WHR, waist-hip ratio.

was that genistein enhances *CPT1* transcription and activates PPAR-α, which is involved in fatty acid beta-oxidation [39]. In the same trial design with 60 subjects, *Cheonggukjang* supplementation (26 g/day) for 12 weeks in overweight adults showed potential antiatherosclerotic and antiobesogenic effects. *Cheonggukjang* treatment led to a significant improvement in apolipoprotein B (ApoB) levels ($P < 0.05$) compared to the placebo group, but there was no significant reduction in visceral fat compared to *Doenjang* [83]. *Doenjang* has more beneficial properties, including anticancer, antihypertensive, and antimutagenic activities, than raw soybeans, cooked soybeans, and other fermented soybeans (including *Cheonggukjang*) [84–86]. The anticancer and antimetastatic properties of *Doenjang* increased with time during a 24-month fermentation [84]. In addition, some compounds derived from *Doenjang* have been shown to have a high activity in reducing blood pressure through inhibition of angiotensin-converting enzyme (ACE) [87].

Some reports have examined whether the effects of *Doenjang* on antiobesity are sustained in subjects harboring polymorphisms in antiobesity genes [88,89]. Genes encoding beta-3 adrenergic receptor, ApoA5, PPAR-γ, and mitochondrial brown fat uncoupling protein 1 (UCP 1) were selected because of the similar frequencies of their polymorphisms in Koreans. The relative frequency of the *UCP1* G allele was 0.61 (an average of 0.53 in Korean) in this study [88]. This *UCP1* polymorphism is associated with increased body weight and body fat gain over time [90] and also with resistance to weight loss during a controlled energy diet [91]. However, *Doenjang* supplementation significantly reduced visceral fat and increased free fatty acid concentrations in subjects harboring the *UCP1* G allele, suggesting that the effects of *Doenjang* may be related to increased free fatty acid levels caused by elevated hormone-sensitive lipase activity in obese subjects. In the case of PPAR-γ, relative frequencies of the *PPARG* genotypes CC, TC, and TT in 51 subjects were 70%, 25.9%, and 3.4%, respectively, whereas those of C and T alleles were 81.6% and 18.4%. Visceral fat was significantly decreased by *Doenjang* supplementation in subjects with the *PPARG* T allele compared to those with the wild-type C allele after adjusting for age, sex, and BMI [89]. *Doenjang* pills significantly increased the oxygen radical absorbance capacity and reduced oxidative DNA damage in subjects with the C allele [89]. Our study suggests that *Doenjang* has antiobesity and antioxidative effects in overweight individuals with mutant *UCP1* and *PPARG* alleles. Many *Doenjang* studies have attempted to show improvements in inflammatory diseases such as osteoporosis and cancer because the antiobesity factors found in fermented soybean paste also have anti-inflammatory effects [11,61,92]. Compared to *Doenjang*, capsaicin in *Kochujang*, a fermented soybean-based red pepper paste, has long been known to have biological effects on thermogenesis, fat oxidation, and antiinflammation. Capsaicin suppresses obesity-induced inflammatory responses and macrophage migration induced by adipose tissue and macrophage activation by reducing TNF-α, IL-6, and MCP-1 levels and thus enhances adiponectin in adipose tissue and liver [93,94]. The reduction of visceral fat following *Kochujang* dietary supplementation (10.6 g/day) was similar to that observed in a previous study, but this effect was not sustained in subjects with *PPARG*, *UCP1*, and *APOA5* polymorphisms.

We will now describe several limitations of previous clinical trials of soy products and improvements in design that can be taken to address these. Although a 12-week randomized double-blind, placebo-controlled design is sufficiently powered to assess weight control, the side effects of soy-product intake may require longer-term studies. Due to the short duration, a phase of negative energy balance occurred in many subjects. It is known that negative energy balance can influence certain metabolic factors, sometimes in the opposite direction of the effects expected with weight loss. The long-term effects of the treatment on study outcomes should be evaluated by increasing the trial duration. Second, the dietary recommendation allowance of soybeans should be reevaluated. A daily intake of 25 g soybeans, equivalent to 6.25 g soy-protein-containing foods, is allowed by U.S. Food and Drug Administration to prevent cardiovascular diseases for Americans. Most nutrients also have a tolerable upper intake level to prevent the risk of adverse effects from excessive nutrient intakes. Using an intervention study, appropriate dietary reference intakes (DRIs) should be proposed. In addition, the enhanced weight loss with soybean consumption may be caused by different meal formats for the treatment and control diets. It is currently unknown whether a single component of the soy product or the whole soy meal including trace components such as phytosterols, including phytoestrogen, are responsible for improvements in the observed weight loss [10,28,95–97]. Many studies on soy-product interventions have not included an analysis of serum levels of specific components such as isoflavones. Moreover, the absorption rates and bioactivity of isoflavones are heavily dependent on the production conditions such as fermentation or the age of subjects, such as infants, elderly people, or postmenopausal women. When comparing different clinical trials, the underlying causes of conflicting results may be related to variations in experimental designs and exposure protocols (e.g. route of administration, composition, dose, and duration). Standardized studies are therefore needed to further evaluate these putative beneficial effects.

CONCLUSION AND FUTURE RESEARCH PERSPECTIVES

A possible reason for the lower incidence of inflammatory diseases including obesity, diabetes, or even breast cancers among Asians is that they have consumed traditional fermented soybean products such as *Cheonggukjang*, *Doenjang*, *Kochujang*, *Miso*, and *Tofu* for thousands of years. Although we agree that the creation of a national policy for obesity should prioritize prevention over treatment, the strategy for obesity research remains unclear. Methods appropriate to the prevention and treatment of obesity are critically different. Research into differentiation and expression of relevant factors using 3T3L-1 cells or in vivo models of diet-induced obesity has focused on developing treatments. Since obese status is influenced by the environment, cell differentiation, beta-oxidation, thermogenesis, insulin-glucose transportation, and inflammatory adipogenesis are altered by environmental factors. How systemic mechanisms interact with one another in complicated tissues should be systematically evaluated to prevent obesity. This could provide basic evidence to develop intervention studies for natural therapeutic sources; without this process, the future development of antiobesity drugs is at risk.

As good examples of natural antiobesity factors, the roles of phytochemicals on antioxidation, activation of immune system, antiinflammation, inhibition of platelet aggregation, and hormonal control are of great interest. Soybeans fermented for both short and long periods contain more beneficial components to ameliorate metabolic disorders than do unfermented soybeans. Changes in nutritive and non-nutritive biofactors during fermentation and changes in their capacity to ameliorate metabolic disorders have been reported in several Asian countries, especially in Korea. [98] Although the antiobesity mechanisms of isoflavonoids, phenols, and terpenes have been investigated, the active targeting mechanism must be identified to enable drug development. Currently, soybean bioactive peptides with inhibitory action against ACE and HMG-CoA reductase are the subjects of investigation for new drugs and functional food ingredients to improve gut health and modulate the intestinal absorption of nutrients [87]. Identifying the long-term side effects of natural therapeutic sources of antiobesity drugs must be a primary aim of the competitive pharmaceutical industry. At the moment, Korean fermented soybean products have the potential to be good competitive drug sources as long as their beneficial effects are supported by systematic research.

We suggest that future research into preventing obesity should focus on high-technology interdisciplinary research in the areas of nutrition, physiology, molecular biology, chemistry, medicine, pharmacy, and statistics. In addition, new biomarkers or potential drug mechanisms should be confirmed by systematic obesity research that includes evidence-based interventions. It will also be important to avoid deleterious changes in lipid profiles that are not associated with major changes in body weight or the disappearance of long-term benefits. Furthermore, there are essential differences between the rodents and humans; for example, probiotics found in humans may modulate the absorption and bioavailability of soybeans products and metabolize active compounds into inactive ones, and vice versa [99,100]. Moreover, how cellular metabolism regulates drug absorption in different ethnic groups is also unclear. In addition, PPAR-α-dependent lipolysis in the liver may be species dependent because the expression of PPAR-α receptors and PPAR-α differs between mice and humans [101]. Lastly, bioinformatics technologies must be improved and simplified to make them more useful tools for improving general public health. As mentioned before, it is necessary to develop DRIs for use in the general population using bioinformatics technologies. In addition to DRIs, individualized nutrition depends on a consideration of ethnicity; thus, nutrigenomics technology may also contribute to the prevention of obesity among different populations.

Acknowledgments

This work was supported by a grant from the Cooperative Research Program for Agriculture Science & Technology Development (Project No. PJ907089) in Korea. The authors have no conflict of interest for the information presented in this review.

References

[1] Jenkins DJ, Kendall CW, Jackson CJ, Connelly PW, Parker T, Faulkner D, et al. Effects of high- and low isoflavone soyfoods on blood lipids, oxidized LDL, homocysteine, and blood pressure in hyperlipidemic men and women. Am J Clin Nutr 2002;76:365–72.

[2] Kim JI, Kim JC, Kang MJ, Lee MS, Kim JJ, Cha IJ. Effects of pinitol isolated from soybeans on glycaemic control and cardiovascular risk factors in Korean patients with type II diabetes mellitus: a randomized controlled study. Eur J Clin Nutr 2005;59:456–8.

[3] Coward L, Barnes NC, Setchell KDR, Barnes S. Genistein, daidzein, and their β-glycoside conjugates: Antitumor isoflavones in soybean foods from American and Asian diets. J Agric FoodChem 1993;41:1961–7.

[4] Park Y, Moon HJ, Paik DJ, Kim DY. Effect of dietary legume on bone-specific gene expression in ovariectomized rats. Nutr Res Pract 2013;7:185–91.

[5] Record IR, Dreosti IE, McInerney JK. The antioxidant activity of genistein in vitro. J Nutr Biochem 1995;6:481–5.

[6] Song TT, Hendrich S, Murphy PA. Estrogenic activity of glycitein, a soy isoflavone. J Agric FoodChem 1999;47:1607–10.

[7] Sugano M, Gatchalian-Yee M, Arimura Y, Ochiai E, Yamada K. Soybean protein lowers serum cholesterol levels in hamsters: effect of debittered undigested fraction. Nutrition 1997;13:633–9.

[8] Velasquez MT, Bhathena SJ. Role of dietary soy protein in obesity. Int J Med Sci 2007;4:72–82.

[9] Cornwell T, Cohick W, Raskin I. Dietary phytoestrogens and health. Phytochemistry 2004;65:995–1016.

[10] Setchell KD. Phytoestrogens: the biochemistry, physiology, and implications for human health of soy isoflavones. Am J Clin Nutr 1998;68:1333S–46S.

[11] Park KY, Jung KO, Rhee SH, Choi YH. Antimutagenic effects of *Doenjang* (Korean fermented soypaste) and its active compounds. Mutation Res 2003;523–524:43–53.

[12] Kwon DY, Daily 3rd JW, Kim HJ, Park S. Antidiabetic effects of fermented soybean products on type 2 diabetes. Nutr Res 2010;30:1–13.

[13] Jang CH, Park CS, Lim JK. Metabolism of isoflavone derivatives during manufacturing of traditional meju and *Doenjang*. Food Sci Biotechnol 2008;17:442–5.

[14] Busby MG, Jeffcoat AR, Bloedon LT, Koch MA, Black T, Dix KJ, et al. Clinical characteristics and pharmacokinetics of purified soy isoflavones: single-dose administration to healthy men. Am J Clin Nutr 2002;75:126–36.

[15] Kwon DY, Jang JS, Hong SM, Lee JE, Sung SR, Park HR, et al. Long-term consumption offermented soybean-derived *Cheonggukjang* enhances insulin tropic action unlike soybeans in 90% pancreatectomized diabetic rats. Eur J Nutr 2007;46:44–52.

[16] Kim Y, Cho JY, Kuk JH, Moon JH, Cho JI, Kim YC, et al. Identification and antimicrobialactivity of phenyl acetic acid produced by Bacillus licheniformis isolated from fermented soybean, *Cheonggukjang*-Jang. CurrMicrobiol 2004;48:312–7.

[17] Nakajima N, Nozaki N, Ishihara K, Ishikawa A, Tsuji H. Analysis of isoflavone content in tempeh, a fermented soybean, and preparation of a new isoflavone-enriched tempeh. J Biosci Bioeng 2005;1006:685–7.

[18] Slavin JL, Karr SC, Hutchins AM, Lampe JW. Influence of soybean processing, habitual diet, and soy dose on urinary isoflavonoid excretion. Am J Clin Nutr 1998;68:1492S–5S.

[19] Naaz A, Yellayi S, Zakroczymski MA, Bunick D, Doerge DR, Lubahn DB, et al. The soy isoflavone genistein decreases adipose deposition in mice. Endocrinology 2003;144:3315–20.

[20] Mikkelsen PB, Toubro S, Astrup A. Effect of fat reduced diets on 24-h energy expenditure: comparisons between animal protein vegetable protein, and carbohydrates. Am J Clin Nutr 2000;72:1135–41.

[21] Guthrie JR, Ball M, Murkies A, Dennerstein L. Dietary phytoestrogen intake in mid-life Australian-born women: relationship to health variables. Climacteric 2000;3:254–6.

[22] Goodman-Gruen D, Kritz-Silverstein D. Usual dietary isoflavone intake and body composition in postmenopausal women. Menopause 2003;10:427–32.

[23] Wu J, Oka J, Higuchi M, Tabata I, Toda T, Fujioka M, et al. Cooperative effects of isoflavones and exercise on bone and lipid metabolism in postmenopausal Japanese women: a randomized placebo-controlled trial. Metabolism 2006;55:423–33.

[24] Allison DB, Gadbury G, Schwartz LG, Murugesan R, Kraker JL, Heshka S, et al. A novel soy-based meal replacement formula for weight loss among obese individuals: a randomized controlled clinical trial. Eur J Clin Nutr 2003;57:514–22.

[25] Ikeda Y, Iki M, Morita A, Kajita E, Kagamimori S, Kagawa Y, et al. Intake of fermented soybeans, natto, is associated with reduced bone loss in postmenopausal women: Japanese Population-Based Osteoporosis (JPOS) Study. J Nutr 2006;136:1323–8.

[26] de Kleijn MJ, van der Schouw YT, Wilson PW, Grobbee DE, Jacques PF. Dietary intake of phytoestrogens is associated with a favorable metabolic cardiovascular risk profile in postmenopausal U.S. women: the Framingham study. J Nutr 2002;132:276–82.

[27] Anderson JW, Fuller J, Patterson K, Blair R, Tabor A. Soy compared to casein meal replacement shakes with energy-restricted diets for obese women: randomized controlled trial. Metabolism 2007;56:280–8.

[28] Cederroth CR, Nef S. Soy, phytoestrogens and metabolism: a review. Mol Cell Endocrinol 2009;304:30–42.

[29] Hwang CS, Kwak HS, Lim HJ, Lee SH, Kang YS, Choe TB, et al. Isoflavone metabolites and their in vitro dual functions: they can act as an estrogenic agonist or antagonist depending on the estrogen concentration. J Steroid Biochem Mol Biol 2006;101:246–53.

[30] Cooke PS, Heine PA, Taylor JA, Lubahn DB. The role of estrogen and estrogen receptor-alpha in male adipose tissue. Mol Cell Endocrinol 2001;178:147–54.

[31] Ahmed-Sorour H, Bailey CJ. Role of ovarian hormones in the long-term control of glucose homeostasis. Interaction with insulin, glucagon and epinephrine. Horm Res 1980;13:396–403.

[32] Bailey CJ, Ahmed-Sorour H. Role of ovarian hormones in the long-term control of glucose homeostasis. Effects of insulin secretion. Diabetologia 1980;19:475–81.

[33] Godsland IF. Oestrogens and insulin secretion. Diabetologia 2005;48:2213–20.

[34] Case AM, Reid RL. Menstrual cycle effects on common medical conditions. Compr Ther 2001;27:65–71.

[35] Carani C, Qin K, Simoni M, Faustini-Fustini M, Serpente S, Boyd J, et al. Effect of testosterone and estradiol in man with aromatase deficiency. N Engl J Med 1997;337:91–5.

[36] Choi MS, Jung UJ, Yeo J, Kim MJ, Lee MK. Genistein and daidzein prevent diabetes onset by elevating insulin level and altering hepatic gluconeogenic and lipogenic enzyme activities in non-obese diabetic (NOD) mice. Diabetes Metab Res Rev 2008;24:74–81.

[37] Kwon DY, Hong SM, Ahn IS, Kim MJ, Yang HJ, Park S. Isoflavonoids and peptides from meju, long term fermented soybeans, increase insulin sensitivity and exert insulin tropic effects in vitro. Nutrition 2011;27:244–52.

[38] Szkudelska K, Nogowski L, Szkudelski T. Genistein affects lipogenesis and lipolysis in isolated rat adipocytes. J Steroid Biochem Mol Biol 2000;75:265–71.

[39] Kim S, Shin HJ, Kim SY, Kim JH, Lee YS, Kim DH, et al. Genistein enhances expression of genes involved in fatty acid catabolism through activation of PPAR alpha. Mol Cell Endocrinol 2004;220:51–8.

[40] Yang JY, Lee SJ, Park HW, Cha YS. Effect of genistein with carnitine administration on lipid parameters and obesity in C57Bl/6J mice fed a high-fat diet. J Med Food 2006;9:459–67.

[41] Soh J, Kwon DY, Cha YS. Hepatic gene expression profiles are altered by dietary unsalted Korean fermented soybean (*Cheonggukjang*) consumption in mice with diet-induced obesity. J Nutr Metab 2011;2011:260214.

[42] Cederroth CR, Vinciguerra M, Kuhne F, Madani R, Doerge DR, Visser TJ, et al. A phytoestrogen-rich diet increases energy expenditure and decreases adiposity in mice. Environ Health Perspect 2007;115:1467–73.

[43] Lephart ED, Rhees RW, Setchell KD, Bu LH, Lund TD. Estrogens and phytoestrogens: brain plasticity of sexually dimorphic brain volumes. J Steroid Biochem MolBio 2003;85:299–309.

[44] Stutz AM, Morrison CD, Argyropoulos G. The Agouti-related protein and its role in energy homeostasis. Peptides 2005;26:1771–81.

[45] Makimura H, Mizuno TM, Mastaitis JW, Agami R, Mobbs CV. Reducing hypothalamic AGRP by RNA interference increases metabolic rate and decreases body weight without influencing food intake. BMC Neurosci 2002;3:18.

[46] Wortley KE, Anderson KD, Yasenchak J, Murphy A, Valenzuela D, Diano S, et al. Agouti-related protein deficient mice display an age-related lean phenotype. Cell Metab 2005;2:421–7.

[47] Schwartz MW, Woods SC, Porte Jr D, Seeley RJ, Baskin DG. Central nervous system control of food intake. Nature 2002;404:661–71.

[48] Cederroth CR, Vinciguerra M, Gjinovci A, Kühne F, Klein M, Cederroth M, et al. Dietary phytoestrogens activate AMP-activated protein kinase with improvement in lipid and glucose metabolism. Diabetes 2008;57:1176–85.

[49] Park S, Kim S, Kim JH, Kim JS, Kim HJ. Glyceollin-containing fermented soybeans improve glucose homeostasis in diabetic mice. Nutrition 2012;28:204–11.

[50] Yang HJ, Kim HJ, Kim MJ, Kang S, Kim da S, Daily JW, et al. Standardized *Cheonggukjang*, short-term fermented soybeans with Bacillus lichemiformis, improves glucose homeostasis as much as traditionally made *Cheonggukjang* in diabetic rats. J Clin Biochem Nutr 2013;52:49–57.

[51] Ouchi N, Parker JL, Lugus JJ, Walsh K. Adipokines in inflammation and metabolic disease. Nat Rev Immunol 2011;11(2):85–97.

[52] Gonzalez-Castejon M, Rodriguez-Casado A. Dietary phytochemicals and their potential effects on obesity: a review. PharmacolRes 2011;64:438–55.

[53] Rayalama S, Della-Fera MA, Baile CA. Phytochemicals and regulation of the adipocyte life cycle; review. J Nutr Biochem 2008;19:717–26.

[54] Kim MH, Park JS, Seo MS, Jung JW, Lee YS, Kang KS. Genistein and daidzeinrepress adipogenic differentiation of human adipose tissue-derived mesenchymal stem cellsvis Wnt/β catenin signaling or lipolysis. Cell Prolif 2010;43(60):594–605.

[55] Lim SY, Park KY, Bae MS, Kim KH. Effect of *Doenjang* with black soybean on cytokine production and inhibition of tumor metastasis. J Life Sci 2009;19(2):264–70.

[56] Wu J, Wang X, Chiba H, Higuchi M, Nakatani T, Ezaki O. Combined intervention of soy isoflavone and moderate exercise prevents body fat elevation and bone loss in ovariectomized mice. Metabolism 2004;53:942–8.

[57] Bu LH, Lephart ED. Effects of dietary phytoestrogens on core body temperature during the estrous cycle and pregnancy. Brain Res Bull 2005;65:219–23.

[58] Penza M, Montani C, Romani A, Vignolini P, Pampaloni B, Tanini A, et al. Genistein affects adipose tissue deposition in a dose-dependent and gender-specific manner. Endocrinology 2006;147:5740–51.

[59] Kwak CS, Park SC, Song KY. *Doenjang*, a fermented soybean paste, decreased visceral fat accumulation and adipocyte size in rats fed with high fat diet more effectively than non-fermented soybeans. J Med Food 2012;15:1–9.

[60] Park NY, Rico CW, Lee SC, Kang MY. Comparative effects of *Doenjang* prepared from soybean and brown rice on the body weight and lipid metabolism in high fat-fed mice. J Clin Biochem Nutr 2012;51:235–40.

[61] Choi J, Kwon SH, Park KY, Yu BP, Kim ND, Jung JH, et al. The anti-inflammatory action of fermented soybean products in kidney of high-fat-fed rats. J Med Food 2011;14:232–9.

[62] Yang HJ, Kwon DY, Kim MJ, Kang S, Park S. Meju, unsalted soybeans fermented with Bacillus subtilis and Aspergilusoryzae, potentiates insulin tropic actions and improves hepatic insulin sensitivity in diabetic rats. Nutr Metab (Lond) 2012;9:37.

[63] Lee MH, Park YH, Oh HS, Kwak TS. Isoflavone content in soybean and its processed products. Korean J Food Sci Technol 2002;34:365–9.

[64] Kwon DY, Hong SM, Lee JE, Sung SR, Park S. Long-term consumption of fermented soybean-derived Chungkookjang attenuates hepatic insulin resistance in 90% pancreatectomized diabetic rats. Horm Metab Res 2007;39:752–7.

[65] Kwon DY, Jang JS, Lee JE, Kim YS, Sin DW, Park S. The isoflavonoid aglycone-rich fractions of *Cheonggukjang*, fermented unsalted soyneans, enhance insulin signaling and peroxisome proliferator-activated receptor-γ activity in vitro. Biofactors 2006;26:245–58.

[66] Pyo YH, Seong KS. Hypolipidemic effects of Monascus-fermented soybean extracts in rats fed a high-fat and -cholesterol diet. J Agric Food Chem 2009;57:8617–22.

[67] Anderson JW, Kendall CWC, Jenkins DJA. Meta-analysis of effects of soyprotein intakes on serum lipids in human. New Eng J Med 1995;333:276–82.

[68] Crouse III JR, Morgan T, Terry JG, Ellis J, Vitolins M, Burke GL. A randomized trial comparing the effects of casein with that of soy protein containing varying amounts of isoflavones on plasma concentration of lipids and lipoproteins. Arch Intern Med 1999;159:2070–6.

[69] Bosello O, Cominacini L, Zocca I, et al. Short- and long-term effects of hypocaloric diets containing proteins of different sources on plasma lipids and apoproteins of obese subjects. Ann Nutr Metab 1998;32:206–14.

[70] Fisler JS, Drenick EJ, Yoshimura NN, Swendseid ME. Plasma concentration of amino acids in obese men consuming low-calorie diets composed of soy or collagen protein. Int J Obes 1985;9:335–46.

[71] Yamashita T, Sasahara T, Pomeroy SE, Collier G, Nestel PJ. Arterial compliance, blood pressure, plasma leptin, and plasma lipids in women are improved with weight reduction equally with a meat based diet and a plant-based diet. Metabolism 1998;47:1308–14.

[72] Anderson JW, Hoie LH. Weight loss and lipid changes with low-energy dets: Comparison of milk based vs soy-based liquid meal replacement interventions. J Am Coll Nutr 2005;24:210–6.

[73] Li Z, Hong K, Saltsman P, De Shields S, Bellman M, Thames G, et al. Long-term efficacy of soy-based meal replacements vs an individualized diet plan in obese type II DM patients: relative effects on weight loss, metabolic parameters. Eur J Clin Nutr 2005;59:411–8.

[74] Cheung SY, Shaw NS, Tsai KS, Chen CY. The Hypoglycemic effects of soy isoflavones on postmenopausal women. J Women's Health 2004;13(10):1080–6.

[75] Hsu CS, Shen WW, Hsueh YM, Yeh SL. Soy isoflavone supplementation in postmenopausal women. Effects on plasma lipids, antioxidant enzyme activities and bone density. J Reprod Med 2001;46(3):221–6.

[76] Weickert MO, Reimann M, Otto B, Hall WL, Vafeiadou K, Hallund J, et al. Soy isoflavones increase preprandial peptide YY (PYY), but have no effect on ghrelin and body weight in healthy postmenopausal women. J Negat Results Biomed 2006;5:11.

[77] Hall WL, Vafeiadou K, Hallund J, Bugel S, Reimann M, Koebnick C, et al. Soy-isoflavone-enriched foods and markers of lipid and glucose metabolism in postmenopausal women: interactions with genotype and equol production. Am J Clin Nutr 2006;83(3):592–600.

[78] Taku K, Umegaki K, Sato Y, Taki Y, Endoh K, Watanabe S. Soy isoflavones lower serum total and LDL cholesterol in humans: a meta-analysis of 11 randomized controlled trials. Am J Clin Nutr 2007;85(4):1148–56.

[79] Zhuo XG, Melby MK, Watanable S. Soy isoflavone intake lowers serum LDL cholesterol: a meta-analysis of 8 randomized controlled trials in humans. J Nutr 2004;134(9):2395–400.

[80] Song KB, Atkinson C, Frankenfeld CL, Jokela T, Wähälä K, Thomas WK, et al. Prevalence of daidzein-metabolizing phenotypes differs between Caucasian and Korean American women and girls. J Nutr 2006;136(5):1347–51.

[81] Cha YS, Yang JA, Back HI, Kim SR, Kim MG, Jung SJ, et al. Visceral fat and body weight are reduced in overweight adults by the supplementation of *Doenjang*, a fermented soybean paste. Nutr Res Prac 2012;6(6):520–6.

[82] Sung JH, Choi SJ, Lee SW, Park KH, Moon TW. Isoflavones found in Korean soybean paste as 3-hydroxy- 3-methylglutaryl coenzyme a reductase inhibitors. Biosci Biotechnol Biochem 2004;68:1051–8.

[83] Back HI, Kim SR, Yang JA, Kim MG, Chae SW, Cha YS. Effects of Chungkookjang supplementation on obesity and atherosclerotic indices in overweight/obese subjects: a 12-week, randomized, double-blind, placebo-controlled clinical trial. J Med Food 2011;14:532–7.

[84] Jung KO, Park SY, Park KY. Longer aging time increases the anticancer and antimetastatic properties of *Doenjang*. Nutrition 2006;22:539–45.

[85] Yang JL, Lee SH, Song YS. Improving effect of powders of cooked soybean and chongkukjang on blood pressure and lipid metabolism in spontaneously hypertensive rats. J Korean Soc Food Sci Nutr 2003;32:899–905.
[86] Soh JR, Shin DH, Kwon DY, Cha YS. Effect of *Cheonggukjang* supplementation upon hepatic acyl-CoA synthase, carnitine palmitoyltransferase I, acyl-CoA oxidase and uncoupling protein 2 mRNA levels in C57BL/6J mice fed with high fat diet. Genes Nutr 2008;2:365–9.
[87] Kim SH, Lee YJ, Kwon DY. Isolation of angiotensin converting enzyme Inhibitor from *Doenjang*. Korean J Food Sci Technol 1999;31(3):848–54.
[88] Lee M, Chae S, Cha YS, Park Y. Supplementation of Korean fermented soy paste *Doenjang* reduces visceral fat in overweight subjects with mutant uncoupling protein-1 allele. Nutr Res 2012;32:8–14.
[89] ChaYS, Park Y, Lee M, ChaeSW, Park K, Kim Y, et al. *Doenjang*, a Korean fermented soy food, exerts anti-obesity and antioxidative activities in overweight subjects with the PPARγ2 C1431T polymorphism: 12 weeks double blind randomized clinical trial, J Medicinal Foods, in press.
[90] Clément K, Ruiz J, Cassard-Doulcier AM, Bouillaud F, Ricquier D, Basdevant A, et al. Additive effect of A→G (−3826) variant of the uncoupling protein gene and the Trp64Arg mutation of the beta 3-adrenergic receptor gene on weight gain in morbid obesity. Int J Obes Relat Metab Disord 1996;20:1062–6.
[91] Fumeron F, Durack-Bown I, Betoulle D, Cassard-Doulcier AM, Tuzet S, Bouillaud F, et al. Polymorphisms of uncoupling protein (UCP) and beta 3 adrenoreceptor genes in obese people submitted to a low calorie diet. Int J Obes Relat Metab Disord 1996;20:1051–4.
[92] Cho KM, Hong SY, Math RK, Lee JH, Kambiranda DM, Kim JM, et al. Biotransformation of phenolics (isoflavones, flavanols and phenolic acids) during the fermentation of *Cheonggukjang* by Bacillus pumilus HY1. Food Chemistry 2009;114:413–9.
[93] Kang JH, Tsuyoshi G, Han IS, Kawada T, Kim YM, Yu R. Dietary capsaicin reduces obesity-induced insulin resistance and hepatic steatosis in obese mice fed a high-fat diet. Obesity 2010;18(4):780–7.
[94] Joo JI, Kim DH, Choi JW, Yun JW. Proteomic analysis for anti-obesity potential of capsaicin on white adipose tissue in rats fed with a high fat diet. J Proteome Res 2010;9(6):2977–87.
[95] Kuriyan R, Raj T, Srinivas SK, Vaz M, Rajendran R, Kurpad AV. Effect of Caralluma Fimbriata extract on appetite, food intake and anthropometry in adult Indian men and women. Appetite 2007;48:338–44.
[96] Oben J, Kuate D, Agbor G, Momo C, Talla X. The use of a Cissus quadrangularis formulation in the management of weight loss and metabolic syndrome. Lipids Health Dis 2006;5:24.
[97] Cederroth Christopher R, Nef. Serge. Soy, phytoestrogens and metabolism: a review. Mol Cell Endocrinol 2009;304:30–42.
[98] Yang HJ, Park S, Pak V, Chung KR, Kwon DY. Fermented soybean products, and their bioactive compounds, In: El-Shemy H, editor. Soybean and Health. InTech 2011, p. 21–58, http://dx.doi.org/10.5772/10670
[99] Fernandez-Raudales D, Hoeflinger JL, Bringe NA, Cox SB, Dowd SE, Miller MJ, et al. Consumption of different soymilk formulations differentially affects the gut microbiomes of overweight and obese men. Gut Microbes 2012;3(6):490–500.
[100] McMullen MH, Hamilton-Reeves JM, Bonorden MJ, Wangen KE, Phipps WR, Feirtag JM, et al. Consumption of *Lactobacillus acidophilus* and *Bifidobacterium longum* does not alter phytoestrogen metabolism and plasma hormones in men: a pilot study. J Altern Complement Med 2006;12(9):887–94.
[101] Stienstra R, Duval C, Müller M, Kersten S. PPARs, obesity, and inflammation. PPAR Res 2007;2007:95974.

CHAPTER

23

Alcohol Intake and Hormonal Dysregulation of Food Intake in Visceral Fat Accumulation

Gustavo D. Pimentel and Thayana O. Micheletti

Department of Internal Medicine, Faculty of Medical Sciences, University of Campinas (UNICAMP), São Paulo, Brazil

BACKGROUND

The consumption of alcoholic beverages with meals or as an appetizer has been studied worldwide. Furthermore, alcohol is considered a topic of great interest to health professionals. Thus, several studies have demonstrated that alcohol intake is related to modulation of appetite and visceral fat gain [1,2].

Alcohol intake increases thermogenesis in the short term and modulates several neuronal systems in peripheral tissues that are related to appetite control, including inhibition of glucagon-like peptide 1 (GLP-1), leptin, and serotonin [5-hydroxytryptamine(5-HT)], and increases in γ-aminobutyric acid (GABA), ghrelin, neuropeptide Y (NPY), and opioids [2,3]. Likewise, some studies have found that alcohol use increases the risk of development of obesity [4].

Chronic alcohol consumption is positively associated with changes in hypothalamic receptors and in adipose tissue levels of two hormones, leptin, and resistin [5–7]. In addition, low plasma concentrations of leptin following ethanol administration may be due to the suppression of leptin secretion from adipose tissue into the systemic circulation [8], resulting in the accumulation of visceral fat.

Collectively, these mechanisms may lead to an increase in food consumption, resulting in a positive energy balance. However, the mechanisms by which alcohol (ethanol) consumption leads to hunger are still uncertain, mainly due to the small number of studies with an adequate design on this subject. Therefore, in this chapter we highlight the relationships between acute or chronic intake of alcohol on the modulation of energy homeostasis, anorexigenic and orexigenic hormone levels, and visceral fat accumulation.

ALCOHOL METABOLISM

Alcohol is characterized as a highly caloric macronutrient [2,9] that has pharmacological action on the central nervous system by altering numerous neurochemical systems. Furthermore, it cannot be stored, since its use is prioritized for metabolization and utilization compared to others macronutrients [2].

In the short term, the pharmacological effects of alcohol can have both direct and indirect effects on the food intake [10], which occur 30–60 min after consumption and metabolization. Likewise, ethanol metabolism generates energy; therefore, the maximum number of calories derived from the metabolism of alcohol occurs after the pharmacological action peak. Thus, these pharmacological and metabolic effects on appetite and hormonal dysregulation may be dissociated by the action time; pharmacological effects are represented by increased energy production from ethanol metabolism [2] that may increase hormonal and metabolic activity (until a plateau is reached) after ethanol consumption, especially chronic consumption.

Ethanol is absorbed rapidly by the gut and reaches the blood a few minutes after ingestion. Moreover, it can reach cells in all tissues, including the brain. The liver is the main organ that converts ethanol to acetaldehyde, which is catalyzed by the alcohol dehydrogenase enzyme; after that, acetaldehyde conversion to acetate is accompanied by the reduction of NAD^+ to NADH by the

Nutrition in the Prevention and Treatment of Abdominal Obesity
http://dx.doi.org/10.1016/B978-0-12-407869-7.00023-4

aldehyde dehydrogenase enzyme [11]. Increased acetate leads to activation of acetyl coenzyme A (acetyl-CoA) by the action of an acyl-CoA synthetase enzyme. After its formation, acetyl-CoA can be metabolized through two pathways: the first is to provide energy in the citric acid cycle, and the second is to synthesize fatty acids. In fact, the metabolism of ethanol is similar to that of carbohydrates, proteins, and lipids, which also generate acetyl-CoA and NADH.

Ethanol oxidation leads to increased levels of NADH in the cytosol of liver cells, in which normal NAD^+ concentrations are much higher than those of NADH. Mitochondrial NADH levels also rise after acetaldehyde oxidation, causing inhibition of the Krebs cycle (citric acid cycle) and the Lynen cycle. Initially, the accumulated acetyl-CoA is converted to ketone bodies, leading to metabolic acidosis. Subsequently, fatty acids are not degraded and, by mechanisms that remain unclear, ethanol synthesis is increased, leading to hepatic steatosis [11]. Therefore, chronic consumption of alcohol associated with other nutrients from the diet provides excess energy and induces a greater accumulation of visceral fat and serum triacylglycerols, and leads to hepatic steatosis [11].

Moderate alcohol intake (340 mL/day of wine or beer) increases food intake, when compared with a control meal (with the same energy and volume), in both normal and overweight individuals [4]. These results suggest that ethanol metabolism contributes to adiposity. Furthermore, alcohol consumed at levels comprising 2% of total caloric intake can lead to serious metabolic problems, including weight and fat gain, fatty liver, and cirrhosis [11].

ALCOHOL INTAKE AND APPETITE CONTROL

The control of food intake is classically regulated by the brain-gut axis, which includes two hypothalamic centers with opposite functions: the lateral hypothalamic area (known as the *feeding* or *appetite center*) and the ventromedial hypothalamic area (known as the *satiety center*) [12].

It has been shown in animals that hypothalamic lesions in the ventromedial portion cause loss of appetite, anorexia, and cachexia. Thus, it has been suggested that the satiety center works by inhibiting the feeding center [3]. Furthermore, it has been proposed that the feeding center is chronically active under fasting conditions, although this center may be rapidly inhibited with the onset of caloric consumption.

The thermogenic effect of macronutrients differs somewhat with respect to energy homeostasis. For example, protein has a larger and prolonged thermogenic effect (20–30%) than carbohydrate (10%) and fat (0–3%) [13]. However, Stubbs et al. [14] found that the macronutrient oxidation rate during the postprandial period is alcohol > protein > carbohydrate > fat. Accordingly, it has been suggested that alcohol intake may acutely increase food intake because it is metabolized rapidly compared with other macronutrients. Nevertheless, a hyperprotein diet could be useful in weight loss due to its high thermogenic effect (three times greater than carbohydrates or fats), i.e. more energy is required to metabolize protein from the diet.

ALCOHOL CONSUMPTION AND HORMONAL DEREGULATION

The gastrointestinal hormone, ghrelin, is a 28-amino-acid peptide produced mainly in the stomach during fasting by the oxyntic cells of the gastric fundus. Its discovery raised the possibility of a signaling system between the gastrointestinal tract (GI) and brain, with implications for energy homeostasis [15]. Ghrelin is also found in the gut, kidney, placenta, pituitary, and hypothalamus, where it acts as an "initiator meal"; although its blood levels are elevated 1–2 h before a meal, they are reduced afterwards (in the postprandial state) [16].

Ghrelin may stimulate food intake through neuropeptide Y (NPY)/agouti-related protein (AgRP)-mediated activation of neurons in the arcuate nucleus (ARC) of the hypothalamus [17]. In addition, excessive production of this hormone leads to obesity by decreasing energy expenditure and lipid oxidation.

Obese patients have lower ghrelin levels compared with people of normal weight. Moreover, lower amounts of alcohol appear to stimulate the appetite in obese individuals by increasing the secretion of gastric acid (H^+) [2] and the expression of ghrelin by gastric mucosal cells [17]. In addition, ghrelin is also known to antagonize the action of leptin, a neuropeptide with an important role in the pathophysiology of alcoholism [18]. Ghrelin-induced leptin antagonism appears to be mediated by NPY- and AgRP-expressing neurons, which are key centers in the central regulation of energy homeostasis. Besides, in rodents, acute alcohol withdrawal modulates NPY expression in orexigenic neurons in the hypothalamus, which increases food intake.

In humans, a moderate intake of ethanol (0.45 g/kg) three times per day decreases leptin levels [19]. However, Roth et al. [20] showed that moderate alcohol consumption (15–30 g/day) increases serum leptin concentrations in postmenopausal women.

In a clinical study, Raben et al. [9] investigated the effects of ethanol intake on appetite, food intake, energy expenditure, and the energy substrate used. The authors evaluated four different meals: a hyperprotein diet (32% of total calories); a diet containing normal amounts of carbohydrates (65% of total calories); a diet rich in fat (65% of total calories); and a diet rich in alcohol (23% of total calories). After the consumption of a meal plus ethanol, lower fat oxidation and leptin concentrations were observed; however, the concentrations of gastric inhibitory polypeptide (GIP), GLP-1, and GLP-2 did not change when compared to the other three types of meals. Therefore, it was suggested that alcohol is absorbed almost completely by the stomach. Moreover, blood GIP, GLP-1, and GLP-2 concentrations cannot be modified by gut hormones, and the amount of alcohol that reached the intestine was probably insufficient to modulate the production of these anorexigenic hormones.

With respect to wine intake, it was found that the consumption of 150 mL/day three times/week leads to increased leptin levels [10]. Furthermore, in humans, the consumption of 0.45 g/kg of alcohol at 0900 and 1200 hours (Test A) and the consumption of 40 mg propranolol (a catecholamine inhibitor) plus alcohol at 0800 hours and 20 mg at 1200 hours (Test B) did not modify the levels of insulin and insulin-like growth factor I (IGF-I), but did decrease leptin concentrations in approximately 29% of subjects evaluated in both the tests. Therefore, decrease leptin levels after acute alcohol consumption does not seem to be mediated by catecholamine or by changing insulin and IGF-I levels. Thus, two mechanisms may contribute to the decreased secretion of leptin: first, a direct inhibitory effect of alcohol on adipocyte hormonal production; and second, the increased release of leptin for peripheral metabolism or renal excretion [21].

In healthy men, Calissendorff et al. [22] showed that alcohol inhibits the secretion of ghrelin, although this hormone cannot modulate the orexigenic effects of alcohol. However, it is notable that this inhibition was seen in healthy young men with a moderate consumption of alcohol at social events. Therefore, we cannot consider the results of this study to be particularly relevant to clinical practice.

Collectively, it is known that moderate-to-high alcohol consumption (more than two doses equivalent to 30 g ethanol/day) may decrease the oxidation of fatty acids, primarily in the liver [23], modulate the energy expenditure [24], increase NPY expression or steady state levels [25], activate the release of ghrelin [3,7], and inhibit leptin [9], 5-HT [2], GLP-1 [9], and IGF-I [26]. Additionally, withdrawal and alcohol dependency increase the desire to eat sweet foods [27], resulting in the accumulation of body fat. However, no clinical study has demonstrated that the effects of alcohol intake alone lead to weight gain. Nevertheless, alcohol consumption is associated with higher adiposity (waist circumference compared to body mass index). Parallel to this, there is evidence [7–10,18,28,29] to indicate that ethanol/alcohol intake, even in small amounts, can stimulate several highly orexigenic peptides and inhibit anorexigenic hormones, thus increasing the food intake (Fig. 23.1)

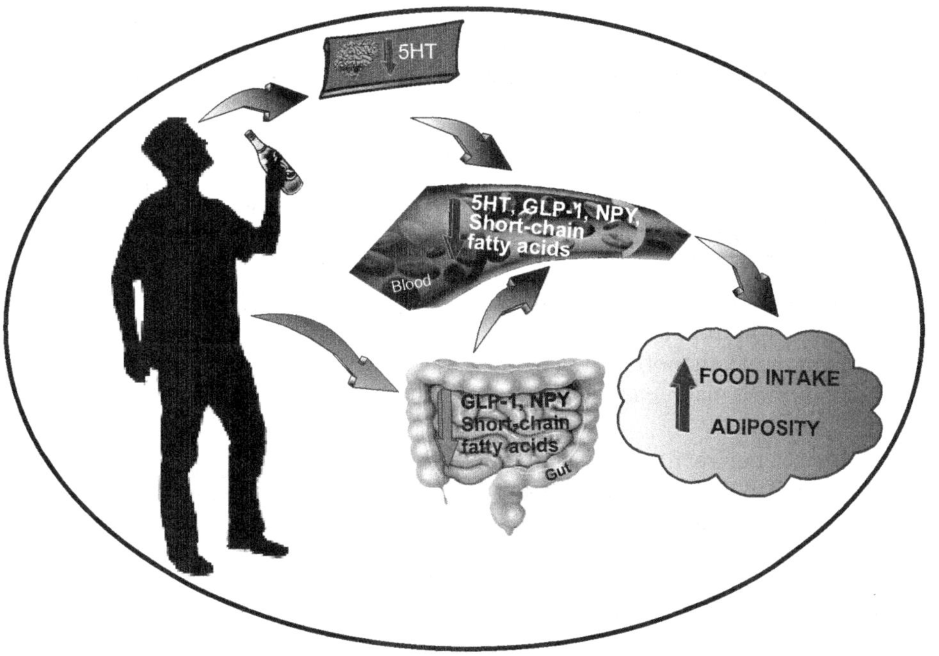

FIGURE 23.1 Schematic diagram showing the effects of ethanol on serotonin [5-hydroxytryptamine (5-HT)], anorexigenic and orexigenic hormones, and short-chain fatty acids, and thus on adiposity and food intake. (See color plate at the back of the book.)

EFFECTS OF ALCOHOL CONSUMPTION AND ABSTINENCE ON APPETITE REGULATION

The effect of alcohol consumption on appetite regulation occurs through a complex metabolic system [2], since they depend on metabolic and psychological effects, including those caused by specific foods [30].

A study by Raben et al. [9] compared the effects of four different macronutrients on appetite and noted that after a meal including alcohol, fat oxidation was greatly suppressed. According to Siler et al. [23], this is probably due to the fact that acetate is released into the circulation and rapidly oxidized, probably with priority over other energy substrates (i.e. carbohydrates, proteins, and fats). Furthermore, it is known that the release of acetate into the circulation inhibits lipolysis. Likewise, Krahn et al. [27] observed in a randomized study that individuals undergoing alcohol withdrawal and dependence showed a strong desire for sweet foods, which may favor weight gain.

With chronic alcoholism, individuals may present with changes in body composition and glucose homeostasis compared to healthy subjects. Therefore, research that takes into account the duration of abstinence can minimize other nutritional and metabolic disorders. Additionally, this would help to improve the interpretation of the clinical assessments, including the neurobiological effects of AgRP, insulin, ghrelin, leptin, and NPY, as well as alcohol, which predisposes patients to metabolic abnormalities, such as increased food intake and body fat gain.

Wurst et al. [31] suggest that there should be further research into the hormones cholecystokinin, insulin, leptin, NPY, and peptide YY, since they all play important metabolic roles in alcohol metabolism and obesity.

CONCLUSIONS

Collectively, several studies have shown that moderate-to-high alcohol consumption (more than two doses/day of approximately 30 g ethanol) is related to increased food intake, body adiposity gain, and hormonal dysregulation.

Therefore, the relationship between alcohol intake and obesity represents a challenge for the health-care professional, as well as for patients who are vulnerable to the misinformation that exists regarding alcohol and appetite regulation. With this in mind, health-care providers should simplify the findings from scientific investigations.

References

[1] Kokavec A. Is decreased appetite for food a physiological consequence of alcohol consumption? Appetite 2008;51(2):233–43.
[2] Yeomans MR, Caton S, Hetherington MM. Alcohol and food intake. Curr Opin Clin Nutr Metab Care. 2003;6(6):639–44.
[3] Konturek SJ, Konturek JW, Pawlik T, Brzozowski T. Brain-gut axis and its role in the control of food intake. J Phys Pharmacol Official J Polish Physiolo Soc 2004;55(1 Pt 2):137–54.
[4] Hetherington MM, Cameron F, Wallis DJ, Pirie LM. Stimulation of appetite by alcohol. Physiol Behav 2001;74(3):283–9.
[5] Obradovic T, Meadows GG. Chronic ethanol consumption increases plasma leptin levels and alters leptin receptors in the hypothalamus and the perigonadal fat of C57BL/6 mice. Alcohol Clin Exp Res 2002;26(2):255–62.
[6] Santolaria F, Perez-Cejas A, Aleman MR, Gonzalez-Reimers E, Milena A, de la Vega MJ, et al. Low serum leptin levels and malnutrition in chronic alcohol misusers hospitalized by somatic complications. Alcohol Alcohol 2003;38(1):60–6.
[7] Kim DJ, Yoon SJ, Choi B, Kim TS, Woo YS, Kim W, et al. Increased fasting plasma ghrelin levels during alcohol abstinence. Alcohol Alcohol 2005;40(1):76–9.
[8] Otaka M, Konishi N, Odashima M, Jin M, Wada I, Matsuhashi T, et al. Effect of alcohol consumption on leptin level in serum, adipose tissue, and gastric mucosa. Dig Dis Sci 2007;52(11):3066–9.
[9] Raben A, Agerholm-Larsen L, Flint A, Holst JJ, Astrup A. Meals with similar energy densities but rich in protein, fat, carbohydrate, or alcohol have different effects on energy expenditure and substrate metabolism but not on appetite and energy intake. Am J Clin Nutr 2003;77(1):91–100.
[10] Djurovic S, Berge KE, Birkenes B, Braaten O, Retterstol L. The effect of red wine on plasma leptin levels and vasoactive factors from adipose tissue: a randomized crossover trial. Alcohol Alcohol 2007;42(6):525–8.
[11] Marzzoco A TB. Bioquímica básica. 3ªed Rio de Janeiro (RJ): Guanabara Koogan; 2007.
[12] Bray GA. Drug insight: appetite suppressants. Nat Clin Prac Gastroenterol Hepatol 2005;2(2):89–95.
[13] Tappy L. Thermic effect of food and sympathetic nervous system activity in humans. Reprod Nutr Dev 1996;36(4):391–7.
[14] Stubbs JRA, Westerterp-Plantenga MS. Substrate metabolism and appetite in humans. In: Westerterp-Plantenga MS, , Steffens AB, Tremblay A, editors. Regulation of food intake and energy expenditure. Milan: Editora; 1999.
[15] Sakata I, Nakamura K, Yamazaki M, Matsubara M, Hayashi Y, Kangawa K, et al. Ghrelin-producing cells exist as two types of cells, closed- and opened-type cells, in the rat gastrointestinal tract. Peptides 2002;23(3):531–6.
[16] Cummings DE, Purnell JQ, Frayo RS, Schmidova K, Wisse BE, Weigle DS. A preprandial rise in plasma ghrelin levels suggests a role in meal initiation in humans. Diabetes 2001;50(8):1714–9.
[17] Peeters TL. Central and peripheral mechanisms by which ghrelin regulates gut motility. J Physiol Pharmacol Official J Polish Physiol Soc 2003;54(Suppl. 4):95–103.
[18] Nicolas JM, Fernandez-Sola J, Fatjo F, Casamitjana R, Bataller R, Sacanella E, et al. Increased circulating leptin levels in chronic alcoholism. Alcohol Clin Exp Res 2001;25(1):83–8.
[19] Rojdmark S, Calissendorff J, Brismar K. Alcohol ingestion decreases both diurnal and nocturnal secretion of leptin in healthy individuals. Clin Endocrinol 2001;55(5):639–47.
[20] Roth MJ, Baer DJ, Albert PS, Castonguay TW, Dorgan JF, Dawsey SM, et al. Relationship between serum leptin levels and alcohol consumption in a controlled feeding and alcohol ingestion study. J Natl Cancer Inst 2003;95(22):1722–5.

[21] Calissendorff J, Brismar K, Rojdmark S. Is decreased leptin secretion after alcohol ingestion catecholamine-mediated? Alcohol Alcohol 2004;39(4):281–6.
[22] Calissendorff J, Danielsson O, Brismar K, Rojdmark S. Inhibitory effect of alcohol on ghrelin secretion in normal man. Eur J Endocrinol/Eur Federation Endocrine Soc 2005;152(5):743–7.
[23] Siler SQ, Neese RA, Hellerstein MK. De novo lipogenesis, lipid kinetics, and whole-body lipid balances in humans after acute alcohol consumption. Am J Clin Nutr 1999;70(5):928–36.
[24] Suter PM, Jequier E, Schutz Y. Effect of ethanol on energy expenditure. Am J Physiol 1994;266(4 Pt 2):R1204–12.
[25] Clark JT, Keaton AK, Sahu A, Kalra SP, Mahajan SC, Gudger JN. Neuropeptide Y (NPY) levels in alcoholic and food restricted male rats: implications for site selective function. Regul Pept 1998;75–76:335–45.
[26] Lavigne JA, Baer DJ, Wimbrow HH, Albert PS, Brown ED, Judd JT, et al. Effects of alcohol on insulin-like growth factor I and insulin-like growth factor binding protein 3 in postmenopausal women. Am J Clin Nutr 2005;81(2):503–7.
[27] Krahn D, Grossman J, Henk H, Mussey M, Crosby R, Gosnell B. Sweet intake, sweet-liking, urges to eat, and weight change: relationship to alcohol dependence and abstinence. Addict Behav 2006;31(4):622–31.
[28] Leibowitz SF. Overconsumption of dietary fat and alcohol: mechanisms involving lipids and hypothalamic peptides. Physiol Behav 2007;91(5):513–21.
[29] Kraus T, Schanze A, Groschl M, Bayerlein K, Hillemacher T, Reulbach U, et al. Ghrelin levels are increased in alcoholism. Alcohol Clin Exp Res 2005;29(12):2154–7.
[30] Buemann B, Toubro S, Astrup A. The effect of wine or beer versus a carbonated soft drink, served at a meal, on ad libitum energy intake. Int J Obesity Related Metab Dis J Int Assoc Study Obesity 2002;26(10):1367–72.
[31] Wurst FM, Rasmussen DD, Hillemacher T, Kraus T, Ramskogler K, Lesch O, et al. Alcoholism, craving, and hormones: the role of leptin, ghrelin, prolactin, and the pro-opiomelanocortin system in modulating ethanol intake. Alcohol Clin Exp Res 2007;31(12): 1963–7.

CHAPTER

24

Coffee Intake and Obesity

Gustavo D. Pimentel[a], Thayana O. Micheletti[a], and Astrid Nehlig[b]

[a]Department of Internal Medicine, Faculty of Medical Sciences, University of Campinas (UNICAMP), Campinas, São Paulo, Brazil; [b]French Medical Research Institute, INSERM U 663, Faculty of Medicine, Strasbourg, France

OBESITY, COFFEE CONSUMPTION, AND ACTIVE COMPOUNDS

Obesity is classified as an excess body fat and is defined as a body mass index of 30 mg/kg^2 or above. Estimates of the prevalence and secular trend for obesity from 1960 to 2025 are increasing in many countries; for example, it is estimated that by 2025 45% of the population of the United States population will be obese and that this figure will reach 28% in England and 25% in Brazil [1].

Among the consequences of obesity are insulin resistance, inflammation, dyslipidemia, high blood pressure, and liver injury. In addition, these disturbances can be aggravated by the consumption of excess calories and both saturated and *trans* fatty acids [2–6], leading to cardiovascular diseases [7].

Although genetic factors may play a role in the etiology of obesity [8–10], there is now convincing evidence that obesity is strongly associated with modifiable factors, such as diet and exercise. In the 1950s, Linus Pauling established an inverse correlation between obesity and longevity [11]. At same time, the first evidence for a link between coffee intake and body weight was published. However, reports were contradictory: first, it was observed that coffee intake decreased the total liquid intake and led to a body weight reduction [12]; however, nowadays the relationship between reduced body weight and a low coffee intake-induced reduction in fluid consumption is merely speculative.

In the 1960s, two other studies [13,14] also showed contradictory effects, but these contained methodological errors: in the first study, the lean group was treated with 400 mg/kg caffeine and the obese/hyperglycemic group with only 80 mg/kg [13]; in the second study, diabetic humans treated with caffeine had increased serum glucose levels, but some individuals frequently consumed a hypoglycemiant drink [14].

In the mid-1960s and 1970s, the beneficial actions of coffee and caffeine intake on glucose homeostasis and atherosclerotic disease were first reported [15–17]. After 1970, several epidemiological, physiological, and molecular studies tried to understand how coffee and its compounds improve the metabolic consequences of obesity.

Large amounts of coffee are consumed by the population of many countries [18–21]. According to International Coffee Organization [22], the current annual coffee consumption is highest in Europe (2.4–12.0 kg/person/year); followed by South America (0.8–6.8 kg/person/year), North America, and Oceania (2.4–4.5 kg/person/year); Central America (0.8–4.5 kg/person/year); Asia (≤0.8–4.5 kg/person/year); and Africa (≤0.8–2.4 kg/person/year; Fig. 24.1).

When considering caffeine (the main component of coffee) intake, the mean caffeine intake per capita in Western society reaches 300 mg/day, coming mainly from dietary sources such as coffee, tea, cola drinks, and chocolate [23]. Data from the National Health and Nutrition Examination Surveys (NHANES III) showed that the American population consumes roughly 236 mg caffeine/day from coffee and tea [18]. However, data from Brazil are scarce [24]. Thus, coffee consumption is largely thought to involve dietetic compounds that are potentially able to reduce chronic diseases risk, for instance obesity and its complications [25–28].

The beneficial effects of different kinds of coffee are probably a result of the combined action of various compounds such as caffeine, antioxidant phenolic compounds, minerals, vitamins, and fibers. Consequently, coffee constituents might have the potential to improve the deleterious effects of obesity, such as dyslipidemia,

Nutrition in the Prevention and Treatment of Abdominal Obesity
http://dx.doi.org/10.1016/B978-0-12-407869-7.00024-6

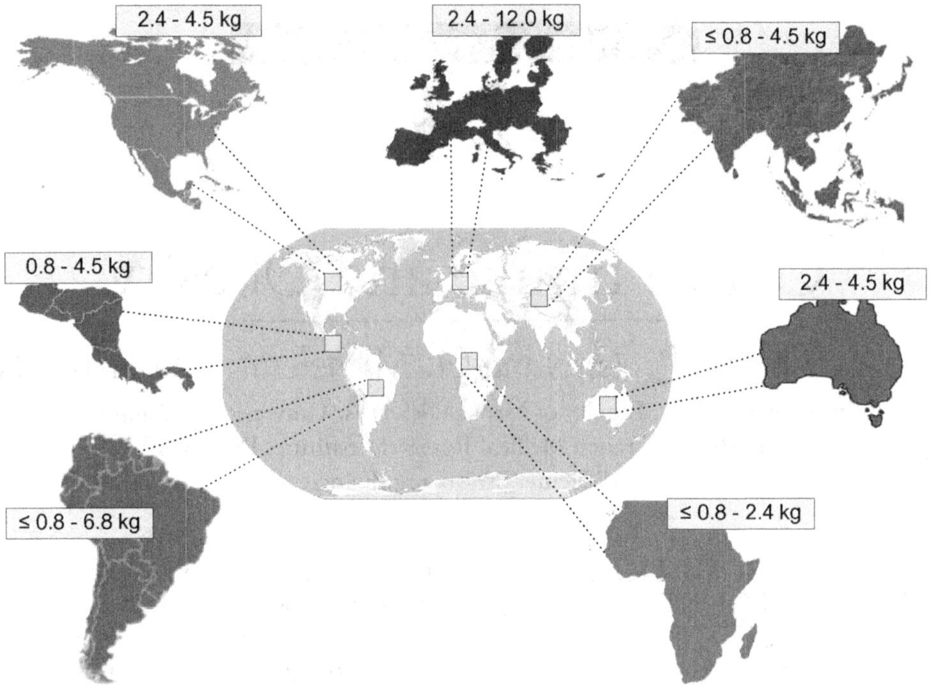

FIGURE 24.1 Current annual coffee consumption per capita per year throughout the world. Gray, South America; red, Central America; blue, North America; dark blue, Europe; green, Asia; purple, Oceania; orange, Africa. (See color plate at the back of the book.)

inflammation, hypertension, insulin and leptin resistance, and modified gut microbiota.

COFFEE AND REDUCTION OF OBESITY RISK: A VISION FROM EPIDEMIOLOGICAL STUDIES

The association between coffee intake and the risk of developing obesity has been repeatedly studied. Data from prospective and cohort studies indicate an inverse association between coffee consumption and the consequences of obesity, independent of race, age, or gender.

When considering a link between coffee intake and type 2 diabetes mellitus (T2DM), since 2002 several epidemiological studies [19,26,27,29–38] have shown that regular coffee consumption reduces the risk of developing T2DM. Indeed, as outlined in Table 24.1, subjects who drank between 2 and 3 cups of coffee daily had an approximately 25% lower risk of developing T2DM than those who did not drink more than one cup per day. Those who drank more than 4–6 cups per day had a risk reduction of 35%, which increased with the number of cups up to 55% in those who drank more than 10 cups per day. Additionally, most studies showed that the protective effects of coffee can be found in caffeinated, decaffeinated, and filtered coffee. The risk reduction of T2DM by coffee is observed after long-term consumption, i.e. >12 consecutive months [39–41]. Thus, epidemiological studies indicate that coffee consumption has a protective role against the development of T2DM.

Regarding coffee consumption and the reduction of metabolic syndrome indicators, several studies have reported that the main causes of improvement are weight and adiposity loss [42–46], while changes in caloric

TABLE 24.1 Summary of all Prospective and Cohort Studies that Showed a Reduction of Type 2 Diabetes Mellitus Risk With Coffee Intake

Dose (cups[a] per day)	Reduction in T2DM risk (%)[b]
0–1	No protection
≥2–3	25
≥4–6	35
≥6	42
≥10	55

[a]*Cup of 150 mL, containing an average of 60 mL of caffeine, as well as other coffee compounds.* [b]*Approximate values.*
T2DM, type 2 diabetes mellitus.

intake have less or no significance [47]. Besides, it is likely that the reduction in body weight by coffee consumption is one of the main factors responsible for the reduction in T2DM risk. In this respect, we have shown in adults and adolescents that a lifestyle program leads to weight loss and consequent reductions in serum levels of cholesterol, endotoxin, insulin, leptin, and triacylglycerols, and increased adiponectin; hence, metabolic syndrome indicators are reduced [4,48–50].

Some epidemiological studies also support the hypothesis that habitual coffee consumption is associated with the reduction of a variety of obesity indicators, in particular with improved glucose tolerance, lipid profile, and resistance to adiponectin, insulin, and leptin hormones.

COFFEE AND ITS COMPONENTS

Among the coffee components, caffeine has received the most attention due to its physiological and pharmacological properties, mainly its effects on type 2 diabetes mellitus, obesity, and cardiovascular diseases [26,27,32,37,39,41,43], as well as on other diseases unrelated to obesity [51–55].

Physiologically, caffeine can be entirely absorbed by the stomach and small intestine within 45 min after consumption, and it reaches a maximal concentration in the bloodstream in 15–120 min [56]. Recently, it was shown that caffeine and its metabolites are present in the blood after moderate coffee intake [57]. Once absorbed, caffeine is distributed throughout the body [58]. A linear correlation was observed between the concentrations of caffeine in the blood and brain ($r=0.86$) and between caffeine concentrations in plasma and the kidney ($r=0.91$) [59]. Furthermore, caffeine can cross the placenta and is available in mother's milk [60].

Caffeine metabolism takes place in the liver, starting with the removal of the methyl 1 and 7 groups in a reaction catalyzed by cytochrome P450 to form three methylxanthines: paraxanthine (84%), theobromine (12%), and theophylline (4%). Each of these has a different role in human physiology: paraxanthine increases lipolysis; theobromine stimulates blood vessel dilatation and increases urine volume; and theophylline controls glucose metabolism [61].

Blood levels of caffeine or its metabolites reflect coffee intake over the preceding hours [57,62]. Nevertheless, caffeine intake may not correlate strongly with coffee intake, as it also depends on the intake of other sources of caffeine, such as chocolate, energy drinks, cola soft drinks, and others. Caffeine concentrations in coffee are higher than those in tea, soft drinks, and energy drinks [63]. After coffee, yerba mate tea (*Ilex paraguariensis*) contains the most caffeine; for example, 237 mL of yerba mate tea contains 78 mg of caffeine, and 237 mL of black or green tea contain 55 and 35 mg of caffeine, respectively [64,65]. The approximated caffeine content of some foods and drinks is summarized in Table 24.2.

The Canadian Clinical Practice Guidelines [66] reported that for the average adult, a daily caffeine intake of 400–450 mg is not associated with any adverse effects. The recommendation for pregnant women and those who are breastfeeding is reduced to 300 mg/day; for children, it depends on age (Table 24.3).

TABLE 24.2 Caffeine Levels in Selected Foods and Drinks

Food or drink	Caffeine (mg)
Regular coffee, brewed from grounds, caffeinated[a]	95
Regular coffee, brewed from grounds, decaffeinated[a]	2
Coffee, brewed, espresso[a]	509
Regular instant coffee[a]	62
Decaffeinated instant coffee[a]	2
Carbonated beverage, cola[b]	29
Energy drink[b]	108
Milk chocolate bar[c]	9
Yerba mate tea[a]	78
Black tea[a]	55
Green tea[a]	35

Source: U.S. Department of Agriculture Agricultural Research Service, 2007 [145] and others [64,65].

[a]237 mL (or 8 fl oz.) cup. [b]355 mL (or 12 fl oz.) can. [c]44 g or (1.55 oz.) bar.

TABLE 24.3 Recommendation of Daily Caffeine Intake According to Age

Individuals	Caffeine (mg)
Children	–
4–6 year old	45.0
7–9 year old	62.5
10–12 year old	85.0
Adults	400
Pregnant/breastfeeding women	300

Source: Canadian Clinical Practice Guidelines [66].

COFFEE AND THE MECHANISMS THAT UNDERLIE ITS PROTECTIVE EFFECTS AGAINST OBESITY

At the moment, several mechanisms of action have been proposed to underlie the potential role of coffee and its components in improving the metabolic consequences of obesity. Mechanistic studies are discussed below.

Appetite Regulation, Satiety, and Hormone Sensitivity

The hypothesis that habitual coffee consumption improves peripheral metabolism consequences is related to numerous mechanisms, as it is likely to have effects on hormones, adiposity, and appetite regulation, which are important modulators of obesity.

Lopez-Garcia et al. [67], in a 12-year follow-up study of both men and women showed that individuals who consumed coffee lost more weight than those who did not. A randomized placebo-controlled, double-blind study of overweight men and women showed that a high-caffeine diet (524mg/day) reduces body weight, fat mass, and waist circumference, and increases satiety compared with a low-caffeine diet (151mg/day) [68]. Increased caffeine consumption (511mg/day) leads to higher satiety than that obtained with low caffeine intake (149mg/day) [69]. Recently, an American study demonstrated that consuming a beverage containing caffeine and catechins from green tea in combination with soluble fiber reduced caloric consumption at the next meal [70]. Furthermore, other studies suggest that yerba mate, a type of tea with a high caffeine content, reduces food intake and increases serum glucagon-like peptide 1 (GLP-1) levels [5,71].

Additionally, coffee affects the secretion of gastrointestinal peptides, gastric inhibitory polypeptide (GIP) and GLP-1, thus lowering glucose absorption in the small intestine [72–74] and activating central anorexigenic proopiomelanocortin (POMC)/cocaine- and amphetamine-regulated transcript (CART) neurons. Moreover, the secretion of these gut hormones seems to reach the hypothalamus and inhibit orexigenic neurons [neuropeptide Y/agouti-related protein (NPY/AgRP) [75–77]. Likewise, McCarty [78] reported higher GLP-1 release after the consumption of drinks containing chlorogenic acid, such as coffee. Another suggested mechanism is the direct stimulation of pancreatic beta cells by caffeine and theophylline [79]. Recently, van Dam's group observed an increase in GLP-1 concentrations 30min after the consumption of 12g decaffeinated coffee, 1g chlorogenic acid, and 500mg trigonelline compared to the placebo group [80]. The same was observed in healthy volunteers, i.e. increased postprandial secretion of GLP-1 after decaffeinated coffee compared with control group (without coffee) [74]. In Fig. 24.2, we schematically show the effects of coffee and its compounds on appetite regulation, adiposity, beta cell damage, and hormone sensitivity.

The beneficial effects of coffee compounds other than caffeine on obesity should be noted. Coffee is a major source of the polyphenol, chlorogenic acid, in the human diet and may modulate glucose metabolism by various mechanisms: these include increasing insulin sensitivity [81]; attenuating intestinal glucose absorption [74]; inhibiting tyrosine-protein phosphatase non-receptor type 1B [protein-tyrosine phosphatase 1B (PTP-1B)], a negative modulator of the insulin pathway [82]; inhibiting or retarding the action of alpha-glucosidase [83]; inhibiting intestinal glucose transporters [84]; reducing or inhibiting hepatic glucose-6-phosphatase (G6Pase) hydrolysis, which may reduce plasma glucose output, leading to reduced plasma glucose concentration [85–87]; stimulating glucose transport in the soleus muscle and increasing the phosphorylation of 5′-AMP-activated protein kinase (AMPK) and acetyl-CoA carboxylase (ACC), as well as activating Akt and inducing the translocation of glucose transporter member 4 (GLUT4) to the plasma membrane [88]; and increasing GLP-1 and GIP levels in the blood, and improving the oral glucose tolerance test [71,74,78, 80,89]. Moreover, chlorogenic acid neutralizes the deleterious effects of free fatty acids on the function of beta cells in insulin-resistant overweight subjects [78]. The effects of coffee and its compounds on glucose metabolism are summarized in Fig. 24.3. Nevertheless, it is important to take into account potential confounders in other food sources of chlorogenic acid, such as apples and other fruits [81].

Thus, it is suggested that the beneficial effects of coffee on appetite regulation and hormone sensitivity are obtained by ingestion of caffeine or the phenolic compound, chlorogenic acid.

Thermogenesis, Lipid Metabolism, and Lipolysis

Among the possible therapeutic targets of coffee are increased metabolic rate and energy expenditure [90,91]. It has been shown that an intake of 300mg/day of caffeine increased energy expenditure by 79kcal/day, thus maintaining a stable weight body [92]. Moreover, other evidence suggests that coffee intake can increase energy expenditure, as well as lipid and carbohydrate oxidation [93]. However, in the 1980s, a study showed that caffeine stimulates the metabolic rate in both lean and obese subjects, but induced greater fat oxidation in lean than obese subjects [90]. Another study done at the end of the 1980s

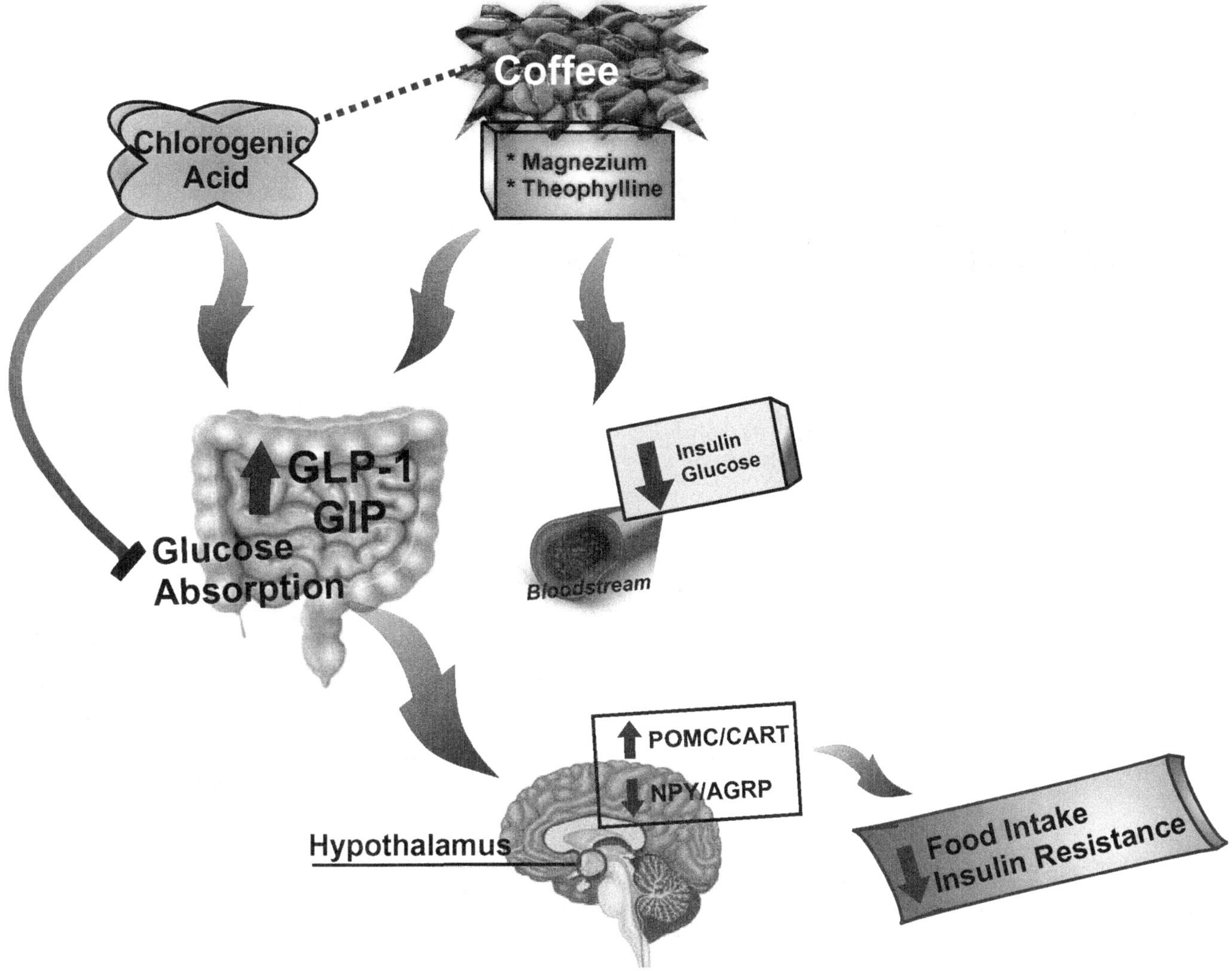

FIGURE 24.2 Schematic diagram showing the effects of coffee and its compounds on reducing food intake and improving insulin resistance. The consumption of coffee, theophylline, and chlorogenic acid has several beneficial actions: it (1) increases serum glucagon-like peptide 1 (GLP-1) and gastric inhibitory polypeptide (GIP) levels; (2) reduces beta cell damage; (3) increases C-peptide levels; (4) inhibits glucose absorption; and (5) reduces blood insulin and glucose concentrations. These effects may activate the neuropeptides proopiomelanocortin (POMC)/cocaine- and amphetamine-regulated transcript (CART) and reduce neuropeptide Y/agouti-related protein (NPY/AgRP), hence decreasing food intake and insulin resistance. (See color plate at the back of the book.)

showed that a single dose of 100mg caffeine could raise the resting metabolic rate in lean, but not in obese, individuals [94]. Although the thermogenic effects are larger in lean than in obese individuals, it is clear that stimulating energy expenditure in the treatment of obesity is an appropriate strategy of nutritional education in clinical practice.

Considering that an individual may become overweight with a daily overintake of approximately 50–100kcal, an increased energy expenditure of 80–150kcal/day should counterbalance weight gain [92,93]. In addition, an increased energy expenditure of 5% in obese and 7% in lean subjects can control body weight. Additionally, changes in metabolic rate with caffeine consumption also occur through increased skin and internal temperature [91,95].

The potential relationship between coffee and energy expenditure emerged in the 1980s, but has been attributed more recently to mechanisms that may explain the thermogenic effects of coffee. Among these mechanisms are (1) inhibition of phosphodiesterase-induced degradation of intracellular cyclic AMP (cAMP), leading to cAMP activation of lipolytic pathway proteins such as protein kinase A (PKA), which phosphorylates hormone-sensitive lipase (HSL) and perilipin, thus releasing free fatty acids and glycerol to stimulate the adrenoceptor,

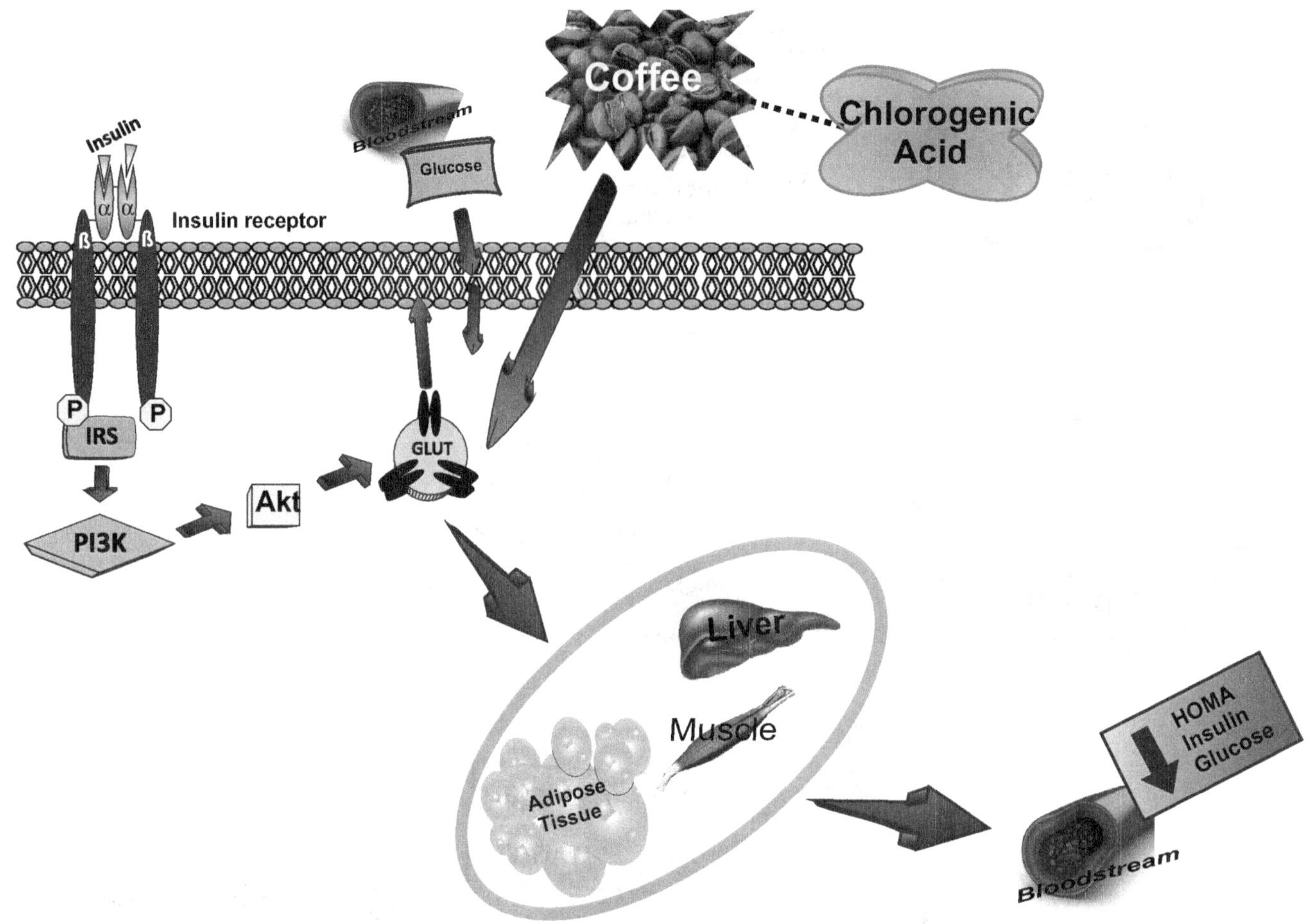

FIGURE 24.3 Diagram showing the effects of coffee and its compounds on glucose metabolism and insulin signaling. In healthy subjects, insulin binds to it receptors, which phosphorylates tyrosine residues in its substrates [insulin receptor substrate (IRS) 1 and 2], which activate phosphoinositide 3-kinase (PI3K), leading to Akt serine phosphorylation, which increases glucose transporters to the plasmatic membrane, which in turn favors the uptake of glucose by liver cells, muscle, and adipose tissue for use as an energy source. Glucose uptake can also be enhanced via 5′-AMP-activated protein kinase (AMPK). However, insulin signaling is blocked or impaired and AMPK is inactivated in obese individuals. Thus, coffee consumption (≥3 cups of 150 mL/day) or chlorogenic acid can activate GLUT proteins and induce AMPK phosphorylation, mainly in adipose tissue, the liver, and skeletal muscle. (See color plate at the back of the book.)

leading to thermogenesis [96–100]; (2) stimulation of norepinephrine secretion and activation of thermogenesis [101,102]; and (3) upregulation of uncoupling protein (UCPs 1, 2, and 3) expression in brown adipose tissue. The latter effect has been shown both for UCP 2 and UCP 3 in murine skeletal muscle [102] and for UCP 2 in cultured cells [103] after the administration of either caffeine or coffee. These UCPs are located inside the mitochondrial membrane and are responsible for dissipating the electrochemical gradient generated by respiratory activity. Thus, UCPs uncouple mitochondrial respiration from oxidative phosphorylation, thus causing energy to be dispersed as heat instead of being used for adenosine triphosphate (ATP) synthesis [96].

Similarly, studies in differentiated 3T3-L1 adipocytes [104] and in humans found a higher rate of lipolysis after caffeine treatment, independent of physical activity level and active [105] or sedentary [106,107] lifestyle. Moreover, a recent in vitro study reported that triacylglycerol content and cholesterol levels were depleted in HepG2 (a human hepatocellular liver carcinoma cell line) cells through inhibition of lipogenesis, mainly through downregulation of genes encoding sterol response element-binding proteins 1c and 2 (SREBP 1c and 2), fatty acid synthase (FAS), and acyl-CoA desaturase [stearoyl-CoA desaturase (SCD1)], and stimulation of lipolysis via expression of AMPK and ACC [108]. However, no changes in lipolysis indicators are found following the consumption of decaffeinated coffee [105,109]. Therefore, caffeine represents a potential target for inducing lipolysis and preventing metabolic syndrome in diet-induced obese rats [110].

Taken together, it is possible that both caffeine and coffee increase thermogenesis and lipolysis, acting as key modulators of obesity disturbances. Fig. 24.4 illustrates the main mechanisms of action of coffee and caffeine in the regulation of these mechanisms.

Anti-inflammatory Actions

Recently, the use of coffee as a source of polyphenols and anti-inflammatory activity has been widely recognized [111,112]. These phenolic compounds are derived from plant metabolites that are beneficial against oxidative stress and inflammation-related diseases. The European Prospective Investigation into Cancer and Nutrition (EPIC) study of 36,037 individuals evaluated the consumption of different sources of phenolic acids and found that coffee was the main food source of phenolic acids compared to fruits, vegetables, and nuts [113]. A cross-sectional study of 2554 male and 763 female Japanese workers showed that coffee intake was negatively associated with blood leptin, triacylglycerols and C-reactive protein (CRP) levels [112]. Another recent cohort study performed in 4455 Japanese men and 5942 Japanese women demonstrated lower serum CRP concentrations in individuals with regular coffee intake [114].

In humans, it was also reported that habitual coffee intake may ameliorate alcohol-induced hepatic inflammation, mainly via reducing CRP levels [115]. Furthermore, it was observed in rodents that treatment with coffee prevents liver fibrosis by inhibiting the expression of genes encoding inducible nitric oxide synthase (iNOS), transforming growth factor beta (TGF-β), tumor necrosis factor (TNF-α), interleukin-1 β (IL-1 β), and platelet-derived growth factor beta (PDGF-β) in liver tissue and iNOS in macrophages [116].

In addition, Kempf et al. [57] demonstrated in 2010 that habitual coffee consumption of an average of 8 cups (150 mL/cup) of filtered coffee per day reduced levels of IL-18 and 8-isoprostane and increased adiponectin levels compared with individuals who did not consume coffee. Therefore, it is possible that a moderate-to-high coffee consumption reduces subclinical inflammation and increases adiponectin, an adipokine linked to cardiovascular disease. Once activated, adiponectin binding to its receptors (AdipoR1 and AdipoR2) leads to AMPK phosphorylation at 172-threonine, which activates peroxisome proliferator-activated receptors gamma (PPAR-γ), thus blocking nuclear factor-kappa-B (NF-κB) translocation into the nucleus and reducing inflammatory cytokine levels (Figs. 24.5 and 24.6). Similarly, in humans, NF-κB activity is suppressed by PPAR-γ activation [117].

In an attempt to understand the effects of chlorogenic acid on inflammation, Shi et al. [118] found that this acid downregulated toll-like receptor 4 (TLR4), Myeloid differentiation primary response protein (MyD88), iNOS, prostaglandin G/H synthase 2 [cyclooxygenase-2 (COX-2)], inhibited NF-κB activation and various proinflammatory cytokines in rats with carbon tetrachloride-induced liver fibrosis. In addition, a cross-sectional American study carried out with 730 healthy women and 663 women with type 2 diabetes mellitus from the Nurses' Health Study I cohort showed that approximately 63–75% of healthy or type 2 diabetes mellitus women consumed ≥1 cup (237 mL) of caffeinated or decaffeinated coffee per month. Additionally, in women with type 2 diabetes mellitus, a higher caffeinated coffee intake was associated with lower plasma CRP levels; in healthy women, only decaffeinated coffee led to a reduction in CRP. Thus, it seems that both caffeinated and decaffeinated coffee, as well as coffee compounds, are responsible for modulating the inflammatory process and blocking inflammatory signaling, thus preventing or treating obesity-associated metabolic disturbances. Inflammatory pathways and the role of coffee in the modulation of proinflammatory proteins are summarized in Figs. 24.5 and 24.6.

Cardiovascular Protection

In the 90's, two meta-analyses reported that the consumption of 5 or more cups of coffee per day may increase the risk of myocardial infarction and coronary death in approximately 40–60% of the population [119,120]. However, more recent data shows that habitual coffee intake reduces cardiovascular disease risk [67,121,122]. Similarly, acute caffeine intake (200 mg) could improve endothelial function and reduce proinflammatory cytokines [122].

In a Netherland cohort study of 37,514 individuals, those who drank 2.1–3 cups of coffee per day decreased their risk of developing coronary heart disease by 21% [123]. Furthermore, in a study performed with 93,676 postmenopausal women from the Women's Health Initiative Observational Study, it was observed that total caffeine, regular coffee, decaffeinated coffee, and regular tea intakes were not associated with the risk of sudden cardiac death [121]. Thus, there is strong evidence that both coffee caffeinated and decaffeinated and their constituents can reduce or at least not increase cardiovascular disease risk factors.

In rodents, the administration of caffeine (25 mg per kg/day) before myocardial ischemia/reperfusion surgery reduced myocardial injury by inhibiting inflammatory and apoptotic indicators, such as iNOS, IL-6, poly (ADP-ribose)-polymerase (PARP), and TNF-α [124]. In addition, a recent study suggested that chlorogenic acids may provide an attractive opportunity for decreasing inflammation, blood pressure, type 2 diabetes mellitus indicators, and platelet aggregation. In addition,

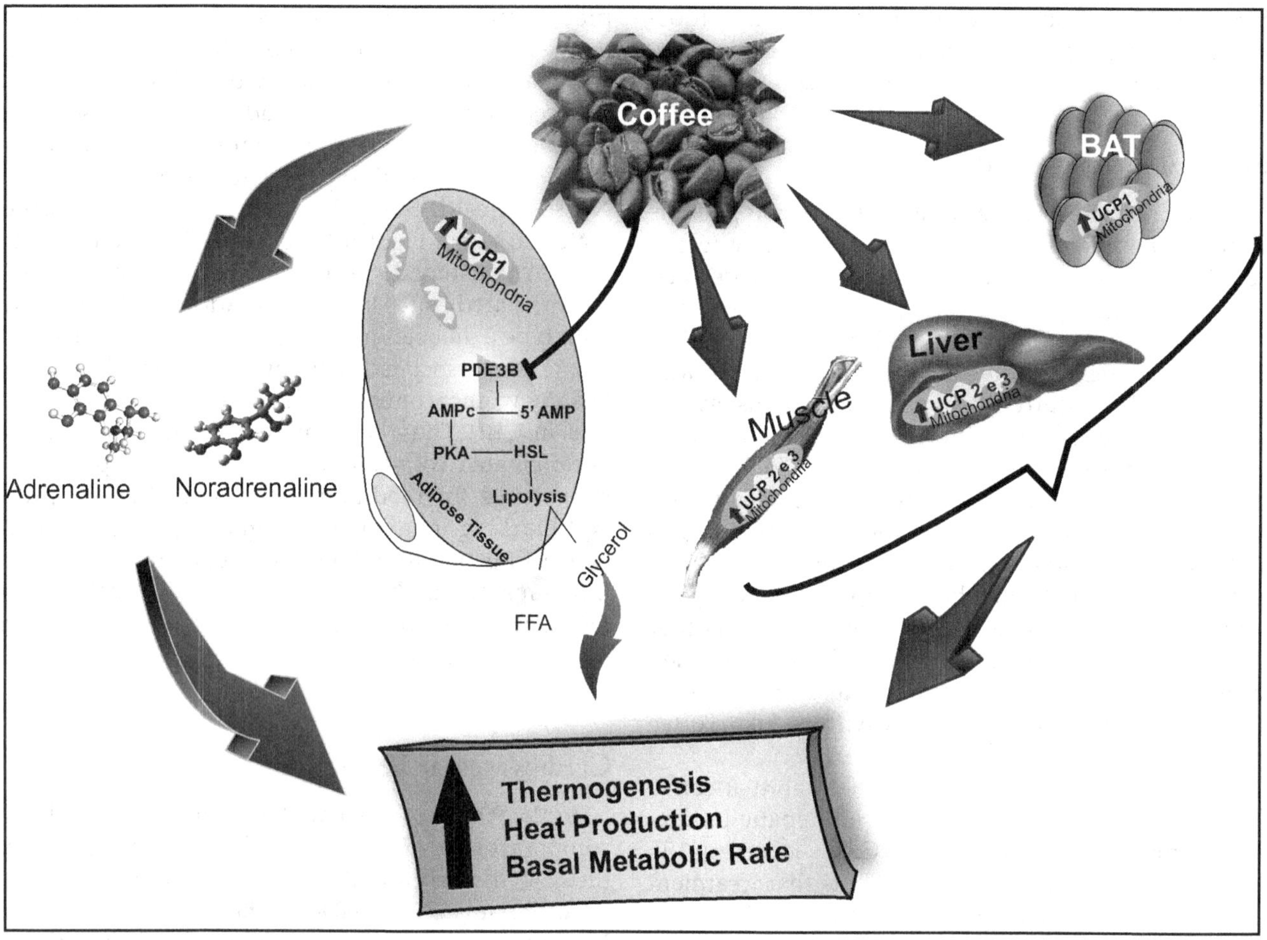

FIGURE 24.4 Main mechanisms of action of coffee and caffeine in increasing thermogenesis. Coffee and caffeine consumption may increase thermogenesis by (1) activating uncoupling proteins (UCPs 1, 2, and 3) in brown adipose tissue (BAT), liver, or skeletal muscle; (2) releasing noradrenaline and adrenaline and increasing lipolysis; and (3) inhibiting phosphodiesterase-induced degradation of intracellular cyclic AMP (cAMP). cAMP activates lipolysis pathway proteins such as protein kinase A (PKA), which phosphorylates hormone-sensitive lipase (HSL) and perilipin, releasing free fatty acids and glycerol to stimulate adrenoceptors, leading to thermogenesis. (See color plate at the back of the book.)

caffeine was reported to increase flow-induced arterial dilation [42].

Microbiota and Other Possible Mechanisms

The gut microbiota modulates energy homeostasis and the digestion and metabolism of nutrients. Thus, low-grade inflammation-related diseases, such as obesity, have emerged as an attractive opportunity for researchers to understand how nutrients may modify the gut microbiota and improve health [76,125–127]. Consequently, some authors have suggested that coffee may have prebiotic- and probiotic-like properties, leading to modifications in the gut microbiota [128,129].

Recently, Nakayama et al. [129] demonstrated in A/J mice (specific pathogen-free rodents) treated with coffee (500 μL/day) that antibiotic actions were indicated by the inhibition of bacterial growth, such as *Escherichia coli* and *Clostridium* spp., an increase in *Bifidobacterium* spp., and no significant change in *Bacteroidetes* and *Lactobacillus* spp. in the proximal colon. Furthermore, these authors observed increased aquaporin-8 expression in both the proximal colon and distal small intestine. These findings are extremely fascinating since they suggest that coffee consumption can modulate the gut microbiota and improve intestinal balance in individuals with impaired gut microbiota, such as individuals with metabolic syndrome, inflammatory bowel disease, and cancer.

Another factor that may contribute to a healthy gut is increased aquaporin-8 expression in the intestine. This protein is mainly expressed in hepatocytes and the intestine [130,131]. According to Yamamoto et al. [131], it is a transmembrane water-channel protein that facilitates

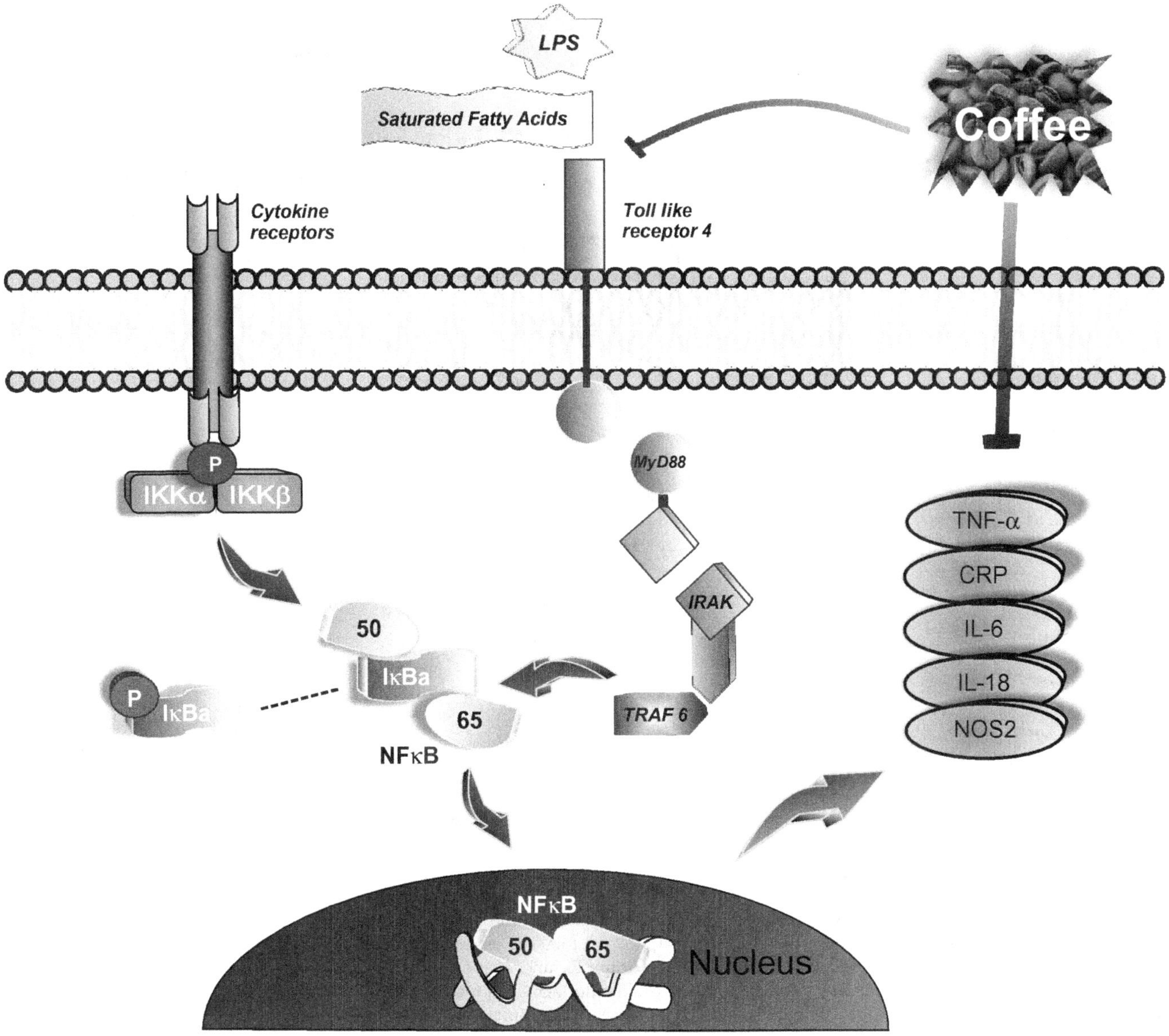

FIGURE 24.5 Schematic diagram showing the effects of coffee on the levels of proinflammatory molecules. In obese patients, inflammatory signaling is activated. A high intake of *trans* or saturated fatty acids, as well as a high lipopolysaccharide (LPS) content in the blood, has been demonstrated to induce proinflammatory cytokine production through the nuclear factor-kappa-B (NFκB) pathway after activation of the toll-like receptor 4 (TLR4). Activation of TLR4 initiates the myeloid differentiation primary response protein (MyD88)-dependent signaling pathway. MyD88 binding to the cytoplasmic domain of TLR4 activates TNF receptor-associated factor 6 (TRAF6), which is recruited by interleukin-1 receptor-associated kinase 1 (IRAK-1). Following IRAK-1 phosphorylation, the TRAF6 complex dissociates from the TLRs and TRAF6 interacts with various proteins to form a large complex that activates of transforming growth factor-beta-activated kinase 1 (TAK1). TAK1 phosphorylates the inhibitor of nuclear factor kappa-B (IκB) kinase (IKK) complex, and phosphorylated IκB is targeted for proteasomal degradation. Thus, the p65 subunit of NFκB is activated and translocates to the nucleus, where it binds to its target genes to produce proinflammatory cytokines, such as tumor necrosis factor (TNF-α), interleukin-6 (IL-6), interleukin-1β (IL-1β), interleukin-13 (IL-13), inducible nitric oxide synthase (iNOS/NOS2) and C-reactive protein (CRP). On the other hand, coffee and chlorogenic acid consumption can reduce proinflammatory cytokines in the blood, brain, and peripheral tissues and inhibit TLR4 expression, thus reducing inflammation and obesity. (See color plate at the back of the book.)

water transport. Low aquaporin-8 expression is related to impaired gut health in mice with food allergy and diarrhea [131] and in patients with ulcerative colitis [132].

In addition to the beneficial effects of coffee, it has been observed that iron absorption is blocked by polyphenol compounds in coffee, such as chlorogenic acid; this may be one of the mechanisms underlying

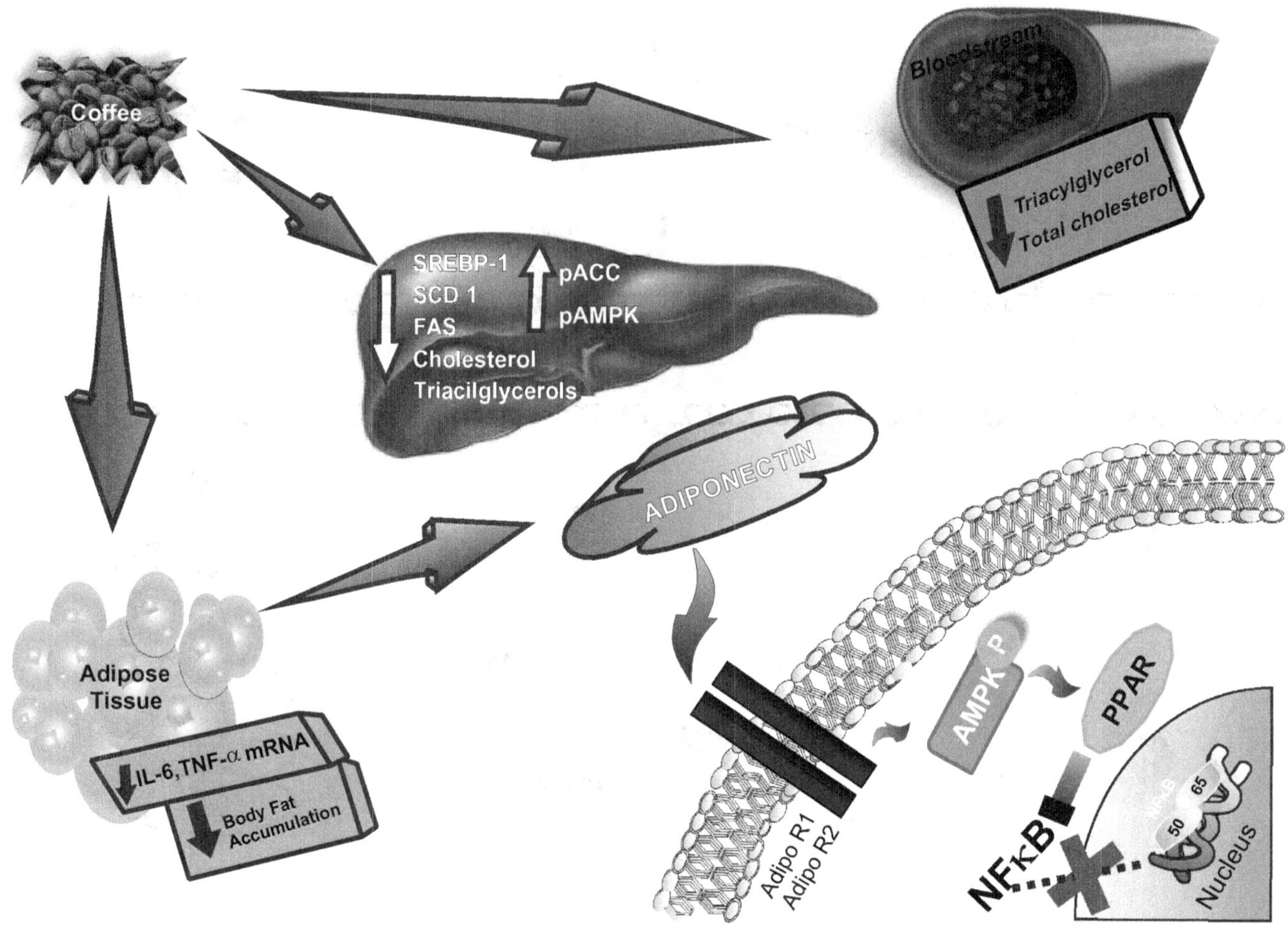

FIGURE 24.6 Schematic diagram showing the effects of coffee on cardiovascular disease indicators and inflammatory parameters in the bloodstream, liver, and white adipose tissue. Obese patients frequently have large amounts of adipose tissue and hepatic steatosis, accompanied by increased proinflammatory protein expression. Thus, coffee intake reduces adiposity and steatosis, as well as inflammation, by inhibiting tumor necrosis factor (TNF-α), interleukin-6 (IL-6), interleukin-1β (IL-1β), total cholesterol, triacylglycerols, glycemia, and insulin, and increasing blood adiponectin levels. Adiponectin binding to its receptors (Adipo R1 and Adipo R2) leads to 5′-AMP-activated protein kinase (AMPK) phosphorylation at threonine-172, which activates peroxisome proliferator-activated receptor gamma (PPAR-γ). This blocks the translocation of nuclear factor-kappa-B (NFκB) into the nucleus and thus reduces levels of inflammatory cytokines. (See color plate at the back of the book.)

the protective effects of coffee on glucose metabolism [133–135], as there is some evidence that iron accumulation and type 2 diabetes mellitus risk increases with increased body weight [136]. A review has shown that the induction of iron deficiency in impaired glucose-tolerant subjects improves insulin sensitivity [137]. Moreover, phenolic acids are also found in other nutrients, teas, such as chamomile (*Matricaria recutita* L.), vervain (*Verbena officinalis* L.), lime flower (*Tilia cordata* Mill.), pennyroyal (*Mentha pulegium* L.), peppermint (*M. piperita* L.) and black tea, as well as in products rich in cocoa [134]. These compounds may decrease iron content by 47–94%, depending on the period between their intake and that of iron.

In summary, changes in the gut microbiota and reduced iron absorption are possible mechanisms by which habitual coffee intake can improve the metabolic consequences of obesity.

POTENTIAL ADVERSE EFFECTS OF COFFEE

Effects on Blood Pressure

Coffee is thought to trigger hypertension. In a meta-analysis published in 2005 [138], the authors compiled all data concerning coffee intake, caffeine intake, and hypertension published between January 1966 and January 2003. Sixteen studies were included, comprising a total of 1010 subjects. For all studies, a mean significant increase of 2.04 mmHg [95% confidence interval(CI)]

1.10–2.99 mmHg systolic blood pressure (BP), and 0.73 mmHg (95% CI 0.14–1.31) diastolic BP was found. When data on coffee ($n = 18$; mean quantity ingested, 725 mL/day) and caffeine ($n = 7$; mean quantity of caffeine ingested, 410 mg/day) were analyzed separately, increases in BP were larger for caffeine alone (systolic BP, 4.16 mmHg 95% CI 2.13–6.20; diastolic BP, 2.41 mmHg, 95% CI 0.98–3.84) than for coffee alone (systolic BP, 1.22 mmHg, 95% CI 0.52–1.92; diastolic BP, 0.49 mmHg, 95% CI 0.06–1.04). The difference between data for coffee and caffeine suggests that other components in coffee can compensate for the increase in BP linked to caffeine intake.

The potential hypotensive role for chlorogenic acids in coffee was recently reviewed [139]. Chlorogenic acid supplementation, both acute and chronic, decreased BP in a rat model of hypertension [140,141]. In two human studies, chlorogenic acids (vs. placebo) also appeared to significantly decrease both systolic and diastolic BP [142,143]. This effect could be attributed to chlorogenic acids and their metabolites that attenuate oxidative stress and thus act by improving endothelial function and NO bioavailability at the arterial level. The authors hypothesized that a diet rich in chlorogenic acids could constitute a nonpharmacological approach in the prevention or treatment of arterial hypertension. The presence of a large amount of chlorogenic acids in coffee could explain differences between the effects of coffee and caffeine on BP. Thus, for people at risk of hypertension, such as obese subjects or those with metabolic syndrome, it is preferable to consume caffeine in the form of coffee to avoid or limit the transient increases in BP that may be generated by the consumption of caffeine alone. Moreover, the regular consumption of caffeinated coffee was reported not to increase the risk of hypertension [144].

Effects of Coffee on Cholesterol

Cholesterol linked to low-density lipoprotein (LDL) and triglycerides has a high atherogenic potential, and its increase is potentially harmful: obese people are particularly at risk in this respect. Coffee is a bean and, as such, is rich in lipids. In earlier studies, the acute ingestion of coffee was reported to increase total cholesterol, and especially total cholesterol linked to triglycerides. This effect is generally observed only after the ingestion of more than 3 cups of boiled unfiltered coffee per day and is due to the action of diterpenes (mainly cafestol and kahweol). Classically, filtered, instant, and espresso coffee do not significantly affect lipid metabolism. The consumption of relatively high quantities of coffee was also associated with increased plasma levels of homocysteine, which may also be associated with an increased risk of cardiovascular disease. However, the consumption or adequate supplementation of folic acid prevents the increase in plasma homocysteine [144,145].

The cardiovascular risk of coffee is not supported by recent studies. In populations at risk, the primary lifestyle advice is to stop smoking and increase physical activity and diet quality.

CONCLUSION

In summary, since the 1950s the habitual intake of coffee and its compounds have provided attractive areas of research for scientific investigators and clinical health professionals. Several epidemiological studies have demonstrated that the consumption of ≥3 cups of coffee per day or its phenolic compounds may reduce the risk of obesity. Furthermore, numerous mechanisms that underlie the actions of coffee have proven to improve insulin resistance, inflammation, and body weight, and provide protection from cardiovascular diseases.

References

[1] Kopelman PG. Obesity as a medical problem. Nature 2000;404(6778):635–43.
[2] Friedman JM. A tale of two hormones. Nat Med 2010;16(10):1100–6.
[3] Cunha CA, Lira FS, Rosa Neto JC, Pimentel GD, Souza GI, da Silva CM, et al. Green tea extract supplementation induces the lipolytic pathway, attenuates obesity, and reduces low-grade inflammation in mice fed a high-fat diet. Mediators Inflamm 2013;2013:635470.
[4] Lira FS, Rosa JC, Pimentel GD, Santos RV, Carnier J, Sanches PL, et al. Long-term interdisciplinary therapy reduces endotoxin level and insulin resistance in obese adolescents. Nutr J 2012;11:74.
[5] Pimentel GD, Lira FS, Rosa JC, Caris AV, Pinheiro F, Ribeiro EB, et al. Yerba mate extract (Ilex paraguariensis) attenuates both central and peripheral inflammatory effects of diet-induced obesity in rats. J Nutr Biochem 2013;24(5):809–18.
[6] Pimentel GD, Lira FS, Rosa JC, Oliveira JL, Losinskas-Hachul AC, Souza GI, et al. Intake of trans fatty acids during gestation and lactation leads to hypothalamic inflammation via TLR4/NFkappaBp65 signaling in adult offspring. J Nutr Biochem 2012;23(3):265–71.
[7] Flegal KM, Kit BK, Orpana H, Graubard BI. Association of all-cause mortality with overweight and obesity using standard body mass index categories: a systematic review and meta-analysis. JAMA 2013;309(1):71–82.
[8] Ebbeling CB, Ludwig DS. Sugar-sweetened beverages, genetic risk, and obesity. N Engl J Med 2013;368(3):287.
[9] Qi Q, Chu AY, Kang JH, Jensen MK, Curhan GC, Pasquale LR, et al. Sugar-sweetened beverages and genetic risk of obesity. N Engl J Med 2012;367(15):1387–96.
[10] Farooqi IS, Wangensteen T, Collins S, Kimber W, Matarese G, Keogh JM, et al. Clinical and molecular genetic spectrum of congenital deficiency of the leptin receptor. N Engl J Med 2007;356(3):237–47.
[11] Pauling L. The relation between longevity and obesity in human beings. Proc Natl Acad Sci USA 1958;44(6):619–22.
[12] Janis LB. Coffee and obesity. Ohio Med 1957;53(6):659–60.
[13] Kuftinec DM, Mayer J. Extreme sensitivity of obese hyperglycemic mice to caffeine and coffee. Metabolism 1964;13:1369–75.

[14] Jankelson OM, Beaser SB, Howard FM, Mayer J. Effect of coffee on glucose tolerance and circulating insulin in men with maturity-onset diabetes. Lancet 1967;1(7489):527–9.
[15] Hankiewicz J. Effect of the use of caffeine on the level of glucose in the blood. Pol Tyg Lek 1960;15:742–5.
[16] Goldman JA, Ovadia J. The effect of coffee on glucose tolerance in normal and prediabetic pregnant women. Obstet Gynecol 1969;33(2):214–8.
[17] Dawber TR, Kannel WB, Gordon T. Coffee and cardiovascular disease. Observations from the framingham study. N Engl J Med 1974;291(17):871–4.
[18] Duffey KJ, Popkin BM. Shifts in patterns and consumption of beverages between 1965 and 2002. Obesity (Silver Spring) 2007;15(11):2739–47.
[19] Freedman ND, Park Y, Abnet CC, Hollenbeck AR, Sinha R. Association of coffee drinking with total and cause-specific mortality. N Engl J Med 2012;366(20):1891–904.
[20] Mure K, Maeda S, Mukoubayashi C, Mugitani K, Iwane M, Kinoshita F, et al. Habitual coffee consumption inversely associated with metabolic syndrome-related biomarkers involving adiponectin. Nutrition 2013;29(7–8):982–7.
[21] Park S, Onufrak S, Blanck HM, Sherry B. Characteristics associated with consumption of sports and energy drinks among US adults: National Health Interview Survey, 2010. J Acad Nutr Diet 2013;113(1):112–9.
[22] ICO. International coffee organization, statistics. <http://www.ico.org/trade_statistics.asp> [accessed 18.04.13].
[23] Barone JJ, Roberts HR. Caffeine consumption. Food Chem Toxicol 1996;34(1):119–29.
[24] de Souza RA, Sichieri R. Caffeine intake and food sources of caffeine and prematurity: a case-control study. Cadernos de saude publica 2005;21(6):1919–28.
[25] Paynter NP, Yeh HC, Voutilainen S, Schmidt MI, Heiss G, Folsom AR, et al. Coffee and sweetened beverage consumption and the risk of type 2 diabetes mellitus: the atherosclerosis risk in communities study. Am J Epidemiol 2006;164(11):1075–84.
[26] van Dam RM, Feskens EJ. Coffee consumption and risk of type 2 diabetes mellitus. Lancet 2002;360(9344):1477–8.
[27] Tuomilehto J, Hu G, Bidel S, Lindstrom J, Jousilahti P. Coffee consumption and risk of type 2 diabetes mellitus among middle-aged Finnish men and women. JAMA 2004;291(10):1213–9.
[28] Takami H, Nakamoto M, Uemura H, Katsuura S, Yamaguchi M, Hiyoshi M, et al. Inverse correlation between coffee consumption and prevalence of metabolic syndrome: baseline survey of the Japan Multi-Institutional Collaborative Cohort (J-MICC) Study in Tokushima, Japan. J Epidemiol 2013;23(1):12–20.
[29] Saremi A, Tulloch-Reid M, Knowler WC. Coffee consumption and the incidence of type 2 diabetes. Diabetes Care 2003;26(7):2211–2.
[30] Carlsson S, Hammar N, Grill V, Kaprio J. Coffee consumption and risk of type 2 diabetes in Finnish twins. Int J Epidemiol 2004;33(3):616–7.
[31] Salazar-Martinez E, Willett WC, Ascherio A, Manson JE, Leitzmann MF, Stampfer MJ, et al. Coffee consumption and risk for type 2 diabetes mellitus. Ann Intern Med 2004;140(1):1–8.
[32] van Dam RM, Dekker JM, Nijpels G, Stehouwer CD, Bouter LM, Heine RJ. Coffee consumption and incidence of impaired fasting glucose, impaired glucose tolerance, and type 2 diabetes: the Hoorn Study. Diabetologia 2004;47(12):2152–9.
[33] van Dam RM, Hu FB. Coffee consumption and risk of type 2 diabetes: a systematic review. JAMA 2005;294(1):97–104.
[34] Smith B, Wingard DL, Smith TC, Kritz-Silverstein D, Barrett-Connor E. Does coffee consumption reduce the risk of type 2 diabetes in individuals with impaired glucose? Diabetes Care 2006;29(11):2385–90.
[35] Sartorelli DS, Fagherazzi G, Balkau B, Touillaud MS, Boutron-Ruault MC, de Lauzon-Guillain B, et al. Differential effects of coffee on the risk of type 2 diabetes according to meal consumption in a French cohort of women: the E3N/EPIC cohort study. Am J Clin Nutr 2010;91(4):1002–12.
[36] Boggs DA, Rosenberg L, Ruiz-Narvaez EA, Palmer JR. Coffee, tea, and alcohol intake in relation to risk of type 2 diabetes in African American women. Am J Clin Nutr 2010;92(4):960–6.
[37] Bhupathiraju SN, Pan A, Malik VS, Manson JE, Willett WC, van Dam RM, et al. Caffeinated and caffeine-free beverages and risk of type 2 diabetes. Am J Clin Nutr 2013;97(1):155–66.
[38] Doo T, Morimoto Y, Steinbrecher A, Kolonel LN, Maskarinec G. Coffee intake and risk of type 2 diabetes: the Multiethnic Cohort. Public Health Nutr 2013:1–9.
[39] van Dam RM, Willett WC, Manson JE, Hu FB. Coffee, caffeine, and risk of type 2 diabetes: a prospective cohort study in younger and middle-aged U.S. women. Diabetes Care 2006;29(2):398–403.
[40] Pereira MA, Parker ED, Folsom AR. Coffee consumption and risk of type 2 diabetes mellitus: an 11-year prospective study of 28 812 postmenopausal women. Arch Intern Med 2006;166(12):1311–6.
[41] Wu T, Willett WC, Hankinson SE, Giovannucci E. Caffeinated coffee, decaffeinated coffee, and caffeine in relation to plasma C-peptide levels, a marker of insulin secretion, in U.S. women. Diabetes Care 2005;28(6):1390–6.
[42] Montagnana M, Favaloro EJ, Lippi G. Coffee intake and cardiovascular disease: virtue does not take center stage. Semin Thromb Hemost 2012;38(2):164–77.
[43] Pimentel GD, Zemdegs JC, Theodoro JA, Mota JF. Does long-term coffee intake reduce type 2 diabetes mellitus risk? Diabetol Metabol Syndr 2009;1(1):6.
[44] Vinson JA, Burnham BR, Nagendran MV. Randomized, double-blind, placebo-controlled, linear dose, crossover study to evaluate the efficacy and safety of a green coffee bean extract in overweight subjects. Diab Metab Syndr Obes 2012;5:21–7.
[45] Choi EY, Park SY, Cho YO. Freeze-dried instant coffee can promote the activities of antioxidant enzymes and induce weight loss but also aggravate the plasma cholesterol profile in rats. Nutrition 2011;27(11–12):1202–5.
[46] Greenberg JA, Boozer CN, Geliebter A. Coffee, diabetes, and weight control. Am J Clin Nutr 2006;84(4):682–93.
[47] Han LK, Takaku T, Li J, Kimura Y, Okuda H. Anti-obesity action of oolong tea. Int J Obes Relat Metab Disord 1999;23(1):98–105.
[48] Lira FS, Rosa JC, Pimentel GD, Souza HA, Caperuto EC, Carnevali Jr LC, et al. Endotoxin levels correlate positively with a sedentary lifestyle and negatively with highly trained subjects. Lipids Health Dis 2010;9:82.
[49] Pimentel GD, Zemdegs JC. Foods and nutrients modulates the release of anorexigenic gastrointestinal hormones. Acta Med Port 2010;23(5):891–900.
[50] Pimentel GD, Arimura ST, de Moura BM, Silva ME, de Sousa MV. Short-term nutritional counseling reduces body mass index, waist circumference, triceps skinfold and triglycerides in women with metabolic syndrome. Diabetol Metabol Syndr 2010;2:13.
[51] Nehlig A. Are we dependent upon coffee and caffeine? A review on human and animal data. Neurosci Biobehav Rev 1999;23(4):563–76.
[52] Graham DM. Caffeine—its identity, dietary sources, intake and biological effects. Nutr Rev 1978;36(4):97–102.
[53] Vercambre MN, Berr C, Ritchie K, Kang JH. Caffeine and cognitive decline in elderly women at high vascular risk. J Alzheimers Dis 2013;35(2):413–21.
[54] Lee KW, Im JY, Woo JM, Grosso H, Kim YS, Cristovao AC, et al. Neuroprotective and anti-inflammatory properties of a coffee

component in the MPTP model of Parkinson's disease. Neurotherapeutics 2013;10(1):143–53.

[55] Wang S, Yoon YC, Sung MJ, Hur HJ, Park JH. Antiangiogenic properties of cafestol, a coffee diterpene, in human umbilical vein endothelial cells. Biochem Biophys Res Commun 2012;421(3):567–71.

[56] Sinclair CJ, Geiger JD. Caffeine use in sports. A pharmacological review. J Sports Med Phys Fitness 2000;40(1):71–9.

[57] Kempf K, Herder C, Erlund I, Kolb H, Martin S, Carstensen M, et al. Effects of coffee consumption on subclinical inflammation and other risk factors for type 2 diabetes: a clinical trial. Am J Clin Nutr 2010;91(4):950–7.

[58] Newton R, Broughton LJ, Lind MJ, Morrison PJ, Rogers HJ, Bradbrook ID. Plasma and salivary pharmacokinetics of caffeine in man. Eur J Clin Pharmacol 1981;21(1):45–52.

[59] Biaggioni I, Davis SN. Caffeine: a cause of insulin resistance? Diabetes Care 2002;25(2):399–400.

[60] Eskenazi B. Caffeine—filtering the facts. N Engl J Med 1999;341(22):1688–9.

[61] Kalow W, Tang BK. The use of caffeine for enzyme assays: a critical appraisal. Clin Pharmacol Ther 1993;53(5):503–14.

[62] Blanchard J, Sawers SJ. Comparative pharmacokinetics of caffeine in young and elderly men. J Pharmacokinet Biopharm 1983;11(2):109–26.

[63] McCusker RR, Goldberger BA, Cone EJ. Caffeine content of specialty coffees. J Anal Toxicol 2003;27(7):520–2.

[64] dE Kennedy A. The effects of natural caffeine versus synthetic caffeine on rat body weight and food intake. University of IllinoisUrbana-Champaign, Food Science and Human Nutrition; 2007.

[65] Heckman MA, Weil J, Gonzalez de Mejia E. Caffeine (1, 3, 7-trimethylxanthine) in foods: a comprehensive review on consumption, functionality, safety, and regulatory matters. J Food Sci 2010;75(3):R77–87.

[66] Canadian clinical practice guidelines: originating associations 2008.

[67] Lopez-Garcia E, van Dam RM, Rajpathak S, Willett WC, Manson JE, Hu FB. Changes in caffeine intake and long-term weight change in men and women. Am J Clin Nutr 2006;83(3):674–80.

[68] Westerterp-Plantenga MS, Lejeune MP, Kovacs EM. Body weight loss and weight maintenance in relation to habitual caffeine intake and green tea supplementation. Obes Res 2005;13(7):1195–204.

[69] Kovacs EM, Lejeune MP, Nijs I, Westerterp-Plantenga MS. Effects of green tea on weight maintenance after body-weight loss. Br J Nutr 2004;91(3):431–7.

[70] Carter BE, Drewnowski A. Beverages containing soluble fiber, caffeine, and green tea catechins suppress hunger and lead to less energy consumption at the next meal. Appetite 2012;59(3):755–61.

[71] Hussein GM, Matsuda H, Nakamura S, Hamao M, Akiyama T, Tamura K, et al. Mate tea (Ilex paraguariensis) promotes satiety and body weight lowering in mice: involvement of glucagon-like peptide-1. Biol Pharm Bull 2011;34(12):1849–55.

[72] Nauck MA, Heimesaat MM, Orskov C, Holst JJ, Ebert R, Creutzfeldt W. Preserved incretin activity of glucagon-like peptide 1 [7-36 amide] but not of synthetic human gastric inhibitory polypeptide in patients with type-2 diabetes mellitus. J Clin Invest 1993;91(1):301–7.

[73] Meier JJ, Hucking K, Holst JJ, Deacon CF, Schmiegel WH, Nauck MA. Reduced insulinotropic effect of gastric inhibitory polypeptide in first-degree relatives of patients with type 2 diabetes. Diabetes 2001;50(11):2497–504.

[74] Johnston KL, Clifford MN, Morgan LM. Coffee acutely modifies gastrointestinal hormone secretion and glucose tolerance in humans: glycemic effects of chlorogenic acid and caffeine. Am J Clin Nutr 2003;78(4):728–33.

[75] Scott R, Tan T, Bloom S. Gut hormones and obesity: physiology and therapies. Vitam Horm 2013;91:143–94.

[76] Pimentel GD, Micheletti TO, Pace F, Rosa JC, Santos RV, Lira FS. Gut-central nervous system axis is a target for nutritional therapies. Nutr J 2012;11:22.

[77] Rasoamanana R, Darcel N, Fromentin G, Tome D. Nutrient sensing and signalling by the gut. Proc Nutr Soc 2012;71(4):446–55.

[78] McCarty MF. A chlorogenic acid-induced increase in GLP-1 production may mediate the impact of heavy coffee consumption on diabetes risk. Med Hypotheses 2005;64(4):848–53.

[79] Tuomilehto J, Tuomilehto-Wolf E, Virtala E, LaPorte R. Coffee consumption as trigger for insulin dependent diabetes mellitus in childhood. BMJ 1990;300(6725):642–3.

[80] Olthof MR, van Dijk AE, Deacon CF, Heine RJ, van Dam RM. Acute effects of decaffeinated coffee and the major coffee components chlorogenic acid and trigonelline on incretin hormones. Nutr Metab 2011;8:10.

[81] Clifford MN, Wu W, Kirkpatrick J, Kuhnert N. Profiling the chlorogenic acids and other caffeic acid derivatives of herbal chrysanthemum by LC-MSn. J Agric Food Chem 2007;55(3):929–36.

[82] Baskaran SK, Goswami N, Selvaraj S, Muthusamy VS, Lakshmi BS. Molecular dynamics approach to probe the allosteric inhibition of PTP1B by chlorogenic and cichoric acid. J Chem Inf Model 2012;52(8):2004–12.

[83] Matsui T, Ueda T, Oki T, Sugita K, Terahara N, Matsumoto K. α-Glucosidase inhibitory action of natural acylated anthocyanins. 1. Survey of natural pigments with potent inhibitory activity. J Agric Food Chem 2001;49(4):1948–51.

[84] Kobayashi Y, Suzuki M, Satsu H, Arai S, Hara Y, Suzuki K, et al. Green tea polyphenols inhibit the sodium-dependent glucose transporter of intestinal epithelial cells by a competitive mechanism. J Agric Food Chem 2000;48(11):5618–23.

[85] Newgard CB, Foster DW, McGarry JD. Evidence for suppression of hepatic glucose-6-phosphatase with carbohydrate feeding. Diabetes 1984;33(2):192–5.

[86] Youn JH, Youn MS, Bergman RN. Synergism of glucose and fructose in net glycogen synthesis in perfused rat livers. J Biol Chem 1986;261(34):15960–9.

[87] Arion WJ, Canfield WK, Ramos FC, Schindler PW, Burger HJ, Hemmerle H, et al. Chlorogenic acid and hydroxynitrobenzaldehyde: new inhibitors of hepatic glucose 6-phosphatase. Arch Biochem Biophys 1997;339(2):315–22.

[88] Ong KW, Hsu A, Tan BK. Chlorogenic acid stimulates glucose transport in skeletal muscle via AMPK activation: a contributor to the beneficial effects of coffee on diabetes. PloS One 2012;7(3):e32718.

[89] Beaudoin MS, Robinson LE, Graham TE. An oral lipid challenge and acute intake of caffeinated coffee additively decrease glucose tolerance in healthy men. J Nutr 2011;141(4):574–81.

[90] Acheson KJ, Zahorska-Markiewicz B, Pittet P, Anantharaman K, Jequier E. Caffeine and coffee: their influence on metabolic rate and substrate utilization in normal weight and obese individuals. Am J Clin Nutr 1980;33(5):989–97.

[91] Tagliabue A, Terracina D, Cena H, Turconi G, Lanzola E, Montomoli C. Coffee induced thermogenesis and skin temperature. Int J Obes Relat Metab Disord 1994;18(8):537–41.

[92] Rudelle S, Ferruzzi MG, Cristiani I, Moulin J, Mace K, Acheson KJ, et al. Effect of a thermogenic beverage on 24-hour energy metabolism in humans. Obesity (Silver Spring) 2007;15(2):349–55.

[93] Bracco D, Ferrarra JM, Arnaud MJ, Jequier E, Schutz Y. Effects of caffeine on energy metabolism, heart rate, and methylxanthine metabolism in lean and obese women. Am J Physiol 1995;269(4 Pt 1):E671–8.

[94] Dulloo AG, Geissler CA, Horton T, Collins A, Miller DS. Normal caffeine consumption: influence on thermogenesis and daily energy expenditure in lean and postobese human volunteers. Am J Clin Nutr 1989;49(1):44–50.

[95] Koot P, Deurenberg P. Comparison of changes in energy expenditure and body temperatures after caffeine consumption. Ann Nutr Metab 1995;39(3):135–42.

[96] Scherer T, O'Hare J, Diggs-Andrews K, Schweiger M, Cheng B, Lindtner C, et al. Brain insulin controls adipose tissue lipolysis and lipogenesis. Cell Metab 2011;13(2):183–94.

[97] Cocchi M, Siniscalchi C, Rogato F, Valeriani A. Free fatty acid levels in habitual coffee drinkers in relation to quantities consumed, sex and age. Ann Nutr Metab 1983;27(6):477–80.

[98] Hawkins GE, Davis WE. Changes in plasma free fatty acids and triglycerides in dairy cattle after dosing with coffee or caffeine. J Dairy Sci 1970;53(1):52–5.

[99] Granneman JG, Moore HP, Granneman RL, Greenberg AS, Obin MS, Zhu Z. Analysis of lipolytic protein trafficking and interactions in adipocytes. J Biol Chem 2007;282(8):5726–35.

[100] Granneman JG, Moore HP, Krishnamoorthy R, Rathod M. Perilipin controls lipolysis by regulating the interactions of AB-hydrolase containing 5 (Abhd5) and adipose triglyceride lipase (Atgl). J Biol Chem 2009;284(50):34538–44.

[101] Westerterp-Plantenga M, Diepvens K, Joosen AM, Berube-Parent S, Tremblay A. Metabolic effects of spices, teas, and caffeine. Physiol Behav 2006;89(1):85–91.

[102] Kogure A, Sakane N, Takakura Y, Umekawa T, Yoshioka K, Nishino H, et al. Effects of caffeine on the uncoupling protein family in obese yellow KK mice. Clin Exp Pharmacol Physiol 2002;29(5–6):391–4.

[103] Riedel A, Pignitter M, Hochkogler CM, Rohm B, Walker J, Bytof G, et al. Caffeine dose-dependently induces thermogenesis but restores ATP in HepG2 cells in culture. Food Funct 2012;3(9):955–64.

[104] Hashimoto T, Sato K, Iemitsu M. Exercise-inducible factors to activate lipolysis in adipocytes. J Appl Physiol 2013;115(2):260–7.

[105] Costill DL, Dalsky GP, Fink WJ. Effects of caffeine ingestion on metabolism and exercise performance. Med Sci Sports 1978;10(3):155–8.

[106] Keijzers GB, De Galan BE, Tack CJ, Smits P. Caffeine can decrease insulin sensitivity in humans. Diabetes Care 2002;25(2):364–9.

[107] Bellet S, Kershbaum A, Finck EM. Response of free fatty acids to coffee and caffeine. Metabolism 1968;17(8):702–7.

[108] Quan HY, Kim do Y, Chung SH. Caffeine attenuates lipid accumulation via activation of AMP-activated protein kinase signaling pathway in HepG2 cells. BMB Rep 2013;46(4):207–12.

[109] Shearer J, Farah A, de Paulis T, Bracy DP, Pencek RR, Graham TE, et al. Quinides of roasted coffee enhance insulin action in conscious rats. J Nutr 2003;133(11):3529–32.

[110] Panchal SK, Wong WY, Kauter K, Ward LC, Brown L. Caffeine attenuates metabolic syndrome in diet-induced obese rats. Nutrition 2012;28(10):1055–62.

[111] Tangney CC, Rasmussen HE. Polyphenols, inflammation, and cardiovascular disease. Curr Atheroscler Rep 2013;15(5):324.

[112] Yamashita K, Yatsuya H, Muramatsu T, Toyoshima H, Murohara T, Tamakoshi K. Association of coffee consumption with serum adiponectin, leptin, inflammation and metabolic markers in Japanese workers: a cross-sectional study. Nutr Diab 2012;2:e33.

[113] Zamora-Ros R, Rothwell JA, Scalbert A, Knaze V, Romieu I, Slimani N, et al. Dietary intakes and food sources of phenolic acids in the European Prospective Investigation into Cancer and Nutrition (EPIC) study. Br J Nutr 2013:1–12.

[114] Pham NM, Wang Z, Morita M, Ohnaka K, Adachi M, Kawate H, et al. Combined effects of coffee consumption and serum gamma-glutamyltransferase on serum C-reactive protein in middle-aged and elderly Japanese men and women. Clin Chem Lab Med 2011;49(10):1661–7.

[115] Maki T, Pham NM, Yoshida D, Yin G, Ohnaka K, Takayanagi R, et al. The relationship of coffee and green tea consumption with high-sensitivity C-reactive protein in Japanese men and women. Clin Chem Lab Med 2010;48(6):849–54.

[116] Shin JW, Wang JH, Kang JK, Son CG. Experimental evidence for the protective effects of coffee against liver fibrosis in SD rats. J Sci Food Agric 2010;90(3):450–5.

[117] Remels AH, Langen RC, Gosker HR, Russell AP, Spaapen F, Voncken JW, et al. PPARγ inhibits NF-κB-dependent transcriptional activation in skeletal muscle. Am J Physiol Endocrinol Metab 2009;297(1):E174–83.

[118] Shi H, Dong L, Jiang J, Zhao J, Zhao G, Dang X, et al. Chlorogenic acid reduces liver inflammation and fibrosis through inhibition of toll-like receptor 4 signaling pathway. Toxicology 2013;303:107–14.

[119] Greenland S. A meta-analysis of coffee, myocardial infarction, and coronary death. Epidemiology 1993;4(4):366–74.

[120] Kawachi I, Colditz GA, Stone CB. Does coffee drinking increase the risk of coronary heart disease? Results from a meta-analysis. Br Heart J 1994;72(3):269–75.

[121] Bertoia ML, Triche EW, Michaud DS, Baylin A, Hogan JW, Neuhouser ML, et al. Long-term alcohol and caffeine intake and risk of sudden cardiac death in women. Am J Clin Nutr 2013;97(6):1356–63.

[122] Shechter M, Shalmon G, Scheinowitz M, Koren-Morag N, Feinberg MS, Harats D, et al. Impact of acute caffeine ingestion on endothelial function in subjects with and without coronary artery disease. Am J Cardiol 2011;107(9):1255–61.

[123] de Koning Gans JM, Uiterwaal CS, van der Schouw YT, Boer JM, Grobbee DE, Verschuren WM, et al. Tea and coffee consumption and cardiovascular morbidity and mortality. Arterioscler Thromb Vasc Biol 2010;30(8):1665–71.

[124] Li XY, Xu L, Lin GS, Jiang XJ, Wang T, Lu JJ, et al. Protective effect of caffeine administration on myocardial ischemia/reperfusion injury in rats. Shock 2011;36(3):289–94.

[125] Ley RE, Backhed F, Turnbaugh P, Lozupone CA, Knight RD, Gordon JI. Obesity alters gut microbial ecology. Proc Natl Acad Sci USA 2005;102(31):11070–5.

[126] Turnbaugh PJ, Ley RE, Mahowald MA, Magrini V, Mardis ER, Gordon JI. An obesity-associated gut microbiome with increased capacity for energy harvest. Nature 2006;444(7122):1027–31.

[127] Cani PD, Amar J, Iglesias MA, Poggi M, Knauf C, Bastelica D, et al. Metabolic endotoxemia initiates obesity and insulin resistance. Diabetes 2007;56(7):1761–72.

[128] Tunnicliffe JM, Shearer J. Coffee, glucose homeostasis, and insulin resistance: physiological mechanisms and mediators. Appl Physiol Nutr Metab (Physiologie appliquee, nutrition et metabolisme) 2008;33(6):1290–300.

[129] Nakayama TOK. Influence of coffee (Coffea arabica) and galacto-oligosaccharide consumption on intestinal microbiota and the host responses. FEMS Microbiol Lett 2013:1–8.

[130] Suh HN, Lee SH, Lee MY, Heo JS, Lee YJ, Han HJ. High glucose induced translocation of Aquaporin8 to chicken hepatocyte plasma membrane: involvement of cAMP, PI3K/Akt, PKC, MAPKs, and microtubule. J Cell Biochem 2008;103(4):1089–100.

[131] Yamamoto T, Kuramoto H, Kadowaki M. Downregulation in aquaporin 4 and aquaporin 8 expression of the colon associated with the induction of allergic diarrhea in a mouse model of food allergy. Life Sci 2007;81(2):115–20.

[132] Zahn A, Moehle C, Langmann T, Ehehalt R, Autschbach F, Stremmel W, et al. Aquaporin-8 expression is reduced in ileum and induced in colon of patients with ulcerative colitis. World J Gastroenterol 2007;13(11):1687–95.

[133] Mascitelli L, Pezzetta F, Sullivan JL. Inhibition of iron absorption by coffee and the reduced risk of type 2 diabetes mellitus. Arch Intern Med 2007;167(2):204–5. [author reply 5]

[134] Hurrell RF, Reddy M, Cook JD. Inhibition of non-haem iron absorption in man by polyphenolic-containing beverages. Br J Nutr 1999;81(4):289–95.

[135] Morck TA, Lynch SR, Cook JD. Inhibition of food iron absorption by coffee. Am J Clin Nutr 1983;37(3):416–20.

[136] Jiang R, Manson JE, Meigs JB, Ma J, Rifai N, Hu FB. Body iron stores in relation to risk of type 2 diabetes in apparently healthy women. JAMA 2004;291(6):711–7.

[137] Facchini FS, Saylor KL. Effect of iron depletion on cardiovascular risk factors: studies in carbohydrate-intolerant patients. Ann NY Acad Sci 2002;967:342–51.

[138] Noordzij M, Uiterwaal CS, Arends LR, Kok FJ, Grobbee DE, Geleijnse JM. Blood pressure response to chronic intake of coffee and caffeine: a meta-analysis of randomized controlled trials. J Hypertens 2005;23(5):921–8.

[139] Zhao Y, Wang J, Ballevre O, Luo H, Zhang W. Antihypertensive effects and mechanisms of chlorogenic acids. Hypertens Res 2012;35(4):370–4.

[140] Suzuki A, Kagawa D, Ochiai R, Tokimitsu I, Saito I. Green coffee bean extract and its metabolites have a hypotensive effect in spontaneously hypertensive rats. Hypertens Res 2002;25(1):99–107.

[141] Suzuki A, Yamamoto N, Jokura H, Yamamoto M, Fujii A, Tokimitsu I, et al. Chlorogenic acid attenuates hypertension and improves endothelial function in spontaneously hypertensive rats. J Hypertens 2006;24(6):1065–73.

[142] Kozuma K, Tsuchiya S, Kohori J, Hase T, Tokimitsu I. Antihypertensive effect of green coffee bean extract on mildly hypertensive subjects. Hypertens Res 2005;28(9):711–8.

[143] Watanabe T, Arai Y, Mitsui Y, Kusaura T, Okawa W, Kajihara Y, et al. The blood pressure-lowering effect and safety of chlorogenic acid from green coffee bean extract in essential hypertension. Clin Exp Hypertens 2006;28(5):439–49.

[144] Geleijnse JM. Habitual coffee consumption and blood pressure: an epidemiological perspective. Vasc Health Risk Manag. 2008;4(5):963–70.

[145] USDA. Agricultural research service. National nutrient database for standard reference 2007.

CHAPTER

25

Bread Intake and Abdominal Fat

Inmaculada Bautista-Castaño, Almudena Sanchez-Villegas, and Luis Serra-Majem

Department of Clinical Sciences, University of Las Palmas de Gran Canaria, Las Palmas de Gran Canaria, Spain; CIBER Fisiopatología de la Obesidad y Nutrición (CIBERobn), Instituto de Salud Carlos III (ISCIII), Madrid, Spain

INTRODUCTION

Dietary habits play a pivotal role in the development of overweight and obesity [1]. Because abdominal obesity is more closely associated with type 2 diabetes mellitus (T2DM), cardiovascular disease (CVD), and all-cause mortality than is adipose tissue accumulation in other regions of the body [2,3], several epidemiological studies have investigated the relationship between diet and general or abdominal obesity, with differing results [4]. It seems that dietary factors such as low energy density and low glycemic index (GI) may be associated with a lower abdominal adiposity gain. A better understanding of which food groups or items contribute to these associations is necessary [5,6].

Some of these studies have specifically investigated associations between cereal consumption and body mass index (BMI) or abdominal fat. They have shown inverse associations between anthropometric variables and whole-grain cereals but conflicting results for refined cereals [7]. Factors such as postprandial insulin responses, gastric emptying after consuming a high-GI meal, and other factors may be implicated in a potential differential effect of refined vs. whole-grain cereals on adiposity [8]. Within the cereals group, bread is an important dietary constituent from a nutritional point of view. However, a long-standing belief held by the general public is that bread fattens. This encourages many people to restrict or even eliminate bread from their diet.

The present chapter assesses whether or not eating patterns that include bread and bread consumption itself are associated with overall obesity, and mainly with excess abdominal adiposity, either in the general population or in subjects undergoing obesity management. This knowledge will assist efforts to provide public health messages and recommendations regarding healthy eating habits to help individuals maintain an appropriate BMI and prevent abdominal obesity. Achieving better nutritional health for the general population is an additional beneficial outcome.

SCIENTIFIC EVIDENCE

We recently published a systematic review about the influence of bread intake on body weight and abdominal fat distribution [9]. In this chapter, we have included the main results of some of the studies included in this review and other more recently published studies that have investigated the relationship between abdominal adiposity and dietary patterns that include bread or the consumption of bread itself. These studies were classified into three groups according to the study design: cross-sectional, prospective cohort, and intervention studies.

CROSS-SECTIONAL STUDIES

Table 25.1 shows the methodology, clinical characteristics, principal results, and conclusions from the cross-sectional design studies.

The analysis of principal components and cluster analysis are two statistical techniques that have been used increasingly in the examination and description of complex dietary patterns. Different studies that have investigated the relationship between cereals consumption (including several types of bread) and abdominal or general obesity have used these techniques [10].

One of these studies, conducted by Ledikwe et al. [11] in a sample of 179 subjects aged between 66 and 87 years (which was part of the Geisinger Rural Aging Study)

Nutrition in the Prevention and Treatment of Abdominal Obesity
http://dx.doi.org/10.1016/B978-0-12-407869-7.00025-8

TABLE 25.1 Methodology, Clinical Characteristics, Principal Results, and Conclusions from the Cross-Sectional Design Studies

Author, Year [Reference], Country	Subjects	Measures of the Bread Variable	Outcome Variable Related to Abdominal Obesity	Study Methods	Results and Conclusions
Ledikwe et al. 2004 [11], USA	179 adult subjects (66–87 y) from the GRAS	5 × 24-h recalls; the items were classified into 6 groups (based on the USDA Food Pyramid) and subsequently into 29 groups (based on similarities of nutrient content); portions of food items were calculated according to USDA guidelines; diets were scored using the Healthy Eating Index as a measure of dietary quality Cluster 1: pattern of low-density nutrients (including the consumption of bread) Cluster 2: pattern of high-density nutrients Bread type was not differentiated	WC	Logistic regression analysis to compare dietary pattern with obesity or WC adjusted for energy intake, age, gender, and habitual consumption of alcohol	Individuals with pattern of low-density nutrients (including the consumption of bread) have double the risk of presenting with obesity or increased WC compared to the risk of the other patterns
Haveman-Nies et al. 2001 [12], USA and Europe	828 subjects from the US FHS and 1282 subjects from the European SENECA study (70 ± 77 y)	FHS cohort: FFQ (self-administered) SENECA cohort: interview with the modified dietary history, 3 × 24 h recall and listing of frequency of food items adapted to each country 12 groups of principal items (bread included in the group of grains); cluster analysis used to select 5 dietary patterns (bread included in the pattern of "fish and grains")	WC	Logistic regression analysis to compare clusters with BMI and WC; variables adjusted for age, gender, smoking habit, PA, and country	BMI and WC tend to be lower in the "fish and grain" group that included bread
Wirfält et al. 2001 [13], Sweden	2400 males and 2959 females from the Malmö Diet and Cancer study (45–68 y)	7 × 24-h recall and 1 questionnaire of dietary history; 43 groups of food items; 6 food patterns identified using cluster analysis (one pattern, whole-grain bread; another pattern, refined bread)	WC (as a component of MS)	Logistic regression analysis to relate the risk of each component of MS in relation to each pattern of food compared to the other dietary patterns; controlled for age, energy intake, % body fat, interviewer, past dietary changes, and sociodemographic status	In males a decrease in abdominal obesity associated with the dietary pattern that included whole-grain bread

Panagiotakos et al. 2007 [14], Greece	1514 males (18–87 y) and 1528 females (18–89 y) from the ATTICA study	FFQ: 156 items, classified into 6 dietary patterns; bread included in the pattern "bread, pasta"	WC	Logistic regression analysis, with the outcome variable being each component of the MS and the independent variables being the dietary patterns adjusted for age, gender, PhA, tobacco habit, education level, medication, special diets, and BMI	The dietary pattern that includes bread (and pasta) was not related to the prevalence of MS in general, nor with any of its components, including WC following adjustment for several variables including BMI
Jacobs et al. 1998 [15], USA	34,492 postmenopausal women from the Iowa Women's Health Study (55–69 y)	FFQ: 127 items; "wholemeal grains" was defined as containing >25% whole grain or bran and included whole-grain bread and group of refined grains that included refined bread	WHR	The intake of whole-grain or refined items distributed in quintiles; comparison adjusted for age and energy intake with BMI and WHR (linear regression)	High consumption of wholemeal grains associated with lower BMI and WHR The consumption of refined grains was not associated with BMI but led to a slight increase in WHR
McKeown et al. 2002 [16], USA	2941 (1338 males and 1603 females) from the Framingham Offspring Study cohort (mean age 54 y)	FFQ: 126 items; consumption of cereals based on Jacobs' definition; distribution in quintiles of portions/week of whole-grain (including whole-grain bread) or refined (including refined bread) cereals	ICC, WC	Comparison of measures of BMI, WC, and WHR in quintiles of (whole-grain or refined) cereal consumption adjusted, or not, for age, gender, tobacco habit, antihypertension medication, alcohol, use of multivitamins, estrogens, and PhA; other added adjustments were BMI (in the case of WHR and WC), polyunsaturated fatty acids, and intake of fish, fruit, and vegetables	Intake of whole-grain cereals inversely correlated with BMI and WHR (following adjustment for confounding factors) No difference between refined-cereal consumption and anthropometric measurements (an inverse relationship also between whole-grain cereals and Chol, LDLc, and fasting insulin)
Esmaillzadeh et al. 2005 [17], Iran	827 individuals (357 males and 470 females; 18–74 y), a subsample of the TLGS	FFQ: whole-grain bread in the group of wholemeal grains and refined bread in the group of refined grains (Jacobs' classification); intake classified into quintiles	Abdominal obesity (WC >102 cm in males and >88 cm in females), WC, and WHR	Logistic regression analysis relating quartiles of cereal intake (whole grain or refined) with obesity and WC, adjusted for total energy, age, energy from fats, antihypertension medication, use of estrogens, tobacco, PA, consumption of meat, fish, fruit, and vegetables	No relationship observed between obesity and cereal group (whole grain or refined); no relationship between group of cereals and WC; relationship between quartiles of higher intake of whole-grain cereals and the lower prevalence of abdominal obesity
Azadbakht et al. 2005 [18], Iran	775 individuals (20–70 y), subsample of the TLGS	FFQ and 2 × 24-h recall; nutrients and food items classified into quartiles In males, bread included in the groups of whole-grain or refined grains. In females, refined bread was included in its own group of refined bread, and whole-grain bread in the group of wholemeal grains and bread	WC, WHR	Logistic regression analysis adjusted for confounding variables: age, gender, civic status, PhA, education level, dietary intake, general and central obesity, tobacco habit, oral contraceptives, and antithyroid medication	No relationship observed between groups that included bread (refined or whole grain) with general obesity (for males, BMI >24; for females, BMI >25) nor with abdominal obesity

(continued)

TABLE 25.1 Continued

Author, Year [Reference], Country	Subjects	Measures of the Bread Variable	Outcome Variable Related to Abdominal Obesity	Study Methods	Results and Conclusions
Newby et al. 2007 [19], USA	1516 adults from the BLSA	7 × 24-h recall; organized into 3 consumption groups that included the different types of bread (wholemeal grains, refined grains, and fiber from cereals), distributed in quintiles of consumption	WC	Liner regression analysis adjusted for age, gender, total energy, decade of clinical visit, ethnicity, education, use of vitamin supplements, tobacco habit,% energy derived from saturated fats, alcohol, refined grains (in case of wholemeal grain) and wholemeal grains (in the case of refined grains)	Wholemeal grains and fiber from cereals were inversely related to BMI, body weight, and WC; refined grains not related to these measure
McKeown et al. 2009 [20], USA	434 free-living adults (177 men and 257 women; 60–80 y)	FFQ: 126 items; organized into 3 consumption groups that included the 2 different types of bread (whole-grain food, refined-grain food), and fiber from cereals, distributed in quartiles of consumption	Percentage trunk fat mass	Comparison of measures of BMI,% body fat and% trunk fat mass in quartiles of cereal consumption (whole-grain or refined) or fiber consumption (by testing for linear trend across quartile categories), adjusted for age, sex, total energy intake,% energy from fat, PhA, smoking, alcohol intake, and multivitamin use	Whole-grain intake was inversely associated with BMI,% body and% trunk fat mass; refined-grain intake was not associated with any measure of body fat distribution Cereal fiber was inversely associated with BMI,% body and% trunk fat mass; no significant association was observed between intakes of total fiber, vegetable or fruit fiber, and body composition measurements
McKeown et al. 2010 [21], USA	2834 (1434 men and 1400 women; 32–83 y) from the FHS cohort	FFQ: 126 items, distribution into quintiles of servings/day in a whole-grain category (including dark bread) or refined-grain categories (including refined bread)	SAT, VAT, WC	Comparison (by testing for a linear trend across quintiles) of measures of SAT, VAT, and WC in quintiles of whole-grain or refined-grain intake, adjusted for age, sex, smoking status, total energy, and alcohol intake	Whole-grain intake was inversely associated with SAT, VAT, and WC; refined-grain intake was positively associated with SAT and VAT; when SAT and VAT were evaluated jointly, only VAT remained associated with both whole grains and refined grains
O'Neil et al. 2010 [22], USA	Analysis of 1999–2004 NHANES data was conducted using adults 19–50 y (*n*, 7039) and >51 y (*n*, 6237)	24-h dietary recalls; participants were categorized into one of four whole-grain (bread included) consumption groups: 0 to <0.6 servings; ≥0.6 to <1.5 servings; ≥1.5 to <3.0 servings; and ≥3.0 servings/day (in oz. equivalents)	WC	Least-square means and standard errors were calculated for body weight measures Two regression models were developed and compared; model 1 covariates included age, gender, ethnicity, and total energy intake; model 2 was extended to include cereal fiber Trend analysis was conducted to test for differences between least-square means	A significant trend was observed in both age groups for increased consumption of whole grains with lower BMI, WC, and% overweight/obese (model 1); however, a significant trend was not observed when cereal fiber was added as a covariate (model 2)

Kim et al. [23], 2012 Korea	Analysis of 3742, women from baseline data from the Korean Health and Genome Study	FFQ: 103 items, grouped into 34 predefined food groups; four dietary patterns were identified using factor analysis of data; bread was included in the "bread-dairy" patterns (greater intake of bread, breakfast cereals, pizza, hamburgers, snacks, eggs, dairy products, coffee, carbonated drinks, and tea)	WC, WHR, abdominal obesity prevalence (WC ≥80 cm)	General linear regression analysis was done to assess the relationships between dietary patterns and continuous variables such as age, height, weight, WC, hip circumference, and BMI; energy-adjusted nutrient intake was calculated using the regression residual method To determine the associations between dietary patterns and obesity or abdominal obesity, the ORs and 95% CIs from unconditional logistic regression models were calculated, which were controlled for age, occupation, family income, education level, and energy intake	There was no relationship between these dietary patterns and BMI; people who preferred "bread-dairy" dietary patterns had a lower WC
Kanerba et al. 2013 [24], Finland	4720 Finns (25–74 y) from the National FINRISK 2007 study	FFQ: 131 items; bread (mainly rye bread) included in the cereals group (compound of the BSDS)	WC	An association between the adherence to the Baltic Sea diet and decreased risk of abdominal adiposity was tested using logistic regression analysis; for the risk analyses, the final score was divided into quintiles, with the highest quintile representing high adherence to the Baltic Sea diet; the likelihood ratio test was used to test the significance of each variable in the model; multivariable-adjusted models controlled for the following potential confounders: age, energy intake, and PhA	In a multivariable model, men in the highest vs. lowest BSDS quintile were more likely to have a normal WC (OR 0·48, 95% CI 0.29–0.80); in women, this association was similar but not significant (OR 0·65, 95% CI 0.39–1.09) Nordic cereals and alcohol were found to be the most important BSDS components related to WC

BLSA, Baltimore Longitudinal Study of Aging; BSDS, Baltic Sea Diet Score; Chol, total plasma cholesterol; CI, confidence interval; FFQ, food frequency questionnaire; FHS, Framingham Heart Study; GI, glycemic index; GRAS, Geisinger Rural Aging Study; ICC, intradass correlation coefficient; LDLc, low-density lipoprotein cholesterol; MS, metabolic syndrome; NHANES, National Health and Nutrition Examination Survey; OR, odds ratio; PhA, physical activity; SAT, subcutaneous adipose tissue; TLGS, Tehran Lipid and Glucose Study; USDA, United States Department of Agriculture; VAS, visual analog scales; VAT, visceral adipose tissue; WC, waist circumference; WHR, waist-hip ratio; y, years.

showed that the cluster that included the consumption of bread (a low-density nutrient pattern) compared to the cluster that did not include bread (a high-density nutrient pattern) showed a greater risk of general and abdominal obesity.

Other authors such as Haveman-Nies et al. [12] conducted a study of subjects from two different cohorts (age range, 70–77 years): 828 subjects from the US Framingham Heart Study (FHS) and 1282 subjects from the European SENECA study. Using cluster analysis, five dietary patterns were found (bread was included in the "fish and grain"-labeled pattern). After adjusting for confounding variables, they observed that BMI and waist circumference (WC) tended to be lower in the "fish and grain" group.

A study conducted in Sweden by Wirfält et al. [13] in a sample of 2040 males and 2959 females from the Malmö Diet and Cancer study identified six food patterns (one pattern was labeled "brown bread" and another "refined bread") using cluster analysis. The study analyzed the association between the adherence to the different dietary patterns and each component of the metabolic syndrome (MS). The results indicated that, among males, abdominal obesity was inversely associated with the food pattern that included bread.

In Greece, Panagiotakos et al. [14] investigated 1514 males and 1528 females aged >18 years as part of the ATTICA study, the aim which was to analyze the role of several dietary patterns in the prevalence of MS and its components. The food items were classified into six dietary patterns, with bread included in the pattern named "bread and pasta." This dietary pattern was not related to the prevalence of MS in general nor with any of its components, including WC, following adjustment for several variables including BMI. The study carried out by Jacobs et al. [15] studied 34,492 postmenopausal women from the Iowa Women's Health Study (age range, 55–69 years). The "whole-grain" group (>25% whole-grain or bran) included whole-grain bread and the "refined-grain" group included refined bread. Intakes of whole-grain or refined food items were distributed in quintiles and compared against BMI and waist-hip ratio (WHR). The results showed that high whole-grain consumption was associated with lower BMI and WHR. The consumption of refined food items was not related to BMI, but was associated with a slight increase in the WHR.

McKeown et al. [16] analyzed 2941 subjects (1338 males and 1603 females) from the Framingham Offspring Study cohort. They studied the consumption of cereals based on Jacobs' definition [15] and compared the quintiles of whole-grain cereals (including whole-grain bread) or refined cereals (including refined bread) with BMI, WHR, and WC. The study found that the intake of whole-grain cereals was inversely associated with BMI and WHR (after adjusting the data for confounding factors). There were no significant differences between the consumption of refined cereals and anthropometric measurements. Furthermore, the study found an inverse relationship between the consumption of whole-grain cereals and fasting plasma cholesterol, low-density lipoprotein (LDL) cholesterol, and insulinemia.

Within the group of cross-sectional studies, Esmaillzadeh et al. [17] analyzed a subsample from the Tehran Lipid and Glucose Study that included 827 Iranian individuals (357 males and 470 females, aged 18–74 years). Jacobs' classification of whole-grain grains (including whole-grain bread) [15] was used and the distribution of consumption was categorized in quartiles. An association between the quartiles of high intake of whole-grain cereals and lower prevalence of abdominal obesity was observed. There were no differences in general obesity prevalence between any of the groups studied.

Azadbakht et al. [18] studied 775 Iranian individuals in a subsample from the same study. The nutrients and food groups were classified into quartiles and compared against BMI, WC and WHR. There were no significant relationships between the groups that included bread (refined or brown) with respect to general obesity (male BMI >24 kg/m^2, female BMI >25 kg/m^2) nor to abdominal obesity.

Newby et al. [19] studied 1516 adults from the Baltimore Longitudinal Study of Aging (BLSA). Food item consumption was organized into three groups that included the different types of bread: whole-grain grains, refined grains, and fiber from cereals categorized into quintiles of consumption. The variables compared were BMI, body weight, and WC. The whole-grain grains and fiber from cereals food groups were inversely related to BMI, body weight, and WC. None of these relationships were found for refined grains.

McKeown et al. [20] studied 434 free-living adults (177 men and 257 women) aged 60–80 years. Three groups of food items that included different types of bread were studied (whole-grain foods, including different types of dark bread; refined-grain foods, including refined bread; and fiber from cereals). As outcomes, BMI, percentage body fat, and percentage trunk fat mass were considered. Two of the three food groups, i.e. whole-grain foods and fiber from cereals, were inversely related to BMI, body fat, and percentage trunk fat mass. None of these relationships were found for refined grains.

The same author, McKeown et al. [21], in a sample of 2834 adult subjects from the FHS cohort, studied the relationship between the intake of whole-grain foods (including several types of dark bread) and refined-grain foods (including refined bread) and WC, subcutaneous adipose tissue (SAT), and visceral adipose tissue (VAT). They found that a higher intake of whole-grain foods was associated with lower VAT in adults, whereas a higher intake of refined grains was associated with higher VAT.

O'Neil et al. [22] carried out an analysis of the 1999–2004 National Health and Nutrition Examination Survey (NHANES) data from 13,276 adults. Participants were categorized into one of four whole-grain (bread included) consumption groups. Adults who consumed the most servings of whole grains (whole-grain bread included) had lower body weight measures and abdominal perimeters.

As a consequence of the prevalence of obesity in Korean adults increasing from 13.9% in 1995 to 30.6% in 2001, Kim et al. [23] designed a study using 3742 women with baseline data from the Korean Health and Genome Study. The aim of the study was to classify dietary patterns and investigate relationships between dietary patterns, sociodemographic and lifestyle-related issues, and obesity in Korean women. Four dietary patterns were identified: (1) "animal food" (greater intake of meats and fish); (2) "rice-vegetable" (greater intake of steamed rice, tofu, kimchi, vegetables, dried anchovy, and seaweeds); (3) "bread-dairy" (greater intake of bread, eggs, milk, and dairy products); and (4) "noodle" (greater intake of ramyun, noodles, and Chajangmyeon). The results showed that, among Korean women, dietary patterns were related to abdominal obesity but not to overall obesity. The "rice-vegetable" and "noodle" dietary patterns were associated with an increased risk of abdominal obesity; however, the "bread-dairy" dietary pattern had an inverse relationship with abdominal obesity. This information enabled the authors to recommend a healthy dietary pattern to prevent obesity in Korean women.

Of particular interest was the study conducted by Kanerva et al. [24]. These authors studied the relationship between the Baltic Sea Diet Score (BSDS) and abdominal obesity in a population of 4720 Finns (aged 25–74 years) from the National FINRISK 2007 study. The score included Nordic fruits and berries, vegetables, cereals, the ratio of polyunsaturated to saturated fatty acids, *trans* fatty acids, low-fat milk, fish, red and processed meat, total fat (percentage energy), and alcohol. The results of the study suggested that the combination of Nordic foods, especially cereals and moderate alcohol consumption, is likely to be inversely associated with abdominal obesity. Nordic cereals included in the BSDS were rye, oats, and barley. In Nordic countries, almost all rye is consumed as rye bread (made from rye flour), which is very rich in dietary fiber. The Finnish population obtains over half of their dietary fiber by eating rye bread. This could be the reason for rye being linked to a normal WC. Other Nordic cereals such as oats and barley are also used as whole grains in several types of bread, but they are more commonly used in porridges.

LONGITUDINAL STUDIES

Table 25.2 shows the methodology, clinical characteristics, principal results, and conclusions from the longitudinal design studies. It is worth mentioning two studies in particular, each with 10 years of follow-up conducted in 459 healthy individuals of both genders participating in the BLSA. In these, data on intake were obtained every 12–24 months between 1984 and 1991. Newby et al. [25] performed the first analysis in which five cluster solutions were selected. Refined bread was a food item included in one of the clusters. Two other clusters (named "healthy" and "meat and potatoes" dietary patterns) included whole-grain bread. The outcome variables were weight, BMI, and WC. The results indicated that refined bread was associated with a higher increase in WC. Whole-grain bread consumption, which was included in two groups, showed an inverse effect on WC increase. The same early study was later analyzed by Newby et al. [26] using six different clusters. The results indicated that dietary patterns including whole-grain bread prevented the increase in BMI and WC, while no effect was observed for the pattern including refined bread.

Another study was performed in 2300 middle-aged Danish males and females who were part of the MONICA Project. The follow-up period of the cohort was 6 years, with data acquisition at three time points: 1982, 1987, and 1993. In the analysis carried out by Halkjaer et al. [27], relationships were investigated between the diet in 1987 (M-87) and variations in the WC from 1987 to 1993. All results were adjusted for various confounding factors, including changes in BMI. In females, a high intake of refined bread was associated with an increase in WC.

Halkjaer et al. [28] performed another study involving 22,570 females and 20,126 males (age ranged 50–64 years). The participants belonged to the Danish Diet, Cancer and Health Study, with 4 years of follow-up (1993–1997). Dietary habits were collected using a food frequency questionnaire (FFQ). In the carbohydrate (CHO) subgroups, refined bread was included in the subgroup of refined cereals and whole-grain bread in the group of whole-grain cereals. The associations between basal diet and changes in WC were analyzed and adjusted for WC, BMI, age, tobacco habit, alcohol intake, and physical activity. Moreover, macronutrient subgroups were adjusted for other macronutrients and for total energy. The results indicated that whole-grain bread was in the group that had no influence on WC changes, while refined bread was in the group that was associated positively with WC increase (but only in women).

In 2011, Romaguera et al. [4] studied the association between the consumption of several food groups or items and annual changes in "WC for a given BMI"

TABLE 25.2 Methodology, Clinical Characteristics, Principal results, and Conclusions of the Studies of Longitudinal Design

Author, Year [Reference], Country	Subjects	Measure of the Bread Variable	Outcome Variable Related to Ponderal Status	Study Design	Results and Conclusions
Newby et al. 2003 [25], USA	459 healthy individuals of both genders participating in the BLSA (10 y of follow-up)	7 × 24-h recall; 1984–1991 (data collected every 12–24 months) 41 food item groups in cluster analysis; refined bread included in group of "refined bread and refined grains" and whole-grain bread in the group "nonrefined breads"; 5 cluster groups were selected for analysis: healthy, refined bread, alcohol, sweets, meat and potatoes Whole-grain bread included in healthy pattern and in the pattern of meat and potatoes	WC	Regression analysis; covariables for adjustment were collected in the first visit: ethnicity, PhA, tobacco habit, education, vitamin supplements	Refined bread included in the group associated with increased WC; of the two groups included whole-grain bread, one had a smaller increase in WC than the other
Newby et al. 2004 [26], USA	Same as above	Same as above, using 6 distinct clusters; bread type was differentiated	Same as above	Same as above, except that 6 distinct clusters were examined instead of 5; comparisons of changes in BMI and WC were made among quintiles, adjusting for several covariables	The dietary pattern that includes whole-grain bread prevents increases in BMI and WC
Halkjaer et al. 2004 [27], Denmark	2300 males and females of middle age taking part in the MONICA study, with 6 y of follow-up; data obtained in 1982, 1987, 1993	Diet data collected in the second stage (1987) FFQ: 26 items, two groupings Food item group: 24 of the 26 food items grouped into 10 "groups" of items (1 group, whole-grain bread and another refined bread) Factor scores: 21 of the 26 items; three factor scores in males and two in females; traditional (includes refined-wheat bread), green (includes whole-grain bread positive and refined-wheat bread negative) and sweet factor in males; traditional/sweet (includes refined-wheat bread) and green factor (includes whole-grain bread positive and refined-wheat bread negative) in females	WC, changes in WC at the second relative to the third follow-up (WC was not included in the first measurement), adjusted for changes in BMI	Multiple linear regression analysis; relationships studied between diet (1987) and changes in WC (1987 and 1993), adjusted for several factors including changes in BMI	In females, high intake of refined bread was associated with increased WC; no relationship was observed with food item scores This same study was published by Togo et al. in 2004 [49], who also observed that the food factors did not predict changes in BMI or the development of obesity (sample slightly larger, 2436 individuals)

Halkjaer et al. 2006 [28], Denmark	22,570 females and 20,126 males (50–64 y; 1993–1997); Danish Diet, Cancer and Health Study; 4 y of follow-up	FFQ: 192 items; in the carbohydrate subgroups, refined bread was included in the subgroup of refined cereals and whole-grain bread in the group of whole-grain cereals;% contribution to total energy	WC, changes in WC	Cohort study; 5-y follow-up; linear regression analysis for association of baseline diet with changes in WC; adjustment for WC, BMI, age, tobacco, alcohol, PhA; the subgroups of the macronutrients were adjusted for other macronutrients and for total energy	Whole-grain bread included in a group does not influence WC changes; refined bread included in a group is associated with increased WC (in females)
Romaguera et al. 2011 [4], Europe	48,631 men and women from 5 countries participating in the EPIC study; median follow-up time of 5.5 y	Usual food intakes were measured using country-specific FFQ; bread and nonrefined bread were analyzed (included in the cereal products group)	WC, WCBMI	Anthropometric measurements were obtained at baseline and follow-up; the association between food groups/items and annual change in WCBMI was modeled using center-specific adjusted linear regression, and random-effects meta-analyses to obtain pooled estimates, adjusting for several covariables	Higher fruit and dairy product consumption was associated with a lower gain in WCBMI, whereas the consumption of refined bread, processed meat, margarine, and soft drinks was positively associated with an annual change in WCBMI; no relation was found with nonrefined bread
Bautista-Castaño et al. 2012 [29], Spain	2213 men and women (50–80 y) from the PREDIMED trial; 4 y of follow-up	Semiquantitative FFQ: 137 items; basal total, refined, and whole-grain bread at baseline and in every follow-up assessment was adjusted for total energy intake using the residuals method	WC, changes in WC at 4-y follow-up	Multivariate means and their 95% CI for anthropometric measures at baseline according to quartiles of initial consumption of total, refined, and whole-grain bread, and increases in anthropometric measures according to quartiles of change in the consumption of total, refined, and whole-grain bread were calculated using generalized linear models; ordinal logistic regression analyses were fitted to assess the association between the change in each type of bread consumption (quartiles) and a clinically meaningful gain or loss (>2 kg) in body weight and WC (>2 cm) after 4 y of follow-up	Over 4 y, participants in the highest quartile of change in refined bread intake gained 0·76 kg more than those in the lowest quartile, and 1·28 cm more in WC than those in the lowest quartile Participants in the highest quartile of changes in refined bread intake had a reduction of 33% in the odds of losing weight (>2 kg) and a reduction of 36% in the odds of losing WC (<2 cm) No relationships were observed for change in whole-grain bread consumption

BLSA, Baltimore Longitudinal Study of Aging; BMI, body mass index; EPIC, European Prospective Investigation into Cancer and Nutrition; FFQ, food frequency questionnaire; PhA, physical activity; WC, waist circumference; WCBMI, residuals of WC regressed on BMI; y, years.

(WCBMI), a proxy for abdominal adiposity. The authors analyzed data from 48,631 men and women from five countries participating in the European Prospective Investigation into Cancer and Nutrition study. Higher fruit and dairy product consumption was associated with a lower gain in WCBMI, whereas the consumption of refined bread, processed meat, margarine, and soft drinks was positively associated with an annual change in WCBMI. No relationship with non-white-bread was found.

We recently published a longitudinal study [29], which was the first prospective cohort study to report significant associations between an increase in bread consumption (in g/day) and weight or gains in a sample of participants at high cardiovascular risk (the PREDIMED trial). We analyzed 2213 participants. Dietary habits were assessed using a validated FFQ at baseline and repeatedly every year during 4 years of follow-up. Using multivariate models to adjust for covariates, long-term weight and WC changes according to quartiles of change in energy-adjusted refined and whole-grain bread consumption were calculated. The results of the study showed that over 4 years, participants in the highest quartile of change in refined bread intake gained 0.76 kg more than those in the lowest quartile (*P* for trend, 0.003) and 1.28 cm more in WC than those in the lowest quartile (*P* for trend, <0.001). No significant dose-response relationships were observed for changes in whole-bread consumption and anthropometric measures. Gaining weight (>2 kg) and gaining WC (>2 cm) during follow-up was not associated with increased bread consumption, but participants in the highest quartile of changes in refined bread intake had a reduction of 33% in the odds of losing weight (≥2 kg) and a reduction of 36% in the odds of losing WC (≥2 cm). These results suggested that reducing refined bread, but not whole-grain bread consumption, within a Mediterranean-style food pattern setting was associated with lower gains in weight and abdominal fat.

INTERVENTION STUDIES

There are only a few intervention studies in which the intake of bread and its relation with abdominal fat was specifically assessed (Table 25.3).

In the UK, Lean et al. [30] conducted an intervention study in 110 healthy females with BMI >25 kg/m^2 (age range, 18–68 years) with the objective of comparing the effects of two diets of 1200 calories daily: one low in CHOs (35%) and the other high in CHO (58%). The low-CHO diet contained four interchanges of bread/day and the high-CHO diet had seven interchanges of bread/day (unspecified type of bread). The analyses were carried out in the overall sample and in a subgroup of 23 pairs of postmenopausal women. Outcome variables selected were BMI, weight, WC, WHR, and percentage body fat. No differences were observed in anthropometric variables between the two diets, except in the subgroup, in which the loss in ponderal status was greater at 3, 6, and 12 months among those participants assigned to the low-CHO diet.

McAuley et al. [31] conducted an intervention study in 96 normoglycemic females with BMI >27 kg/m^2 and insulin resistance in New Zealand. Three kinds of diets for weight loss were compared: (1) a high-CHO diet, which included at least six portions of bread and cereals (preferably whole grain); (2) a high-fat diet; and (3) a high-protein diet. The 8-week dietary intervention was followed by a maintenance diet for another 8 weeks, and results were evaluated 8 weeks after the end of the intervention (i.e. 24 weeks after the start of the study). A weight change of 3 kg was considered to be clinically important. Weight loss and decreased WC were the outcomes analyzed. The results indicated that the high-fat and high-protein diets produced a greater weight loss and WC reduction than did the high-CHO diet (i.e. the diet with the high bread content).

Aston el al. [32] conducted an intervention study in the UK in 19 overweight or stably obese women with moderate hyperinsulinemia. The study involved two crossover interventions of 12 weeks each. The objective was to assess the effect of the CHO intake with high or low GI, including refined versus whole-grain bread, on body weight, body composition, and appetite. No differences in energy intake, body weight, WC, or body fat were found between the two interventions.

No differences in body weight change were observed in a more recent randomized controlled trial (12-weeks duration) performed in obese individuals with MS, which was conducted by Katcher et al. [33]. In this study, participants were assigned to receive one of two low-calories diets (reduced by 500 kcal/day): one based on whole-grain products (including whole-grain bread; about 5 servings/day of whole grains); and the other, the refined-cereal diet group, with a reduced whole-grain food intake (<0.2 servings/day). In the absence of differences in body weight loss between the two treatments, the whole-grain group showed a higher percentage of abdominal fat loss and a decrease in plasma C-reactive protein (CRP) levels compared to the refined-cereal diet group.

Venn et al. [34] conducted an 18-month randomized controlled trial study in 18 overweight volunteers in New Zealand. Diets were based on the guidelines published by the National Heart Foundation of New Zealand, which included a recommendation to eat at least 6 servings of breads and cereals each day. The intervention group was advised to consume 2 servings of pulses and 4 servings of whole-grain foods (including

TABLE 25.3 Methodology, Clinical Characteristics, Principal Results, and Conclusions from Intervention Studies

Author, Year [Reference], Country	Subjects	Measurement of the Bread Variable	Outcome Variable Related with Ponderal Status	Design of the Study: Intervention	Results	Conclusions
Lean et al. 1997 [30], UK	110 healthy females with BMI >25, aged 51.5 y (range 18–68 y)	Compare the effects of 2 diets of 1200 kcal, one low in carbohydrates (35%) and the other high (58%); the low-carbohydrate diet contained 4 exchanges of bread/day and the HC diet had 7 exchanges of bread/day	BMI, weight, WC, WHR,% body fat	Randomized controlled trial; paired t-test used to compare the means of the two measures in each group of subjects and procedures; t-test for independent samples used to compare differences in the changes in measures between the two groups of subjects; differences in weight loss between the subgroup of the 23 pairs adjusted for menopausal women with diets high or low in carbohydrates were compared using the paired t-test, adjusted for age at menopause and BMI	No difference in anthropometric variables between the two subgroups of 23 pairs of menopausal women in whom the loss in ponderal status was greater at 3, 6, and 12 months with the low-carbohydrates diet	No differences in weight loss, WC, or WHR with diets with more or with less bread
McAuley et al. 2005 [31], New Zealand	96 females with BMI >27 kg/m^2, recruited from local community; normoglycemic and with insulin resistance	Three dietary systems compared: HC [32%, including at least 6 portions of bread and cereals (preferably whole grain)], HF (31%; Atkins diet), and HP (30%) over 8 weeks of diet and 8 weeks of maintenance	BMI, weight, WC	3 kg differences considered to be of clinical importance; outcomes compared were weight loss and decrease in WC	Diets high in fats and high in proteins produce greater loss of weight, ponderal status, and WC than diets high in carbohydrates (rich in bread)	Diet with a higher content of bread produces less weight loss in women with insulin resistance and higher ponderal status
Aston et al. 2008 [32], UK	19 females with obesity/stable overweigh and moderate hyperinsulinemia	Bread of high or low GI (presumably whole-grain or refined) included in the foods rich in carbohydrates of low or high GI (bread, breakfast cereals, rice, and pasta/potatoes), incorporated ad libitum into the habitual diet of subjects; intervention for 12 consecutive weeks for each group (total of 24 weeks); diets were equivalent in energy,% macronutrients, and fiber (difference of 8.4 GI units); 48% carbohydrates	Weight, WC, fat mass (kg), lean mass (kg),% fat mass	Intervention crossover study; 12 weeks each, intended to assess the effect of intake of carbohydrates of high or low energy density on weight, body composition, and appetite	There were no differences between the two interventions in energy intake, body weight (both interventions increased body weight), WC, or body fat	Bread with greater or lesser GI (whole grain or not) did not influence body weight in women with excess ponderal status and hyperinsulinemia

(continued)

TABLE 25.3 Continued

Author, Year [Reference], Country	Subjects	Measurement of the Bread Variable	Outcome Variable Related with Ponderal Status	Design of the Study: Intervention	Results	Conclusions
Katcher 2008 [33], USA	50 obese adults (25 men, 25 women; age range 20–65 y)	Participants in the whole-grain group received whole-grain cereals (including 4–7 servings/day whole-grain bread); participants in the refined-grain group were instructed to avoid whole-grain cereals	BMI, WC,% body fat,% body fat in the abdominal region	Obese adults with MS were randomly assigned to receive dietary advice to either avoid whole-grain foods or obtain all of their grain servings from whole grains for 12 weeks; all participants were given the same dietary advice in other respects for weight loss, a low-calorie diet (reduced by 500 kcal/day)	Body weight, WC, and% body fat decreased significantly in both groups over the study period, but there was a significantly greater decrease in% body fat in the abdominal region in the whole-grain group than in the refined-grain group	There were significantly greater decreases in% body fat in the abdominal region in participants consuming whole grains (whole-grain bread included) than in those consuming refined grains (refined bread included)
Venn 2010 [34], New Zealand	108 volunteers (55 in control group and 53 in intervention group; BMI > 28 kg/m²)	The control group was instructed to follow the guidelines published by the National Heart Foundation of New Zealand, which included recommendations to eat at least 6 servings of breads and cereals each day; the intervention group was given similar advice, except they were specifically instructed to consume 2 servings of pulses as a substitute for 2 servings of bread and cereal, and all other bread and cereals were to be whole grain	BMI, WC	18-months randomized controlled study; data were analyzed according to the modified intention to treat, after the missing values were imputed using chained equations; regression analysis with adjustment for baseline values, sex, and age was used to estimate the differences between treatments at 26 weeks; at 18 months, an additional adjustment was made for the measures obtained at 26 weeks	Weight loss was not different between groups; WC was reduced at 18 months in the intervention group compared with the control group	Incorporation of pulses and whole-grain foods (whole-grain bread included) into a weight loss program resulted in a greater reduction in WC compared with the group consuming a control diet, although no difference in weight loss was noted between groups
Kohen 2011 [35], Spain	122 women (BMI > 25 kg/m² and <40 kg/m²)	The women were randomly assigned to consume one of the two following meals: no-bread meal and bread meal; these had equal caloric and food content, except that the former included bread instead of rice and pasta	BMI, WC,% body fat, muscle mass,% body water, feelings of hunger and satiety	Randomized controlled trial of a hypocaloric diet, with and without bread; Student's t-test or Mann-Whitney U test were used to assess differences in weight, WC,% body fat, muscle mass, and% body water post intervention; the intervention duration was 16 weeks; VAS were used to measure feelings of hunger and satiety	Favorable changes in weight, WC,% body fat, muscle mass, and% body water were similar between both groups; there was a greater sensation of satiety after eating	With equal caloric and foods, incorporation of bread into a hypocaloric diet resulted in the same beneficial results on anthropometric measures and body composition as the same diet without bread; bread increased the feelings of hunger and satiety

BMI, body mass index; GI, glycemic index; HC, high carbohydrate; HF, high fat; HP, high protein; MS, metabolic syndrome; WC, waist circumference; WHR, waist-hip ratio; VAS, visual analog scales.

whole-grain bread) per day, substituting more refined CHOs. Although no difference in weight loss was noted between groups, the incorporation of pulses and whole-grain foods into a weight loss program resulted in a greater reduction in WC compared with the control-diet group.

Finally, Kohen et al. [35] designed a randomized controlled trial in Spain to compare the differences in feelings of hunger and satiety in a group of overweight and obese women after eating a test meal with or without bread. The women were randomly assigned to consume one of two low-calorie meals, "no-bread meals" and a "bread meals," both with equal caloric intake and food types, except that bread was substituted by rice and pasta in the "no-bread meal" group. The authors measured BMI, WC, and body composition prior to the study and after 16 weeks of intervention. They did not find any differences between the groups in relation to anthropometric parameters, but the inclusion of bread in the low-calorie meal resulted in a greater sensation of satiety after eating.

SUMMARY OF THE SCIENTIFIC EVIDENCE ABOUT THE INFLUENCE OF BREAD CONSUMPTION ON ABDOMINAL OBESITY

Table 25.4 summarizes the main results of the studies that have investigated the influence of food groups that include bread on the deposition of abdominal fat.

A total of 14 cross-sectional studies and six longitudinal studies were reviewed. We also analyzed the results of six interventional studies.

INFLUENCE OF BREAD CONSUMPTION ON ABDOMINAL OBESITY PREVENTION

Of the cross-sectional design studies (see Tables 25.1 and 25.4), nine specifically investigated the relationship between the consumption of food patterns that included whole-grain bread and measures of abdominal fat. All showed an inverse relation between the intake of this food item and abdominal obesity distribution. However, three of the nine studies [16,19,20] did not show any influence of the consumption of food groups that included refined bread on abdominal obesity; another two studies [15,21] found a nonfavorable influence on abdominal fat when they analyzed food patterns that included refined bread, but an inverse relationship between whole-grain cereals (including whole-grain bread) and several measures of abdominal adiposity.

Of the five cross-sectional studies in which bread type was not differentiated, two [14,18] did not find any relation between the intake of food groups that included bread and abdominal obesity, while another two [12,24] showed a lower WC tendency in the group that included bread. The study conducted by Ledikwe et al. [11] showed that the cluster that included the consumption of bread compared to the cluster that did not include bread had a greater risk of general and abdominal obesity.

Thus, current data from cross-sectional studies consistently demonstrate that food groups that include whole-grain bread intake are associated with lower abdominal adiposity; however, the cross-sectional nature of these studies does not enable us to infer any causality between dietary exposures and abdominal fat regulation, which can only be demonstrated by prospective studies.

With regard to the observational studies (Tables 25.2 and 25.4), all studies that investigated the influence of the intake of food groups that included refined bread indicated that a dietary pattern low in refined bread might help to prevent abdominal fat accumulation. This association was not observed in the case of whole-grain bread intake: this food item did not show any influence in abdominal adiposity. The study by Newby et al. [26] indicated that the adherence to a dietary pattern in which whole-grain bread was included could prevent WC increment.

Therefore, results from prospective studies consistently suggest that dietary patterns that include refined-grain bread or the consumption of whole refined bread itself have no beneficial effects on abdominal fat regulation; however, only the results of randomized controlled intervention studies can provide evidence for a cause-effect relationship between whole-grain bread intake and body weight.

INFLUENCE OF BREAD CONSUMPTION ON ABDOMINAL OBESITY TREATMENT

Regarding the intervention studies, two [30,35] found that, with equal caloric and food intake, the incorporation of bread to a hypocaloric diet resulted in the same beneficial results on anthropometric measures and body composition as those obtained with the same diet without bread.

Another two studies [33,34] showed that dietary intervention in obese subjects led to a greater loss of percentage body fat in the abdominal region when participants consumed whole grains (including whole-grain bread) than when participants consumed refined grains (refined bread included). However, the study of Aston el al. [32], did not find any differences in changes in WC when several types of bread with different GIs were included in the diet intervention.

TABLE 25.4 Classification of Studies According to the Influence on Abdominal Obesity of Food Groups that Included Bread Consumption

Author, Year [Reference]	Study Conclusions	Relationship with Abdominal Obesity
Conclusions from cross-sectional studies		
Ledikwe et al. 2004 [11]	Bread (type not defined) was included in the group presenting with a higher risk of general and abdominal obesity	Group that included bread, ↑
Haveman-Nies et al. 2001 [12]	Bread included in the group was inversely related to WC	Group that included bread, ↓
Wirfält et al. 2001 [13]	Whole-grain bread consumption was inversely related to abdominal obesity	Group that included whole-grain bread, ↓
Panagiotakos et al. 2007 [14]	The pattern that included bread had no influence on WC	Group that included bread, no change
Jacobs et al. 1998 [15]	Whole-grain bread included in the group was associated with WHR; refined bread included in the group was associated with increased WHR	Group that included whole-grain bread, ↓ Group that included refined bread, ↑
McKeown et al. 2002 [16]	Inverse relationship between whole-grain cereals (including whole-grain bread) and measures of adiposity; no relationship with refined cereals (including refined bread)	Group that included whole-grain bread, ↓. Group that included refined bread, no change
Esmaillzadeh et al. 2005 [17]	Whole-grain bread included in the group with a lower prevalence of abdominal obesity	Group that included whole-grain bread, ↓
Azadbakht et al. 2005 [18]	No relationship between group that included bread and abdominal obesity distribution	Group that included bread, no change
Newby et al. 2007 [19]	Group that included whole-grain bread was inversely related to WC; group that included refined bread, no relationship	Group that included whole-grain bread, ↓ Group that included refined bread, no change
McKeown et al. 2009 [20]	Dark bread in the group correlated with lower trunk fat mass; no relationship between measured variables and the group that included refined bread	Group that included whole-grain bread, ↓ Group that included refined bread, no change
McKeown et al. 2010 [21]	Increasing whole-grain intake is associated with lower VAT in adults, whereas higher intakes of refined grains are associated with higher VAT	Group that included whole-grain bread, ↓ Group that included refined bread, ↑
O'Neil et al. 2010 [22]	Adults who consumed the most servings of whole grains (whole-grain bread included) had a lower abdominal perimeter	Group that included whole-grain bread, ↓
Kim et al. 2012 [23]	In a population of Korean women, a food pattern that included bread showed a negative relation with WC	Group that included whole-grain bread, ↓
Kanerba et al. 2013 [24]	Bread included in the group was inversely related to WC	Group that included bread, ↓
Conclusions from longitudinal studies		
Newby et al. 2003 [25]	Refined bread in the group produces a greater increase in WC	Group that included refined bread, ↑
Newby et al. 2004 [26]	Whole-grain bread included in the groups prevents an increase in WC	Group that included whole-grain bread, ↓
Halkjaer et al. 2004 [27]	In females, a high intake of groups that include refined bread is associated with increased WC	Group that included refined bread (females), ↑ Group that included whole-grain bread, no change

(continued)

TABLE 25.4 Continued

Author, Year [Reference]	Study Conclusions	Relationship with Abdominal Obesity
Halkjaer et al. 2006 [28]	White bread consumption was related to WC gain in females; this association was not observed with whole-grain bread	Group that included refined bread, ↑ Group that included whole-grain bread, no change
Romaguera et al. 2011 [4]	A dietary pattern low in refined bread may help to prevent abdominal fat accumulation; this association not observed with whole-grain bread	Group that included refined bread, ↑ Group that included whole-grain bread, no change
Bautista et al. 2012 [29]	Results suggest a dose-response relationship between the increase in refined bread consumption and WC gain; this association not observed with whole-grain bread	Group that included refined bread, ↑ Group that included whole-grain bread, no change
Conclusions from intervention studies		
Lean et al. 1997 [30]	No difference in WC loss with diets containing lower or greater amounts of bread	No difference in abdominal measures with more or less bread intake
McAuley et al. 2005 [31]	Diet with a high bread content produces lower WC loss in insulin-resistant and overweight women	Minor WC loss with higher content of bread in the diet, ↑
Aston et al. 2008 [32]	Bread with greater or lower GI (whole grain or not) does not influence WC variation in females with excess weight and hyperinsulinemia	There were no differences in changes in WC between different GI of breads
Katcher 2008 [33]	Obese subjects consuming whole grains (whole-grain bread included) lost a greater percentage of body fat in the abdominal region than did subjects consuming refined grains (refined bread included)	Wholemeal bread intake led to a greater loss in% abdominal fat compared to refined bread intake
Venn 2010 [34]	Incorporation of pulses and whole-grain foods (whole-grain bread included) into a weight loss program resulted in a greater reduction in WC compared with a group consuming a control diet	Group that included whole-grain bread, ↓
Kohen 2011 [35]	With equal caloric and foods, incorporation of bread in a hypocaloric diet resulted in no change to the beneficial effects on anthropometric measures and body composition compared to the same diet without bread	No difference in abdominal measures with more or less bread intake

GI, glycemic index; VAT, visceral adipose tissue; WC, waist circumference; WHR, waist-hip ratio.

EFFECTS OF LOW-CARBOHYDRATE VS. LOW-FAT DIETS

One of the studies [30] compared differences between three different diets (high-fat diet, high-protein diet, and high-CHO diet) and found less WC reduction with the high-CHO diet (i.e. with a high bread content). However, the intervention was of short duration (8 weeks of diet and 8 weeks of maintenance). Currently, there is considerable debate about the efficacy of weight loss diets based on the composition of macronutrients (i.e. relative content of CHOs, fats, and proteins). In some studies, low-CHO diets produce greater weight loss in the short term [36,37]. However, until now, all studies evaluating the effect of low-calorie diets with different nutrient composition on body weight loss for up to 1 year have failed to demonstrate a higher effectiveness of one type of diet over another (i.e. low-CHO vs. traditional low-fat or high-protein diets), with no differences in changes in body weight loss, body composition, abdominal fat, or hepatic fat between the assigned macronutrient amounts [38]. Only one study has demonstrated that either a Mediterranean, restricted-calorie diet or a low-CHO, nonrestricted-calorie diet can induce a higher body weight loss after 2 years of intervention compared to a low-fat, restricted-calorie diet. All groups had significant decreases in WC, but the differences among the groups were not significant [39].

HYPOTHESES ON THE MECHANISM OF ACTION BY WHICH BREAD CONSUMPTION INFLUENCES ABDOMINAL OBESITY

We do not know exactly how whole-grain bread may prevent WC increment and how a dietary pattern low in refined bread might help to prevent abdominal fat accumulation. However, possible mechanisms of the action of whole grains (including bread) involve energy density, GI, dietary fiber, and the gut microbiota [40,41].

ENERGY DENSITY

The lower energy density of products based on whole-grain cereals compared to those based on refined cereals, as well as the satiating effect of whole-grain products, may both play an important role in body weight regulation. In the case of bread intake, both types of bread (whole-grain bread vs. refined bread) have similar caloric content; however, whole-grain bread has the greatest satiating power [35], which may result in lower energy intake from other foods.

GLYCEMIC INDEX

Lower plasma glucose and insulin responses to whole-grain cereal intake can also contribute to body weight regulation. Lower plasma glucose and insulin responses have been observed in diabetic and non-diabetic subjects after the ingestion of a low-GI diet containing pumpernickel bread, pasta, and legumes compared with a high-GI diet containing refined bread and potatoes. In fact, several studies have shown that the consumption of foods or meals with a low GI has a higher satiating effect than those with a high GI, irrespective of the evaluation method utilized (direct or indirect) and the possible contribution of confounders (e.g. palatability and fiber content) [42]. The lower rate of nutrient digestion and absorption that is typical of low-GI foods seems to stimulate the gastrointestinal receptors that trigger satiety signals for a longer time, thus protracting the effects on hunger/satiety centers. Therefore, the intact food structure that confers whole-grain cereals with their lower GI can contribute to body weight regulation.

Du et al. [43] carried out a prospective cohort study of 89,432 Europeans aged between 20 and 78 years; subjects were monitored for an average of 6.5 years to assess the effect of GI and glycemic load (GL) on body weight and abdominal circumference. The study did not support an effect of these factors on changes in body weight. The GI (but not the GL) was moderately associated with a larger abdominal circumference. As mentioned previously, MacKeown et al. carried out a study [21] on a sample population from the FHS cohort and found that a higher intake of whole-grain foods to be associated with lower VAT in adults, whereas a higher intake of refined grains was associated with higher VAT. In this study, fasting insulin concentrations were observed to attenuate the associations between refined-grain intake, but not whole-grain intake, and VAT volume, suggesting an intermediary role for insulin on the positive relation between refined-grain intake and VAT volume. The additional adjustment for insulin did not affect the relationship observed between whole-grain intake and VAT.

Finally, in 2013, Giacco et al. [44] designed an interventional study to evaluate the glucose and insulin metabolism in response to long-term consumption of rye and whole wheat compared with a diet containing the same amount of refined-cereal foods, in individuals with MS from two European locations (Kuopio, Finland and Naples, Italy). A total of 146 participants were assigned to a diet based on whole-grain (whole-grain group) or refined-cereal products (control group) for 12 weeks. At the end of the intervention, insulin sensitivity indexes and secretion did not change significantly in the whole-grain and control groups in comparison with baseline and no differences were observed between the two groups.

DIETARY FIBER

The potential mechanism(s) by which whole grains may be related to regional adiposity are speculative. Whole grains are rich in fermentable CHOs such as dietary fiber, resistant starch, and oligosaccharides. Cereal fiber influences body weight by multiple mechanisms depending on its intrinsic properties, hormonal effects, and intestinal fermentation. Intrinsic properties specifically concern the ability of soluble fiber to bind to water and form a viscous solution that delays gastric emptying and intestinal transit and limits glucose absorption, thus leading to a lower blood glucose response [45]. The hormonal effects of fiber are mediated by insulin and gastrointestinal hormones. Fiber decreases insulin secretion and consequently reduces the risk of reactive hypoglycemia during the postabsorption period, thus promoting satiety, increasing fat oxidation, and decreasing fat storage. Fiber also influences gut hormones secretion, which acts on satiety independently of the plasma glucose response or by modifying glucose homeostasis. Cholecystokinin, secreted by small bowel cells, stimulates pancreatic secretion, modulates gastric emptying, and stimulates the hypothalamic satiety center [46].

In the previously mentioned study, McKeown [21] also adjusted for added bran and dietary fiber and the association between both higher intake of whole-grain foods with lower VAT and higher intake of refined grains with higher VAT persisted, suggesting that dietary fiber from grains was not related to body fat distribution.

We carried out a study [29] on a sample group of the PREDIMED trial on the influence of bread intake on WC. However, we did not find any differences in the relationship between a higher intake of refined bread and increasing WC when adjusting for dietary fiber.

GUT MICROBIOTA

A further mechanism by which whole grains may influence body weight regulation is via a probiotic effect modulating the intestinal flora. Available evidence, primarily from investigations in animal models, suggests that the gut microbiota affects nutrient acquisition and energy regulation. Microbiota composition has also been shown to differ in lean vs. obese animals and humans [47]. Among the possible mechanisms, of particular interest is the hypothesis that the metabolic activities of the gut microbiota facilitate the extraction of calories from ingested dietary substances and help to store these calories in host adipose tissue for later use. In fact, the gut bacterial flora of obese mice and humans include fewer Bacteroidetes and correspondingly more Firmicutes than that of their lean counterparts, suggesting that differences in caloric extraction of ingested food substances may be due to the composition of the gut microbiota [47].

In humans, however, it is unknown whether whole grains influence body fat distribution through an effect on gut incretin hormones; however, available data in humans show that a diet rich in whole-wheat cereals compared with a diet based on bran wheat can increase the number of fecal bifidobacteria and lactobacilli, which are the target genera for prebiotic intake [48].

CONCLUSIONS

This chapter indicates that, in the majority of studies, following a food pattern that includes whole-grain bread is more beneficial in relation to abdominal fat distribution than following a food pattern including refined bread. Adherence to dietary patterns that include whole-grain bread or the consumption of whole-grain bread itself do not seems to influence WC gain and may be beneficial in preventing abdominal obesity. With respect to dietary patterns that include refined bread or the consumption of refined bread itself, most well-designed cohort studies indicate that a reduction in refined bread consumption may help to prevent abdominal fat accumulation.

The few clinical trials published on the influence of bread in the effectiveness of weight loss diets have reported controversial results that do not confirm whether (1) the incorporation of bread to a hypocaloric diet affects the outcome of the intervention; or (2) different diets in obese subjects leads to a greater loss in percentage body fat in the abdominal region when participants consume whole-grain bread than when participants consume refined bread. The results discussed in this chapter may have been affected by the small sample sizes or short durations of the interventions. To clarify the relationship between the intake of different types of bread and its influence on WC changes in a weight loss intervention, further studies are needed.

Finally, the mechanisms by which whole-grain or refined bread intake may be related to regional adiposity are speculative; however, factors like energy density, GI, insulin responses, dietary fiber, or the gut microbiota may be involved in this relationship.

References

[1] Beunza JJ, Toledo E, Hu FB, Bes-Rastrollo M, Serrano-Martínez M, Sánchez-Villegas A, et al. Adherence, the Mediterranean diet, long-term weight change, and incident overweight or obesity: the Seguimiento Universidad de Navarra (SUN) cohort. Am J Clin Nutr 2010;92:1–8.

[2] Seidell JC, Perusse L, Despres JP, Bouchard C. Waist and hip circumferences have independent and opposite effects on cardiovascular disease risk factors: the Quebec Family Study. Am J Clin Nutr 2001;74:315–21.

[3] Janssen I, Katzmarzyk PT, Ross R. Waist circumference and not body mass index explains obesity-related health risk. Am J Clin Nutr 2004;79:379–84.

[4] Romaguera D, Ängquist L, Du H, Jakobsen MU, Forouhi NG, Halkjær J, et al. Food composition of the diet in relation to changes in waist circumference adjusted for body mass index. PLoS One 2011;6(8):e23384. http://dx.doi.org/10.1371/journal.pone.0023384. [Epub 2011 Aug 17].

[5] Gaesser GA. Carbohydrate quantity and quality in relation, body mass index. J Am Diet Assoc 2007;107:1768–80.

[6] Bradlee ML, Singer MR, Qureshi MM, Moore LL. Food group intake and central obesity among children and adolescents in the Third National Health and Nutrition Examination Survey (NHANES III). Public Health Nutr 2010;13:797–805.

[7] Williams PG, Grafenauer SJ, O'Shea JE. Cereal grains, legumes, and weight management: a comprehensive review of the scientific evidence. Nutr Rev 2008;66:171–82.

[8] Juntunen KS, Niskanen LK, Liukkonen KH, Poutanen KS, Holst JJ, Mykkänen HM. Postprandial glucose, insulin, and incretin responses to grain products in healthy subjects. Am J Clin Nutr 2002;75:254–62.

[9] Bautista-Castaño I, Serra-Majem L. Relationship between bread consumption, body weight, and abdominal fat distribution: evidence from epidemiological studies. Nutr Rev 2012;70(4):218–33.

[10] Hu F. Dietary pattern analysis: a new direction in nutritional epidemiology. Lipidology 2002;13:3–9.

[11] Ledikwe JH, Smiciklas-Wright H, Mitchell DC, Miller CK, Jensen GL. Dietary patterns of rural older adults are associated with weight and nutritional status. J Am Geriatr Soc 2004;52:589–95.

[12] Haveman-Nies A, Tucker KL, de Groot LC, Wilson PW, van Staveren WA. Evaluation of dietary quality in relationship to nutritional and lifestyle factors in elderly people of the US Framingham Heart Study and the European SENECA study. Eur J Clin Nutr 2001;55:870–80.

[13] Wirfält E, Hedblad B, Gullberg B, Mattisson I, Andrén C, Rosander U, et al. Food patterns and components of the MetS in men and women: a cross-sectional study within the Malmö Diet and Cancer Cohort. Am J Epidemiol 2001;154:1150–9.

[14] Panagiotakos DB, Pitsavos C, Skoumas Y, Stefanadis C. The association between food patterns and the metabolic syndrome using principal components analysis: The ATTICA Study. J Am Diet Assoc 2007;107:979–87.

[15] Jacobs Jr DR, Meyer KA, Kushi LH, Folsom AR. Wholegrain intake may reduce the risk of ischemic heart disease death in postmenopausal women: the Iowa Women's Health Study. Am J Clin Nutr 1998;68:248–57.

[16] McKeown NM, Meigs JB, Liu S, Wilson PW, Jacques PF. Wholegrain intake is favorably associated with metabolic risk factors for type 2 diabetes and cardiovascular disease in the Framingham Offspring Study. Am J Clin Nutr 2002;76:390–8.

[17] Esmaillzadeh A, Mirmiran P, Azizi F. Wholegrain consumption and the metabolic syndrome: a favorable association in Tehranian adults. Eur J Clin Nutr 2005;59:353–62.

[18] Azadbakht L, Mirmiran P, Shiva N, Azizi F. General obesity and central adiposity in a representative sample of Tehranian adults: prevalence and determinants. Int J Vitam Nutr Res 2005;75:297–304.

[19] Newby PK, Maras J, Bakun P, Muller D, Ferrucci L, Tucker KL. Intake of whole grains, refined grains, and cereal fiber measured with 7-d diet records and associations with risk factors for chronic disease. Am J Clin Nutr 2007;86:1745–53.

[20] McKeown NM, Yoshida M, Shea MK, Jacques PF, Lichtenstein AH, Rogers G, et al. Wholegrain intake and cereal fiber are associated with lower abdominal adiposity in older adults. J Nutr 2009;139(10):1950–5.

[21] McKeown NM, Troy LM, Jacques PF, Hoffmann U, O'Donnell CJ, Fox CS. Whole- and refined-grain intakes are differentially associated with abdominal visceral and subcutaneous adiposity in healthy adults: the Framingham Heart Study. Am J Clin Nutr 2010;92(5):1165–71.

[22] O'Neil CE, Zanovec M, Cho SS, Nicklas TA. Wholegrain and fiber consumption are associated with lower body weight measures in US adults: National Health and Nutrition Examination Survey 1999–2004. Nutr Res 2010;30(12):815–22.

[23] Kim JH, Lee JE, Jung IK. Dietary pattern classifications and the association with general obesity and abdominal obesity in Korean women. J Acad Nutr Diet 2012;112(10):1550–9.

[24] Kanerva N, Kaartinen NE, Schwab U, Lahti-Koski M, Männistö S. Adherence to the Baltic Sea diet consumed in the Nordic countries is associated with lower abdominal obesity. Br J Nutr 2012;10:1–9.

[25] Newby PK, Muller D, Hallfrisch J, Qiao N, Andres R, Tucker KL. Dietary patterns and changes in body mass index and waist circumference in adults. Am J Clin Nutr 2003;77:1417–25.

[26] Newby PK, Muller D, Hallfrisch J, Andres R, Tucker KL. Food patterns measured by factor analysis and anthropometric changes in adults. Am J Clin Nutr 2004;80:504–13.

[27] Halkjaer J, Sørensen TI, Tjønneland A, Togo P, Holst C, Heitmann BL. Food and drinking patterns as predictors of 6-year BMI-adjusted changes in waist circumference. Br J Nutr 2004;92:735–48.

[28] Halkjaer J, Tjønneland A, Thomsen BL, Overvad K, Sørensen TI. Intake of macronutrients as predictors of 5-y changes in waist circumference. Am J Clin Nutr 2006;84:789–97.

[29] Bautista-Castaño I, Sánchez-Villegas A, Estruch R, Martínez-González MA, Corella D, Salas-Salvadø J, et al. Changes in bread consumption and 4-year changes in adiposity in Spanish subjects at high cardiovascular risk. Br J Nutr 2012;3:1–10.

[30] Lean ME, Han TS, Prvan T, Richmond PR, Avenell A. Weight loss with high and low carbohydrate 1200 kcal diets in free living women. Eur J Clin Nutr 1997;51:243–8.

[31] McAuley KA, Hopkins CM, Smith KJ, McLay RT, Williams SM, Taylor RW, et al. Comparison of high-fat and high-protein diets with a high-carbohydrate diet in insulin-resistant obese women. Diabetologia 2005;48:8–16.

[32] Aston LM, Stokes CS, Jebb SA. No effect of a diet with a reduced glycemic index on satiety, energy intake and body weight in overweight and obese women. Int J Obes 2008;32:160–5.

[33] Katcher HI, Legro RS, Kunselman AR, Gillies PJ, Demers LM, Bagshaw DM, et al. The effects of a wholegrain-enriched hypocaloric diet on cardiovascular disease risk factors in men and women with metabolic syndrome. Am J Clin Nutr 2008;87(1):79–90.

[34] Venn BJ, Perry T, Green TJ, Skeaff CM, Aitken W, Moore NJ, et al. The effect of increasing consumption of pulses and whole grains in obese people: a randomized controlled trial. J Am Coll Nutr 2010;29(4):365–72.

[35] Loria Kohen V, Gómez Candela C, Fernández Fernández F, Pérez Torres A, Villarino Sanz M, Bermejo LM. Impact of two low-calorie meals with and without bread on the sensation of hunger, satiety and amount of food consumed. Nutr Hosp 2011;26(5):1155–60.

[36] Nordmann AJ, Nordmann A, Briel M, Keller U, Yancy Jr WS, Brehm B, et al. Effects of low-carbohydrate vs. low-fat diets on weight loss and cardiovascular risk factors: a meta-analysis of randomized controlled trials. Arch Intern Med 2006;166:285–93.

[37] Hession M, Rolland C, Kulkarni U, Wise A, Broom J. Systematic review of randomized controlled trials of low-carbohydrate vs. low-fat/low-calorie diets in the management of obesity and its co-morbidities. Obes Rev 2009;10(1):36–50.

[38] de Souza RJ, Bray GA, Carey VJ, Hall KD, LeBoff MS, Loria CM, et al. Effects of 4 weight-loss diets differing in fat, protein, and carbohydrate on fat mass, lean mass, visceral adipose tissue, and hepatic fat: results from the POUNDS LOST trial. Am J Clin Nutr 2012;95(3):614–25.

[39] Shai I, Schwarzfuchs D, Henkin Y, Shahar DR, Witkow S, Greenberg I, et al. Weight loss with a low-carbohydrate, Mediterranean, or low-fat diet. N Engl J Med 2008;359:229e41.

[40] Fardet A. New hypotheses for the health-protective mechanisms of wholegrain cereals: what is beyond fiber? Nutr Res Rev 2010;23:65–134.

[41] Giacco R, Della Pepa G, Luongo D, Riccardi G. Wholegrain intake in relation to body weight: from epidemiological evidence to clinical trials. Nutr Metab Cardiovasc Dis 2011;21(12):901–8.

[42] Bornet FR, Jardy-Gennetier AE, Jacquet N, Stowell J. Glycemic response to foods: impact on satiety and long-term weight regulation. Appetite 2007;49:535–53.

[43] Du H, van der A DL, van Bakel MM, Slimani N, Forouhi NG, Wareham NJ, et al. Dietary glycemic index, glycemic load and subsequent changes of weight and waist circumference in European men and women. Int J Obes (Lond) 2009;33:1280–8.

[44] Giacco R, Lappi J, Costabile G, Kolehmainen M, Schwab U, Landberg R, et al. Effects of rye and whole wheat versus refined cereal foods on metabolic risk factors: a randomized controlled two-centre intervention study. Clin Nutr 2013;6. doi: pii: S0261-5614 (13)00043-5.

[45] Weickert MO, Pfeiffer AF. Metabolic effects of dietary fiber consumption and prevention of diabetes. J Nutr 2008;138:439e42. [Review].

[46] Burton-Freeman BM, Keim NL. Glycemic index, cholecystokinin, satiety and disinhibition: is there an unappreciated paradox for overweight women? Int J Obes (Lond) 2008;31:1647e54. [Epub 2008 Sep 30].

[47] Di Baise JK, Zhang H, Crowell MD, Krajmalnik-Brown R, Decker GA, Rittmann BE. Gut microbiota and its possible relationship with obesity. Mayo Clin Proc 2008;83:460e9.

[48] Costabile A, Klinder A, Fava F, Napolitano A, Fogliano V, Leonard C, et al. Wholegrain wheat breakfast cereal has a prebiotic effect on the human gut microbiota: a double blind, placebo-controlled, crossover study. Br J Nutr 2008;99(1): 110e20.

[49] Togo P, Osler M, Sørensen TIA, Heitmann BL. A longitudinal study of food intake patterns and obesity in adult Danish men and women. Int J Obes Relat Metab Disord 2004;28:583–93.

CHAPTER

26

Role of the Immune System in Obesity-Associated Inflammation and Insulin Resistance

Yoshinori Nagai[a] *and Kiyoshi Takatsu*[a,b]

[a]Department of Immunobiology and Pharmacological Genetics, Graduate School of Medicine and Pharmaceutical Science for Research, University of Toyama, Toyama-shi, Toyama, Japan; [b]Toyama Prefectural Institute for Pharmaceutical Research, Imizu City, Toyama, Japan

Abbreviations

ASC, apoptosis-associated speck-like protein containing a CARD; ATM, adipose tissue macrophage; CCR2, C-C chemokine receptor type 2; CX3CR1, CX3C chemokine receptor 1; DAG, diacylglycerol; DAMP, damage-associated molecular pattern; DHA, docosahexaenoic acid; EPA, eicosapentaenoic acid; eWAT, epididymal white adipose tissue; FA, fatty acid; GPR, G protein-coupled receptor; HFD, high-fat diet; IAPP, islet amyloid polypeptide; IFN-γ, interferon gamma; IKK, inhibitor of nuclear factor kappa-B (IκB) kinas; eIL, interleukin; IRS, insulin receptor substrate; JNK, c-Jun N-terminal kinase; KO, knockout; LPS, lipopolysaccharide; LRR, leucine-rich repeat; LTB4, leukotriene B4; MAPK, mitogen-activated protein kinase; MCP-1, C-C motif chemokine 2/monocyte chemotactic protein 1; MD, myeloid differentiation; MyD88, myeloid differentiation primary response gene 88; NAFLD, nonalcoholic fatty liver disease; NASH, nonalcoholic steatohepatitis; NF-κB, nuclear factor-kappa-B; NKT, natural killer T; NLR, NOD-like receptor; NLRP, NOD-, LRR-, and pyrin domain-containingNOD, nucleotide oligomerization domain; PAMP, pathogen-associated molecular pattern; PGN, peptidoglycan; PPAR-γ, peroxisome proliferator-activated receptor gamma; PRR, pattern recognition receptor; ROS, reactive oxygen species; RP105, radioprotective 105 kDa protein; SVF, stromal vascular fraction; T2DM, type 2 diabetes mellitus; Th, T helper; TLR, toll-like receptor; TNF-α, tumor necrosis factor; Treg, regulatory T; TZD, thiazolidinedione; WT, wild-type

INTRODUCTION

Obesity is a hallmark of the metabolic disorders, which comprise a cluster of disorders that lead to the development of chronic diseases, such as type 2 diabetes mellitus (T2DM) [1,2]. Accumulating evidence indicates that adipose tissues in obesity are in a state of chronic, low-grade inflammation [3]. Inflammatory mediators, including C-C motif chemokine 2 [monocyte chemotactic protein 1 (MCP-1)], interleukin-1β (IL-1β), IL-6, IL-10, and tumor necrosis factor (TNF- α; encoded by *TNF*) are bioactive mediators secreted from obese adipose tissue. Interestingly, the adipose stromal vascular fraction (SVF), which contains nonfat cells, including immune cell, endothelial cells, and stromal cells, plays a more prominent role in the development of obesity-associated inflammation and insulin resistance because cells in this fraction tend to secrete higher levels of inflammatory mediators compared to adipocytes.

An important finding for understanding the pathogenesis of adipose tissue inflammation is that large numbers of macrophages infiltrate into adipose tissue in obese rodents and humans [4,5]. There is considerable evidence for the pathophysiologic role of the MCP-1 chemokine pathway in macrophage infiltration into obese adipose tissue [6]. However, the story of adipose tissue inflammation goes beyond macrophages, and there are many unexpected findings as we learn about the complex interactions between the different immune cells that accumulate in adipose tissue, including T cells, B cells, and natural killer T (NKT) cells [3].

Lipotoxicity is the state of lipid stress associated with elevated lipid content and ectopic lipid storage in tissues, such as the liver. Obesity results in an elevation in circulating fatty acid (FA) levels and, subsequently, an increase in adipose tissue inflammation [7]. FAs probably enter macrophages through plasma membrane transporters.

Nutrition in the Prevention and Treatment of Abdominal Obesity
http://dx.doi.org/10.1016/B978-0-12-407869-7.00026-X

In addition, adipose macrophages play critical roles in immune responses through several FA-sensing mechanisms, such as pattern recognition receptors (PRRs) and G protein-coupled receptors (GPRs). PRRs have provided us with great insights into immune responses against pathogens [8]. Several families of PRRs, such as the toll-like receptors (TLRs) and nucleotide oligomerization domain (NOD)-like receptors (NLRs), have been discovered. It is now becoming ever more apparent that these PRRs are not only able to recognize microbial components but they also mediate immune responses to endogenous molecules, including those induced in metabolic disorders, such as FAs. These endogenous molecules have been termed "danger-associated molecular patterns" (DAMPs) and have similar functions to microbial components in activating proinflammatory pathways [9]. For example, saturated FAs activate TLR2 and TLR4 and drive proinflammatory responses in macrophages by activating the nuclear factor-kappa-B (NF-κB) pathway, leading to increased expression of proinflammatory target genes [10,11]. In contrast, long-chain polyunsaturated omega-3 FAs, such as docosahexaenoic acid (DHA) and eicosapentaenoic acid (EPA), can exert anti-inflammatory effects through GPR120 [12].

Inflammation-induced insulin resistance can be viewed as a two-hit process. First, activated immune cells accumulate in tissues, such as adipose tissue, and release proinflammatory cytokines, such as TNF-α. Second, these cytokines act on neighboring insulin target cells, causing insulin resistance. In the target cells, activation of TLRs and/or TNF receptor (TNFR) leads to the activation of serine kinases, including inhibitor of nuclear factor kappa-B (IκB) kinase (IKK) and c-Jun N-terminal kinase (JNK), which inhibit insulin signaling [3]. Inflammasome-induced IL-1β production can also impair insulin sensitivity and insulin secretion by pancreatic beta cells [13,14].

In this chapter, we will focus on the role of the immune system in the induction of obesity-associated inflammation and highlight links to insulin resistance. We will also offer our view of how cytokines, chemokines, lipids, PRRs, and immune cells work together to cause inflammation and insulin resistance.

INFLAMMATORY CHANGES IN OBESITY AND INSULIN RESISTANCE

Cytokines

Hotamisligil et al. first reported the landmark observation that established the concept of chronic adipose tissue inflammation in obesity [15]: they found that TNF-α is elevated in obese rodents and that neutralizing TNF- α attenuates insulin resistance. TNF-α is excessively secreted from activated macrophages and directly causes insulin resistance by inhibiting insulin receptor signaling in insulin target cells. For example, TNF-α activates IKK and mitogen-activated protein kinases (MAPKs) such as JNK, which inhibit insulin receptor signaling by serine phosphorylation of insulin receptor substrate 1 (IRS-1) [16,17]. It is noteworthy that TNF-α-deficient mice are protected from obesity-induced insulin resistance.

IL-1β can also exert proinflammatory effects [18]. High-fat diet (HFD) treatment induces the secretion of FAs, which activates the inflammasome in macrophages, resulting in IL-1β production and attenuated insulin sensitivity [13]. The inflammasome is composed of the NOD-, LRR- and pyrin domain-containing 3 (NLRP3) protein and the adaptor protein, apoptosis-associated speck-like protein containing a CARD (ASC); NLRP3-deficient or ASC-deficient mice are protected from HFD-induced insulin resistance [14]. Interestingly, IL-1 β is also secreted from inflamed pancreatic beta cells and has detrimental effects on beta cell function [19]. Clinical studies of IL-1β inhibitors suggest that their major effects of improving hyperglycemia are related to improved insulin secretion rather than to improved insulin sensitivity [20,21].

In addition to proinflammatory cytokines, anti-inflammatory cytokines are produced by adipose tissue. Adiponectin, which is secreted exclusively from adipocytes, is markedly downregulated in obese adipose tissue, and supplementation of adiponectin in obese mice effectively reverses insulin resistance. IL-10 inhibits the deleterious effects of proinflammatory signaling on the insulin receptor [22]. In vivo administration of IL-10 prevents the development of lipid-induced insulin resistance [23], and muscle-specific overexpression of IL-10 increases whole-body insulin sensitivity [24].

Chemokines

Although concentrations of many inflammatory chemokines are elevated in obese adipose tissue, some of them appear to be involved in the infiltration of adipose tissue macrophages (ATMs) into inflammatory sites. MCP-1 is an important chemokine secreted by hypertrophic adipocytes and acts with its receptor, C-C chemokine receptor type 2 (CCR2), on macrophages, thus stimulate their migration. In HFD-fed mice, MCP-1 deficiency or CCR2 deficiency attenuates macrophage accumulation in adipose tissue, adipose tissue inflammation, and systemic insulin resistance [6]. In addition, pharmacological antagonism of CCR2 reduces the number of ATMs and improves insulin sensitivity in obese mice. However, there is a contradictory report that MCP-1 and CCR2 are involved in the recruitment of macrophages into adipose tissue [25], and this issue remains to be resolved.

Fractalkine and its receptor CX3C chemokine receptor 1 (CX3CR1) have been implicated in the recruitment of monocytes in atherosclerosis [26]. Fractalkine, which is expressed in adipocytes and macrophages, is markedly upregulated in obese human adipose tissue and contributes to the adhesion of monocytes to adipocytes [27]. Leukotriene B4 (LTB4) is secreted by adipocytes and has a chemotactic activity on neutrophils. Mice lacking LTB4 or its receptor, LTB4-R1, are protected from diet-induced adipose tissue inflammation and insulin resistance [28].

Fatty Acids

Circulating free FAs are elevated in insulin-resistant states, and dietary fat intake influences the composition of these FAs [7]. In addition to circulating FAs, immune cells such as macrophages in adipose tissue are exposed to high local concentrations of FAs, which are released from adipocytes by lipolysis. In this way, immune cells can amplify the effects of saturated FAs within adipose tissue, a lipid-rich environment.

Saturated FAs are proinflammatory lipid compounds that activate inflammatory signaling in various cell types, such as macrophages and adipocytes [29,30]. This leads to stimulation of IKK/NF-κB and JNK/AP1 pathways, as well as cytokine production, through TLR2 and TLR4 [10,11]. Saturated FAs can also stimulate TLR-independent inflammatory pathways. Saturated FA treatment leads to an increase in reactive oxygen species (ROS) production, which can activate a number of stress kinases. Saturated FA-induced ROS may also drive stimulation of the NLRP3 inflammasome and increase IL-1β release [13]. When applied to insulin target cells, IL-1β decreases insulin signaling, thereby providing another mechanism for saturated FA-mediated inflammatory responses to cause insulin resistance. In addition, saturated FAs may be precursors to other lipids, such as diacylglycerols (DAGs) [31]. Increased levels of intracellular DAGs lead to protein kinase C (PKC) activation and decreased insulin signaling [32]. Taken together, these mechanisms may explain an important component of *lipotoxicity*: saturated FA promotion of chronic inflammation and insulin resistance.

Protein Kinases: IKK and JNK Kinases

It is accepted that chronic obesity-induced inflammation leads to activation of protein kinases, including IKKs and JNKs. It is becoming increasingly clear that the NF-κB pathway plays a key role in the pathogenesis of obesity and insulin resistance. This pathway may be activated by TLR4 due to interactions with dietary FAs or bacterial lipopolysaccharide (LPS), or as a consequence of hypoxia [33–35]. An in vivo analysis using HLL mice, a transgenic line bearing the NF-κB-responsive HIV LTR promoter fused to luciferase, revealed that HFD activates NF-κB in adipose tissue and liver, with the greatest increase in adipocytes and ATMs [36]. IKKβ activation during obesity releases NF-κB from its inhibitor, IκB, resulting in increased tissue inflammation. Targeted disruption or pharmacological inhibition of IKKβ can restore insulin sensitivity in obese mice and humans [37–40]. Another NF-κB-related kinase, IKKε, is a direct transcriptional target of the NF-κB pathway and is likely to further amplify inflammatory signals. A recent study showed that HFD induces a specific increase in IKKε expression in the liver and white adipose tissue compared with other IKKs [41]. The cell types responsible for these changes may be adipocytes and macrophages in the SVF. IKKε-deficient mice are resistant to the deleterious effects of HFD on insulin sensitivity, exhibiting normal glucose and insulin tolerance. Blood cholesterol levels are markedly reduced and adiponectin is elevated in IKKε-deficient mice. IKKε knockout (KO) mice do not gain as much weight as wild-type (WT) mice on HFD, probably due to increased energy expenditure. In addition, these mice show improved hepatic steatosis, macrophage accumulation in adipose tissue, and increased proinflammatory gene expression in fat.

JNK1 and JNK2 have been implicated in obesity-induced glucose intolerance; JNK1 is believed to be the major contributor [17,42]. JNK1 is chronically activated in obesity and T2DM, at least in part due to lipotoxic stress [43]. JNK1-deficiency in mice or treatment with pharmacological JNK1 inhibitors protect against obesity-induced insulin resistance [17,42,44]. JNK1 activation induces insulin resistance through direct interference with insulin signaling: JNK1 inhibits phosphorylation of IRS-1 and IRS-2 and prevents their recruitment to activated insulin receptors [45,46]. JNK1 activation in hematopoietic cells has been suggested to be a major contributor to both HFD-induced inflammation and insulin resistance, but has no impact on development of obesity [47].

INFLAMMATORY CHANGES OF ADIPOCYTES AND IMMUNE CELLS IN THE ADIPOSE TISSUE MICROENVIRONMENT

Adipocytes

Adipose tissue was first considered to be a static triglyceride storage depot (for energy), but is now recognized to be an endocrine organ with an important role in local and systemic homeostasis. It has been shown that adipocytes can secrete various bioactive molecules, including cytokines and chemokines called *adipokines*. Adiponectin is a well-known anti-inflammatory adipokine that promotes insulin sensitivity [48,49]. In contrast, several adipokines have been shown to promote insulin resistance in obesity [50]. For example, IL-6, resistin, and TNF-α are inflammatory adipokines that have been linked to the development of insulin resistance and inflammation.

In addition, lipids are secreted and act both locally and systemically. In the lean state, insulin signaling promotes inhibition of lipolysis and FA release from adipocytes. With the progression of obesity, however, decreased insulin sensitivity in adipocytes results in reduced lipolysis and elevated levels of circulating FAs [51]. FAs, such as palmitate, play an important role in the lipotoxic effects associated with adipose tissue inflammation and insulin resistance [52].

Macrophages

Adipose tissue inflammation results from the complex cross talk between adipocytes, macrophages, and other immune cells, with contributions from both the innate and adaptive immune system (Fig. 26.1). The recruitment of macrophages into adipose tissue is the initial event in obesity-induced inflammation and insulin resistance [5]. Hypertrophic adipocytes secrete chemokines such as MCP-1 and LTB4, thus providing a chemotactic gradient that attracts monocytes into adipose tissue [6,53]. Once monocytes migrate into adipose tissue, they can differentiate into macrophages. Macrophage activation is a crucial step in the induction of adipose tissue inflammation and is influenced by adaptive immune cells. T helper 1 (Th1) and Th17 cells produce interferon gamma (IFN-γ) and IL-17, respectively, which stimulate proinflammatory M1 macrophage differentiation, whereas Th2 and regulatory T (Treg) cells promote anti-inflammatory M2 macrophage polarization through the production of IL-4, IL-10, and IL-13 [50].

The proinflammatory state of ATMs is reported to correlate well with insulin resistance [54]. M1 macrophages, also named *classically activated macrophages*, are highly proinflammatory, producing a variety of cytokines such as IL-1β and TNF-α. M1 macrophages can be induced in vitro by treating bone marrow-derived cells with LPS and IFN-γ. Fujisaka et al. showed that the number of $CD11c^+$ M1 macrophages correlates well with insulin sensitivity [55]. Furthermore, IL-1β and TNF-α are secreted locally and have paracrine effects, and possibly also systemic effects, causing decreased insulin sensitivity in insulin target cells, including adipocytes, hepatocytes, and muscle cells. M2 macrophages, also named *alternatively activated macrophages*, are not inflammatory; they produce anti-inflammatory cytokines such as IL-4 and IL-10. M2 macrophages can be induced in vitro by culturing bone marrow-derived cells with IL-4 and macrophage colony-stimulating factor. The phenotype of ATMs can be altered; they can repolarize from one to another. For example, activation of nuclear receptor peroxisome proliferator-activated receptor gamma (PPAR-γ) by pioglitazone, a thiazolidinedione drug, can drive conversion from M1 to M2 phenotype, coincident with increased insulin sensitivity [56]. More knowledge is needed about the factors that direct the polarization state of macrophages toward either the proinflammatory or anti-inflammatory state, as this could provide key information for designing therapeutic interventions.

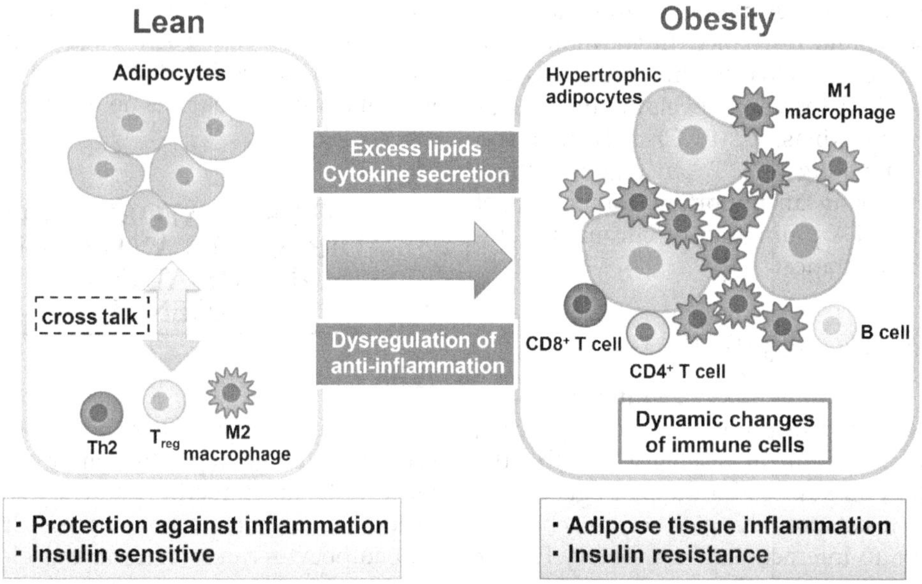

FIGURE 26.1 Functional interactions between adipocytes and immune cells in the lean or obese state. In the lean state, Th2 cells, Treg cells, and M2 macrophages are prominent in adipose tissue. These cells contribute to the suppression of inflammation in adipose tissue. As obesity progresses, excess lipids and proinflammatory cytokines are released and anti-inflammatory regulation by the immune system is impaired. In obese adipose tissue, adipocytes are hypertrophic and infiltrated M1 macrophages, $CD8^+$ T cells, $CD4^+$ T cells, and B cells contribute to induce chronic adipose tissue inflammation and insulin resistance. (See color plate at the back of the book.)

T Cells

Although macrophages are the most important cells in cytokine production leading to insulin resistance, their recruitment to adipose tissue and their subsequent activation is influenced by other types of immune cells, including lymphocytes. HFD-fed *Rag1* (recombination activating gene 1)-deficient mice, which lack T cells, are more insulin resistant than WT mice, indicating that T cells may have a protective role against insulin resistance [57]. The number of Treg cells, which express forkhead box protein P3 (FOXP3), decreases with obesity. Treg cells can secrete anti-inflammatory signals, inhibit macrophage migration, and induce M2-like macrophage differentiation [58]. Boosting the number of Treg cells in obese mice can improve insulin sensitivity, suggesting that Treg cells may have a protective role against insulin resistance. On the other hand, Nishimura et al. found that increased numbers of $CD8^+$ cytotoxic Th1 cells in obese adipose tissue promote the recruitment and activation of macrophages [59,60]. However, another report demonstrates that Th1 cell numbers do not increase until 20 weeks after HFD treatment, which is several months after the increase in macrophages and insulin resistance.

B Cells

The role of B cells in the development of metabolic disorders has been unclear. B cells are recruited to adipose tissue early after the initiation of HFD, and before T cell recruitment [61]. B cells also exacerbate metabolic disorders through immunoglobulin G (IgG) production. B cell-deficient mice fed with a HFD have improved glucose tolerance and insulin resistance regardless of weight gain, compared with WT mice. To reduce glucose tolerance, B cells require $CD4^+$ and $CD8^+$ T cell-mediated induction of proinflammatory cytokine production, which potentiate M1 macrophage polarization and insulin resistance. IgG transfer from HFD-fed mice to B cell-deficient mice enables them to rapidly induce inflammatory cytokine production and insulin resistance. Moreover, IgG autoantibodies, which recognize distinct antigenic targets, are present in insulin-resistant humans.

Natural Killer T Cells

NKT cells are innate-like T cells that recognize glycolipids and rapidly produce a mixture of Th1 and Th2 cytokines, for example, IFN-γ and IL-4, respectively. It has not been determined whether NKT cells are involved in the development of metabolic disorders, despite evidence showing that NKT cells are present at significant levels in the SVF of white adipose tissue. NKT cell-deficient beta2-microglobulin KO mice show HFD-induced glucose intolerance and visceral adipose tissue inflammation with comparable obesity [62]. Injection of alpha-galactosylceramide in HFD-fed WT mice enhances NKT cell infiltration into adipose tissue. Furthermore, NKT cell activation by alpha-galactosylceramide injection exacerbates glucose intolerance and adipose tissue inflammation, including macrophage infiltration and inflammatory cytokine and chemokine expression. Therefore, NKT cells enhance visceral adipose tissue inflammation and contribute to the development of metabolic disorders in obesity.

Other Immune Cells

Feeding a HFD to mice causes an increase in neutrophil infiltration in adipose tissue [63]. Neutrophils secrete various proteases, such as neutrophil elastase. Treatment of hepatocytes or adipocytes with neutrophil elastase causes insulin resistance, and the depletion of neutrophil elastase in HFD-fed mice improves adipose tissue inflammation, with reduced infiltration of neutrophils and macrophages. Therefore, secreted elastase from neutrophils is the key mediator of adipose tissue inflammation.

Eosinophils are typically associated with allergy and helminthic infection. On the other hand, they also regulate the state of macrophage activation in adipose tissue and play an important role in metabolic homeostasis. Eosinophil is the major source of IL-4, which is a crucial cytokine for the induction of alternatively activated M2 macrophages. In the absence of IL-4 or eosinophils in adipose tissue, alternative activation of ATMs is impaired [64].

Mast cells can also accumulate in the visceral adipose tissue of obese mice. A recent study showed that genetic depletion or pharmacological stabilization of mast cells reduces diet-induced obesity, inflammatory responses, and insulin resistance [65].

SIGNALING MOLECULES THAT INDUCE OR REDUCE OBESITY-ASSOCIATED INFLAMMATION AND INSULIN RESISTANCE

Toll-Like Receptors

Exogenous signals can modify inflammatory responses in obesity. TLRs are transmembrane receptors that are important for sensing conserved structural moieties of microorganisms and for the subsequent induction of proinflammatory responses [8]. Following ligand recognition, they activate the NF-κB and MAPK pathways to induce the production of proinflammatory cytokines that are important for evading pathogens. It is well

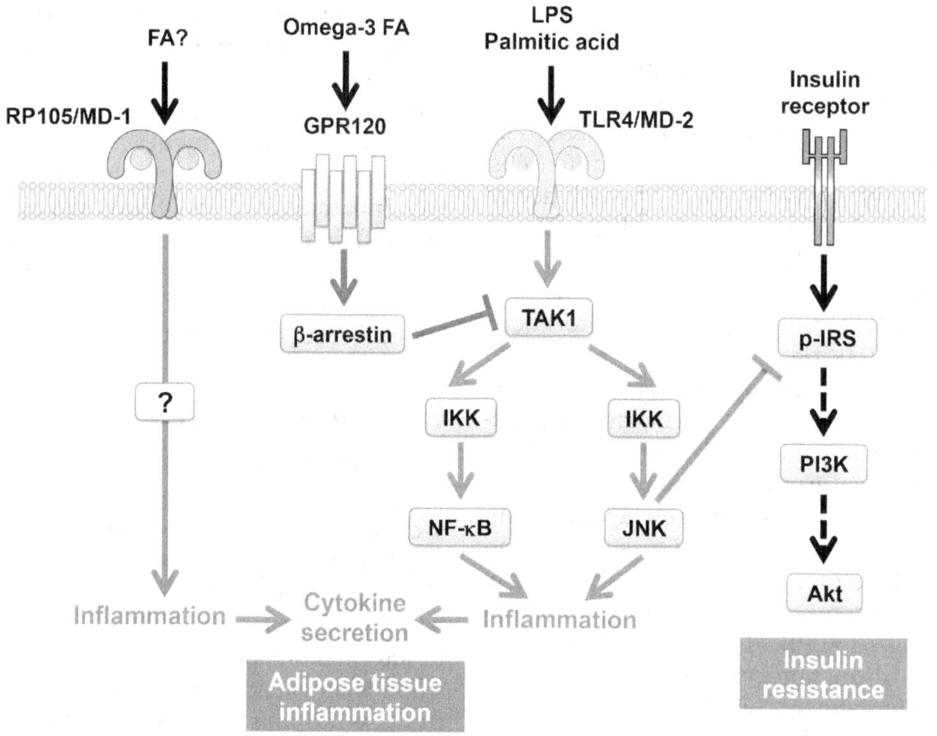

FIGURE 26.2 Inflammatory signaling pathways involved in the development of mechanisms controlling adipose tissue inflammation and insulin resistance. Lipopolysaccharides (LPS) or palmitic acid can signal via TLR4/MD-2 to induce inflammatory responses and inhibit IRS phosphorylation of insulin receptor signaling. Omega-3 fatty acids (FA) signal via GPR120 and inhibit TLR4 signaling via sequestration of TAK1. Signal via RP105/MD-1 may induce inflammatory responses, but the nature of RP105-mediated signaling in adipose tissue inflammation remains unclear. (See color plate at the back of the book.)

known that TLRs also sense nonmicrobial endogenous ligands, such as dietary FAs [9]. Recent advances in deciphering TLR signaling networks reveal that TLR ligation by endogenous ligands activates similar proinflammatory pathways to those activated by microbial ligands in various organs, including adipose tissue, the liver, and the central nervous system (CNS).

TLR4/MD-2 Complex

TLR4 is the most important member of the TLR protein family for LPS recognition and LPS-mediated inflammatory responses [66]. In addition, TLR4 requires lymphocyte antigen 96 [myeloid differentiation 2 (MD-2)] for LPS recognition by its extracellular portion [67]: without MD-2, TLR4 is not expressed on the cell surface [68]. It is established that TLR4/MD-2 complexes are essential for LPS responses, because neither TLR4-deficient nor MD-2-deficient mice respond to LPS [66,68]. Recent crystal structure analyses reveal that LPS can fit into a hydrophobic cavity of MD-2, and this binding leads to homodimerization of the TLR4/MD-2 complex, which results in the activation of TLR4 downstream signaling [69,70].

A body of evidence suggests that TLR4 is an attractive candidate for linking innate immune responses to obesity and insulin resistance (Fig. 26.2). First, TLR4 expression is increased in adipose tissue inflammatory macrophages in obesity [10,29]. Second, TLR4 KO mice or mice with a loss-of-function mutation in the *Tlr4* gene are protected from obesity-induced insulin resistance [10,34]. Third, hematopoietic cell-specific deletion of *Tlr4* ameliorates HFD-induced hepatic and adipose tissue insulin resistance [71]. Fourth, saturated FAs released by adipocyte lipolysis activate the NF-κB pathway in vitro through TLR4 expressed on macrophages [72]. Additionally, LPS derived from the gut microflora can leak into the circulation in obesity, resulting in a higher serum LPS concentration, and LPS signals through TLR4/MD-2 to stimulate the production of proinflammatory cytokines in adipose tissue [73].

Interestingly, recent studies suggest that the TLR4/MD-2 complex may play a key role in nonimmune systems, such as pancreatic islets and the hypothalamus. Within pancreatic islets, TLR4 is expressed in beta cells; palmitate induces inflamed pancreatic beta cell dysfunction in vivo by activating inflammatory responses in islets [74]. In addition, the palmitate-TLR4/MD-2-myeloid differentiation primary response gene 88 (MyD88) axis regulates the production of chemokines such as MCP-1 and CXCL1, which induce the recruitment of M1 macrophages into the islets. This M1 macrophage accumulation is important for beta cell dysfunction in T2DM model *db/db* mice. There is accumulating evidence that saturated FAs activate TLR4 signaling in the hypothalamus, leading to proinflammatory cytokine production and endoplasmic reticulum stress [75]. Another report indicated that an adipokine, resistin, derived from adipose tissue binds directly to TLR4 in the hypothalamus and leads to the activation of MAPK signaling and the promotion of insulin resistance through MyD88 [76]. These results suggest that resistin is an endogenous TLR4 ligand that links hypothalamic inflammation to insulin resistance.

RP105/MD-1 Complex

CD180 antigen [radioprotective 105kDa protein (RP105)] was identified as a leucine-rich repeat (LRR) protein expressed on the surface of B cells [77]. RP105 shares some features with TLR4. First, RP105 is associated with lymphocyte antigen 86 (MD-1), an MD-2 homolog [78]. Second, both RP105 and TLR4 contain 22 LRRs in their extracellular domains, suggesting a possible involvement of RP105/MD-1 in LPS-induced responses. In fact, both RP105-deficient mice and MD-1-deficient mice show reduced LPS-dependent proliferation and CD86 upregulation in B cells, albeit to a lesser extent than that observed in TLR4-deficient mice [79,80]. Third, LPS appears to bind to MD-1 with a lower affinity than to MD-2. We infer from these results that TLR4/MD-2 is indispensable for LPS responses, while RP105/MD-1 is dispensable for these responses.

We have examined whether the RP105/MD-1 complex has a role in sensing an obesity-related endogenous ligand or whether this complex participates in immune responses leading to diet-induced adipose tissue inflammation and insulin resistance [81]. Of interest, murine epididymal white adipose tissue (eWAT) expresses *Cd180* (*Rp105*) mRNA and this expression is markedly increased by HFD treatment. Cell surface expression of RP105 and MD-1 are also increased on inflammatory M1 ATMs but not on anti-inflammatory M2 ATMs by HFD. Using a co-culture system composed of 3T3-L1 adipocytes and macrophage cell lines, we have shown that *Rp105* and *Ly86* (*Md-1*) mRNA expression is increased in macrophages in parallel with upregulated *Tnf* mRNA expression, but smaller increases in *Tlr4* and *Ly96* (*Md-2*) mRNA expression are seen in this system. Furthermore, HFD-induced obesity, adipose tissue inflammation, and insulin resistance are severely attenuated in RP105 KO and MD-1 KO mice compared to WT and TLR4 KO mice. These results clearly suggest that the induction of obesity-related inflammation and metabolic disorders by HFD may require or be dependent on the RP105/MD-1 pathway rather than the TLR4/MD-2 pathway. However, RP105/MD-1 may recognize lipids other than palmitic acid, since RP105-deficient or MD-1-deficient macrophages normally respond to the FA as well as do WT macrophages [81]. Further study is necessary to determine the precise actions of RP105/MD-1 in adipose tissue, including identifying the relevant endogenous ligand and signaling pathway (Fig. 26.2).

Toll-Like Receptor 2

TLR2 recognizes a variety of microbial components derived from Gram-positive bacteria, such as lipopeptides, peptidoglycan, and lipoteichoic acids. TLR2 forms a heterodimeric complex with TLR1 or TLR6 to discriminate among different types of synthetic lipopeptides [82,83]. Interestingly, TLR2 requires RP105/MD-1 to facilitate B cell and macrophage activation by lipopeptides and *Mycobacterium tuberculosis* lipoproteins, respectively [84,85].

The acylated saturated FA moieties in lipopeptides are critical for ligand recognition by TLR2. Deacylated bacterial lipoproteins are unable to both activate TLR2 and induce cytokine production in monocytes. Interestingly, a saturated FA, lauric acid, induces NF-κB activation through TLR2 dimerized with either TLR1 or TLR6 [86]. Another report indicates that palmitate stimulation of a myoblast cell line activates MAPK and NF-κB activation through TLR2/MyD88 signaling, and these inflammatory responses induce insulin resistance in muscles [87,88]. Previous in vivo studies have implicated TLR2 in the pathogenesis of obesity and metabolic disorders. Transient siRNA inhibition of TLR2 in vivo resulted in improved insulin sensitivity in WT mice fed a HFD [88]. TLR2-deficeint mice are substantially protected from diet-induced adiposity, insulin resistance, hypercholesterolemia, and hepatic steatosis [89].

Toll-Like Receptor 5

TLR5 recognizes the conserved domain in flagellin monomers and triggers proinflammatory responses [90]. Uniquely, TLR5 is not expressed in macrophages and conventional dendritic cells in mice. In contrast, TLR5 is highly expressed in intestinal $CD11c^+$ lamina propria dendritic cells, which do not express TLR4 [91]. These cells can detect pathogenic bacteria, such as *Salmonella typhimurium*, and produce proinflammatory cytokines in a TLR5-dependent manner. A previous study in TLR5 KO mice showed that 10% of these mice exhibit severe colitis and an additional 30% exhibit gross and/or histopathological evidence of colitis [92].

Recently, a possible role for the gut microbiota in obesity and metabolic syndrome has been suggested. In both humans and mice, the development of obesity correlates with shifts in the relative abundance of the two dominant bacterial phyla in the gut: Bacteroidetes and Firmicutes spp. [93,94]. Additionally, transfer of the gut microbiota from *ob/ob* mice to germ-free mice leads to an increase in fat weight [95]. TLR5 KO mice show hyperphagia and develop hallmark features of metabolic syndrome, including hyperlipidemia, insulin resistance, and increased adiposity [96]. TLR5 KO mice differ from WT mice regarding intestinal microbiome composition: this is thought to be related to both the metabolic phenotype of these mice and the development of spontaneous colitis in a proportion of them. Indeed, the transfer of the gut microbiota from TLR5 KO mice to WT germ-free mice confers many features of metabolic syndrome in the recipients. However, in contrast to TLR5 KO mice, loss of human TLR5 function by a dominant nonsense polymorphism (R392X) protects from weight gain but predisposes to T2DM [97].

Monocyte Differentiation Antigen CD14

Monocyte differentiation antigen CD14 is a 55-kDa protein that is expressed in two forms: glycosylphosphatidylinositol-anchored membrane form (mCD14) and a soluble form (sCD14) [98,99]. mCD14 is mainly expressed in myeloid cells, whereas sCD14 is secreted from other type of cells, such as hepatocytes and adipocytes [100–102]. Both mCD14 and sCD14 bind to LPS and augment LPS responses. CD14 is also known to cooperate with TLR2 in the response to lipoproteins [103]. CD14 KO mice show attenuated, but still significant, LPS responses [99]. Although CD14 is not essential for LPS recognition and the response, it may have a role in loading LPS onto the TLR4/MD-2 dimer, which shows little binding to LPS in the absence of CD14 [104].

CD14 is suggested to be associated with obesity and insulin resistance. *CD14* gene expression is increased in adipose tissue and adipocytes from obese human subjects. Treatment with recombinant human sCD14 improves glucose tolerance in HFD-fed WT mice and *ob/ob* mice [105]. CD14 KO mice show decreased body fat and do not become obese under normal dietary conditions [106]. Furthermore, analyses of bone marrow chimeric mice reveal that bone marrow-derived macrophages and tissue macrophages may be responsible for CD14-mediated adipose tissue inflammation and insulin resistance [105].

NOD-Like Receptors and Inflammasomes

TLRs are transmembrane proteins located at the membrane surface or in endosomes. In contrast, NLRs and inflammasome are located in the cytoplasm. NLR proteins have an important role in the host defense against microbial infection and in gut homeostasis. Genetic evidence shows that the impaired recognition and killing of commensal bacteria in NLR-deficient mice can contribute to the development of metabolic disorders [107].

NOD-Like Receptors

Peptidoglycan (PGN) is a bacterial cell wall component that stimulates innate immune responses. NOD proteins are currently the only proteins known to propagate inflammatory signals in response to PGN [108]. NOD1 recognizes d-glutamyl-meso-diaminopimelic acid-containing PGN found in Gram-positive bacteria, whereas NOD2 recognizes muramyl dipeptide present in all bacteria [108,109]. NOD1/2 double KO mice are protected from HFD-induced inflammation, lipid accumulation, and insulin resistance in adipose tissue and the liver [110]. Conversely, NOD1 ligands induce profound acute insulin resistance in mice without major systemic inflammation, potentially mediated by a direct action on hepatocytes and adipocytes and an indirect action on skeletal muscle.

NLRP3 Inflammasome

IL-1β has been implicated in various nonmicrobial proinflammatory diseases, including atherosclerosis, gout, and T2DM. The secretion of IL-1β by inflammatory cells is largely dependent on a multiprotein complex termed the *inflammasome*, the hallmark activity of which is caspase-1 (CASP-1) activation [107]. Following inflammasome activation, CASP-1 proteolytically cleaves pro-IL-1β into its active form, IL-1β.

Our understanding of how IL-1β induction occurs during chronic sterile inflammation has been advanced by analyses of the molecular basis of the NLRP3 inflammasome. In general, NLRP3 signaling is regulated by two different steps: the first is controlled by TLR- or cytokine-dependent transcriptional upregulation of NLRP3; and the second step is activation of the NLRP3 inflammasome, which results in CASP-1 activation [107]. NLRP3 activation is regulated by various sterile stimuli, including cholesterol crystals, amyloid-β, palmitate, and ceramides. Islet amyloid polypeptide (IAPP) is deposited in the pancreas and is associated with a loss of beta cell function in T2DM. The observation of NLRP3-dependent IL-1β production by macrophages in response to IAPP implied a potential role for NLRP3 in promoting IL-1β secretion in T2DM [111]. Interestingly, an antidiabetic drug, glyburide, blocks IL-1β production by macrophages in response to IAPP. The direct involvement of NLRP3 in obesity has been confirmed in studies showing that NLRP3 KO mice fed HFD display reduced CASP-1 activation and pro-IL-1β expression in adipose tissue compared with WT mice. Moreover, NLRP3 KO and CASP-1 KO mice are more protected from HFD-induced insulin resistance. The decrease in insulin sensitivity is a consequence of NLRP3 inflammasome-mediated activation of effector T cells that, through release of IFN-γ, mediate downstream pathways resulting in insulin resistance.

Nonalcoholic fatty liver disease (NAFLD) and nonalcoholic steatohepatitis (NASH) are considered to be manifestations of metabolic disorders. A "two-hit" theory is proposed to drive NAFLD and NASH pathogenesis [112]. The first hit is hepatic steatosis, which is closely associated with lipotoxicity-induced mitochondrial abnormalities. The second hit is proinflammatory insults, including enhanced lipid peroxidation and increased generation of ROS. A recent report suggests that NLRP3- and NLRP6-dependent processing of IL-1β and IL-18 may have an important role in the pathogenesis of NAFLD, as well as in multiple aspects of metabolic syndrome via the modulation of the gut microbiota [113]. In the gut of inflammasome-deficient mice, abnormal accumulation of bacterial products is observed in the portal circulation; the liver is exposed to the highest concentration of those bacterial products such as pathogen-associated molecular patterns (PAMPs). The accumulation of PAMPs drives progression of NAFLD and NASH through TLR4 and TLR9, but not TLR5, signaling. These results demonstrate the complex, cooperative effect of two PRRs, NLRs and TLRs, in shaping metabolic events.

GPR120

While saturated FAs are proinflammatory, certain classes of unsaturated FAs, such as the omega-3 FAs DHA and EPA, can exert anti-inflammatory effects [114]. Of interest, GPR120 recognizes those omega-3 FAs and inhibits insulin resistance by suppressing TLR4-mediated macrophage activation. This anti-inflammatory pathway activates β-arrestin2/TAB1 signaling that blocks TLR4/TAK1-mediated IKKβ and JNK1 activation, preserving insulin sensitivity (Fig. 26.2) [12]. This was confirmed in studies of GPR120 KO mice. On a normal diet, GPR120 KO mice show glucose intolerance, hyperlipidemia, and decreased insulin sensitivity in skeletal muscles and the liver. In contrast, on HFD, GPR120 KO mice and WT mice become equally obese and insulin resistant. Furthermore, supplementation of omega-3 FAs markedly increases insulin sensitivity in WT mice but not in GPR120 KO mice.

Interestingly, human obese subjects show higher levels of GPR120 expression in adipose tissue compared with control lean subjects [115]. Moreover, a loss-of-function polymorphism (R270H) in human *GPR120* was identified as a risk of obesity in European populations. These results suggest that GPR120 stimulators may be useful in the development of new therapies for obesity-associated inflammation and insulin resistance.

IMMUNOTHERAPY FOR INSULIN RESISTANCE

From a clinical perspective, any anti-inflammatory therapy must be scrutinized for unwanted immune suppression, which leads to deleterious side effects. This suggests that an anti-inflammatory approach targeted to the inflammatory pathway most directly related to insulin resistance would be preferred.

Thiazolidinedione Therapy

Anti-inflammatory treatments have an obvious potential as insulin-sensitizing therapies. However, current attempts have not been overly successful. A widespread therapeutic approach to modulating the immune system involves thiazolidinediones (TZDs). TZDs are PPAR-γ agonists that have well-known insulin-sensitizing effects in the clinical setting. TZDs have direct effects in adipocytes, liver, macrophages, skeletal muscle, Treg cells, and the CNS; all of these tissue-specific effects can contribute to overall systemic insulin sensitization. These drugs also have potent anti-inflammatory actions on immune cells and contribute to improvements in insulin resistance in T2DM patients [116]. For example, they can promote the M2 polarization state of macrophages and enhance Treg cell differentiation and function. However, TZDs only partially correct insulin resistance. Although TZDs have a robust effect in lowering glucose levels in T2DM subjects, they show a relatively modest effect in improving insulin sensitivity. In addition, TZDs are associated with several adverse effects, including weight gain, edema, and heart disease [117].

Anticytokine and Antichemokine Therapies

Blocking TNF-α improves insulin resistance in rodents [15], but neutralizing antibodies to TNF-α have only partial effects on fasting glucose levels in obese subjects [118]. One potential reason for this is that TNF-α exerts its effects in a paracrine fashion, and interstitial adipose tissue levels are much higher than the circulating TNF-α concentration. Therefore, it is possible that TNF-α-blocking agents have not sufficiently neutralized the relatively high concentrations of TNF-α at its tissue site of action. A recent study demonstrated that patients receiving TNF-α inhibitors for systemic inflammatory conditions have a significantly decreased risk of developing T2DM [20,119]. Thus, TNF-α blocking therapy for T2DM is still a potential goal.

IL-1β inhibitors have also been used in the treatment of T2DM, again with only partial success [20]. Studies in rodents and humans have shown that IL-1β blockade improves glycemia, but insulin sensitivity is not increased. A clinical study of IL-1β inhibitors indicates that the major beneficial effects on glycemia are associated with improved insulin secretion rather than improved insulin sensitivity. Promising preliminary results have been reported in a phase 2 trial treating T2DM patients with an oral CCR2 antagonist. The studies show that administration of the CCR2 antagonist leads to a significant decrease in fasting glucose levels and glycated hemoglobin.

Therapeutic Perspective

So far, therapeutic strategies that target single cytokines or chemokines have had limited success in humans. Therefore, targeting upstream components rather than single cytokines or chemokines may provide a more effective therapeutic approach. For example, inhibition of IKK or JNK could be a useful strategy. However, anti-inflammatory therapy may compromise immune system responses. A more specific approach that selectively targets the proinflammatory M1, but not M2, macrophages may provide therapeutic benefits without inhibiting other immune functions. Targeting a protein expressed on M1 macrophages, such as TLRs, RP105, and GPR120, could provide improved specificity. In contrast, a treatment that boosts the number of resident M2 macrophages could also redirect the ATM balance to a less proinflammatory state and improve inflammation-induced insulin resistance.

CONCLUDING REMARKS

Obesity is now recognized as a state of low-grade, chronic inflammation associated with alterations in immune cell populations, including dynamic fluxes in the number and types of cells found within inflamed tissues. Tremendous progress has been made in recent years in demonstrating the complex relationships between the immune system and obesity that contribute to inflammation and metabolic disorders. The accumulation of proinflammatory cells of the innate and adaptive immune system in adipose tissue in rodents has been shown, illustrating a complex interplay between various cell types in the tissue. There is as yet insufficient data to demonstrate an interaction between the innate and adaptive immune systems contributing to adipose tissue inflammation, and further studies are needed. Targeting different immune cells at different stages of obesity could eventually lead to novel therapeutic approaches for metabolic disorders.

Acknowledgments

This work was supported by grants from Grant-in-Aid for Scientific Research from the Ministry of Education, Culture, Sports, Science and Technology (MEXT) of the Japanese Government (MEXT KAKENHI Grant Number24117708 to Y. N.) and from the Japan Society for the Promotion of Science (JSPS; JSPS KAKENHI Grant Number 24390119 to K. T., and 24590577 to Y. N.), the Hokuriku Innovation Cluster for Health Science, the MEXT Regional Innovation Cluster Program, the Toyama/Ishikawa Region (K. T.), the Takeda Science Foundation (Y. N.), and the Suzuken Memorial Foundation (Y. N.).

We also thank all members of our laboratory in University of Toyama for helpful discussions. The authors sincerely thank Toyama Prefecture for supporting our laboratory.

References

[1] Wellen KE, Hotamisligil GS. Inflammation, stress, and diabetes. J Clin Invest 2005;115(5):1111–9.

[2] Milner JJ, Beck MA. The impact of obesity on the immune response to infection. Proc Nutr Soc 2012;71(2):298–306.

[3] Osborn O, Olefsky JM. The cellular and signaling networks linking the immune system and metabolism in disease. Nat Med 2012;18(3):363–74.

[4] Xu H, Barnes GT, Yang Q, Tan G, Yang D, Chou CJ, et al. Chronic inflammation in fat plays a crucial role in the development of obesity-related insulin resistance. J Clin Invest 2003;112(12):1821–30.

[5] Weisberg SP, McCann D, Desai M, Rosenbaum M, Leibel RL, Ferrante Jr AW. Obesity is associated with macrophage accumulation in adipose tissue. J Clin Invest 2003;112(12):1796–808.

[6] Weisberg SP, Hunter D, Huber R, Lemieux J, Slaymaker S, Vaddi K, et al. CCR2 modulates inflammatory and metabolic effects of high-fat feeding. J Clin Invest 2006;116(1):115–24.

[7] Fielding BA, Callow J, Owen RM, Samra JS, Matthews DR, Frayn KN. Postprandial lipemia: the origin of an early peak studied by specific dietary fatty acid intake during sequential meals. Am J Clin Nutr 1996;63(1):36–41.

[8] Kawai T, Akira S. The roles of TLRs, RLRs and NLRs in pathogen recognition. Int Immunol 2009;21(4):317–37.

[9] Chen GY, Nunez G. Sterile inflammation: sensing and reacting to damage. Nat Rev Immunol 2010;10(12):826–37.

[10] Shi H, Kokoeva MV, Inouye K, Tzameli I, Yin H, Flier JS. TLR4 links innate immunity and fatty acid-induced insulin resistance. J Clin Invest 2006;116(11):3015–25.

[11] Senn JJ. Toll-like receptor-2 is essential for the development of palmitate-induced insulin resistance in myotubes. J Biol Chem 2006;281(37):26865–75.

[12] Oh DY, Talukdar S, Bae EJ, Imamura T, Morinaga H, Fan W, et al. GPR120 is an omega-3 fatty acid receptor mediating potent anti-inflammatory and insulin-sensitizing effects. Cell 2010;142(5):687–98.

[13] Wen H, Gris D, Lei Y, Jha S, Zhang L, Huang MT, et al. Fatty acid-induced NLRP3-ASC inflammasome activation interferes with insulin signaling. Nat Immunol 2011;12(5):408–15.

[14] Stienstra R, Joosten LA, Koenen T, van Tits B, van Diepen JA, van den Berg SA, et al. The inflammasome-mediated caspase-1 activation controls adipocyte differentiation and insulin sensitivity. Cell Metab 2010;12(6):593–605.

[15] Hotamisligil GS, Shargill NS, Spiegelman BM. Adipose expression of tumor necrosis factor-alpha: direct role in obesity-linked insulin resistance. Science 1993;259(5091):87–91.

[16] Gao Z, Hwang D, Bataille F, Lefevre M, York D, Quon MJ, et al. Serine phosphorylation of insulin receptor substrate 1 by inhibitor kappa B kinase complex. J Biol Chem 2002;277(50):48115–21.

[17] Hirosumi J, Tuncman G, Chang L, Gorgun CZ, Uysal KT, Maeda K, et al. A central role for JNK in obesity and insulin resistance. Nature 2002;420(6913):333–6.
[18] Martinon F, Burns K, Tschopp J. The inflammasome: a molecular platform triggering activation of inflammatory caspases and processing of proIL-beta. Mol Cell 2002;10(2):417–26.
[19] Bendtzen K, Mandrup-Poulsen T, Nerup J, Nielsen JH, Dinarello CA, Svenson M. Cytotoxicity of human pI 7 interleukin-1 for pancreatic islets of Langerhans. Science 1986;232(4757):1545–7.
[20] van Asseldonk EJ, Stienstra R, Koenen TB, Joosten LA, Netea MG, Tack CJ. Treatment with Anakinra improves disposition index but not insulin sensitivity in nondiabetic subjects with the metabolic syndrome: a randomized, double-blind, placebo-controlled study. J Clin Endocrinol Metab 2011;96(7):2119–26.
[21] Donath MY, Shoelson SE. Type 2 diabetes as an inflammatory disease. Nat Rev Immunol 2011;11(2):98–107.
[22] Schottelius AJ, Mayo MW, Sartor RB, Baldwin Jr AS. Interleukin-10 signaling blocks inhibitor of kappaB kinase activity and nuclear factor kappaB DNA binding. J Biol Chem 1999;274(45):31868–74.
[23] Kim HJ, Higashimori T, Park SY, Choi H, Dong J, Kim YJ, et al. Differential effects of interleukin-6 and -10 on skeletal muscle and liver insulin action in vivo. Diabetes 2004;53(4):1060–7.
[24] Hong EG, Ko HJ, Cho YR, Kim HJ, Ma Z, Yu TY, et al. Interleukin-10 prevents diet-induced insulin resistance by attenuating macrophage and cytokine response in skeletal muscle. Diabetes 2009;58(11):2525–35.
[25] Chen A, Mumick S, Zhang C, Lamb J, Dai H, Weingarth D, et al. Diet induction of monocyte chemoattractant protein-1 and its impact on obesity. Obes Res 2005;13(8):1311–20.
[26] Imai T, Hieshima K, Haskell C, Baba M, Nagira M, Nishimura M, et al. Identification and molecular characterization of fractalkine receptor CX3CR1, which mediates both leukocyte migration and adhesion. Cell 1997;91(4):521–30.
[27] Shah R, Hinkle CC, Ferguson JF, Mehta NN, Li M, Qu L, et al. Fractalkine is a novel human adipochemokine associated with type 2 diabetes. Diabetes 2011;60(5):1512–8.
[28] Spite M, Hellmann J, Tang Y, Mathis SP, Kosuri M, Bhatnagar A, et al. Deficiency of the leukotriene B4 receptor, BLT-1, protects against systemic insulin resistance in diet-induced obesity. J Immunol 2011;187(4):1942–9.
[29] Nguyen MT, Favelyukis S, Nguyen AK, Reichart D, Scott PA, Jenn A, et al. A subpopulation of macrophages infiltrates hypertrophic adipose tissue and is activated by free fatty acids via Toll-like receptors 2 and 4 and JNK-dependent pathways. J Biol Chem 2007;282(48):35279–92.
[30] Nguyen MT, Satoh H, Favelyukis S, Babendure JL, Imamura T, Sbodio JI, et al. JNK and tumor necrosis factor-alpha mediate free fatty acid-induced insulin resistance in 3T3-L1 adipocytes. J Biol Chem 2005;280(42):35361–71.
[31] Kumashiro N, Erion DM, Zhang D, Kahn M, Beddow SA, Chu X, et al. Cellular mechanism of insulin resistance in nonalcoholic fatty liver disease. Proc Natl Acad Sci USA 2011;108(39):16381–5.
[32] Samuel VT, Petersen KF, Shulman GI. Lipid-induced insulin resistance: unravelling the mechanism. Lancet 2010;375(9733):2267–77.
[33] Kim F, Pham M, Luttrell I, Bannerman DD, Tupper J, Thaler J, et al. Toll-like receptor-4 mediates vascular inflammation and insulin resistance in diet-induced obesity. Circ Res 2007;100(11):1589–96.
[34] Tsukumo DM, Carvalho-Filho MA, Carvalheira JB, Prada PO, Hirabara SM, Schenka AA, et al. Loss-of-function mutation in Toll-like receptor 4 prevents diet-induced obesity and insulin resistance. Diabetes 2007;56(8):1986–98.
[35] Ye J, Gao Z, Yin J, He Q. Hypoxia is a potential risk factor for chronic inflammation and adiponectin reduction in adipose tissue of *ob/ob* and dietary obese mice. Am J Physiol Endocrinol Metab 2007;293(4):E1118–28.
[36] Sadikot RT, Jansen ED, Blackwell TR, Zoia O, Yull F, Christman JW, et al. High-dose dexamethasone accentuates nuclear factor-kappa b activation in endotoxin-treated mice. Am J Respir Crit Care Med 2001;164(5):873–8.
[37] Arkan MC, Hevener AL, Greten FR, Maeda S, Li ZW, Long JM, et al. IKK-beta links inflammation to obesity-induced insulin resistance. Nat Med 2005;11(2):191–8.
[38] Cai D, Yuan M, Frantz DF, Melendez PA, Hansen L, Lee J, et al. Local and systemic insulin resistance resulting from hepatic activation of IKK-beta and NF-kappaB. Nat Med 2005;11(2):183–90.
[39] Zhang X, Zhang G, Zhang H, Karin M, Bai H, Cai D. Hypothalamic IKKbeta/NF-kappaB and ER stress link overnutrition to energy imbalance and obesity. Cell 2008;135(1):61–73.
[40] Yuan M, Konstantopoulos N, Lee J, Hansen L, Li ZW, Karin M, et al. Reversal of obesity- and diet-induced insulin resistance with salicylates or targeted disruption of Ikkbeta. Science 2001;293(5535):1673–7.
[41] Chiang SH, Bazuine M, Lumeng CN, Geletka LM, Mowers J, White NM, et al. The protein kinase IKKepsilon regulates energy balance in obese mice. Cell 2009;138(5):961–75.
[42] Tuncman G, Hirosumi J, Solinas G, Chang L, Karin M, Hotamisligil GS. Functional in vivo interactions between JNK1 and JNK2 isoforms in obesity and insulin resistance. Proc Natl Acad Sci USA 2006;103(28):10741–6.
[43] Solinas G, Naugler W, Galimi F, Lee MS, Karin M. Saturated fatty acids inhibit induction of insulin gene transcription by JNK-mediated phosphorylation of insulin-receptor substrates. Proc Natl Acad Sci USA 2006;103(44):16454–9.
[44] Kaneto H, Nakatani Y, Miyatsuka T, Kawamori D, Matsuoka TA, Matsuhisa M, et al. Possible novel therapy for diabetes with cell-permeable JNK-inhibitory peptide. Nat Med 2004;10(10):1128–32.
[45] Aguirre V, Uchida T, Yenush L, Davis R, White MF. The c-Jun NH(2)-terminal kinase promotes insulin resistance during association with insulin receptor substrate-1 and phosphorylation of Ser(307). J Biol Chem 2000;275(12):9047–54.
[46] Aguirre V, Werner ED, Giraud J, Lee YH, Shoelson SE, White MF. Phosphorylation of Ser307 in insulin receptor substrate-1 blocks interactions with the insulin receptor and inhibits insulin action. J Biol Chem 2002;277(2):1531–7.
[47] Solinas G, Vilcu C, Neels JG, Bandyopadhyay GK, Luo JL, Naugler W, et al. JNK1 in hematopoietically derived cells contributes to diet-induced inflammation and insulin resistance without affecting obesity. Cell Metab 2007;6(5):386–97.
[48] Yamauchi T, Kamon J, Waki H, Terauchi Y, Kubota N, Hara K, et al. The fat-derived hormone adiponectin reverses insulin resistance associated with both lipoatrophy and obesity. Nat Med 2001;7(8):941–6.
[49] Ouchi N, Walsh K. Adiponectin as an anti-inflammatory factor. Clin Chim Acta 2007;380(1–2):24–30.
[50] Johnson AR, Milner JJ, Makowski L. The inflammation highway: metabolism accelerates inflammatory traffic in obesity. Immunol Rev 2012;249(1):218–38.
[51] Staehr P, Hother-Nielsen O, Landau BR, Chandramouli V, Holst JJ, Beck-Nielsen H. Effects of free fatty acids per se on glucose production, gluconeogenesis, and glycogenolysis. Diabetes 2003;52(2):260–7.
[52] Cao H, Gerhold K, Mayers JR, Wiest MM, Watkins SM, Hotamisligil GS. Identification of a lipokine, a lipid hormone linking adipose tissue to systemic metabolism. Cell 2008;134(6):933–44.
[53] Chakrabarti SK, Wen Y, Dobrian AD, Cole BK, Ma Q, Pei H, et al. Evidence for activation of inflammatory lipoxygenase pathways in visceral adipose tissue of obese Zucker rats. Am J Physiol Endocrinol Metab 2011;300(1):E175–87.

[54] Morris DL, Singer K, Lumeng CN. Adipose tissue macrophages: phenotypic plasticity and diversity in lean and obese states. Curr Opin Clin Nutr Metab Care 2011;14(4):341–6.

[55] Fujisaka S, Usui I, Bukhari A, Ikutani M, Oya T, Kanatani Y, et al. Regulatory mechanisms for adipose tissue M1 and M2 macrophages in diet-induced obese mice. Diabetes 2009;58(11): 2574–82.

[56] Odegaard JI, Ricardo-Gonzalez RR, Goforth MH, Morel CR, Subramanian V, Mukundan L, et al. Macrophage-specific PPARgamma controls alternative activation and improves insulin resistance. Nature 2007;447(7148):1116–20.

[57] Winer S, Chan Y, Paltser G, Truong D, Tsui H, Bahrami J, et al. Normalization of obesity-associated insulin resistance through immunotherapy. Nat Med 2009;15(8):921–9.

[58] Feuerer M, Herrero L, Cipolletta D, Naaz A, Wong J, Nayer A, et al. Lean, but not obese, fat is enriched for a unique population of regulatory T cells that affect metabolic parameters. Nat Med 2009;15(8):930–9.

[59] Nishimura S, Manabe I, Nagasaki M, Eto K, Yamashita H, Ohsugi M, et al. CD8+ effector T cells contribute to macrophage recruitment and adipose tissue inflammation in obesity. Nat Med 2009;15(8):914–20.

[60] Strissel KJ, DeFuria J, Shaul ME, Bennett G, Greenberg AS, Obin MS. T-cell recruitment and Th1 polarization in adipose tissue during diet-induced obesity in C57BL/6 mice. Obesity (Silver Spring) 2010;18(10):1918–25.

[61] Winer DA, Winer S, Shen L, Wadia PP, Yantha J, Paltser G, et al. B cells promote insulin resistance through modulation of T cells and production of pathogenic IgG antibodies. Nat Med 2011;17(5):610–7.

[62] Ohmura K, Ishimori N, Ohmura Y, Tokuhara S, Nozawa A, Horii S, et al. Natural killer T cells are involved in adipose tissues inflammation and glucose intolerance in diet-induced obese mice. Arterioscler Thromb Vasc Biol 2010;30(2):193–9.

[63] Talukdar S, Oh da Y, Bandyopadhyay G, Li D, Xu J, McNelis J, et al. Neutrophils mediate insulin resistance in mice fed a high-fat diet through secreted elastase. Nat Med 2012;18(9):1407–12.

[64] Wu D, Molofsky AB, Liang HE, Ricardo-Gonzalez RR, Jouihan HA, Bando JK, et al. Eosinophils sustain adipose alternatively activated macrophages associated with glucose homeostasis. Science 2011;332(6026):243–7.

[65] Liu J, Divoux A, Sun J, Zhang J, Clement K, Glickman JN, et al. Genetic deficiency and pharmacological stabilization of mast cells reduce diet-induced obesity and diabetes in mice. Nat Med 2009;15(8):940–5.

[66] Hoshino K, Takeuchi O, Kawai T, Sanjo H, Ogawa T, Takeda Y, et al. Cutting edge: Toll-like receptor 4 (TLR4)-deficient mice are hyporesponsive to lipopolysaccharide: evidence for TLR4 as the Lps gene product. J Immunol 1999;162(7):3749–52.

[67] Shimazu R, Akashi S, Ogata H, Nagai Y, Fukudome K, Miyake K, et al. MD-2, a molecule that confers lipopolysaccharide responsiveness on Toll-like receptor 4. J Exp Med 1999;189(11): 1777–82.

[68] Nagai Y, Akashi S, Nagafuku M, Ogata M, Iwakura Y, Akira S, et al. Essential role of MD-2 in LPS responsiveness and TLR4 distribution. Nat Immunol 2002;3(7):667–72.

[69] Ohto U, Fukase K, Miyake K, Satow Y. Crystal structures of human MD-2 and its complex with antiendotoxic lipid IVa. Science 2007;316(5831):1632–4.

[70] Kim HM, Park BS, Kim JI, Kim SE, Lee J, Oh SC, et al. Crystal structure of the TLR4-MD-2 complex with bound endotoxin antagonist Eritoran. Cell 2007;130(5):906–17.

[71] Saberi M, Woods NB, de Luca C, Schenk S, Lu JC, Bandyopadhyay G, et al. Hematopoietic cell-specific deletion of toll-like receptor 4 ameliorates hepatic and adipose tissue insulin resistance in high-fat-fed mice. Cell Metab 2009;10(5):419–29.

[72] Suganami T, Tanimoto-Koyama K, Nishida J, Itoh M, Yuan X, Mizuarai S, et al. Role of the Toll-like receptor 4/NF-kappaB pathway in saturated fatty acid-induced inflammatory changes in the interaction between adipocytes and macrophages. Arterioscler Thromb Vasc Biol 2007;27(1):84–91.

[73] Cani PD, Bibiloni R, Knauf C, Waget A, Neyrinck AM, Delzenne NM, et al. Changes in gut microbiota control metabolic endotoxemia-induced inflammation in high-fat diet-induced obesity and diabetes in mice. Diabetes 2008;57(6):1470–81.

[74] Eguchi K, Manabe I, Oishi-Tanaka Y, Ohsugi M, Kono N, Ogata F, et al. Saturated fatty acid and TLR signaling link beta cell dysfunction and islet inflammation. Cell Metab 2012;15(4):518–33.

[75] Kleinridders A, Schenten D, Konner AC, Belgardt BF, Mauer J, Okamura T, et al. MyD88 signaling in the CNS is required for development of fatty acid-induced leptin resistance and diet-induced obesity. Cell Metab 2009;10(4):249–59.

[76] Benomar Y, Gertler A, De Lacy P, Crepin D, Ould Hamouda H, Riffault L, et al. Central resistin overexposure induces insulin resistance through Toll-like receptor 4. Diabetes 2013;62(1):102–14.

[77] Miyake K, Yamashita Y, Ogata M, Sudo T, Kimoto M. RP105, a novel B cell surface molecule implicated in B cell activation, is a member of the leucine-rich repeat protein family. J Immunol 1995;154(7):3333–40.

[78] Miyake K, Shimazu R, Kondo J, Niki T, Akashi S, Ogata H, et al. Mouse MD-1, a molecule that is physically associated with RP105 and positively regulates its expression. J Immunol 1998;161(3):1348–53.

[79] Ogata H, Su I, Miyake K, Nagai Y, Akashi S, Mecklenbrauker I, et al. The toll-like receptor protein RP105 regulates lipopolysaccharide signaling in B cells. J Exp Med 2000;192(1):23–9.

[80] Nagai Y, Shimazu R, Ogata H, Akashi S, Sudo K, Yamasaki H, et al. Requirement for MD-1 in cell surface expression of RP105/CD180 and B-cell responsiveness to lipopolysaccharide. Blood 2002;99(5):1699–705.

[81] Watanabe Y, Nakamura T, Ishikawa S, Fujisaka S, Usui I, Tsuneyama K, et al. The radioprotective 105/MD-1 complex contributes to diet-induced obesity and adipose tissue inflammation. Diabetes 2012;61(5):1199–209.

[82] Takeuchi O, Sato S, Horiuchi T, Hoshino K, Takeda K, Dong Z, et al. Cutting edge: role of Toll-like receptor 1 in mediating immune response to microbial lipoproteins. J Immunol 2002;169(1):10–14.

[83] Takeuchi O, Kawai T, Muhlradt PF, Morr M, Radolf JD, Zychlinsky A, et al. Discrimination of bacterial lipoproteins by Toll-like receptor 6. Int Immunol 2001;13(7):933–40.

[84] Nagai Y, Kobayashi T, Motoi Y, Ishiguro K, Akashi S, Saitoh S, et al. The radioprotective 105/MD-1 complex links TLR2 and TLR4/MD-2 in antibody response to microbial membranes. J Immunol 2005;174(11):7043–9.

[85] Blumenthal A, Kobayashi T, Pierini LM, Banaei N, Ernst JD, Miyake K, et al. RP105 facilitates macrophage activation by Mycobacterium tuberculosis lipoproteins. Cell Host Microbe 2009;5(1):35–46.

[86] Lee JY, Zhao L, Youn HS, Weatherill AR, Tapping R, Feng L, et al. Saturated fatty acid activates but polyunsaturated fatty acid inhibits Toll-like receptor 2 dimerized with Toll-like receptor 6 or 1. J Biol Chem 2004;279(17):16971–9.

[87] Coll T, Palomer X, Blanco-Vaca F, Escola-Gil JC, Sanchez RM, Laguna JC, et al. Cyclooxygenase 2 inhibition exacerbates palmitate-induced inflammation and insulin resistance in skeletal muscle cells. Endocrinology 2010;151(2):537–48.

[88] Jang HJ, Kim HS, Hwang DH, Quon MJ, Kim JA. Toll-like receptor 2 mediates high-fat diet-induced impairment of vasodilator actions of insulin. Am J Physiol Endocrinol Metab 2013;304(10):E1077–88.

[89] Himes RW, Smith CW. Tlr2 is critical for diet-induced metabolic syndrome in a murine model. FASEB J 2010;24(3):731–9.
[90] Hayashi F, Smith KD, Ozinsky A, Hawn TR, Yi EC, Goodlett DR, et al. The innate immune response to bacterial flagellin is mediated by Toll-like receptor 5. Nature 2001;410(6832):1099–103.
[91] Uematsu S, Jang MH, Chevrier N, Guo Z, Kumagai Y, Yamamoto M, et al. Detection of pathogenic intestinal bacteria by Toll-like receptor 5 on intestinal CD11c+ lamina propria cells. Nat Immunol 2006;7(8):868–74.
[92] Vijay-Kumar M, Sanders CJ, Taylor RT, Kumar A, Aitken JD, Sitaraman SV, et al. Deletion of TLR5 results in spontaneous colitis in mice. J Clin Invest 2007;117(12):3909–21.
[93] Ley RE, Turnbaugh PJ, Klein S, Gordon JI. Microbial ecology: human gut microbes associated with obesity. Nature 2006;444(7122):1022–3.
[94] Turnbaugh PJ, Hamady M, Yatsunenko T, Cantarel BL, Duncan A, Ley RE, et al. A core gut microbiome in obese and lean twins. Nature 2009;457(7228):480–4.
[95] Turnbaugh PJ, Ley RE, Mahowald MA, Magrini V, Mardis ER, Gordon JI. An obesity-associated gut microbiome with increased capacity for energy harvest. Nature 2006;444(7122):1027–31.
[96] Vijay-Kumar M, Aitken JD, Carvalho FA, Cullender TC, Mwangi S, Srinivasan S, et al. Metabolic syndrome and altered gut microbiota in mice lacking Toll-like receptor 5. Science 2010;328(5975):228–31.
[97] Al-Daghri NM, Clerici M, Al-Attas O, Forni D, Alokail MS, Alkharfy KM, et al. A nonsense polymorphism (R392X) in TLR5 protects from obesity but predisposes to diabetes. J Immunol 2013;190(7):3716–20.
[98] Wright SD, Ramos RA, Tobias PS, Ulevitch RJ, Mathison JC. CD14, a receptor for complexes of lipopolysaccharide (LPS) and LPS binding protein. Science 1990;249(4975):1431–3.
[99] Pugin J, Heumann ID, Tomasz A, Kravchenko VV, Akamatsu Y, Nishijima M, et al. CD14 is a pattern recognition receptor. Immunity 1994;1(6):509–16.
[100] Pan Z, Zhou L, Hetherington CJ, Zhang DE. Hepatocytes contribute to soluble CD14 production, and CD14 expression is differentially regulated in hepatocytes and monocytes. J Biol Chem 2000;275(46):36430–5.
[101] Fearns C, Kravchenko VV, Ulevitch RJ, Loskutoff DJ. Murine CD14 gene expression in vivo: extramyeloid synthesis and regulation by lipopolysaccharide. J Exp Med 1995;181(3):857–66.
[102] Sewter CP, Digby JE, Blows F, Prins J, O'Rahilly S. Regulation of tumour necrosis factor-alpha release from human adipose tissue in vitro. J Endocrinol 1999;163(1):33–8.
[103] Hirschfeld M, Kirschning CJ, Schwandner R, Wesche H, Weis JH, Wooten RM, et al. Cutting edge: inflammatory signaling by Borrelia burgdorferi lipoproteins is mediated by toll-like receptor 2. J Immunol 1999;163(5):2382–6.
[104] Akashi S, Saitoh S, Wakabayashi Y, Kikuchi T, Takamura N, Nagai Y, et al. Lipopolysaccharide interaction with cell surface Toll-like receptor 4-MD-2: higher affinity than that with MD-2 or CD14. J Exp Med 2003;198(7):1035–42.
[105] Fernandez-Real JM, Perez del Pulgar S, Luche E, Moreno-Navarrete JM, Waget A, Serino M, et al. CD14 modulates inflammation-driven insulin resistance. Diabetes 2011;60(8):2179–86.
[106] Johnson GB, Riggs BL, Platt JL. A genetic basis for the "Adonis" phenotype of low adiposity and strong bones. FASEB J 2004;18(11):1282–4.
[107] De Nardo D, Latz E. NLRP3 inflammasomes link inflammation and metabolic disease. Trends Immunol 2011;32(8):373–9.
[108] Carneiro LA, Magalhaes JG, Tattoli I, Philpott DJ, Travassos LH. Nod-like proteins in inflammation and disease. J Pathol 2008;214(2):136–48.
[109] Carneiro LA, Travassos LH, Philpott DJ. Innate immune recognition of microbes through Nod1 and Nod2: implications for disease. Microbes Infect 2004;6(6):609–16.
[110] Schertzer JD, Tamrakar AK, Magalhaes JG, Pereira S, Bilan PJ, Fullerton MD, et al. NOD1 activators link innate immunity to insulin resistance. Diabetes 2011;60(9):2206–15.
[111] Masters SL, Dunne A, Subramanian SL, Hull RL, Tannahill GM, Sharp FA, et al. Activation of the NLRP3 inflammasome by islet amyloid polypeptide provides a mechanism for enhanced IL-1beta in type 2 diabetes. Nat Immunol 2010;11(10):897–904.
[112] Day CP, James OF. Steatohepatitis: a tale of two "hits"? Gastroenterology 1998;114(4):842–5.
[113] Henao-Mejia J, Elinav E, Jin C, Hao L, Mehal WZ, Strowig T, et al. Inflammasome-mediated dysbiosis regulates progression of NAFLD and obesity. Nature 2012;482(7384):179–85.
[114] Calder PC. N-3 polyunsaturated fatty acids, inflammation, and inflammatory diseases. Am J Clin Nutr 2006;83(6 Suppl.):1505S–19S.
[115] Ichimura A, Hirasawa A, Poulain-Godefroy O, Bonnefond A, Hara T, Yengo L, et al. Dysfunction of lipid sensor GPR120 leads to obesity in both mouse and human. Nature 2012;483(7389):350–4.
[116] Hevener AL, Olefsky JM, Reichart D, Nguyen MT, Bandyopadyhay G, Leung HY, et al. Macrophage PPAR gamma is required for normal skeletal muscle and hepatic insulin sensitivity and full antidiabetic effects of thiazolidinediones. J Clin Invest 2007;117(6):1658–69.
[117] Rizos CV, Elisaf MS, Mikhailidis DP, Liberopoulos EN. How safe is the use of thiazolidinediones in clinical practice? Expert Opin Drug Saf 2009;8(1):15–32.
[118] Stanley TL, Zanni MV, Johnsen S, Rasheed S, Makimura H, Lee H, et al. TNF-alpha antagonism with etanercept decreases glucose and increases the proportion of high molecular weight adiponectin in obese subjects with features of the metabolic syndrome. J Clin Endocrinol Metab 2011;96(1):E146–50.
[119] Solomon DH, Massarotti E, Garg R, Liu J, Canning C, Schneeweiss S. Association between disease-modifying antirheumatic drugs and diabetes risk in patients with rheumatoid arthritis and psoriasis. JAMA 2011;305(24):2525–31.

CHAPTER

27

Metabolic Effects of Abdominal Fats in Animal Models and Humans

Michal M. Masternak

University of Central Florida, Burnett School of Biomedical Sciences, College of Medicine, Orlando, FL, USA

OBESITY

In most developed countries, we face the problems of increasing lack of activity and overnutrition starting from young ages and continuing throughout the life span, which predisposes to growing obesity that affects the healthy metabolic functions of the body. According to the World Health Organization, the population of obese people has almost doubled since 1980 (until 2013); frightening statistics state that 35% of adults aged 20 and over are overweight and about 11% are obese. More alarming is the fact that in 2011 there were over 40 million overweight children under the age of 5 years. These statistics raise serious concerns about the future cost and function of health-care systems and the well-being of human populations worldwide. It is known that in an obese person the regulation of glucose, lipids, and fatty acid metabolism by insulin is attenuated, which causes dysregulation of blood glucose, blood pressure, and lipid balance. The progressive co-occurrence of dysregulated glycemia, dyslipidemia, and hypertension begin the condition known as metabolic syndrome [1], which predisposes to the development of type 2 diabetes mellitus (T2DM). However, studies of metabolic diseases and obesity provide strong evidence that not only is weight important for health but fat tissue distribution and particularly abdominal (also referred to as intra-abdominal, central, or visceral) obesity also appears to present an important risk factor for most metabolic complications, T2DM, cardiovascular diseases, and cancer, as well as a high risk of mortality [2].

ADIPOSE TISSUE: BODY FAT

Adipose tissue, commonly related to body fat, consists of loose connective tissue mostly composed of adipocytes. Beside adipocytes, adipose tissue contains preadipocytes, fibroblasts, vascular endothelial cells, and adipose tissue macrophages. Initially, body fat was known as the main organ to store energy in the form of lipids and to insulate the body. However, studies of adipose tissue in recent years recognized this tissue as a major endocrine organ, producing and releasing different hormones such as adiponectin, estrogen, leptin, and resistin, as well as different kinds of cytokines. The function of adipose tissue and the balance of adipokines and cytokines produced can affect other organ systems and lead to organ dysfunction or diseases, including insulin resistance, metabolic syndrome, diabetes, chronic inflammation, and cancer. This indicates how important the function of adipose tissue can be to whole-body well-being. It is known that we need fat, but too much fat i.e. obesity can be detrimental for our health. There are also two major types of adipose tissue: white adipose tissue (WAT) and brown adipose tissue (BAT). The main function of BAT is to generate body heat, while WAT is used to store energy. However, the latest research divides the WAT in to different adipose depots based on its location and, more importantly, function and the role of particular fat pads on whole-body health. There is also more evidence that different fat depots are responsible for the production and release of different adipokines and cytokines. Despite growing obesity, it is important to better understand the function of adipose tissue and the different roles of fat in storing energy and regulating metabolic function. Excessive caloric intake and lack of physical activity promote the expansion of adipose tissue, leading to conditions classified as overweight, obesity, and finally morbid obesity. These changes are accompanied by alterations in whole-body physiology i.e. increased proinflammatory cytokines, decreased adiponectin level, glucose intolerance, and insulin resistance. However, individuals at different levels of obesity can indicate more or less alarming physiological

Nutrition in the Prevention and Treatment of Abdominal Obesity
http://dx.doi.org/10.1016/B978-0-12-407869-7.00027-1

complications, which seem to be dependent on the location of fat accumulation [3]. Individuals depositing more visceral adipose tissue are at higher risk of metabolic diseases than those depositing more subcutaneous fat [3]. At the same time, antidiabetic medications such as pioglitazone improves insulin sensitivity but also cause weight gain as a side effect in patients usually classified as obese. However, this weight gain does not diminish the beneficial effect of the treatment, probably due to an increase in subcutaneous adipose tissue rather than visceral fat. Unfortunately, the beneficial function of subcutaneous adipose tissue can be compromised by an excess of visceral fat [4]. Clinical studies of women with visceral obesity indicated that excess visceral obesity can impair insulin action in subcutaneous adipose tissue. It seems that, despite of the positive role of different fat pads, visceral adipose tissue can deteriorate the metabolic function of the body by affecting insulin signaling and the physiology of different insulin target organs [4].

BODY SIZE, FUNCTION, AND HEALTH

In clinical practice and research into obesity and metabolic syndrome, weight and size are used as important determinants of a patient's health status. Based on the weight and height of a person, we can calculate the body mass index (BMI) and classify the person as being normal weight, overweight, obese, or morbidly obese [5]. Another important measurement is the size relating to waist circumference measurements, which specifies central obesity and identifies metabolic syndrome [6]. It is known that a higher percentage or accumulation of body fat means a higher incidence of metabolic complications, insulin resistance, and finally risk of diabetes. However, there is not always a direct correlation between obesity and the development of metabolic complications. About 20–30% of obese humans do not develop metabolic disorders [7]. However, the size of the person is not the only factor with an important role in metabolic abnormalities. More in-depth studies indicated that size is also important when studying the biology of adipose tissue. The distribution, location, and amount of WAT are not the main predictors of metabolic disorders. It is known that in obese patients growing fat mass strongly correlates with increased adipocyte number and also increased size of adipocytes [8]. It is also known that obese patients with larger adipocytes have a higher incidence of insulin resistance than equally obese subjects with smaller adipocytes [9–11]. Another study of morbidly obese men indicated a positive correlation between the size of visceral adipocytes and serum triglyceride and C-reactive protein (CRP) levels [12]. This finding explains the 20–30% of obese individuals that do not develop metabolic complications. These individuals are protected from metabolic abnormalities in a way that appears to be related to their ability to maintain smaller sizes of adipocytes.

A study in rodents indicated that growth hormone (GH) receptor/GH binding protein knockout (GHRKO) mice, known also as *Laron dwarf mice*, are obese, yet have low insulin and glucose levels, together with improved sensitivity to injected insulin and enhanced glucose tolerance [13–17]. At the same time, these animals are characterized by smaller sized intra-abdominal adipocytes [18]. This physiological characteristic of WAT in Laron dwarf mice may be critical for maintaining healthy metabolism regardless of increased obesity. It suggests that a genetic condition in humans and animals can prevent increases in the size of adipocytes and at the same time protects from metabolic complications, regardless of obesity. However, in the majority of the population, increased calorie consumption or high-fat diet regimens promote an increase in the size of adipocytes. At the same time, subjecting mice to calorie restriction (CR) has been shown to decrease the size of adipocytes [11]. It was shown in human studies that a small body weight decrease during dieting will almost immediately promote great improvements in metabolic parameters, together with reducing adipocyte size [19]. A study by Varady et al. showed that 5–10% of body weight loss increases the concentration of adiponectin by up to 20%, while decreasing the size of visceral adipose tissue by 41% [19]. These findings indicate that the size plays an important role in terms of the weight of a person, their waist circumference, and the size of adipocytes, which in most cases correlate with one another.

ABDOMINAL OBESITY AND CARDIOVASCULAR DISEASES

It is well accepted that weight is a main marker for determining the risk of potential cardiovascular complications. Nobody will argue with the fact that obesity strongly correlates with an increased risk of cardiovascular disease. However, the question is whether BMI is required to determine the risk or if simply a determination of being overweight can place the person in a risk group. In the 1950s, increased attention was already focused on the pattern of fat distribution, rather than simply the weight of the patient, and their risk of coronary artery disease. The two distinguished models of obesity are known as "Pear" and "Apple" [20,21], where "Apple" results from the deposition of adipose tissue around the abdomen. A person with an "Apple" body shape will have big belly and a waist circumference greater than their hip circumference. In the 1980s, there were two independent 12–13-year follow-up studies of waist circumference and waist-hip ratio, which showed an association between abdominal obesity and coronary heart diseases in both men and women [22,23]. Other studies of visceral adiposity performed using more advanced computed tomography (CT) scanning confirmed an association between abdominal obesity, carotid atherosclerosis, and angiographically documented cardiovascular disease [24–31]. In 2008, a study of over 90,000 ambulant patients in 27 European countries predicted a strong association between abdominal obesity and an increased risk of diabetes and cardiovascular disease in both genders regardless of the region of Europe [32]. All of these studies provide evidence that abdominal obesity is mainly responsible for cardiovascular complications in obese patients. This theory is also supported by studies completed by Nakamura et al., indicating that lean, nonobese men with increased visceral fat accumulation also have an increased risk of cardiovascular diseases [33,34].

ADIPOSE TISSUE AND INFLAMMATION

Many studies have indicated strong correlations between obesity, metabolic complication, and constant low-grade inflammation [35]. In obese subjects, there is a tendency for WAT to be infiltrated by immune cells such as macrophages or T cell [36–38], which will produce and release different proinflammatory cytokines and chemokines. However, the presence of immune cells in WAT is not the only source of inflammation because adipocytes also have the potential to produce and release different pro- or anti-inflammatory adipokines and cytokines [39]. Depending on the function of adipocytes, they can be beneficial by producing and releasing anti-inflammatory and insulin-sensitizing adiponectin or proinflammatory interleukin-6 (IL-6) or tumor necrosis factor (TNF-α).

Infiltration of White Adipose Tissue

The biological role of WAT macrophage infiltration in obesity is still not well understood and remains under intensive investigation. However, most of the available studies correlate abdominal fat with metabolic complications, insulin resistance, and cardiovascular diseases. Adipose-derived inflammation is also believed to be mostly related to macrophages infiltration of abdominal fat. In 2006, Cancello et al. performed an analysis of omental and subcutaneous adipose tissue in morbidly obese men and women [40]. In this study, the authors showed that omental fat contained twice as many macrophages as did subcutaneous adipose tissue [40]. The increased infiltration of intra-abdominal adipose tissue was also positively correlated with hepatic fibroinflammatory lesions in these morbidly obese patients [40]. Moreover, studies on mice showed that in obese mice about 50% of adipose tissue cells express the macrophage marker, EGF-like module-containing mucin-like hormone receptor-like 1 (EMR1), while only about 10% of adipose tissue cells from lean mice showed expression of this marker [36]. Another study showed that not only total fat content in diet but also, more importantly, dietary saturated fat content strongly influences the infiltration of WAT by macrophages, inflammation, and insulin resistance [41]. Other studies in *ob/ob* mice (an obesity experimental model) indicated a role for macrophages in capillary formation in obesity-enhanced adipogenesis for adipose tissue remodeling [42]. The complete mechanism of macrophage action in metabolic complications of obesity is still undetermined; however, in 2006 Lumeng and his collaborators examined direct and indirect interactions between macrophages and adipocytes [43]. They showed that macrophages secrete factors that block insulin action in WAT by the suppression of solute carrier family 2, facilitated glucose transporter member 4 (GLUT4) and insulin receptor substrate 1 (IRS-1), causing a further decrease in Akt phosphorylation and blocking insulin-regulated GLUT4 translocation [43]. The study also showed that this negative regulation of insulin signaling was associated with the production of TNF-α by macrophages [43]. However, a study in high-fat diet-induced obese mice showed that subjecting these mice to exercise training decreased macrophage infiltration [44]. In addition, reducing caloric intake to control body weight was shown to suppress WAT macrophage infiltration in human subjects [45,46].

Proinflammatory Action of Adipose Tissue

During the development of obesity, adipose tissue is infiltrated by macrophages and T cells, which significantly alters the function of adipose tissue. The adipose tissue starts to release different adipokines and cytokines into the circulation, which promotes inflammation in different organs and leads to insulin resistance, arthritis, and cardiovascular complications. This chronic low-grade inflammation is also suspected to promote aging and to be responsible for shortening the life span. The main changes observed in obesity are elevated levels of circulating proinflammatory cytokines such as CRP, IL-6, C-C motif chemokine 2 [monocyte chemoattractant protein 1 (MCP-1)], plasminogen activator inhibitor 1 (PAI-1), and TNF-α [47]. Increased levels of these cytokines, especially IL-6 and TNF-α, strongly correlate with insulin resistance [48–51]. However, decreasing the amount of adipose tissue by controlling weight will decrease the circulating levels of these cytokines [49,52]. The suppression of inflammatory cytokines and adipokines by genetic manipulation or pharmacological interventions in mice provides protection from the negative effect of a high-fat diet on insulin signaling [53–56]. It was also shown that mice characterized by TNF-α deficiency will not develop diabetes when subjected to a high-fat diet [57]. At the same time, studies in obese mice characterized by insulin resistance showed that blocking TNF-α in these mice improves their insulin sensitivity [51]. These data all show that the different profiles and actions of adipokines toward insulin are strongly associated with obesity. However, there are known exceptions, which prove that the function of WAT can be altered regardless of the amount of adipose tissue. In a study of animals overexpressing GH, it was shown that these giant mice have elevated levels of IL-6 and TNF-α in their adipose tissues [58]. Interestingly, these animals are extremely lean, with a very limited amount of intra-abdominal fat, but at the same time are characterized by insulin resistance and a shortened life span [58]. In contrast, Laron dwarf mice (GHRKO) show increased obesity in comparison to normal controls [16,17]. Surprisingly, these long-lived, hyperinsulin-sensitive animals have increased intra-abdominal WAT accumulation [16], however, analysis of both epididymal and perinephric WAT from these healthy obese mice revealed decreased levels of IL-6 [16]. These data clearly show that the inflammatory action of adipose tissue is associated with obesity but that the inflammatory action of WAT can also be triggered in lean subjects.

Anti-Inflammatory and Proinsulin Action of Adipose Tissue

WAT, especially abdominal fat, is mostly related to negative consequences on whole-body metabolism, insulin resistance, cardiovascular health, and other physiological functions. However, our body needs fat and below a healthy percentage fat content we are talking about a condition known as *underfat*, which as implied is *unhealthy*. It is difficult to specify what percentage of fat is really healthy, because it depends on lifestyle i.e. an athlete or regular person, age, and (mostly) gender. However, in 2000, Gallagher at al. reported that for people aged between 20–40 years, a healthy range of fat is approximately 21–33% for women and 8–19% for men [59]. It is known that fat is important not only for storing energy but also for adipose tissue function as an active endocrine organ that produces and releases different hormones into the circulation. Besides proinflammatory cytokines and adipokines, WAT produces adiponectin, leptin, and resistin, which are important hormones for regulating metabolism, insulin action, and glucose homeostasis.

Adiponectin

Adiponectin is recognized as a protein hormone that regulates several metabolic processes including glucose regulation and fatty acid oxidation. Adiponectin is categorized as an insulin sensitizer and anti-inflammatory factor, but it also exhibits antiatherogenic, proapoptotic, and antiproliferative properties. Adiponectin was shown to regulate insulin sensitivity and glucose homeostasis via the activation of 5′-AMP-activated protein kinase (AMPK) in the liver and muscles; this enzyme phosphorylates and inactivates acetyl-coenzyme A carboxylase (ACC) and decreases the production of malonyl-CoA, a substrate for fatty acid synthase (FAS) and a potent inhibitor of mitochondrial transportation of fatty acids [60]. This process decreases fatty acid synthesis, promotes fatty acid oxidation, and reduces the accumulation of triglycerides in the liver and muscles [60]. Adiponectin also reduces the expression of enzymes involved in gluconeogenesis, including glucose-6-phosphatase (G6Pase) and phosphoenolpyruvate carboxykinase (PEPCK) in the liver [61], and directly stimulates glucose uptake in muscle and adipocytes by activating AMPK [62], thus regulating insulin sensitivity and energy homeostasis. Adiponectin is produced and released by WAT and its level is inversely correlated with percentage body fat [63]. The specific regulation of adiponectin is still not well understood: there is some suggestion that it is mainly produced by subcutaneous adipose tissue, although other studies show that it is also synthesized and released by intra-abdominal adipocytes [64]. Studies in GHRKO animals, characterized by high adiponectin levels, show that the surgical removal of visceral fat caused a significant decrease in circulating adiponectin levels [16] However, it is important to remember that more fat does not mean more adiponectin, especially as obese patients with metabolic syndrome and diabetes have decreased levels of adiponectin. In contrast, overexpression of human adiponectin in transgenic mice was shown to decrease adipocyte differentiation and to protect mice from fat accumulation on regular and high-calorie diets [65,66]. Moreover, transgenic mice with elevated adiponectin showed extended life span on a regular diet and were also protected from high-calorie diet-induced premature death [66]. Human studies of centenarians showed that in people exhibiting such extraordinary longevity adiponectin levels were elevated; this effect was independent of sex and BMI [67,68]. Longevity studies in mice indicate that there is a strong correlation between GH, insulin-like growth factor I (IGF-I), and life span [69,70]. GH is known to have lipolytic effects on fat, which causes faster fat burning. This suggests that GH may be beneficial for metabolic function and may improve insulin action in obese patients. However, available data shows that GH treatment causes glucose intolerance and predisposition to diabetes in healthy humans [71–74]. Adiponectin levels are also shown to be negatively associated with GH levels. Studies in long-living GH-deficient Ames dwarf mice and GH-resistant Laron dwarf mice showed that these small animals are characterized by elevated levels of circulating adiponectin [16,58,75–79]. In contrast, giant transgenic animals overexpressing GH have decreased levels of adiponectin and are short lived [58]. Additional studies in GH-deficient Ames dwarf mice indicated that supplementing GH decreases adiponectin levels in these long-living mice and also shortens their life span [76,77]. These data show that well-functioning adipose tissue and the efficient production of adiponectin are as crucial not only for healthy metabolism but also for a long life span.

Leptin

Leptin is another hormone that regulates energy intake, mainly by controlling appetite, hunger, metabolism, and behavior [80]. It was shown that by binding to its receptor, leptin initiates a phosphorylation cascade via the tyrosine-protein kinase JAK/signal transducer and activator of transcription 3 (STAT3) pathway and then phosphorylates and activates AMPK and proliferator-activated receptor peroxisome gamma coactivator-1-alpha (PGC-1α) [81]. Thus, it downregulates lipogenic enzymes such as ACC and FAS, upregulates lipid oxidation-related enzymes such as carnitine *O*-palmitoyltransferase 1 (CPT-1) and acyl-CoA oxidase (ACO), and therefore regulates lipogenesis and fatty acid oxidation [81]. In experimental model studies, it was shown that *ob/ob* mice treated with leptin consumed less food and showed increased energy expenditure with a concomitant improvement in insulin action before any significant alterations in body weight [82–84]. Another study also showed increased glucose turnover in healthy, lean mice [85]. This provides strong evidence that elevated leptin levels are important for metabolic function and that elevated levels of leptin predict healthy metabolism, but lots of available data show that obese patients have high levels of leptin. However, the elevated leptin in obese humans or animals is caused by leptin resistance [86]. Under this condition, adipose tissue produces elevated levels of leptin that is not active due to a lack of proper function of its receptor.

Resistin

Resistin is yet another hormone produced by adipose tissue. The name *resistin* originates from a study in which it was shown that mice injected with resistin develop insulin resistance. The role of this hormone on insulin action is still unknown, and there is still controversy regarding the involvement of resistin in obesity and T2DM [87].

INTRA-ABDOMINAL OBESITY AND DIABETES

T2DM is the most common type of diabetes. According to the American Diabetes Association, over 25 million people ranging from children to adults have diabetes. This represents 8.3% of the total population of the USA, and this number is growing every year. A considerable tendency toward low physical activity and a diet containing high concentrations of fat means that diabetes is a serious health risk factor in all developed countries. Patients with diabetes are at a greater risk of heart disease and stroke, high blood pressure, blindness, kidney disease, neuropathy, limb amputation, and death. It is well known that obese patients represent the main risk group for the development of metabolic syndrome and diabetes. BMI is used most frequently to determine overweight, obesity, and the risk of diabetes. However, in some cases BMI can inaccurately categorize some individuals as being at risk for diabetes because BMI does not account for body composition and fat distribution [88,89]. Therefore, BMI itself is not enough to determine the risk of metabolic syndrome and diabetes, making it necessary to include other clinical measurements such as waist-hip circumference ratio [90]. Intra-abdominal fat accumulation is recognized as a main cause of metabolic complications [91,92]. It is well established that increased amounts of intra-abdominal fat (*central obesity*) is associated with insulin resistance, a higher risk of T2DM, dyslipidemia, atherosclerosis, and mortality [93–96]. In addition, data collected using spinal dual-energy X-ray absorptiometry (DEXA) of women aged 40 years or older for the assessment of osteoporosis revealed the association between fat distribution and the risk of diabetes [97]. This data showed that DEXA-derived measurements of abdominal fat can be helpful in determining the increased risk of diabetes, as well as supporting the evidence that abdominal fat acts as a main contributor to the development of metabolic abnormalities [97]. In contrast to abdominal obesity, increased amounts of subcutaneous peripheral fat are associated with improved insulin sensitivity and a lower risk of developing T2DM, dyslipidemia, and atherosclerosis in comparison to patients with central obesity [98–100]. Thus, liposuction intervention in humans, which removes subcutaneous fat, does not improve any aspect of the metabolic syndrome, while the removal of visceral fat results in a decrease in glucose and insulin levels [101]. Similar studies in mice have shown that surgical removal of visceral fat only can reverse the negative effects of a high-fat diet on insulin signaling as quickly as within 8 days of the surgical procedure [102]. Surgical removal of visceral fat in these mice normalizes the levels of insulin and glucose, and lipid parameters. Another study also indicated that the removal of visceral fat in rats on a normal diet produces improved insulin signaling comparable to the effects of CR [102,103]. All of the available data suggests that the distribution of fat plays a major role in whole-body insulin sensitivity. However, studies performed by Tran et al. indicate that the function of a particular fat pad can be altered by moving it to a different location within the body and changing the secretory pattern. These changes in the fat pad's secretory pattern are more important for insulin sensitivity than its location [104]. The authors transplanted subcutaneous or visceral fat from donor mice into a subcutaneous or visceral region. It is striking that the transplantation of subcutaneous fat into a visceral area produced the strongest improvement in insulin sensitivity. This data indicates that changes in the secretory pattern of this tissue by transplantation into a visceral region were crucial for enhancing whole-body insulin sensitivity [104], and strongly suggests that it is not only important where the adipose tissue is located but also where the initial development of particular adipose tissue took place and its later role in metabolism. Additionally, studies with the antidiabetic drug pioglitazone showed that along with increased insulin sensitivity in T2DM patients there was a concomitant increase in body weight and fat mass [105]. However, a DEXA analysis indicated that there was an increase in subcutaneous fat together with an increase in lean mass and a tendency to decrease liver fat infiltration [105]. Current observations lead to the conclusion that the accumulation of adipose tissue in intra-abdominal regions (rather than BMI) should be considered as a predictor of a high risk of diabetes.

ABDOMINAL OBESITY AND CANCER

Obesity usually is associated with metabolic syndrome, T2DM, and cardiovascular diseases, as discussed above. However, there is currently more focus on the association between obesity and various types of malignancies. It is known that obesity is associated with an increased risk of colon, endometrial, esophageal, gallbladder, kidney, pancreatic, rectal, thyroid, and postmenopausal breast cancer [106]. There is also a possibility that obesity is related to different types of cancer. The mechanism responsible for increased cancer development in obese patients is not fully determined. A Canadian study following 810 histologically confirmed kidney cancer patients and over 3000 controls indicated a strong correlation between excessive caloric intake, obesity, and etiological risk factors for both renal and nonrenal cell cancer [107]. In the same study, the authors included a group with recreational exercise; their findings did not indicate an association between exercise and the risk of kidney cancer [107]. However, although obesity is linked to cancer, there is still some controversy; there is a strong suggestion that abdominal fat rather than overall obesity is critical for cancer risk. Moreover, there is plenty of evidence that abdominal obesity increases cancer-related mortality in both obese and nonobese women, indicating that this risk is independent of BMI but driven by intra-abdominal fat accumulation [108]. The discrepancy between obesity classified by BMI and abdominal obesity has led to conflicting data. There have been controversial reports with regard to a link between prostate cancer and obesity. Wright at al. showed a lack of association between BMI and low-grade prostate cancer but a strong association between fatal prostate cancer and BMI [109]. However, a study by von Hafe et al. suggested a strong correlation between visceral fat accumulation and the risk of prostate cancer [110]. These data again show that the link between obesity with cancer should not relate on BMI, but rather to abdominal obesity because the potential inflammatory action of visceral fat promotes constant low-grade inflammation, which can contribute to prostate carcinogenesis [111,112]. In addition, leptin, the cytokine produced by WAT, is associated with cellular differentiation and prostate cancer progression. Several studies have shown an association between leptin and prostate cancer development and progression [113–117]. Additionally, increased expression of leptin and the leptin receptor is associated with breast cancer progression [118]. It has been suggested that elevated leptin and leptin receptor expression in primary breast cancer can be caused by exposure of these cells to high levels of insulin and IGF-I, conditions that are present in obese patients [118]. However, a study of fatless A-Zip-F1 mice with undetectable adipokine levels indicated that these mice have an increased risk of tumor development in comparison to normal control mice [119]. These findings suggest that obesity and the production of adipokines by WAT are unrelated to the risk of cancer development. Moreover, it is important to understand that although adipose tissue can be detrimental for the healthy function of the body, including a role in cancer development, deficiencies in adiposity can also be unhealthy, as discussed above. WAT can produce proinflammatory adipokines and cytokines, but healthy white adipose tissue can also produce anti-inflammatory adiponectin. As previously discussed, adiponectin levels are decreased in obesity, but deficiencies in adipose tissue also suppress adiponectin levels. Fatless mice have undetectable levels of adipokines together with deficiencies in adiponectin. Importantly, low levels of adiponectin are strongly associated with a high risk of different types of cancer [120]. Additional studies performed in animals showed that tumor growth and tumor angiogenesis are inhibited by exogenous adiponectin [121]. In addition, adiponectin is known to be reduced in transgenic animals overexpressing GH [58]; interestingly, these animals are short lived and have a higher incidence of cancer than do normal controls. In contrast, long-living Ames dwarf mice have high levels of adiponectin and are known to be cancer resistant [122]. Moreover, another long-living dwarf mouse strain, Laron dwarfs, characterized by increased intra-abdominal obesity and concomitant high levels of adiponectin, are also protected from cancer development [123]. This suggests that the healthy function of WAT in promoting the production of anti-inflammatory and antidiabetic adipokines such as adiponectin over proinflammatory factors is beneficial and protective against various types of malignancies. However, to maintain a well-functioning adipose tissue it is important to prevent not only obesity as diagnosed by BMI but also more importantly to control abdominal fat accumulation, which can be detrimental in nonobese patients.

ABDOMINAL OBESITY AND AGING

Aging, independent of obesity, increases the risk of development of T2DM, cardiovascular complications, and cancer. Increasing obesity in aging population accelerates the risk of mortality in elderly people. It is known that obesity, defined as a BMI greater than 30 kg/m^2 significantly increases the risk of specific disease and all-cause mortality [124]. More importantly, Fontaine at al. showed that obesity in middle age (20–30 years), characterized by a BMI > 45 kg/m^2, is expected to decrease life expectancy by 13 years in men and about 8 years in women [125]. The life shortening caused by obesity corresponds to an approximately 22% shorter life span in men. In addition, feeding mice or rats a high-fat diet leads to the development of insulin resistance and diabetes, with associated detrimental effects on both health span and life span. The mechanism by which adipose tissue affects aging and longevity is not well established; however, there is a suggestion that constant low-grade inflammation accelerates aging in humans and animals. It is known that acute infection promotes increased and prolonged inflammatory activity in older people in comparison to young people [126]. A cross-sectional study showed that older persons have two-fold–four-fold higher levels of CRP, IL-1 receptor antagonist (IL-1ra), IL-6, and TNF-α than young or even middle-aged adults [127,128]. This upregulation of inflammatory markers was shown to be strongly associated with diabetes, heart diseases, sarcopenia, disability, and more importantly higher mortality [129–133]. Another study of total and abdominal adiposity in older adults showed a strong association with high levels of inflammatory factors such as CRP, IL-1ra, and IL-6, which further highlights the important role of adipose tissue in inflammation during aging [134]. These data could indicate that an excess of adipose tissue alone should be recognized as one of the factors promoting aging and shortening longevity. However, other reports show that it is not always the quantity or distribution of fat that is important for life span and health span: the characteristics of adipocytes may play a major role in regulating metabolism and protecting against diabetes, cardiovascular diseases, cancer, and mortality. Yet, it is vital to understand that during obesity the accumulation of excess of fat tissue can significantly change the biology and physiology of adipocytes. Transgenic mice expressing bovine GH (bGH) showed increased body growth in comparison to their normal controls. At the same time, GH, known as the hormone that promotes lipolysis, was responsible for decreased fat accumulation in these animals [58]. However, regardless of their lean body type, these transgenic animals are short lived and insulin resistant [58]. Furthermore, it was shown that these animals have decreased circulating adiponectin levels, which could be associated with limited adiposity; however, they also have elevated levels of proinflammatory IL-6 and TNF-α [58]. Interestingly, histological examination of adipose tissue from these giant mice indicated a large number of heterogeneous differentiation phases, mostly presenting as preadipocytes unable to produce insulin-sensitizing hormones such as adiponectin due to excessive lipolysis caused by excessive GH levels [58]. Increased inflammatory pathway activity and insulin resistance is suggested to play a major role in shortening the life span of these lean mice. In contrast, GH-deficient Ames dwarf and Laron (GHRKO) dwarf mice have a tendency to increased obesity in comparison to their normal controls as they age [17], but are characterized by 40–60% extended longevity and high insulin sensitivity [15,16,77,135]. These long-living mice also have elevated levels of adiponectin and show decreased inflammation through their life span [78]. Interestingly, Laron dwarf mice are characterized by increased visceral fat, known to be a *bad* anti-inflammatory and prodiabetic fat [16], which should rather be detrimental for insulin signaling and longevity. It is especially intriguing that surgical removal of visceral fat in rats increased insulin sensitivity, as expected, but also extended longevity [103]. In addition, in another experiment, the same surgical intervention improved insulin sensitivity in mice fed a high-fat diet [102]. Based on these observations, surgical removal of intra-abdominal fat has been proposed as a mimetic of CR [103]. Similar surgical interventions were performed in healthy obese Laron dwarf mice: as expected, removing most of the visceral fat improved glucose tolerance and insulin sensitivity in normal controls; however, the same intervention caused attenuation of insulin signaling in long-living Laron dwarf mice [16]. It is striking that visceral fat removal in Laron dwarf mice caused a decrease in circulating levels of adiponectin, while there were no alterations in adiponectin levels in normal controls after surgery [16]. This result strongly suggests that visceral adipose tissue has different endocrine characteristics in Laron dwarf mice than the same fat in normal animals, and indicates a strong involvement of GH in the physiology of adipose tissue and a role on longevity. During a study of GH-deficient Ames dwarf mice, it was shown that GH treatment decreases adiponectin levels and promotes glucose intolerance and insulin resistance, but more importantly GH treatment decreased the longevity of Ames dwarf mice [135]. A study of CR in *ob/ob* mice provided more evidence that adipose tissue can undergo remodeling to promote a beneficial action on overall health and metabolism [136]. In this study, Harrison et al. showed that reduced caloric intake in *ob/ob* mice extends the life span, while maintaining high adiposity such that fat composed about half of their body weight [136]. These data suggest that well-functioning adipocytes, rather than the amount of fat, are detrimental for healthy obesity.

SUMMARY

In summary, we agree that overall obesity should be considered to increase the risk of elevated inflammation, metabolic syndrome, diabetes, cardiovascular diseases, cancer, and early mortality. However, it is essential to understand that the location of fat can be more important for metabolism than the percentage of total body fat. Intra-abdominal adipose tissue is the type that can be detrimental for a healthy metabolism in patients who are not classified as obese. However, some studies of genetically modified or mutant animals showed that intra-abdominal WAT can also be altered to promote healthy metabolism. It is suggested that the cellular biology of adipocytes and their secretory activity can shift fat into either being "good" or "bad." Unfortunately, excessive caloric intake and a sedentary lifestyle in a healthy person will promote excessive accumulation of abdominal fat leading to obesity and an unhealthy status. Continuous obesity causes molecular changes in adipocytes, altering their physiological function by shifting the balance in the production of proinflammatory vs. anti-inflammatory adipokines, which in time will contribute to development of diabetes, cardiac complications, cancer, or death. Currently, overweight and obesity affect nearly two-thirds of Americans, and there are several pharmaceutical and surgical interventions available to improve the health status of patients with metabolic abnormalities. However, to the best of our knowledge, there is a better way than using modern medicine: a healthy diet with a caloric intake adequate for the personal energy expenditure requirement and the use of regular physical activity to control weight and body fat accumulation.

References

[1] Grundy SM. Inflammation, hypertension, and the metabolic syndrome. JAMA 2003;290(22):3000–2.

[2] Misra A, Khurana L. Obesity and the metabolic syndrome in developing countries. J Clin Endocrinol Metab 2008;93(11 Suppl 1):S9–S30.

[3] Gealekman O, Guseva N, Hartigan C, Apotheker S, Gorgoglione M, Gurav K, et al. Depot-specific differences and insufficient subcutaneous adipose tissue angiogenesis in human obesity. Circulation 2011;123(2):186–94.

[4] Johnson JA, Fried SK, Pi-Sunyer FX, Albu JB. Impaired insulin action in subcutaneous adipocytes from women with visceral obesity. Am J Physiol Endocrinol Metab 2001;280(1):E40–9.

[5] Arnlov J, Sundstrom J, Ingelsson E, Lind L. Impact of BMI and the metabolic syndrome on the risk of diabetes in middle-aged men. Diabetes Care 2011;34(1):61–5.

[6] Ness-Abramof R, Apovian CM. Waist circumference measurement in clinical practice. Nutr Clin Pract 2008;23(4):397–404.

[7] Stefan N, Kantartzis K, Machann J, Schick F, Thamer C, Rittig K, et al. Identification and characterization of metabolically benign obesity in humans. Arch Intern Med 2008;168(15):1609–16.

[8] Salans LB, Cushman SW, Weismann RE. Studies of human adipose tissue. Adipose cell size and number in nonobese and obese patients. J Clin Invest 1973;52(4):929–41.

[9] Koska J, Stefan N, Permana PA, Weyer C, Sonoda M, Bogardus C, et al. Increased fat accumulation in liver may link insulin resistance with subcutaneous abdominal adipocyte enlargement, visceral adiposity, and hypoadiponectinemia in obese individuals. Am J Clin Nutr 2008;87(2):295–302.

[10] Weyer C, Foley JE, Bogardus C, Tataranni PA, Pratley RE. Enlarged subcutaneous abdominal adipocyte size, but not obesity itself, predicts type II diabetes independent of insulin resistance. Diabetologia 2000;43(12):1498–506.

[11] Larson-Meyer DE, Heilbronn LK, Redman LM, Newcomer BR, Frisard MI, Anton S, et al. Effect of calorie restriction with or without exercise on insulin sensitivity, beta-cell function, fat cell size, and ectopic lipid in overweight subjects. Diabetes Care 2006;29(6):1337–44.

[12] De Naeyer H, Ouwens DM, Van Nieuwenhove Y, Pattyn P, t Hart LM, Kaufman JM, et al. Combined gene and protein expression of hormone-sensitive lipase and adipose triglyceride lipase, mitochondrial content, and adipocyte size in subcutaneous and visceral adipose tissue of morbidly obese men. Obes Facts 2011;4(5):407–16.

[13] Bonkowski MS, Rocha JS, Masternak MM, Al Regaiey KA, Bartke A. Targeted disruption of growth hormone receptor interferes with the beneficial actions of calorie restriction. Proc Natl Acad Sci USA 2006;103(20):7901–5.

[14] Bonkowski MS, Dominici FP, Arum O, Rocha JS, Al Regaiey KA, Westbrook R, et al. Disruption of growth hormone receptor prevents calorie restriction from improving insulin action and longevity. PLoS One 2009;4(2):e4567.

[15] Masternak MM, Panici JA, Bonkowski MS, Hughes LF, Bartke A. Insulin sensitivity as a key mediator of growth hormone actions on longevity. J Gerontol A Biol Sci Med Sci 2009;64(5): 516–21.

[16] Masternak MM, Bartke A, Wang F, Spong A, Gesing A, Fang Y, et al. Metabolic effects of intra-abdominal fat in GHRKO mice. Aging Cell 2012;11(1):73–81.

[17] Bonkowski MS, Pamenter RW, Rocha JS, Masternak MM, Panici JA, Bartke A. Long-lived growth hormone receptor knockout mice show a delay in age-related changes of body composition and bone characteristics. J Gerontol A Biol Sci Med Sci 2006;61(6):562–7.

[18] Flint DJ, Binart N, Boumard S, Kopchick JJ, Kelly P. Developmental aspects of adipose tissue in GH receptor and

prolactin receptor gene disrupted mice: site-specific effects upon proliferation, differentiation and hormone sensitivity. J Endocrinol 2006;191(1):101–11.
[19] Varady KA, Tussing L, Bhutani S, Braunschweig CL. Degree of weight loss required to improve adipokine concentrations and decrease fat cell size in severely obese women. Metabolism 2009;58(8):1096–101.
[20] Mitka M. Obesity's role in heart disease requires apples and pears comparison. JAMA 2005;294(24):3071–2.
[21] Wingard DL. Sex differences and coronary heart disease. A case of comparing apples and pears? Circulation 1990;81(5):1710–2.
[22] Larsson B, Svardsudd K, Welin L, Wilhelmsen L, Bjorntorp P, Tibblin G. Abdominal adipose tissue distribution, obesity, and risk of cardiovascular disease and death: 13 year follow up of participants in the study of men born in 1913. Br Med J (Clin Res Ed) 1984;288(6428):1401–4.
[23] Lapidus L, Bengtsson C, Larsson B, Pennert K, Rybo E, Sjostrom L. Distribution of adipose tissue and risk of cardiovascular disease and death: a 12 year follow up of participants in the population study of women in Gothenburg. Sweden Br Med J (Clin Res Ed) 1984;289(6454):1257–61.
[24] Bonora E, Tessari R, Micciolo R, Zenere M, Targher G, Padovani R, et al. Intimal-medial thickness of the carotid artery in nondiabetic and NIDDM patients. Relationship with insulin resistance. Diabetes Care 1997;20(4):627–31.
[25] Yamamoto M, Egusa G, Hara H, Yamakido M. Association of intraabdominal fat and carotid atherosclerosis in non-obese middle-aged men with normal glucose tolerance. Int J Obes Relat Metab Disord 1997;21(10):948–51.
[26] Folsom AR, Prineas RJ, Kaye SA, Munger RG. Incidence of hypertension and stroke in relation to body fat distribution and other risk factors in older women. Stroke 1990;21(5):701–6.
[27] Rexrode KM, Carey VJ, Hennekens CH, Walters EE, Colditz GA, Stampfer MJ, et al. Abdominal adiposity and coronary heart disease in women. JAMA 1998;280(21):1843–8.
[28] Pouliot MC, Despres JP, Lemieux S, Moorjani S, Bouchard C, Tremblay A, et al. Waist circumference and abdominal sagittal diameter: best simple anthropometric indexes of abdominal visceral adipose tissue accumulation and related cardiovascular risk in men and women. Am J Cardiol 1994;73(7):460–8.
[29] Arad Y, Newstein D, Cadet F, Roth M, Guerci AD. Association of multiple risk factors and insulin resistance with increased prevalence of asymptomatic coronary artery disease by an electron-beam computed tomographic study. Arterioscler Thromb Vasc Biol 2001;21(12):2051–8.
[30] Hartz A, Grubb B, Wild R, Van Nort JJ, Kuhn E, Freedman D, et al. The association of waist hip ratio and angiographically determined coronary artery disease. Int J Obes 1990;14(8):657–65.
[31] Hauner H, Stangl K, Schmatz C, Burger K, Blomer H, Pfeiffer EF. Body fat distribution in men with angiographically confirmed coronary artery disease. Atherosclerosis 1990;85(2–3):203–10.
[32] Fox KA, Despres JP, Richard AJ, Brette S, Deanfield JE. Does abdominal obesity have a similar impact on cardiovascular disease and diabetes? A study of 91,246 ambulant patients in 27 European countries. Eur Heart J 2009;30(24):3055–63.
[33] Nakamura T, Tokunaga K, Shimomura I, Nishida M, Yoshida S, Kotani K, et al. Contribution of visceral fat accumulation to the development of coronary artery disease in non-obese men. Atherosclerosis 1994;107(2):239–46.
[34] Nakamura T, Kobayashi H, Yanagi K, Nakagawa T, Nishida M, Kihara S, et al. Importance of intra-abdominal visceral fat accumulation to coronary atherosclerosis in heterozygous familial hypercholesterolaemia. Int J Obes Relat Metab Disord 1997; 21(7):580–6.
[35] Hotamisligil GS. Inflammation and metabolic disorders. Nature 2006;444(7121):860–7.
[36] Weisberg SP, McCann D, Desai M, Rosenbaum M, Leibel RL, Ferrante Jr AW. Obesity is associated with macrophage accumulation in adipose tissue. J Clin Invest 2003;112(12):1796–808.
[37] Wu H, Ghosh S, Perrard XD, Feng L, Garcia GE, Perrard JL, et al. T-cell accumulation and regulated on activation, normal T cell expressed and secreted upregulation in adipose tissue in obesity. Circulation 2007;115(8):1029–38.
[38] Kintscher U, Hartge M, Hess K, Foryst-Ludwig A, Clemenz M, Wabitsch M, et al. T-lymphocyte infiltration in visceral adipose tissue: a primary event in adipose tissue inflammation and the development of obesity-mediated insulin resistance. Arterioscler Thromb Vasc Biol 2008;28(7):1304–10.
[39] Lago F, Dieguez C, Gomez-Reino J, Gualillo O. Adipokines as emerging mediators of immune response and inflammation. Nat Clin Pract Rheumatol 2007;3(12):716–24.
[40] Cancello R, Tordjman J, Poitou C, Guilhem G, Bouillot JL, Hugol D, et al. Increased infiltration of macrophages in omental adipose tissue is associated with marked hepatic lesions in morbid human obesity. Diabetes 2006;55(6):1554–61.
[41] Enos RT, Davis JM, Velazquez KT, McClellan JL, Day SD, Carnevale KA, et al. Influence of dietary saturated fat content on adiposity, macrophage behavior, inflammation, and metabolism: composition matters. J Lipid Res 2013;54(1):152–63.
[42] Pang C, Gao Z, Yin J, Zhang J, Jia W, Ye J. Macrophage infiltration into adipose tissue may promote angiogenesis for adipose tissue remodeling in obesity. Am J Physiol Endocrinol Metab 2008;295(2):E313–22.
[43] Lumeng CN, Deyoung SM, Saltiel AR. Macrophages block insulin action in adipocytes by altering expression of signaling and glucose transport proteins. Am J Physiol Endocrinol Metab 2007;292(1):E166–74.
[44] Kawanishi N, Yano H, Yokogawa Y, Suzuki K. Exercise training inhibits inflammation in adipose tissue via both suppression of macrophage infiltration and acceleration of phenotypic switching from M1 to M2 macrophages in high-fat-diet-induced obese mice. Exerc Immunol Rev 2010;16:105–18.
[45] Jolly CA. Dietary restriction and immune function. J Nutr 2004;134(8):1853–6.
[46] Capel F, Klimcakova E, Viguerie N, Roussel B, Vitkova M, Kovacikova M, et al. Macrophages and adipocytes in human obesity: adipose tissue gene expression and insulin sensitivity during calorie restriction and weight stabilization. Diabetes 2009;58(7):1558–67.
[47] Fantuzzi G. Adipose tissue, adipokines, and inflammation. J Allergy Clin Immunol 2005;115(5):911–9. quiz 20
[48] Bluher M, Fasshauer M, Tonjes A, Kratzsch J, Schon MR, Paschke R. Association of interleukin-6, C-reactive protein, interleukin-10 and adiponectin plasma concentrations with measures of obesity, insulin sensitivity and glucose metabolism. Exp Clin Endocrinol Diabetes 2005;113(9):534–7.
[49] Christiansen T, Richelsen B, Bruun JM. Monocyte chemoattractant protein-1 is produced in isolated adipocytes, associated with adiposity and reduced after weight loss in morbid obese subjects. Int J Obes (Lond) 2005;29(1):146–50.
[50] Spiegelman BM, Hotamisligil GS. Through thick and thin: wasting, obesity, and TNF alpha. Cell 1993;73(4):625–7.
[51] Hotamisligil GS, Shargill NS, Spiegelman BM. Adipose expression of tumor necrosis factor-alpha: direct role in obesity-linked insulin resistance. Science 1993;259(5091):87–91.
[52] Clement K, Viguerie N, Poitou C, Carette C, Pelloux V, Curat CA, et al. Weight loss regulates inflammation-related genes in white adipose tissue of obese subjects. FASEB J 2004;18(14): 1657–69.
[53] Arkan MC, Hevener AL, Greten FR, Maeda S, Li ZW, Long JM, et al. IKK-beta links inflammation to obesity-induced insulin resistance. Nat Med 2005;11(2):191–8.

[54] Cai D, Yuan M, Frantz DF, Melendez PA, Hansen L, Lee J, et al. Local and systemic insulin resistance resulting from hepatic activation of IKK-beta and NF-kappaB. Nat Med 2005;11(2):183–90.

[55] Kim JK, Kim YJ, Fillmore JJ, Chen Y, Moore I, Lee J, et al. Prevention of fat-induced insulin resistance by salicylate. J Clin Invest 2001;108(3):437–46.

[56] Yuan M, Konstantopoulos N, Lee J, Hansen L, Li ZW, Karin M, et al. Reversal of obesity- and diet-induced insulin resistance with salicylates or targeted disruption of Ikkbeta. Science 2001;293(5535):1673–7.

[57] Uysal KT, Wiesbrock SM, Marino MW, Hotamisligil GS. Protection from obesity-induced insulin resistance in mice lacking TNF-alpha function. Nature 1997;389(6651):610–4.

[58] Wang Z, Masternak MM, Al-Regaiey KA, Bartke A. Adipocytokines and the regulation of lipid metabolism in growth hormone transgenic and calorie-restricted mice. Endocrinology 2007;148(6):2845–53.

[59] Gallagher D, Heymsfield SB, Heo M, Jebb SA, Murgatroyd PR, Sakamoto Y. Healthy percentage body fat ranges: an approach for developing guidelines based on body mass index. Am J Clin Nutr 2000;72(3):694–701.

[60] Kadowaki T, Hara K, Yamauchi T, Terauchi Y, Tobe K, Nagai R. Molecular mechanism of insulin resistance and obesity. Exp Biol Med (Maywood) 2003;228(10):1111–7.

[61] Lochhead PA, Salt IP, Walker KS, Hardie DG, Sutherland C. 5-aminoimidazole-4-carboxamide riboside mimics the effects of insulin on the expression of the 2 key gluconeogenic genes PEPCK and glucose-6-phosphatase. Diabetes 2000;49(6):896–903.

[62] Yamauchi T, Kamon J, Minokoshi Y, Ito Y, Waki H, Uchida S, et al. Adiponectin stimulates glucose utilization and fatty-acid oxidation by activating AMP-activated protein kinase. Nat Med 2002;8(11):1288–95.

[63] Ukkola O, Santaniemi M. Adiponectin: a link between excess adiposity and associated comorbidities? J Mol Med (Berl) 2002;80(11):696–702.

[64] Motoshima H, Wu X, Sinha MK, Hardy VE, Rosato EL, Barbot DJ, et al. Differential regulation of adiponectin secretion from cultured human omental and subcutaneous adipocytes: effects of insulin and rosiglitazone. J Clin Endocrinol Metab 2002;87(12):5662–7.

[65] Bauche IB, El Mkadem SA, Pottier AM, Senou M, Many MC, Rezsohazy R, et al. Overexpression of adiponectin targeted to adipose tissue in transgenic mice: impaired adipocyte differentiation. Endocrinology 2007;148(4):1539–49.

[66] Otabe S, Yuan X, Fukutani T, Wada N, Hashinaga T, Nakayama H, et al. Overexpression of human adiponectin in transgenic mice results in suppression of fat accumulation and prevention of premature death by high-calorie diet. Am J Physiol Endocrinol Metab 2007;293(1):E210–8.

[67] Atzmon G, Pollin TI, Crandall J, Tanner K, Schechter CB, Scherer PE, et al. Adiponectin levels and genotype: a potential regulator of life span in humans. J Gerontol A Biol Sci Med Sci 2008;63(5):447–53.

[68] Arai Y, Takayama M, Gondo Y, Inagaki H, Yamamura K, Nakazawa S, et al. Adipose endocrine function, insulin-like growth factor-1 axis, and exceptional survival beyond 100 years of age. J Gerontol A Biol Sci Med Sci 2008;63(11):1209–18.

[69] Brown-Borg HM, Borg KE, Meliska CJ, Bartke A. Dwarf mice and the ageing process. Nature 1996;384(6604):33.

[70] Coschigano KT, Holland AN, Riders ME, List EO, Flyvbjerg A, Kopchick JJ. Deletion, but not antagonism, of the mouse growth hormone receptor results in severely decreased body weights, insulin, and insulin-like growth factor I levels and increased life span. Endocrinology 2003;144(9):3799–810.

[71] Corpas E, Harman SM, Blackman MR. Human growth hormone and human aging. Endocr Rev 1993;14(1):20–39.

[72] Blackman MR, Sorkin JD, Munzer T, Bellantoni MF, Busby-Whitehead J, Stevens TE, et al. Growth hormone and sex steroid administration in healthy aged women and men: a randomized controlled trial. JAMA 2002;288(18):2282–92.

[73] Christmas C, O'Connor KG, Harman SM, Tobin JD, Munzer T, Bellantoni MF, et al. Growth hormone and sex steroid effects on bone metabolism and bone mineral density in healthy aged women and men. J Gerontol A Biol Sci Med Sci 2002;57(1):M12–8.

[74] Munzer T, Harman SM, Sorkin JD, Blackman MR. Growth hormone and sex steroid effects on serum glucose, insulin, and lipid concentrations in healthy older women and men. J Clin Endocrinol Metab 2009;94(10):3833–41.

[75] Al-Regaiey KA, Masternak MM, Bonkowski M, Sun L, Bartke A. Long-lived growth hormone receptor knockout mice: interaction of reduced insulin-like growth factor i/insulin signaling and caloric restriction. Endocrinology 2005;146(2):851–60.

[76] Panici JA, Wang F, Bonkowski MS, Spong A, Bartke A, Pawlikowska L, et al. Is altered expression of hepatic insulin-related genes in growth hormone receptor knockout mice due to GH resistance or a difference in biological life spans? J Gerontol A Biol Sci Med Sci 2009;64(11):1126–33.

[77] Masternak MM, Panici JA, Wang F, Wang Z, Spong A. The effects of growth hormone (GH) treatment on GH and insulin/IGF-1 signaling in long-lived Ames dwarf mice. J Gerontol A Biol Sci Med Sci 2010;65(1):24–30.

[78] Masternak MM, Bartke A. Growth hormone, inflammation and aging. Pathobiol Aging Age Relat Dis 2012;2.

[79] Lubbers ER, List EO, Jara A, Sackman-Sala L, Cordoba-Chacon J, Gahete MD, et al. Adiponectin in mice with altered GH action: links to insulin sensitivity and longevity? J Endocrinol 2013;216(3):363–74.

[80] Brennan AM, Mantzoros CS. Drug Insight: the role of leptin in human physiology and pathophysiology—emerging clinical applications. Nat Clin Pract Endocrinol Metab 2006;2(6):318–27.

[81] Unger RH. Minireview: weapons of lean body mass destruction: the role of ectopic lipids in the metabolic syndrome. Endocrinology 2003;144(12):5159–65.

[82] Considine RV, Considine EL, Williams CJ, Hyde TM, Caro JF. The hypothalamic leptin receptor in humans: identification of incidental sequence polymorphisms and absence of the db/db mouse and fa/fa rat mutations. Diabetes 1996;45(7):992–4.

[83] Pelleymounter MA, Cullen MJ, Baker MB, Hecht R, Winters D, Boone T, et al. Effects of the obese gene product on body weight regulation in *ob/ob* mice. Science 1995;269(5223):540–3.

[84] Campfield LA, Smith FJ, Guisez Y, Devos R, Burn P. Recombinant mouse OB protein: evidence for a peripheral signal linking adiposity and central neural networks. Science 1995;269(5223):546–9.

[85] Kamohara S, Burcelin R, Halaas JL, Friedman JM, Charron MJ. Acute stimulation of glucose metabolism in mice by leptin treatment. Nature 1997;389(6649):374–7.

[86] Considine RV, Sinha MK, Heiman ML, Kriauciunas A, Stephens TW, Nyce MR, et al. Serum immunoreactive-leptin concentrations in normal-weight and obese humans. N Engl J Med 1996;334(5):292–5.

[87] Lazar MA. Resistin- and Obesity-associated metabolic diseases. Horm Metab Res 2007;39(10):710–6.

[88] Gelber RP, Gaziano JM, Orav EJ, Manson JE, Buring JE, Kurth T. Measures of obesity and cardiovascular risk among men and women. J Am Coll Cardiol 2008;52(8):605–15.

[89] Storti KL, Brach JS, FitzGerald SJ, Bunker CH, Kriska AM. Relationships among body composition measures in

community-dwelling older women. Obesity (Silver Spring) 2006;14(2):244–51.

[90] Seidell JC, Perusse L, Despres JP, Bouchard C. Waist and hip circumferences have independent and opposite effects on cardiovascular disease risk factors: the Quebec Family Study. Am J Clin Nutr 2001;74(3):315–21.

[91] von Eyben FE, Mouritsen E, Holm J, Montvilas P, Dimcevski G, Suciu G, et al. Intra-abdominal obesity and metabolic risk factors: a study of young adults. Int J Obes Relat Metab Disord 2003;27(8):941–9.

[92] Jensen MD. Role of body fat distribution and the metabolic complications of obesity. J Clin Endocrinol Metab 2008;93(11 Suppl 1):S57–63.

[93] Carey VJ, Walters EE, Colditz GA, Solomon CG, Willett WC, Rosner BA, et al. Body fat distribution and risk of non-insulin-dependent diabetes mellitus in women. The Nurses' Health Study. Am J Epidemiol 1997;145(7):614–9.

[94] Wang Y, Rimm EB, Stampfer MJ, Willett WC, Hu FB. Comparison of abdominal adiposity and overall obesity in predicting risk of type 2 diabetes among men. Am J Clin Nutr 2005;81(3):555–63.

[95] Nicklas BJ, Cesari M, Penninx BW, Kritchevsky SB, Ding J, Newman A, et al. Abdominal obesity is an independent risk factor for chronic heart failure in older people. J Am Geriatr Soc 2006;54(3):413–20.

[96] Ross R, Berentzen T, Bradshaw AJ, Janssen I, Kahn HS, Katzmarzyk PT, et al. Does the relationship between waist circumference, morbidity and mortality depend on measurement protocol for waist circumference? Obes Rev 2008;9(4):312–25.

[97] Leslie WD, Ludwig SM, Morin S. Abdominal fat from spine dual-energy x-ray absorptiometry and risk for subsequent diabetes. J Clin Endocrinol Metab 2010;95(7):3272–6.

[98] Misra A, Garg A, Abate N, Peshock RM, Stray-Gundersen J, Grundy SM. Relationship of anterior and posterior subcutaneous abdominal fat to insulin sensitivity in nondiabetic men. Obes Res 1997;5(2):93–9.

[99] Snijder MB, Dekker JM, Visser M, Bouter LM, Stehouwer CD, Kostense PJ, et al. Associations of hip and thigh circumferences independent of waist circumference with the incidence of type 2 diabetes: the Hoorn Study. Am J Clin Nutr 2003;77(5):1192–7.

[100] Tanko LB, Bagger YZ, Alexandersen P, Larsen PJ, Christiansen C. Peripheral adiposity exhibits an independent dominant antiatherogenic effect in elderly women. Circulation 2003;107(12): 1626–31.

[101] Thorne A, Lonnqvist F, Apelman J, Hellers G, Arner P. A pilot study of long-term effects of a novel obesity treatment: omentectomy in connection with adjustable gastric banding. Int J Obes Relat Metab Disord 2002;26(2):193–9.

[102] Gabriely I, Ma XH, Yang XM, Atzmon G, Rajala MW, Berg AH, et al. Removal of visceral fat prevents insulin resistance and glucose intolerance of aging: an adipokine-mediated process? Diabetes 2002;51(10):2951–8.

[103] Muzumdar R, Allison DB, Huffman DM, Ma X, Atzmon G, Einstein FH, et al. Visceral adipose tissue modulates mammalian longevity. Aging Cell 2008;7(3):438–40.

[104] Tran TT, Yamamoto Y, Gesta S, Kahn CR. Beneficial effects of subcutaneous fat transplantation on metabolism. Cell Metab 2008;7(5):410–20.

[105] Shah PK, Mudaliar S, Chang AR, Aroda V, Andre M, Burke P, et al. Effects of intensive insulin therapy alone and in combination with pioglitazone on body weight, composition, distribution and liver fat content in patients with type 2 diabetes. Diabetes Obes Metab 2011;13(6):505–10.

[106] Reeves GK, Pirie K, Beral V, Green J, Spencer E, Bull D. Cancer incidence and mortality in relation to body mass index in the million women study: cohort study. BMJ 2007;335(7630):1134.

[107] Pan SY, DesMeules M, Morrison H, Wen SW. Obesity, high energy intake, lack of physical activity, and the risk of kidney cancer. Cancer Epidemiol Biomarkers Prev 2006;15(12):2453–60.

[108] Zhang C, Rexrode KM, van Dam RM, Li TY, Hu FB. Abdominal obesity and the risk of all-cause, cardiovascular, and cancer mortality: sixteen years of follow-up in US women. Circulation 2008;117(13):1658–67.

[109] Wright ME, Chang SC, Schatzkin A, Albanes D, Kipnis V, Mouw T, et al. Prospective study of adiposity and weight change in relation to prostate cancer incidence and mortality. Cancer 2007; 109(4):675–84.

[110] von Hafe P, Pina F, Perez A, Tavares M, Barros H. Visceral fat accumulation as a risk factor for prostate cancer. Obes Res 2004;12(12):1930–5.

[111] Nelson WG, De Marzo AM, DeWeese TL, Isaacs WB. The role of inflammation in the pathogenesis of prostate cancer. J Urol 2004;172(5 Pt 2):S6–S11. discussion S-2

[112] Platz EA, De Marzo AM. Epidemiology of inflammation and prostate cancer. J Urol 2004;171(2 Pt 2):S36–40.

[113] Hsing AW, Chua Jr S, Gao YT, Gentzschein E, Chang L, Deng J, et al. Prostate cancer risk and serum levels of insulin and leptin: a population-based study. J Natl Cancer Inst 2001;93(10):783–9.

[114] Saglam K, Aydur E, Yilmaz M, Goktas S. Leptin influences cellular differentiation and progression in prostate cancer. J Urol 2003;169(4):1308–11.

[115] Stattin P, Soderberg S, Hallmans G, Bylund A, Kaaks R, Stenman UH, et al. Leptin is associated with increased prostate cancer risk: a nested case-referent study. J Clin Endocrinol Metab 2001;86(3):1341–5.

[116] Lagiou P, Signorello LB, Trichopoulos D, Tzonou A, Trichopoulou A, Mantzoros CS. Leptin in relation to prostate cancer and benign prostatic hyperplasia. Int J Cancer 1998;76(1):25–8.

[117] Kaaks R, Lukanova A, Rinaldi S, Biessy C, Soderberg S, Olsson T, et al. Interrelationships between plasma testosterone, SHBG, IGF-I, insulin and leptin in prostate cancer cases and controls. Eur J Cancer Prev 2003;12(4):309–15.

[118] Garofalo C, Koda M, Cascio S, Sulkowska M, Kanczuga-Koda L, Golaszewska J, et al. Increased expression of leptin and the leptin receptor as a marker of breast cancer progression: possible role of obesity-related stimuli. Clin Cancer Res 2006;12(5): 1447–53.

[119] Hursting SD, Nunez NP, Varticovski L, Vinson C. The obesity-cancer link: lessons learned from a fatless mouse. Cancer Res 2007;67(6):2391–3.

[120] Dalamaga M, Diakopoulos KN, Mantzoros CS. The role of adiponectin in cancer: a review of current evidence. Endocr Rev 2012;33(4):547–94.

[121] Brakenhielm E, Veitonmaki N, Cao R, Kihara S, Matsuzawa Y, Zhivotovsky B, et al. Adiponectin-induced antiangiogenesis and antitumor activity involve caspase-mediated endothelial cell apoptosis. Proc Natl Acad Sci USA 2004;101(8):2476–81.

[122] Ikeno Y, Bronson RT, Hubbard GB, Lee S, Bartke A. Delayed occurrence of fatal neoplastic diseases in ames dwarf mice: correlation to extended longevity. J Gerontol A Biol Sci Med Sci 2003;58(4):291–6.

[123] Ikeno Y, Hubbard GB, Lee S, Cortez LA, Lew CM, Webb CR, et al. Reduced incidence and delayed occurrence of fatal neoplastic diseases in growth hormone receptor/binding protein knockout mice. J Gerontol A Biol Sci Med Sci 2009;64(5):522–9.

[124] Bender R, Jockel KH, Trautner C, Spraul M, Berger M. Effect of age on excess mortality in obesity. JAMA 1999;281(16): 1498–504.

[125] Fontaine KR, Redden DT, Wang C, Westfall AO, Allison DB. Years of life lost due to obesity. JAMA 2003;289(2):187–93.

[126] Krabbe KS, Bruunsgaard H, Hansen CM, Moller K, Fonsmark L, Qvist J, et al. Ageing is associated with a prolonged fever response in human endotoxemia. Clin Diagn Lab Immunol 2001;8(2):333–8.
[127] Ferrucci L, Corsi A, Lauretani F, Bandinelli S, Bartali B, Taub DD, et al. The origins of age-related proinflammatory state. Blood 2005;105(6):2294–9.
[128] Bruunsgaard H, Andersen-Ranberg K, Jeune B, Pedersen AN, Skinhoj P, Pedersen BK. A high plasma concentration of TNF-alpha is associated with dementia in centenarians. J Gerontol A Biol Sci Med Sci 1999;54(7):M357–64.
[129] Penninx BW, Kritchevsky SB, Newman AB, Nicklas BJ, Simonsick EM, Rubin S, et al. Inflammatory markers and incident mobility limitation in the elderly. J Am Geriatr Soc 2004;52(7):1105–13.
[130] Pai JK, Pischon T, Ma J, Manson JE, Hankinson SE, Joshipura K, et al. Inflammatory markers and the risk of coronary heart disease in men and women. N Engl J Med 2004;351(25): 2599–610.
[131] Pradhan AD, Manson JE, Rifai N, Buring JE, Ridker PM. C-reactive protein, interleukin 6, and risk of developing type 2 diabetes mellitus. JAMA 2001;286(3):327–34.
[132] Harris TB, Ferrucci L, Tracy RP, Corti MC, Wacholder S, Ettinger Jr WH, et al. Associations of elevated interleukin-6 and C-reactive protein levels with mortality in the elderly. Am J Med 1999;106(5):506–12.
[133] Cesari M, Kritchevsky SB, Baumgartner RN, Atkinson HH, Penninx BW, Lenchik L, et al. Sarcopenia, obesity, and inflammation—results from the Trial of Angiotensin Converting Enzyme Inhibition and Novel Cardiovascular Risk Factors study. Am J Clin Nutr 2005;82(2):428–34.
[134] Brinkley TE, Hsu FC, Beavers KM, Church TS, Goodpaster BH, Stafford RS, et al. Total and abdominal adiposity are associated with inflammation in older adults using a factor analysis approach. J Gerontol A Biol Sci Med Sci 2012;67(10):1099–106.
[135] Panici JA, Harper JM, Miller RA, Bartke A, Spong A, Masternak MM. Early life growth hormone treatment shortens longevity and decreases cellular stress resistance in long-lived mutant mice. FASEB J 2010;24(12):5073–9.
[136] Harrison DE, Archer JR, Astle CM. Effects of food restriction on aging: separation of food intake and adiposity. Proc Natl Acad Sci USA 1984;81(6):1835–8.

CHAPTER

28

Appetite and Reward Signals in the Brain: Sugar Intake Effects on Brain Activity as Measured by Functional Magnetic Resonance Imaging

Samantha M. Hudgins, Anna Schlappal, and Thomas W. Castonguay

Department of Nutrition and Food Science, University of Maryland, College Park, MD, USA

INTRODUCTION

The objective of this chapter is to introduce the reader to a new approach to the study of food intake and its control. Functional magnetic resonance imaging (fMRI) is now being used to study the neural mechanisms controlling hunger and appetite. Rather than attempt to summarize the entire field (which is growing exponentially), we hope to summarize a subset of that literature by focusing on the effects of sugars on brain activity as measured by fMRI. We start this brief overview with an attempt to place this work in context. The control of food intake has a long and rich history. Contemporary students of the neural controls of hunger and appetite recognize that multiple systems within the brain act in concert with one another to a common end. Hypothalamic controls, hind brain integration of peripheral signals, and taste and reward systems all contribute to our ability to monitor and control caloric intake.

The scientific study of the control of food intake has a history that spans the last 100 years. The pioneering works of C.P. Richter, Jean Mayer, Gordon Kennedy, Eliot Stellar, Jacques LeMagnen, and dozens of others have all contributed to our understanding of the biological bases of hunger and satiety. Rather than attempt to review the entire area here, we offer the reader two excellent recent reviews that summarize contemporary hypotheses about hunger and satiety. Guyenet and Schwartz [1] and Choi et al. [2] have not only clearly outlined the role of the hypothalamus in the regulation of energy balance but also noted that a segment of that region (specifically the ventromedial nucleus) plays several interactive roles in maintaining intake. They also note that energy regulation results from not only an interaction of hypothalamic neurons but also includes input from brain reward as well as brainstem-sensory systems (reviewed in [3]).

We have chosen to focus on sugar solutions because of their relative simplicity, from a nutrition perspective, and because sweetened beverages constitute a major source of calories in the American diet. By studying the mechanisms involved with sugar solution intake, we hope to develop a better understanding of how and why our usual appetite mechanisms fail to adequately protect us from overeating when we are presented with sweetened beverages. Such an understanding could be instrumental in reversing the obesity epidemic facing the country.

Obesity Epidemic

Recent statistics from the Center for Disease Control reveal that the obesity epidemic is continuing to spread throughout the USA, with obesity rates in most states greater than 30% of adults. Even more troubling is that in some segments of the American population an even greater percentage of people are affected. For example, more that 80% of adult African-American women are

Nutrition in the Prevention and Treatment of Abdominal Obesity
http://dx.doi.org/10.1016/B978-0-12-407869-7.00028-3

currently either overweight or obese. Perhaps most discouraging of all the recent statistics is that no single factor or combination of factors has been definitively identified as the cause or causes of the recent epidemic. Failure in determining these root causes only leads to the persistence of the condition, and has resulted in the prediction that, for the first time, today's U.S. children will not be expected to live as long as their parents.

Recent Controversy About Fructose and High Fructose Corn Syrup

Researchers have an ample number of hypotheses to consider in guiding their efforts in determining the causes of obesity. One such hypothesis is that the composition of the American diet has shifted from a diet low in sugars and high in complex carbohydrates to one that is high in sugar. Bray and colleagues [4] have noted that the typical American now consumes >1000% more sugar than only one generation ago (Figure 28.1). Several lines of evidence have linked high sugar diets with insulin resistance and subsequent obesity, and several researchers have identified specific sugars suspected of being effective in promoting obesity. In particular, high fructose corn syrup has been linked to a myriad of metabolic changes conducive to promoting obesity.

Effects of Single Nutrients on Gene Expression

Mindful of these developments, we examined the short-term effects of sugar consumption on liver and adipose tissue corticosteroid 11-beta-dehydrogenase isozyme 1 [11β-hydroxysteroid dehydrogenase 1 (11β-HSD1)] and glucose-6-phosphate 1-dehydrogenase (G6PD) message and expression [5]. These two enzymes have been linked to obesity (and in particular to omental obesity) in both humans and animal models. The question posed was: "Could any one sugar affect the regulation and/or expression of these enzymes?" We reported that rats given 24-h access to dilute fructose solutions dramatically increased hepatic 11β-HSD1 and G6PD message and protein, whereas controls given access to the same concentration of glucose had no effect on either enzyme. We went on to show that 7-day access to sucrose had a comparable effect on hepatic 11β-HSD1. Again, 7-day access to glucose failed to induce any significant effect on either enzyme, despite comparable sugar intake in both sucrose- and fructose-fed rats. Clearly, different sugars can influence these critical components of sugar-induced obesity.

Specific Effect of Fructose

More recently, we repeated one of London et al.'s experiments by giving rats 24-h access to one of four different dilute sugar solutions in addition to unrestricted access to a standard diet [6]. Hypothalamic samples taken from the brains of these animals were then probed using gene expression arrays. Several differences in appetite-regulating genes between sugar-fed and control rats were noted, including a dramatic suppression of cholecystokinin that was specific to fructose-fed rats. Differences in gene expression could be attributed to several factors, such as overeating, novelty, and differences in sensory and reward factors that accompany sugar intake. However fructose (and not high-fructose corn syrup or any other sugar tested) promoted several

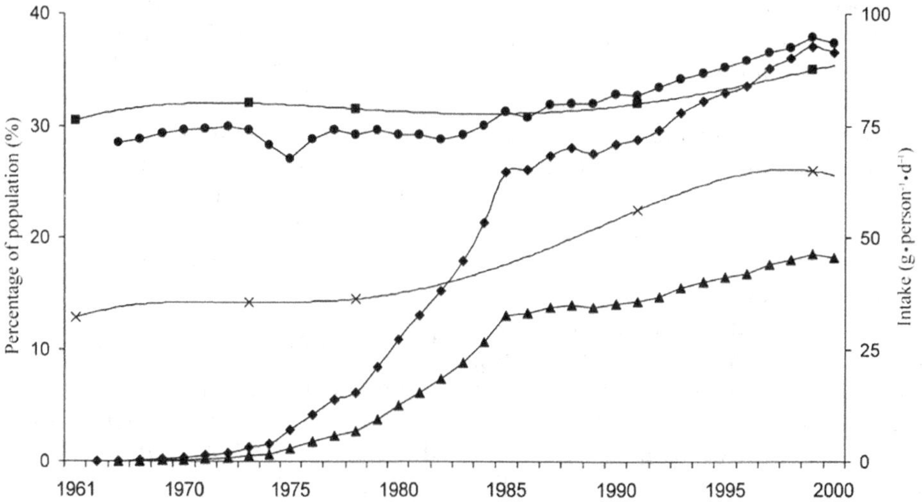

FIGURE 28.1 ***Fructose Consumption, 1961-2000.*** Graphical representation of estimated total fructose (•), free fructose (▲), and high-fructose corn syrup (HFCS; ◆) intake in relation to increasing prevalence of overweight (■) and obesity (x) in the United States from 1961–2000. *Adapted from Bray GA, et al. [4].*

unique changes in hypothalamic controls and was the only sugar tested that additionally produced a pronounced increase in circulating triglycerides. Although Storlien et al. [7] and others have reported that long-term exposure to fructose can induce hypertriglyceridemia, to our knowledge we were the first to demonstrate that this effect could be produced with as short a period as overnight access. These studies provide convincing evidence that fructose is uniquely suited to promote both the regulatory and metabolic conditions that cause obesity.

Glucose Affects Hypothalamic Signaling

The main function of carbohydrate metabolism is to modulate postprandial blood glucose to avoid high or low glucose concentrations—both of which cause cellular damage. Postprandial carbohydrates, disaccharides and polysaccharides, are broken down by enzymes on intestinal villi into one-unit sugars called *monosaccharides*. Glucose, a monosaccharide, is considered to be the physiologically preferred sugar for energy use and storage. From the intestine, glucose is absorbed into the bloodstream. The brain uses about 25% of blood glucose as its primary fuel source. The glucose-rich blood travels through the hepatic portal vein, which stimulates a biphasic insulin secretion from pancreatic beta cells proportional to the concentration of blood glucose. Insulin then travels through the bloodstream, facilitating glucose uptake into cells for storage or energy use. Within the hypothalamus, insulin can bind and inhibit the action of neuropeptide Y/agouti-related protein (NPY/AGRP) neurons, known modulators of food intake. Additionally, glucose-sensing neurons of the hypothalamus are inhibited by a rise in blood glucose. As a consequence, glucose ingestion and subsequent insulin secretion reduce neuronal activity within the hypothalamus.

Functional Magnetic Resonance Imaging

Functional magnetic resonance imaging (fMRI) is a noninvasive method for measuring changes in the brain. Prior to the inception of functional imaging, MRI had been used almost exclusively for the clinical imaging of abnormal or damaged tissues. True to its namesake, MRI uses magnetic resonance to image particular tissues when set to a particular frequency (Figure 28.2). A proton normally spins about its own axis, but when a magnetic field is introduced that axis will align with the field. The alignment of the protons with the magnet creates a "resting" energy state, which can be disrupted by radio frequencies. The application of the radio-frequency wave increases the energy state of the protons. When the radio-frequency wave is removed, the protons return to their original magnetic alignment; doing so releases energy frequencies, which are integrated through the radio-frequency coils to create an image. A series of multiple images that reveal moment-to-moment changes in

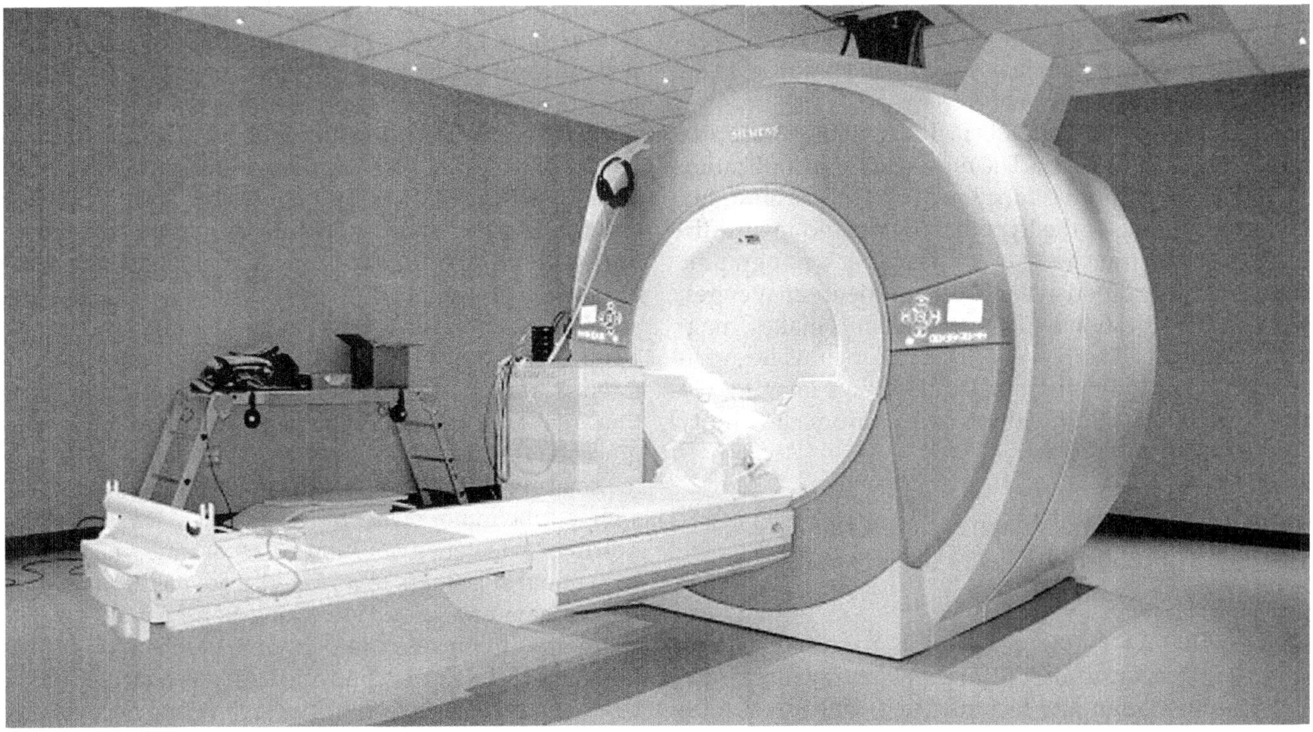

FIGURE 28.2 Image of the fMRI 3-Tesla Magnet used at the University of Maryland, Neuroimaging Center.

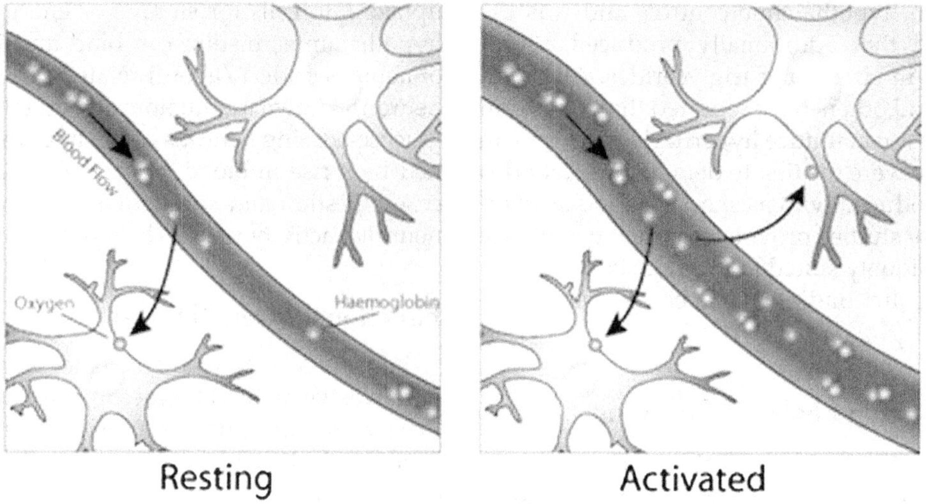

FIGURE 28.3 ***BOLD fMRI Signal.*** When blood hemoglobin is oxygenated, it contains no unpaired electrons and is thus not attracted to a magnetic field. However, it becomes paramagnetic (has unpaired electrons) when deoxygenated. This difference in magnetic properties makes it possible to detect small differences in the magnetic resonance signal of blood. Thus, the changes in oxygenation reflect levels of neural activity. This form of functional magnetic resonance imaging fMRI is known as blood oxygenation level dependent (BOLD) fMRI. (See color plate at the back of the book.)

the brain is called fMRI. Blood oxygen level dependent (BOLD) fMRI takes measuring changes within the brain a step further. BOLD fMRI is based on the imaging property of blood in its oxygenated or deoxygenated state (Figure 28.3). When imaged at a particular frequency, oxygenated blood appears almost black on a gray scale, while deoxygenated blood appears light gray. When a neuron becomes active, oxygen is required; therefore, changes in blood flow occur to supply the neuron with oxygen. This translates into BOLD fMRI, which measures blood oxygenation levels within the brain to determine differences in neuronal activity.

The development of BOLD fMRI technology has promoted its use in research. The most common application is to measure cognitive functions such as learning and memory. Imaging of the hypothalamus could reveal differences in substrate metabolism as well as demographic variations in responsiveness to nutrient challenges. However, the location of the hypothalamus makes imaging challenging. The presence of a major sinus immediately adjacent to the hypothalamus makes imaging the region particularly difficult, as echoes from the empty sinus interfere with imaging.

Applying Functional Magnetic Resonance Imaging to Study the Effects of Sugars on the Hypothalamus

Using BOLD fMRI, a decrease in hypothalamic activity in response to both oral and intravenous glucose administration has been reported. Smeets et al. [8] observed that oral consumption of a 25 g or 75 g glucose solution elicited a 1–2.5% signal decrease in the hypothalamus shortly after consumption. Furthermore, the 75-g dose induced a greater reduction in hypothalamic activity compared to the 25-g dose; the effects of the 75-g dose were also significantly different from control for at least 5 min longer than those of the 25-g dose. When analyzed regionally, only the upper anterior hypothalamus (UAH) and upper posterior hypothalamus (UPH) showed a reduction in signal due to glucose administration; only the UAH responded to glucose in a dose-dependent manner. Smeets et al. [9] was able to repeat his previous results of a 1.5–2% hypothalamic signal decrease in response to a 75-g glucose solution administered orally. When they compared oral and intravenous glucose administration, an equivalent glucose infusion resulted in a transient 1% hypothalamic signal decrease. Furthermore, the signal reduction extended from an onset time of 9 min to at least 20 min when glucose was administered orally versus an onset time of 4 min to 17 min for intravenous glucose administration. The difference in magnitude is probably a result of gastrointestinal regulatory mechanisms that are stimulated when glucose is orally administered. Smeets et al. [8] sought to determine whether hypothalamic signal decreases were a function of sweet taste or caloric density. A nonnutritive sweetened solution of aspartame was created with equal sweetness to a 75-g glucose solution in addition to having an equicaloric solution of maltodextrin. Neither solution decreased hypothalamic activity; nor did they differ from control. Regional analysis of the UPH showed inconsistent but significant decreases in response to the maltodextrin solution. These results suggest that hypothalamic signal decrease is dependent on both calories and sweet taste.

Extrahypothalamic signal changes also occur in response to glucose administration. Liu et al. [10] analyzed the whole-brain response to oral glucose administration. This study looked at clusters of activity change over a period and noted two peaks in activity. The first peak was observed in the supplementary motor area, somatosensory cortex, cerebellum, anterior cingulate, and orbitofrontal cortex. This peak is most likely the result of sensory and visceral signaling, but is not considered a result of "eating" because a control did not produce the same peak. The second peak of activity was observed as a decrease in signal within the hypothalamus around 7.7–12.8 min postingestion. These results are consistent with previously discussed effects of glucose on hypothalamic activity and serve to validate research into hypothalamic brain activity changes in response to sugar solutions.

Altered glucose and insulin levels in response to a glucose solution are believed to be the predominating factor driving changes in hypothalamic activity when a glucose solution is consumed. However, several signaling pathways respond to the consumption of either glucose solutions or an equal volume of water. Matsuda et al. [11] was among the first to observe a decrease in hypothalamic activity in response to the water control. By using obese and lean subjects they sought to determine differences in hypothalamic signal changes in response to a glucose solution. To measure controls 8 of the 20 subjects were randomly chosen to consume an equal volume of water as the glucose treatment solution. When analyzed regionally the consumption of the water elicited a signal decrease in hypothalamic activity that was reportedly "virtually identical to that of glucose." This result suggests that gastric motility may attenuate hypothalamic signals. It is important to note that this is the only study that observed a response to water consumption.

Increases in hypothalamic activity can be observed when subjects undergo hyperinsulinemic clamp sessions. Page et al. [12] demonstrated that a decrease in blood glucose results in a two-fold increase in hypothalamic activity that is dependent on counter-regulatory hormones like glucagon, epinephrine, and somatotropin/growth hormone. Subjects showed an increase in hypothalamic activity following 77.2 ± 2 mg/dL. Musen et al. [13] observed hypothalamic activation in nondiabetic subjects when blood glucose dropped to 68 ± 9 mg/dL; the same results were seen in insulin-dependent diabetic subjects at 76 ± 8 mg/dL. Note that these numbers are not significantly different.

Specificity: Glucose Versus Fructose

Glucose is not the only monosaccharide that is metabolized by the body. Fructose is another monosaccharide that the body metabolizes—but through an unregulated pathway. Almost all absorbed fructose is quickly taken up by the liver. Fructose, unlike glucose, is immediately converted to two glyceraldehyde-3-phosphate (G3P) molecules, with minimal regulatory mechanisms. This is where the term *instant triose* originates. The metabolic processes that take place after this are highly controversial. Many believe that the influxes of G3Ps are eventually metabolized into acetyl coenzyme A (acetyl-CoA), which in turn increases de novo lipogenesis. Others believe that fructose is simply incorporated in to the metabolic pathway of glucose. Page et al. [12] performed a study to determine whether fructose could cross the blood-brain barrier to be metabolized within the brain. Using rats, a 20% fructose infusion raised plasma fructose levels more than 20-fold. As a result, Page observed an increase in the amount of fructose found in dialysis fluid taken from the ventral medial hypothalamic region. Additionally, *Slca5* [encoding solute carrier family 2, facilitated glucose transporter member 5 (GLUT5)] and *Khk* (encoding ketohexokinase) mRNA was expressed in the hypothalamus, which indicates that fructose could be metabolized within the hypothalamus. These results suggest that fructose can be used as an energy source within the brain. It is important to note that the fructose was infused and not orally administered, and in that way bypassed hepatic uptake mechanism. We are left to conclude that fructose may be used in the brain as an energy source, but that the amount of fructose that reaches the brain is probably negligible.

Other appetite regulatory mechanisms can be differentially altered by glucose and fructose. For example, Page et al. [12] demonstrated that a fructose solution affects the hypothalamus differently than a glucose solution. Consistent with several other previously reported studies, they found a decrease in hypothalamic activity in response to consumption of a glucose solution. They also reported that 15 min after subjects consumed a glucose solution, a reduction in hypothalamic cerebral blood flow of −6.84 mL/g was observed. Hypothalamic cerebral blood flow (CBF) increased by 5.10 mL/g in response to an equal concentration fructose solution. An overall decrease in hypothalamic CBF averaged −5.45 mL/g in response to a glucose solution and 2.84 mL/g in response to a fructose solution. Several other differences between glucose and fructose treatments were also reported. Glucose administration increased plasma glucose, insulin, and glucagon-like peptide 1 (GLP-1) levels, whereas fructose administration increased circulating lactate and peptide YY (PYY). There were no differences in circulating leptin or ghrelin between glucose- and fructose-treated subjects. In an earlier study, Purnell et al. [14] attempted to find a difference between glucose and fructose following intravenous delivery. However, their results were inconclusive and showed fructose decreasing hypothalamic activity and glucose increasing hypothalamic activity in the control region. Smeets et al. [9] demonstrated that hypothalamic signal changes are difficult to measure when glucose is administered intravenously rather than orally. Additionally, the hypothalamus is difficult to image using fMRI technology due to its size and placement.

The hypothalamus is not the sole regulator of appetite in the brain. There are many pathways that the hypothalamus communicates with to respond to changes in appetite. Page et al. [12] measured the functional connectivity between the hypothalamus and the rest of the brain when subjects were given either a glucose or fructose solution. After glucose administration, subjects' functional connectivity increased in the thalamus, caudate, and putamen, whereas connectivity increased only to the thalamus after fructose consumption. In addition to a reduction in CBF in the hypothalamus, reductions were seen in the thalamus, insula, anterior cingulate, and striatum after glucose consumption. In response to consumption of the fructose solution, CBF decreased in the thalamus, hippocampus, posterior cingulate cortex, fusiform gyrus, and visual cortex. The changes in activity observed when a glucose solution was administered are conducive to a satiety response for both homeostatic and reward centers. The response to fructose consumption suggests an inability to properly regulate appetite for both homeostatic and reward centers.

TASTE AND REWARD

Reward Pathway

The reward pathway is a brain circuit that plays a critical role in motivating reward-based learning, the development of goal-directed behaviors, responses to food intake, and monetary rewards [15–17]. This network is part of the corticobasal ganglia that includes the prefrontal cortex, nucleus accumbens (NAcc), ventral tegmental area, and the medial dorsal nucleus of the thalamus [15]. The reward pathway uses dopamine as one of its main neurotransmitters to mediate signals in response to rewards [18]. This pathway also responds to drugs of abuse such as cocaine and heroin [19]. Recently, sugar has also been suggested to stimulate the reward pathway and possibly to bring about sugar "addiction" or addiction-related behaviors [20,21].

Gustatory (Taste) Pathway

The gustatory (taste) pathway involves signals that originate from taste receptors in the mouth and throat [22]. The five main taste sensations are sweet, salty, bitter, sour, and umami [23]. These signals travel to the brain via nerves, including the chorda tympani and glossopharyngeal nerves, through the nucleus of the solitary tract in the medulla, the thalamus, and primary taste cortex to the amygdala and hypothalamus [22,24]. The taste pathway is important in discriminating not only taste but also postingestive consequences regarding caloric content to the brain [25]. Additionally, sweet and bitter taste receptors (T1R and T2R, respectively) have been identified in the gastrointestinal tract, indicating that taste signals are not limited to the mouth and throat region [26,27]. Taste perception can be disrupted in obese people, resulting in reward system activation in response to any, not just palatable, taste cues [28]. Furthermore, artificial sweeteners can also play a role in disrupting the natural homeostatic taste mechanisms responsible for regulating taste and food ingestion [29].

Reward and Calorie Content

Two recurring questions asked by researchers over the years have been "How does the reward value of a food item relate to its calorie content?" and "What is the connection between a reward received and the ability of the brain to discern its caloric content?" In a study focusing on the caloric content of food, Killgore and associates [30] reported that amygdalar activation as measured by fMRI was high following presentation of food pictures when compared to nonfood pictures. High-calorie foods produced increased activation of the hypothalamus and frontal cortex areas [30], thereby contributing to the brain's ability to evaluate the reward value of higher-calorie foods.

This natural mechanism can be complicated by the use of artificial sweeteners such as saccharin, a non-nutritive sweetener. Green et al. [29] reported that there are differences in brain activity between subjects who commonly consume diet soda when compared to subjects who regularly consume soda sweetened with caloric sweeteners. In diet-soda drinkers, there was a large response in the dopaminergic midbrain as measured by fMRI when consuming either saccharin or sucrose [29]. These results indicate that the reward system has modified itself within the diet-soda drinker to respond to both caloric and noncaloric sweet taste, and does not discriminate based on caloric content. Green speculated that this change may in fact lead to changes in body weight because a person may not be able to evaluate caloric content and may overeat. These findings are consistent with those of Davidson and Swithers [31] who reported that rats intermittently given sweet taste and calories were unable to compensate for a sweet and caloric pre-meal compared to rats consistently given sweet taste and calories. While rats are much better at tightly regulating their caloric intake, similar changes may still be seen in human populations.

Rudenga et al. [32] has reported that fMRI-measured activation of the amygdala was affected differently between people who drink artificially sweetened drinks and those who drink sugar-sweetened beverages. They reported a negative correlation between the regular use of artificial sweetener and the amygdala response to sucrose. The amygdala has been shown to be involved in flavor-nutrient conditioning, which allows for preference of flavor previously paired with sucrose over saline [33]. Reduced amygdalar activation as measured by fMRI resulted from treatment with a μ-opioid receptor inverse agonist in subjects consuming palatable food [34]. As already noted, disruptions in flavor sensing and the ability to judge caloric content have the potential to impact regulation of caloric intake.

Taste and Reward in Obese vs. Nonobese People

The brain activity of obese people is significantly different from that of normal weight controls. Some of these differences include the reward pathway. In an fMRI study, people with high body mass index measurements showed activation in their reward pathway in response to high-calorie taste cues [35]. Furthermore, people showing high reward pathway activity also had a greater number of binge-eating symptoms. These two observations make it tempting to suspect that reward pathway activation links reward processing with binge eating [35]. In another fMRI study, obese subjects had high levels of activation in the NAcc for all samples that provided a taste (sweet, fatty, or quinone), whereas controls varied their response depending on taste cues [28]. This study suggests the obese subjects did not discriminate among tastes, but instead discriminated against a lack of taste. Leptin-deficient obese subjects treated with leptin had lower activation in the striatum in response to food images compared to controls [36]. Additionally, in obese women there is widespread activation of the reward system in response to high-calorie food pictures [37]. These results indicate that changes might occur within the reward system either as a result of or as a correlate to obesity, which represses the natural taste and reward systems.

Obesity and Type 2 Diabetes Mellitus

Obesity and type 2 diabetes mellitus (T2DM) are polygenic diseases for which a cause is still unknown. However, T2DM is often preceded by obesity through a genetic component that can be exacerbated by environmental factors. One environmental factor is diet and, as previously mentioned, sugar intake has been shown to be a potential contributor to these diseases. Obesity in general results from the inability of the body to properly maintain energy homeostasis. Matsuda et al. [11] sought to determine differences in hypothalamic activity in response to a glucose solution between lean and obese subjects. They observed an attenuated and delayed response in the obese group. Although both groups experienced a decrease in hypothalamic activity, the obese group showed a 4.8% decrease whereas the lean group exhibited a 7.9% decreased. Additionally, obese subjects did not exhibit a significant reduction in hypothalamic activity until 9.4 min postingestion whereas the lean group responded sooner, at 6.4 min postingestion. This delay was observed in two different regions of the hypothalamus: the lateral posterior hypothalamus (LPH) and the UAH. Plasma glucose concentrations were not different between groups during the fMRI session. However, fasting plasma insulin and mean plasma insulin levels were significantly higher in this same obese group. Additionally, fasting plasma leptin was 21 μg/L higher in the obese group than in the lean group.

Smeets et al. [9] compared hypothalamic activity in response to the consumption of an oral glucose solution between T2DM subjects and healthy controls. The control group demonstrated a reduction in hypothalamic activity congruent with previous studies. In contrast, the T2DM group's BOLD signal in all hypothalamic areas was unaffected. Additionally, when the T2DM group consumed water, hypothalamic activity was significantly increased in the lateral anterior hypothalamus (LAH) and LPH. These results suggest that subjects with T2DM may lack a regulatory mechanism required for energy homeostasis within the hypothalamus. However, the results do not give any indication as to what regulatory mechanism is missing and whether this response contributed to or was caused by T2DM.

CONCLUSIONS

fMRI is providing new perspectives into how the brain controls food intake and energy metabolism. This chapter offers only a limited insight into the extent to which this new technology is contributing to a better understanding of how and why we eat what we eat. Here, we have focused on the effects of sugars on brain regions that are known to participate in hunger and appetite. Early reports in this field make it clear that sugar affects several neural systems that can be monitored by fMRI. Hypothalamic, sensory, and reward pathways are all influenced by sugar. It remains to be determined how different sugars influence the activities of each pathway. Early evidence supports the speculation that not all sugars act alike. The application of this technology also serves to test in humans hypotheses about regulatory mechanisms that originated in animal models. For example, can the suppressive effect of fructose on hypothalamic cholecystokinin be observed using fMRI?

Future applications of this technology will undoubtedly advance our understanding of these effects and in that way support the need for better approaches to the treatment and prevention of diet-induced obesity.

Acknowledgments

This work was supported in part by grants from the Maryland Agricultural Experiment Station, the Office of the Vice President for Research and USDA Cooperative Agreement # 58-1235-2-112 to TWC.

References

[1] Guyenet SJ, Schwartz MW. Clinical review: regulation of food intake, energy balance, and body fat mass: implications for the pathogenesis and treatment of obesity. J Clin Endocrinol Metab 2012;97:745–55.

[2] Choi YH, Fujikawa T, Lee J, Reuter A, Kim KW. Revisiting the ventral medial nucleus of the hypothalamus: the roles of SF-1 neurons in energy homeostasis. Front Neurosci 2013;7:1–9.

[3] Grill HJ, Hayes MR. Hindbrain neurons as an essential hub in the neuroanatomically distributed control of energy balance. Cell Metab 2012;16:296–309.

[4] Bray GA, Nielsen SJ, Popkin BM. Consumption of high-fructose corn syrup in beverages may play a role in the epidemic of obesity. Am J Clin Nutr 2004;79:537–43.

[5] London E, Castonguay T. High fructose diets increase 11β-hydroxysteroid dehydrogenase type 1 in liver and visceral adipose in rats within 24-h exposure. Obesity (Silver Spring) 2011;19:925–32.

[6] Colley D, London E, Jiang B, Khural J, Castonguay TW. Fructose and the control of food intake. In: Johnston BM, Collins AB, editors. Fructose and the Synthesis, Functions and Health Implications. NY: Nova Science Publishers Hauppage; 2012. pp. 129–43.

[7] Storlein LH, Oakes ND, Pan DA, Kusunoki M, Jenkins AB. Syndromes of insulin resistance in the rat. Inducement by diet and amelioration with benfluorex. Diabetes 1993;42:457–62.

[8] Smeets PA, de Graaf C, Stafleu A, van Osch MJ, van der Grond J. Functional MRI of human hypothalamic responses following glucose ingestion. Neuroimage 2005;24:363–8.

[9] Smeets PA, de Graaf C, Stafleu A, van Osch MJ, Viergever MA, et al. Oral glucose intake inhibits hypothalamic neuronal activity more effectively than glucose infusion. Am J Physiol Endocrinol Metab 2007;293:E754–8.

[10] Lie K, Xu L, Szalkowski D, Li Z, Ding V, Kwei G, et al. Discovery of a potent, highly selective and orally efficacious small-molecule activator of the insulin receptor. J Med Chem 2000;43:3487–94.

[11] Matsuda M, Liu Y, Mahankali S, Pu Y, Mahankali A, Wang J, et al. Altered hypothalamic function in response to glucose ingestion in obese humans. Diabetes 1999;48:1801–6.

[12] Page KA, Chan O, Arora J, Belfort-Deaguiar R, Dzuira J, Roehmholdt B, et al. Effects of fructose vs glucose on regional cerebral blood flow in brain regions involved with appetite and reward pathways fructose consumption and weight gain. JAMA 2013;309:63–70.

[13] Musen G, Simsonson DC, Bolo NR, Driscoll A, Weinger K, Raji A, et al. Regional brain activation during hypoglycemia in type 1 diabetes. J Clin Endocrinol Metab 2008;93:1450–7.

[14] Purnell JQ, Klopfenstein BA, Stevens AA, Havel PJ, Adams SH, Dunn TN, et al. Brain functional magnetic resonance imaging response to glucose and fructose infusions in humans. Diabetes Obes Metab 2011;13:229–34.

[15] Haber SN, Knutson B. The reward circuit: linking primate anatomy and human imaging. Neurophychopharmacology 2010;35:4–26.

[16] D'Adrenne K, McClure SM, Nystrom LE, Cohen JD. BOLD responses reflecting dopaminergic signals in the human ventral tegmental area. Science 2008;319:1264–7.

[17] Knutson B, Cooper JC. Functional magnetic resonance imaging of reward prediction. Curr Opin Neurol 2005;18:411–7.

[18] Carr KD, Tsimberg Y, Berman Y, Yamamoto N. Evidence of increased dopamine receptor signaling in food-restricted rats. Neuroscience 2003;119:1157–67.

[19] Hoebel BG, Hernandez L, McClelland RC, Schwarts D. Dexfenfluramine and feeding reward. ClinNeuropharmacol 1988;11:S72–85.

[20] Avena NM, Rada P, Hoebel BG. Evidence for sugar addiction: behavioral and neurochemical effects intermittent, excessive sugar intake. Neurosci Biobehav Rev 2008;32:20–39.

[21] Colantuoni C, Rada P, McCarthy J, Patten C, Avena NM, Chadeayne A, et al. Evidence that intermittent excessive sugar intake causes endogenous opioid dependence. Obes Res 2002;10:478–88.

[22] Kobayashi M. Functional organization of the human gustatory cortex. J Oral Biosci 2006;48:244–60.

[23] Chandrashekar J, Hoon MA, Ryba NJ, Zuker CS. The receptors and cells for mammalian taste. Nature 2006;444:288–94.

[24] Rolls ET. Taste, olfactory, and food textures processing in the brain, and the control of food intake. Physiol Behav 2005;85:45–56.

[25] Sclafani A. Learned controls of ingestive behaviour. Appetite 1997;29:153–8.

[26] Wu SV, Rozengurt N, Yang M, Young SH, Sinnett-Smith J, Rozengurt E. Expression of bitter taste receptors of the T2R family in the gastrointestinal tract and enteroendocrine STC-1 cells. Proc Natl Acad Sci USA 2002;99:2392–7.

[27] Rozengurt E. Taste receptors in the gastrointestinal tract. I. Bitter taste receptors and alpha-gustducin in the mammalian gut. Am J Physiol Gastrointest Liver Physiol 2006;291:G171–7.

[28] Szalay C, Aradi M, Schwarcz A, Orsi G, Perlaki G, Németh L, et al. Gustatory perception alterations in obesity: an fMRI study. Brain Res 2012;1473:131–40.

[29] Green E, Murphy C. Altered processing of sweet taste in the brain of diet soda drinkers. Physiol Behav 2012;107:560–7.

[30] Killgore WD, Young AD, Femia LA, Bogordzki P, Rogowska J, Yurgelun-Todd DA. Cortical and limbic activation during viewing of high- versus low-calorie foods. Neuroimage 2003;19:1381–94.

[31] Davidson TL, Swithers SE. A Pavlovian approach to the problem of obesity. Intl J Obes Rleat Metab Disord 2004;28:933–5.

[32] Rudenga KJ, Small DM. Amygdala response to sucrose consumption is inversely related to artificial sweetener use. Appetite 2012;58:504–7.

[33] Sclafani A, Clare RA. Female rats show a bimodal preference response to the artificial sweetener sucralose. Chem Senses 2004;29:523–8.

[34] Rabiner EA, Beaver J, Makwana A, Searle G, Long C, Nathan PJ, et al. Pharmacological differentiation of opioid receptor antagonists by molecular and functional imaging of target occupancy and food reward-related brain activation in humans. Mol Psychiatry 2011;16:826–35.

[35] Filbey FM, Myers US, Dewitt S. Rewarding circuit function in high BMI individuals with compulsive overeating: similarities with addiction. Neuroimage 2012;63:1800–6.

[36] Farooqi IS, Bullmore E, Keogh J, Gillard J, O'Rahilly S, Fletcher PC. Leptin regulates striatal regions and human eating behavior. Science 2007;317:1355.

[37] Stoeckel LE, Weller RE, Cook 3rd EW, Tweig DB, Knowlton RC, Cox JE. Widespread reward-system activation in obese women in response to pictures of high-calorie foods. Neuroimage 2008;41:636–47.

PART F

DIETARY SUPPLEMENTS AND VISCERAL OBESITY

CHAPTER

29

Flaxseed Secoisolariciresinol Diglucoside and Visceral Obesity

A Closer Look at its Chemical Properties, Absorption, Metabolism, Bioavailability, and Effects on Visceral Fat, Lipid Profile, Systemic Inflammation, and Hypertension

Jae B. Park

Diet, Genomics, and Immunology Laboratory, Beltsville Human Nutrition Research Center, United States Department of Agriculture, Agricultural Research Service, Beltsville, MD, USA

INTRODUCTION

Linum usitatissimum (flax), which belongs to the Linaceae family, is an important flowering crop that is cultivated worldwide. Although the genus *Linum* consists of more than 100 species, *L. usitatissimum* (flax) has long been considered as a valuable agricultural crop plant due to the production of oil, fiber, lignan, and other products [1–3]. Traditionally, flax products and compounds have also been prescribed for treating several human chronic diseases such as diabetes, high cholesterol, cardiovascular diseases, and related conditions [4–7]. Although flaxseed contains various bioactive compounds, it contains a relatively high amount of lignans such as secoisolariciresinol diglucoside (SDG), which has been reported to have numerous biological activities and health benefits [8–13]. Obesity is a serious, rampant health problem closely associated with multiple contributing factors such as unhealthy or unbalanced diets, a sedentary lifestyle, and genetic factors [14–16]. Obesity causes many physiological changes in humans; visceral obesity, manifested by increased adiposity around the waist, is a hallmark physical change [17–19]. In fact, visceral obesity is strongly associated with the development and progression of several chronic diseases such as diabetes, cardiovascular diseases, hypertension, and kidney diseases [20–26]. In the marketplace, many flaxseed-related products are currently available. SDG lignan-enriched flaxseed powder was recently introduced as a dietary ingredient in the marketplace, but the potential effects of the powder on obesity and hypertension have not been examined in detail. Therefore, in this chapter, the potential effects of SDG lignan-enriched flaxseed powder on obesity are reviewed via closely examining the chemical properties, absorption, metabolism, and bioavailability of SDG, as well as its effects on body weight, visceral fat, lipid profiles, systemic inflammation, and blood pressure. Particularly, the potential effects of SDG lignan powder on systemic inflammation induced by adipokines are thoroughly reviewed because increased adiposity is closely associated with systemic inflammation manifested by increased production of cytokines [C-C motif chemokine 2/monocyte chemoattractant protein 1 (MCP-1), interleukin-6 (IL-6), and tumor necrosis factor (TNF-α)], as well as decreased production of anti-inflammatory and antidiabetic adiponectin [27–33]. The overall aim of this review is to provide scientific information to enable a better understanding of the potential effects of SDG on obesity and its related conditions.

FLAXSEED CHEMICALS

The nutritional composition of flaxseed is about 30% carbohydrate, 18% protein, and 39% fat [34–35]. Most of the carbohydrate in flaxseed is in the form of fiber and more than 45% of the oil comprises omega-3 fatty acids [34]. Other compounds include coumaric acid ferulic acid glucoside, glucoside, herbacetin diglucoside,

Nutrition in the Prevention and Treatment of Abdominal Obesity
http://dx.doi.org/10.1016/B978-0-12-407869-7.00029-5

TABLE 29.1 Composition of Flaxseed Products

	Flaxseed	Flaxseed Oil	Defatted Flaxseed	SDG Powder[a]
Carbohydrate	30%	–	48%	–
Fiber	27%	–	45%	–
Protein	18%	–	30%	–
Fat	39%	100%	<3%	–
Lignan	0.3%	–	0.4%	<35%

Source: Data were taken from Refs [34,35].
[a]*Indicates SDG-enriched powder used in [66].*
–, amounts are negligible or unknown.

lariciresinol, matairesinol, pinoresinol, and secoisolariciresinol (Table 29.1) [35]. Currently, many flaxseed products such as whole flaxseeds, milled flaxseeds, flaxseed oil, (defatted) flaxseed cakes, and lignan-enriched flaxseed powder are available on the market. Among them, SDG lignan-enriched flaxseed powder is a relatively new flaxseed product. As shown in Table 29.1, SDG-enriched powder contains approximately 35% SDG complex, with 15.1% coumaric acid glucoside, 8.1% ferulic acid glucoside, and 15.6% hydroxymethylglutaric acid [35].

Since any potential effects of SDG should be understood within the context of its chemical properties, absorption, and metabolism, these topics are reviewed first.

CHEMICAL PROPERTIES, ABSORPTION, AND METABOLISM OF SECOISOLARICIRESINOL DIGLUCOSIDE

Lignans belong to a class of diphenolic compounds that occur widely in nature, which are often classified into several major subgroups: dibenzocyclooctadiene-type, dibenzylbutane-type, dibenzylbutyrolactone-type, naphthalene-type, neo-type tetrahydrofuran-type, and tetralin-type lignans. In plants; lignans are synthesized from phenylpropanoic acids (caffeic, cinnamic, coumaric, and ferulic acids) via oxidative coupling and other processes [36]. As shown in Table 29.2, lignans are found in a variety of food sources [37–39].

Among the lignans, SDG (empirical formula, $C_{32}H_{46}O_{16}$; molecular weight, 686.7) is a dibenzylbutane-type lignan and a major lignan component in flaxseed products [38–39]. The total proportion of lignans in flaxseeds is about 0.335%, and most are in the form of secoisolariciresinol (SECO; 0.32%) [1]. In flaxseeds, SECO (empirical formula, $C_{20}H_{26}O_6$; molecular weight, 362.4) is synthesized via a radical-initiated dimerization process that converts coniferyl alcohols to pinoresinol (PINO), which is then converted into a dibenzylbutane-type SECO (Fig. 29.1) [36]. SECO is then glycosylated into SDG by the addition of UDP-glucose (Fig. 29.1) [40].

After SDG intake, the lignan is believed to be deglycosylated in the small intestine by glucosidase, either in the brush border of the gut mucosa or in gut bacteria, back into SECO. SECO is then converted by the gut microflora into mammalian lignans such as enterodiol

TABLE 29.2 Amounts of Lignans in Plant Sources[a]

Sources	SECO	MATA	LARI	PINO
Seeds/Grains				
Flax	323.6	5.202	3.670	2.460
Sesame	0.014	0.734	5.389	25.88
Wheat	0.035	0.003	0.062	0.037
Barley	0.030	0.003	0.085	0.072
Rye	0.038	0.027	0.324	0.381
Oat	0.019	0.071	0.018	0.019
Rice	0.003	0.002	0.028	0.007
Vegetables				
Broccoli	0.038	–	0.970	0.310
Garlic	0.050	–	0.280	0.200
French bean	0.028	–	0220	0.022
Carrot	0.092	–	0.060	0.018
Pumpkin	0.971	0.003	3.913	0.235
Asparagus	0.183	0.002	0.047	0.049
Eggplant	0.005	–	0.068	0.028
Fruits				
Strawberry	2.305	0.005	0.970	0.817
Lingonberry	1.402	0.005	0.308	2.625
Mango	0.265	0.011	0.561	0.080
Kiwi	0.116	–	0.010	0.008
Avocado	0.081	0.011	0.076	0.494
Grape	0.032	–	0.037	0.028
Orange	0.011	–	0.019	0.009
Pineapple	0.007	0.010	0.067	0.004
Lemon	0.004	–	0.025	0.185
Tomato	0.001	–	0.011	0.005

Source: Data were taken from Refs [1,38].
[a]*In mg/100 g*
–, amounts are negligible or unknown. LARI, lariciresinol; MATA, matairesinol; PINO, pinoresinol; SECO, secoisolariciresinol.

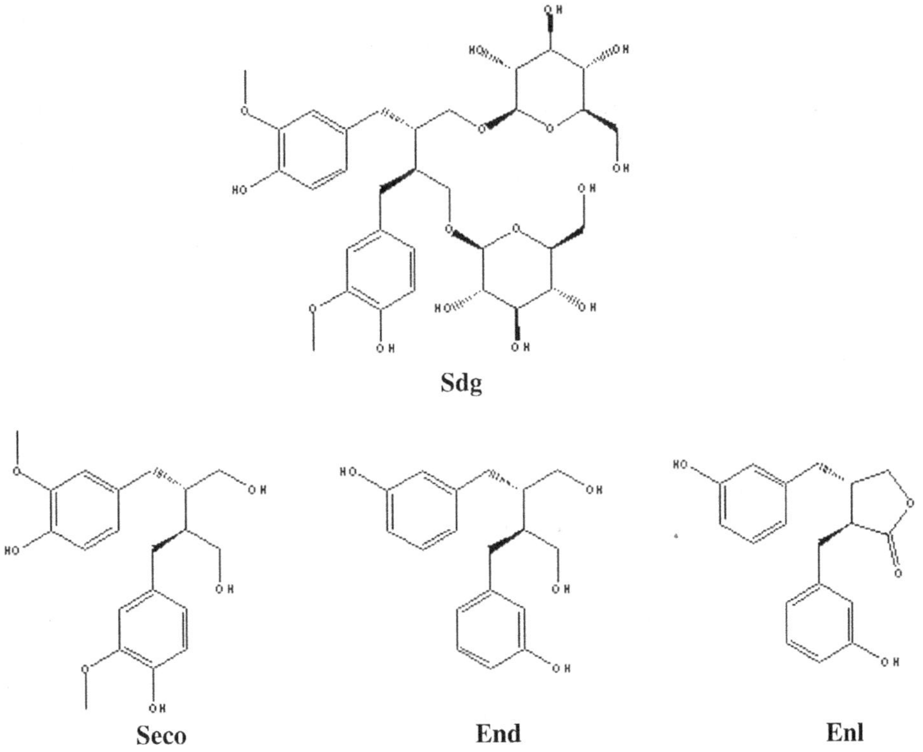

FIGURE 29.1 **Chemical structures.** END, enterodiol; ENL, enterolactone; SDG, secoisolariciresinol diglucoside; SECO, secoisolariciresinol.

(END; empirical formula, $C_{18}H_{22}O^4$; molecular weight, 302.3) and enterolactone (ENL; empirical formula, $C_{18}H_{18}O_4$; molecular weight, 298.3) probably via multiple processes including demethylation, dehydroxylation, and dehydrogenation (Fig. 29.1) [41,42]. ENL and END generated in the intestine are then absorbed into the bloodstream and reach the liver, where they may be conjugated with glucuronic acid or sulfate [43]. In fact, most of ENL and END appear as conjugates in various body fluids in humans and animals [44,45], and the main END and ENL metabolites found in plasma and urine are glucuronide conjugates [45–47]. In addition it is possible for oxidative metabolism of ENL and END to occur in liver microsomes, whereby additional hydroxylation is added to the *para* and *ortho* positions of the original hydroxy position in the phenolic moiety [43]. From the antioxidant perspective, these hydroxylation processes may be important because ENL and END then contain a catechol-like structure that can be reversibly oxidized to an *O*-quinone structure upon oxidation. In fact, a catechol-like structure is usually found in well-known antioxidant compounds, and is believed to be involved in scavenging the radical oxygen species (ROS) generated in cells. Another property of enterolignans (ELs; including ENL and END) is that they are relatively stable in biological fluids. Therefore, they are commonly used as biomarkers, as described below [48].

BIOAVAILABILITY OF SECOISOLARICIRESINOL DIGLUCOSIDE

Bioavailability is the term used to describe the physiological availability of a compound in a given amount; it depends mainly on the amount initially administered, as well as absorption, metabolism, tissue distribution, and excretion. Studies often use several different doses and different administration routes to determine the bioavailability of a compound. To evaluate the potential effects of SDG on human health, it is critical to determine its bioavailability. As mentioned above, due to its relative stability in biological fluids, EL is commonly used as a biomarker for determining SDG bioavailability [49]. Several reported bioavailability studies are worth examining. First, SDG bioavailability was investigated in healthy human subjects who consumed 30 g milled flaxseeds (equivalent to 90 mg SDG lignan) daily for 4 weeks. This study reported that the total EL concentration was about 513 nM, and average END and ENL concentrations were 209 nM and 304 nM, respectively [49,50]. Another human study investigated the possible effects of different types of flaxseed products (whole flaxseed, crushed flaxseed, and ground flaxseed) on SDG lignan bioavailability. In this study, the total EL concentration of ELs was approximately 270 nM, and average concentrations of END and ENL were 103 nM and 167 nM, respective, following the consumption of about 20 g ground flaxseed (equivalent to 60 mg lignan) [51]. The latter study also reported that plasma EL concentrations following the consumption of crushed flaxseed and whole flaxseed were lower than those observed in the ground flaxseed group. Data showed that the relative bioavailability of ELs from whole flaxseed was about 28% that of ground flaxseed, whereas the relative bioavailability of ELs from crushed flaxseeds was about 43% [51]. Although a number of studies have clearly shown that the intake of lignan-rich foods leads to increased plasma EL levels in most subjects, there are growing concerns that the bioavailability of ELs may be significantly influenced by food matrix, gut microbial action, and other factors, thereby being subject to large interpersonal, foodstuff-derived, and other variations. For examples, a continuous increase serum EL concentration was observed over a 4-month intervention with flaxseed (33, 52, and 70 nM at baseline and after 2 and 4 months, respectively) [52]. In another study, a dose-response urinary excretion of SDG metabolites was reported (with no plateau) after the daily consumption of 5, 15, and 25 g flaxseed products for 7 days [53]. These data indicate that the amount of ELs produced by intestinal bacteria may increase linearly, but that blood levels of ELs may largely depend on an individual-specific threshold, caused by adaptation to metabolic and excretory mechanisms. This indicates that future intervention studies in human subjects should comprehensively assess the effects of several different lignan concentrations on the digestive system, blood, and urine. As noted, variations and individual limitations in EL concentrations are expected; this point should be considered when interpreting potential in vivo biological activities.

EFFECTS OF SECOISOLARICIRESINOL DIGLUCOSIDE ON OBESITY AND LEVELS OF REACTIVE OXYGEN SPECIES

So far, we have looked at the chemical properties, absorption, metabolism, and bioavailability of SDG. Now, it is time to turn our attention to the potential effects of SDG on obesity because (1) obesity is a serious global health problem affecting many people and (2) flaxseed products have often been used to treat obesity-related conditions [14–18]. In fact, obesity is a result of multiple contributing factors such as unhealthy or unbalanced diets, eating habits, lifestyle, and genetic factors [14,15]. Particularly, modern sedentary lifestyles, lack of exercise, and/or unhealthy diets that often contain high levels of daily calories have been blamed for the increase in obesity worldwide [16–18]. Although obesity is associated with many physiological changes, visceral obesity is a noticeable physical change that is strongly associated with "bad" lipid profiles and low-level systemic inflammation, which are the main causes of the development and progression of several chronic diseases including diabetes, cardiovascular diseases, hypertension, and kidney disease [16–19]. Although the cellular and molecular events related to obesity are still being elucidated, a high-calorie diet coupled with the lack of physical activity is believed to be a leading cause of the increased body weight associated with significant visceral fat accumulation, high triglyceride and cholesterol levels, and systemic inflammation (Fig. 29.2) [20–23]. Currently, there are only a limited number of studies relating the effects of SDG on body weight, particularly in humans. Therefore, more studies should be performed in the future to determine the potential effects and mechanisms of SDG in obesity. Nonetheless, there are some reports that flaxseed compounds including SDG possess a broad spectrum of biological properties, thus paving the way to endorsing their positive effects on risk factors associated with several obesity-related chronic diseases such as diabetes, cardiovascular diseases, and hypertension [4,6,7,14–17,54,55]. In fact, some epidemiological studies also suggest that flaxseeds containing SDG may protect against obesity-related diseases [17–19]. As mentioned previously, SDG and its mammalian metabolites (SECO, END, and ENL) have good antioxidant properties [56].

Oxidative stress is a major concern in obesity because increased levels are seen in obese subjects; these are considered to be a major cause of diabetes, cardiovascular disease, hypertension, kidney disease, and neuronal disorders [57,58]. Oxidative stress is mainly caused by ROS, produced as normal or abnormal by-products from several sources such as mitochondria, xanthine oxidase, and NADPH oxidase [59,60]. Along with insufficient antioxidant defense systems and/or some types of disease conditions, elevated ROS can cause grave damage to cellular components such as carbohydrates, lipids, proteins, and DNA, thus leading to homeostatic changes, cellular transformation, and/or apoptosis [61,62]. SDG is reported to restore antioxidant capacity in diabetic rats and to deliver positive effects on obesity in mice fed a high-fat diet [63,64]. The latter study showed that both oral administration of (−)-SECO and subcutaneous injection of SECO significantly suppressed the gain of body weight in mice [64]. Also, the subcutaneous injection of (−)-SECO, (−)-END, or (−)-ENL was reported to upregulate the expression of several genes such as those encoding acyl-CoA oxidase (ACO), carnitine *O*-palmitoyltransferase 1 (CPT-1; encoded by *Cpt1b*), and peroxisome proliferator-activated receptor alpha (PPAR-α), suggesting that (−)-SECO may be able to reduce body weight gain in mice fed a high-fat diet, possibly by inducing changes the expression of genes related to fatty acid synthesis and beta-oxidation [64,65]. Similarly, our study showed that 0.02% SDG-enriched flaxseed power (SEFP) was effective in reducing body weight in rats [66]. In this study, after feeding a control, a high-fat diet, or a high-fat diet containing SEFP (equivalent to 200 mg/day in body weight of 60 kg) for 12 weeks, the body weight of rats fed the high-fat diet containing SEFP was comparable to those on the control diet and significantly lower than that of rats fed the high-fat diet, although the initial body weights and feed intakes of rats in the three groups were similar. In other words, body weight gain per day was significantly lower in rats fed both the control and the high-fat diet supplemented with SEFP compared to those fed the high-fat diet alone. These data indicates that SDG supplementation may have positive effects on body weight reduction in rats fed a high-fat diet. Although these data are limited, a human study also reported that the daily consumption of a flaxseed lignan complex (600 mg SDG) for 3 months leads to a reduction of abdominal fat accumulation along with other benefits in older type 2 diabetics [67]. However, the potential effects of SDG on body weight reduction are still limited, so more studies should be performed in the future.

EFFECTS OF SECOISOLARICIRESINOL DIGLUCOSIDE ON ADIPOSE TISSUES

If SDG is truly able to suppress body weight gain, then this may result mainly from a reduction in adipose tissue, because adipose tissues are major sites of fat storage that contribute to nonmuscular body weight gain (Fig. 29.2). In an in vitro study, (−)-SECO was reported to reduce lipid accumulation in adipocytic 3T3-L1 cells [68]. In this study, mRNA expression of adipogenesis-related genes and DNA-binding activity of PPAR-γ to

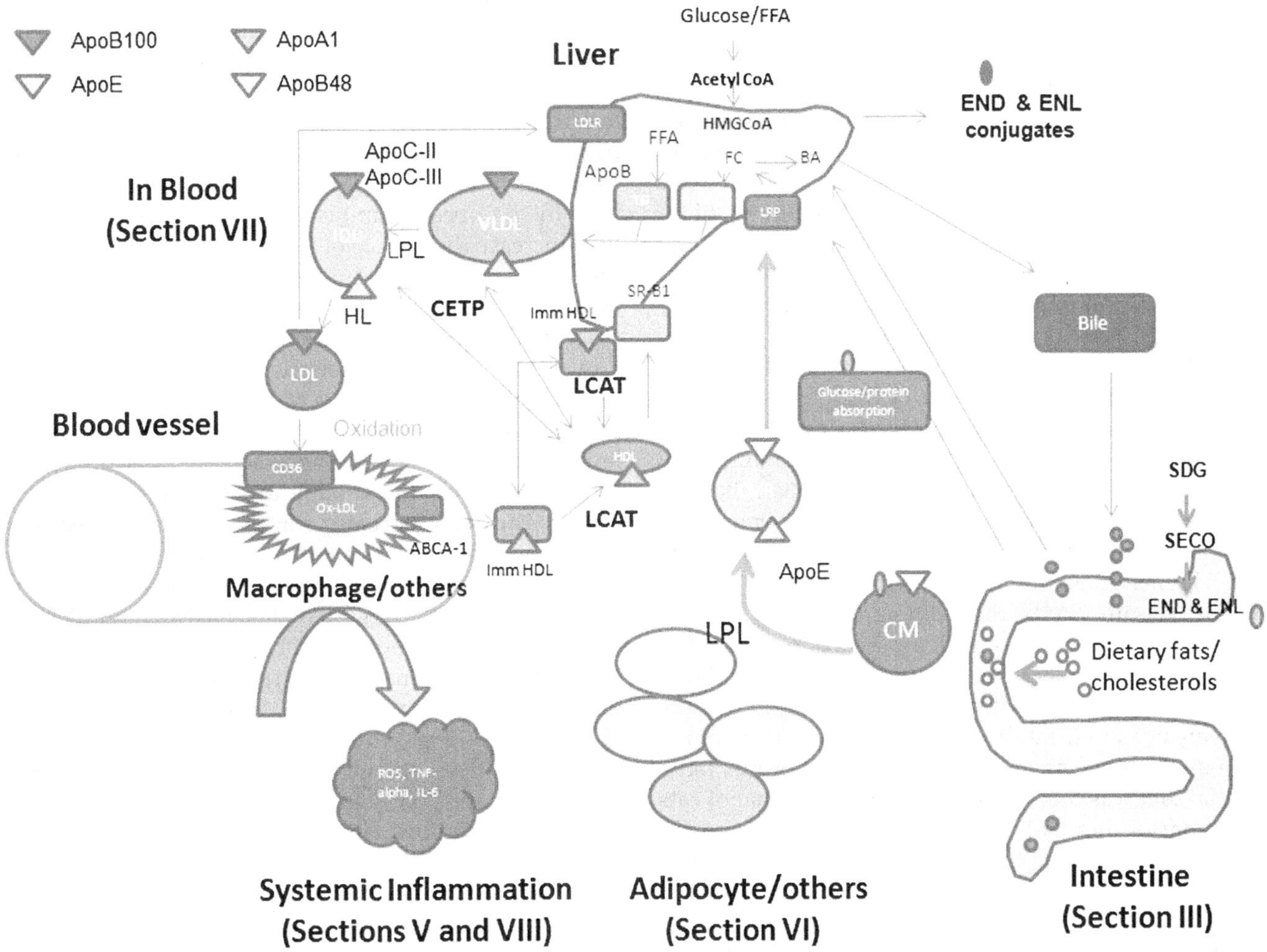

FIGURE 29.2 Diagram of lignan, cholesterol, and lipid absorption, cholesterol metabolism, and systemic inflammation. BA, bile acids; CETP, cholesteryl ester transfer protein; CM, chylomicrons; CMR, chylomicron remnants; END, enterodiol; ENL, enterolactone; FFA, free fatty acids; FC, free cholesterol; HDL, high-density lipoprotein; HL, hepatic lipase; Imm, inner mitochondrial membrane; LCAT, lecithin cholesterol acyl transferase; LPL, lipoprotein lipase; LRP, lipoprotein receptor-related proteins; Ox-LDL, oxidized low-density lipoprotein; SDG, secoisolariciresinol diglucoside; SECO, secoisolariciresinol. (See color plate at the back of the book.)

PPAR response elements were investigated in differentiated 3T3-L1 adipocytes treated with several doses of END. END induced the mRNA expression of several adipogenesis-related genes, such as those encoding adiponectin, leptin, solute carrier family 2, facilitated glucose transporter member 4 (GLUT4), and PPAR-γ, and also increased the DNA-binding activity of PPAR-γ to the PPAR response sequence [68]. These in vitro data are supported to some extent by an in vivo study showing that (−)-SECO has positive effects on obesity in C57BL/6 male mice fed a high-fat diet, even though this study did not specifically investigate effects on adipose tissue [64]. As mentioned previously, subcutaneous injection of (−)-SECO increases the expression of genes related to fat metabolism, suggesting that this lignan may suppress fat accumulation in adipocytes via altering the gene expression of various enzymes related to fatty acid synthesis and beta-oxidation. In another study, body weight, visceral fat weight, liver fat content, and other parameters were investigated in mice fed a low-fat diet (5%), a high-fat diet (30%), or high-fat diet containing 0.5% and 1.0% SDG for 4 weeks. In this study, SDG significantly reduced high-fat diet-induced visceral and liver fat accumulation [68]. Likewise, our study showed that a high-fat diet was clearly a major factor in obesity in rats; the high-fat diet increased the average rat body weight by 10% more than the control diet and the high-fat diet containing SEFP. Therefore, in this study, the fat sources contributing to body weight gain were investigated by measuring the weights of the major organs (liver, heart, and kidney) and adiposes tissues (epididymal, subdiaphragmatic, and visceral) [66]. Although no significant change in the weight of hearts was found in any of the three groups, the average liver weight of rats fed the high-fat diet and high-fat diet containing SEFP were slightly but not significantly higher than those of rats fed a control diet [66]. However, the average kidney weight of rats fed the high-fat diet were significantly (20%) higher than those of rates fed the control diet [66]. In the same study, three different types of adipose fats were also measured and compared as potential fat-contributing sources of body weight gain. Although the average weights of epididymal and subdiaphragmatic fats were not significantly different in rats fed any of the three diets, the average visceral fat weight of rats fed a high-fat diet was more than 40% higher than that of rats fed a control diet [66]. However, the increased weight was reduced by more than 40% in rats fed the high-fat diet containing SEFP. Similarly, the average weight of combined adipose fats (epididymal, subdiaphragmatic, and visceral) from rats fed a high-fat diet was 27% higher than in rats fed a control diet, but the average weight was reduced by more than 50% in rats fed the high-fat diet containing SEFP. These data indicate that rats fed both a high-fat diet and a high-fat diet containing SEFP gained weight particularly in visceral fat, but that SDG lignan supplementation significantly lowered the average visceral fat weight. Since rat visceral fat is considered to be equivalent to abdominal fat in humans, these data suggest that SDG supplementation may alleviate central obesity-related conditions in humans. However, there is still limited information about changes in fat accumulation in human adipose tissues and organs, although SDG has been reported to have some positive effects on central obesity.

EFFECTS OF SECOISOLARICIRESINOL DIGLUCOSIDE ON PLASMA LIPIDS AND CHOLESTEROLS

Hyperlipidemia and hypercholesterolemia are often associated with the onset of obesity, leading to the initiation and progression of several chronic diseases such as atherosclerosis and cardiovascular disease (Fig. 29.2) [69]. In humans, dyslipidemia is manifested by high total cholesterol (TC; >240 mg/dL), low high-density lipoprotein cholesterol (HDLc; <40 mg/dL), high low-density lipoprotein cholesterol (LDLc; >160 mg/dL), and high triglyceride (>200 mg/dL) levels, all of which are significant contributors to plaque formation in blood vessels [69]. In the obese, diminished antioxidants and rising ROS increase the chance of LDL oxidation, thus promoting the increased production of the proinflammatory cytokines IL-6, TNF-α, and others (Fig. 29.2), which are associated with the progressions of atherosclerosis, cardiovascular disease, hypertension, and kidney disease [58]. In animal studies, dietary flaxseed supplementation was associated with significant reductions in plasma TC levels and TC:HDLc ratio and increased plasma HDLc, compared to animals without the supplementation [70,71]. The first report also pointed out that flaxseed significantly reduced hepatic cholesterol and triglyceride levels in chemically induced diabetic hamsters [70], and the second report suggested that flaxseed supplementation has positive effects on hypertriglyceridemia and hypercholesterolemia in SHR rats, although the effects were not solely derived from SDG [71]. In a rabbit model, similar results were obtained: rabbits fed CDC-flaxseed (i.e. type II flaxseed) with a very low omega-linolenic acid content for 4-8 weeks showed lower plasma TC and LDLc concentrations [54]. Similarly, SDG supplementation was reported to reduce hyperlipemia, hypercholesterolemia, hyperinsulinemia, and hyperleptinemia in mice fed a high-fat diet [68]. In this study, SDG also suppressed the expression of info *Srebf1* mRNA (encoding sterol response element-binding protein 1c (SREBP-1c)] in the liver and increased the expression of *Cpt1b* mRNA in the skeletal muscle [68]. Our study showed similar results: plasma triglycerides and LDL concentrations in rats fed a high-fat diet containing SEFP were lower than in those fed a high-fat diet and similar to in those on a control diet [66]. In addition SDG supplementation restored plasma HDL concentration in rats fed a high-fat diet containing SEFP, indicating that supplementation may improve serum LDL and HDL levels and increase the HDL:TC ratio [66]. These data suggest that SDG supplementation may improve the plasma lipid profile in animals, compared to those fed on a high-fat diet alone. Dyslipidemia is also profoundly associated with obesity in humans [69]. In a human study, diets supplemented with partially defatted flaxseed were reported to lower TC and LDLc, possibly due to the fiber and other components present in defatted flaxseed [72]. However, this study hinted that the hypocholesterolemic effect may be attributed to flaxseed components other than omega-linolenic acid (such as SDG) because partially defatted flaxseed is low in this fatty acid. This hypothesis is actually supported by another human study reporting that SDG (600 mg/day for 8 days) decreases cholesterol, LDL, and TC levels in humans with hypercholesterolemia and hypertriglyceridemia [73]. However, human studies often provided contradictory or outcomes showing no effect. For example, SDG (20 mg/day for 12 weeks) was reported to have no effect on lipid parameters, and only a small drop in the LDL:HDL ratio [10]. Another human study reported that although flaxseed may be able to reduce circulating TC and LDLc concentrations, these changes were often dependent on the type of intervention, gender, and initial lipid profiles of the subjects participating in the study [74]. Therefore, more studies are required to determine the dose-dependent efficiency of SDG on lipid profiles in men and women in order to determine its potential benefits in obesity.

EFFECTS OF SECOISOLARICIRESINOL DIGLUCOSIDE ON ADIPONECTIN, TNF-α, IL-6, AND SYSTEMIC INFLAMMATION

As discussed above, obesity is often associated with dyslipidemia and hypercholesterolemia. Excessive fats and cholesterols in the obese often accumulate in adipocytes and other cells (Fig. 29.2). Besides their fat-storage capacity, adipose tissues can produce a wide range of hormones and cytokines such as adiponectin, leptin, IL-6, and TNF-α as a result of adipocyte hypertrophy, and these molecules greatly affect the metabolism and function of many organs and tissues including muscle, liver, vasculature, kidney, and brain [28,30]. Leptin is considered to be a key signaling molecule in communicating long-term nutritional and fat mass status to the brain (hypothalamus), and its production is remarkably increased in large adipocytes [27,75,76]. Like leptin, adiponectin is an adipocyte-derived hormone with antidiabetic, anti-atherogenic, and anti-inflammatory functions. However, plasma adiponectin decreases with obesity and insulin resistance. In an in vitro study, (−)-SECO was reported to reduce lipid accumulation and induce adiponectin production in 3T3-L1 adipocytes [65]. In another study, lignan was also reported to increase the expression of adiponectin mRNA in white adipose tissue [10]. Similarly, in our animal study, average plasma adiponectin levels in the control group were higher than those in the high-fat group, and the average plasma adiponectin levels in rats fed a high-fat diet containing SEFP were slightly higher than those in rats fed a high-fat diet, indicating that the supplementation can increase adiponectin levels to those found in the control group [66]. In the same study, the levels of inflammatory cytokines such as IL-6 and TNF-α were also investigated. TNF-α is a cytokine that is critically involved in normal host resistance to infection and to the growth of malignant tumors; it is produced by activated macrophages and other cell types such as T and B cells, natural killer cells, endothelial cells, and muscle cells [77–79]. In fact, macrophages are more prevalent in the adipose tissue of obese subjects than in lean subjects, and macrophage quantity correlates well with the severity of insulin resistance and obesity [77]. However, in our study, no significant difference in plasma TNF-α level was observed among all three groups. IL-6 is another inflammatory cytokine related to obesity that is involved in the acute-phase reactions, inflammation, hematopoiesis, and cancer [27,80,81]. Like TNF-α, IL-6 levels are often higher in obese subjects than in lean subjects [27]. However, no significant change in IL-6 levels was observed among all three groups. These observations are actually consistent with other studies, indicating that changes in the levels of these two molecules (IL-6 and TNF-α) are not often followed by a moderate body weight gain [82–84]. Therefore, it is likely that the level of obesity plays a critical role in changing the expression of inflammatory cytokines. In a human study, C-reactive protein (CRP), IL-6, thiobarbituric acid reactive substance (TBARS), and TNF-α levels and homeostatic model assessment of insulin resistance (HOMA-IR) were measured before and after a daily intake of 40 g ground flaxseed (equivalent to 120 mg SDG) for 3 months. This study showed that flaxseed supplementation decreased TBARS and HOMA-IR, although the flaxseed supplement in this study included more components than SDG alone. In another human study, flaxseed lignan complex (about 600 mg SDG/day) for 3 months was reported to reduce central obesity, dyslipidemia, and inflammation, although the levels of adiponectin, leptin, IL-6, and TNF-α were not specifically investigated [67]. In addition the daily consumption of a low-fat muffin enriched with a lignan complex for 6 weeks may reduce CRP concentrations compared to a low-fat muffin without supplementation, although no data about

IL-6 and TNF-α were reported [85]. Taken together, the evidence shows that SDG supplementation is likely to attenuate systemic inflammation via lowering inflammatory cytokine levels. However, further comprehensive studies should be conducted in order to fully determine its effects on systemic inflammation in humans.

EFFECTS OF SECOISOLARICIRESINOL DIGLUCOSIDE ON OBESITY-RELATED HYPERTENSION

As discussed, obesity and hypertension (high blood pressure) are strongly correlated, indicating that a small amount of weight loss may significantly lower blood pressure, despite the cause of hypertension in obesity being complex and multifactorial [86,87]. Hypertension is a serious widespread health condition. Left untreated, hypertension leads to severe damage to many organs, eventually causing organ failure in the heart, lung, kidneys, and brain [88]. Therefore, weight reduction is strongly recommended to improve hypertension and related conditions in humans. In fact, weight loss is highly recommended in the obese, and commonly results in improved lipid profile, insulin sensitivity, as well as heart, lung, and kidney function [89,90]. In our animal study, significant body weight reduction and a moderate reduction in systolic blood pressure were observed in rats fed a high-fat diet containing SEFP compared to rats fed a high-fat diet alone, even though the average blood pressure of rats fed a high-fat diet containing SEFP remained higher than that of the control group [66]. However, we did not observe any significant change in diastolic blood pressure among all three groups. These data indicate that SDG supplementation may lower systolic blood pressure in the rats fed a high-fat diet containing SEFP compared to rats fed a high-fat diet alone. Although no specific mechanism is known to be involved in this effect, improved endothelial dysfunction by SDG antioxidant activity was suggested as a possible mechanism. This is echoed by a previous study showing that a high-flaxseed diet improves endothelial vascular relaxation through a pressure-independent mechanism in spontaneously hypertensive rats [91]. Regarding the potential effects of SDG on hypertension, few reports are currently available. However, one human study reported that daily consumption of flaxseed lignan complex (about 600 mg SDG) for 3 months reduced blood pressure along with improvements in other areas such as central obesity, hyperglycemia, dyslipidemia, and LDL oxidation [67]. Another human study suggested that flaxseed omega-3 polyunsaturated fatty acid may prevent hypertension induced by its deficiency, although this was not directly linked to SDG [92]. Another report indicates effects of flaxseed peptide mixture on hypertension [93]: a flaxseed peptide mixture prepared from flaxseed protein hydrolysates was reported to have antihypertensive properties by inhibiting angiotensin-converting enzyme (ACE) [93]. With respect to nitric oxide (NO) production, a report indicates that cationic protein hydrolysate fractions may reduce activity of calmodulin-dependent endothelial NO synthase (eNOS) in vitro [94]. Again, all these data provide only limited information about the potential effects of SDG on hypertension, and more studies are required in the future.

CONCLUSION

In this chapter, we have taken a close look at the potential health benefits of SDG on obesity, body weight, visceral fat, lipid profile, systemic inflammation, and hypertension. As mentioned, the overall effects of SDG on obesity should be interpreted and understood as part of a comprehensive milieu because (1) obesity is closely clustered with other chronic diseases such as diabetes, cardiovascular disease, and kidney disease and (2) most flaxseed products available on the market may contain other components in addition to SDG such as fiber and omega-3 fatty acid (e.g. α-linolenic acid). Therefore, potential effects of flaxseed products should be evaluated and validated in a broad setting, including potential effects of active ingredients and pre-existing disease conditions. Nonetheless, this review provides valuable information about the potential health benefits of SDG on body weight, visceral fat, lipid profile, systemic inflammation, and blood pressure obtained from both in vitro and in vivo models.

Acknowledgments

The mention of trade names or commercial products in this chapter is solely for the purpose of providing specific information and does not imply recommendation or endorsement by the U.S. Department of Agriculture.

The USDA is an equal opportunity provider and employer.

References

[1] Adlercreutz H. Lignans and human health. Crit Rev Clin Lab Sci 2007;44:483–525.

[2] Singh KK, Mridula D, Rehal J, Barnwal P. Flaxseed: a potential source of food, feed and fiber. Crit Rev Food Sci Nutr 2011;51:210–22.

[3] Basch E, Bent S, Collins J, Dacey C, Hammerness P, Harrison M, et al. Natural standard resource collaboration. Flax and flaxseed oil (*Linum usitatissimum*): a review by the Natural standard research collaboration. J Soc Integr Oncol 2007;5:92–105.

[4] Rhee Y, Brunt A. Flaxseed supplementation improved insulin resistance in obese glucose intolerant people: a randomized crossover design. Nutr J 2011;10:44.

[5] Prasad K. Flaxseed and cardiovascular health. J Cardiovasc Pharmacol 2009;54:369–77.

[6] Thakur G, Mitra A, Pal K, Rousseau D. Effect of flaxseed gum on reduction of blood glucose and cholesterol in type 2 diabetic patients. Int J Food Sci Nutr 2009;22:1–11.

[7] Rodriguez-Leyva D, Dupasquier CM, McCullough R, Pierce GN. The cardiovascular effects of flaxseed and its omega-3 fatty acid, alpha-linolenic acid. Can J Cardiol 2010;26:489–96.

[8] Adolphe JL, Whiting SJ, Juurlink BH, Thorpe LU, Alcorn J. Health effects with consumption of the flax lignan secoisolariciresinol diglucoside. Br J Nutr 2010;103:929–38.

[9] Hu C, Yuan YV, Kitts DD. Antioxidant activities of the flaxseed lignan secoisolariciresinol diglucoside, its aglycone secoisolariciresinol and the mammalian lignans enterodiol and enterolactone in vitro. Food Chem Toxicol 2007;45:2219–27.

[10] Fukumitsu S, Aida K, Shimizu H, Toyoda K. Flaxseed lignan lowers blood cholesterol and decreases liver disease risk factors in moderately hypercholesterolemic men. Nutr Res 2010;30:441–6.

[11] Felmlee MA, Woo G, Simko E, Krol ES, Muir AD, Alcorn J. Effects of the flaxseed lignans secoisolariciresinol diglucoside and its aglycone on serum and hepatic lipids in hyperlipidaemic rats. Br J Nutr 2009;102:361–9.

[12] Zhang W, Wang X, Liu Y, Tian H, Flickinger B, Empie MW, et al. Effects of dietary flaxseed lignan extract on symptoms of benign prostatic hyperplasia. J Med Food 2008;11:207–14.

[13] Penumathsa SV, Koneru S, Thirunavukkarasu M, Zhan L, Prasad K, Maulik N. Secoisolariciresinol diglucoside: relevance to angiogenesis and cardioprotection against ischemia-reperfusion injury. J Pharmacol Exp Ther 2007;320:951–9.

[14] Hill JO, Peters JC. Environmental contributions to the obesity epidemic. Science 1998;280:1371–4.

[15] Schrauwen P, Westerterp KR. The role of high-fat diets and physical activity in the regulation of body weight. Br J Nutr 2000;84:417–27.

[16] Hamilton MT, Hamilton DG, Zderic TW. Role of low energy expenditure and sitting in obesity, metabolic syndrome, type 2 diabetes, and cardiovascular disease. Diabetes 2007;56:2655–67.

[17] Misra A, Singhal N, Khurana L. Obesity, the metabolic syndrome, and type 2 diabetes in developing countries: role of dietary fats and oils. J Am Coll Nutr 2010;29:289. S–301. S.

[18] Ritchie SA, Connell JM. The link between abdominal obesity, metabolic syndrome and cardiovascular disease. Nutr Metab Cardiovasc Dis 2007;17:319–26.

[19] Tailor AM, Peeters PH, Norat T, Vineis P, Romaguera D. An update on the prevalence of the metabolic syndrome in children and adolescents. Int J Pediatr Obes 2010;5:202–13.

[20] Natali A, Pucci G, Boldrini B, Schillaci G. Metabolic syndrome: at the crossroads of cardiorenal risk. J Nephrol 2009;22:29–38.

[21] Guize L, Pannier B, Thomas F, Bean K, Jégo B, Benetos A. Recent advances in metabolic syndrome and cardiovascular disease. Arch Cardiovasc Dis 2008;101:577–83.

[22] Després JP, Arsenault BJ, Côté M, Cartier A, Lemieux I. Abdominal obesity: the cholesterol of the 21st century? Can J Cardiol 2008;24:7. D–12. D.

[23] Gallagher EJ, Leroith D, Karnieli E. Insulin resistance in obesity as the underlying cause for the metabolic syndrome. Mt Sinai J Med 2010;77:511–23.

[24] Horita S, Seki G, Yamada H, Suzuki M, Koike K, Fujita T. Insulin resistance, obesity, hypertension, and renal sodium transport. Int J Hypertens 2011:391762.

[25] Bakris GL. Current perspectives on hypertension and metabolic syndrome. J Manag Care Pharm 2007;13:S3–S5.

[26] Wahba IM, Mak RH. Obesity and obesity-initiated metabolic syndrome: mechanistic links to chronic kidney disease. Clin J Am Soc Nephrol 2007;2:550–62.

[27] Hajer GR, van Haeften TW, Visseren FL. Adipose tissue dysfunction in obesity, diabetes, and vascular diseases. Eur Heart J 2008;29:2959–71.

[28] Galic S, Oakhill JS, Steinberg GR. Adipose tissue as an endocrine organ. Mol Cell Endocrinol 2010;316:129–39.

[29] Suganami T, Ogawa Y. Adipose tissue macrophages: their role in adipose tissue remodeling. J Leukoc Biol 2010;88:33–9.

[30] Rasouli N, Kern PA. Adipocytokines and the metabolic complications of obesity. J. Clin Endocrinol Metab 2008;93:S64–73.

[31] Onat A, Hergenç G. Low-grade inflammation, and dysfunction of high-density lipoprotein and its apolipoproteins as a major driver of cardiometabolic risk. Metabolism 2011;60:499–512.

[32] Deng Y, Scherer PE. Adipokines as novel biomarkers and regulators of the metabolic syndrome. Ann NY Acad Sci 2010;1212:E1–E19.

[33] Cui J, Panse S, Falkner B. The role of adiponectin in metabolic and vascular disease. Clin Nephrol 2011;75:26–33.

[34] USDA National Nutrient Database. <http://ndb.nal.usda.gov/>, Accessed 29 September 2013.

[35] Hosseinian FS, Beta T. Patented techniques for the extraction and isolation of secoisolari-ciresinol diglucoside from flaxseed. Recent Pat Food Nutr Agric 2009;1:25–31.

[36] Davin LB, Lewis NG. Dirigent proteins and dirigent sites explain the mystery of specificity of radical precursor coupling in lignan and lignin biosynthesis. Plant Physiol 2000;123:453–62.

[37] Hemmati S, von Heimendahl CB, Klaes M, Alfermann AW, Schmidt TJ, Fuss E. Pinoresinol-lariciresinol reductases with opposite enantiospecificity determine the enantiomeric composition of lignans in the different organs of *Linum usitatissimum* L. Planta Med 2010;76:928–34.

[38] Schmidt TJ, Klaes M, Sendker J. Lignans in seeds of Linum species. Phytochemistry 2012;82:89–99.

[39] Penalvo JL, Haajanen KM, Botting NP, Adlercreutz H. Quantification of lignan in food using isotope dilution gas chromatography-mass spectrometry. J Agric Food Chem 2005;53:9342–7.

[40] Hano C, Martin I, Fliniaux O, Legrand B, Gutierrez L, Arroo RR, et al. Pinoresinol-lariciresinol reductase gene expression and secoisolariciresinol diglucoside accumulation in developing flax (*Linum usitatissimum*) seeds. Planta 2006;224:1291–301.

[41] Wang LQ, Meselhy MR, Li Y, Qin GW, Hattori M. Human intestinal bacteria capable of transforming secoisolariciresinol diglucoside to mammalian lignans, enterodiol and enterolactone. Chem Pharm Bull 2000;48:1606–10.

[42] Jin JS, Zhao YF, Nakamura N, Akao T, Kakiuchi N, Min BS, et al. Enantioselective dehydroxylation of enterodiol and enterolactone precursors by human intestinal bacteria. Biol Pharm Bull 2007;30:2113–9.

[43] Niemeyer HB, Honig D, Lange-Böhmer A, Jacobs E, Kulling SE, Metzler M. Oxidative metabolites of the mammalian lignans enterodiol and enterolactone in rat bile and urine. J Agric Food Chem 2000;48:2910–9.

[44] Atkinson DA, Hill HH, Shultz TD. Quantification of mammalian lignans in biological fluids using gas chromatography with ion mobility detection. J Chromatogr 1993;617:173–9.

[45] Knust U, Hull WE, Spiegelhalder B, Bartsch H, Strowitzki T, Owen RW. Analysis of enterolignan glucuronides in serum and urine by HPLC-ESI-MS. Food Chem Toxicol 2006;44:1038–49.

[46] Jacobs E, Metzler M. Oxidative metabolism of the mammalian lignans enterolactone and enterodiol by rat, pig, and human liver microsomes. J Agric Food Chem 1999;47:1071–7.

[47] Gagnon N, Côrtes C, da Silva D, Kazama R, Benchaar C, dos Santos G, et al. Ruminal metabolism of flaxseed (*Linum usitatissimum*) lignans to the mammalian lignan enterolactone and its concentration in ruminal fluid, plasma, urine and milk of dairy cows. Br J Nutr 2009;102:1015–23.

[48] Eeckhaut E, Struijs K, Possemiers S, Vincken JP, Keukeleire DD, Verstraete W. Metabolism of the lignan macromolecule into enterolignans in the gastrointestinal lumen as determined in the

simulator of the human intestinal microbial ecosystem. J Agric Food Chem 2008;56:4806–12.

[49] Edel AL, Aliani M, Pierce GN. Supported liquid extraction in the quantitation of plasma enterolignans using isotope dilution GC/MS with application to flaxseed consumption in healthy adults. J Chromatogr B. Analyt Technol Biomed Life Sci 2013;912:24–32.

[50] Clavel T, Doré J, Blaut M. Bioavailability of lignans in human subjects. Nutr Res Rev 2006;19:187–96.

[51] Kuijsten A, Arts IC, Van't Veer P, Hollman PC. The relative bioavailability of enterolignans in humans is enhanced by milling and crushing of flaxseed. J Nutr 2005;135:2812–6.

[52] Tarpila S, Aro A, Salminen I, Tarpila A, Kleemola P, Akkila J, et al. The effect of flaxseed supplementation in processed foods on serum fatty acids and enterolactone. Eur J Clin Nutr 2002;56:157–65.

[53] Nesbitt PD, Lam Y, Thompson LU. Human metabolism of mammalian lignan precursors in raw and processed flaxseed. Am J Clin Nutr 1999;69:549–55.

[54] Prasad K, Mantha SV, Muir AD, Westcott ND. Reduction of hypercholesterolemic atherosclerosis by CDC-flaxseed with very low alpha-linolenic acid. Atherosclerosis 1998;136:367–75.

[55] Reilly JJ, Penpraze V, Hislop J, Davies G, Grant S, Paton JY. Objective measurement of physical activity and sedentary behavior: review with new data. Arch Dis Child 2008;93:614–9.

[56] Moree SS, Rajesha J. Investigation of in vitro and in vivo antioxidant potential of secoisolariciresinol diglucoside. Mol Cell Biochem 2013;373:179–87.

[57] Bondia-Pons I, Ryan L, Martinez JA. Oxidative stress and inflammation interactions in human obesity. J Physiol Biochem 2012;68:701–11.

[58] Khan SR. Is oxidative stress, a link between nephrolithiasis and obesity, hypertension, diabetes, chronic kidney disease, metabolic syndrome? Urol Res 2012;40:95–112.

[59] Wei YH, Lu CY, Lee HC, Pang CY, Ma YS. Oxidative damage and mutation to mitochondrial DNA and age-dependent decline of mitochondrial respiratory function. Ann NY Acad Sci 1998;854:155–70.

[60] Richter C, Gogvadze V, Laffranchi R, Schlapbach R, Schweizer M, Suter M, et al. Oxidants in mitochondria: from physiology to diseases. Biochim Biophys Acta 1995;1271:67–74.

[61] Cutler RG, Plummer J, Chowdhury K, Heward C. Oxidative stress profiling: Theory, technology, and practice. Ann NY Acad Sci 2005;1055:136–58.

[62] Mena S, Ortega A, Estrela JM. Oxidative stress in environmental-induced carcinogenesis. Mutat Res 2009;674:36–44.

[63] Moree SS, Kavishankar GB, Rajesha J. Antidiabetic effect of secoisolariciresinol diglucoside in streptozotocin-induced diabetic rats. Phytomedicine 2013;20:237–45.

[64] Tominaga S, Nishi K, Nishimoto S, Akiyama K, Yamauchi S, Sugahara T. (−)-Secoisolariciresinol attenuates high-fat diet-induced obesity in C57. BL/6 mice. Food Funct 2012;3:76–82.

[65] Tominaga S, Sugahara T, Nishimoto S, Yamawaki M, Nakashima Y, Kishida T, et al. The Effect of Secoisolariciresinol on 3. T3-L1. Adipocytes and the Relationship between Molecular Structure and Activity. Biosci Biotechnol Biochem 2009;73:35–9.

[66] Park JB, Velasquez MT. Potential effects of lignan-enriched flaxseed powder on bodyweight, visceral fat, lipid profile, and blood pressure in rats. Fitoterapia 2012;83:941–6.

[67] Barre DE, Mizier-Barre KA, Stelmach E, Hobson J, Griscti O, Rudiuk A, et al. Flaxseed lignan complex administration in older human type 2 diabetics manages central obesity and prothrombosis-an invitation to further investigation into polypharmacy reduction. J Nutr Metab 2012;585:170–5.

[68] Fukumitsu S, Aida K, Ueno N, Ozawa S, Takahashi Y, Kobori M. Flaxseed lignan attenuates high-fat diet-induced fat accumulation and induces adiponectin expression in mice. Br J Nutr 2008;100:669–76.

[69] Kwiterovich Jr PO. Recognition and management of dyslipidemia in children and adolescents. J Clin Endocrinol Metab 2008;93:4200–9.

[70] Haliga R, Mocanu V, Oboroceanu T, Stitt PA, Luca VC. The effects of dietary flaxseed supplementation on lipid metabolism in streptozotocin-induced diabetic hamsters. Rev Med Chir Soc Med Nat Iasi 2007;111:472–6.

[71] Bhathena SJ, Ali AA, Haudenschild C, Latham P, Ranich T, Mohamed AI, et al. Dietary flaxseed meal is more protective than soy protein concentrate against hypertriglyceridemia and steatosis of the liver in an animal model of obesity. J Am Coll Nutr 2003;22:157–64.

[72] Jenkins DJ, Kendall CW, Vidgen E, Agarwal S, Rao AV, Rosenberg RS, et al. Health aspects of partially defatted flaxseed, including effects on serum lipids, oxidative measures, and ex vivo androgen and progestin activity: a controlled crossover trial. Am J Clin Nutr 1999;69:395–402.

[73] Zhang W, Wang X, Liu Y. Dietary flaxseed lignan extract lowers plasma cholesterol and glucose concentrations in hypercholesterolaemic subjects. Br J Nutr 2008;99:1301–9.

[74] Pan A, Yu D, Demark-Wahnefried W, Franco OH, Lin X. Meta-analysis of the effects of flaxseed interventions on blood lipids. Am J Clin Nutr 2009;90:288–97.

[75] Villanueva EC, Myers Jr MG. Leptin receptor signaling and the regulation of mammalian physiology. Int J Obes (Lond) 2008;32:S8–12.

[76] de Luis DA, Perez Castrillón JL, Dueñas A. Leptin and obesity. Minerva Med 2009;100:229–36.

[77] Maury E, Brichard SM. Adipokine dysregulation, adipose tissue inflammation and metabolic syndrome. Mol Cell Endocrinol 2010;314:1–16.

[78] Cawthorn WP, Sethi JK. TNF-alpha and adipocyte biology. FEBS Lett 2008;582:117–31.

[79] Warne JP. Tumour necrosis factor alpha: a key regulator of adipose tissue mass. J Endocrinol 2003;177:351–5.

[80] Gurevich-Panigrahi T, Panigrahi S, Wiechec E, Los M. Obesity: pathophysiology and clinical management. Curr Med Chem 2009;16:506–21.

[81] Forsythe LK, Wallace JM, Livingstone MB. Obesity and inflammation: the effects of weight loss. Nutr Res Rev 2008;21:117–33.

[82] Klempel MC, Varady KA. Reliability of leptin, but not adiponectin, as a biomarker for diet-induced weight loss in humans. Nutr Rev 2011;69:145–54.

[83] Varady KA, Tussing L, Bhutani S, Braunschweig CL. Degree of weight loss required to improve adipokine concentrations and decrease fat cell size in severely obese women. Metabolism 2009;58:1096–101.

[84] Romeo J, Martinez-Gomez D, Diaz LE, Gómez-Martinez S, Marti A, Martin-Matillas M, et al. Changes in cardiometabolic risk factors, appetite-controlling hormones and cytokines after a treatment program in overweight adolescents. Pediatr Diabetes 2011;12:372–80.

[85] Hallund J, Tetens I, Bügel S, Tholstrup T, Bruun JM. The effect of a lignan complex isolated from flaxseed on inflammation markers in healthy postmenopausal women. Nutr Metab Cardiovasc Dis 2008;18:497–502.

[86] Ibrahim HN, Weber ML. Weight loss: a neglected intervention in the management of chronic kidney disease. Curr Opin Nephrol Hypertens 2010;19:534–8.

[87] Wallace JP. Exercise in hypertension. A clinical Rev Sports Med 2003;33:585–98.

[88] Keith 3rd TA. Systemic hypertension: prevention and treatment of target organ catastrophe. Compr Ther 1983;9:6–26.

[89] Lambert GW, Straznicky NE, Lambert EA, Dixon JB, Schlaich MP. Sympathetic nervous activation in obesity and the metabolic syndrome—causes, consequences and therapeutic implications. Pharmacol Ther 2010;126:159–72.

[90] Niswender K. Diabetes and obesity: therapeutic targeting and risk reduction—a complex interplay. Diabetes Obes Metab 2010;12:267–87.

[91] Talom RT, Judd SA, McIntosh DD, McNeill JR. High flaxseed (linseed) diet restores endothelial function in the mesenteric arterial bed of spontaneously hypertensive rats. Life Sci 1999;64:1415–25.

[92] Begg DP, Sinclair AJ, Stahl LA, Premaratna SD, Hafandi A, Jois M, et al. Hypertension induced by omega-3 polyunsaturated fatty acid deficiency is alleviated by alpha-linolenic acid regardless of dietary source. Hypertens Res 2010;33:808–13.

[93] Udenigwe CC, Aluko RE. Antioxidant and angiotensin converting enzyme-inhibitory properties of a flaxseed protein-derived high Fischer ratio peptide mixture. J Agric Food Chem 2010;58: 4762–8.

[94] Omoni AO, Aluko RE. Effect of cationic flaxseed protein hydrolysate fractions on the in vitro structure and activity of calmodulin-dependent endothelial nitric oxide synthase. Mol Nutr Food Res 2006;50:958–66.

CHAPTER

30

Carotenoids as a Nutraceutical Therapy for Visceral Obesity

Kazuo Miyashita and Masashi Hosokawa

Faculty of Fisheries Sciences, Hokkaido University, Hakodate, Japan

INTRODUCTION

Obesity is defined as a condition of excess body fat that is associated with a large number of metabolic disorders that induce cardiovascular and other kinds of noncommunicable diseases such as diabetes. It also contributes to increased mortality rates of most diseases, including cancer. The obesity prevalence rate is increasing in most industrialized countries, as well as in developing countries that adopt a similar lifestyle, owing to the reduction in physical exercise and the increased consumption of tasty, affordable food that has a high energy density. Since cardiovascular disease (CVD), diabetes, and cancers are the leading causes of death worldwide, tremendous interest is now focusing on obesity control.

It is clear that there are only two ways to treat obesity: reducing energy intake or increasing energy expenditure. However, homeostatic energy regulation in humans is strongly biased toward weight gain and the storage of fat, with only a few mechanisms that encourage weight loss. Humans are generally accepted to have a particular genotype, which is the result of evolution, and store energy in lipid form. This genotype has remained unchanged for thousands of years and the increased prevalence of obesity is considered to be the result of an interaction between this genotype and the current lifestyle. Understanding the genetic and environmental factors involved in the tendency to increase body weight should lead to improvements in obesity therapy.

Lifestyle interventions, i.e. changed dietary habits and increased physical activity, are fundamentally important to obesity therapy [1]. The promotion of long-term lifestyle changes in diet and physical activity provides a realistic chance of success in combating the obesity epidemic.

In addition to this essential concept, much attention has been paid to nutritional and dietary factors, as well as relevant metabolically active food compounds that may address the energy imbalance issue [2–4]. Major molecular mechanisms for obesity control are reducing food intake through the control of signals from the gut and adipose tissue; inhibiting of nutrient absorption; increasing thermogenesis to dissipate food energy as heat; and modulating fat synthesis/lipolysis or adipose differentiation/apoptosis [5,6]. Many functional food components have been shown to alter energy metabolism by influencing fat absorption, substrate utilization rate, and thermogenesis.

Upregulation of sympathetically mediated thermogenesis by food component is one of the main targets in developing functional foods for obesity therapy. Several natural compounds such as caffeine and capsaicin, a major pungent principle in hot red peppers, have been reported to activate the sensory nervous system, induce norepinephrine (NE) release, stimulate β-adrenoceptors, and enhance both substrate oxidation and heat production [4,7,8]. Caffeine enhances sympathetic neuronal release of NE, which mediates thermogenesis through stimulation of β-adrenoceptors [4,7,8]. Increased NE secretion by activation of the central nervous system makes it possible to increase the usage of adenosine triphosphate (ATP) through ion pumping and substrate cycling and to increase the rate of mitochondrial oxidation with poor coupling of ATP synthesis, leading to increased heat production. Capsaicin has also been reported to increase thermogenesis by a dose-dependent enhancement of catecholamine secretion followed by β3-adrenergic stimulation [9–11].

A major thermogenic tissue is brown adipose tissue (BAT). BAT has an enormous capacity to produce heat by adaptive thermogenesis [12–15]. BAT has been predominantly found in hibernating animals, small rodents, and newborns that require active thermogenesis to protect them from cold exposure and maintain body

Nutrition in the Prevention and Treatment of Abdominal Obesity
http://dx.doi.org/10.1016/B978-0-12-407869-7.00030-1

temperature. Uncoupling protein 1 (UCP 1) expression is a major factor of the BAT thermogenic process. UCP 1 allows BAT to dissipate the mitochondrial proton electrochemical gradient that is normally used to drive ATP synthesis. Since BAT is also found in healthy adults, which provides the possibility of inducing BAT-mediated dissipation of excess energy in adult humans [13], a great deal of interest has been focused on the functionality of food components that induce thermogenesis through UCP 1 activation. This chapter deals with the antiobesity effect of carotenoids, especially focusing on the brown seaweed carotenoid, fucoxanthin, from the viewpoint of its regulatory effect on UCP 1 induction and related molecular changes.

CAROTENOIDS

Carotenoids belong to the tetraterpene family that is principally found in plants, algae, photosynthetic bacteria, and animals. These are the most important pigments in determining the various colors of plants and animals. Several carotenoids such as β-carotene and β-cryptoxanthin are well known as provitamin A carotenoids. In addition, dietary carotenoids, including non-provitamin A carotenoids, are considered to play a role in the prevention of common chronic diseases such as CVD, age-related macular degeneration, and cancers [16,17]. Further, epidemiological studies have established a positive correlation between carotenoid consumption and a reduced risk of cancer [18,19].

Several carotenoids have been reported to decrease the risk of diseases and disorders by reducing oxidative stress in target tissues, since they can be present in sufficient amounts and the correct location to have antioxidant function. For example, lutein and zeaxanthin have been studied widely and proven to show diverse beneficial effects on human health, particularly in optimizing eye health [20]. The biological mechanisms for the protective effects of both these carotenoids may include their powerful blue-light filtering activities and antioxidant properties. There have been several studies into the relationship between astaxanthin antioxidant activity and the prevention of CVD [21–23]. The prevention of atherosclerosis by astaxanthin intake can be explained by its protective effects on low-density lipoprotein (LDL) and vein endothelial cells against oxidative injury and dysfunction.

There is little doubt that, under the right conditions, carotenoids can show health beneficial effects by protecting cells, tissues, and other structures such as lipoproteins against oxidative damage. On the other hand, we can understand that not all of the biological activities ascribed to carotenoids are necessarily linked to their ability to scavenge free radicals and reactive oxygen species [24,25]. Other mechanisms of action that are independent of the antioxidant activity are also likely to be important. To obtain a better understanding of the physiological effects of carotenoids, efforts have been made to define the modulatory effects of carotenoids or their metabolites on specific gene and protein expressions in biological systems. Their effects are usually based on an interaction between the carotenoid or its metabolite and a biological key molecule such as a receptor protein or coactivator, in which the specific chemical structure of the carotenoid may be essential for binding to these biomolecules. From this viewpoint, the unique mechanism for the antiobesity effect of the brown seaweed carotenoid, fucoxanthin, is interesting, since it is based on the induction of UCP 1 in abdominal white adipose tissue (WAT) mitochondria, leading to fatty acid oxidation and heat production in WAT [25–28].

ANTIOBESITY EFFECT OF FUCOXANTHIN

There has been little information on the antiobesity effect of carotenoids, except for fucoxanthin and astaxanthin. Astaxanthin is a carotenoid commonly found in red fish and crustaceans such as crab, krill, lobster, prawn, and shrimp [29,30]. Recent research has suggested beneficial applications for astaxanthin to improve obesity, diabetes, and insulin resistance [31–34]. The antidiabetic effect of astaxanthin may be caused in part by its strong antioxidant activity, since oxidative stress induced by hyperglycemia is involved in the induction of insulin resistance. However, the main mechanism for the antiobesity and antidiabetic effects of astaxanthin is suggested to be independent of its antioxidant activity, although the detailed mechanism involved and its molecular targets have not been elucidated [35]. More research will be needed to confirm the antiobesity effect of astaxanthin.

On the other hand, there have been many studies on the antiobesity effect of fucoxanthin in animal models [25–28,36–39]. The first finding of the antiobesity effect of fucoxanthin was carried out using brown seaweed lipids from Wakame (*Undaria pinnatifida*), containing 10% fucoxanthin [40]. The effect has been confirmed using another preparation of brown seaweed lipids rich in fucoxanthin [41–44] and purified fucoxanthin in vivo [45–47] and in vitro [48,49] systems.

After feeding fucoxanthin to obese diabetic KK-A^y mice, the body weight gain was significantly reduced compared with that of controls, although there was no difference in food intake [41,45]. This reduction was consistent with decreases in the weight of mesentery, perirenal, retroperitoneal, and uterine WAT normalized for body weight. On the other hand, BAT weight normalized for body weight was increased by fucoxanthin intake. Fucoxanthin supplementation also significantly suppressed body weight and attenuated excess fat accumulation in abdominal WAT of obese mice given a high-fat (HF) diet. Dietary administration of the HF diet resulted in hyperglycemia, hyperinsulinemia, and hyperleptinemia in the mouse model. These perturbations were completely normalized by fucoxanthin supplementation.

Animal experiments using both obese KK-A^y mice and lean C57BL/6J mice have demonstrated the specificity of fucoxanthin. Fucoxanthin attenuated excess fat accumulation in abdominal WAT of obese KK-A^y mice, while no effect was found in lean C57BL/6J mice fed a normal-fat (NF) diet [46]. In contrast, fucoxanthin significantly suppressed abdominal WAT weight in C57BL/6J mice fed a HF diet to the level found in the normal diet group [50]. These results suggest that the suppressive effect of fucoxanthin on WAT weight gain is specific for adiposity in the development of obesity in mice. This specificity will be important for the safe application of fucoxanthin therapy in human obesity.

Fucoxanthin is a major carotenoid present in the chloroplasts of brown seaweeds: it is the most abundant of all carotenoids, accounting for >10% of the estimated total natural production of carotenoids [30]. It forms a complex with chlorophyll protein and plays an important role in light harvesting and photoprotection for effective light utilization and photosynthesis upregulation. Fucoxanthin has a unique structure that includes an unusual allene bond and 5,6-monoepoxide (Fig. 30.1). Of the approximately 700 naturally occurring carotenoids, about 40 contain an allene bond. The principal allenic carotenoids are fucoxanthin (from brown seaweed), perinijin (from microalgae), neoxanthin (present in higher plants), and fucoxanthin metabolites, such as fucoxanthinol and amarouciaxanthin A [51]. The specific structure of fucoxanthin might be related to its antiobesity effect; this hypothesis has informed attempts at screening for antiobesity activity in different carotenoids [48,49,52].

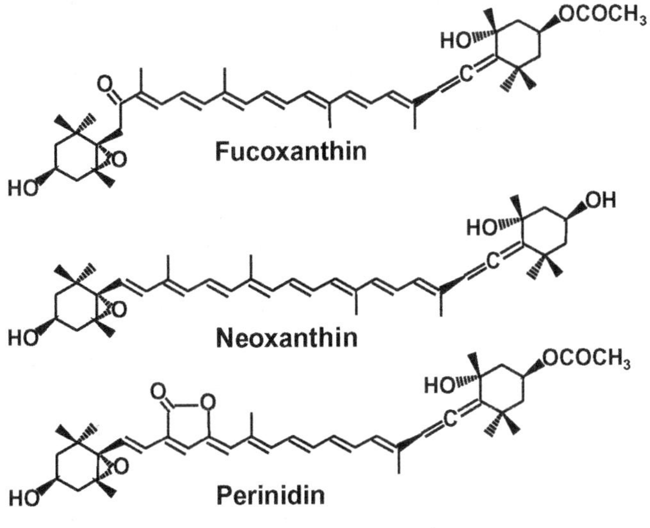

FIGURE 30.1 Structure of allenic carotenoids.

To screen the antiobesity activity of natural compounds, their effect on preadipocyte differentiation and adipogenesis in adipose cell are evaluated together with the analysis of key biomolecules related to changes in genetic programming for lipid synthesis and storage in adipose cell affecting the expression of CCAAT/enhancer-binding proteins (C/EBPs) and peroxisome proliferator-activated receptor gamma (PPAR-γ). When various carotenoids were screened for potential suppression effects on adipocyte differentiation [48,49,52], only fucoxanthin, neoxanthin, and two fucoxanthin metabolites (fucoxanthinol and amarouciaxanthin A) showed an encouraging suppressive effect on the differentiation of 3T3-L1 adipose cells, while other carotenoids did not show such an effect (Fig. 30.2). These four active carotenoids significantly inhibited intercellular lipid accumulation during adipocyte differentiation of 3T3-L1 cells and significantly decreased levels of glycerol-3-phosphate, an indicator of adipocyte differentiation, as compared with the control cells. Moreover, the levels of C/EBPα and PPAR-γ expression were decreased by the treatment of 3T3-L1 cell with fucoxanthin, fucoxanthinol, and amarouciaxanthin A. A structure-function analysis suggested that carotenoids containing an allene bond may have suppressive effects on adipocyte differentiation in 3T3-L1 cells. The importance of allene in carotenoid activity has been confirmed by a comparison of amarouciaxanthin A and amarouciaxanthin B [52]: although both carotenoids have a similar structure (Fig. 30.2), only amarouciaxanthin A inhibited 3T3-L1 differentiation, fat accumulation, and gene expressions of C/EBPα and PPAR-γ. Further studies on the active site of allenic carotenoids may help to produce a new compound for antiobesity therapy.

ACCUMULATION OF FUCOXANTHIN METABOLITES IN ABDOMINAL WHITE ADIPOSE TISSUE

Several food components are currently being promoted for weight management and obesity therapy [53,54]. Their potential biological mechanisms include increased energy expenditure, increased fat oxidation, decreased fat absorption, and increased satiety through the regulation of related signaling pathways and specific molecular targets, mainly in adipose tissue and liver. A major target of fucoxanthin is abdominal WAT. When a diet containing 0.1% purified fucoxanthin (100 mg fucoxanthin/100 g food) was given to mice, more than 80% of

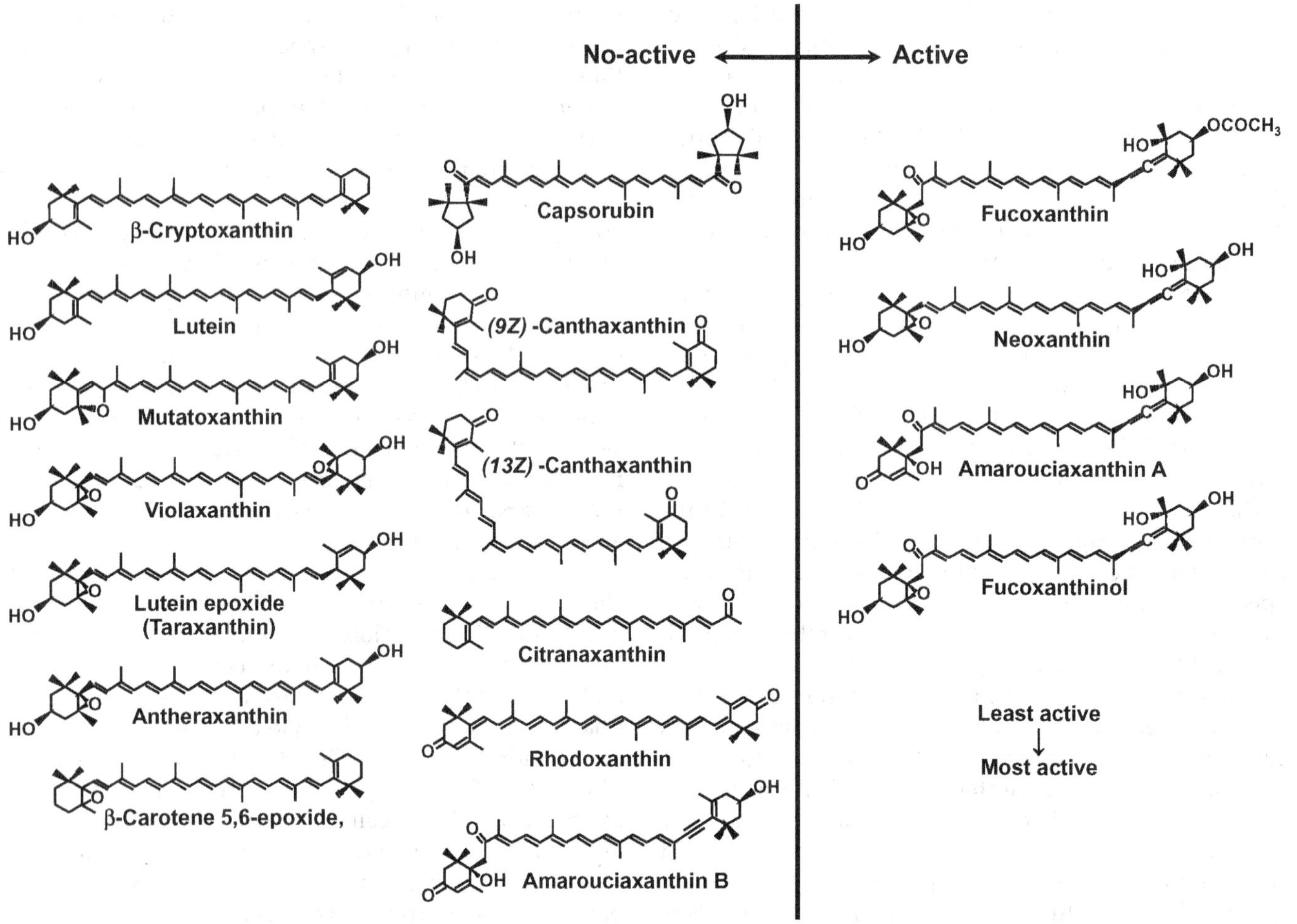

FIGURE 30.2 Suppressive effect of various carotenoids on 3T3-L1 adipocyte differentiation and/or fat accumulation.

fucoxanthin metabolites accumulated in abdominal WAT (Fig. 30.3) [55], suggesting a direct action of fucoxanthin metabolites on abdominal WAT. Dietary fucoxanthin preferentially accumulates as amarouciaxanthin A in abdominal WAT and as fucoxanthinol in the tissues (Fig. 30.3) [55–57]; therefore, the main active form of fucoxanthin in abdominal WAT is amarouciaxanthin A.

Dietary fucoxanthin is hydrolyzed to fucoxanthinol in the gastrointestinal tract by digestive enzymes such as lipase and cholesterol esterase [56]. When a duodenal infusion of 1 mL of test oil emulsion containing 2 mg of fucoxanthin was administered to portal cannulated rats through the lymph duct, intact fucoxanthin was not detected in either lymph fluid or portal blood at any time point, while fucoxanthinol was detected in the lymph, but not in portal blood [58]. This result indicates a quick conversion of fucoxanthin to fucoxanthinol during lymphatic absorption from the intestine. Some fucoxanthinol is also converted to amarouciaxanthin A in the liver [59,60].

Fucoxanthin supplementation in an obese mouse model effectively decreases excess fat accumulation in abdominal WAT. This activity has been reported to appear following doses of at least 60 mg fucoxanthin intake/kg mouse/day [55]. On the other hand, a recent study demonstrated a significant reduction in abdominal WAT in obese female volunteers following an intake of fucoxanthin of <0.024 mg/kg/day (2.4 mg intake/day for volunteers with an average weight of 100 kg) [61]. The difference in effectiveness observed between rodents and human may be due to differences in absorption rate and/or their differential sensitivity to fucoxanthin.

UCP 1 INDUCTION IN ABDOMINAL WHITE ADIPOSE TISSUE BY FUCOXANTHIN

UCP 1 is a major factor involved in the thermogenic process in BAT [14,15,62–65]. The UCP 1 expression allows BAT to dissipate the electrochemical gradient that is normally used to drive ATP synthesis; BAT therefore generates heat by uncoupling oxidative phosphorylation. The thermogenic activity of BAT is dependent on UCP 1 expression that is controlled by the sympathetic

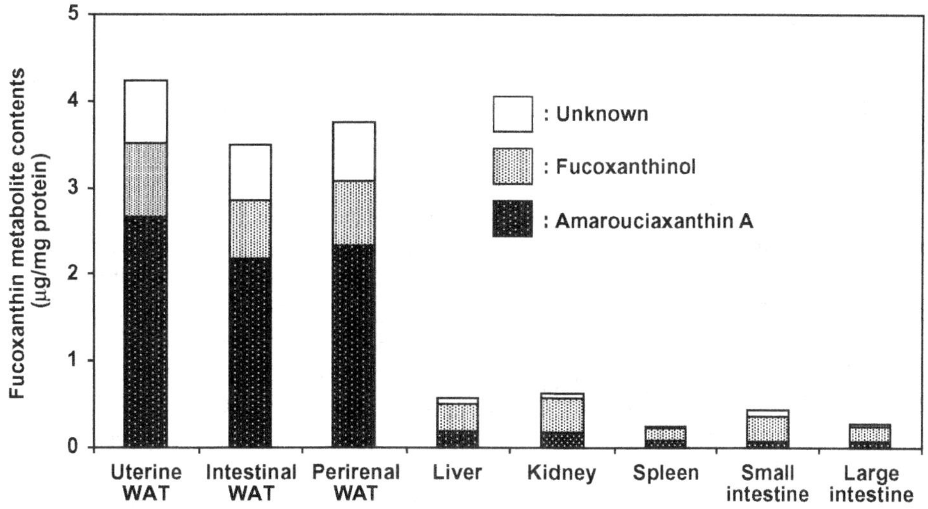

FIGURE 30.3 Accumulation of fucoxanthin metabolites in the tissues of mice fed fucoxanthin.Fucoxanthin metabolites were analyzed using high performance liquid chromatography. Three peaks appeared in the chromatogram: two were identified as fucoxanthinol and amarouciaxanthin A by nuclear magnetic resonance and mass spectral analyses. The third peak could not be identified because of its low concentration. Judging from the retention time and the ultraviolet absorption curve, it is thought to be a *cis*-isomer of fucoxanthinol or amarouciaxanthin A.*Source: adapted from Airanthi et al.* [55].

nervous system via noradrenaline, which is stimulated by cold, adrenergic stimulation, β3-agonists, retinoids, and thyroid hormone [64,66–69]. As a consequence of noradrenaline binding to the β3-adrenergic receptor on the adipocyte plasma membrane, β3-adrenergic receptors are coupled to heterotrimeric G-proteins and adenylate cyclase, resulting in elevated levels of intracellular cyclic adenosine monophosphate (cAMP), activation of cAMP-dependent protein kinase (PKA), and of cAMP-responsive element-binding protein (CREB) (Fig. 30.4). PKA activation induces hormone-sensitive lipase (HSL) expression that stimulates lipolysis and the liberated free fatty acids (FFAs) serve as substrate in BAT thermogenesis. They also act as cytosolic second messengers that activate UCP 1 as a PPAR-γ ligand. In addition to PPAR-γ, PPAR-γ (PGC-1) is a key molecule BAT thermogenesis [6]. PGC-1 can bind to a variety of nuclear receptors, including the retinoic acid and thyroid hormone receptors, both of which positively regulate UCP 1 expression. Moreover, mitochondrial biogenesis is induced by PGC-1 activation.

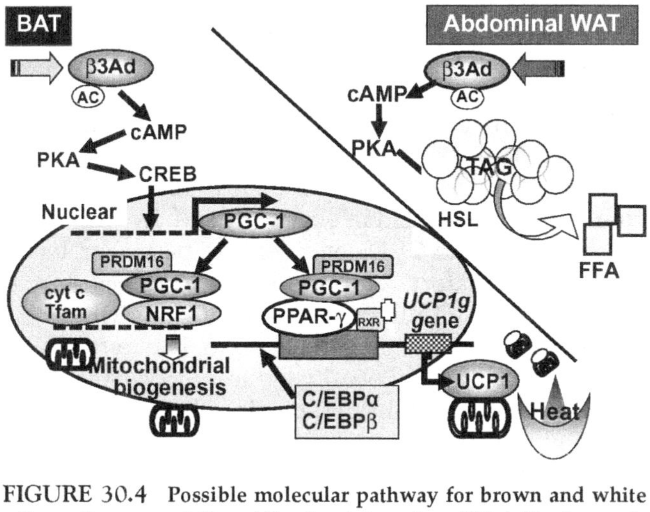

FIGURE 30.4 Possible molecular pathway for brown and white adipose tissue regulation. AC, adenylate cyclase; β3Ad, β3-adrenergic receptor; BAT, brown adipose tissue; cAMP, cyclic adenosine monophosphate; cyt c, cytochrome C; FFA, free fatty acids; TAG, triacylglycerides; WAT, white adipose tissue.

Its capacity for uncoupled mitochondrial respiration caused BAT to be considered an important site of facultative energy expenditure in small rodents. This led to speculation that BAT normally functions to prevent obesity. In fucoxanthin-fed mice, BAT weight was significantly greater than that of control mice, while abdominal WAT weight was decreased by fucoxanthin feeding [40,41,45,46]. Interestingly, fucoxanthin supplementation also induced UCP 1 expression even in abdominal WAT (Fig. 30.5) [40,41,45]. These findings show that the decrease in abdominal WAT weight caused by fucoxanthin intake in rodents is mainly due to the upregulation of thermogenesis through UCP 1 expression in both BAT and abdominal WAT.

UCP 1 is mainly expressed in BAT through the upregulation or stimulation of several key biomolecules such as β3-adrenergic receptor, PGC-1, and PPAR-γ (Fig. 30.4). Although UCP 1 expression is a signature of BAT, it has been also found in the WAT of mice overexpressing *Foxc2* (a winged helix gene encoding forkhead box protein C2), linked to a change in steady-state levels of several WAT- and BAT-derived mRNAs [70]. This result suggests that

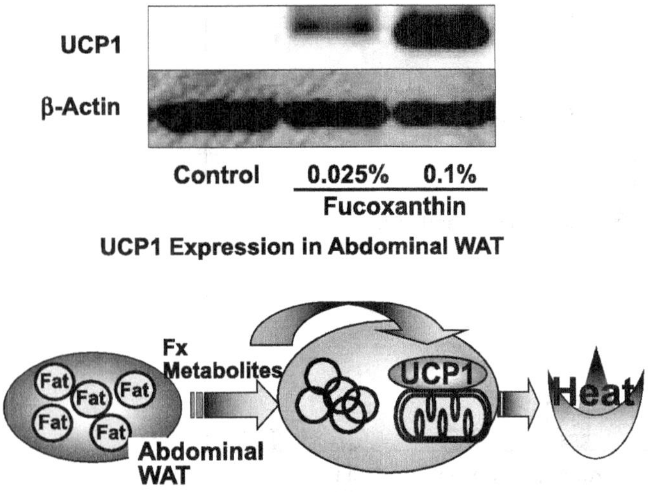

FIGURE 30.5 UCP 1 induction and heat production in abdominal white adipose tissue. Fx, fucoxanthin; WAT, white adipose tissue. *Source: adapted from Maeda et al.* [40].

UCP 1 expression may occur in WAT; this would be an attractive target for the development of antiobesity therapies. As key molecular components become defined, screening for food constituents that increase energy dissipation is becoming a more attainable goal. In this regard, it is noteworthy that fucoxanthin induces both protein and mRNA expressions of UCP 1 in WAT [40,41,45]. Although the mechanism for inducing UCP 1 expression in abdominal WAT by fucoxanthin supplementation is not yet clear, the upregulation of several factors such as β3-adrenergic receptor and PGC-1 may be involved [50,71]. Overexpression of the β1-adrenergic receptor increases PKA pathway signaling. Transgenic overexpression of FOXC2 in the RIIβ-PKA knockout mouse also augments PKA signaling by upregulating the RIα-regulatory subunit, which increases activity of the differentiation pathway for brown adipocytes in white fat depots by lower the affinity constant for cAMP [70,72,73]. UCP 1-expressing brown-like adipocytes are recruited to WAT by prolonged cold exposure or treatment with β-adrenergic agonists [74]. Fucoxanthin activity may be related to the induction of this brown adipose-like cell formation in abdominal WAT.

DOWNREGULATION OF INSULIN RESISTANCE-INDUCING ADIPOCYTOKINES IN ABDOMINAL WHITE ADIPOSE TISSUE BY FUCOXANTHIN

Type 2 diabetes mellitus (T2DM) and CVD are twin epidemics that are escalating globally. Metabolic syndrome is a cluster of risk factors for both diseases. Abdominal obesity is the most obvious symptom of diseases linked to metabolic syndrome such as T2DM [75]. Although not all overweight and obese individuals are insulin resistant [76], it is apparent that the increasing global prevalence of T2DM is linked to rising rates of obesity [77]. Indeed, most T2DM patients are obese [78] and have several modifiable cardiovascular factors, thus emphasizing the need for lifestyle modification as an essential component of metabolic syndrome care.

Several clinical trials have demonstrated the benefits of lifestyle modification in reducing T2DM morbidity and mortality [79]. Lifestyle interventions, mainly diet and/or physical activity, are effective in delaying or preventing T2DM induced by obesity. The increased availability of refined foods, which are often cheaper than traditional foods, and limited physical activity, which is typical of modern civilizations, have been recognized as the main causes of obesity. An initial nutritional approach to protection against obesity and T2DM should, therefore, be focused on reversing the root causes of a high-calorie diet and sedentary lifestyle. Epidemiological evidence suggests that a lower prevalence of metabolic syndrome is associated with dietary patterns rich in fruit, vegetables, whole grains, dairy products, and polyunsaturated fats [80,81]. In addition to this basic treatment, several nutraceuticals have also been shown to reduce the risk of T2DM.

The most desirable nutraceuticals in the fight against T2DM are those that improve a cluster of metabolic abnormalities induced by abdominal obesity. Much attention has therefore been paid to the biological activities of fucoxanthin. Fucoxanthin can not only attenuate the excess accumulation of fat in abdominal WAT but also downregulate the overexpression of proinflammatory and insulin resistance-inducing adipocytokines [45,50]. Abdominal WAT has been recognized as an active endocrine organ in addition to its role as the main storage depot for triacylglycerols. A characteristic imbalance of adipocytokine secretion from WAT is found in individuals that are obese and/or suffer from metabolic syndrome [82]. With the exception of adiponectin and adipsin (complement factor D), most other adipocytokines are hypersecreted in obesity, T2DM, hypertension, inflammatory, and CVD conditions. In particular, levels of proinflammatory adipocytokines such as tumor necrosis factor (TNF-α) and interleukin-6 (IL-6) are strongly correlated to insulin resistance in obesity.

The development of obesity induces macrophage infiltration into abdominal WAT, causing chronic low-grade inflammation that is characterized by upregulation of pro-inflammatory adipocytokines and downregulation of anti-inflammatory adiponectin. Interaction between adipose and macrophage cells following their infiltration into adipose tissue upregulates the production of proinflammatory and insulin resistance-inducing adipocytokines

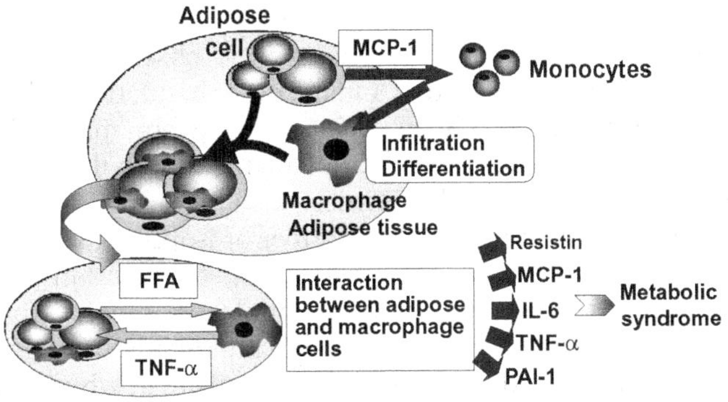

FIGURE 30.6 Macrophage infiltration into abdominal white adipose tissue, interaction between adipose and macrophage cells, and induction of proinflammatory and insulin resistance-inducing adipocytokines. FFA, free fatty acids.

(Fig. 30.6). In abdominal WAT of obese/diabetes model mice, fucoxanthin supplementation significantly inhibited monocyte infiltration into adipose tissues and the differentiation of monocytes to macrophage cells and reduced proinflammatory the expression and secretion of adipocytokines such as IL-6, C-C motif chemokine 2 [monocyte chemoattractant protein-1 (MCP-1); encoded by *CCL2*], plasminogen activator inhibitor 1 (PAI-1), and TNF-α [46]. In addition, fucoxanthin decreased *Nos2* (encoding inducible nitric oxide synthase) and *Ptgs2* (encoding prostaglandin G/H synthase 2/cyclooxygenase-2) mRNA expression in macrophage-like cell model [46].

Downregulation of proinflammatory adipokine secretion from visceral WAT by fucoxanthin is specific for the obese/diabetic state but not for the normal state [46]. When fucoxanthin was given to two mouse lines, diabetic/obese KK-A^y mice and lean C57BL/6J mice, the blood glucose level of obese/diabetic mice was decreased following fucoxanthin intake to the level present of control C57BL/6J mice; however, fucoxanthin did not affect blood glucose levels in C57BL/6J lean mice. In addition, fucoxanthin supplementation normalized *Ccl2*, *Pai1*, and *Tnf* mRNA levels in KK-A^y mice, but had no effect on *Ccl2* and *Tnf* mRNA levels in WAT of lean C57BL/6J mice. MCP-1 recruits macrophages to adipose tissue in obese mice [83] and humans [84]. Downregulation of MCP-1 expression in the visceral WAT of obese subjects by fucoxanthin may be based on the inhibitory effect of fucoxanthin on macrophage infiltration into adipose tissue. Suganami et al. [85] further demonstrated a paracrine loop involving TNF-α and FFA between infiltrated macrophages and adipocytes (Fig. 30.6). Adipose cells and macrophages secrete large amounts of TNF-α. TNF-α and other proinflammatory adipokines promote lipolysis of triacylglycerols and release FFAs. These FFAs activate macrophages within WAT, which then enhances TNF-α production [86]. Fucoxanthin effectively stops this adverse feedback loop between adipose cells and macrophages [46].

FUCOXANTHIN UPREGULATES GLUT4 IN SKELETAL MUSCLE

Skeletal muscle [expressing solute carrier family 2, facilitated glucose transporter member 4 (GLUT4)] accounts for up to 40–60% of body mass and thus regulates glucose homeostasis. The regulatory effect of fucoxanthin on glucose utilization in muscle is also strongly related to its antidiabetic activity. Insulin increases the uptake of glucose into fat or muscle cells through redistribution of glucose transport proteins at the cell surface. GLUT4 is the predominant glucose transporter isoform expressed in skeletal muscle and adipose tissue [87]. Since the discovery of GLUT4, mechanisms that regulate the GLUT4 expression have been intensively studied. Studies using transgenic mouse models have demonstrated that modifying GLUT4 expression profoundly affects whole-body insulin action and, consequently, glucose and lipid metabolism [88,89]. Mice overexpressing the *Glut4* gene in skeletal muscle or adipose tissue show enhanced insulin responsiveness and peripheral glucose utilization [90].

On the other hand, a significant reduction in GLUT4 protein and mRNA levels in skeletal muscle is found in mice fed a HF diet [91,92]. When mice were fed a HF or NF diet, the HF group developed hyperglycemia, hyperinsulinemia, and hyperleptinemia, along with a significant decrease in *Glut4* mRNA levels in skeletal muscle, compared to the NF group [50]. However, these perturbations were completely normalized by the addition of fucoxanthin to the HF diet: *Glut4* mRNA levels in the HF group fed fucoxanthin were restored to levels observed in the NF group. Increased GLUT4 levels following fucoxanthin intake has been also reported in obese/diabetes model KK-A^y mice. This increase has been found in the extensor digitorum longus (EDL) muscle of the mice, together with upregulated PGC-1α expression [71]. PGC-1α is an important coactivator implicated in the regulation of mitochondrial biogenesis and the oxidative metabolism of muscle [93]. PGC-1α has been reported to activate GLUT4 expression in myocytes [94]. Overexpression of PGC-1α in muscle led to increased GLUT4 expression and insulin-stimulated glucose uptake [95]. Increased PGC-1α level following fucoxanthin intake is a main mechanism of GLUT4 upregulation.

Following insulin and other stimuli, GLUT4 is quickly moved to plasma membranes from intracellular depots, and thus promotes glucose uptake in skeletal muscle [96]. Insulin-stimulated glucose uptake is linearly related to levels of GLUT4 plasma membrane expression [97,98]. On the other hand, in T2DM, insulin signaling is impaired and GLUT4 translocation to the plasma membrane is attenuated [99]. Therefore, another important method for increasing the effective utilization of glucose is to increase the GLUT4 translocation to the cell membrane. When fucoxanthin was given to KK-A^y mice, GLUT4 translocation to plasma membrane from the cytosol was significantly upregulated in the soleus muscle. Upregulation of GLUT4 translocation has been also found in EDL muscle, although the effectiveness of fucoxanthin was lower on the EDL muscle than on the soleus muscle [71]. The levels of insulin receptor mRNA expression and Akt phosphorylation, upstream components of the insulin signaling pathway regulating GLUT4 translocation, were also enhanced in the soleus and EDL muscles of mice fed fucoxanthin.

FUCOXANTHIN INTAKE IMPROVES GLUCOSE LEVEL AND HAS IN VIVO ANTIOXIDANT ACTIVITY

As a consequence of downregulating several adipocytokines in abdominal WAT and upregulating GLUT4 activity in skeletal muscle, fucoxanthin improves insulin resistance to normalize glucose levels. When fucoxanthin was given to obese/diabetes model KK-A^y mice, it significantly decreased blood glucose and plasma insulin levels, compared with control KK-A^y mice [45]. The same results were obtained in normal C57BL/6J mice fed HF diet [50,100]. Dietary administration of a HF diet resulted in hyperglycemia, hyperinsulinemia, and hyperleptinemia in the mouse model, while these perturbations were completely normalized in the fucoxanthin-fed group.

Fucoxanthin intake significantly increases the arachidonic acid (AA; 20:4n-6) and docosahexaenoic acid (DHA; 22:6n-3) content of the liver, probably due to upregulation of delta-6-desaturase expression [66,101]. AA and DHA are known to be very easily oxidized in model systems because the oxidative stability of each polyunsaturated fatty acid (PUFA) is inversely proportional to its degree of unsaturation [102,103]. Therefore, the higher levels of these PUFAs in the liver of mice fed fucoxanthin might induce the peroxidation of liver lipids. However, lipid peroxidation was significantly reduced by fucoxanthin feeding [55].

In vivo antioxidant activity of fucoxanthin has been also observed in obese/diabetes KK-A^y mice [104]. A significant increase in oxidative stress has been observed in obese subjects [105–107]. Hyperglycemia and fundamental abnormalities found in diabetes can also induce oxidative stress [107–110]. Therefore, the obese, diabetic status of KK-A^y mice results in oxidative stress that produces higher levels of lipid hydroperoxides than those found in normal controls. When lipid hydroperoxide levels in the liver and abdominal WAT of obese/diabetic KK-A^y mice were compared with those of normal ICR mice, more lipid hydroperoxides were observed in the obese/diabetic mice [104]. On the other hand, the higher hydroperoxide levels in KK-A^y mice were markedly decreased by fucoxanthin supplementation, to the same level as that of control ICR mice.

Due to the presence of a number of isoprenoid structures with conjugated double bonds, fucoxanthin can scavenge singlet oxygen ($^1O_2$), similar to other carotenoids. The quenching of $^1O_2$ by carotenoids has been mainly attributed to a physical mechanism, in which the excess energy of singlet oxygen is transferred to the carotenoid. With the added energy, the carotenoid is excited to a triplet state; upon losing the energy as heat, it relaxes to a singlet state without a change in structure [111–113]. The quenching efficacy of carotenoids increases with the number of conjugated double bonds within the molecule. The number of conjugated double bonds in fucoxanthin is nine (Fig. 30.1); this is lower than the number present in lutein (10), β-carotene (11), lycopene (11), and astaxanthin (13). Therefore, fucoxanthin is less reactive than these other carotenoids toward $^1O_2$.

On the other hand, several studies have reported that fucoxanthin has free-radical quenching ability of [114–118]. Fucoxanthin has di(phenyl)-(2,4,6-trinitrophenyl) iminoazanium (DPPH), 2,2′-azino-bis (3-ethylbenzothiazoline-6-sulfonic acid) (ABTS), and hydroxyl radical-scavenging activity. The scavenging activity of fucoxanthin is higher than that of α-tocopherol, as measured by a chemiluminescence technique. A similar trend was observed when hydroxyl radical scavenging was assessed by an electron spin resonance (ESR) technique [117]. ESR analysis of superoxide radical scavenging also showed a high activity for fucoxanthin. The electron-rich status of carotenoids makes capable of reacting with free radicals. Although the reactions of carotenoids with free radicals are much more complex than with $^1O_2$, this mainly depends on the nature of the free radicals rather than the carotenoids [112,119]. Miller et al. [120] reported that carotenoid activity generally increases with the presence of terminal ring functional groups, as seen in fucoxanthin.

The radical-scavenging activity of fucoxanthin may be related to its in vivo antioxidant activity. However, dietary fucoxanthin had little effect on lipid hydroperoxide levels of both the liver and abdominal WAT of normal ICR mice fed a normal diet [104]. The in vivo antioxidant activity of fucoxanthin was only observed under diabetic and/or hepatic hyperlipidemic conditions, as found in KK-A^y mice. On the other hand, blood glucose levels of KK-A^y mice were significantly reduced by fucoxanthin supplementation, while no significant difference in glucose level was found in ICR mice following fucoxanthin intake. These results suggest that the well-known ability of fucoxanthin to scavenge active oxygen species and/or free radicals is not the main explanation for its in vivo antioxidant activity. In general, it is difficult to explain all of the physiological effects of carotenoids by their antioxidant activity [24,25]. The in vivo antioxidant activity of fucoxanthin is not a direct effect of fucoxanthin on active oxygen species and/or free radicals; instead, fucoxanthin regulatory effects on target molecules lead to improvements in metabolic disorders such as hyperglycemia.

Dietary fucoxanthin also significantly reduces hepatic liver lipids of KK-A^y mice to the same level as those found in ICR control mice [104]. The decrease in lipid substrates available for oxidation could result in the lower lipid hydroperoxide levels present in the liver of KK-A^y mice. Woo et al. [100] reported that fucoxanthin improves the hepatic lipid profiles of C57BL/6N mice fed a HF diet containing 39% of calories as fat. Both 0.05% and 0.2% fucoxanthin supplementation significantly lowered triacylglycerol levels by 38% and 24%, respectively, and cholesterol levels by 26% and 24%, respectively, compared to the control group. From an analysis of its enzymatic activities, they demonstrated that the effect of fucoxanthin on lipid metabolism is due to the suppression of hepatic lipogenesis and stimulation of hepatic lipolysis through regulation of the nuclear receptors, PPAR-α and PPAR-γ.

CONCLUSION

Although seaweeds are significantly behind marine fish in lipid content, due to their large availability in coastal waters, seaweeds are still a prospective source of functional lipids. While the lipid content of oily fish has been reported to be generally around 20% and sometimes reaches 50% dry weight (DW), seaweeds can contain up to 1–5% DW of total lipids [121–125]. However, our recent study found that the lipid content of *Sargassum* species of brown seaweed changes seasonally, reaching more than 14–15% DW in the spring, with high concentration of omega 3 PUFAs (>40 wt% of total fatty acids) and fucoxanthin (>4% of total lipids) [126]. Brown seaweed oil is now commercially available for fucoxanthin supplement. The chemical synthesis of fucoxanthin is possible; however, it costs too much money and its recovery level is very low. On the other hand, several brown seaweeds can be used for the production of nutraceutical and functional food materials containing high amounts of fucoxanthin.

As shown in this chapter, a characteristic function of fucoxanthin is the promotion of adaptive thermogenesis through UCP 1 upregulation in the mitochondria of abdominal WAT that leads to fatty acid oxidation and heat production. Another key function of fucoxanthin is the regulation of adipocytokine secretion from both abdominal adipose and macrophage cells [25]. This fucoxanthin effect improves insulin resistance and decreases blood glucose levels. The antidiabetic activity of fucoxanthin is also promoted by its regulatory effect on GLUT4 expression and translocation [71]. Although more efforts should be made to elucidate the molecular mechanism of antiobesity fucoxanthin effects, it is clear that fucoxanthin is a promising marine gift for managing obesity and its related disorders.

References

[1] Saha S, Gerdtham U-G, Johansson P. Economic evaluation of lifestyle interventions for preventing diabetes and cardiovascular diseases. Int J Environ Res Public Health 2010;7:3150–95.

[2] Kovacs EMR, Mela DJ. Metabolically active functional food ingredients for weight control. Obes Rev 2005;7:59–78.

[3] St-Onge M-P. Dietary fats, teas, dairy, and nuts: potential functional foods for weight control? Am J Clin Nutr 2005;81:7–15.

[4] Hursel R, Westerterp-Plantenga MS. Thermogenic ingredients and body weight regulation. Int J Obes 2010;34:659–69.

[5] Bray GA, Tartaglia LA. Medicinal strategies in the treatment of obesity. Nature 2000;404:672–7.

[6] Lowell BB, Spiegelman BM. Towards a molecular understanding of adaptive thermogenesis. Nature 2000;404:6452–660.

[7] Diepvens K, Westerterp KR, Westerterp-Plantenga MS. Obesity and thermogenesis related to the consumption of caffeine, ephedrine, capsaicin, and green tea. Am J Physiol Regul Integr Comp Physiol 2005;292:R77–85.

[8] Westerterp-Plantenga M, Diepvens K, Joosen AMCP, Berube-Parent S, Tremblay A. Metabolic effects of spices, teas, and caffeine. Physiol Behav 2006;89:85–91.

[9] Kawada T, Watanabe T, Takaishi T, Tanaka T, Iwai K. Capsaicin-induced beta-adrenergic action on energy metabolism in rats: influence of capsaicin on oxygen consumption, the respiratory quotient, and substrate utilization. Proc Soc Exp Biol Med 1986;183:250–6.

[10] Watanabe T, Kawada T, Yamamoto M, Iwai K. Capsaicin, a pungent principle of hot red pepper, evokes catecholamine secretion from the adrenal medulla of anesthetized rats. Biochem Biophys Res Commun 1987;142:259–64.

[11] Jimenez M, Leger B, Canola K, Lehr L, Arboit P, Seydoux J, et al. $\beta_1/\beta_2/\beta_3$ adrenoceptor knockout mice are obese and cold-sensitive but have normal lipolytic responses to fasting. FEBS Lett 2002;530:37–40.

[12] Obregon M-J. Thyroid hormone and adipocyte differentiation. Thyroid 2008;18:185–95.

[13] Enerbäck S. Brown adipose tissue in humans. Int J Obes 2010;34:S43–6.

[14] Kozak LP. Brown fat and the myth of diet-induced thermogenesis. Cell Metab 2010;11:263–7.

[15] Seale P. Transcriptional control of brown adipocyte development and thermogenesis. Int J Obes 2010;34:S17–22.

[16] Cooper DA, Eldridge AL, Peters JC. Dietary carotenoids and lung cancer: a review of recent research. Nutr Rev 1999;57:133–45.

[17] Cooper DA, Eldridge AL, Peters JC. Dietary carotenoids and certain cancers, heart disease and age related macular degeneration: a review of recent research. Nutr Rev 1999;57:201–14.

[18] Willett WC. Diet and cancer: one view at the start of the millennium. Cancer Epidemiol Biomark Prev 2001;2001(10):3–8.

[19] Riboli E, Norat T. Epidemiiologic evidence of the protective effect of fruit and vegetables on cancer risk. Am J Clin Nutr 2003;78:559S–69S.
[20] Ma L, Lin X-M. Effects of lutein and zeaxanthin on aspects of eye health. J Sci Food Agric 2010;90:2–12.
[21] Fredric JP, David GW, Charles LC. Astaxanthin: a novel potential treatment for oxidative stress and inflammation in cardiovascular disease. Am J Cardiol 2008;101:58D–68D.
[22] Fassett RG, Coombes JS. Astaxanthin, oxidative stress, inflammation and cardiovascular disease. Future Cardiol 2009;5:333–42.
[23] Yuan J-P, Peng J, Yin K, Wang J-H. Potential health-promoting effects of astaxanthin: a high-value carotenoid mostly from microalgae. Mol Nutr Food Res 2011;55:150–65.
[24] Erdman Jr JW, Ford NA, Lindshield BL. Are the health attributes of lycopene related to its antioxidant function? Arch Biochem Biophys 2009;483:229–35.
[25] Miyashita K, Nishikawa S, Beppu F, Tsukui T, Abe M, Hosokawa M. Allenic carotenoid, fucoxanthin, as a novel marine nutraceutical from brown seaweed. J Sci Food Agric 2011;91:1166–74.
[26] Miyashita K. Function of marine carotenoids. Forum Nutr 2009;61:136–46.
[27] Miyashita K. The carotenoid fucoxanthin from brown seaweed affects obesity. Lipid Tech 2009;21:186–90.
[28] Miyashita K, Maeda H, Okada T, Abe M, Hosokawa M. Anti-obesity and anti-diabetic effects of allenic carotenoid, fucoxanthin. Agro Food 2010;21:24–7.
[29] Goodwin TW. Metabolism, nutrition, and function of carotenoids. Ann Rev Nutr 1986;6:273–97.
[30] Matsuno T. Aquatic animal carotenoids. Fisheries Sci 2001;67:771–83.
[31] Hussein G, Nakagawa T, Goto H, Shimada Y, Matsumoto K, Sankawa U, et al. Astaxanthin ameliorates features of metabolic syndrome in SHR/NDmcr-*cp*. Life Sci 2007;80:522–9.
[32] Ikeuchi M, Koyama T, Takahashi J, Yazawa K. Effects of Astaxanthin in obese mice fed a high-fat diet. Biosci Biotechnol Biochem 2007;71:893–9.
[33] Arunkumar E, Bhuvaneswari S, Anuradha CV. An intervention study in obese mice with astaxanthin, a marine carotenoid—effects on insulin signaling and pro-inflammatory cytokines. Food Funct 2012;3:120–6.
[34] Preuss HG, Echard B, Yamashita E, Perricone NV. High dose astaxanthin lowers blood pressure and increases insulin sensitivity in rats: are these effects interdependent? Int J Med Sci 2011;8:126–38.
[35] Inoue M, Tanabe H, Matsumoto A, Takagi M, Umegaki K, Amagaya S, et al. Astaxanthin functions differently as a selective peroxisome proliferator-activated receptor γ modulator in adipocytes and macrophages. Biochem Pharmacol 2012;84:692–700.
[36] Peng J, Yuan J-P, Wu C-F, Wang J-H. Fucoxanthin, a marine carotenoid present in brown seaweeds and diatoms: metabolism and bioactivities relevant to human health. Mar Drugs 2011;9:1806–28.
[37] Riccioni G, D'Orazio N, Franceschelli S, Speranza L. Marine carotenoids and cardiovascular risk markers. Mar Drugs 2011;9:1166–75.
[38] D'Orazio N, Gemello E, Gammone MA, de Girolamo M, Ficoneri C, Riccioni G. Fucoxantin: a treasure from the sea. Mar Drugs 2012;10:604–16.
[39] Mohamed S, Hashim SN, Rahman HA. Seaweeds: a sustainable functional food for complementary and alternative therapy. Trends Food Sci Tech 2012;23:83–96.
[40] Maeda H, Hosokawa M, Sashima T, Funayama K, Miyashita K. Fucoxanthin from edible seaweed, *Undaria pinnatifida*, shows antiobesity effect through UCP1 expression in white adipose tissues. Biochem Biophys Res Commun 2005;332:392–7.
[41] Maeda H, Hosokawa M, Sashima T, Funayama K, Miyashita K. Effect of medium-chain triacylglycerols on anti-obesity effect of fucoxanthin. J Oleo Sci 2007;56:615–21.
[42] Woo M-N, Jeon S-M, Shin YC, Lee M-K, Kang MA, Choi M-S. Anti-obese property of fucoxanthin is partly mediated by altering lipid-regulating enzymes and uncoupling proteins of visceral adipose tissue in mice. Mol Nutr Food Res 2009;53:1603–11.
[43] Hu X, Li Y, Li C, Fu Y, Cai F, Chen Q, et al. Combination of fucoxanthin and conjugated linoleic acid attenuates body weight gain and improves lipid metabolism in high-fat diet-induced obese rats. Arch Biochem Biophys 2012;519:59–65.
[44] Kang S-I, Shin H-S, Kim H-M, Yoon S-A, Kang S-W, Kim J-H, et al. *Petalonia binghamiae* extract and its constituent fucoxanthin ameliorate high-fat diet-induced obesity by activating AMP-activated protein kinase. J Agric Food Chem 2012;60:3389–95.
[45] Maeda H, Hosokawa M, Sashima T, Miyashita K. Ditary combination of fucoxanthin and fish oil attenuates the weight gain of white adipose tissue and decrease blood glucose in obese/diabetic KK-A^y mice. J Agric Biol Chem 2007;55:7701–6.
[46] Hosokawa M, Miyashita T, Nishikawa S, Emi S, Tsukui T, Beppu F, Miyashita K. Fucoxanthin regulates adipocytokine mRNA expression in white adipose tissue of diabetic/obese KK-A^y mice. Arch Biochem Biophys 2010;504:17–25.
[47] Beppu F, Hosokawa M, Yim M-J, Shinoda T, Miyashita K. Down-regulation of hepatic stearoyl-CoA desaturase-1 expression by Fucoxanthin via leptin signaling in diabetic/obese KK-A^y mice. Lipids 2013;48:449–55.
[48] Maeda H, Hosokawa M, Sashima T, Takahashi N, Kawada T, Miyashita K. Fucoxanthin and its metabolite, fucoxanthinol, suppress sdipocyte differentiation in 3T3-L1 cells. Int J Mole Med 2006;18:147–52.
[49] Okada T, Nakai M, Maeda H, Hosokawa M, Sashima T, Miyashita K. Suppressive effect of neoxanthin on the differentiation of 3T3-L1 adipose cells. J Oleo Sci 2008;57:345–51.
[50] Maeda H, Hosokawa M, Sashima T, Murakami-Funayama K, Miyashita K. Anti-obesity and anti-diabetic effects of fucoxanthin on diet-induced obesity conditions in a murine model. Mol Med Rep 2009;2:897–902.
[51] Dembitsky VM, Maoka T. Allenic and cumulenic lipids. Prog Lipid Res 2007;46:328–75.
[52] Yim M-J, Hosokawa M, Mizushina Y, Yoshida H, Saito Y, Miyashita K. Suppressive effects of amarouciaxanthin A on 3T3-L1 adipocyte differentiation through down-regulation of PPARγ and C/EBP mRNAα expression. J Agric Food Chem 2011;59:1646–52.
[53] Pittler MH, Ernst E. Dietary supplements for body-weight reduction: a systematic review. Am J Clin Nutr 2004;79:527–8.
[54] Onakpoya IJ, Wider B, Pittler MH, Ernst E. Food supplements for body weight reduction: a systematic review of systematic reviews. Obesity 2011;19:239–44.
[55] Airanthi MKWA, Sasaki N, Iwasaki S, Baba N, Abe M, Hosokawa M, et al. Effect of brown seaweed lipids on fatty acid composition and lipid hydroperoxide levels of mouse liver. J Agric Food Chem 2011;59:4156–63.
[56] Sugawara S, Baskaran V, Tsuzuki W, Nagao A. Brown algae fucoxanthin is hydrolyzed to fucoxanthinol during absorption by Caco-2 human intestinal cells and mice. J Nutr 2002;132:946–51.
[57] Hashimoto T, Ozaki Y, Taminato M, Das SK, Mizuno M, Yoshimura K, et al. The distribution and accumulation of fucoxanthin and its metabolites after oral administration in mice. Br J Nutr 2009;102:242–8.
[58] Matsumoto M, Hosokawa M, Matsukawa N, Hagio M, Shinoki A, Nishimukai M, et al. Suppressive effects of the marine carotenoids, fucoxanthin and fucoxanthinol on triglyceride absorption in lymph duct-cannulated rats. Eur J Nutr 2010;49:243–9.

[59] Asai A, Sugawara T, Ono H, Nagao A. Biotransformation of fucoxanthinol into amarouciaxanthin A in mice and HepG2 cells: formation and cytotoxicity of fucoxanthin metabolites. Drug Metab Dispos 2004;32:205–11.

[60] Tsukui T, Baba T, Hosokawa M, Sashima T, Miyashita K. Enhancement of hepatic docosahexaenoic acid and arachidonic acid contents in C57BL/6J mice by dietary fucoxanthin. Fisheries Sci 2009;75:261–3.

[61] Abidov M, Ramazanov Z, Seifulla R, Grachev S. The effects of Xanthigen™ in the weight management of obese premenopausal women with non-alcoholic fatty liver disease and normal liver fat. Diabetes Obes Metab 2010;12:72–81.

[62] Smith RE, Horwitz BA. Brown fat and thermogenesis. Physiol Rev 1969;49:330–425.

[63] Rothwell NJ, Stock MJ. A role for brown adipose tissue in diet-induced thermogenesis. Nature 1979;281:31–5.

[64] Nedergaard J, Golozoubova V, Matthias A, Asadi A, Jacobsson A, Cannon B. UCP1: the only protein able to mediate adaptive non-shivering thermogenesis and metabolic inefficiency. Biochim Biophys Acta 2001;1504:82–106.

[65] Collins S, Yehuda-Shnaidman E, Wang H. Positive and negative control of Ucp1 gene transcription and the role of β-adrenergic signaling networks. Int J Obesity 2010;34:S28–33.

[66] Silva JE, Rabelo R. Regulation of the uncoupling protein gene expression. Eur J Endocrinol 1997;136:251–64.

[67] Del Mar Gonzalez-Barroso M, Ricquier D, Cassard-Doulcier AM. The human uncoupling protein-1 gene (UCP1): present status and perspectives in obesity research. Obesity Rev 2000;1:61–72.

[68] Argyropoulos G, Harper M-L. Molecular biology of thermoregulation. Invited review: uncouling proteins and thermoregulation. J Appl Physiol 2002;92:2187–98.

[69] Mozo J, Emre Y, Bouillaud F, Ricquier D, Criscuolo F. Thermoregulation: what role for UCPs in mammals and birds? Biosci Rep 2005;25:227–49.

[70] Cederberg A, Grønning LM, Ahrén B, Taskén K, Carlsson P, Enerbäck S. *FOXC2* is a winged helix gene that counteracts obesity, hypertriglyceridemia, and diet-induced insulin resistance. Cell 2001;106:563–73.

[71] Nishikawa S, Hosokawa M, Miyashita K. Fucoxanthin promotes translocation and induction of glucose transporter 4 in skeletal muscles of diabetic/obese KK-A(y) mice. Phytomedicine 2012;19:389–94.

[72] Cummings DE, Brandon EP, Planas JV, Motamed K, Idzerda RL, McKnight GS. Genetically lean mice result from targeted disruption of the RII beta subunit of protein kinase A. Nature 1996;382:622–6.

[73] Soloveva V, Graves RA, Rasenick MM, Spiegelman BM, Ross SR. Transgenic mice overexpressing the beta 1-adrenergic receptor in adipose tissue are resistant to obesity. Mol Endocrinol 1997;11:27–38.

[74] Himms-Hagen J, Melnyk A, Zingaretti MC, Ceresi E, Barbatelli G, Cinti S. Multilocular fat cells in WAT of CL-316243-treated rats derive directly from white adipocytes. Am J Physiol Cell Physiol 2000;279:C670–81.

[75] Gade W, Schmit J, Collins M, Gade J. Beyond obesity: the diagnosis and pathophysiology of metabolic syndrome. Clin Lab Sci 2010;23:51–61.

[76] Reaven GM. Themetabolic syndrome: time to get off the merry-go-round? J Intern Med 2010;269:127–36.

[77] Teixeira ME, Budd GM. Obesity stigma: a newly recognized barrier to comprehensive and effective type 2 diabetes management. J Am Acad Nurse Pract 2010;22:527–33.

[78] Leibson CL, Williamson DF, Melton LJ, Palumbo PJ, Smith SA, Ransom JE, et al. Temporal trends in BMI among adults with diabetes. Diabetes Care 2001;24:1584–9.

[79] Bloomgarden ZT. Approaches to treatment of pre-diabetes and obesity and promising new approaches to type 2 diabetes. Diabetes Care 2008;31:1461–6.

[80] Rudkowska I. Functional foods for health: focus on diabetes. Maturitas 2009;62:263–9.

[81] Abete I, Astrup A, Martinez JA, Thorsdottir I, Zulet MA. Obesity and the metabolic syndrome: role of different dietary macronutrient distribution patterns and specific nutritional components on weight loss and maintenance. Nutr Rev 2010;68:214–31.

[82] Deng Y, Scherer PE. Adipokines as novel biomarkers and regulators of the metabolic syndrome. Ann NY Acad Sci 2010;1212:E1–E19.

[83] Xu H, Barnes GT, Yang Q, Tan G, Yang D, Chou CJ, et al. Chronic inflammation in fat plays a crucial role in the development of obesity-related insulin resistance. J Clin Invest 2003;112:1821–30.

[84] Curat CA, Miranville A, Sengenès C, Diehl M, Tonus C, Busse R, et al. From blood monocytes to adipose tissue-resident macrophages: induction of diapedesis by human mature adipocytes. Diabetes 2004;53:1285–92.

[85] Suganami T, Nishida J, Ogawa Y. A paracrine loop between adipocytes and macrophages aggravates inflammatory changes: role of free fatty acids and tumor necrosis factor α. Arterioscler Thromb Vasc Biol 2005;25:2062–8.

[86] Kennedy A, Martinez K, Chuang CC, LaPoint K. McIntosh M. Saturated fatty acid-mediated inflammation and insulin resistance in adipose tissue: mechanisms of action and implications. J Nutr 2008;139:1–4.

[87] Joost HG, Bell GI, Best JD, Birnbaum MJ, Charron MJ, Chen YT, et al. Nomenclature of the GLUT/SLC2A family of sugar/polyol transport facilitators. Am J Physiol Endocrinol Metab 2002;282:E974–6.

[88] Charron MJ, Katz EB. Metabolic and therapeutic lessons from genetic manipulation of GLUT4. Mol Cell Biochem 1998;182:143–52.

[89] Minokoshi Y, Kahn CR, Kahn BB. Tissue-specific ablation of the GLUT4 glucose transporter or the insulin receptor challenges assumptions about insulin action and glucose homeostasis. Tissue-specific ablation of the GLUT4 glucose transporter or the insulin receptor challenges assumptions about insulin action and glucose homeostasis. J Biol Chem 2003;278:33609–12.

[90] Charron MJ, Ellen B, Katz EB, Olson AL. GLUT4 gene regulation and manipulation. J Biol Chem 1999;274:3253–6.

[91] Kahn BB, Pedersen O. Suppression of GLUT4 expression in skeletal muscle of rats that are obese from high fat feeding but not from high carbohydrate feeding or genetic obesity. Endocrinology 1993;132:13–22.

[92] Kim Y, Tamura T, Iwashita S, Tokuyama K, Suzuki M. Effect of high-fat diet on gene expression of and insulin receptor in soleus muscle. Biochem Biophys Res Commun 1994;202:519–26.

[93] Bonen A. PGC-1α-induced improvements in skeletal muscle metabolism and insulin sensitivity. Appl Physiol Nutr Metab 2009;34:307–14.

[94] Michael LF, Wu Z, Cheatham RB, Puigserver P, Adelmant G, Lehman JJ, et al. Restoration of insulin-sensitive glucose transporter (GLUT4) gene expression in muscle cells by the transcriptional coactivator PGC-1. Proc Natl Acad Sci USA 2001;98:3820–5.

[95] Benton CR, Nickerson JG, Lally J, Han X-X, Holloway GP, Glatz JFC, et al. Modest PGC-1α overexpression in muscle in vivo is sufficient to increase insulin sensitivity and palmitate oxidation in subsarcolemmal, not intermyofibrillar, mitochondria. J Biol Chem 2008;283:4228–40.

[96] Huang S, Czech MP. The GLUT4 glucose transporter. Cell Metab 2007;5:237–52.

[97] Goodyear LJ, King PA, Hirshman MF, Thompson CM, Horton ED, Horton ES. Contractile activity increases plasma membrane glucose transporters in absence of insulin. Am J Physiol 1990;258:E667–72.

[98] Henriksen EJ, Bourey RE, Rodnick KJ, Koranyi L, Permutt MA, Holloszy JO. Glucose transporter protein content and glucose transport capacity in rat skeletal muscles. Am J Physiol 1999;259:E593–8.

[99] Shepherd PR, Kahn BB. Glucose transporters and insulin action-implications for insulin resistance and diabetes mellitus. N Engl J Med 1999;341:248–57.

[100] Woo M-N, Jeon S-M, Kim H-J, Lee M-K, Shin S-K, Shin YC, et al. Fucoxanthin supplementation improves plasma and hepatic lipid metabolism and blood glucose concentration in high-fat fed C57BL/6N mice. Chem Biol Interact 2010;186:316–22.

[101] Tsukui T, Konno K, Hosokawa M, Maeda H, Sashima T, Miyashita K. Fucoxanthin and fucoxanthinol enhance the amount of docosahexaenoic acid in the liver of KKAy obese/diabetic mice. J Agric Food Chem 2007;55:5025–9.

[102] Cho SY, Miyashita K, Miyazawa T, Fujimoto K, Kaneda T. Autoxidation of ethyl eicosapentaenoate and docosahexaenoate. J Am Oil Chem Soc 1987;64:876–9.

[103] Cosgrove JP, Church DF, Pryor WA. The kinetics of the autoxidation of polyunsaturated fatty acids. Lipids 1987;1987(22): 299–304.

[104] Iwasaki S, Airanthi MKWA, Koide A, Kaga T, Nakano S, Beppu F, et al. *In vivo* antioxidant activity of fucoxanthin on obese/diabetes KK-*A*^{y} mice. Food Nutr Sci 2012;3:1491–9.

[105] Vincent HK, Taylor AG. Biomarkers and potential mechanisms of obesity-induced oxidant stress in humans. Int J Obesity 2006;30:400–18.

[106] Vincent HK, Innes KE, Vincent KR. Oxidative stress and potential interventions to reduce oxidative stress in overweight and obesity. Diabetes Obes Metab 2007;9:813–39.

[107] Andrikopoulos A. Obesity and type 2 diabetes: slow down!-can metabolic deceleration protect the islet beta cell from excess nutrient-induced damage? Mol Cell Endocrinol 2010;316: 140–6.

[108] Grattagliano I, Palmieri VO, Portincasa P, Moschetta A, Palasciano G. Oxidative stress-induced risk factors associated with the metabolic syndrome: a unifying hypothesis. J Nutr Biochem 2008;19:491–504.

[109] Yang H, Jin X, Lam CWK, Yan S-K. Oxidative stress and diabetes mellitus. Clin Chem Lab Med 2011;49:1773–82.

[110] Shi Y-C, Pan T-M. Red mold, diabetes, and oxidative stress: a review. Appl Microbiol Biotechnol 2012;94:47–55.

[111] Namitha KK, Negi PS. Chemistry and biotechnology of carotenoids. Crit Rev Food Sci Nutr 2010;50:728–60.

[112] Böhm F, Edge R, Truscott G. Interactions of dietary carotenoids with activated (singlet) oxygen and free radicals: potential effects for human health. Mol Nutr Food Res 2012;56:205–16.

[113] Stahl W, Sies H. Photoprotection by dietary carotenoids: concept, mechanisms, evidence and future development. Mol Nutr Food Res 2012;56:287–95.

[114] Nomura T, Kikuchi M, Kubodera A, Kawakami Y. Proton-donative antioxidant activity of fucoxanthin with 1,1-diphenyl-2-picrylhydrazyl (DPPH). Biochem Mol Biol Intl 1997;42:361–70.

[115] Nishino H. Cancer prevention by carotenoids. Mut Res 1998;402:159–63.

[116] Yan X, Chuda Y, Suzuki M, Nagata T. Fucoxanthin as the major antioxidant in *Hijikia fusiformis*, a common edible seaweed. Biosci Biotechnol Biochem 1999;63:605–7.

[117] Sachindra NM, Sato E, Maeda H, Hosokawa M, Niwano Y, Kohno M, et al. Radical scavenging and singlet oxygen quenching activity of marine carotenoid fucoxanthin and its metabolites. J Agric Food Chem 2007;55:8516–22.

[118] Zaragozá MC, López D, Sáiz MP, Poquet M, Pérez J, Puig-Parellada P, et al. Toxicity and antioxidant activity in vitro and in vivo of two *Fucus vesiculosus* extracts. J Agric Food Chem 2008;56:7773–80.

[119] Krinsky NI, Yeum KJ. Carotenoid-radical interactions. Biochem Biophys Res Commu 2003;305:754–60.

[120] Miller NJ, Sampson J, Candeias LP, Bramley PM, Rice-Evans CA. Antioxidant activities of carotenes and xanthophylls. FEBS Lett 1996;384:240–2.

[121] Arao T, Yamada M. Positional distribution of fatty acids in galactolipids of algae. Phytochemistry 1989;28:805–10.

[122] Vaskovsky VE, Khotimchenko SV, Xia B, Hefang L. Polar lipids and fatty acids of some marine macrophytes from the Yellow Sea. Phytochemistry 1996;42:1347–56.

[123] Li X, Fan X, Han L, Lou Q. Fatty acids of some algae from the Bohai Sea. Phytochemistry 2002;59:157–61.

[124] Bhaskar N, Hosokawa M, Miyashita K. Comparitive evaluation of fatty acid composition of different *Sargassum* (Fucales, Phaeophyta) species harvested from temperate and tropical waters. J Aquatic Product Tech 2004;13:53–70.

[125] Terasaki M, Baba Y, Yasui H, Saga N, Hosokawa M, Miyashita K. Evaluation of recoverable functional lipid components with special reference to fucoxanthin and fucosterol contents of several brown seaweeds of Japan. J Phycol 2009;45:974–80.

[126] Nomura M, Kamogawa H, Susanto E, Kawagoe C, Yasui H, Saga N, Hosokawa M, Miyashita K. Seasonal variations of total lipids, fatty acid composition, and fucoxanthin contents of *Sargassum horneri* (Turner) and *Cystoseira hakodatensis* (Yendo) from north seashore of Japan. J Appl Phycol 2013;25:1159–69.

CHAPTER

31

Nutritional Deficiencies in Obese Sleeve Gastrectomy Patients

Antje Damms-Machado and Stephan C. Bischoff

Institute of Nutritional Medicine, University of Hohenheim, Stuttgart, Germany

INTRODUCTION

There has been a rapid increase in bariatric operations since the late twentieth century in terms of frequency but also in the evolution of operation types and techniques. Since 2000, sleeve gastrectomy (SG), which is usually performed as laparoscopic surgery, has been gaining popularity as one-stage revision operation. The first clinical trials proved this procedure to be a simple and safe technique with promising short- and mid-term efficacy, resulting in excess weight loss and remission of comorbidities comparable to those of other acknowledged procedures, such as the combined malabsorptive/restrictive Roux-en-Y gastric bypass (RYGB) [1–3].

SLEEVE GASTRECTOMY: DIETARY RESTRICTION AND ASSOCIATED MECHANISMS

SG is usually classified as a restrictive, "food limiting" procedure. By resecting the greater curvature of the gastric body, a narrow, tubular stomach is formed. The reduction in stomach size restricts distention and increases the sensation of fullness, thus resulting in the ingestion of smaller meals. Additionally, the natural band effect of the pylorus is maintained in SG, which facilitates restriction. Hence, the incidence of nutritional deficiencies, which are often observed in malabsorptive or combined restrictive/malabsorptive procedures, were not expected.

The latest evidence indicates a more sophisticated mechanism for SG, involving alterations to gut hormones such as ghrelin, glucagon-like peptides (GLPs), and peptide YY (PYY) [4]. One example is the reduction in hunger drive thought to be due to resection of ghrelin-secreting cells lining the fundus [5,6]. Moreover, recent studies demonstrate accelerated gastric emptying caused by faster peristaltic folds [7–10]. Thus, the mechanism of action and the physiological impact of gastric volume restriction, decreased dilatation, alterations in the gastric tube gradient and pressure, hormone influence, and gastric motility still need to be unraveled. Another point is that the improved glycemic control observed after this bariatric operation supports the "hindgut theory" [11]. This hypothesis suggests that an expedited delivery of unabsorbed, incompletely digested nutrients to the distal intestine results in the stimulation of hormonal changes, leading to positive effects associated with insulin resistance and type 2 diabetes mellitus. This observation also indicates that nutrient processing and absorption may be incomplete. Hence, SG seems to be a metabolic operation instead of a purely restrictive mechanism leading to weight loss.

At present, the complex mechanisms resulting in beneficial effects of SG and the impact of surgically modified food ingestion and digestion remain poorly understood. In particular, there is little information on whether a faster passage of food through the gastrointestinal tract promotes nutrient deficiencies and protein malnutrition after SG.

PREOPERATIVE NUTRITIONAL DEFICIENCIES IN BARIATRIC SURGERY CANDIDATES

Regarding the influence of a bariatric procedure on nutritional status, it should be considered that nutritional deficiencies may also exist preoperatively in the bariatric patient population. Indeed, evidence obtained over the past few years has shown that obesity itself (without previous bariatric treatment) can be associated with substantial nutrient deficiencies [12–15]. The prevalence of

Pylorus connects the stomach to the duodenum.

phyloric sphincter

Nutrition in the Prevention and Treatment of Abdominal Obesity
http://dx.doi.org/10.1016/B978-0-12-407869-7.00031-3

TABLE 31.1 Clinical Trials Assessing Preoperative Micronutrient Deficiencies in Obese Bariatric Surgery Candidates

Reference	No. of Patients	BMI [kg/m²]	Deficiencies (%)								
			Ferritin	Zinc	Selenium	Vitamin B1	Folate	Vitamin B12	Vitamin A	Vitamin E	25(OH) D 3
Brolin et al. [58]	$n=56$	89-189 kg	–	–	–	–	14.3	8.9	–	–	–
Skroubis et al. [59]	$n=79$	<50	8.3	–	–	–	–	16.4	–	–	–
	$n=95$	>50	3.2	–	–	–	–	6.5	–	–	–
Madan et al. [60]	$n=100$	≥35	6.0	28.0	58.0	–	2.0	5.0	7.0	–	40.0
Kimmons et al. [16]	Male, n $n=1244$	≥30	–	–	2.8	–	25.2	14.2	0.4	21.1	7.2
	Female, $n=1320$	≥30	–	–	6.1	–	31.6	17.0	1.7	25.8	19.0
Flancbaum et al. [61]	$n=379$	52	8.4	–	–	29.0	–	0	–	–	68.1
Ernst et al. [15]	$n=232$	≥35	6.9	24.6	–	–	3.4	18.1	–	–	89.7
	$n=89$				32.6	0			0	2.2	
Damms-Machado et al. [28]	$n=54$	51	18.0	0	14.0	–	5.5	9.3	2.0	–	83.0

micronutrient deficiencies in obese individuals is higher compared to normal-weight controls of the same age and sex [16,17], and affects several micronutrients such as folate, selenium, vitamin A, vitamin B1, vitamin B12, 25-hydroxyvitamin D3 [25(OH)D3], vitamin E, and zinc (Table 31.1); this might lead to diet-related complications in the postoperative period.

Besides the common clinical manifestations of substantial micronutrient deficits, imbalances or insufficiencies of essential micronutrients significantly influence the day-to-day performance, behavior, and emotional state, as well as the intellectual and physical activity of obese individuals [18–20]. Toxic by-products of incomplete biochemical reactions resulting from excessive intake of kilocalories and simultaneous micronutrient deficiencies could lead to further weight gain and the development of associated metabolic diseases [18].

For the micronutrient deficiencies observed in obese individuals, several mechanisms can be considered. First, energy-dense foods are mainly preferred by obese individuals; these are characterized by low micronutrient density, poor fatty acid dispersal, increased simple carbohydrate content, and low fiber content [18,21]. Second, this can be aggravated by an elevated need for essential micronutrients due to increased rates of absorption and dispersal, as well as a high turnover and increased excretion of micronutrients [16]. One example is vitamin D: the increased amount of subcutaneous fat with a high storage capacity for lipophilic compounds observed in obese individuals may explain why serum pools are deprived of 25(OH)D [14,22,23]. Furthermore, particular micronutrient deficiencies in obesity might result from increased systemic and adipose tissue-specific oxidative stress [16]. Iron deficiency might also result from impaired absorption caused by activation of inflammatory pathways [24]. In view of these interactions, low micronutrient concentrations in obesity are probably not only a result of inadequate supply.

In this context, it should be considered that the reference values for daily micronutrient supply, i.e. the Dietary Reference Intake (DRI), apply to healthy, normal-weight individuals. They account for individual variations and distinguish between age groups and sex. However, they do not necessarily apply to patients with metabolic alterations or other diseases, especially those with regular medication use. Hence, DRIs do not meet the metabolic needs of obese individuals. Obese patients may need different amounts of micronutrients from non-obese individuals, especially under conditions of physiologic stress, like significant weight loss or weight cycling, but also after bariatric operations including restrictive procedures.

POSTOPERATIVE NUTRITIONAL DEFICIENCIES AFTER SLEEVE GASTRECTOMY

Little is known about the postoperative nutritional consequences of SG. In this procedure, gastric emptying is accelerated but the food contact is still made throughout all segments of the gastrointestinal tract. SG patients are potentially at a high risk of nutrient deficiencies for several reasons: (1) they have a substantially reduced dietary intake; (2) stomach resection leads to decreased levels of hydrochloric acid and intrinsic factor; (3) patients may suffer from nausea and vomiting

TABLE 31.2 Overview of Studies Assessing Postoperative Micronutrient Deficiencies in Sleeve Gastrectomy Patients

Reference	Patient no. (n) and supplement intake	Zinc	Iron	Ferritin	Vitamin B12	Vitamin B1	Folate	25(OH) Vitamin D	Calcium
Hakeam et al. [37]	$n=61$ Iron-free multivitamin + cyanocobalamin	–	4.9	–	26.2	–	9.8	–	–
Toh et al. 2009 [62]	$n=46$ Multivitamin and mineral supplement	–	11	0	0	–	0	–	–
Gehrer et al. 2010 [25]	$n=50$ Targeted treatment of deficiencies	34	18	–	18	0	22	32	0
Sallé et al. 2010 [47]	$n=33$ Zinc and iron supplementation	14.3 (6) 18.8 (12)	32.1 (6) 25.0 (12)	–	–	–	–	–	–
Kehagias et al. 2011 [42]	$n=28$ No supplementation	–	18	18	4	–	0	–	0
Pech et al. 2012[a] [63]	$n=100$ Targeted treatment of deficiencies	14	–	–	42	–	19	–	–
Damms-Machado et al. 2012 [28]	$n=54$ No general supplementation	–	38 (6) 4 (12)	–	10 (6) 14 (12)	–	10 (6) 17 (12)	70 (6) 70 (12)	0 (6) 4 (12)
Ruiz-Tovar et al. 2012 [26]	$n=30$ Standard multivitamin supplements	0	6.6	3.3	0	–	0	3.3	0
Moizé et al. 2013 [30]	$n=61$ Universal supplementation	31.8 (6) 39.3 (12) 25.0 (24) 47.6 (48) 12.5 (60)	4.3 (6) 10.3 (12) 9.4 (24) 9.5(48) 12.5 (60)	0 (6) 6.5 (12) 20.6 (24) 23.8 (48) 0 (60)	3.7 (6) 3.2 (12) 5.9 (24) 0 (48) 12.5 (60)	4.8 (6) 9.1 (12) 25.0 (24) 0 (48) 0 (60)	–	90 22.7 (6) 37 (12) 66.7 (24) 44.4 (48) 0 (60)	0 (6) 3.6 (12) 3.1 (24) 4.8 (48) 12.5 (60)

[a] *Frequencies of patients treated with supplements due to deficiency.*
Numbers in parenthesis indicate the number of months after operation.

directly after surgery; and (4), SG often results in poor food choices and food avoidance due to intolerances.

An overview of published studies analyzing nutrient deficiencies after SG is provided in Table 31.2. Following SG, patients are mainly at risk of developing deficiencies in folate, vitamin B12, vitamin D, vitamin B1, calcium, iron (and associated indexes of iron status), and zinc. These substances and the possible SG-associated mechanisms that lead to their deficiencies are described in detail in the following sections.

Vitamin D and Calcium

The prevalence of vitamin D deficiency is higher in obese individuals compared to those of normal weights. Insufficient serum 25(OH)D is a common condition in obese subjects before bariatric surgery. Most authors indicate high levels of vitamin D deficiency in preoperative obese patients ranging from 33% to 97% [25,26]. Several studies have reported an inverse correlation between 25(OH)D serum concentration and body mass index or fat mass [27,28]. This observation can be explained by the high storage capacity of body fat for lipophilic compounds, such as vitamin D. The higher amount of fat tissue in obesity could lead to increased accumulation of vitamin D in fat stores, which in turn leads to a deficit in the serum pool.

Interestingly, some studies showed that bariatric surgery can increase 25(OH)D serum concentrations or decrease the frequency of vitamin D deficiency [26,28,29].

This might be explained by the fact that the reduction in adiposity caused by surgery potentiates the bioavailability of vitamin D. This observation should be addressed in further studies.

However, several studies showed that the doses of vitamin D contained in multivitamin preparations seem to be insufficient to correct vitamin D levels in subjects with deficiency before surgery. There seems to be no difference between gastric bypass and SG regarding postoperative deficiencies [30]. This may be due to malnutrition secondary to food restrictions, but may also indicate an insufficient supply through using DRI reference values for obese individuals because of the increased requirements of this patient population. It can also be related to lower sunlight exposure caused by obese individuals having little or no physical activity, as well as their tendency to live indoors due to psychological reasons.

Normal levels of vitamin D are essential for adequate intestinal calcium uptake. Calcium levels must then be maintained mainly from bone resorption. Thus, low levels of vitamin D lead to a negative calcium balance and cause a compensatory rise in parathyroid hormone (PTH) to promote bone resorption [31]. Secondary parathyroidism causes muscle weakness, bone disease, and various other health problems associated with the vitamin D deficiency.

It has been shown that bone metabolism can change during the first year after SG, resulting in a decline in bone mineral density [31]. On the one hand, this change can be explained by the weight loss itself due to the decreased pressure on weight-bearing bones, which serves as a potent stimulant for bone preservation.

Consequently, an assessment of calcium and vitamin D status before and at least 6 months after bariatric surgery should be performed in order to select subjects who need specific treatments.

Thiamine

Thiamine (vitamin B1) deficiency leads to Wernicke encephalopathy, which can develop after any type of gastrectomy operation, usually within 6 months [32]. Several reports indicate that Wernicke encephalopathy was due to gastrectomy to remove benign or malign tumors in the stomach. In recent years, also case reports of thiamine deficiency after SG for the treatment of obesity have increased in quantity [32–34]. Not only in this context, however, has Wernicke encephalopathy been linked to prolonged fasting, starvation, malnutrition, and an unbalanced diet [35].

The absorption of thiamine takes mainly place in the duodenum and small intestine, in particular the ileum and jejunum. The onset of clinical manifestation occurs rapidly because thiamine can be depleted from the human body in only 18 days.

Thiamine is an essential cofactor for several enzymes involved in carbohydrate metabolism. Moreover, these enzymes are also important for the biosynthesis of neurotransmitters. Thiamine deficiency causes a disorder of energy metabolism in brain cells that leads to mobility impairments of neurotransmitters, thus resulting in neurological symptoms like those seen in Wernicke encephalopathy.

Regarding SG, the restriction of energy intake imposed by the stomach "sleeve" leads to periodic vomiting in 36% of patients, and a lack of supplementation may contribute to the onset of Wernicke encephalopathy caused by thiamine deficiency.

Iron

There are two forms of dietary iron: heme and nonheme. In the stomach and small intestine, proteolytic enzymes induce the release of heme iron from hemoglobin and myoglobin. The heme molecule is taken up by a specific transporter on the apical surface of the enterocyte and is later degraded, returning iron to the soluble iron pool. A cation transporter takes up dietary nonheme iron in the ferrous form [36].

Iron absorption is largely accomplished in the duodenum and the first sections of the jejunum, which is kept intact in SG. However, a reduction in stomach volume decreases parietal cell mass, resulting in a reduction in hydrochloric acid (HCl) production and thus gastric acid [37]. HCl plays an important role in iron absorption through two mechanisms: (1) HCl assists in protein denaturation, thus liberating protein-bound iron; and (2) HCl reduces ferric ions from dietary resources to the ferrous state, which is the form in which it can be absorbed. Iron is an important constituent of hemoglobin, myoglobin, and many iron-containing enzymes such as cytochromes. Iron deficiency is associated with reduced immune function and enhanced susceptibility to infectious diseases [38]. Iron deficiency has been shown to impact cognition and cause fatigue [39]. A severe deficiency may negatively influence collagen production and wound healing. Uncorrected, prolonged iron deficiency can progress to anemia.

One study addressed the question whether restrictive (SG) and restrictive/malabsorptive (RYGB) procedures have differential effects on iron absorption and iron status, and analyzed whether these types of surgery affect heme- and non-heme-iron absorption differently [36]. An important feature of the two procedures is the resultant drastic reduction in stomach size. Accordingly, this anatomical change leads to an immediate reduction in food-gastric juice interaction. Gastric juice is an essential factor supporting the release of heme from dietary hemoglobin and myoglobin. Moreover, it is involved in the release of non-heme iron from its protein matrix and in the solubilization and ionization of dietary ion. In a similar way to RYGB, SG resulted in a decreased capacity to absorb iron. Moreover, the results did not show differences in iron absorption between both bariatric procedures.

Consequently, the recommended iron intake may need to be increased to effectively prevent postoperative iron-status impairment.

Cobalamin

Vitamin B12 (cobalamin) is usually absorbed from the small bowel at the terminal ileum in the presence of intrinsic factor, which is secreted by parietal cells in the gastric body. Resection of a significant proportion of the stomach during SG may reduce the production of intrinsic factor, which is essential for the release of 99% of vitamin B12 derived from food sources.

Severe vitamin B12 deficiency can manifest as macrocytic anemia [40]. Vitamin B12-deficient patients also may develop symptoms of neurologic deficit [41]. Even restrictive operations such as SG seem to have an effect on vitamin B12 and folate blood concentrations. In the postoperative period, the incidence of vitamin B12 deficiency ranges from 9% to 20% [37,42]. Vitamin B12 inadequacy can be aggravated by restrictive surgeries if patients have a low intake of meat or dairy products.

If vitamin B12 deficiency is detected early, it can be treated with oral supplements or intramuscular injections without any difficulty.

Folate

Vitamin B12 is an important cofactor in folate metabolism. Low serum concentrations of folate have been associated with atherosclerotic diseases [43], cancer [44], psychiatric disorders [45], and cognitive impairment [46]. Folate deficiency following laparoscopic SG can hardly be ascribed to anatomical or physiological changes in the gastrointestinal tract. Instead, the primary cause of this deficit is assigned to food choice following the intervention: it is linked to a low intake of sources rich in this vitamin, such as legumes and green leafy vegetables.

Zinc

Zinc deficiency can be caused by malabsorption and protein malnutrition. Pre- and early postsurgery differences in plasma zinc concentrations may be secondary to an inadequate protein status. One study showed that plasma zinc levels correlate with indirect markers of protein nutritional status such as prealbumin and with other markers of protein-related nutrients such as iron [47]. Additionally, patients often dislike the taste of meat products, from which a great portion of dietary zinc is derived, thus resulting in the inadequate dietary intake of zinc.

Unlike many other micronutrients, the body is not able to store zinc and has no functional reserves. The long-term effects of mild deficiency are unclear but seem to be linked to delayed wound healing, suboptimal immune function, increased plasma lipid peroxides, reduced taste and smell acuity, and alopecia [48,49].

The requirement for zinc supplementation after bariatric surgery is not widely recognized. There are currently no guidelines for zinc supplementation after bariatric surgery. However, it has been shown that specific zinc supplementation after bariatric surgery can be effective and is quantitatively sufficient [47].

Protein

Following SG, protein energy malnutrition can occur due to the decreased volume of dietary intake. Following restrictive procedures like gastric banding, protein loss has been demonstrated but it is lower than in malabsorptive procedures [50,51]. After SG, adequate protein intake is difficult to accomplish due to a common intolerance to protein-rich food such as dairy products and meat, which may lead to net protein loss. Patients might profit from protein supplements to improve the quality of fat-free mass and counteract a catabolic state. However, the efficiency of added protein intake after surgery needs to be proven in further studies.

In summary, in the majority of cases, SG itself has only a modest effect on micronutrient status, at least within the first 1–2 years postoperation, especially when accounting for patients who already had poor concentrations of the corresponding micronutrients before surgery. Moreover, insufficient concentrations of the nutrients discussed in this section are common in the general population.

Even if SG does not affect micronutrient status as severely as do malabsorptive bariatric or combined malabsorption-restriction procedures, some SG patients are at risk of developing deficiencies. These patients need to be identified and treated to avoid diet-related complications during the postoperative period. Hence, micronutrient status should be assessed before surgery in order to start an early treatment. Several studies assessing preoperative nutritional status report that more than half of patients were deficient in at least one nutrient before surgery [25,28]. If not treated adequately, those patients will remain deficient in the postoperative period and may even manifest clinical symptoms. In those patients, postoperative deficiencies may be prevented by starting targeted supplementation before the intervention.

MICRONUTRIENT SUPPLEMENTATION

Data from clinical trials indicate that self-organized intake of multivitamin supplements by the patient is not efficient in the prevention of some nutritional deficits

[26,28,30]. Our own experience showed that about a quarter of the patients who reported taking supplements developed micronutrient deficiencies [28].

Patients are mainly advised to use over-the-counter multivitamin products, which do not necessarily include some micronutrients of concern, like iron. In addition, after other bariatric procedures, standard multivitamin supplementation could not prevent nutritional deficiencies [52,53]. However, this might be explained by irregular supplement consumption. Moreover, standard multivitamin supplements contain the maximal nutrient levels suggested by the DRI, which apply to healthy, normal-weight individuals. In obese patients, micronutrient requirements might be enhanced due to metabolic alterations and elevated oxidative stress [14,16,24], especially during a period of major weight loss. Furthermore, supplementation of vitamins that rarely cause deficiencies, like vitamins A and E, might lead to excessive concentrations [54]. Thus, general recommendations to take standard multivitamin products may be insufficient to prevent deficits. The intake of supplements targeted to the specific deficiency should follow a medical diagnosis and should be carefully supervised.

RECOMMENDATIONS FOR NUTRITION CARE AFTER SLEEVE GASTRECTOMY

Only a few protocols for nutrition care following SG are available; these mainly include general recommendations and are not evidence based. A registered dietician plays an important role in postoperative nutrition care, and should ideally form part of a multidisciplinary team that attends the patient before and during the first months after SG.

It is commonly recommended that SG patients should adhere to a high-protein diet, along with routine follow-up focused on the evaluation of electrolyte and nutritional status at 3, 6, and 12 months. Subsequently, annual check-ups should be performed [55]. At each visit, nutritional symptoms, food tolerance, and weight loss should be assessed. Moreover, the patient should be counseled on the nutritional adequacy of their food intake and diet progression [56]. Postoperative food intake should follow a gradual return to solid food within a maximum of 6 weeks. During this time, fatty foods as well as fruit acid derived from fruit juice or fruits should be avoided.

The daily consumption of protein-rich foods is explicitly recommended. There are currently no standard recommendations for protein intake after bariatric surgery. For SG patients, 1.1 g/kg ideal body weight is suggested to estimate daily protein needs [56]. These needs should be met by the daily consumption of liquid protein supplements.

To maintain adequate hydration following SG, liquids should be consumed with a goal of 1.5 L/day [56]. The consumption of liquids should be separated from eating to avoid gastrointestinal symptoms as well as to fill the sleeved stomach to enable nutrient-rich food ingestion. The nutritional goal is for patients to consume a balanced diet that includes adequate servings from all food classes while avoiding added sugar, sweets, fruit juice, fried foods, caffeine, and alcohol. Regarding macronutrient intake, patients should aim to meet the minimal needs for carbohydrate and fat according to DRI.

SG patients typically do not require an aggressive regimen of supplementation, compared to patients who have undergone bariatric procedures including malabsorptive components. Recent clinical trials indicate a need for lifelong multivitamin supplementation following restrictive SG. However, no controlled trials that provide evidence of the type and dosage of vitamin and mineral supplements are currently available. Table 31.3 lists the recommended micronutrient intakes following SG to maintain an adequate micronutrient status [57]. Supplements should be administered as chewable or liquid formulations. However, individual requirements may vary depending on the pre- to postoperative micronutrient status, assessed by laboratory analysis. Snyder-Marlow et al. [56] also published recommendations serving as general guidelines for micronutrient supplement intake. These include a daily intake of chewable multivitamin/

TABLE 31.3 Requirement for Additional Micronutrient Supplements

Micronutrient	Suggested Intake After Sleeve Gastrectomy (% DRI)
Vitamin A	100
Vitamin B1 (thiamin)	150
Vitamin B2 (riboflavin)	150
Vitamin B3 (niacin)	100
Vitamin B6	150
Vitamin B9 (Folate)	150
Vitamin B12	300
Vitamin C	200
Vitamin D	100
Vitamin E	100
Vitamin K	25
Calcium	100
Iron (fumerate)	50
Zinc	33
Copper	50
Selenium	33

DRI, Dietary Reference Intake.

mineral supplements including copper, iron, and zinc, which provide 200% of DRI daily values. Additionally, patients should take chewable or liquid calcium citrate (1000–1500 mg calcium) containing vitamin D (400–800 mg vitamin D3), as well as 500 μg sublingual vitamin B12. If patients exhibit clinical indications of anemia, supplementation with chewable elemental iron is also recommended.

In conclusion, controlled trials are needed to define the exact type and dosage of micronutrients for general postoperative care. Deficiencies should be assessed at regular check-up visits (3, 6, and 12 months postoperation, with subsequent yearly routine check-ups) and additional targeted supplementation therapies should be provided to correct discovered deficiencies.

References

[1] Abu-Jaish W, Rosenthal RJ. Sleeve gastrectomy: a new surgical approach for morbid obesity. Expert Rev Gastroenterol Hepatol 2010;4(1):101–19.

[2] Chambers AP, Jessen L, Ryan KK, Sisley S, Wilson-Perez HE, Stefater MA, et al. Weight-independent changes in blood glucose homeostasis after gastric bypass or vertical sleeve gastrectomy in rats. Gastroenterology 2011;141(3):950–8.

[3] Peterli R, Wolnerhanssen B, Peters T, Devaux N, Kern B, Christoffel-Courtin C, et al. Improvement in glucose metabolism after bariatric surgery: comparison of laparoscopic Roux-en-Y gastric bypass and laparoscopic sleeve gastrectomy: a prospective randomized trial. Ann Surg 2009;250(2):234–41.

[4] Akkary E. Bariatric surgery evolution from the malabsorptive to the hormonal era. Obes Surg 2012;22(5):827–31.

[5] Ariyasu H, Takaya K, Tagami T, Ogawa Y, Hosoda K, Akamizu T, et al. Stomach is a major source of circulating ghrelin, and feeding state determines plasma ghrelin-like immunoreactivity levels in humans. J Clin Endocrinol Metab 2001;86(10):4753–8.

[6] Langer FB, Reza Hoda MA, Bohdjalian A, Felberbauer FX, Zacherl J, Wenzl E, et al. Sleeve gastrectomy and gastric banding: effects on plasma ghrelin levels. Obes Surg 2005;15(7):1024–9.

[7] Melissas J, Daskalakis M, Koukouraki S, Askoxylakis I, Metaxari M, Dimitriadis E, et al. Sleeve gastrectomy-a food limiting operation. Obes Surg 2008;18(10):1251–6.

[8] Braghetto I, Davanzo C, Korn O, Csendes A, Valladares H, Herrera E, et al. Scintigraphic evaluation of gastric emptying in obese patients submitted to sleeve gastrectomy compared to normal subjects. Obes Surg 2009;19(11):1515–21.

[9] Shah S, Shah P, Todkar J, Gagner M, Sonar S, Solav S. Prospective controlled study of effect of laparoscopic sleeve gastrectomy on small bowel transit time and gastric emptying half-time in morbidly obese patients with type 2 diabetes mellitus. Surg Obes Relat Dis 2010;6(2):152–7.

[10] Baumann T, Kuesters S, Grueneberger J, Marjanovic G, Zimmermann L, Schaefer AO, et al. Time-resolved MRI after ingestion of liquids reveals motility changes after laparoscopic sleeve gastrectomy—preliminary results. Obes Surg 2011;21(1):95–101.

[11] Chandarana K, Batterham RL. Shedding pounds after going under the knife: Metabolic insights from cutting the gut. Nat Med 2012;18(5):668–9.

[12] Schneider A. Malnutrition with Obesity. Aktuelle Ernährungsmedizin 2008;33(6):280–3.

[13] Grzybek A, Klosiewicz-Latoszek L, Targosz U. Changes in the intake of vitamins and minerals by men and women with hyperlipidemia and overweight during dietetic treatment. Eur J Clin Nutr 2002;56(12):1162–8.

[14] Aasheim ET, Hofso D, Hjelmesaeth J, Birkeland KI, Bohmer T. Vitamin status in morbidly obese patients: a cross-sectional study. Am J Clin Nutr 2008;87(2):362–9.

[15] Ernst B, Thurnheer M, Schmid SM, Schultes B. Evidence for the necessity to systematically assess micronutrient status prior to bariatric surgery. Obes Surg 2009;19(1):66–73.

[16] Kimmons JE, Blanck HM, Tohill BC, Zhang J, Khan LK. Associations between body mass index and the prevalence of low micronutrient levels among US adults. MedGenMed 2006;8(4):59.

[17] Kaidar-Person O, Person B, Szomstein S, Rosenthal RJ. Nutritional deficiencies in morbidly obese patients: a new form of malnutrition? Part B: minerals. Obes Surg 2008;18(8):1028–34.

[18] Kaidar-Person O, Person B, Szomstein S, Rosenthal RJ. Nutritional deficiencies in morbidly obese patients: a new form of malnutrition? Part A: vitamins. Obes Surg 2008;18(7):870–6.

[19] Bourre JM. Effects of nutrients (in food) on the structure and function of the nervous system: update on dietary requirements for brain. Part 1: micronutrients. J Nutr Health Aging 2006;10(5):377–85.

[20] Reynolds E. Vitamin B12, folic acid, and the nervous system. Lancet Neurol 2006;5(11):949–60.

[21] Markovic TP, Natoli SJ. Paradoxical nutritional deficiency in overweight and obesity: the importance of nutrient density. Med J Aust 2009;190(3):149–51.

[22] Mawer EB, Backhouse J, Holman CA, Lumb GA, Stanbury SW. The distribution and storage of vitamin D and its metabolites in human tissues. Clin Sci 1972;43(3):413–31.

[23] Wortsman J, Matsuoka LY, Chen TC, Lu Z, Holick MF. Decreased bioavailability of vitamin D in obesity. Am J Clin Nutr 2000;72(3):690–3.

[24] McClung JP, Karl JP. Iron deficiency and obesity: the contribution of inflammation and diminished iron absorption. Nutr Rev 2009;67(2):100–4.

[25] Gehrer S, Kern B, Peters T, Christoffel-Courtin C, Peterli R. Fewer nutrient deficiencies after sleeve gastrectomy (LSG) than after laparoscopic Roux-Y-gastric bypass (LRYGB)-a prospective study. Obes Surg 2010;20(4):447–53.

[26] Ruiz-Tovar J, Oller I, Tomas A, Llavero C, Arroyo A, Calero A, et al. Mid-term effects of sleeve gastrectomy on calcium metabolism parameters, vitamin D and parathormone (PTH) in morbid obese women. Obes Surg 2012;22(5):797–801.

[27] Lin E, Armstrong-Moore D, Liang Z, Sweeney JF, Torres WE, Ziegler TR, et al. Contribution of adipose tissue to plasma 25-hydroxyvitamin D concentrations during weight loss following gastric bypass surgery. Obesity (Silver Spring) 2011;19(3):588–94.

[28] Damms-Machado A, Friedrich A, Kramer KM, Stingel K, Meile T, Kuper MA, et al. Pre- and postoperative nutritional deficiencies in obese patients undergoing laparoscopic sleeve gastrectomy. Obes Surg 2012;22(6):881–9.

[29] Coupaye M, Breuil MC, Riviere P, Castel B, Bogard C, Dupre T, et al. Serum vitamin D increases with weight loss in obese subjects 6 months after Roux-en-Y gastric bypass. Obes Surg 2013;23(4):486–93.

[30] Moize V, Andreu A, Flores L, Torres F, Ibarzabal A, Delgado S, et al. Long-term dietary intake and nutritional deficiencies following sleeve gastrectomy or Roux-En-Y gastric bypass in a mediterranean population. J Acad Nutr Diet 2013;113(3):400–10.

[31] Pluskiewicz W, Buzga M, Holeczy P, Bortlik L, Smajstrla V, Adamczyk P. Bone mineral changes in spine and proximal femur in individual obese women after laparoscopic sleeve gastrectomy: a short-term study. Obes Surg 2012;22(7):1068–76.

[32] Jeong HJ, Park JW, Kim YJ, Lee YG, Jang YW, Seo JW. Wernicke's encephalopathy after sleeve gastrectomy for morbid obesity—a case report. Ann Rehabil Med 2011;35(4):583–6.

[33] Makarewicz W, Kaska L, Kobiela J, Stefaniak T, Krajewski J, Stankiewicz M, et al. Wernicke's syndrome after sleeve gastrectomy. Obes Surg 2007;17(5):704–6.

[34] Moize V, Ibarzabal A, Sanchez Dalmau B, Flores L, Andreu A, Lacy A, et al. Nystagmus: an uncommon neurological manifestation of thiamine deficiency as a serious complication of sleeve gastrectomy. Nutr Clin Pract 2012;27(6):788–92.
[35] Andreu A, Moize V, Rodriguez L, Flores L, Vidal J. Protein intake, body composition, and protein status following bariatric surgery. Obes Surg 2010;20(11):1509–15.
[36] Ruz M, Carrasco F, Rojas P, Codoceo J, Inostroza J, Basfi-Fer K, et al. Heme- and nonheme-iron absorption and iron status 12 mo after sleeve gastrectomy and Roux-en-Y gastric bypass in morbidly obese women. Am J Clin Nutr 2012;96(4):810–7.
[37] Hakeam HA, O'Regan PJ, Salem AM, Bamehriz FY, Eldali AM. Impact of laparoscopic sleeve gastrectomy on iron indices: 1 year follow-up. Obes Surg 2009;19(11):1491–6.
[38] Oppenheimer SJ. Iron and its relation to immunity and infectious disease. J Nutr 2001;131(2S-2):616S–33S.
[39] Verdon F, Burnand B, Stubi CL, Bonard C, Graff M, Michaud A, et al. Iron supplementation for unexplained fatigue in non-anaemic women: double blind randomised placebo controlled trial. BMJ 2003;326(7399):1124.
[40] Pfeiffer CM, Johnson CL, Jain RB, Yetley EA, Picciano MF, Rader JI, et al. Trends in blood folate and vitamin B-12 concentrations in the United States, 1988 2004. Am J Clin Nutr 2007;86(3):718–27.
[41] Stabler SP, Allen RH. Vitamin B12 deficiency as a worldwide problem. Annu Rev Nutr 2004;24:299–326.
[42] Kehagias I, Karamanakos SN, Argentou M, Kalfarentzos F. Randomized clinical trial of laparoscopic Roux-en-Y gastric bypass versus laparoscopic sleeve gastrectomy for the management of patients with BMI <50 kg/m^2. Obes Surg 2011;21(11):1650–6.
[43] Haynes WG. Hyperhomocysteinemia, vascular function and atherosclerosis: effects of vitamins. Cardiovasc Drugs Ther 2002;16(5): 391–9.
[44] Kennedy DA, Stern SJ, Moretti M, Matok I, Sarkar M, Nickel C, et al. Folate intake and the risk of colorectal cancer: a systematic review and meta-analysis. Cancer Epidemiol 2011;35(1):2–10.
[45] Stanger O, Fowler B, Piertzik K, Huemer M, Haschke-Becher E, Semmler A, et al. Homocysteine, folate and vitamin B12 in neuropsychiatric diseases: review and treatment recommendations. Expert Rev Neurother 2009;9(9):1393–412.
[46] Malouf M, Grimley EJ, Areosa SA. Folic acid with or without vitamin B12 for cognition and dementia. Cochrane Database Syst Rev 2003(4):CD004514.
[47] Salle A, Demarsy D, Poirier AL, Lelievre B, Topart P, Guilloteau G, et al. Zinc deficiency: a frequent and underestimated complication after bariatric surgery. Obes Surg 2010;20(12):1660–70.
[48] Fortes C, Agabiti N, Fano V, Pacifici R, Forastiere F, Virgili F, et al. Zinc supplementation and plasma lipid peroxides in an elderly population. Eur J Clin Nutr 1997;51(2):97–101.
[49] Neve HJ, Bhatti WA, Soulsby C, Kincey J, Taylor TV. Reversal of hair loss following vertical gastroplasty when treated with zinc sulphate. Obes Surg 1996;6(1):63–5.
[50] Giusti V, Suter M, Heraief E, Gaillard RC, Burckhardt P. Effects of laparoscopic gastric banding on body composition, metabolic profile and nutritional status of obese women: 12-months follow-up. Obes Surg 2004;14(2):239–45.
[51] Strauss BJ, Marks SJ, Growcott JP, Stroud DB, Lo CS, Dixon JB, et al. Body composition changes following laparoscopic gastric banding for morbid obesity. Acta Diabetol 2003;40(Suppl 1):S266–9.
[52] Gasteyger C, Suter M, Gaillard RC, Giusti V. Nutritional deficiencies after Roux-en-Y gastric bypass for morbid obesity often cannot be prevented by standard multivitamin supplementation. Am J Clin Nutr 2008;87(5):1128–33.
[53] Ledoux S, Msika S, Moussa F, Larger E, Boudou P, Salomon L, et al. Comparison of nutritional consequences of conventional therapy of obesity, adjustable gastric banding, and gastric bypass. Obes Surg 2006;16(8):1041–9.
[54] Aarts EO, Janssen IM, Berends FJ. The gastric sleeve: losing weight as fast as micronutrients? Obes Surg 2011;21(2):207–11.
[55] Moy J, Pomp A, Dakin G, Parikh M, Gagner M. Laparoscopic sleeve gastrectomy for morbid obesity. Am J Surg 2008;196(5): e56–9.
[56] Snyder-Marlow G, Taylor D, Lenhard MJ. Nutrition care for patients undergoing laparoscopic sleeve gastrectomy for weight loss. J Am Diet Assoc 2010;110(4):600–7.
[57] Pournaras DJ, le Roux CW. After bariatric surgery, what vitamins should be measured and what supplements should be given? Clin Endocrinol (Oxf) 2009;71(3):322–5.
[58] Brolin RE, Gorman JH, Gorman RC, Petschenik AJ, Bradley LJ, Kenler HA, et al. Are vitamin B12 and folate deficiency clinically important after roux-en-Y gastric bypass? J Gastrointest Surg 1998;2(5):436–42.
[59] Skroubis G, Sakellaropoulos G, Pouggouras K, Mead N, Nikiforidis G, Kalfarentzos F. Comparison of nutritional deficiencies after Roux-en-Y gastric bypass and after biliopancreatic diversion with Roux-en-Y gastric bypass. Obes Surg 2002;12(4):551–8.
[60] Madan AK, Orth WS, Tichansky DS, Ternovits CA. Vitamin and trace mineral levels after laparoscopic gastric bypass. Obes Surg 2006;16(5):603–6.
[61] Flancbaum L, Belsley S, Drake V, Colarusso T, Tayler E. Preoperative nutritional status of patients undergoing Roux-en-Y gastric bypass for morbid obesity. J Gastrointest Surg 2006;10(7): 1033–7.
[62] Toh SY, Zarshenas N, Jorgensen J. Prevalence of nutrient deficiencies in bariatric patients. Nutrition 2009;25(11–12):1150–6.
[63] Pech N, Meyer F, Lippert H, Manger T, Stroh C. Complications, reoperations, and nutrient deficiencies two years after sleeve gastrectomy. J Obes 2012;2012:828737.

PART G

MACROMOLECULES IN FOODS AND DIETS AND ABDOMINAL OBESITY

CHAPTER

32

Dairy Whey Proteins and Obesity

Sebely Pal, Simone Radavelli-Bagatini, Suleen Ho, Jenny-Lee McKay, Martin Hagger, and Monica Jane

School of Public Health; Curtin Health Innovation Research Institute; Curtin University of Technology, Perth, Western Australia, Australia

INTRODUCTION

Obesity has become a major public health issue in recent years [1]. The prevalence of obesity has reached epidemic proportions worldwide, with approximately 35% of adults aged 20 years or older being overweight in 2008 [2].

Obesity significantly increases the risk of developing metabolic syndrome (MS), which is associated with increased cardiovascular morbidity and mortality, and has been implicated in the development of atherosclerosis [3]. MS comprises a number of physiological abnormalities [4], such as abdominal obesity, atherogenic dyslipidemia, insulin resistance, glucose intolerance, elevated blood pressure, impaired endothelial function [5], arterial stiffness [6], and inflammation [7]. According to the National Health and Nutrition Examination Survey (NHANES) 2003-2006, 34% of Americans had MS and the prevalence increased up to 50% with age [8]. Those who have MS are three times more likely to having a heart attack or stroke and five times more at risk of developing type 2 diabetes mellitus (T2DM) compared with those without the syndrome [9].

Studies trying to find prevention and treatment strategies for different components of MS have focused their attention on macronutrients in recent decades. It is now well known that when the energy contents of diets are equal, the consumption of a high-protein diet produces a greater loss of body fat and a reduced loss of lean body mass [10–13]. However, these beneficial effects can vary according to the different protein sources [14,15]. In recent years, dairy whey protein consumption has been found to have many health benefits. Therefore, the aim of this chapter is to examine the effects of dairy whey protein on several MS risk factors, such as glucose and insulin homeostasis, satiety, body weight and composition, hypertension, vascular function, and lipids and lipoproteins.

WHEY PROTEINS AND HEALTH

Both animal and human studies [16–19] have indicated that whey protein and its components may exert an effect on antimicrobial and antiviral activity, immune-modulating activity, anticancer activity, and cardiovascular health benefits [20], as well as improving mood and preserving lean body mass during normal or energy-restricted diets [21]. Evidently, the consumption of whey proteins can have an array of benefits not associated with other protein sources such as egg and soy [14]. Milk is synthesized in mammary secretory epithelial cells and contains two major protein groups: caseins, which account for around 80% of the total protein in milk; and whey, which accounts for the other 20% [22].

Whey, a by-product of the cheese-making process, contains a heterogeneous, polymorphic group of proteins consisting of five main protein fractions with ratios varying from 8% to 35% (Table 32.1). Beta-lactoglobulin (β-Lg), alpha-lactalbumin (α-LA), glycomacropeptide, proteose peptones, and immunoglobulin have been shown to exert biological activities in vitro and/or in animal studies [23]. Other minor constituents such as bovine serum albumin (BSA), lactoferrin, lactoperoxidase, and other nonprotein fractions such as lactose, minerals (e.g. calcium, magnesium, phosphorus, and zinc), vitamins, and traces of milk fat [24,25] are present in whey. The primary casein components in milk are alpha-caseins, beta-casein, and kappa-casein [26]. Whey proteins are globular (secondary, tertiary, and quaternary) structures that are neither phosphorylated nor extensively glycosylated, but are sensitive to heat. The main proteins in whey, α-LA and β-Lg, appear to be responsible for whey's functional properties such as foaming and gel formation [20,22]. In addition, the composition of whey differs according to the milk source, type of cheese, and manufacturing process.

Nutrition in the Prevention and Treatment of Abdominal Obesity
http://dx.doi.org/10.1016/B978-0-12-407869-7.00042-8

TABLE 32.1 Constituents of Whey and Casein

Whey	Casein
Beta-lactoglobulin (35%)	Alpha-s1-casein
Alpha-lactalbumin (12%)	Alpha-s2-casein
Glycomacropeptide (12%)	Beta-casein
Proteose peptone 3 (12%)	Kappa-casein
Immunoglobulin (8%)	
Bovine serum albumin (5%)	
Lactoferrin (1%)	
Lactoperoxidase (0.5%)	
Branched chain amino acids	
Other components (lactose)	
Vitamins and minerals (Ca, Fe, K, P, Mg, Zn)	
Traces of milk fat	

Whey contains a greater proportion of proteins that are thought to participate in biological activities that are beneficial to health [31,32]. Values are % by energy. Ca, calcium; Fe, iron; K, potassium; Mg, magnesium; P, phosphorus; Zn, zinc.

The efficiency in metabolizing whey proteins is thought to result from their branched chain amino acid (BCAA) content (isoleucine, leucine, and valine). Whey proteins are also known as "fast" proteins because they are rapidly emptied from the stomach and delivered intact to the small intestine. Casein, however, is referred to as a "slow" protein because gastric emptying is delayed: it is precipitated in the stomach by gastric acids and consequently coagulated, which results in a reduction in postprandial plasma amino acids [20,27].

The biological compounds found in whey are thought to be responsible for the effect of whey on health. An examination of the available evidence for whey, casein, and soy proteins indicates that these proteins do not have many common biological activities. Therefore, the effects of these proteins are probably due to the unique features of each type of protein.

Depending on the desired use and effects, whey can be used as a fresh pasteurized liquid or in the form of condensed products: whey protein concentrate (WPC), whey protein isolate (WPI), reduced-lactose whey, hydrolyzed whey proteins, and demineralized whey. The condensed forms preserve desirable components such as the protein content, and contain reduced amounts of unnecessary components such as lactose and fat [20].

WPC and WPI are manufactured from whey using ultrafiltration, spray drying, and evaporation techniques [28]. WPC consists of approximately 34–85% protein and moderate amounts of lactose, fats, and minerals [20]. WPI is composed of 90% protein and little or no lactose or fat [20,29,30]. The latter product provides more protein and eliminates the effects of other components, thus enhancing its functionality. Whey hydrolyzates are peptides derived from hydrolyzing whey proteins derived from milk in a process that includes their fermentation with proteolytic enzymes [24].

METABOLIC EFFECTS OF WHEY PROTEINS

Appetite

It is well known that protein ingestion is a strong factor promoting satiety and energy intake [31–35], with a greater satiating effect than carbohydrate and fat [36,37] under isoenergetic conditions. Current evidence indicates that it is not only the amount of protein consumed but also the protein source [14] that produces the satiating effect; however, results are still contradictory on this issue [14,15,31,38–41].

Several short-term studies show that whey is more satiating than other proteins. WPI has been demonstrated to be more satiating than other dietary proteins such as casein [15] or egg [14] in adults. A study of young lean men (BMI 20–25 kg/m^2) given either water control or preloads of 45–50 g of WPI, soy, or egg albumen in beverages (400 mL) followed by a pizza meal 1-2 h later reported that whey (2766 ± 238 kJ, $P<0.05$) and soy protein (3054 ± 301 kJ, $P<0.05$), but not egg albumen (3816 ± 280 kJ), suppressed pizza consumption 1 h later compared to control (3557 ± 284 kJ) [41]. Another study in healthy lean volunteers ($n=22$, BMI < 25 kg/m^2) tested two liquid preloads consisting of either whey or casein (48 g). Energy intake from an ad libitum buffet meal was significantly decreased 1 min and 30 min after whey preload, compared to casein (3676 ± 359 kJ vs. 4537 ± 528 kJ, $P<0.05$) and satiety was greater following the whey test meal ($P<0.05$) [15]. Pal et al. have shown that 50 g WPI was significantly more satiating than egg, fish, or meat in lean men (mean BMI 22.6 ± 0.8 kg/m^2) [41]. Subjects consumed these four protein liquid test meals on separate occasions and were then offered a buffet meal 4 h later. This study tested the palatability of the test meals, which were matched as closely as possible for appearance, texture, and taste. The area under the curve (AUC) rating of hunger was significantly lower after the whey meal (174.6 ± 16) than after the tuna (201.6 ± 17, $P=0.033$), turkey (237.0 ± 18, $P<0.001$), and egg (253.6 ± 18, $P<0.001$) meals. Mean energy intake at the ad libitum meal was significantly lower with the whey meal (2950.1 ± 98.1 kJ) than with the tuna (3275.2 ± 104.4 kJ), egg (3513.7 ± 110.7 kJ), and turkey (3534.8 ± 113.6 kJ) meals (all $P<0.001$). A review examining the role of proteins in the regulation of food intake found whey protein to have a stronger effect on short-term food intake in humans compared to casein, soy protein, and egg albumin [31].

In contrast, three studies by Bowen et al. found that whey protein did not significantly lower energy intake compared to other protein sources or found no significant differences in energy intake between whey protein and other preloads [38–40]. One of these studies included 25 lean (mean BMI 23.3 ± 0.2 kg/m^2) and 47 obese (mean BMI 30.1 ± 0.5 kg/m^2) subjects. Energy intake was shown to be 10% ($P < 0.05$) lower after all protein preloads containing 50 g of WPI, soy, or gluten compared with a glucose treatment, independent of BMI status and protein type [38], but there was no difference between lean and obese subjects in response to 50 g whey protein. A behavioral effect may account for the lack of difference between groups because lean and overweight subjects were randomly mixed into groups to have their buffet meals together. In addition, as there was no effect of weight on energy intake or appetite, the authors acknowledge that overweight subjects may present reduced sensitivity to glucagon-like peptide 1 (GLP-1) because overweight subjects had higher GLP-1, which is believed to reduce appetite [38]. In a study of 28 obese men (mean BMI 32.5 ± 0.6 kg/m^2), beverages containing 50 g WPI, fructose, or glucose or 25 g whey plus 25 g fructose had similar effects on appetite ($P > 0.05$) [39]. Acute appetite and energy intake were similarly reduced after consumption of beverages containing 55 g WPI or casein or 56 g lactose in a study of 19 obese men (mean BMI 32.1 ± 0.9 kg/m^2), compared with 56 g glucose, as measured by a visual analog scale every 15 min for 2 h [40]. The contradictory results of these studies may indicate that a higher amount of protein is required to promote satiety in obese individuals compared to those that are lean or of lower body weight, as reported in the previous paragraph. It appears that 50 g WPI is adequate to promote satiety in lean individuals, but may not be adequate for those with a BMI > 30 kg/m^2. Therefore, body weight and WPI dose may need to be taken into consideration in future studies.

Some mechanisms have been proposed to explain the effects of whey protein on satiety. The differential effects of whey and casein on satiety may be related to the digestive properties of whey as a "fast protein" and casein as a "slow protein" [27]. The appearance of dietary amino acids in plasma following a meal with whey protein is fast, high, and transient [27]. Whey proteins are rapidly emptied from the stomach, reaching the jejunum as intact proteins. Compared to other proteins, hydrolysis of whey peptides in the small intestine is fast, with their digestion and absorption taking place over a greater length of intestine [27,40]. Whey contains higher amounts of BCAAs [42], which might explain the faster rate of digestion and absorption of whey compared to other proteins. The effect of whey protein on satiety [15,27] and its insulinotropic effect [16,43–45] are thought to be caused by the rapid appearance of essential amino acids in plasma [43]. Whey protein seem to influence gut hormones, stimulating anorexigenic hormones involved in satiety, such as gastric inhibitory polypeptide (GIP), GLP-1, cholecystokinin (CCK), and peptide YY (PYY) [15,43,44,46], or inhibiting ghrelin [47,48]. However, findings in this area are inconsistent. The release of CCK into the blood is promoted by the presence of fat or protein in the duodenum. CCK has been proposed as a suitable biomarker for satiation because it is involved in the events leading to appetite suppression and meal termination [49]. Commercial whey products prepared by ultrafiltration [50] contain 15–20% caseinomacropeptide, which seems to stimulate CCK release [31]. This may be a possible explanation for the emerging benefits of whey protein on satiety. However, whey protein, rather than casein, has been found to increase CCK in some [15] but not all [40] studies. In humans, whey protein ingestion resulted in higher plasma concentrations of GLP-1 for up to 3 h compared to casein [15]. In addition, the orexigenic gut hormone ghrelin [39] is released into the circulation, reaching a peak just before meals, and is suppressed by food ingestion [51]. Whey has been shown to decrease ghrelin for over 3 h [38,40], an effect that correlates with greater suppression of subsequent energy intake [40].

Collectively, the positive postprandial effects of whey protein on satiety and energy intake [14,15,31,41] appear to be related to body weight. The studies presented above using lean participants showed a positive effect of whey on energy intake and satiety with a WPI dose ranging from 45 to 50 g. However, this amount of WPI may not be adequate for overweight or obese individuals, as demonstrated in the Bowen studies [38–40]. Additional studies are needed to investigate whether whey has a greater satiating effect compared to other proteins in overweight and obese subjects and thus to clarify whether a dose-dependent effect of whey is related to an individuals' BMI.

Glucose and Insulin Concentrations

Postprandial studies in animals [16], healthy individuals [41,44,52–55], and those with T2DM [46,56] show that whey proteins may significantly decrease the postprandial glucose response because of the insulinotropic effect of its amino acids [16,44–46,56–58]. In rat studies [16], WPC promoted a lower plasma insulin concentration and insulin:glucose ratio, indicating an improvement in insulin sensitivity. Animal studies have shown that the chronic consumption of WPC (for 6 weeks) also reduced plasma insulin concentrations, indicating an increase in insulin sensitivity [35]. A study by Pal et al. found that supplementation with 55 g WPI for 12 weeks resulted in a significantly lower fasting insulin level (41.71 ± 3.80 pM) compared with the control group (54.77 ± 5.18 pM, $P=0.049$), in the absence of weight loss in overweight and obese individuals without diabetes [33]. Therefore, a daily intake of whey may be beneficial in lowering plasma insulin levels in those with the MS.

Pal et al. investigated the postprandial effects of 50 g WPI on glucose and insulin levels, compared to other protein sources such as egg, turkey, and fish in healthy lean men [41]. WPI led to a significantly lower AUC for plasma glucose (8.69 ± 0.32) than did turkey (9.62 ± 0.35, $P<0.023$) and egg (9.63 ± 0.54, $P<0.001$) meals; and a higher AUC for insulin (46.73 ± 2.4) compared to tuna (34.41 ± 1.9), turkey (29.69 ± 1.9), and egg (23.09 ± 1.5) meals ($P<0.001$ for all) [41]. These effects are consistent with another postprandial study that reported that WPI (0.81 ± 0.07 g/kg) significantly increased insulin response compared with a glucose control (154%, $P=0.02$), casein (143%, $P=0.07$), and soy (151%, $P=0.03$) in lean individuals [57]. In addition, two crossover trials with healthy young adults investigated the postprandial effects of whey protein using two experiments: experiment 1, with 10–40 g intact whey; and experiment 2, with 5–40 g intact whey plus 10 g whey protein hydrolyzate [50]. The study found that whey (10–40 g) significantly reduced blood glucose concentrations and AUC ($P<0.05$) in experiment 1; in experiment 2, whey significantly reduced the AUC for glucose and increased the insulin response at 30 min ($P<0.05$) immediately before the meal, compared with the control, achieving the highest response after doses of 20 g and 40 g whey protein [50].

Another study showed that the consumption of peptides and intact whey protein [doses of 0, 5, 10, and 20 g glycemic index lowering peptide (GILP) fraction from whey added to a 50 g glucose drink] reduced the glucose response in a dose-dependent manner in healthy subjects [54]. The average reduction in glucose response was 4.6 ± 1.4 mM/min/g ingested GILP, as shown by a significant postprandial decrease in the glucose incremental AUC, which was suggested to be due to increased insulin secretion (and thus increased insulin activity). A study of participants with T2DM investigated the postprandial response to a dietary challenge of soup followed by a potato meal, where 55 g WPI was added to either the soup or the potato meal, or no whey was added [56]. WPI in the soup and in the potato meal significantly reduced the glucose AUC compared to the no-whey control [56]. Another study involving diabetic subjects found that 27.6 g whey significantly reduced the postprandial AUC for blood glucose (21%, $P<0.05$) and significantly increased the insulin response to both breakfast (31%, $P<0.05$) and lunch (57%, $P<0.05$) after the consumption of a high-glycemic-index lunch compared to the same meal without whey protein [46].

In the absence of carbohydrates, amino acids seem to be the major insulin secretagogues [59]. Whey protein has been shown to promote a faster increase in plasma amino acids compared to other proteins [15,27]. Evidence suggests that various protein sources have different digestion and absorption rates, and this could impact on the postprandial amino acid responses [44]. This may explain to some extent why whey proteins, which are digested quickly, have a greater insulinotropic effect than other protein sources. The high BCAA content of whey proteins may also promote a higher insulin response [44,60] compared to other proteins and nonprotein sources. Specific amino acids appear to influence insulin release differently [59,60], both acutely and chronically, through their effects on pancreatic beta cells [61].

The effects of insulin generally oppose glucagon secretion; therefore, it is likely that certain proteins and amino acids that increase the insulin response induce a reduction in glucagon levels. In contrast, proteins that lower insulin responses would promote higher glucagon concentrations [53]. Whey protein hydrolyzate has been suggested to decrease glucagon synthesis and consequently enhance insulin secretion, corresponding to a low plasma glucose response due to an increase in GLP-1 and GIP levels [53,55].

Interestingly, chronic consumption of 55 g/day WPI resulted in reduced plasma insulin concentrations in overweight and obese individuals after 12 weeks of intervention [62], indicating an increase in insulin sensitivity [16].

Overall, WPC and WPI have been shown to improve postprandial glucose levels and insulin response in both animals and humans. A dose lower than 10 g of intact whey or its peptides seems to be insufficient to promote postprandial benefits on glucose and insulin levels, as observed by two studies that tested lower dosages of whey [52,54]. A dose of around 50 g WPI has been used in most postprandial studies, which seems to be suitable to promote immediate health benefits. In previous studies, improvements in glucose and insulin concentrations and AUCs were seen in both healthy participants and subjects with T2DM [41,46,52,54,56,57]. Most studies have attributed an influence on insulin release to the specific amino acids present in whey; however, further studies are needed to determine the exact mechanism responsible for the insulinotropic effect of whey proteins, as well as to investigate the effects of acute and chronic whey ingestion in those with MS.

Body Composition

Studies have found that WPC may improve weight loss in both animals and humans [16]. A double-blind, randomized clinical trial compared the effects of 56 g/day WPC or soy protein and an isoenergetic amount of carbohydrate supplementation on body weight and composition in 90 overweight individuals (mean BMIs:

control 31.1 ± 2.5; whey 31.1 ± 2.2; soy 30.9 ± 2.3 kg/m^2) for 23 weeks. Body weight and fat mass were significantly lower in the group consuming the whey protein (−1.8 kg, $P = 0.006$ and −2.3 kg, $P = 0.005$, respectively) than the group consuming carbohydrate, but not compared to soy protein [63]. Another study of 31 overweight and obese postmenopausal women (BMI 33.7 ± 4.9 kg/m^2) randomly assigned the participants to either two doses of 25 g/day of either WPI or maltodextrin supplementation for 6 months, along with a reduced calorie diet [64]. Those on the whey diet lost considerably more weight (−8.0 ± 6.2%, $P = 0.059$) than those on the maltodextrin diet (−4.1 ± 3.6%) [64].

Two other studies reported a decrease in body fat in individuals consuming whey protein [65,66], but found no reduction in body weight. A randomized, double-blind study of 158 overweight and obese subjects (BMI 30–42 kg/m^2) found weight loss to be similar between those consuming a Prolibra supplement (high in leucine, bioactive peptides, and milk calcium, and containing 10 g whey as a combination of intact whey protein and peptides) or an isocaloric ready-to-mix beverage containing maltodextrin 20 min before breakfast and 20 min before dinner for 12 weeks [66]. Caloric intake was reduced by 500 kcal/day. However, subjects in the Prolibra group lost significantly more body fat for both the completers (all subjects who completed the study; 2.81 kg vs. 1.62 kg, $P = 0.03$) and responders (subjects who lost at least 2.25 kg body weight; 3.63 kg vs. 2.11 kg, $P = 0.01$), compared to control subjects. In addition, Prolibra subjects lost significantly less lean muscle mass in the responder group (1.07 kg vs. 2.41 kg, $P = 0.02$) [66]. The lack of weight change in the Prolibra group in this study may be related to the short treatment period of 12 weeks and the low dose of whey compared to other studies showing an effect (20 g/day vs. 50 g/day used in other studies). In another study, 18 participants were randomized to one of the three diets: control [15% protein (64 g); mean BMI 29.9 ± 0.6 kg/m^2], mixed protein [30% mixed protein (124 g), including protein from bread, meat, chicken, fruit and vegetables; mean BMI 30.3 ± 0.7 kg/m^2), or whey protein diet (15% mixed protein plus 15% WPI (124 g); mean BMI 30.6 ± 0.6 kg/m^2) [65]. Subjects were enrolled in a 5-month study, with 8 weeks of controlled food intake followed by 12 weeks of ad libitum intake [65]. The study found no statistically significant differences between those consuming a high-whey-protein diet and the control groups in total weight loss (−9.7 ± 1.27 kg vs. −6.1 ± 0.82 kg, $P = 0.198$) or total fat loss (−8.77 ± 1.3 kg vs. −5.45 ± 1.1 kg, $P = 0.216$) [65]. Although the study may not have been powerful enough to detect significant differences in weight status, a significant difference in regional fat loss in midlife adults was observed between treatments [65].

In summary, a dose of 50 g WPC or WPI for about 6 months was effective in reducing body weight in overweight and obese subjects on either a normal diet [63] or an energy-restricted diet [64], compared to maltodextrin but not to soy protein [63]. Two other studies with overweight and obese participants used supplementation with 20 g/day intact whey protein and peptides [66] or 63 g/day WPI [65] over a 3- or 5-month intervention. Although these studies did not find a greater weight loss in the whey group compared to control groups, they did observe greater fat loss. The low dosages and low power of the studies may explain the lack of observed weight loss in the two latter studies. Collectively, WPC and WPI show a positive effect on body weight and body composition when supplements of approximately 50 g/day are taken for at least 6 months.

Blood Lipids

Recently, human and animal models have suggested that dairy proteins may provide cardiovascular benefits [16,18,67–70]. Increasing dietary protein intake may cause positive changes in circulating lipid and lipoprotein levels, including reductions in low-density lipoprotein (LDL) cholesterol, serum triglycerides (TGs), and serum total cholesterol levels, and an increase in high-density lipoprotein (HDL) concentrations, all of which are independent risk factors for cardiovascular disease (CVD) if not modulated [10,71].

Animal experiments investigating the potential benefits of whey protein on lipid metabolism have been mostly undertaken on rats [18,70,72–74]. A study showed that serum cholesterol levels of rats were reduced after supplementation with WPC compared with casein [74]. Female weanling rats consuming a diet containing whey protein, casein, or amino acid mixtures simulating these proteins for 3 weeks showed a significant reduction in cholesterol and TG concentrations [70]. The hypocholesterolemic effect of whey protein in this study was associated with a reduction in very-low-density lipoprotein cholesterol [70]. Improvements in lipid status were observed in Fisher rats consuming a mixture of WPI, WPC, and partially hydrolyzed whey peptides, compared with casein protein [75]. This study also found a positive relationship between paraoxonase (PON) activity and HDL cholesterol levels in the whey protein group. PON is an esterase/lactonase with cardioprotective properties [76], and has been shown to protect LDL cholesterol and HDL cholesterol from oxidation. PON also has the ability to destroy biologically active peroxidized lipids in lipoproteins and arterial cells [77]. Physiological, pathological, and even dietetic factors can affect PON activity [77]. A whey protein diet promotes increases in HDL cholesterol levels as well as PON activity, with many studies supporting a hypocholesterolemic activity for whey protein in rats [18,70,72]. In addition, whey protein has been shown to reduce hepatic cholesterol levels in aged, but not in young, rats [73].

In 1990, Tseng et al. conducted the first human chronic feeding study investigating the beneficial effects of whey protein on plasma lipid profiles [78]; however, the results of this study were restricted to infants. Pal et al. demonstrated that supplementation with 54 g WPI for 12 weeks improved fasting lipids in 70 overweight and obese individuals [79]. Fasting TG levels (baseline 1.07 ± 0.08 mM) were significantly lowered in the whey group at 6 weeks (0.93 ± 0.05 mM, $P = 0.008$) and 12 weeks (0.93 ± 0.07 mM, $P = 0.003$), compared with the glucose control group (baseline 1.21 ± 0.08; 6 weeks 1.21 ± 0.08; and 12 weeks 1.20 ± 0.09 mM). At 12 weeks, there was a significant decrease in the whey group in total cholesterol (baseline 5.36 ± 0.17 mM) by 9% (4.97 ± 0.16 mM at 12 weeks) compared to casein (baseline 5.34 ± 0.23 mM; 12 weeks 5.30 ± 0.23 mM, $P = 0.026$) and by 11% compared to control (baseline 5.43 ± 0.17 mM; 12 weeks 5.58 ± 0.18 mM, $P < 0.001$). LDL cholesterol significantly decreased in the whey group (baseline 3.31 ± 0.17; 12 weeks 3.08 ± 0.12 mM) compared with the casein (baseline 3.32 ± 0.24; 12 weeks 3.36 ± 0.22 mM, $P = 0.045$) and control (baseline 3.25 ± 0.15; 12 weeks 3.41 ± 0.16 mM, $P = 0.003$) groups [79]. Pal et al. suggested that chronic whey consumption may have long-term benefits in reducing total cholesterol, LDL, and arterial exposure to TGs [9].

The ingestion of dietary fat leads to the appearance of chylomicrons (CMs) in the form of enlarged TG-rich particles. These particles are hydrolyzed by lipoprotein lipase (LPL) to form smaller, cholesterol-rich CM remnants (CMRs). Under normal conditions, CMRs bind mainly to LDL receptors in the liver and are rapidly cleared in the postprandial state; however, under conditions of obesity and/or insulin resistance, the clearing process is impaired and/or CMR production increases [80]. The resultant increase in plasma CMs and CMRs enhances the exposure of TG and cholesterol to the arterial wall, consequently increasing the risk of CVD [80]. Pal et al. examined the acute effects of adding 45 g WPI, casein, or glucose control to a meal on apolipoprotein B-48 (ApoB-48; a marker of CM) in overweight and obese postmenopausal women. The results showed a significant decrease in arterial exposure to smaller TG-enriched lipoprotein particles after the whey meal compared to the glucose control (by 21%, $P = 0.032$) and casein (by 27%, $P < 0.001$). Following consumption of the whey meal (0.15 ± 0.02), there was a reduction by 27% (0.20 ± 0.01, $P = 0.033$) and 32% (0.22 ± 0.02, $P = 0.019$) in the AUC for the TG:ApoB-48 ratio in the whey group compared to the glucose and casein groups, respectively [81]. These results are consistent with a previous acute study that found that the addition of 45 g whey protein to a fat-rich meal significantly lowered the TG response (205 ± 86 mM) when compared to casein (282 ± 132 mM, $P < 0.005$), cod (296 ± 111 mM, $P < 0.005$), and gluten (299 ± 75 mM, $P < 0.005$) protein in individuals with T2DM [82].

Pal et al. suggested [79] that the reduction in circulating TG-rich CMs during whey protein supplementation could be due to the rapid rates of digestion or absorption [15,44] of whey, caused by its higher BCAA content. Other mechanisms include the possible inhibition of cholesterol absorption by β-Lg in the intestine [70], as well as the inhibition of gene expression involved in the absorption and synthesis of intestinal fatty acid and cholesterol [83] and increased fecal steroid excretion [84]. Mortensen et al. [82] proposed that the whey protein meal may have resulted in a reduced production of CM when compared to the casein and cod meals because there was a lower retinyl palmitate response in the CM-rich fraction of the plasma. Vitamin A esters, especially retinyl palmitate, have been used in humans as an endogenous label of the core of CMRs. Retinyl palmitate can then be used as a marker to examine CM kinetics in plasma. Whey may stimulate LPL, which in turn accelerates CM clearance because the retinyl palmitate response in the CM-poor fraction was significantly higher after the whey meal compared to the cod and gluten meals [82].

The mechanisms involved in the beneficial effects of whey on the metabolism of lipids and lipoprotein may include a role for whey proteins in de novo cholesterol synthesis in the liver [70] through inhibiting the activity of 3-hydroxy-3-methylglutaryl-coenzyme A reductase (HMG-CoA reductase; a rate-limiting enzyme in cholesterol synthesis). Whey, casein, skim milk, and some amino acids (isoleucine, leucine, and valine) have been demonstrated to downregulate the expression of genes involved in cholesterol metabolism and lipogenesis in an in vitro study [83]. Whey and isoleucine also appear to downregulate the expression of genes involved in fatty acid transport and cholesterol absorption [83], which suggests an involvement of BCAAs in lipid metabolism. The different effects of whey and casein on lipid metabolism may be due to their specific influence on intestinal digestion and absorption, and their amino acid content [27,85].

Overall, whey protein seems to reduce cardiovascular risk factors by improving the lipid profile in both animals and humans. A dose of 45 g WPI added to a meal seems to lower the postprandial TG response in overweight, postmenopausal women and individuals with T2DM. Few studies have investigated the chronic effect of whey on lipids without the confounding effects of weight loss. A dose of 54 g/day WPI has been shown to reduce TGs, total cholesterol, and LDL cholesterol, but had no effect on HDL cholesterol, in overweight individuals after 12 weeks. However, there is a need for ongoing research to elucidate the exact mechanism of action of whey proteins to fully understand their role in the progression of hyperlipidemia.

Blood Pressure

By modifying environmental factors such as diet, physical activity, and social activity, a small reduction in blood pressure (BP) of 2-5 mmHg can be achieved. It has been proposed that diet may play a more important role in lowering BP [86–88]. A reduction in hypertension is beneficial; it would result in a decrease in total mortality because it is a major contributor to the development of CVD and one of the components of MS [89].

There have been limited human studies into the potential effects of whey protein on BP [18,90], although dairy proteins [91] have been suggested to possess antihypertensive properties. An acute study by Pal et al. demonstrated that a meal containing 45 g casein or WPI led to a postprandial decrease in both systolic BP (SBP) and diastolic BP (DBP) in overweight and obese postmenopausal women without hypertension [92].

Chronic studies have also investigated the effect of whey on hypertension. A study in borderline hypertensive humans ($SBP \geq 120/80$ mmHg and $DBP \leq 155/95$ mmHg) randomized to a whey protein hydrolyzate (active treatment) or an unmodified whey protein (control treatment) found that the ingestion of whey protein hydrolyzate for 6 weeks significantly reduced SBP by 8.0 mmHg ($P<0.05$) and DBP by 5.5 mmHg ($P<0.05$) [93]. Another study in nonhypertensive overweight individuals demonstrated that supplementation with 54 g WPI and 54 g casein protein for 12 weeks decreased DBP to similar levels when compared with a glucose control group [67]. However, there was no significant difference in SBP at 12 weeks, possibly because nonhypertensive subjects were used [67].

The process by which whey protein and its components improve hypertension [91] seems to occur specifically through inhibition of angiotensin-converting enzyme (ACE), the enzyme that catalyzes the conversion of angiotensin I to angiotensin II and leads to arterial vasoconstriction [94]. BP decreases [95] as a result of the action of certain peptides such as α-LA, β-Lg, and BSA, which restricts the action of ACE [94,96,97]. Whey contains lactokinins that inhibit ACE, whereas casokinins are casein-derived ACE inhibitors [98]. Lactokinins and casokinins haven been shown to significantly reduce BP in spontaneously hypertensive animals, with SBP decreasing by 2–34 mmHg [99,100].

Chronic intake of 20 g whey hydrolyzate seems to improve BP in individuals with hypertension. In addition, both acute and chronic WPI intake reduced BP in nonhypertensive subjects. Further studies should be conducted to evaluate the effect of WPI on BP in hypertensive individuals. Overall, it seems that increasing the consumption of dairy WPI or whey protein hydrolyzate may promote a reduction in BP and reduce the risk of hypertension.

Vascular Function

As people age, their central arteries gradually stiffen [101,102] and the rate of progression is influenced by hypertension, diabetes, and atherosclerosis [103]. The augmentation index (AI) is an indicator of arterial stiffness that has been shown to be higher in those with hypercholesterolemia [104]. Arterial stiffening is an independent risk factor for CVD [105,106].

A postprandial study evaluating the effects of 45-g WPI supplementation on BP and vascular function [92] found the AI to remain unchanged immediately after the consumption of whey protein ($175.1 \pm 5.71\%$, $P>0.05$) compared to casein ($172.32 \pm 5.73\%$) and control ($180.33 \pm 5.73\%$) in overweight individuals [92]. Pal and Ellis [92] suggested that whey consumption may need to be continued for several weeks to observe a reduction in AI and, consequently, arterial stiffness. A chronic study conducted thereafter by Pal and Ellis [67] demonstrated that supplementation with 54 g/day WPI for 12 weeks resulted in a significant (21%, $P=0.006$) decrease in AI compared with the control group and a 23% reduction ($P=0.006$) when compared with the casein group in overweight and obese subjects.

The different effects of whey and casein proteins on the AI may be related to their effect on BP. An increase in arterial stiffness has been associated with increases in SBP and DBP [107–109]. Although the mechanisms involved in this process remain to be fully clarified, evidence suggests that components of the renin-angiotensin system, matrix metalloproteinases, intracellular signaling, and extracellular matrix components may be involved [107–109]. As dairy proteins play a role in the rennin-angiotensin system [99,110], they are also likely to affect processes that improve AI [67]. Additionally, the whey peptides α-LA, β-Lg, and BSA can all inhibit the action of ACE [94,96,97] and, as a result, decrease BP [95], hence affecting the AI.

In summary, the consumption of whey protein may lead to a reduction in arterial stiffness. A dose of 54 g WPI has been shown to decrease the AI after 12 weeks of supplementation. More studies are required to elucidate whether these bioactive components, the BCAAs in whey, and/or their effects on the angiotensin system may be responsible for beneficial effect on the AI.

CONCLUSION

Scientific evidence supports the positive health benefits of whey protein and its constituents, especially on several components of MS. Whey protein has been shown to improve lipid profiles glucose levels and insulin response, promote a reduction in BP and arterial stiffness, thereby reducing most cardiovascular risk factors. Research highlighted in this chapter suggests that whey, rather than casein and/or mixed protein, is the dairy component that has a positive effect on MS and other risk markers.

A number of components of whey have been found to produce beneficial effects in animals and humans. Of particular significance is the high BCAA content (isoleucine, leucine, and valine) in whey protein. Whey protein seems to participate in a number of bioactivities in both the gut and circulation. It is rapidly emptied from the stomach and delivered to the small intestine in its intact form. It is still unknown whether consumption of the different condensed products of whey used in the studies (i.e. WPC, WPI, or hydrolyzate) would have distinct effects on reducing risk factors for MS. WPI provides a greater amount of protein (90% protein) and no lactose or fat, thus enhancing its functionality, while the protein content of WPC is lower (34-85%) and it contains moderate amounts of lactose, fats, and minerals.

The current knowledge is sufficient to propose doses of whey protein that would be beneficial for those with MS. Approximately 50 g WPI has been shown to improve glucose and insulin postprandially and chronically. WPC and WPI showed a positive effect on body weight and body composition when supplemented at approximately 50 g/day for at least 6 months. Postprandially, the positive effects of whey protein on satiety and energy intake seem to be related to an individual's body weight, since a dose of WPI ranging from 45 to 50 g was beneficial for lean, but not for obese, subjects. Increasing the whey protein content of the diet may promote a reduction in BP and reduce the risk of developing hypertension, as well as improving the lipid profile and thereby reducing cardiovascular risk factors. Consumption of whey protein also seems to reduce arterial stiffness. A dose of 54 g WPI has been shown to decrease the AI after 12 weeks of supplementation. Research to date provides supportive evidence that the consumption of whey protein improves many components of MS; however, further studies are required to clarify the exact mechanisms of action.

Acknowledgments

Dr Pal participated in the conception, design, writing, and critical revision of this chapter. Dr Radavelli-Bagatini participated in the writing and revision of the chapter. Dr Ho, Mrs McKay, Dr Hagger and Ms Jane participated in the revision of this chapter.

SP has received research grants from Dairy Australia (2007-2012); SRB, MJ, JN, and SH have no conflict of interest to declare.

References

[1] Mokdad AH, Ford ES, Bowman BA, et al. Prevalence of obesity, diabetes, and obesity-related health risk factors, 2001. J Am Med Assoc 2003;289(1):76–9.

[2] WHO. Obesity: preventing and managing the global epidemic. Report of a WHO consultation. World Health Organization technical report series 2000; 894: i–xii, 1–253.

[3] Cook S, Hugli O, Egli M, et al. Clustering of cardiovascular risk factors mimicking the human metabolic syndrome X in eNOS null mice. Swiss Med Wkly 2003;133(25–26):360–3.

[4] Isomaa B, Almgren P, Tuomi T, et al. Cardiovascular morbidity and mortality associated with the metabolic syndrome. Diabetes Care 2001;24(4):683–9.

[5] Alessi MC, Juhan-Vague I. Metabolic syndrome, haemostasis and thrombosis. Thromb Haemost 2008;99(6):995–1000.

[6] Stehouwer CD, Henry RM, Ferreira I. Arterial stiffness in diabetes and the metabolic syndrome: a pathway to cardiovascular disease. Diabetologia 2008;51(4):527–39.

[7] Grundy SM. What is the contribution of obesity to the metabolic syndrome? Endocrin Metab Clin North Am 2004;33(2):267–82. table of contents.

[8] Ervin RB. Prevalence of metabolic syndrome among adults 20 years of age and over, by sex, age, race and ethnicity, and body mass index: United States, 2003–2006. Natl Health Stat Rep 2009;13:1–7.

[9] Alberti KG, Zimmet P, Shaw J. Metabolic syndrome—a new world-wide definition. A Consensus Statement from the International Diabetes Federation. Diabetic Med J Br Diabetic Assoc 2006;23(5):469–80.

[10] Farnsworth E, Luscombe ND, Noakes M, Wittert G, Argyiou E, Clifton PM. Effect of a high-protein, energy-restricted diet on body composition, glycemic control, and lipid concentrations in overweight and obese hyperinsulinemic men and women. Am J Clin Nutr 2003;78(1):31–9.

[11] Layman DK, Baum JI. Dietary protein impact on glycemic control during weight loss. J Nutr 2004;134(4):968S–73S.

[12] Layman DK, Boileau RA, Erickson DJ, et al. A reduced ratio of dietary carbohydrate to protein improves body composition and blood lipid profiles during weight loss in adult women. J Nutr 2003;133(2):411–7.

[13] Noakes M, Keogh JB, Foster PR, Clifton PM. Effect of an energy-restricted, high-protein, low-fat diet relative to a conventional high-carbohydrate, low-fat diet on weight loss, body composition, nutritional status, and markers of cardiovascular health in obese women. Am J Clin Nutr 2005;81(6):1298–306.

[14] Anderson GH, Tecimer SN, Shah D, Zafar TA. Protein source, quantity, and time of consumption determine the effect of proteins on short-term food intake in young men. J Nutr 2004;134(11):3011–5.

[15] Hall WL, Millward DJ, Long SJ, Morgan LM. Casein and whey exert different effects on plasma amino acid profiles, gastrointestinal hormone secretion and appetite. Br J Nutr 2003;89(2):239–48.

[16] Belobrajdic DP, McIntosh GH, Owens JA. A high-whey-protein diet reduces body weight gain and alters insulin sensitivity relative to red meat in wistar rats. J Nutr 2004;134(6):1454–8.

[17] Zhang X, Beynen AC. Lowering effect of dietary milk-whey protein v. casein on plasma and liver cholesterol concentrations in rats. Br J Nutr 1993;70(1):139–46.

[18] Kawase M, Hashimoto H, Hosoda M, Morita H, Hosono A. Effect of administration of fermented milk containing whey protein concentrate to rats and healthy men on serum lipids and blood pressure. J Dairy Sci 2000;83(2):255–63.

[19] Sautier C, Dieng K, Flament C, Doucet C, Suquet JP, Lemonnier D. Effects of whey protein, casein, soya-bean and sunflower proteins on the serum, tissue and faecal steroids in rats. Br J Nutr 1983;49(3):313–9.

[20] Walzem RL, Dillard CJ, German JB. Whey components: millennia of evolution create functionalities for mammalian nutrition: what we know and what we may be overlooking. Crit Rev Food Sci Nutr 2002;42(4):353–75.
[21] Zemel MB, Richards J, Milstead A, Campbell P. Effects of calcium and dairy on body composition and weight loss in African-American adults. Obes Res 2005;13(7):1218–25.
[22] Aimutis WR. Bioactive properties of milk proteins with particular focus on anticarcinogenesis. J Nutr 2004;134(4):989S–95S.
[23] Pannemans DL, Halliday D, Westerterp KR, Kester AD. Effect of variable protein intake on whole-body protein turnover in young men and women. Am J Clin Nutr 1995;61(1):69–74.
[24] Krissansen GW. Emerging health properties of whey proteins and their clinical implications. J Am Nutr 2007;26(6):713S–23S.
[25] Marshall K. Therapeutic applications of whey protein. Altern Med Rev J Clin Ther 2004;9(2):136–56.
[26] Rose D, Brunner JR, Kalan EB, et al. Nomenclature of the proteins of cow's milk: third revision. J Dairy Sci 1970;53(1):1–17.
[27] Boirie Y, Dangin M, Gachon P, Vasson MP, Maubois JL, Beaufrere B. Slow and fast dietary proteins differently modulate postprandial protein accretion. Proc Natl Acad Sci USA 1997;94(26):14930–5.
[28] Etzel MR. Manufacture and use of dairy protein fractions. J Nutr 2004;134(4):996S–1002S.
[29] Bastian E, Harper WJ. Emerging health benefits of whey. Dairy Counc Dig 2003;74(6):31–6.
[30] Qi PX, Onwulata CI. Physical properties, molecular structures, and protein quality of texturized whey protein isolate: effect of extrusion moisture content. J Dairy Sci 2011;94(5):2231–44.
[31] Anderson GH, Moore SE. Dietary proteins in the regulation of food intake and body weight in humans. J Nutr 2004;134(4):974S–9S.
[32] Anderson GH, Tecimer SN, Shah D, Zafar TA. Protein source, quantity, and time of consumption determine the effect of proteins on short-term food intake in young men. J Nutr 2004;134(11):3011–5.
[33] Bertenshaw EJ, Lluch A, Yeomans MR. Dose-dependent effects of beverage protein content upon short-term intake. Appetite 2009;52(3):580–7.
[34] Veldhorst MA, Nieuwenhuizen AG, Hochstenbach-Waelen A, et al. Comparison of the effects of a high- and normal-casein breakfast on satiety, 'satiety' hormones, plasma amino acids and subsequent energy intake. Br J Nutr 2009;101(2):295–303.
[35] Westerterp-Plantenga MS, Smeets A, Lejeune MP. Sensory and gastrointestinal satiety effects of capsaicin on food intake. Int J Obes 2005;29(6):682–8.
[36] Poppitt SD, McCormack D, Buffenstein R. Short-term effects of macronutrient preloads on appetite and energy intake in lean women. Physiol Behav 1998;64(3):279–85.
[37] Weigle DS, Breen PA, Matthys CC, et al. A high-protein diet induces sustained reductions in appetite, ad libitum caloric intake, and body weight despite compensatory changes in diurnal plasma leptin and ghrelin concentrations. Am J Clin Nutr 2005;82(1):41–8.
[38] Bowen J, Noakes M, Clifton PM. Appetite regulatory hormone responses to various dietary proteins differ by body mass index status despite similar reductions in ad libitum energy intake. J Clin Endocrinol Metab 2006;91(8):2913–9.
[39] Bowen J, Noakes M, Clifton PM. Appetite hormones and energy intake in obese men after consumption of fructose, glucose and whey protein beverages. Int J Obes 2007;31(11):1696–703.
[40] Bowen J, Noakes M, Trenerry C, Clifton PM. Energy intake, ghrelin, and cholecystokinin after different carbohydrate and protein preloads in overweight men. J Clin Endocrinol Metab 2006;91(4):1477–83.
[41] Pal S, Ellis V. The acute effects of four protein meals on insulin, glucose, appetite and energy intake in lean men. Br J Nutr 2010;104(8):1241–8.
[42] Layman DK, Shiue H, Sather C, Erickson DJ, Baum J. Increased dietary protein modifies glucose and insulin homeostasis in adult women during weight loss. J Nutr 2003;133(2):405–10.
[43] Nilsson M, Holst JJ, Bjorck IM. Metabolic effects of amino acid mixtures and whey protein in healthy subjects: studies using glucose-equivalent drinks. Am J Clin Nutr 2007;85(4): 996–1004.
[44] Nilsson M, Stenberg M, Frid AH, Holst JJ, Bjorck IM. Glycemia and insulinemia in healthy subjects after lactose-equivalent meals of milk and other food proteins: the role of plasma amino acids and incretins. Am j Clin Nutr 2004;80(5):1246–53.
[45] Ostman EM, Liljeberg Elmstahl HG, Bjorck IM. Inconsistency between glycemic and insulinemic responses to regular and fermented milk products. Am J Clin Nutr 2001;74(1):96–100.
[46] Frid AH, Nilsson M, Holst JJ, Bjorck IM. Effect of whey on blood glucose and insulin responses to composite breakfast and lunch meals in type 2 diabetic subjects. Am J Clin Nutr 2005;82(1): 69–75.
[47] Cummings DE, Overduin J. Gastrointestinal regulation of food intake. J Clin Invest 2007;117(1):13–23.
[48] Lang V, Bellisle F, Alamowitch C, et al. Varying the protein source in mixed meal modifies glucose, insulin and glucagon kinetics in healthy men, has weak effects on subjective satiety and fails to affect food intake. Eur J Clin Nutr 1999;53(12):959–65.
[49] de Graaf C, Blom WA, Smeets PA, Stafleu A, Hendriks HF. Biomarkers of satiation and satiety. Am J Clin Nutr 2004;79(6):946–61.
[50] Brody EP. Biological activities of bovine glycomacropeptide. Br J Nutr 2000;84(Suppl. 1):S39–46.
[51] Badman MK, Flier JS. The gut and energy balance: visceral allies in the obesity wars. Science 2005;307(5717):1909–14.
[52] Akhavan T, Luhovyy BL, Brown PH, Cho CE, Anderson GH. Effect of premeal consumption of whey protein and its hydrolysate on food intake and postmeal glycemia and insulin responses in young adults. Am J Clin Nutr 2010;91(4):966–75.
[53] Claessens M, Calame W, Siemensma AD, van Baak MA, Saris WH. The effect of different protein hydrolysate/carbohydrate mixtures on postprandial glucagon and insulin responses in healthy subjects. Eur J Clin Nutr 2009;63(1):48–56.
[54] Petersen BL, Ward LS, Bastian ED, Jenkins AL, Campbell J, Vuksan V. A whey protein supplement decreases post-prandial glycemia. Nutr J 2009;8:47.
[55] Veldhorst MA, Nieuwenhuizen AG, Hochstenbach-Waelen A, et al. Effects of complete whey-protein breakfasts versus whey without GMP-breakfasts on energy intake and satiety. Appetite 2009;52(2):388–95.
[56] Ma J, Stevens JE, Cukier K, et al. Effects of a protein preload on gastric emptying, glycemia, and gut hormones after a carbohydrate meal in diet-controlled type 2 diabetes. Diabetes Care 2009;32(9):1600–2.
[57] Acheson KJ, Blondel-Lubrano A, Oguey-Araymon S, et al. Protein choices targeting thermogenesis and metabolism. Am J Clin Nutr 2011;93(3):525–34.
[58] Labayen I, Forga L, Martinez JA. Nutrient oxidation and metabolic rate as affected by meals containing different proportions of carbohydrate and fat, in healthy young women. Eur J Nutr 1999;38(3):158–66.
[59] Schmid R, Schulte-Frohlinde E, Schusdziarra V, et al. Contribution of postprandial amino acid levels to stimulation of insulin, glucagon, and pancreatic polypeptide in humans. Pancreas 1992;7(6):698–704.

[60] von Post-Skagegard M, Vessby B, Karlstrom B. Glucose and insulin responses in healthy women after intake of composite meals containing cod-, milk-, and soy protein. Eur J Clin Nutr 2006;60(8):949–54.
[61] Newsholme P, Brennan L, Rubi B, Maechler P. New insights into amino acid metabolism, beta-cell function and diabetes. Clin Sci 2005;108(3):185–94.
[62] Pal S, Ellis V, Dhaliwal S. Effects of whey protein isolate on body composition, lipids, insulin and glucose in overweight and obese individuals. Br J Nutr 2010;104(5):716–23.
[63] Baer DJ, Stote KS, Paul DR, Harris GK, Rumpler WV, Clevidence BA. Whey protein but not soy protein supplementation alters body weight and composition in free-living overweight and obese adults. J Nutr 2011;141(8):1489–94.
[64] Mojtahedi MC, Thorpe MP, Karampinos DC, et al. The effects of a higher protein intake during energy restriction on changes in body composition and physical function in older women. J Gerontol A Biol Sci Med Sci 2011;66(11):1218–25.
[65] Aldrich ND, Reicks MM, Sibley SD, Redmon JB, Thomas W, Raatz SK. Varying protein source and quantity do not significantly improve weight loss, fat loss, or satiety in reduced energy diets among midlife adults. Nutr Res 2011;31(2):104–12.
[66] Frestedt JL, Zenk JL, Kuskowski MA, Ward LS, Bastian ED. A whey-protein supplement increases fat loss and spares lean muscle in obese subjects: a randomized human clinical study. Nutr Metab 2008;5:8.
[67] Pal S, Ellis V. The chronic effects of whey proteins on blood pressure, vascular function, and inflammatory markers in overweight individuals. Obesity 2010;18(7):1354–9.
[68] Pal S, Ellis V. Acute effects of whey protein isolate on blood pressure, vascular function and inflammatory markers in overweight postmenopausal women. Br J Nutr 2011;105(10):1512–9.
[69] Pins JJ, Keenan JM. Effects of whey peptides on cardiovascular disease risk factors. J Clin Hypertens 2006;8(11):775–82.
[70] Zhang X, Beynen AC. Lowering effect of dietary milk-whey protein v. casein on plasma and liver cholesterol concentrations in rats. Br J Nutr 1993;70(1):139–46.
[71] Parker B, Noakes M, Luscombe N, Clifton P. Effect of a high-protein, high-monounsaturated fat weight loss diet on glycemic control and lipid levels in type 2 diabetes. Diabetes Care 2002;25(3):425–30.
[72] Beena A, Prasad V. Effect of yogurt and bifidus yogurt fortified with skim milk powder, condensed whey and lactose-hydrolysed condensed whey on serum cholesterol and triacylglycerol levels in rats. J Dairy Res 1997;64(3):453–7.
[73] Choi YS, Goto S, Ikeda I, Sugano M. Interaction of dietary protein, cholesterol and age on lipid metabolism of the rat. Br J Nutr 1989;61(3):531–43.
[74] Sautier C, Dieng K, Flament C, Doucet C, Suquet JP, Lemonnier D. Effects of whey protein, casein, soya-bean and sunflower proteins on the serum, tissue and faecal steroids in rats. Br J Nutr 1983;49(3):313–9.
[75] Haraguchi FK, Pedrosa ML, Paula H, Santos RC, Silva ME. Evaluation of biological and biochemical quality of whey protein. J Med Food 2010;13(6):1505–9.
[76] Durrington PN, Mackness B, Mackness MI. Paraoxonase and atherosclerosis. Arterioscler Thromb Vasc Biol 2001;21(4):473–80.
[77] Aviram M. Introduction to the serial review on paraoxonases, oxidative stress, and cardiovascular diseases. Free Radic Biol Med 2004;37(9):1301–3.
[78] Tseng E, Potter SM, Picciano MF. Dietary protein source and plasma lipid profiles of infants. Pediatrics 1990;85(4):548–52.
[79] Pal S, Ellis V, Dhaliwal S. Effects of whey protein isolate on body composition, lipids, insulin and glucose in overweight and obese individuals. Br J Nutr 2010;104(5):716–23.
[80] Alipour A, Elte JW, van Zaanen HC, Rietveld AP, Cabezas MC. Postprandial inflammation and endothelial dysfuction. Biochem Soc Trans 2007;35(Pt 3):466–9.
[81] Pal S, Ellis V, Ho S. Acute effects of whey protein isolate on cardiovascular risk factors in overweight, post-menopausal women. Atherosclerosis 2010;212(1):339–44.
[82] Mortensen LS, Hartvigsen ML, Brader LJ, et al. Differential effects of protein quality on postprandial lipemia in response to a fat-rich meal in type 2 diabetes: comparison of whey, casein, gluten, and cod protein. Am J Clin Nutr 2009;90(1):41–8.
[83] Chen Q, Reimer RA. Dairy protein and leucine alter GLP-1 release and mRNA of genes involved in intestinal lipid metabolism in vitro. Nutrition 2009;25(3):340–9.
[84] Lovati MR, West CE, Sirtori CR, Beynen AC. Dietary animal proteins and cholesterol metabolism in rabbits. Br J Nutr 1990;64(2):473–85.
[85] Pal S, Ellis V. The acute effects of four protein meals on insulin, glucose, appetite and energy intake in lean men. Br J Nutr 2010;104(8):1241–8.
[86] Streppel MT, Arends LR, van 't Veer P, Grobbee DE, Geleijnse JM. Dietary fiber and blood pressure a meta-analysis of randomized placebo-controlled trials. Arch Intern Med 2005; 165(2):150–6.
[87] Greger JL. Nondigestible carbohydrates and mineral bioavailability. J Nutr 1999;129(7 Suppl):1434S–5S.
[88] Coudray C, Demigne C, Rayssiguier Y. Effects of dietary fibers on magnesium absorption in animals and humans. J Nutr 2003;133(1):1–4.
[89] Appel LJ, Brands MW, Daniels SR, Karanja N, Elmer PJ, Sacks FM. Dietary approaches to prevent and treat hypertension: a scientific statement from the American heart association. Hypertension 2006;47(2):296–308.
[90] Wu X, Tolvanen JP, Hutri-Kahonen N, et al. Comparison of the effects of supplementation with whey mineral and potassium on arterial tone in experimental hypertension. Cardiovasc Res 1998;40(2):364–74.
[91] Zemel MB. Mechanisms of dairy modulation of adiposity. J Nutr 2003;133(1):252S–6S.
[92] Pal S, Ellis V. Acute effects of whey protein isolate on blood pressure, vascular function and inflammatory markers in overweight postmenopausal women. Br J Nutr 2011;105(10): 1512–9.
[93] Pins JJ, Keenan JM. Effects of whey peptides on cardiovascular disease risk factors. J Clin Hypertens (Greenwich) 2006;8(11):775–82.
[94] FitzGerald RJ, Meisel H. Lactokinins: whey protein-derived ACE inhibitory peptides. Nahrung 1999;43(3):165–7.
[95] Murakami M, Tonouchi H, Takahashi R, et al. Structural analysis of a new anti-hypertensive peptide (beta-lactosin B) isolated from a commercial whey product. J Dairy Sci 2004;87(7): 1967–74.
[96] Layman DK. The role of leucine in weight loss diets and glucose homeostasis. J Nutr 2003;133(1):261S–7S.
[97] Pihlanto-Leppala A, Koskinen P, Piilola K, Tupasela T, Korhonen H. Angiotensin I-converting enzyme inhibitory properties of whey protein digests: concentration and characterization of active peptides. J Dairy Res 2000;67(1):53–64.
[98] FitzGerald RJ, Meisel H. Milk protein-derived peptide inhibitors of angiotensin-I-converting enzyme. Br J Nutr 2000;84(Suppl. 1):S33–7.
[99] Abubakar A, Saito T, Kitazawa H, Kawai Y, Itoh T. Structural analysis of new antihypertensive peptides derived from cheese whey protein by proteinase K digestion. J Dairy Sci 1998;81(12):3131–8.
[100] Nurminen ML, Sipola M, Kaarto H, et al. Alpha-lactorphin lowers blood pressure measured by radiotelemetry in

normotensive and spontaneously hypertensive rats. Life Sci 2000;66(16):1535–43.
[101] Greenwald SE. Ageing of the conduit arteries. J Pathol 2007;211(2):157–72.
[102] McEniery CM, Wilkinson IB, Avolio AP. Age, hypertension and arterial function. Clin Exp Pharmacol Physiol 2007;34(7):665–71.
[103] Benetos A, Waeber B, Izzo J, et al. Influence of age, risk factors, and cardiovascular and renal disease on arterial stiffness: clinical applications. Am J Hypertens 2002;15(12):1101–8.
[104] Wilkinson IB, Prasad K, Hall IR, et al. Increased central pulse pressure and augmentation index in subjects with hypercholesterolemia. J Am Cardiol 2002;39(6):1005–11.
[105] Casey DP, Pierce GL, Howe KS, Mering MC, Braith RW. Effect of resistance training on arterial wave reflection and brachial artery reactivity in normotensive postmenopausal women. Eur J Appl Physiol 2007;100(4):403–8.
[106] Qureshi G, Brown R, Salciccioli L, et al. Relationship between aortic atherosclerosis and non-invasive measures of arterial stiffness. Atherosclerosis 2007;195(2):e190–4.
[107] Blacher J, Safar ME. Large-artery stiffness, hypertension and cardiovascular risk in older patients. Nat Clin Pract Cardiovasc Med 2005;2(9):450–5.
[108] Schiffrin EL. Remodeling of resistance arteries in essential hypertension and effects of antihypertensive treatment. Am J Hypertens 2004;17(12 Pt 1):1192–200.
[109] Tomiyama H, Hashimoto H, Hirayama Y, et al. Synergistic acceleration of arterial stiffening in the presence of raised blood pressure and raised plasma glucose. Hypertension 2006;47(2):180–8.
[110] Hata Y, Yamamoto M, Ohni M, Nakajima K, Nakamura Y, Takano T. A placebo-controlled study of the effect of sour milk on blood pressure in hypertensive subjects. Am J Clin Nutr 1996;64(5):767–71.

CHAPTER

33

Probiotics to Treat Visceral Obesity and Related Liver Disease

Pietro Vajro, Marco Poeta, Luca Pierri, Cristina Pizza, Roberta D'Aniello, Maria Sangermano, Grazia Massa, and Giulia Paolella

Department of Medicine and Surgery, Medical School of Salerno, Baronissi, Salerno, and the European Laboratory for the Investigation of Food-Induced Diseases, University of Naples Federico II, Naples, Italy

INTRODUCTION

Obesity is the main cause of morbidity and mortality, surpassing cigarette smoke and alcohol consumption in its deleterious effects on health [1]. This problem has reached such huge proportions that the World Health Organization has defined it as a global epidemic [2]. Most recently the American Medical Association switched the term obesity condition into "disease". Nowadays, there are estimated to be 1.46 billion overweight around the world, of which over 500 million are obese [3]. Over 170 million school-age children are overweight [4], of which 35–40 million are classified as obese [5]. Accordingly, obesity-related metabolic conditions such as metabolic syndrome (MS) and its hepatic manifestations [e.g. nonalcoholic fatty liver disease (NAFLD)] have increased in people of all ages.

The size of the problem, the consequences on health, and the economic burden on health-care system make the prevention and the treatment of obesity and its related conditions very important issues.

The definition of ponderal excess in adulthood is based on the body mass index (BMI), calculated as the weight in kilograms divided by the square of the height in meters. BMI values of <24.9 kg/m^2 are defined as normal, values between 25 and 29.9 kg/m^2 identify overweight subjects, and values $\geq$30 kg/m^2 are diagnostic for obesity [6].

In children, data are assessed by means of auxological curves and age- and sex-adjusted BMI percentiles. Childhood obesity is defined as $\geq$95th percentile BMI, while overweight is defined as $\geq$85th percentile BMI and <94th percentile [7].

In addition to BMI evaluation, waist circumference (WC) is commonly used in clinical practice as an accurate indicator of the amount of visceral fat (central adiposity). Normal values in male and female adults are <102 cm and <88 cm, respectively [8]. In children, specific percentiles according to age and gender are commonly used [9].

Visceral fat is positively related with obesity complications, particularly MS and NAFLD [10].

METABOLIC SYNDROME

MS is characterized by the presence of multiple risk factors for cardiovascular disease [11] and type 2 diabetes mellitus (T2DM) [12], including obesity (especially visceral obesity, evaluated by WC), impaired glucose tolerance, dyslipidemia (high triglycerides and low high-density lipoprotein cholesterol), and high blood pressure. In 2001, the National Cholesterol Education Program (NCEP) proposed that having at least three of the five defined criteria should be sufficient to diagnose MS (Table 33.1) [13].

Concerning children, there isn't yet a standard, universally accepted definition of MS. However several studies have proposed the same criteria as for adults, although with cutoff points established on age- and sex-adjusted percentile-charts [14–16].

Nonalcoholic Fatty Liver Disease

NAFLD is considered to be the hepatic manifestation of MS and is usually associated with at least one of its components [17]. It comprises a large spectrum of liver diseases, including simple steatosis (fatty liver) and its progressive condition, steatohepatitis (NASH), which

Nutrition in the Prevention and Treatment of Abdominal Obesity
http://dx.doi.org/10.1016/B978-0-12-407869-7.00033-7

TABLE 33.1 Definition of Metabolic Syndrome Criteria

✓ *Waist Circumference*	≥102 cm (men)
	≥88 cm (women)
✓ Triglycerides blood level	≥150 mg/dL
✓ HDL-C blood level	<40 mg/dL (men)
	<50 mg/dL (women)
✓ Blood Pressure	≥130/85 mmHg
✓ Fasting glucose blood level	>100 mg/dL

HDL-C, high-density lipoprotein cholesterol. *Source: modified from the Expert Panel on Detection, Evaluation, and Treatment of High Blood Cholesterol in Adults [13].*

can evolve into fibrosis and cirrhosis, thus increasing the risk of hepatocellular carcinoma [18]. Obesity is the major factor related to the genesis of this liver disorder. WC plays a pivotal role in obesity and correlates with liver disease more often than does BMI [19]. In addition, higher alanine aminotransferase (ALT; a biochemical marker used to identify liver damage) plasma levels were found to be associated with the development of MS after a 20-year follow-up period [20]. NAFLD is also the most common chronic liver disease in the pediatric population, as a consequence of the global epidemic of childhood obesity [21].

The main mechanisms involved in both the pathogenesis and progression of the disease are hepatic free fatty acid accumulation, insulin resistance, oxidative stress, and hepatocyte apoptosis, probably working in a multi-hit mode [22,23]. In overweight and obese subjects, increased visceral fat (larger WC) is linearly correlated with both the grade of hepatic steatosis and the number of MS components. Therefore, abdominal adiposity reduction may represent a relevant therapeutic target to treat both conditions [10].

OBESITY PATHOGENESIS

The pathogenesis of obesity is classically linked to increased energy input (hypercaloric dietary pattern, poor in fiber and rich in fat) [24] and/or reduced energy output (increased sedentary behavior) [25]. Consequently, prevention programs are focused on both main risk factors by promoting a healthy diet and physical activity. Nevertheless, most intervention programs are ineffective due to poor compliance; the obesity problem remains serious and the epidemic continues to expand even further. Therefore, in recent years a number of studies have attempted to identify additional pathogenic mechanisms that may be involved.

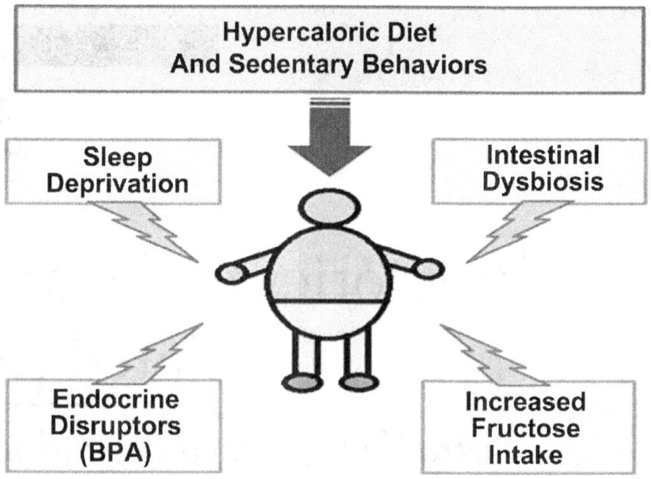

FIGURE 33.1 **Classical and novel obesity risk factors.** BPA, bisphenol A.

In particular, attention has focused on sleep deprivation, endocrine disruption, and increased fructose intake (Fig. 33.1).

Sleep Deprivation

A number of studies have identified a positive correlation between a reduction in the quality and/or quantity of sleep and increased BMI. This is probably due to an imbalance of the neuropeptides that regulate appetite, with increased levels of orexigenic ghrelin and decreased levels of anorexigenic leptin [26]. Furthermore, alterations in sleep duration or sleep fragmentation are associated with insulin resistance, impaired lipid profile, and high C-reactive protein (CRP) levels [27]. Most recently, it has been shown that weekday sleep duration in adolescents potentially mediates the effects of some technologies (computer use, TV viewing and video gaming) on their BMI z-score. If confirmed, improving sleep through better management of technology use could be an achievable intervention for attenuating obesity [28]. Obstructive sleep apnea syndrome (OSAS) in addition to obesity is also associated with an increased risk of MS including NAFLD, NASH, and liver fibrosis. OSAS patients should therefore be screened for the presence and severity of NAFLD [29]

Endocrine Disruptors

Recently, several studies have focused on environmental pollutants, such as bisphenol A (BPA), and their interference with endocrine metabolic pathways through binding to nuclear and membrane-associated estrogen receptors [30]. BPA is an essential component of polycarbonate plastic (used for production of a number of food containers, baby bottles, reusable bottles) and epoxy resins (used for the internal lining of metal food containers, dental materials, etc) [31]. BPA is likely to promote the genesis of obesity: many studies have demonstrated a relationship between BPA exposure (measured primarily in the urine) and overweight/obesity in adults [32–34]. Data in children are still scarce [35,36].

Increased Fructose Intake

The obesity epidemic has coincided with an increased tendency to the excessive consumption of fructose/sucrose in earlier years, mainly due to an augmented intake of sweetened beverages (e.g. soft drinks and sugar-added commercial fruit juices) [37]. As will be discussed in more depth in the following sections, sugary drinks are obesogenic mainly because, despite their high levels of calories, they do not induce satiety. [38].

In 2012, three studies published in the New England Journal of Medicine provided new data on the association between the consumption of sweetened beverages and the development of obesity [39–41]. The role of fructose has also been recognized to specifically increase the risk of NAFLD [42], and to induce both the development of liver disease to steatohepatitis (NASH) and the severity of fibrosis [43].

Gut-Liver Axis

The two major protagonists of this particular axis are mucosal integrity and alterations in the gut microbiota.

Dysregulation of the mucosal barrier is involved in insulin resistance, hepatic steatosis, and the progression of NAFLD to NASH. This will be discussed in the next section.

A growing body of evidence in animal models and humans suggests a role for the intestinal microbiota (IM) in the development of obesity. In general, it has been shown that specific microbiota (mostly related to Western dietary habits) are associated with higher energy extraction from diet. A number of intestinal microorganisms are in fact able to ferment usually undigestible plant polysaccharides into monosaccharides and short-chain fatty acids (SCFAs), leading to an overall enhanced intestinal recovery of calories [44,45]. Furthermore, the microbiota may play a definite role in the specific occurrence of NAFLD/NASH and liver fibrosis [23,46]. Interestingly, it seems that there may be active cross talk among all of these pathomechanisms. Examples are provided in the following sections.

Bisphenol A, Fructose, and Liver Fat Accumulation

A recent study investigated liver fat accumulation in rats by administering drinking water containing 5% fructose ± BPA. There was a significantly higher liver fat content in BPA-exposed rats than in fructose controls. BPA in combination with fructose therefore appears to induce fat infiltration into the liver at doses close to the current tolerable daily intake [47].

Fructose, Intestinal Microbiota, and the Gut-Liver Axis

Bergheim's group in Germany evaluated several aspects of fructose-induced damage and its prevention. She showed that hepatic fat accumulation in fructose-fed mice is associated with the induction of toll-like receptors (TLRs) 1–4 and 6–8 [48]. This effect is halted or prevented by the use of probiotics or antibiotics (e.g. polymyxin B and neomycin) [49]. Similar results were also obtained with the use of metformin, which seemed to act by altering intestinal permeability and subsequently the endotoxin-dependent activation of hepatic Kupffer cells [50]. As summarized by Vajro et al. [51], specific Kupffer cell activation through TLRs (TLR4) determines the production of proinflammatory and profibrogenetic mediators, while hepatic stellate cells determine fibrogenesis of the extra cellular matrix (Fig. 33.2).

Polycarbonate, Intestinal Microbiota, and Physical Exercise

Interestingly, recent data suggest that oral exposure to polycarbonate induces changes in the mouse gut microbiome, primarily decreasing Proteobacteria levels. These changes may be attenuated by physical exercise [52].

In the next section, we will show whether and, if so, how intestinal dysbiosis is a possible target to treat obesity and related hepatometabolic conditions in a minimally invasive and sufficiently safe manner through dietary supplementation with pro-, pre-, and symbiotics [23,51,53].

INTESTINAL MICROBIOTA AND THE GUT-LIVER AXIS

Gut Microbiota

The human gut microbiota consists of trillions of microorganisms that are essential for preserving the integrity of the mucosal barrier. The microbiota plays an important role in the development of gut-associated lymphoid tissue (GALT), IgA secretion, and the production of antimicrobial peptides.

Several large-scale tools and associated projects such as Human Microbiome Project [54] or MetaHIT consortium [55] have enabled major advancements in the understanding of gut microbiota composition and function. It also appears that some metabolic disorders (e.g.

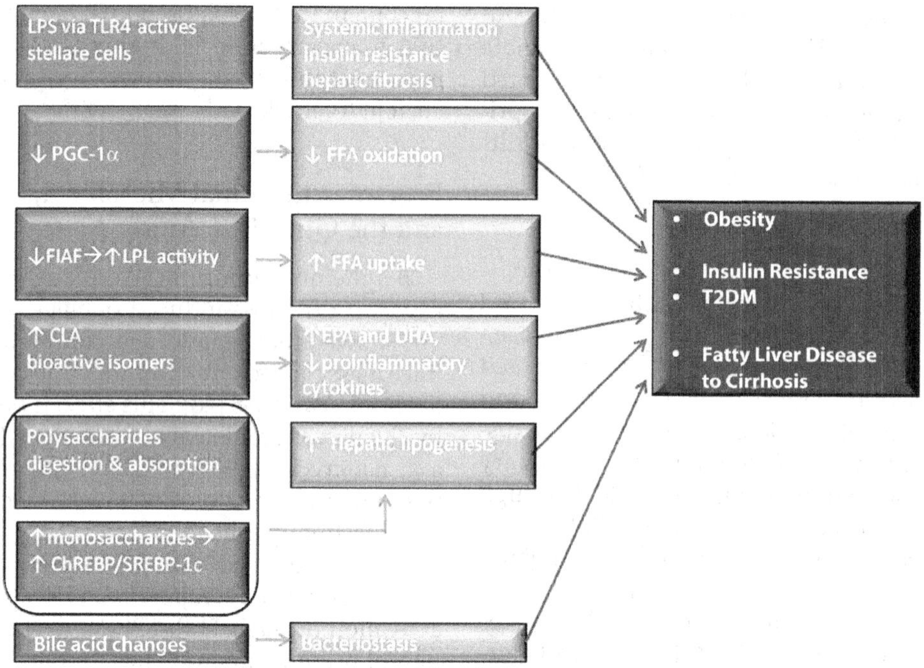

FIGURE 33.2 Mechanisms by which intestinal bacteria may interact on proximal and distal organs or systems. The gut microbiota may be implicated in the pathogenesis of obesity, diabetes, and nonalcoholic fatty liver disease (NAFLD). Gut dysbiosis is associated with an induction of toll-like receptor 4 (TLR4) in patients with NAFLD that causes hepatic fibrogenesis and systemic inflammation. The gut microbiota interferes with free fatty acid (FFA) oxidation and uptake via peroxisomal proliferator-activated receptor gamma coactivator-1-alpha (PGC-1α) and fasting-induced adipose factor/angiopoietin-related protein 4 (FIAF) changes. Gut bacteria produce isomers of conjugated linoleic acid (CLA), which reduce the expression of proinflammatory cytokines and increase the intestinal content of eicosapentaenoic acid (EPA) and docosahexaenoic acid (DHA). The microbiota also converts nondigestible carbohydrates into monosaccharides, thus determining carbohydrate-responsive element-binding protein (ChREBP) and sterol regulatory element-binding protein 1c (SREPB-1c) transcriptional activation that promotes hepatic lipogenesis. Properties of bile acids, which have bacteriostatic activity, are therefore modified. LPS, lipopolysaccharide; T2DM, type 2 diabetes mellitus. *Source: Vajro et al. [51].*

obesity and T2DM) have a strict correlation with the IM composition.

Thanks to modern molecular microbiology techniques [e.g. denaturing gradient gel electrophoresis (DGGE), fluorescence in situ hybridization (FISH), polymerase chain reaction (PCR), and pyrosequencing], it has been possible to accurately profile the IM. The taxonomic evaluation of the IM has led to the recognition of three distinct enterotypes: one dominated by Bacteroides, the second dominated by Prevotella, and the third by Ruminococcus [56,57].

IM studies have enabled us to quantify and qualify their composition. The first feature can be defined as *richness*, which describes the number of different species in a specific ecosystem, not taking into account their relative abundance; the second feature is termed *evenness* and indicates the relative abundance of each species in a specific ecosystem [58]. The main divisions that dominate the IM are Bacteroidetes and Firmicutes, which represent 92.6% of all sequences recognized in fecal samples of healthy subjects [59].

Despite interindividual differences in human gut composition, the presence of a *core microbiota* has been hypothesized, composed of members of several different phyla: Firmicutes (*Eubacterium* and *Ruminococcus*), Bacteroidetes (*Alistipes* and *Bacteroides*), and Actinobacteria (*Bifidobacterium*) [60]. The role of another important phylum, Archaea (represented by *Methanobrevibacter smithii*) is still unclear (Table 33.2).

An imbalance between energy intake and energy expenditure is, of course, the central determining cause of obesity pathogenesis, together with the altered function of adipose tissue, which releases adipokines with pro- and anti-inflammatory properties. It was recently shown that the IM is also a main protagonist in obesity development [61]. The IM was first studied in animal models by Gordon's group, which used microbiota transplantation from obese mice to germ-free mice. They showed that strain-specific composition of the gut microbiota (decreased Bacteroidetes and a corresponding increase in Firmicutes) was one of the "transmissible" causes of obesity (Table 33.3) [62]. Since then, several studies have confirmed that obese gut microbiota has an increased capacity to harvest energy from usually indigestible food residues such as resistant starch, leading to its conversion to specific SCFAs (propionate, butyrate, and acetate) by fermentation and absorption across the colonic mucosa. As shown in Fig. 33.3, carbohydrates are substrates for the synthesis of SCFAs. Some important "propionate-producer" bacteria convert succinate into propionate. Multiple pathways are involved in butyrate synthesis:

TABLE 33.2 Most Important Phyla of the "Core Microbiota"

Phyla	Genera	Species
Firmicutes	Clostridia	*C.Coccoides/C.fragile/ C.leptum*
		Lactobacillus (L.paracasei, L.sakei, L.reuteri)
	Bacilli	*Enterococcus*
		Staphylococcus aureus
Bacteroidetes	Bacteroides	*Bacteroides fragilis*
Actinobacteria	Bifidobacteria	*B.longum/B.breve/B.adolescentis/B.bifidum*
Archaea	Methanobrevi bacteria	*Methanabrevibacter Smithil*

TABLE 33.3 Gut Dysbiosis in Obese Individuals (Adults and Children)

Phyla	Genera	[]Obese Patient	References **Pediatric Obese Patients*
Bacteroidetes	*Bacteroides*	↓	[59] Ley RE et al. Nature (2006). Armougom F et al. PLOS ONE (2009)(A)
Actinobacteria	*Bifidobacterium*	↑	*[70] Santacruz A et al. Obesity [Silver Spring] (2009) [54] Turnbaugh PJ et al. Nature (2009)
		*↓	*[61] Bervoets L et al. Gut Pathog (2013)
Firmicutes	*Clostridia Coccoides / Lituseburense/Histolyticum*	*↑	*[70] Santacruz A et al. Obesity (Silver Spring) (2009) *Nadal I et al. Int J Obes (2009)(B)
	Faecaliabacterium Prausnitzii	*↑	*Balamurugan R et al. Br J Nutr (2010).(C)
	Eubacterium rectale	*↑	*Nadal I et al. Int J Obes (2009)(B)
	Lactobacillus	↑	Million M et al. Int J Obes (2011)(D) [61] Bervoets L. et al. Gut Pathog (2013)
	Staphylococcus	↑	Kalliomäki M et al. Am J Clin Nutr (2008)(E)
Archaea	*Methanobrevibacter smithii*	↓	Zhang H et al. Proc. natl Acad Sci (2009)(F) Million et al. Int J Obes (2013)(G)
		↓	Armougom F et al. PLOS ONE (2009). (A)

(A) Armougom et al. [147]. (B), Nadal et al. [148]. (C), Balamurugan R et al. [149]. (D), Million et al. [150]. (E), Kalliomäki et al. [151]. (F), Zhang et al. [73]. (G), Million et al. [152].

butyryl-CoA: acetate CoA-transferase, lactate-utilizing butyrate-producing bacteria, and butyrate kinases. Acetogen bacteria are responsible for acetate production.

The additional energy provided by bacterial SCFAs is estimated to represent 10% of daily caloric intake. The de novo synthesis pathway of lipids and glucose is accelerated by the augmented availability of substrates (SCFAs) [63]. SCFAs are also ligands for two G protein-coupled receptors [free fatty acid receptor 2 (GPR43) and free fatty acid receptor 3 (GPR41)] that are expressed in

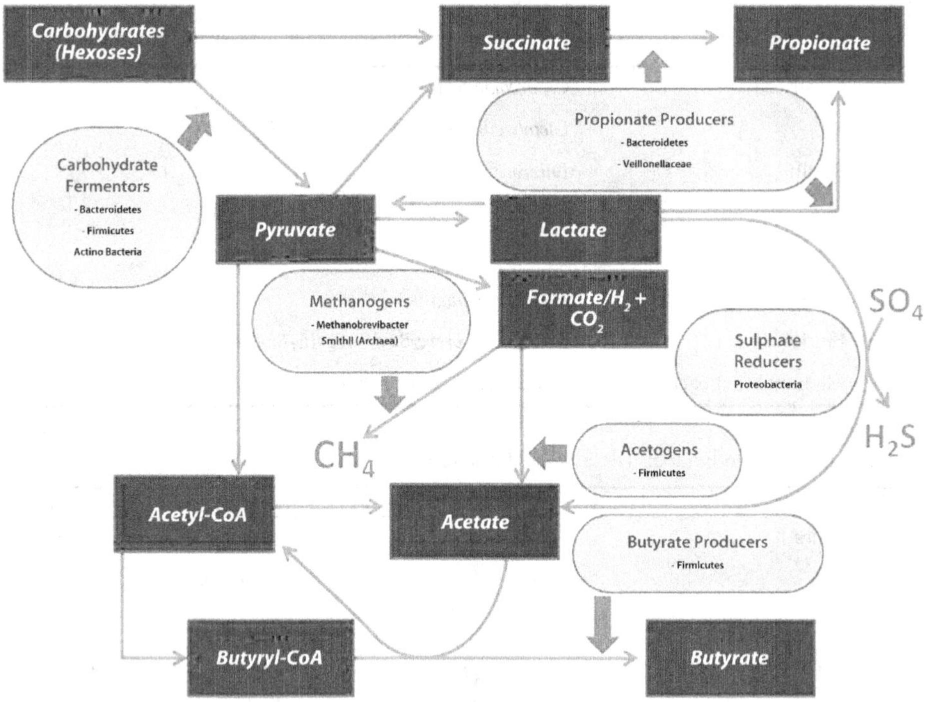

FIGURE 33.3 **Production of short-chain fatty acids by intestinal microbiota.** Carbohydrates are the substrates for the synthesis of short-chain fatty acids; some important "propionate-producer" bacteria converted succinate into propionate. Multiple pathways are involved in butyrate synthesis: butyryl-CoA:acetate CoA-transferase, lactate-utilizing butyrate-producing bacteria, and butyrate kinases. Acetogen bacteria are responsible for acetate production.

several tissues such as the small intestine, colon, adipose tissue, and immune cells. These receptors also have an important role in adipogenesis [64]. Significant evidence links the pro- and anti-inflammatory properties of specific bacterial strains to an augmented risk of developing obesity [65]. Activation of the lipopolysaccharide (LPS) pathway, an essential component of the cell walls of Gram-negative bacteria (Bacteroidetes), appears to lead to an inflammatory state that involves expression of a number of TLRs by certain immune and intestinal cells [66].

Metabolic activity in obese children is higher than in lean ones. Despite IM composition not being significantly different between these two groups, SCFA levels measured in fecal sample were incredibly high in obese and overweight children [67]. These data suggest that high butyrate concentrations can be explained by an increased activation of butyrate-producing pathway, regulated by butyryl-CoA:acetate CoA-transferase expression [68]. Most Firmicutes can produce butyrate using some unusual substrates such as lactate; moreover, the higher prevalence of Firmicutes vs. Bacteroidetes provides increased IM energy extraction. [69].

The IM composition of obese and overweight children after a 10-week diet and physical activity treatment showed some important differences in those who lost more than 4 kg (increased proportion of Bacteroides and Lactobacillus, decreased Bifidobacteria) *vs.* those who lost less than 2 kg (Clostridia and Bifidobacterium bifidum were the predominant species), suggesting that only a significant weight loss intervention appears to be linked to a favorable and healthy IM modification [70].

Another study focusing on the Firmicutes:Bacteroides ratio showed that the gut microbiota in obese children contains high levels of *Lactobacillus* spp. and low levels of Bacteroides *vulgatus*. Moreover the presence of *Lactobacillus* spp. was positively correlated with higher high-sensitivity CRP (hs-CRP) plasma levels. Bervoets's group recently found a correlation between *Staphylococcus* spp. and energy intake (kcal/day), independent of BMI status [61].

Interestingly, IM changes may also happen after Roux-en-Y gastric bypass surgery (RYGB) [71], as recently reviewed by Sweeny [72], with a reduction in Firmicutes and an increase in Enterobacteriaceae (phylum Proteobacteria) [73,74] confirming data obtained in animal models [75].

Studies in obese and lean twins suggested that a core gut microbiome exists, and that obese individuals exhibit reduced diversity and metabolic pathway alteration in their microbiota. [76]. More recently, Tims's group [77] demonstrated, through a phylogenetic study using microarray based on 16S rRNA genes, that monozygotic human twins have more similar microbiotas compared with unrelated subjects. Twin pairs with discordant BMIs revealed an inverse correlation between *Clostridium* cluster IV diversity and BMI. Lower BMI was associated with a more abundant network of primary fiber degraders, while a network of butyrate producers was more prominent in subjects with a higher BMI. Combined with the higher butyrate and valerate contents present in the fecal matter of higher BMI subjects, the difference in microbial networks suggests a shift in fermentation patterns at the end of the colon, which could affect human energy homeostasis. Of course, diet plays an important role in the modulation of the stool microbiota [78].

MICROBIOTA, GUT-LIVER AXIS, AND NONALCOHOLIC FATTY LIVER DISEASE

Intestinal Microbiota

IM can be influenced by several factors (Fig. 33.4), and strain modulation could either prevent or cause important complications involving the liver and cardiovascular system [79]. Concerning hepatic involvement, recently Vajro et al. accurately reviewed the role of IM in the development of hepatic steatosis and its proinflammatory effects [51].

First, the modifications in IM can promote hepatic lipogenesis, owing to an augmented uptake of free fatty acids (FFAs) by the liver [80]. Second, a growing body of evidence has confirmed that SCFAs derived from bacterial activity induce the secretion of peptide YY (PYY) by entero cells, thus slowing down intestinal motility. This event may even promote the development of small intestinal bacterial overgrowth (SIBO), favoring colonization of the upper intestinal tract by several bacterial strains.

Small Intestinal Bacterial Overgrowth

SIBO is a syndrome characterized by bacterial colonization of small intestine, normally almost sterile, that increases its permeability ("leaky gut") and prejudices the integrity of intestinal mucosa tight junctions (TJs) [81]. This condition leads to impairment of the intestinal barrier, with subsequently increased trafficking of fat and waste materials (i.e. parasites, fungi, LPS bacterial products, or undigested proteins) from the intestinal lumen to circulating blood through submucosal absorption (Fig. 33.5). Wigg's group showed, in a much-debated randomized controlled trial (RCT) on the prevalence of SIBO in NASH patients, an increased intestinal permeability, with trafficking of bacterial by-products and high levels of tumor necrosis factor (TNF-α) in patients affected by NASH *vs.* controls [82].

Gut Dysbiosis

Gut dysbiosis is considered to be related to a loss of mucosal integrity and to represent the major cause of the inflammatory state seen in obesity. In animal models, the basic mechanism appears to be linked to decreased

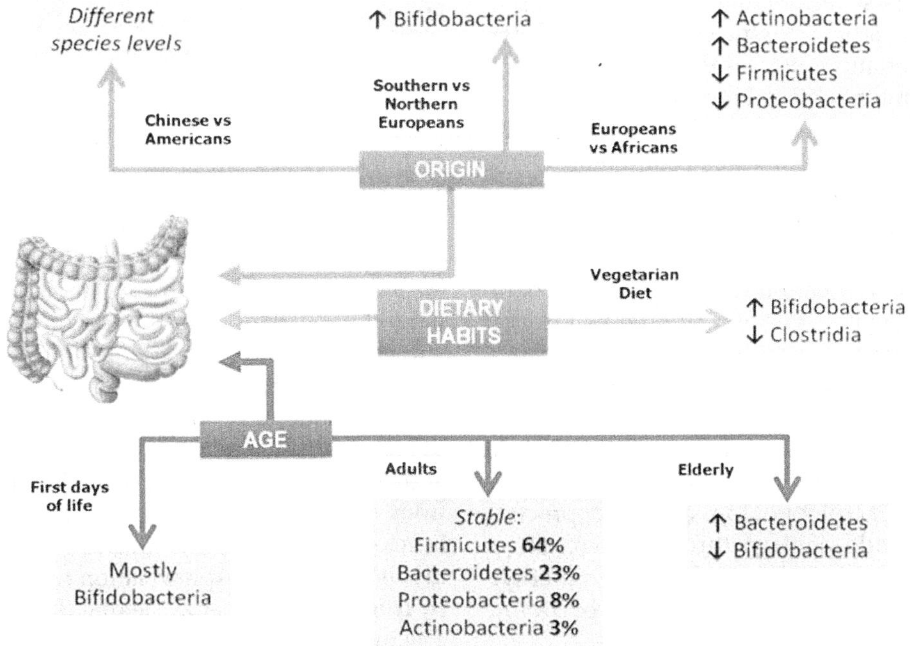

FIGURE 33.4 Factors that influence the gut microbiota. The main factors determining the intestinal microbiota are geographical and ethnic origins, dietary habits, and age. (See color plate at the back of the book.)

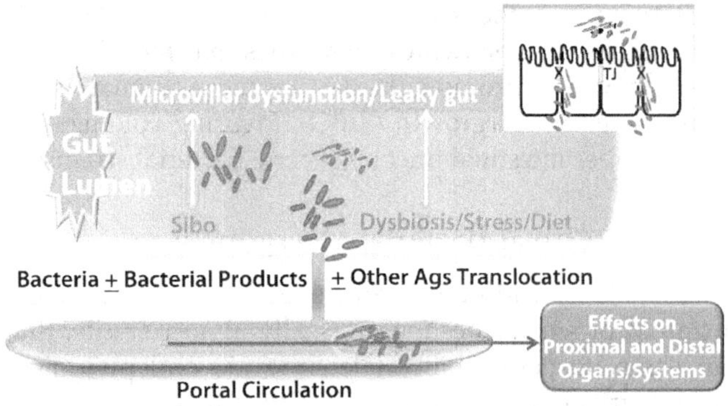

FIGURE 33.5 Events leading to bacterial and bacterial product translocation from the gut lumen to the portal circulation in the presence of microvillar dysfunction/leaky gut, small intestinal bacterial overgrowth (SIBO), gut dysbiosis, stress, or a high-fat diet. Note that tight junction (TJ) malfunction is a critical event. AGs, antigens. *Source: Vajro et al. [51].* (See color plate at the back of the book.)

levels of glucagon-like peptide 2 (GLP-2), an enterotrophic peptide responsible for TJ integrity and intestinal permeability [83]. The first important step of NAFLD/NASH pathogenesis is related to interplay between intestinal permeability and LPS, whose absorption is promoted by a high-fat diet [84]. Altered mucosal permeability induces an endotoxemic metabolic state [48,51,85]. This pattern easily leads to insulin resistance, hepatic steatosis, and the progression of NAFLD to NASH with hepatic inflammation and fibrogenesis.

In other words, the increased level of orexigenic adipokine, leptin, blood glucose, and insulin, as well as intestinal expression of the lipoprotein lipase (LPL)-related fasting-induced adipose factor [angiopoietin-related protein 4 (FIAF)], favors adipose tissue expansion and interplay with FFA oxidation processes mediated by the peroxisome proliferator-activated receptor (PPAR) [86].

One additional, intensely studied feature is the influence of ethanol on proinflammatory hepatic state. Obese people show high levels of endogenous intestinal ethanol related to the presence of specific bacterial strains that cause increased ethanol production [87]. Inflammation is also supported by a number of ethanol metabolic pathway by-products (acetaldehyde and acetate) that trigger the proinflammatory cascade and oxidative stress [88].

IM also has an important role in the catabolism of choline, an important precursor molecule in the hepatic synthesis of very-low-density lipoprotein for lipid excretion. The intestinal dysbiosis of obese patients has been suggested to accelerate the catabolic process, bringing about hepatic damage through accretion of the hepatotoxicity of choline by-products (dimethylamine and trimethylamine) and the depletion of choline [89,90].

The interplay between IM and bile acids represents another important function of intestinal microorganisms and their implications in NAFLD/NASH pathogenesis [91]. Bile acids are ligands for the bile acid receptor [farnesoid X-activated receptor (FXR)], an important nuclear receptor family responsible for lipids homeostasis, glucose homeostasis, hepatic inflammation, and fibrogenesis control. It is proposed that altered IM composition may be implicated in steatosis damage through alteration of the bile acids pathway. In this context, it seems that FXR may also be considered a new therapeutic target for patients with NAFLD [23,92].

FRUCTOSE, OBESITY, AND LIVER INVOLVEMENT

The obesity pandemic coincides with a large increase in the consumption of added refined carbohydrates (including dietary fructose and sucrose in soft drinks) to many foods [37]. The most important sources of fructose are sucrose corn syrup and sweeteners used by the food industry all over the world [93]. Some important RCTs suggest:

(1) a correlation between sweetened beverage intake and obesity development (also based on the presence of some BMI loci) in adults [39];
(2) that a moderate reduction of fructose and sugar intake significantly improves BMIs in obese and overweight children [94];
(3) that children administered a sugar-free diet for 18 months exhibit decreased weight gain and fat accumulation vs. a sugar-containing diet group [40]; and
(4) that obese children receiving a preventive dietary intervention with sugar-free beverages showed a lower increase in BMI than controls after 1 year [41].

As expected, in contrast to glucose, fructose does not stimulate pancreatic beta cells to secrete insulin [95]. This prevents (1) an increase in the circulating levels of leptin [96] and (2) the suppression of orexigenic ghrelin secretion, with the resulting lack of satiety induction [97,98]. Fructose also appears to disrupt serotonin reuptake, thus altering intestinal motility and permeability and causing SIBO [99].

From a molecular point of view, the proinflammatory and lipogenic effect of fructose seems to be due to the depletion of intracellular adenosine triphosphate (ATP) and increased circulating levels of uric acid, resulting from the specific hepatic metabolism of this sugar. Fructose metabolism, unlike glucose metabolism, involves sugar phosphorylation to fructose 1-phosphate by fructokinase, an enzyme that uses ATP as a substrate. The increased activity of fructokinase in fructose metabolism may consequently result in the depletion of cellular ATP [100], and subsequent liver necroinflammation.

This mechanism appears to fit well with the correlation existing between fructose intake and the severity of liver damage. In this regard, it has also been shown that patients with NAFLD and NASH present a higher expression of the fructokinase enzyme in liver biopsies, compared to controls [42].

INTESTINAL MICROBIOTA AND GUT-LIVER AXIS MANIPULATION BY PROBIOTICS

Probiotics are live microorganisms that confer a health benefit to the host when consumed in adequate amounts [101,102]. Their effects can be enhanced by the use of some nondigestible food ingredients (e.g. inulin and fructooligosaccharides), the so-called *prebiotics*. Prebiotics are beneficial for the host by selectively stimulating the growth and/or modifying the metabolic activity of specific intestinal bacteria. [103]. The combination of a probiotic with a prebiotic is defined as *symbiotic* [104].

Probiotics, in particular, mainly act by changing the microflora of the host to the benefit of proximal and distal organ systems (Fig. 33.6). As far as obesity and obesity-related conditions are concerned, probiotics appear to (1) counteract the dysbiotic IM-mediated increased production of metabolic by-products, such as SCFAs, which participate in obesity by increasing of lipogenesis (Fig. 33.3) and (2) to act as immune modulators that influence the gut immune responses [105].

Although probiotics have always been part of the human diet in the form of different fermented foods, there is now a growing body of evidence on their influence on different physiologic functions in the host [28]. The antiobesity potential of probiotics depends on the obesogenic nature of specific IM. Probiotics appear to be able to interact with the resident bacterial members of the gut and alter their properties, including interfering with metabolic pathways involved in the regulation of fat metabolism. Although the underlying molecular pathways driving the possible interference of probiotics on body weight remain unclear, extensive research is ongoing in this field. Most studies have so far dealt with

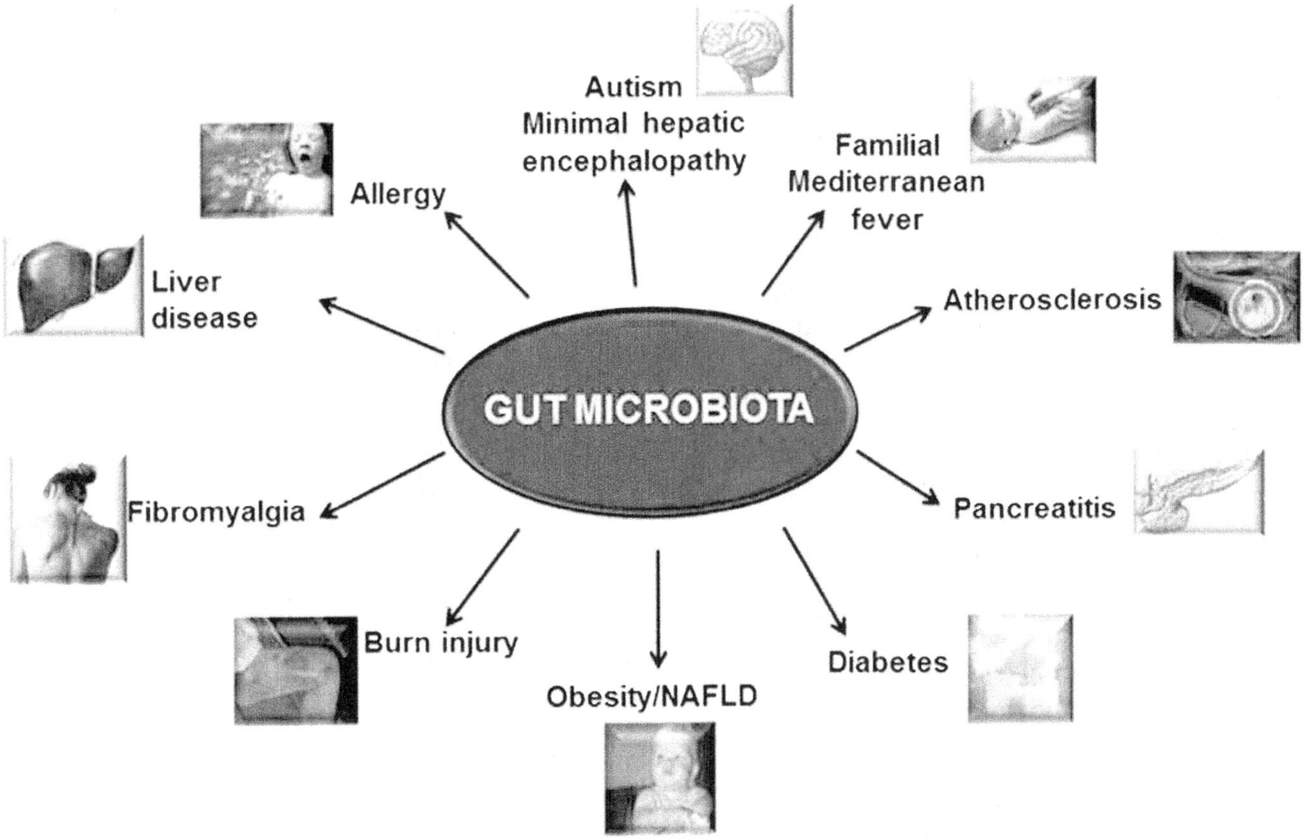

FIGURE 33.6 Proximal and distal organ diseases in which the intestinal microbiota is involved. NAFLD, nonalcoholic fatty liver disease. *Source: Vajro et al. [51].* (See color plate at the back of the book.)

the *Lactobacillus*, *Bifidobacterium*, *Streptococcus* spp. *L. rhamnosus*, *B. lactis*, and *S. thermophilus* [105].

PROBIOTICS, OBESITY, AND VISCERAL FAT DISORDERS

Cani recently reviewed the possible association between the presence of specific taxa in IM and host weight changes. Recent results have also been discussed in the context of interactions between the gut microbiota and host metabolism [106].

Animal Studies

Below are summarized the results of a series of studies conducted in high-fat diet-induced obese mice; all studies show promising results.

- The administration of *L. rhamnosus* PL60 for 8 weeks resulted in a reduction of body weight and white adipose tissue (epididymal and perirenal), probably mediated by the production of conjugated linoleic acid, which plays a role as an antiobesity agent [107].
- Our group showed that a 4-week administration of VSL#3 (a multistrain mixture of Bifidobacteria, Lactobacilli, and Streptococci; with equal food intake) reduced serum and liver triglyceride concentrations, along with a reduction of fat mass [108]. It was suggested that VSL#3 decreases dietary fat absorption by reducing long-chain fatty acid availability.
- The administration of the bacteriocin-producing probiotic *Lactobacillus salivarius* UCC118 Bac(+) was associated with increased proportions of Bacteroidetes and Proteobacteria, and a reduction in Actinobacteria, while Firmicutes remained unchanged. These alterations were not observed after administration of a bacteriocin-nonproducing probiotic. In both cases, however, no changes in metabolic biochemical parameters were detected, in contrast to the use of vancomycin [109].
- Similar results were found with the administration of *Lactobacillus acidophilus* NCDC 13, which was followed by an increase of Bifidobacterium but no significant changes in body weight gain and adiposity [110].
- A 10-week treatment with *Lactobacillus curvatus* HY7601 and *Lactobacillus plantarum* KY1032 was associated with reduced weight gain, fat accumulation, and some biochemical parameters, such as insulin, leptin, total cholesterol, and liver toxicity markers. Downregulation of proinflammatory genes in adipose tissue [such as interleukin-1β (IL-1β), IL-6, and TNF-α] and upregulation of fatty acid oxidation genes were also observed [111].

Akkermansia muciniphila, a Gram-negative bacterium that constitutes 3–5% of the gut microbial community and colonizes the mucosal layer, was recently reported to be reduced in high-fat diet-induced obese mice with metabolic endotoxemia, adipose tissue inflammation, and insulin resistance. Prebiotic (oligofructose) administration was associated with normalization of bacteria levels and improved metabolic profile, total fat mass, and body weight. Using heat-killed bacteria instead of viable ones led to a loss of beneficial effects. These results are probably caused by an increase in the levels of endocannabinoids, which control inflammation, the gut barrier, and gut peptide secretion [112].

Human Studies

Results are quite different among studies. In children, there is a growing body of evidence that early postnatal nutrition is a determinant for the development of obesity later in life, with epigenetic mechanisms probably being involved in this *metabolic programming* process. It has been suggested that breast and formula feeding epigenetically program the developing organs via modulation of the gut microbiota and thus influence the body weight phenotype, including predisposition to adult obesity via microbial metabolites (e.g. SCFAs) [113] For all *Lactobacilli* strains used, the studies reported in this age group (Table 33.4, upper) appear to agree upon their enhancement of body weight gain and/or better growth [114–118].

In lean adults (Table 33.4, lower), two studies [119,120] investigating the effect of probiotics on cardiovascular disease risk factors and serum lipids did not find effects on metabolic parameters, body weight, or BMI, whereas another study [121] noticed a statistically significant reduction in BMI, body weight, and low-density lipoprotein (LDL) cholesterol. However, because of other dietary ingredients and/or possible concomitant lifestyle changes, one cannot definitely assert a cause-effect relationship be due to probiotics alone.

Studies in obese individuals (Table 33.5) also have methodological problems (reviewed by Sanz et al. and Leber et al. [122,123], which are summarized below.

- Primary outcomes either referred mainly to biochemical and inflammatory markers of metabolic disorder and obesity rather than to body weight or were not clearly defined.
- In most cases, the duration of probiotic administration may have been too short to observe an effect.
- The population size was not always estimated.
- The presence of confounders may have affected results.

As shown in Table 33.4, a number of studies did not detect significant body weight changes during probiotic treatment [52,124–129].

TABLE 33.4 Effects of Different *Lactobacilli* Strains in Infants and Lean Adults Studies

Study Reference	Subjects Included	Probiotlc; Treatment Duration	Obesity Parameters; Weight Change
A. Healthy Infants (Age <2 Years)			
[116] Robinson et al. 1952	• Bottle fed • Partially breast fed • Bottle fed + folic acid • Partially breast fed + folic acid	• *L. acidophilus* ATCC4962 + ATCC4963, • 1–6 days	• Weight gain at one month
[118] Vendt et al. 2006	• Formula fed	• *L. rhamnosus* GG; • 6 months	✓ Growth and fecal flora at 6 mos: Better growth (W & L) ✓ Flora: more Lactobacilli
[114] Chouraqui et al. 2008	• Formula fed	• *L. rhamnosus* LPR + *B. longum* BL999 • 4 months	• Daily weight gain at 4 months
[117] Scalabrin et al. 2009	• Formula fed	• Formula (extensively hydrolysed casein) ± *L. rhamnosus* GG; • 120 days	• Weight gain at 120 d
[115] Maldonado et al. 2010	• Breast-fed	• *L. salivarius* CECT5713 • 6 months	• Multiple outcomes: antibiotic susceptibility of the strain, growth parameters, microbiota • Weight gain at 6 months
B. Normal Lean Adults			
[119] De Roos et al. 1999	• 50% of the enrolled volunteers cholesterol levels > 5 mmol/L	• *L. acidophilus* L-1 • 6 weeks	• Lipid profile: no statistical changes • Modest weight gain
(B) Fabian et al. 2007	• Healthy adult women	• Actimel (L. paracasei subsp. Paracasei (L. casei DN-114 001) • 4 weeks	• Antioxidants in plasma ↓ • Oxidants in plasma ↑ • Body weight: NSC
[120] Sadrzadeh-Yeganeh et al. 2010	• Cholesterol < 6mmol/l • TAG < 2.3 mmol/l	• *L. acidophilus* La1 + *Bifidobacterium* lactis Bb12 • 6 weeks	• Lipid profile: NSC • Body weight: NSC
[121] Chang BJ et al. 2011	• Healthy individuals	• *L. acidophilus, S. thermophilus,* B.infantis + B. breve + E. faecalis • 8 weeks	• Weight, BMI, and LDL-cholesterol reduction

(A) Million et al. [153]. (B) Fabian et al. [154].

Among studies that aimed to evaluate changes in markers of cardiovascular disease risk (e.g. fibrinogen, blood pressure, and serum lipids), *S. thermophilus* [124] appeared to be associated with decreased levels of LDL cholesterol and increased levels of fibrinogen. Two other studies [127,128] reported metabolic and anthropometric parameters changes in pregnant women. In the postpartum period, the group who received *L. rhamnosus* GG and *B. lactis* Bb12 probiotics showed a lower risk of central adiposity compared to the placebo control group, but not vs. the diet group (which was given alimentary education). Gobels's group [129] found no encouraging results with the *L. salivarius* Ls-33 probiotic: no changes in inflammation, MS biomarkers, or anthropometric parameters were detected. Aller et al. and Vajro et al. [52,130] observed hepatic changes in adult and pediatric obesity-related NAFLD, respectively (see next section on liver disease), although they did not observe weight change differences vs. controls.

Contrary to the previous series of studies, other groups have reported antiobesogenic results, generally associated with metabolic and hepatic improvements vs. respective controls (Table 33.5, lower). Jung' s group [131] noticed a decrease in body weight and in WC and hip circumference, although not reaching a statistical significance. Another trial [132] detected a decrease in visceral, subcutaneous, and total fat, and even a reduction in weight, BMI, WC and hip circumference, and waist-hip ratio. Safavi's group studied a pediatric population aged 6–18 years [104], and detected a decrease in BMI *z*-score, WC, and waist-hip ratio. They also noticed a reduction in triglycerides and LDL cholesterol.

TABLE 33.5 Effects of Different Lactobacilli Strains in Overweight/Obese Children and Adults Studies

Study Reference	Subjects Included	Probiotlc; Treatment Duration	Obesity Parameters; Weight Change
		Overweight/Obese Children/Adults	
A. No Significant Weight Change			
[125] Bukowska H et al. 1998	• Moderately elevated blood cholesterol	• *L. plantarum* 299v • 6 weeks	• Lipid profile: NSC • Body weight: NSC
[124] Agerholm-Larsen et al. 2000	• Healthy weight-stable overweight and obese	• 2 strains *L. acidophilus* + 1 strain S. thermoph. • 2 strains of *S. thermophilus* +1 strain of *L. rhamnosus* • 8 weeks	• levels of LDL-cholesterol ↓ • levels of fibrinogen ↑ • Little weight gain
[126] Naruszewicz M et al. 2002	• Smokers with elevated fibrinogen	• *L. plantarum* 299 v • 6 weeks	• Lipid profile: NSC • BMI: NSC
[127] Laitinen K et al. 2009	• Normoglycemic women from 1st trimester of pregnancy onward	• *L. rhamnosus* GG + B. lactis Bb12 • 6 months	• Risk of central adiposity ↓ • NSC weight↑ over pregnancy
[130] Aller R et al. 2011	• Adults with NAFLD	• *Lactobacillus bulgaricus* and *Streptococcus thermophiles* • 3 months	• Serum aminotransferases ↓ • Anthropometric parameters and cardiovascular risk factors: NSC
[53] Vajro P et al. 2011	• Obese children with NAFLD	• *Lactobacillus* Rh.GG • 8 weeks	• Serum aminotransferases ↓ • Antipeptidoglycan-polysaccharide antibodies ↓ • TNF-α & US bright liver: NSC • BMI z score & visceral fat: NSC
[129] Gobel RJ et al. 2012	• Obese adolescents	• *L. salivarius* Ls-33 • 12 weeks	• Metabolic syndrome and inflammation parameters: NSC • Anthropometrics: NSC
B. Weight Loss			
[71] Woodard et al. 2009	• Morbidly obese patients undergoing Roux-en-Y gastric bypass (RNYGB)	• Puritan's Pride:1 pill a day;no characterization of Lactobacillus strains; • 6 months	• Bacterial overgrowth ↓ • Vitamin B12 levels ↑ • Weight loss improved at 3mos, borderline effect at 6 mos, and NS at 8 months
[132] Kadooka et al. 2010	• Abdominal visceral fat area: 81.2 – 178.5 cm^2	• *L. gasseri* SBT2055 • 12 weeks	• Abdominal adiposity ↓ • Weight loss
[131] Jung SP et al. 2013	• Fasting blood sugar ≥ 100 mg/dl	• *L. gasseri* BNR17 • 12 weeks	• Weight, waist & hip↓: NSC
[104] Safavi M et al. 2013	• BMI ≥ 85 percentile	• Symbiotics • 8 weeks	• BMI Z-score, waist, waist-to-hip ratio, TG, LDL- cholesterol ↓.

(A) Million et al. [153].(B) Sanz et al. [122].

In conclusion, we believe that some of these findings suggest that gut-liver axis modulation is a target for obesity treatment.

PROBIOTICS USE IN FATTY LIVER DISEASE

Animal Studies

In recent years, several studies in animal models have aimed to investigate a direct role for IM on NAFLD and NASH, independent of body weight changes. Encouraging results have emerged, reinforcing the existence of a link between IM and the development of NAFLD and/or NASH [133]. These data also suggest the prospective use of probiotics to treat these conditions. VSL#3 and *Lactobacilli* are the most frequently used probiotic strains; results obtained with these probiotics are summarized next.

VSL#3

VSL#3, a multistrain mixture of *Bifidobacteria*, *Lactobacilli*, and *Streptococci*, is one of the most studied agents in NAFLD animal models.

One of the first relevant studies dating back to 2003 [86] used VSL#3 in *ob/ob* genetically obese mice suffering from NASH; it was possible to detect a decrease in serum ALT levels, decreased liver fatty acid content, and improved liver histology. These effects were related to a decrease of c-Jun N-terminal kinase (JNK) and nuclear factor-kappa-B (NF-κB) activity, both involved in insulin resistance.

Similar results were obtained in two studies using the same probiotics in diet-induced obese rats. The first [134] showed an increase in liver natural killer T cells, which had been reduced by a high-fat diet, and a decrease in TNF-α. These changes may explain the improvements in insulin resistance and liver steatosis. In the second, our group detected a reduction in other inflammatory markers, such as matrix metalloproteinase-2 (MMP-2) and MMP-9, inducible nitric oxide synthase (iNOS) and prostaglandin G/H synthase 2 [cyclooxygenase-2 (COX-2)] and a rise in PPAR-α [108].

Changes in MMPs and PPAR-α were also reported in another study [135] of a methionine-choline-deficient (MCD) diet-induced mouse model of NASH. Effects on MCD-induced liver steatosis or inflammation prevention were negligible, whereas liver fibrosis was halted, probably by altering collagen expression and transforming growth factor beta (TGF-β) signaling.

More recently, another study [136] showed that VSL#3 modulates the expression of nuclear receptors, improves insulin resistance in liver and adipose tissues, and protects against the development of steatohepatitis and atherosclerosis.

Lactobacilli

Lactobacillus strains also appear to have beneficial effects on animal models of obesity-related hepatic damage, but have been the object of fewer studies [137]. Some normalization of hepatic steatosis occurred after *L. rhamnosus* PL60 administration to diet-induced obese mice [107]. *Bifidobacterium longum* administration in a rat NAFLD model significantly attenuated hepatic fat accumulation; the effect was greater than that of *L. acidophilus*. Neither of these strains appeared to cause improvements in intestinal permeability [138]. *L. plantarum* KY1032 and *L. curvatus* HY7601 had beneficial effects on lipid metabolism and inflammation in high-fat diet-induced obese mice. A combination of both was more effective than a single agent on fat accumulation in adipose tissue and the liver [139].

Human Studies

Research into human NAFLD is scarce, but interesting beneficial preliminary results have been obtained.

The 2007 Cochrane meta-analysis carried out to elucidate the possible beneficial and harmful effects of probiotics on NAFLD and NASH did not provide clear indications because of the lack of RCTs [140]. The only two pilot nonrandomized studies available at that time (both by Loguercio's group, showed that probiotic mixtures were well tolerated and could improve conventional hepatic function tests and reduce markers of lipid peroxidation and/or TNF-α. The results of the first one [141], anyway, are confounded by cotreatment with other NAFLD therapeutic agents (i.e. *L. acidophilus*, *L. bifidus*, *L. bulgaricus*, *L. casei*, *L. rhamnosus*, *L. plantarum*, *L. salivarius*, *Lactococcus lactis*, and *Bifidobacterium breve* plus fructooligosaccharides as prebiotics plus vitamins B6, B2, B12, C, D3 plus folic acid, zinc oxide, ferrous gluconate and potassium iodide, BioFlora capsules and Dermo Duemila Italia antioxidants). A second study investigated the effects of the probiotic VSL#3 on several categories of adult chronic liver diseases, including a small representative NAFLD sample, the results of which were not shown [142].

Since the publication of the Cochrane [140] and subsequent European Society of Paediatric Gastroenterology, Hepatology and Nutrition (ESPGHAN) meta-analysis [143], two new RCTs have appeared.

(1) A double-blind RCT evaluating the efficacy of a 3-month treatment with *L. bulgaricus* and *Streptococcus thermophiles* in adult patients with NAFLD. A significant reduction in serum aminotransferases was reported, while anthropometric parameters and cardiovascular risk factors remained unchanged in both treated and control groups [130].

(2) In the same year, our group performed the first RCT study in children and obtained similar results [53], Obese children with NAFLD (mean age, 10.7 years) and unable to comply with lifestyle interventions were given *Lactobacillus* GG (12 billion colony-forming units/day) for 8 weeks. In this case, a significant decrease in ALT (with normalization in 80% of cases) was also detected. Again, no changes in BMI, z-score, and visceral fat were noted. TNF-α and ultrasound bright liver parameters were also unchanged. A significant reduction in anti-peptidoglycan and anti-polysaccharide serum antibodies (i.e. SIBO markers) was considered to indicate improved intestinal dysbiosis and/or gut barrier.

A symbiotic (*B. longum* probiotic plus fructooligosaccharide prebiotic) treatment vs. a control group prescribed lifestyle modification showed a statistical significant reduction in aspartate aminotransferase, LDL cholesterol, CRP, TNF-α, serum endotoxin, insulin resistance, steatosis, and NASH activity index in the treated group [144]. In 2013 another small RCT in obese adults with NAFLD confirmed probiotics' beneficial role upon the liver disease [155]. These 4 studies have been included in a most recent meta-analysis appearing while proof-checking this chapter [156].

Despite evidence that the IM is involved in the pathogenesis of obesity, its composition in NAFLD patients has only recently been characterized [145], showing an inverse, diet- and BMI-independent association between the presence of NASH and the percentage of Bacteroidetes in stools. Studies looking at changes in these measures after probiotic treatment are urgently needed.

In the light of recent evidence, IM modulation by probiotics an interesting therapeutic tool that should be further investigated for NAFLD and NASH treatment.

CONCLUSIONS

The issues discussed in this chapter highlight the advantage of further investigating the modulation of visceral and hepatic fatty deposition with novel tools, in addition to classical methods of improving diet quality and quantity and reducing sedentary behavior.

We have reviewed the current knowledge of the pathomechanisms of obesity and its related diseases. A number of promising and pioneering topics have emerged, such as gut dysbiosis, sleep deprivation, fructose intake, and endocrine disruptors (e.g. BPA). The cross talk that exists among them could be an important starting point for further therapeutic investigation.

First, intestinal bacteria have been shown to influence gut permeability, systemic inflammation levels, and host metabolism. The contribution of the gut microbiota to obesity and T2DM, steatosis, cardiovascular diseases, and inflammatory bowel diseases is becoming increasingly clear, although causality remains to be proven in humans.

The accurate evaluation of the specific gut microbiota composition in lean and obese individuals is likely to be necessary to enable the modulation of intestinal microflora through pro-, pre-, and symbiotics. Probiotics appear to be a safe, noninvasive treatment option for NAFLD and NASH patients because of their balancing role on gut microflora and beneficial effects on hepatotoxic oxidative injury. Since different probiotic species may have different effects on the IM, further studies are needed.

A. muciniphila, the dominant commensal bacterium in the intestinal mucosal layer, has recently received particular attention because its abundance inversely correlates with BMI and dysmetabolism, at least in mice [112]. The development of a treatment focusing on this mucus colonizer for the prevention or treatment of human obesity and its associated metabolic disorders therefore appears to be very appealing. Mucus colonizers are particularly important if one also considers the development of fecal transplantation strategies [54], which have shown positive effects on insulin resistance and glucose metabolism in humans, although no information on body weight or fat is yet available [146].

The excessive intake of fructose and sucrose is related to obesity, hepatic fat accumulation, insulin resistance, and eventually to gut-liver axis malfunction. The use of pro- and prebiotics and antibiotics may therefore limit the adverse effects of fructose by reducing TLR4 receptor activation.

Sleep alterations are also linked to the insulin resistance, impaired lipid profile, increased BMI, and high CRP levels typical of the chronic low-grade inflammatory status present in obesity and MS. Sleep improvement may therefore have beneficial effects on obesity and its related conditions.

References

[1] Adams KF, Schatzkin A, Harris TB, Kipnis V, Mouw T, Ballard-Barbash R, et al. Overweight, obesity, and mortality in a large prospective cohort of persons 50 to 71 years old. N Engl J Med 2006;355:763–78.

[2] World Health Organization. Obesity: preventing and managing the global epidemic. Report of a WHO consultation. World Health Organ Tech Rep Ser 2000;894:i-xii, 1–253.

[3] Finucane MM, Stevens GA, Cowan MJ, Danaei G, Lin JK, Paciorek CJ, et al. National, regional, and global trends in body-mass index since 1980: systematic analysis of health examination surveys and epidemiological studies with 960 country-years and 9·1 million participants. Lancet 2011;377:557–67.

[4] Lobstein T, Baur L, Uauy R. Obesity in children and young people: a crisis in public health. Obes Rev 2004;5(Suppl. 1):4–104.

[5] Wang Y, Lobstein T. Worldwide trends in childhood overweight and obesity. Int J Pediatr Obes 2006;1:11–25.

[6] National Institutes of Health. Clinical guidelines on the identification, evaluation, and treatment of overweight and obesity in adults: the evidence report. Obes Res 1998;6:51–209.

[7] Cole TJ, Bellizzi MC, Flegal KM, Dietz WH. Establishing a standard definition for child overweight and obesity worldwide: international survey. BMJ 2000;320:1240–3.

[8] Janssen I, Katzmarzyk PT, Ross R. Body mass index, waist circumference, and health risk: evidence in support of current National Institutes of Health guidelines. Arch Intern Med 2002;162:2074–9.

[9] McCarthy HD, Jarrett KV, Crawley HF. The development of waist circumference percentiles in British children aged 5.0-16.9 y. Eur J Clin Nutr 2001;55:902–7.

[10] Jeong SK, Kim YK, Park JW, Shin YJ, Kim DS. Impact of visceral fat on the metabolic syndrome and nonalcoholic fatty liver disease. J Korean Med Sci 2008;23:789–95.

[11] Isomaa B, Almgren P, Tuomi T, Forsén B, Lahti K, Nissén M, et al. Cardiovascular morbidity and mortality associated with the metabolic syndrome. Diabetes Care 2001;24:683–9.

[12] Laaksonen DE, Lakka HM, Niskanen LK, Kaplan GA, Salonen JT, Lakka TA. Metabolic syndrome and development of diabetes mellitus: application and validation of recently suggested definitions of the metabolic syndrome in a prospective cohort study. Am J Epidemiol 2002;156:1070–7.

[13] Expert panel on detection, evaluation, and treatment of high blood cholesterol in adults. Executive summary of the third report of the National Cholesterol Education Program (NCEP) expert panel on detection, evaluation, and treatment of high blood cholesterol in adults (adult treatment panel III). JAMA 2001;285:2486–97.

[14] Cook S, Weitzman A, Auinger P, Nguyen M, Dietz WH. Prevalence of a metabolic syndrome phenotype in adolescents: findings from the Third National Health and Nutrition

Examination Survey, 1988–1994. Arch Pediatr Adolesc Med 2003;157:821–7.
[15] Weiss R, Dziura J, Burgert TS, Tamborlane WV, Taksali SE, Yeckel CW, et al. Obesity and the metabolic syndrome in children and adolescents. N Engl J Med 2004;350:2362–74.
[16] Cruz ML, Goran MI. The metabolic syndrome in children and adolescents. Curr Diab Rep 2004;4:53–62.
[17] Sundaram SS, Zeitler P, Nadeau K. The metabolic syndrome and nonalcoholic fatty liver disease in children. Curr Opin Pediatr 2009;21:529–35.
[18] Chalasani N, Younossi Z, Lavine JE, Diehl AM, Brunt EM, Cusi K, et al. The diagnosis and management of non-alcoholic fatty liver disease: practice guideline by the American Gastroenterological Association, American Association for the Study of Liver Diseases, and American College of Gastroenterology. Gastroenterology 2012;142:1592–609.
[19] Willner IR, Waters B, Patil SR, Reuben A, Morelli J, Riely CA. Ninety patients with nonalcoholic steatohepatitis: insulin resistance, familial tendency, and severity of disease. Am J Gastroenterol 2001;96:2957–61.
[20] Goessling W, Massaro JM, Vasan RS, D'Agostino Sr RB, Ellison RC, Fox CS. Aminotransferase levels and 20-year risk of metabolic syndrome, diabetes, and cardiovascular disease. Gastroenterology 2008;135:1935–44.
[21] Loomba R, Sirlin CB, Schwimmer JB, Lavine JE. Advances in pediatric nonalcoholic fatty liver disease. Hepatology 2009;50:1282–93.
[22] Nobili V, Svegliati-Baroni G, Alisi A, Miele L, Valenti L, Vajro P. A 360-degree overview of paediatric NAFLD: recent insights. J Hepatol 2013;58:1218–29.
[23] Vajro P, Lenta S, Pignata C, Salerno M, D'Aniello R, De Micco I, et al. Therapeutic options in pediatric non-alcoholic fatty liver disease: current status and future directions. Ital J Pediatr 2012;17(38):55.
[24] Johnson L, Mander AP, Jones LR, Emmett PM, Jebb SA. Energy-dense, low-fiber, high-fat dietary pattern is associated with increased fatness in childhood. Am J Clin Nutr 2008;87:846–54.
[25] Hills AP, King NA, Armstrong TP. The contribution of physical activity and sedentary behaviours to the growth and development of children and adolescents: implications for overweight and obesity. Sports Med 2007;37:533–45.
[26] Gozal D, Kheirandish-Gozal L. Childhood obesity and sleep: relatives, partners, or both?—a critical perspective on the evidence. Ann N Y Acad Sci 2012;1264:135–41.
[27] Spruyt K, Molfese DL, Gozal D. Sleep duration, sleep regularity, body weight, and metabolic homeostasis in school-aged children. Pediatrics 2011;127:e345–52.
[28] Arora T, Singh S, Sharma RK. Probiotics: interaction with gut microbiome and antiobesity potential. Nutrition 2013;29:591–6.
[29] Musso G, Cassader M, Olivetti C, Rosina F, Carbone G, Gambino R. Association of obstructive sleep apnoea with the presence and severity of non-alcoholic fatty liver disease. A systematic review and meta-analysis. Obes Rev 2013;14:417–31.
[30] Wetherill YB, Akingbemi BT, Kanno J, McLachlan JA, Nadal A, Sonnenschein C, et al. In vitro molecular mechanisms of bisphenol A action. Reprod Toxicol 2007;24:178–98.
[31] Vandenberg LN, Hauser R, Marcus M, Olea N, Welshons WV. Human exposure to bisphenol A (BPA). Reprod Toxicol 2007;24:139–77.
[32] Carwile JL, Michels KB. Urinary bisphenol A and obesity: NHANES 2003–2006. Environ Res 2011;111:825–30.
[33] Wang T, Li M, Chen B, et al. Urinary Bisphenol A (BPA) concentration associates with obesity and insulin resistance. J Clin Endocrinol Metab 2012;97:E223–7.
[34] Shankar A, Teppala S, Sabanayagam C. Urinary bisphenol a levels and measures of obesity: results from the national health and nutrition examination survey 2003–2008. ISRN Endocrinol 2012;2012:965243.
[35] Trasande L, Attina TM, Blustein J. Association between urinary bisphenol A concentration and obesity prevalence in children and adolescents. JAMA 2012;308:1113–21.
[36] Bhandari R, Xiao J, Shankar A. Urinary bisphenol A and obesity in US children. Am J Epidemiol 2013;177:1263–70.
[37] Duffey KJ, Popkin BM. Shifts in patterns and consumption of beverages between 1965 and 2002. Obesity (Silver Spring) 2007;15:2739–47.
[38] Johnson RK, Frary C. Choose beverages and foods to moderate your intake of sugars: the 2000 Dietary Guidelines for Americans—what's all the fuss about? J Nutr 2001;131:2766S–71S.
[39] Qi Q, Chu AY, Kang JH, Jensen MK, Curhan GC, Pasquale LR, et al. Sugar-sweetened beverages and genetic risk of obesity. N Engl J Med 2012;367:1387–96.
[40] De Ruyter JC, Olthof MR, Seidell JC, Katan MB. A trial of sugar-free or sugar-sweetened beverages and body weight in children. N Engl J Med 2012;367:1397–406.
[41] Ebbeling CB, Feldman HA, Chomitz VR, Antonelli TA, Gortmaker SL, Osganian SK, et al. A randomized trial of sugar-sweetened beverages and adolescent body weight. N Engl J Med 2012;367:1407–16.
[42] Ouyang X, Cirillo P, Sautin Y, McCall S, Bruchette JL, Diehl AM, et al. Fructose consumption as a risk factor for non-alcoholic fatty liver disease. J Hepatol 2008;48:993–9.
[43] Abdelmalek MF, Suzuki A, Guy C, Unalp-Arida A, Colvin R, Johnson RJ, et al. Increased fructose consumption is associated with fibrosis severity in patients with non- alcoholic fatty liver disease. Hepatology 2010;51:1961–71.
[44] Million M, Lagier JC, Yahav D, Paul M. Gut bacterial microbiota and obesity. Clin Microbiol Infect 2013;19:305–13.
[45] Harris K, Kassis A, Major G, Chou CJ. Is the gut microbiota a new factor contributing to obesity and its metabolic disorders? J Obes 2012;2012:879151.
[46] Machado MV, Cortez-Pinto H. Gut microbiota and nonalcoholic fatty liver disease. Ann Hepatol 2012;11:440–9.
[47] Ronn M, Kullberg J, Karlsson H, Berglund J, Malmberg F, Orberg J, et al. Bisphenol A exposure increases liver fat in juvenile fructose-fed Fischer 344 rats. Toxicology 2013;303:125–32.
[48] Wagnerberger S, Spruss A, Kanuri G, Volynets V, Stahl C, Bischoff SC, et al. Toll-like receptors 1–9 are elevated in livers with fructose-induced hepatic steatosis. Br J Nutr 2012;107:1727–38.
[49] Bergheim I, Weber S, Vos M, Krämer S, Volynets V, Kaserouni S, et al. Antibiotics protect against fructose-induced hepatic lipid accumulation in mice: role of endotoxin. J Hepatol 2008;48:983–92.
[50] Spruss A, Kanuri G, Stahl C, Bischoff SC, Bergheim I. Metformin protects against the development of fructose-induced steatosis in mice: role of the intestinal barrier function. Lab Invest 2012;92:1020–32.
[51] Vajro P, Paolella G, Fasano A. Microbiota and gut-liver axis: a mini-review on their influences on obesity and obesity related liver disease. J Pediatr Gastroenterol Nutr 2013;56:461–8.
[52] Choi JJ, Eum SY, Rampersaud E, Daunert S, Abreu MT, Toborek M. Exercise attenuates PCB-induced changes in the mouse gut microbiome. Environ Health Perspect 2013;121:725–30.
[53] Vajro P, Mandato C, Licenziati MR, Franzese A, Vitale DF, Lenta S, et al. Effects of Lactobacillus rhamnosus strain GG in pediatric obesity-related liver disease. J Pediatr Gastroenterol Nutr 2011;52:740–3.
[54] Turnbaugh PJ, Ley RE, Hamady M, Fraser-Liggett CM, Knight R, Gordon JI. The human microbiome project. Nature 2007;449:804–10.

[55] Qin J, Li R, Raes J, Arumugam M, Burgdorf KS, Manichanh C, et al. Human gut microbial gene catalogue established by metagenomic sequencing. Nature 2010;464:59–65.
[56] Huse SM, Ye Y, Zhou Y, Fodor AA. A core human microbiome as viewed through 16S rRNA sequence clusters. PLoS One 2012;7:34242.
[57] Arumugam M, Raes J, Pelletier E, Le Paslier D, Yamada T, Mende DR, et al. Enterotypes of the human gut microbiome. Nature 2011;473:174–80.
[58] Gerritsen J, Smidt H, Rijkers GT, de Vos WM. Intestinal microbiota in human health and disease: the impact of probiotics. Genes Nutr 2011;6:209–40.
[59] Ley RE, Bäckhed F, Turnbaugh P, Lozupone CA, Knight RD, Gordon JI. Obesity alters gut microbial ecology. Proc Natl Acad Sci USA 2005;102:11070–5.
[60] Tap J, Mondot S, Levenez F, Pelletier E, Caron C, Furet JP, et al. Towards the human intestinal microbiota phylogenetic core. Environ Microbiol 2009;11:2574–84.
[61] Bervoets L, Van Hoorenbeeck K, Kortleven I, Van Noten C, Hens N, Vael C, et al. Differences in gut microbiota composition between obese and lean children: a cross-sectional study. Gut Pathog 2013;5:10.
[62] Turnbaugh PJ, Ley RE, Mahowald MA, Magrini V, Mardis ER, Gordon JI. An obesity-associated gut microbiome with increased capacity for energy harvest. Nature 2006;444:1027–31.
[63] Schwiertz A, Taras D, Schäfer K, Beijer S, Bos NA, Donus C, et al. Microbiota and SCFA in lean and overweight healthy subjects. Obesity (Silver spring) 2010;18:190–5.
[64] Macfarlane GT, Macfarlane S. Fermentation in the human large intestine its physiologic consequences and the potential contribution of prebiotics. J Clin Gastroenterol 2011;45(Suppl.):S120–7.
[65] Hotamisligil GS. Inflammation and metabolic disorders. Nature 2006;444:860–7.
[66] Cani PD, Amar J, Iglesias MA, Poggi M, Knauf C, Bastelica D, et al. Metabolic endotoxemia initiates obesity and insulin resistance. Diabetes 2007;56:1761–72.
[67] Payne AN, Chassard C, Zimmermann M, Müller P, Stinca S, Lacroix C. The metabolic activity of gut microbiota in obese children is increased compared with normal-weight children and exhibits more exhaustive substrate utilization. Nutr Diabetes 2011;1:e12.
[68] Louis P, Duncan SH, McCrae SI, Millar J, Jackson MS, Flint HJ. Restricted distribution of the butyrate kinase pathway among butyrate-producing bacteria from the human colon. J Bacteriol 2004;186:2099–106.
[69] Duncan SH, Louis P, Flint HJ. Lactate-utilizing bacteria, isolated from human feces, that produce butyrate as a major fermentation product. Appl Environ Microbiol 2004;70:5810–7.
[70] Santacruz A, Marcos A, Wärnberg J, Martí A, Martin-Matillas M, Campoy C, et al. Interplay between weight loss and gut microbiota composition in overweight adolescents. Obesity (Silver Spring) 2009;17:1906–15.
[71] Woodard GA, Encarnacion B, Downey JR, et al. Probiotics improve outcomes after Roux-en-Y gastric bypass surgery: a prospective randomized trial. J Gastrointest Surg 2009;13:1198–204.
[72] Sweeney TE, Morton JM. The human gut microbiome: a review of the effect of obesity and surgically induced weight loss. JAMA Surg 2013;9:1–7.
[73] Zhang H, DiBaise JK, Zuccolo A, Kudrna D, Braidotti M, Yu Y, et al. Human gut microbiota in obesity and after gastric bypass. Proc Natl Acad Sci USA 2009;106:2365–70.
[74] Li JV, Ashrafian H, Bueter M, Kinross J, Sands C, le Roux CW, et al. Metabolic surgery profoundly influences gut microbial-host metabolic cross-talk. Gut 2011;60:1214–23.
[75] Li JV, Reshat R, Wu Q, Ashrafian H, Bueter M, le Roux CW, et al. Experimental bariatric surgery in rats generates acytotoxic chemical environment in the gut contents. Front Microbiol 2011;2:183.
[76] Turnbaugh PJ, Hamady M, Yatsunenko T, Cantarel BL, Duncan A, Ley RE, et al. A core gut microbiome in obese and lean twins. Nature 2009;22(457):480–4.
[77] Tims S, Derom C, Jonkers DM, Vlietinck R, Saris WH, Kleerebezem M, et al. Microbiota conservation and BMI signatures in adult monozygotic twins. ISME J 2013;7:707–17.
[78] Simões CD, Maukonen J, Kaprio J, Rissanen A, Pietiläinen KH, Saarela M. Habitual dietary intake is associated with stool microbiota composition in monozygotic twins. J Nutr 2013;143:417–23.
[79] Koren O, Spor A, Felin J, Fåk F, Stombaugh J, Tremaroli V, et al. Human oral, gut, and plaque microbiota in patients with atherosclerosis. Proc Natl Acad Sci USA 2011;108(Suppl. 1):4592–8.
[80] Cani PD, Delzenne NM. Gut microflora as a target for energy and metabolic homeostasis. Curr Opin Clin Nutr Metab Care 2007;10:729–34.
[81] Ilan Y. Leaky gut and the liver: a role for bacterial translocation in nonalcoholic steatohepatitis. World J Gastroenterol 2012;18:2609–18.
[82] Wigg AJ, Roberts-Thomson IC, Dymock RB, McCarthy PJ, Grose RH, Cummins AG. The role of small intestinal bacterial overgrowth, intestinal permeability, endotoxaemia, and tumour necrosis factor alpha in the pathogenesis of non-alcoholic steatohepatitis. Gut 2001;48:206–11.
[83] Cani PD, Possemiers S, Van de Wiele T, Guiot Y, Everard A, Rottier O, et al. Changes in gut microbiota control inflammation in obese mice through a mechanism involving GLP-2-driven improvement of gut permeability. Gut 2009;58:1091–103.
[84] Laugerette F, Vors C, Peretti N, Michalski MC. Complex links between dietary lipids, endogenous endotoxins and metabolic inflammation. Biochimie 2011;93:39–45.
[85] Cani PD, Osto M, Geurts L, Everard A. Involvement of gut microbiota in the development of low-grade inflammation and type 2 diabetes associated with obesity. Gut Microbes 2012;3:279–88.
[86] Li Z, Yang S, Lin H, Huang J, Watkins PA, Moser AB, et al. Probiotics and antibodies to TNF inhibit inflammatory activity and improve nonalcoholic fatty liver disease. Hepatology 2003;37:343–50.
[87] Zhu L, Baker SS, Gill C, Liu W, Alkhouri R, Baker RD, et al. Characterization of the gut microbiome in non-alcoholic steatohepatitis (NASH) patients: a connection between endogenous alcohol and NASH. Hepatology 2012;57:6019.
[88] Nair S, Cope K, Risby TH, Diehl AM. Obesity and female gender increase breath ethanol concentration: potential implications for the pathogenesis of nonalcoholic steatohepatitis. Am J Gastroenterol 2001;96:1200–4.
[89] Compare D, Coccoli P, Rocco A, Nardone OM, De Maria S, Cartenì M, et al. Gut-liver axis: the impact of gut microbiota on non alcoholic fatty liver disease. Nutr Metab Cardiovasc Dis 2012;22:471–6.
[90] Dumas ME, Barton RH, Toye A, Cloarec O, Blancher C, Rothwell A, et al. Metabolic profiling reveals a contribution of gutmicrobiota to fatty liver phenotype in insulin-resistant mice. Proc Natl Acad Sci USA 2006;103:12511–6.
[91] Claus SP, Tsang TM, Wang Y, Cloarec O, Skordi E, Martin FP, et al. Systemic multicompartmental effects of the gut microbiome on mouse metabolic phenotypes. Mol Syst Biol 2008;4:219.
[92] Fuchs M. Non-alcoholic fatty liver disease: the bile acid-activated farnesoid x receptor as an emerging treatment target. J Lipids 2012;2012:934396.

[93] Basciano H, Federico L, Adeli K. Fructose, insulin resistance, and metabolic dyslipidemia. Nutr Metab (Lond) 2005;2:5.

[94] Maier IB, Stricker L, Ozel Y, Wagnerberger S, Bischoff SC, Bergheim I. A low fructose diet in the treatment of pediatric obesity: a pilot study. Pediatr Int 2011;53:303–8.

[95] Curry DL. Effects of mannose and fructose on the synthesis and secretion of insulin. Pancreas 1989;4:2–9.

[96] Dekker MJ, Su Q, Baker C, Rutledge AC, Adeli K. Fructose: a highly lipogenic nutrient implicated in insulin resistance, hepatic steatosis, and the metabolic syndrome. Am J Physiol Endocrinol Metab 2010;299:E685–94.

[97] Flanagan DE, Evans ML, Monsod TP, Rife F, Heptulla RA, Tamborlane WV, et al. The influence of insulin on circulating ghrelin. Am J Physiol 2003;284:E313–6.

[98] Teff KL, Elliott SS, Tschöp M, Kieffer TJ, Rader D, Heiman M, et al. Dietary fructose reduces circulating insulin and leptin, attenuates postprandial suppression of ghrelin, and increases triglycerides in women. J Clin Endocrinol Metab 2004;89:2963–72.

[99] Haub S, Kanuri G, Volynets V, Brune T, Bischoff SC, Bergheim I. Serotonin reuptake transporter (SERT) plays a critical role in the onset of fructose-induced hepatic steatosis in mice. Am J Physiol Gastrointest Liver Physiol 2010;298:G335–44.

[100] Havel PJ. Dietary fructose: implications for dysregulation of energy homeostasis and lipid/ carbohydrate metabolism. Nutr Rev 2005;63:133–57.

[101] Schrezenmeir J, de Vrese M. Probiotics, prebiotics, and synbiotics—approaching a definition. Am J Clin Nutr 2001;73:361S–4S.

[102] Guarner F, Schaafsma GJ. Probiotics. Int J Food Microbiol 1998;39:237–8.

[103] Roberfroid M. Prebiotics: the concept revisited. J Nutr 2007;137:830S–7S.

[104] Safavi M, Farajian S, Kelishadi R, Mirlohi M, Hashemipour M. The effects of synbiotic supplementation on some cardio-metabolic risk factors in overweight and obese children: a randomized triple-masked controlled trial. Int J Food Sci Nutr 2013;64(6):687–93.

[105] Thomas DW, Greer FR. American academy of pediatrics committee on nutrition; American academy of pediatrics section on gastroenterology, hepatology, and nutrition. Probiotics and prebiotics in pediatrics. Pediatrics 2010;126:1217–31.

[106] Cani PD. Gut microbiota and obesity: lessons from the microbiome. Brief Funct Genomics 2013;2(4):381–7.

[107] Lee HY, Park JH, Seok SH, Baek MW, Kim DJ, Lee KE, et al. Human originated bacteria, Lactobacillus rhamnosus PL60, produce conjugated linoleic acid and show anti-obesity effects in diet induced obese mice. Biochim Biophys Acta 2006;1761:736–44.

[108] Esposito E, Iacono A, Bianco G, Autore G, Cuzzocrea S, Vajro P, et al. Probiotics reduce the inflammatory response induced by a highfatdiet in the liver of young rats. J Nutr 2009;139:905–11.

[109] Murphy EF, Cotter PD, Hogan A, o'Sullivan O, Joyce A, Fouhy F, et al. Divergent metabolic outcomes arising from targeted manipulation of the gut microbiota in diet induced obesity. Gut 2013;62:220–6.

[110] Arora T, Anastasovska J, Gibson G, Tuohy K, Sharma RK, Bell J, et al. Effect of Lactobacillus acidophilus NCDC 13 supplementation on the progression of obesity in diet-induced obese mice. Br J Nutr 2012;108:1382–9.

[111] Park DY, Ahn YT, Park SH, Huh CS, Yoo SR, Yu R, et al. Supplementation of Lactobacillus curvatus HY7601 and Lactobacillus plantarum KY1032 in diet-induced obese mice is associated with gut microbial changes and reduction in obesity. PLoS One 2013;8:e59470.

[112] Everard A, Belzer C, Geurts L, Ouwerkerk JP, Druart C, Bindels LB, et al. Cross-talk between Akkermansia muciniphila and intestinal epithelium controls diet-induced obesity. Proc Natl Acad Sci USA 2013;110:9066–71.

[113] Mischke M, Plosch T. More than just a gut instinct—The potential interplay between a baby's nutrition, its gut microbiome and the epigenome. Am J Physiol Regul Integr Comp Physiol 2013;304:R1065–9.

[114] Chouraqui JP, Grathwohl D, Labaune JM, Hascoet JM, de Montgolfier I, Leclaire M, et al. Assessment of the safety, tolerance, and protective effect against diarrhea of infant formulas containing mixtures of probiotics or probiotics and prebiotics in a randomized controlled trial. Am J Clin Nutr 2008;87:1365–73.

[115] Maldonado J, Lara-Villoslada F, Sierra S, Sempere L, Gómez M, Rodriguez JM, et al. Safety and tolerance of the human milk probiotic strain Lactobacillus salivarius CECT5713 in 6-month-old children. Nutrition 2010;26:1082–7.

[116] Robinson EL, Thompson WL. Experimental feeding tests with Lactobacillus acidophilus. Am J Dis Child 1952;84:757–8.

[117] Scalabrin DM, Johnston WH, Hoffman DR, P'Pool VL, Harris CL, Mitmesser SH. Growth and tolerance of healthy term infants receiving hydrolyzed infant formulas supplemented with Lactobacillus rhamnosus GG: randomized, double-blind, controlled trial. Clin Pediatr (Phila) 2009;48:734–44.

[118] Vendt N, Grünberg H, Tuure T, Malminiemi O, Wuolijoki E, Tillmann V, et al. Growth during the first 6 months of life in infants using formula enriched with Lactobacillus rhamnosus GG: double-blind, randomized trial. J Hum Nutr Diet 2006;19:51–8.

[119] de Roos NM, Schouten G, Katan MB. Yoghurt enriched with Lactobacillus acidophilus does not lower blood lipids in healthy men and women with normal toborderline high serum cholesterol levels. Eur J Clin Nutr 1999;53:277–80.

[120] Sadrzadeh-Yeganeh H, Elmadfa I, Djazayery A, Jalali M, Heshmat R, Chamary M. The effects of probiotic and conventional yoghurt on lipid profile in women. Br J Nutr 2010;103:1778–83.

[121] Chang BJ, Park SU, Jang YS, Ko SH, Joo NM, Kim SI, et al. Effect of functional yogurt NY-YP901 in improving the trait of metabolic syndrome. Eur J Clin Nutr 2011;65:1250–5.

[122] Sanz Y, Rastmanesh R, Agostoni C. Understanding the role of gut microbes and probiotics in obesity: how far are we? Pharmacol Res 2013;69:144–55.

[123] Leber B, Tripolt NJ, Blattl D, Eder M, Wascher TC, Pieber TR, et al. The influence of probiotic supplementation on gut permeability in patients with metabolic syndrome: an open label, randomized pilot study. Eur J Clin Nutr 2012;66:1110–5.

[124] Agerholm-Larsen L, Raben A, Haulrik N, Hansen AS, Manders M, Astrup A. Effect of 8 week intake of probiotic milk products on risk factors for cardiovascular diseases. Eur J Clin Nutr 2000;54:288–97.

[125] Bukowska H, Pieczul-Mroz J, Jastrzebska M, Chełstowski K, Naruszewicz M. Decrease in fibrinogen and LDL-cholesterol levels upon supplementation of diet with Lactobacillus plantarumin subjects with moderately elevated cholesterol. Atherosclerosis 1998;137:437–8.

[126] Naruszewicz M, Johansson ML, Zapolska-Downar D, Bukowska H. Effect of Lactobacillus plantarum299v on cardiovascular disease risk factors in smokers. Am J Clin Nutr 2002;76:1249–55.

[127] Laitinen K, Poussa T, Isolauri E. Nutrition, allergy, mucosal immunology and intestinal microbiota group. Probiotics and dietary counselling contribute to glucose regulation during and after pregnancy: a randomised controlled trial. Br J Nutr 2009;101:1679–87.

[128] Ilmonen J, Isolauri E, Poussa T, Laitinen K. Impact of dietary counseling and probiotic intervention on maternal anthropometric measurements during and after pregnancy: a randomized placebo-controlled trial. Clin Nutr 2011;30:156–64.

[129] Gobel RJ, Larsen N, Jakobsen M, Molgaard C, Michaelsen KF. Probiotics to obese adolescents; RCT examining the effects on inflammation and metabolic syndrome. J Pediatr Gastroenterol Nutr 2012;55:673–8.
[130] Aller R, De Luis DA, Izaola O, Conde R, Gonzalez Sagrado M. Effect of a probiotic on liver aminotransferases in nonalcoholic fatty liver disease patients: a double blind randomized clinical trial. Eur Rev Med Pharmacol Sci 2011;15:1090–5.
[131] Jung SP, Lee KM, Kang JH, Yun SI, Park HO, Moon Y, et al. Effect of Lactobacillus gasseri BNR17 on overweight and obese adults: a randomized, double-blind clinical trial. Korean J Fam Med 2013;34:80–9.
[132] Kadooka Y, Sato M, Imaizumi K, Ogawa A, Ikuyama K, Akai Y, et al. Regulation of abdominal adiposity by probiotics (Lactobacillus gasseriSBT2055) in adults with obese tendencies in a randomized controlled trial. Eur J Clin Nutr 2010;64:636–43.
[133] Li DY, Yang M, Edwards S, Ye SQ. Nonalcoholic fatty liver disease: for better or worse, blame the gut microbiota? JPEN J Parenter Enteral Nutr 2013 [Epub ahead of print].
[134] Ma X, Hua J, Li Z. Probiotics improve high fat diet-induced hepatic steatosis and insulin resistance by increasing hepatic NKT cells. J Hepatol 2008;49:821–30.
[135] Velayudham A, Dolganiuc A, Ellis M, Petrasek J, Kodys K, Mandrekar P, et al. VSL#3 probiotic treatment attenuates fibrosis without changes in steatohepatitis in a diet-induced nonalcoholic steatohepatitis model in mice. Hepatology 2009;49:989–97.
[136] Mencarelli A, Cipriani S, Renga B, Bruno A, D'Amore C, Distrutti E, et al. VSL#3 resets insulin signaling and protects against NASH and atherosclerosis in a model of genetic dys lipidemia and intestinal inflammation. PLoS One 2012;7:e45425.
[137] Yadav H, Jain S, Sinha PR. Antidiabetic effect of probiotic dahi containing Lactobacillus acidophilus and Lactobacillus casei in high fructose fed rats. Nutrition 2007;23:62–8.
[138] Xu RY, Wan YP, Fang QY, Lu W, Cai W. Supplementation with probiot ics modifies gut flora and attenuates liver fat accumulation in rat nonalco holic fatty liver disease model. J Clin Biochem Nutr 2012;50:72–7.
[139] Yoo SR, Kim YJ, Park DY, Jung UJ, Jeon SM, Ahn YT, et al. Probiotics L. plantarum and L. curvatus in combination alter hepatic lipidmetabolism and suppress diet-induced obesity. Obesity (Silver Spring) 2013 [Epub ahead of print].
[140] Lirussi F, Mastropasqua E, Orando S, Orlando R. Probiotics for non-alcoholic fatty liver disease and/or steatohepatitis. Cochrane Database Syst Rev 2007:CD005165.
[141] Loguercio C, De Simone T, Federico A, Terracciano F, Tuccillo C, Di Chicco M, et al. Gut-liver axis: a new point of attack to treat chronic liver damage? Am J Gastroenterol 2002;97:2144–6.
[142] Loguercio C, Federico A, Tuccillo C, Terracciano F, D'Auria MV, De Simone C, et al. Beneficial effects of a probiotic VSL#3 on parameters of liver dysfunction in chronic liver diseases. J Clin Gastroenterol 2005;39:540–3.
[143] Socha P, Horvath A, Vajro P, Dziechciarz P, Dhawan A, Szajewska H. Pharmacological interventions for nonalcoholic fatty liver disease in adults and in children: a systematic review. J Pediatr Gastroenterol Nutr 2009;48:587–96.
[144] Malaguarnera M, Vacante M, Antic T, Giordano M, Chisari G, Acquaviva R, et al. Bifidobacterium longum with fructo-oligosaccharides in patients with non alcoholic steatohepatitis. Dig Dis Sci 2012;57:545–53.
[145] Mouzaki M, Comelli EM, Arendt BM, Bonengel J, Fung SK, Fischer SE, et al. Intestinal microbiota in patients with nonalcoholic fatty liver disease. Hepatology 2013;58(1):120–7.
[146] Vrieze A, Van Nood E, Holleman F, Salojärvi J, Kootte RS, Bartelsman JF, et al. Transfer of intestinal microbiota from lean donors increases insulin sensitivity in individuals with metabolic syndrome. Gastroenterology 2012;143:913-6e7.
[147] Armougom F, Henry M, Vialettes B, Raccah D, Raoult D. Monitoring bacterial community of human gut microbiota reveals an increase in Lactobacillus in obese patients and Methanogens in anorexic patients. PLoS One 2009;4:e7125.
[148] Nadal I, Santacruz A, Marcos A, Warnberg J, Garagorri JM, Moreno LA, et al. Shifts in clostridia, bacteroides and immunoglobulin-coating fecal bacteria associated with weight loss in obese adolescents. Int J Obes (Lond) 2009;33:758–67.
[149] Balamurugan R, George G, Kabeerdoss J, Hepsiba J, Chandragunasekaran AM, Ramakrishna BS. Quantitative differences in intestinal Faecalibacterium prausnitzii in obese Indian children. Br J Nutr 2010;103:335–8.
[150] Million M, Maraninchi M, Henry M, Armougom F, Raoult D. Obesity-associated Gut microbiota is enriched in Lactobacillus reuteri and depleted in Bifidobacterium animalis and Methanobrevibacter smithii. Int J Obes 2011;36:817–25.
[151] Kalliomäki M, Collado MC, Salminen S, Isolauri E. Early differences in fecal microbiota composition in children may predict overweight. Am J Clin Nutr 2008;87:534–8.
[152] Million M, Angelakis E, Maraninchi M, Henry M, Giorgi R, Valero R, et al. Correlation between body mass index and gut concentrations of Lactobacillus reuteri, Bifidobacterium Animalis, Methanobrevibacter smithii and Escherichia coli. Int J Obes 2013:1–7.
[153] Million M, Angelakis E, Paul M, Armougom F, Leibovici L, Raoult D. Comparative meta-analysis of the effect of Lactobacillus species on weight gain in humans and animals. Microb Pathog 2012;53:100–8.
[154] Fabian E, Elmadfa I. The effect of daily consumption of probiotic and conventional yoghurt on oxidant and antioxidant parameters in plasma of young healthy women. Int J Vitam Nutr Res 2007;77:79–88.
[155] Wong VW, Won GL, Chim AM, Chu WC, Yeung DK, Li KC, et al. Treatment of nonalcoholic steatohepatitis with probiotics. A proof-of-concept study. Ann Hepatol 2013;12:256–62.
[156] Ma YY, Li L, Yu CH, Shen Z, Chen LH, Li YM. Effects of probiotics on nonalcoholic fatty liver disease: A meta-analysis. World J Gastroenterol 2013;19:6911–8.

CHAPTER

34

Beta-Cryptoxanthin, a Novel Carotenoid Derived from Satsuma Mandarin, Prevents Abdominal Obesity

Katsuhiko Takayanagi and Katsuyuki Mukai

R&D Center, UNITIKA Ltd., Uji, Kyoto, Japan

INTRODUCTION

Citrus is a common term and a genus of flowering plants of the rue family, Rutaceae. Citrus plants are believed to have originated in Northwest India, where they have been cultivated in an ever-widening area for the last 4200 years. Citrus is now the world's most popular fruit. More than 600 species of citrus have been identified worldwide and include bergamot orange, calamondin, citron, grapefruit, lemon, lime, pomelo, tangelo, and tangerine. Although there are so many species already, the number is still increasing because citrus trees hybridize readily; this may help in the development of new citrus varieties.

The satsuma mandarin (*Citrus unshiu* Marc.), also known as the satsuma or table orange in Western countries, is one of the local citrus fruits originally found in Kagoshima, Japan, more than 400 years ago. It is now one of the most popular and widely consumed fruits in Japan. The satsuma mandarin is not only sweet and tasty but it also contains a number of nutrients such as vitamin C, hesperidin (also known as vitamin P), pectin, and synephrine. One of the characteristic nutritive compounds found in the satsuma mandarin is a carotenoid typically found in blood, known as beta-cryptoxanthin (β-CRX).

Carotenoids are a group of natural pigments produced from eight isoprene molecules and contain 40 carbon atoms. Besides being simple pigments, carotenoids are important nutrients that need to be acquired through the diet because they are not endogenously synthesized. For example, vitamin A, also known as retinal, is an essential nutrient that is synthesized from four types of carotenoids: α-carotene, β-carotene, γ-carotene, and β-CRX. A number of other carotenoids are also beneficial for health because they can function as antioxidants, macular protectors, or anticancer agents [1,2].

Although more than 700 carotenoids have been found in plants and photosynthetic organisms like algae, bacteria, and fungi, only six of them are found in human blood: α-carotene, β-carotene, lutein and zeaxanthin (isomers), lycopene, and β-CRX. Except for β-CRX, they are all commercially available in supplements or drinks.

β-CRX is a carotenoid classified as a xanthophyll: its chemical structure is similar to that of β-carotene except for the addition of a hydroxyl group at the number 3 carbon atom (Fig. 34.1). Unlike other abundant carotenoids, β-CRX is not found in most fruits or vegetables; only in specific ones such as hot peppers, persimmons, and satsuma mandarins [3].

β-CRX is particularly abundant in satsuma mandarins; no other fruits or vegetables, including other citrus fruits, contain such high amounts of β-CRX. The edible part of the satsuma mandarin contains approximately 1.8 mg β-CRX per 100 g, while that of the Valencia orange contains approximately 0.2 mg per 100 g. In contrast, the grapefruit contains no β-CRX. The serum β-CRX concentration in the Japanese population is higher than that in the Western population, probably because of the presence of good sources of β-CRX such as satsuma mandarin. Satsuma mandarin consumption is also considered a good index of serum β-CRX concentrations in the Japanese population [4,5].

In most cases, the term *carotenoid* refers to abundant carotenoids such as α-carotene, β-carotene, lycopene, and lutein/zeaxanthin. The absorption, metabolism, and nutritional functions of these carotenoids have been well studied [6–10]. In contrast, analyses of minor carotenoids have not been sufficiently reported.

Nutrition in the Prevention and Treatment of Abdominal Obesity
http://dx.doi.org/10.1016/B978-0-12-407869-7.00034-9

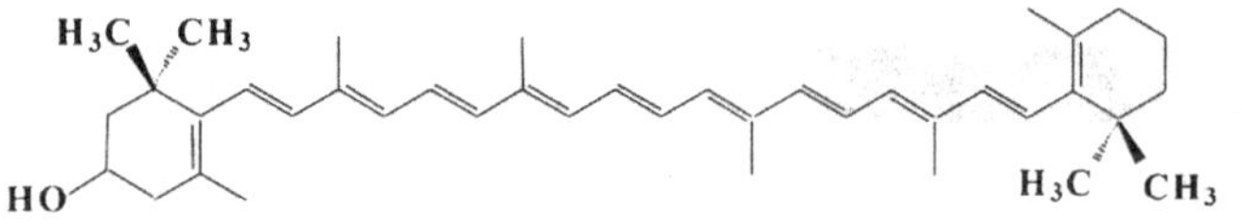

FIGURE 34.1 Chemical structure of beta-cryptoxanthin.

Although the functions of β-CRX have not been examined in detail, several important features of β-CRX have been reported. Studies have shown a significant inverse correlation between satsuma mandarin consumption, which is representative of serum β-CRX concentrations, and disease morbidities such as those for liver disorders [11,12], cancer [13–15], postmenopausal osteoporosis [16–18], and diabetes [19,20]. These results strongly suggest that high satsuma mandarin consumption is beneficial for human health, probably because of elevated serum β-CRX concentrations. Sugiura et al. also reported that serum β-CRX concentrations negatively correlate with serum lipid levels [21], which suggests that β-CRX has some effect on obesity.

Obesity is a major cause of metabolic syndrome, since accumulation of visceral fat results in a number of adverse health effects. We have previously reported that a regular oral intake of satsuma mandarin-derived β-CRX results in a reduction in visceral adipose tissue, body weight, and waist circumference in mildly obese males [22]. Reductions in visceral fat were reproduced in an obese mouse model [23,24], and further investigations revealed the molecular mechanism of the β-CRX effect on adipocytes that reduces visceral fat.

Here, we show how citrus-derived β-CRX affects adipocytes and contributes to reduced abdominal obesity.

EPIDEMIOLOGY OF BETA-CRYPTOXANTHIN

β-CRX is found in human blood together with other abundant carotenoids, even though high levels are not consumed. Wallqvist et al. showed that the daily intake of β-CRX from food is 0.2–0.3 mg and that the serum concentration is 11.7 μg/dL and 20.3 μg/dL in Australian men and women, respectively [25]. In contrast, the daily intake of β-carotene is 4.7 mg in men and 3.6 mg in women, and their serum concentrations are 13.9 μg/dL and 12.6 μg/dL, respectively [25]. Michaud et al. also reported that although the daily β-CRX intake was <100 μg in an American population, the plasma β-CRX concentration was almost 13 mg/dL; in contrast, the daily intake of β-carotene was >5 mg/day and the serum concentration was 25–30 mg/dL [26]. These results suggest that the bioavailability of β-CRX is higher than that of other abundant carotenoids.

Many epidemiological studies have demonstrated a strong correlation between food consumption and reduced disease risk. It is well known that a daily intake of fruits and vegetables is beneficial for human health [27–30] and that serum concentrations of carotenoids and vitamins are good indexes of their consumption [26,31–35].

The majority of cohort studies have reported an inverse correlation between serum carotenoid levels and disease risk. However, most of these studies have focused on major carotenoids such as β-carotene, lycopene, and lutein/zeaxanthin. A few studies found that β-CRX consumption has significant health benefits.

Little attention has so far been paid to the nutritional importance of β-CRX because there are only a few sources of β-CRX in Western countries. However, the importance of β-CRX is now being recognized and several studies focusing on β-CRX have been reported.

Nakamura et al. reported an inverse association between brachial-ankle pulse wave velocity and serum β-CRX, which was independent of the hyperglycemic state. This result indicates that β-CRX can reduce the risk of arteriosclerosis induced by hyperglycemia [36]. Montonen et al. showed that β-CRX intake was significantly associated with a reduced risk of type 2 diabetes mellitus (T2DM) [37]. Sugiura et al. reported that the homeostasis model assessment of insulin resistance (HOMA-IR) index was inversely associated with the serum β-CRX concentration, which suggests that high serum β-CRX levels prevent T2DM [19]. As hyperglycemia and arteriosclerosis are well-known symptoms of metabolic syndrome, these reports strongly support the idea that β-CRX can reduce the risk of developing metabolic syndrome.

Metabolic syndrome comprises a set of symptoms induced by obesity; preventing obesity could therefore improve overall health. Body mass index (BMI) is the most commonly used index for measuring obesity. Michaud et al. found plasma β-CRX to be negatively correlated with BMI in American populations, especially in women [26]. Sugiura et al. also found BMI to be a negative predictor of serum β-CRX in Japanese [5]. Moreover, Suzuki et al. reported similar results, i.e. serum levels of β-CRX are lower in obese Japanese individuals, especially in women [38]. The inverse correlation between serum β-CRX and BMI raises the possibility that β-CRX intake reduces BMI. In other words, β-CRX intake could prevent obesity.

INDUSTRIAL PRODUCTION OF BETA-CRYPTOXANTHIN

Although the satsuma mandarin is one of the best sources of β-CRX, the β-CRX content of satsuma mandarins is still lower than that of other major carotenoids in fruits or vegetables, e.g. β-carotene in carrots. To enable its scientific functional evaluation and industrial application, a consistent quality of β-CRX product is needed. As a result, we prepared two β-CRX formulations: either powder or liquid form. The powder form was enzyme-processed satsuma mandarin, which is made from satsuma mandarin pulp after juicing. In this preparation, β-CRX is enriched by the reduction of water-insoluble dietary fiber. The powder form contains at least 0.2% (w/w) β-CRX, which is almost 200 times the concentration found in satsuma mandarin. The liquid form, on the other hand, is an emulsified satsuma mandarin extract. It contains at least 0.04% (w/w) β-CRX; a test drink for human trials was produced using this formulation.

These formulations dramatically improve the bioavailability of β-CRX. Clinical trials showed that the serum transfer efficiency of β-CRX derived from the powder type is 30 times higher than that of satsuma mandarin. The liquid type also improved β-CRX serum transfer. Takaishi et al. also reported that the liquid type of β-CRX is transferred to the serum faster and stays elevated for longer compared to β-CRX derived from satsuma mandarin fruits or juice. Caco-2 cell experiments revealed that a co-administered emulsifier elevated the intestinal absorption of β-CRX, especially for non-fatty acid-esterified β-CRX [39].

BETA-CRYPTOXANTHIN AND OBESITY

Tsumura Suzuki Obese Diabetes (TSOD) inbred mice [23,24] and their genetic controls, Tsumura Suzuki Nonobese Diabetes (TSNO) were used to evaluate the effects of β-CRX in powder form. TSOD mice accumulate visceral fat after 4 weeks of age and show symptoms similar to those of human metabolic syndrome.

Three-week-old male TSOD and TSNO mice were obtained from the Institute for Animal Reproduction (Ibaraki, Japan). After an acclimatization period of 1 week, mice were divided into four test and control groups (six mice in each group): TSOD experimental group (TSOD-E); TSOD control group (TSOD-C); TSNO experimental group (TSNO-E); and TSNO control group (TSNO-C).

During the 8-week test period, experimental groups received oral administration of satsuma mandarin-derived β-CRX (powder type) suspended in olive oil at a dose of 400 mg/kg/day (equivalent to 0.8 mg/kg/day β-CRX), whereas control groups received olive oil only. Each group of mice was housed in a single cage under a 12-h light:dark cycle and fed with Labo MR Stock (Nosan, Kanagawa, Japan). Body weight and food and water consumption were monitored throughout the experimental period. Following the experimental period, three adipose tissues (epididymal, mesenteric, and perirenal), liver, femoral muscle, and serum were harvested.

The average body weight for each group is shown in Fig. 34.2. No differences in the body weights were observed between TSNO-E and TSNO-C mice. The average weight of TSOD-C mice was significantly higher than that of TSNO-C mice, presumably because of differences in their genetic backgrounds. In contrast, the body weight of TSOD-E mice was notably reduced compared to TSOD-C mice, with the differences becoming statistically significant after the second week. As the food and water consumption of both TSOD groups was almost the same during the experimental period, these differences were probably not due to differences in food consumption but instead to the administration of β-CRX. Moreover, β-CRX consumption did not affect the body weight of nonobese mice, suggesting that β-CRX contributes to body weight reduction only in obese individuals.

Liver weights were also compared among groups (Fig. 34.3). No differences in the liver weight were observed between TSNO groups; however, the liver weight of TSOD-C mice was significantly higher than that of TSNO-E mice. Although liver weight was higher in TSOD-E mice than in TSNO mice, it was significantly lower in TSOD-E mice than in TSOD-C mice. This indicates that obesity-induced liver hypertrophy was repressed by β-CRX administration.

A similar trend was observed in the three adipose tissues (epididymal, mesenteric, and perirenal; Fig. 34.4). The weights of the epididymal, perirenal, and mesenteric tissues of TSOD-E mice were reduced to 86%, 80%, and 74%, respectively, compared to equivalent tissues

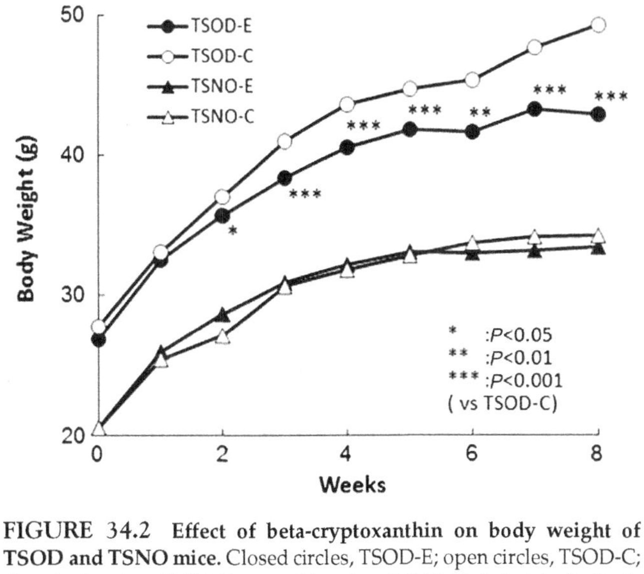

FIGURE 34.2 Effect of beta-cryptoxanthin on body weight of TSOD and TSNO mice. Closed circles, TSOD-E; open circles, TSOD-C; closed triangles, TNSO-E; open triangles, TSNO-C. Asterisks indicate statistical significance between the TSOD-E and TSOD-C groups. TSNO, Tsumura Suzuki Nonobese Diabetes; TSOD, Tsumura Suzuki Obese Diabetes. TSNO-C, TSNO in the control group; TSNO-E, TSNO in the experimental group; TSOD-C, TSOD in the control group; TSOD-E, TSOD in the experimental group.

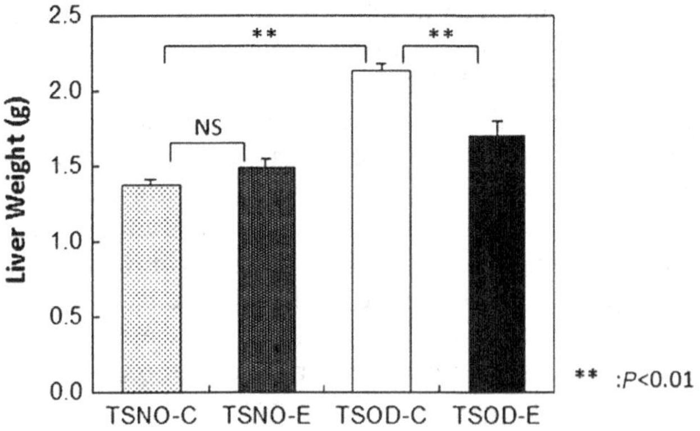

FIGURE 34.3 **Effect of beta-cryptoxanthin on liver weight.** TSNO, Tsumura Suzuki Nonobese Diabetes; TSOD, Tsumura Suzuki Obese Diabetes. TSNO-C, TSNO in the control group; TSNO-E, TSNO in the experimental group; TSOD-C, TSOD in the control group; TSOD-E, TSOD in the experimental group.

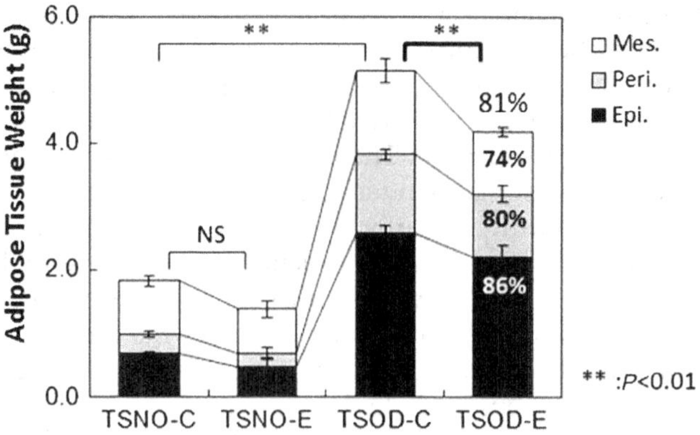

FIGURE 34.4 **Effect of beta-cryptoxanthin on the visceral adipose tissue weight.** Epi., epididymal; Mes., mesenteric; Peri., perirenal. TSNO, Tsumura Suzuki Nonobese Diabetes; TSOD, Tsumura Suzuki Obese Diabetes. TSNO-C, TSNO in the control group; TSNO-E, TSNO in the experimental group; TSOD-C, TSOD in the control group; TSOD-E, TSOD in the experimental group.

from TSOD-C mice. The weight reduction in mesenteric adipose tissue, commonly called *intraperitoneal adipose tissue*, was the highest among the three tissues. Moreover, the total weight of the three adipose tissues from TSOD-E mice was reduced to 81% that of TSOD-C mice.

Histological specimens were prepared from epididymal adipose tissues for microscopic examination (Fig. 34.5). Adipocyte size was nearly the same in TSNO-E and TSNO-C mice. However, adipocytes from TSOD-C mice were enlarged relative to those of TSNO-C mice, and significantly smaller in TSOD-E mice.

The average areas of the adipocyte cells in the different groups were calculated (Fig. 34.6); results were consistent with visual assessments. Taken together, these data show that mature adipocytes from TSOD mice are hypertrophic compared to those of TSNO mice and that β-CRX administration may prevent adipocyte hypertrophy.

The serum triglyceride (TG), total cholesterol (TC), and nonesterified fatty acid (NEFA) concentrations were assayed; results are shown in Fig. 34.7. No differences were observed in the serum lipid concentrations between TSNO-C and TSNO-E mice. In contrast, the levels of all three lipids were significantly elevated in the TSOD-C group compared to the other three groups. TG and NEFA

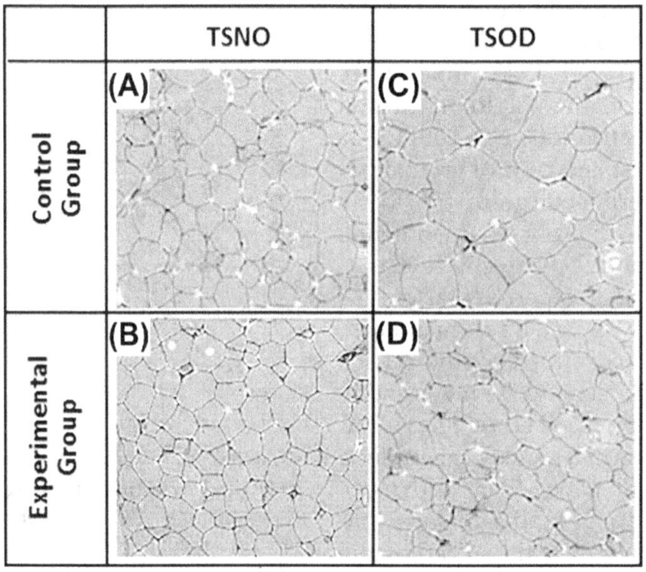

FIGURE 34.5 **Effect of beta-cryptoxanthin on the size of the adipocytes.** A, TSNO-C; B, TSNO-E; C, TSOD-C; D, TSOD-E. TSNO, Tsumura Suzuki Nonobese Diabetes; TSOD, Tsumura Suzuki Obese Diabetes. TSNO-C, TSNO in the control group; TSNO-E, TSNO in the experimental group; TSOD-C, TSOD in the control group; TSOD-E, TSOD in the experimental group.

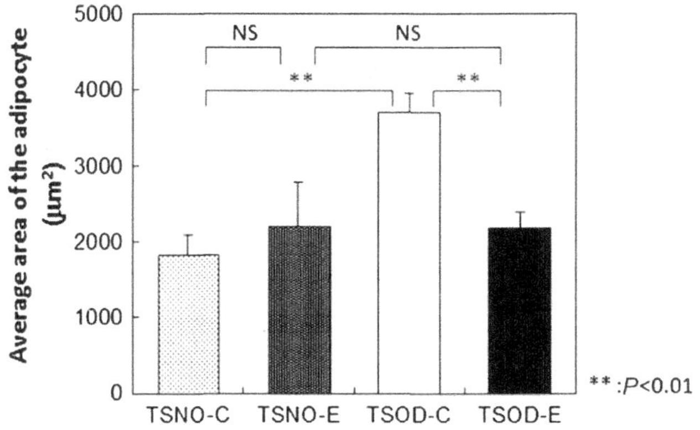

FIGURE 34.6 Average area of individual adipocytes in each group. TSNO, Tsumura Suzuki Nonobese Diabetes; TSOD, Tsumura Suzuki Obese Diabetes. TSNO-C, TSNO in the control group; TSNO-E, TSNO in the experimental group; TSOD-C, TSOD in the control group; TSOD-E, TSOD in the experimental group.

concentrations in TSOD-E mice were significantly reduced compared to those in TSOD-C mice; levels in TSOD-E mice were similar to those observed in TSNO-C mice. Although the TC concentration in TSOD-E mice was also significantly repressed compared to TSOD-C mice, it was still significantly higher than that of TSNO-E mice. β-CRX administration significantly repressed the elevation of serum lipids in TSOD mice but had no discernible effect on nonobese TSNO mice. These results indicate that β-CRX administration does not simply reduce serum lipid levels; instead, it normalizes them by repressing their elevation.

The effect of β-CRX on gene expression in TSOD mice was evaluated by DNA microarray analysis. Total RNA was isolated from epididymal adipose tissue, liver, and femoral muscle using an RNeasy kit (QIAGEN, Duesseldorf, Germany). RNA was then biotin labeled and fragmented using a GeneChip 3′-IVT labeling kit (Affymetrix, Santa Clara, CA). The resulting fragmented cRNA was hybridized at 45°C for 16h to a GeneChip Mouse Genome 430A 2.0 Array (Affymetrix; containing approximately 14,000 well-characterized genes), washed, and stained using a fluid station and then scanned using a GeneChip scanner (Affymetrix). Data were analyzed using an Expression Console (Affymetrix) and imported into the ArrayStar software program (DNAstar, Madison, MI). Data were then normalized and gene expression levels were compared using ArrayStar. The Database for Annotation, Visualization and Integrated Discovery (DAVID) v6.2 (http://david.abcc.ncifcrf.gov/) was used for the biological interpretation of differentially expressed genes [40]. Changes in gene ontology biological processes with a P value of <0.01 were considered to be statistically significant. Moreover, differentially expressed genes were categorized and mapped onto pathways using KEGG tools (http://www.genome.jp/kegg/) [41].

Results of the gene expression analysis are summarized in Table 34.1. The number of genes showing > two-fold expression changes between the TSOD-C and TSNO-C groups and the TSOD-C and TSNO-E groups in the liver, adipocyte, and muscle were 270, 217, and 56, respectively.

TABLE 34.1 Summary of Microarray Analysis of Changes in Gene Expression in Mice Fed Beta-Cryptoxanthin

Organ/Cell	TSNO-C vs. TSOD-C			TSOD-C vs. TSOD-E			Overall Total (Both Groups)
	Up	Down	Total	Up	Down	Total	
Liver	920	424	1344	146	260	406	270
Adipocyte	728	1229	1957	71	181	252	217
Muscle	190	677	867	30	59	89	56

TSNO, Tsumura Suzuki Nonobese Diabetes; TSOD, Tsumura Suzuki Obese Diabetes.

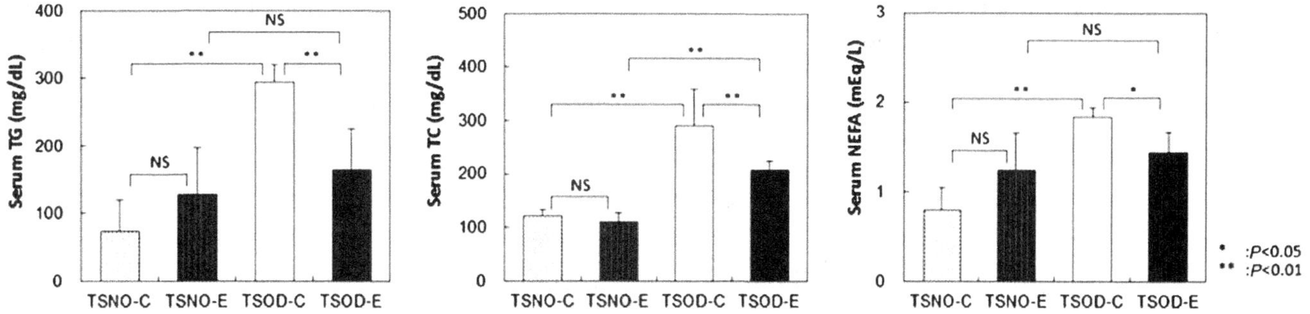

FIGURE 34.7 Effect of beta-cryptoxanthin on serum lipid markers. TG, serum triglyceride level; TC, total cholesterol levels; NEFA, non-esterified fatty acid level. TSNO, Tsumura Suzuki Nonobese Diabetes; TSOD, Tsumura Suzuki Obese Diabetes. TSNO-C, TSNO in the control group; TSNO-E, TSNO in the experimental group; TSOD-C, TSOD in the control group; TSOD-E, TSOD in the experimental group.

TABLE 34.2 Gene Ontology Biological Processes Affected by Oral Ingestion of Beta-Cryptoxanthin

	GO ID	GO Biological Process	Changed Genes	Total Genes	%	P Value[a]
Liver						
1	GO:0006270	DNA replication initiation	4	20	20.0	3.10×10^{4}
2	GO:0045455	Steroid metabolic process	9	224	4.0	2.00×10^{3}
3	GO:0045859	Regulation of protein kinase activity	10	372	2.7	2.10×10^{3}
4	GO:0019220	Regulation of phosphate metabolic process	16	611	2.6	2.50×10^{5}
5	GO:0006468	Protein amino acid phosphorylation	19	1020	1.9	4.20×10^{3}
Adipocytes						
1	GO:0050000	Chromosome localization	4	17	23.5	8.60×10^{5}
2	GO:0007049	Cell cycle	36	1000	3.6	3.40×10^{15}
3	GO:0006935	Chemotaxis	10	291	3.4	5.40×10^{6}
4	GO:0002520	Immune system development	12	466	2.6	7.40×10^{4}
5	GO:0042981	Regulation of apoptosis	16	988	1.6	2.20×10^{3}
Muscle						
1	GO:0060048	Cardiac muscle contraction	4	33	12.1	6.20×10^{3}
2	GO:0006633	Fatty acid biosynthetic process	4	122	3.3	1.70×10^{3}
3	GO:0006869	Lipid transport	5	159	3.1	4.00×10^{4}
4	GO:0042060	Wound healing	3	187	1.6	4.30×10^{2}
5	GO:0010817	Regulation of hormone levels	4	295	1.4	6.30×10^{3}

[a]*Determined using the Database for Annotation, Visualization and Integrated Discovery (DAVID) v6.2 (http://david.abcc.ncifcrf.gov).*
GO, gene ontology; ID, identification number.

The results of a functional clustering analysis are shown in Table 34.2. Nine genes involved in steroid metabolism were affected by β-CRX in the liver of TSOD mice. Among them, the expression levels of genes encoding hydroxymethylglutaryl-CoA synthase (*Hmgcs1*), lanosterol 14-alpha demethylase (*Cyp51a1/Cyp51*), and isopentenyl-diphosphate delta isomerase 1 (*Idi1*), which are involved in the synthesis of steroids, were upregulated by β-CRX in TSOD mice. In contrast, their mRNA levels were decreased in TSOD-C mice relative to those in TSNO-C mice (Table 34.3). Moreover, the expression levels of genes encoding vigilin [high-density lipoprotein-binding protein (*Hdlbp*)] and ATP-binding cassette subfamily A member 1 (*Abca1*), which are involved in the transport of steroids, were downregulated by β-CRX in TSOD mice, whereas their expression was higher in TSOD-C mice than in TSNO-C mice. Four genes involved in DNA replication initiation, the first step of cell proliferation, were also affected by β-CRX. In addition, the expression levels of genes encoding members of the minichromosome maintenance (MCM) replication initiating complex, *Mcm2*, *Mcm4*, *Mcm5*, and *Mcm6*, were repressed in the liver by β-CRX in TSOD mice, although their mRNA levels were increased in TSOD-C mice relative to levels in TSNO-C mice.

In adipocytes, the expression of genes involved in the cell cycle, chemotaxis, and immune system development were affected by β-CRX (Table 34.2). Genes encoding cyclin-dependent kinase 1 (*Cdk1*) and cyclins (*Ccna2*, *Ccnb1*, and *Ccnb2*), which are well-known key regulators of the cell cycle, were downregulated by β-CRX, although their mRNA levels were increased in the TSOD-C group compared to the TSNO-C group (Table 34.4). Moreover, genes encoding CXCL (*Cxc12* and *Cxc110*) and CCL (*Cc12*, *Cc13*, *Cc14*, *Cc17*, and *Cc112*) chemokines were also repressed by β-CRX. However, their mRNA levels were increased in TSOD-C mice relative to those in TSNO-C mice.

TABLE 34.3 Genes Regulated in the Liver by Oral Ingestion of Beta-Cryptoxanthin in TSOD Mice

Gene Symbol	Gene Name	Fold Change	
		TSOD-C vs. TSNO-C	TSOD-E vs. TSOD-C
GO:0006270 DNA replication initiation			
Mcm2	minichromosome maintenance deficient 2	3.25	0.45
Mcm4	minichromosome maintenance deficient 4	3.32	0.45
Mcm5	minichromosome maintenance deficient 5	4.82	0.28
Mcm6	minichromosome maintenance deficient 6	4.82	0.29
GO:0045455 Steroid metabolic process			
Sult2a2	sulfotransferase family 2A2	3.70	0.28
Pctp	phosphatidylcholine transfer protein	5.85	0.31
Hdlbp	high-density lipoprotein-binding protein	4.26	0.33
Mbtps1	membrane-bound transcription factor peptidase, site 1	4.22	0.37
Nr3c1	nuclear receptor subfamily 3, group C, member 1	4.05	0.44
Abca1	ATP-binding cassette, subfamily A, member 1	3.58	0.45
Cyp51	cytochrome P450, family 51	0.48	2.07
Hmgcs1	3-hydroxy-3-methylglutaryl-Coenzyme A synthase 1	0.39	2.16
Idi1	isopentenyl-diphosphate delta isomerase	0.25	3.95
GO:0045859 Regulation of protein kinase activity			
Aplp2	amyloid beta (A4) precursor-like protein 2	4.69	0.36
Hgf	hepatocyte growth factor	3.14	0.37
Met	met proto-oncogene	2.54	0.40
Ceacam1	carcinoembryonic antigen-related cell adhesion molecule 1	4.12	0.42
Ptpn11	protein tyrosine phosphatase, nonreceptor type 11	2.17	0.47
Shc1	src homology 2 domain-containing transforming protein C1	2.50	0.48
Nf2	neurofibromatosis 2	2.41	0.49
Tgfbr2	transforming growth factor, beta receptor II	2.12	0.49
Lats2	large tumor suppressor 2	0.43	2.17
Gtpbp4	GTP binding protein 4	0.35	2.91

GO, gene ontology; TSNO, Tsumura Suzuki Nonobese Diabetes; TSOD, Tsumura Suzuki Obese Diabetes.

TABLE 34.4 Genes Regulated in Adipocytes by Oral Ingestion of Beta-Cryptoxanthin in TSOD Mice

Gene Symbol	Gene Name	Fold Change	
		TSOD − β-CRX vs. TSNO − β-CRX	TSOD + β-CRX vs. TSOD − β-CRX
GO:0007049 Cell cycle			
Ereg	epiregulin	8.44	0.14
Birc5	baculoviral IAP repeat-containing 5	6.78	0.25
Mki67	antigen identified by monoclonal antibody Ki 67	4.85	0.27
Cenpf	centromere protein F	3.21	0.28
Cdk1	cell division cycle 2 homolog A	4.62	0.29
Ccnb2	cyclin B2	4.15	0.29
Mcm6	minichromosome maintenance deficient 6	4.26	0.30
Bub1	budding uninhibited by benzimidazoles 1	4.69	0.32
Cdca5	cell division cycle associated 5	4.56	0.32
Cep55	centrosomal protein 55	6.53	0.33
Ccna2	cyclin A2	3.83	0.34
Kif11	kinesin family member 11	4.01	0.35
Prc1	protein regulator of cytokinesis 1	3.78	0.36
Aspm	asp (abnormal spindle)-like, microcephaly associated	3.75	0.37
Nusap1	nucleolar and spindle associated protein 1	3.25	0.40
Hells	helicase, lymphoid specific	2.64	0.40
Ccdc99	coiled-coil domain-containing 99	2.25	0.40
Brca1	breast cancer 1	2.53	0.42
Spag5	sperm associated antigen 5	2.41	0.42
Ccnb1	cyclin B1	2.73	0.43
Tpx2	TPX2, microtubule-associated protein	2.82	0.43
C79407	expressed sequence C79407	2.82	0.44
Ska1	RIKEN cDNA 2810433K01 gene	2.44	0.44
Nuf2	NDC80 kinetochore complex component	3.11	0.45
Mad2l1	mitotic arrest deficient-like 1	2.48	0.45
Spc25	SPC25, NDC80 kinetochore complex component	4.45	0.45
Trip13	thyroid hormone receptor interactor 13	3.09	0.45
Plk2	polo-like kinase 2	3.23	0.46
Uhrf1	ubiquitin-like, containing PHD and RING finger domains, 1	2.27	0.46
Aurkb	aurora kinase B	4.03	0.46
Cdca3	cell division cycle associated 3	2.99	0.47
Cdt1	chromatin licensing and DNA replication factor 1	2.42	0.47
Dbf4	DBF4	3.14	0.47
Ndc80	NDC80 homolog, kinetochore complex component	2.35	0.48
Ckap2	cytoskeleton associated protein 2	2.01	0.49
Pttg1	pituitary tumor-transforming gene 1	3.94	0.49

(Continued)

TABLE 34.4 Continued

Gene Symbol	Gene Name	Fold Change	
		TSOD − β-CRX vs. TSNO − β-CRX	TSOD + β-CRX vs. TSOD − β-CRX
GO:0006935 Chemotaxis			
Cxcl10	chemokine (C-X-C motif) ligand 10	12.58	0.31
Ccl12	chemokine (C-C motif) ligand 12	2.46	0.33
Ccl7	chemokine (C-C motif) ligand 7	30.74	0.33
Ccl2	chemokine (C-C motif) ligand	22.65	0.33
S100a8	S100 calcium binding protein A8	2.15	0.36
Ccl3	chemokine (C-C motif) ligand 3	4.56	0.46
C5ar1	complement component 5a receptor 1	4.77	0.46
Cxcl2	chemokine (C-X-C motif) ligand 2	2.76	0.46
Ccl4	chemokine (C-C motif) ligand 4	3.02	0.47
C3ar1	complement component 3a receptor 1	2.85	0.49
GO:0002520 Immune system development			
Timp1	tissue inhibitor of metalloproteinase 1	5.98	0.24
Ccnb2	cyclin B2	4.15	0.29
Stap1	signal transducing adaptor family member 1	8.90	0.32
Il7r	interleukin-7 receptor	4.96	0.40
Hells	helicase, lymphoid specific	2.64	0.40
Tnfrsf11a	tumor necrosis factor receptor superfamily, member 11a	2.63	0.45
Runx1	runt related transcription factor 1	3.29	0.46
Bcl3	B-cell leukemia/lymphoma 3	3.40	0.47
Vav1	vav 1 oncogene	3.03	0.48
Tiparp	TCDD-inducible poly(ADP-ribose) polymerase	0.29	2.08
Zbtb16	zinc finger and BTB domain containing 16	0.36	2.41
Pik3r1	phosphatidylinositol 3-kinase, regulatory subunit, polypeptide 1	0.31	2.90

β-CRX, beta-cryptoxanthin; TSNO, Tsumura Suzuki Nonobese Diabetes; TSOD, Tsumura Suzuki Obese Diabetes.

The expression of important adipokines, adiponectin (encoded by *Adipoq*), C-C motif chemokine 2 [monocyte chemoattractant protein 1 (MCP-1), encoded by *Ccl2*] and tumor necrosis factor (TNF-α; encoded by *Tnf*), were precisely measured by quantitative reverse transcription polymerase chain reaction (RT-PCR) analysis. The sequence of the primers used for the experiment is shown in Table 34.5 [42–44] and the results are shown in Table 34.6. *Adipoq* mRNA expression was significantly upregulated by β-CRX in the TSOD group, whereas *Ccl2* was significantly downregulated. *Tnf* expression was also downregulated, but not significantly.

The expression in skeletal muscle cells of genes involved in (cardiac) muscle contraction, fatty acid biosynthesis, lipid transport, and the wound response were modulated by β-CRX (Table 34.2). Genes involved in muscle contraction (*Myh7*, *My2*, *Tpm3*, and *Tnnc1*) were upregulated by β-CRX. Furthermore, their mRNA levels were increased in the TSOD-C group relative to those in the TSNO-C group (Table 34.7). The expression levels of genes encoding elongation of very long chain fatty acids protein 6 (*Elovl6*), acyl-CoA desaturase (*Scd1*), and fatty acid synthase (*Fasn*), which are involved in fatty acid synthesis, were downregulated by β-CRX. In contrast, their mRNA levels were decreased in the TSOD-C group

TABLE 34.5 Primer Sequences used for Adipocyte Analysis

Gene	Sense	Antisense	Reference
Adipoq	5′-AGAGAAGGGAGAGAAAGGAGATGC-3′	5′-TGAGCGATACACATAAGCGGC-3′	[42]
Ccl2	5′-TTAAAAACCTGGATCGGAACCAA -3′	5′-GCATTAGCTTCAGATTTACGGGT-3′	[43]
Tnf	5′- TCCCCAAAGGGATGAGAAGTTC -3′	5′-TCATACCAGGGTTTGAGCTCAG-3′	[44]

TABLE 34.6 Messenger RNA Expression in Adipocytes

Gene	TSNO			TSOD			
	−β-CRX	+β-CRX	*P* value	−β-CRX	+β-CRX	*P* value	
Adipoq	1.00 ± 0.01	1.52 ± 0.65	0.358	0.59 ± 0.07	1.13 ± 0.21	0.022	*
Ccl2	1.00 ± 0.31	1.00 ± 0.06	0.998	60.56 ± 6.10	16.67 ± 9.33	0.031	*
Tnf	1.00 ± 0.24	1.47 ± 0.14	0.141	5.05 ± 0.07	2.92 ± 0.71	0.051	–

**P value <0.05 for the difference between −CRX and +CRX.*
β-CRX, beta-cryptoxanthin; TSNO, Tsumura Suzuki Nonobese Diabetes; TSOD, Tsumura Suzuki Obese Diabetes.

TABLE 34.7 Genes Regulated in the Muscle by Oral Ingestion of Beta-Cryptoxanthin in TSOD Mice

Gene Symbol	Gene Name	Fold Change	
		TSOD-C vs. TSNO-C	TSOD-E vs. TSOD-C
GO:0060048 Cardiac muscle contraction			
Myh7	myosin, heavy polypeptide 7, cardiac muscle, beta	4.67	5.03
My12	myosin, light polypeptide 2, regulatory, cardiac, slow	5.35	8.87
Tpm3	tropomyosin 3, gamma	2.87	7.15
Tnnc1	troponin C, cardiac/slow skeletal	2.59	8.76
GO:0006633 Fatty acid biosynthetic process			
Elov16	ELOVL family member 6	0.08	0.29
Scd1	stearoyl-Coenzyme A desaturase 1	0.09	0.33
Fasn	fatty acid synthase	0.05	0.48
My05a	myosin VA	0.50	2.32
GO:0006869 Lipid transport			
Apoa1	apolipoprotein A-I	2.74	0.27
Apoa2	apolipoprotein A-II	2.34	0.36
Apoc3	apolipoprotein C-III	2.31	0.38
Apoc1	apolipoprotein C-I	0.28	0.44
Rbp4	retinol-binding protein 4, plasma	0.20	0.48
GO:0042060 Wound healing			
Fga	fibrinogen alpha chain	4.35	0.22
Kng1	kininogen 1	2.57	0.35
Serpinc1	serine peptidase inhibitor, clade C, member 1	2.42	0.48

compared to the TSNO-C group. Further, genes encoding apolipoprotein A (ApoA; *Apoa1* and *Apoa2*) and ApoC (*Apoc1* and *Apoc3*) were downregulated by β-CRX in TSOD mice. The wound healing-related genes (*Fga*, *Kng*, and *Serpinc1*) were similarly downregulated by β-CRX in TSOD mice. However, their mRNA levels were increased in the TSOD-C group relative to those in the TSNO-C group.

Obesity is closely associated with chronic diseases such as diabetes, cardiovascular disease, hyperlipidemia, and hypertension, which are well-known comorbidities of metabolic syndromes.

TSOD was recently established as an animal model of obese T2DM mellitus by the selective breeding of ddY mice. The adiposity and significantly high BMI in TSOD mice can be detected as early as 4 weeks of age and are maintained until at least 18 months of age [45,46].

As cohort studies have indicated a negative relationship between serum β-CRX levels and BMI, we thought that oral administration of β-CRX might affect body weight and BMI. To identify the mechanism by which β-CRX exerts its antiobesity effects, we initially focused on visceral adipose tissue. Adipose tissue has two roles: energy storage and endocrine function, with both of these roles being closely related to each other. When mature adipocytes accumulate adequate amounts of TG, they secrete several beneficial adipokines, including adiponectin and leptin. Obesity leads to the hyperaccumulation of TG in adipocytes, with hypertrophic adipocytes subsequently secreting inflammatory messengers such as interleukin-1β (IL-1β), IL-10 and TNF-α, instead of beneficial ones [47]. This evokes a strong immune response, which is exacerbated by the resultant inflammation of adipocytes. Finally, these events can result in insulin resistance, the development of diabetes, or worsened obesity.

In this section, we have demonstrated that oral administration of β-CRX represses body weight and adipocyte hypertrophy in a mouse model of obesity. These changes may prevent the decline of beneficial adipokines and the escalation of inflammatory messengers. Microarray and RT-PCR analyses indicate that these changes are caused by modulating the expression of a number of genes.

Adipocyte differentiation is known to be regulated by peroxisome proliferator-activated receptor gamma (PPAR-γ). PPAR is a nuclear receptor originally identified in *Xenopus* spp. [48]. There are three PPAR subtypes, α, β, and γ, which are differentially expressed in different organs. Among the three PPARs, PPAR-γ is specifically expressed in preadipocytes, where it accelerates their maturation [49]. Further investigations revealed that PPAR-γ activation is the key step in preadipocyte maturation.

PPARs are also expressed in muscles, where they control several important genes. For example, *Apoa1*, *Apoa2*, *Apoc3*, and *Scd1* (listed in Table 34.7) are transcriptionally regulated by PPAR-γ [50]; these data indicate that β-CRX can modulate muscular lipid transport and its metabolism via the PPAR-γ signaling pathway, and implicates the PPAR pathway as a target of β-CRX in both muscle and adipose tissue.

PPAR-γ has recently been recognized as a major target for the treatment of metabolic syndrome or diabetes. For example, thiazolidinedione, a well-known synthetic PPAR-γ agonist, is widely used as a drug to treat diabetes [51]. PPAR-γ is also thought to be a regulator of inflammation because thiazolidinedione has also been reported to suppress the secretion of inflammatory cytokines and chemokines [52].

Taken together, these results suggest that β-CRX may act to modulate PPAR-γ signaling, resulting in the repression of adipocyte hypertrophy, adipocyte chronic inflammation, and visceral fat accumulation.

BETA-CRYPTOXANTHIN REDUCES THE VISCERAL FAT IN MILDLY OBESE HUMANS

A placebo-controlled, double-blind test was designed to evaluate the effect of β-CRX on mildly obese humans. Subjects were pre-informed adult men aged 45.6 ± 9.7 years, with a BMI of 27.9 ± 1.5 kg/m^2 and a waist circumference of 93.3 ± 7.0 cm.

Subjects were divided into a test group and a placebo group and received either a test drink containing 0.25 mg β-CRX in a bottle (100 mL) or a placebo drink without β-CRX for 12 weeks. Both groups consumed two bottles of the test drink or placebo drink daily, mostly after breakfast and supper. Biochemical serum indexes [serum β-CRX, TG, blood glucose, and hemoglobin A1c (HbA1c)] and physical indexes (body weight and waist circumference) were evaluated every 4 weeks. Visceral adipose areas were calculated from computed tomography (CT) cross-sectional images at the beginning and end of the trial.

To secure the validity of the trial, subjects were prohibited from ingesting foods containing β-CRX, such as satsuma mandarins, persimmons, and papaya.

As Fig. 34.8 shows, the serum β-CRX level at the beginning of the trial was not statistically different between the test group and the placebo group. Serum β-CRX levels in the placebo group did not change over the trial period, or rather tended to decrease because of seasonal variation. In contrast, serum β-CRX levels in the test group were significantly higher than those in the placebo group at 4, 8, and 12 weeks owing to the consumption of the test drink. This indicates that β-CRX in the test drink was efficiently transferred to the serum and possibly to body tissues.

Continuous β-CRX consumption induced several physical changes in subjects of the test group, especially in visceral fat accumulation. Visceral fat areas were estimated from the CT cross-sectional images scanned around the L4-L5 intervertebral disks before and after the trial.

The initial visceral fat area on the test group was $130.54 \pm 54.58\,cm^2$ at the beginning and significantly decreased to $117.38 \pm 55.14\,cm^2$ ($P < 0.001$), while the fat area in the placebo group at the beginning of the study period was $109.39 \pm 33.14\,cm^2$ and was $114.50 \pm 37.04\,cm^2$ at the end. Changes in the visceral fat area during the test period are shown in Fig. 34.9. The visceral fat area in the test group decreased by $13.16 \pm 9.31\,cm^2$ over 12 weeks, while that of the placebo group significantly increased to $5.11 \pm 16.18\,cm^2$ ($P < 0.01$).

Typical CT images of the visceral fat area are shown in Fig. 34.10. In this case, the visceral adipose area was $122.9\,cm^2$ at the beginning of the trial and reduced to $89.3\,cm^2$ 12 weeks later. According to the diagnostic criterion for the metabolic syndrome, the upper limit of the visceral fat area was $100\,cm^2$. Oral administration of β-CRX reduced the visceral fat area by 27%; this reached normal levels in >12 weeks.

In accordance with the visceral fat area reduction, the subcutaneous and total fat areas also significantly decreased in the test group compared to the placebo group. Body weight and waist circumference were also significantly decreased in the test group compared to the placebo group at 12 weeks (Figs. 34.11 and 34.12). These results indicate that oral administration of β-CRX derived from satsuma mandarin reduces visceral adipose tissue and improves several physical indexes.

Some serum indexes such as serum TG and HbA1c were also improved by administration of the test drinks.

The average serum TG in the test group was 184.5 ± 72.1 mg/dL at the beginning of the trial. It gradually decreased during the trial and reached 140.8 ± 1.5 mg/dL 12 weeks later, a significant decrease compared to the initial value. In contrast, serum TG levels in the placebo group were not significantly decreased (Fig. 34.13). HbA1c increased to $0.11 \pm 0.13\%$ in the placebo group, but significantly decreased to $0.08 \pm 0.27\%$ in the test group over 12 weeks.

Other serum indexes such as liver and kidney function did not show any abnormalities, suggesting that adverse events did not occur because of the β-CRX. Self-reporting of health status and doctor interviews also indicated no harmful adverse event had occurred.

Although the nutritional importance of β-CRX has been suggested from cohort studies [11–20], a full scientific evaluation of its nutritional role is lacking. We showed that oral administration of β-CRX can reduce body weight and visceral fat accumulation on TSOD mice. The next question is whether these functions can be reproduced in humans.

We showed that the continuous oral administration of satsuma mandarin-derived β-CRX can reduce visceral fat and improve several indexes related to metabolic syndrome. This indicates that β-CRX may prevent the development of metabolic syndrome.

The dose of β-CRX used in this trial was 0.5 mg/day, which was calculated from the concentration of liquid-type β-CRX; it was effectively transferred to the serum and delivered to target tissues, e.g. adipocyte and muscle, in the study participants. However, the question of how β-CRX reduces visceral fat and improves the symptoms of metabolic syndrome remains. DNA microarray and quantitative RT-PCR analyses showed several key findings regarding this mechanism. In the next section, we investigate this mechanism using 3T3 preadipocytes.

THE MECHANISM OF BETA-CRYPTOXANTHIN-DEPENDENT OBESITY PREVENTION

To assess the ability of β-CRX to modulate adipose tissue area, 3T3-L1 cells were cultured in the presence of β-CRX. Briefly, mouse 3T3-L1 preadipocytes were cultured in Dulbecco's modified Eagle medium containing 10% fetal bovine serum, 50 μg/mL penicillin, 50 μg/mL streptomycin, and 125 ng/mL amphotericin at 37°C under 95% humidified air/5% CO_2. Once cells had reached confluency, they were incubated for an additional 48 h, followed by incubation in differentiation medium I (containing 10 μg/mL insulin, 0.5 mM isobutyl-methylxanthine, and 1 μM dexamethasone) for 48 h. The medium was then replaced with differentiation medium II (containing 10 μg/mL insulin) and exchanged every 48 h. Satsuma mandarin-derived purified β-CRX (Shikoku Yashima Pure Chemicals, Tokushima, Japan) was included in differentiation media I and II, and intracellular lipid accumulation was assessed by Oil Red O staining.

As shown in Fig. 34.14, 3T3-L1 cells accumulated intracellular lipid and become hypertrophic (see also Fig. 34.15). Intracellular lipid accumulation was reduced by β-CRX supplementation in the medium, in a dose-dependent manner. Treatment with 1 μM β-CRX resulted in a 25% reduction in intracellular lipids compared to untreated cells, while a reduction of 40% was observed at 10 μM β-CRX, without any cytotoxic effect (data not shown). These results indicate that β-CRX potently inhibits intracellular lipid accumulation in 3T3-L1 cells.

Matsumoto et al. have demonstrated the ability of β-CRX to act as a retinoic acid receptor (RAR) ligand [50]. RAR is a nuclear receptor, which has three isoforms: RARα, RARβ, and RARγ. Of these, RARα and RARγ are reported to be predominantly expressed in preadipocytes [53].

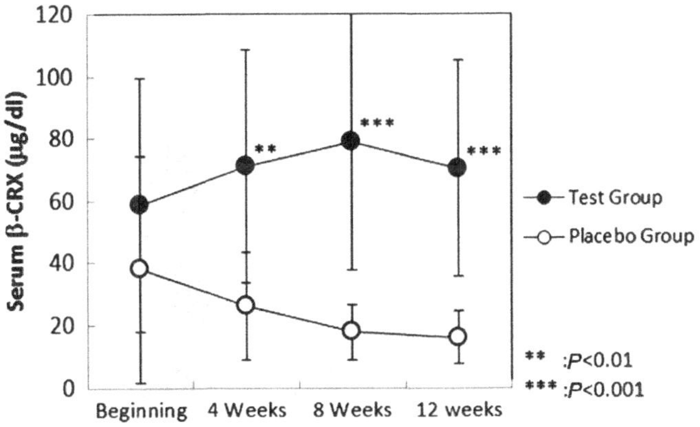

FIGURE 34.8 Serum beta-cryptoxanthin levels during the trial period. Asterisks indicate statistical differences compared to baseline. β-CRX, beta-cryptoxanthin.

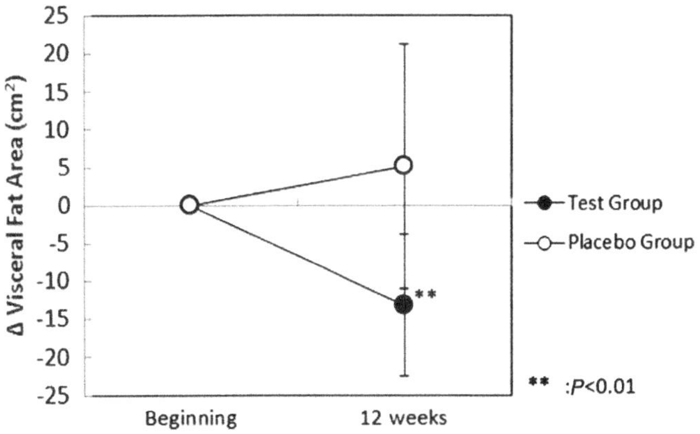

FIGURE 34.9 Variations in visceral fat area during the trial period. Asterisks denote statistical differences between the test group and the placebo group at 12 weeks. Δ, change in.

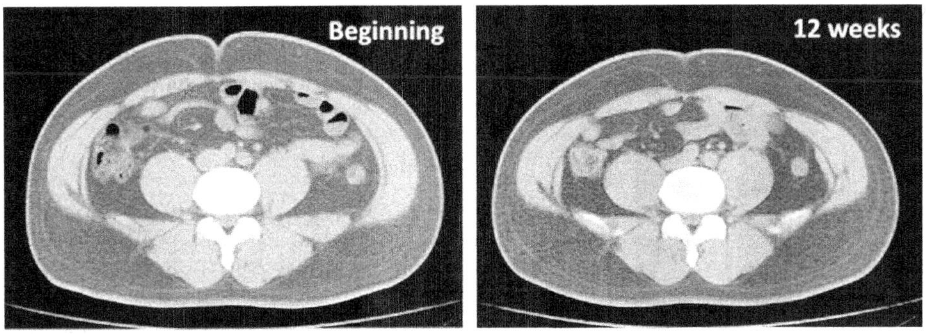

FIGURE 34.10 Typical computed tomography cross-sectional image of a test-group subject. Front of the abdomen facing the top. White, light gray and dark gray areas indicate the spine, internal organs and muscles, and adipose tissue, respectively.

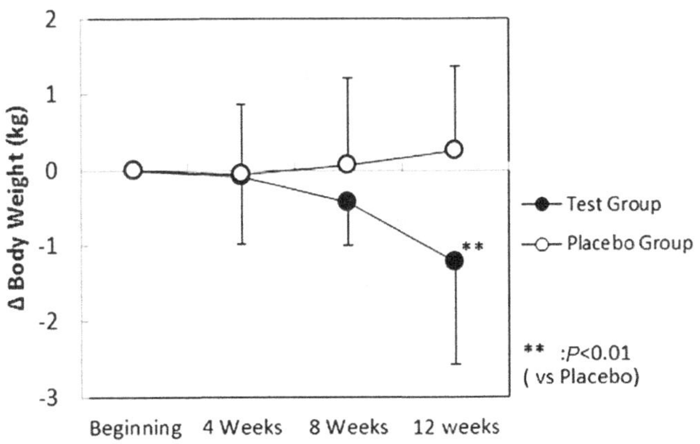

FIGURE 34.11 Variations in body weight during the trial period. Asterisks indicate the statistical differences between the groups at the same time point. Δ, change in.

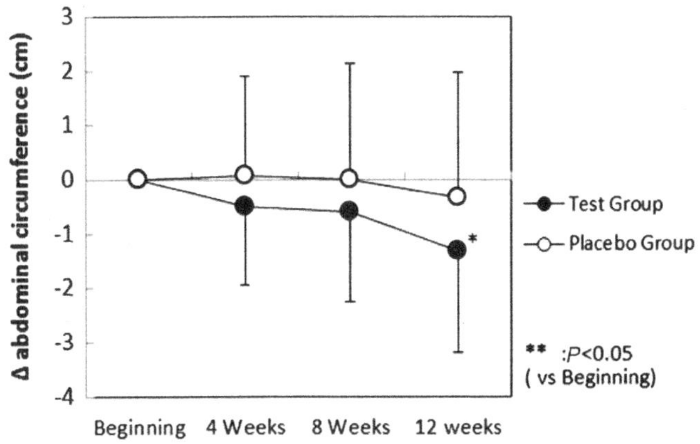

FIGURE 34.12 Variation in waist (abdominal) circumference during the trial period. Asterisks indicate the statistical differences compared to the initial level. Δ, change in.

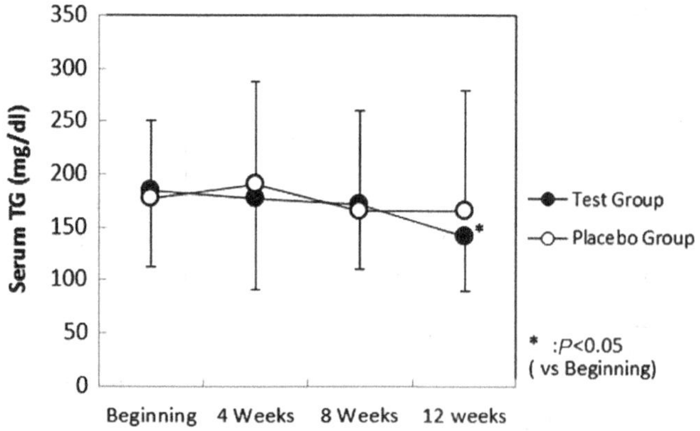

FIGURE 34.13 Variation in serum triglycerides during the trial period. Asterisks indicate the statistical differences compared to the initial level.

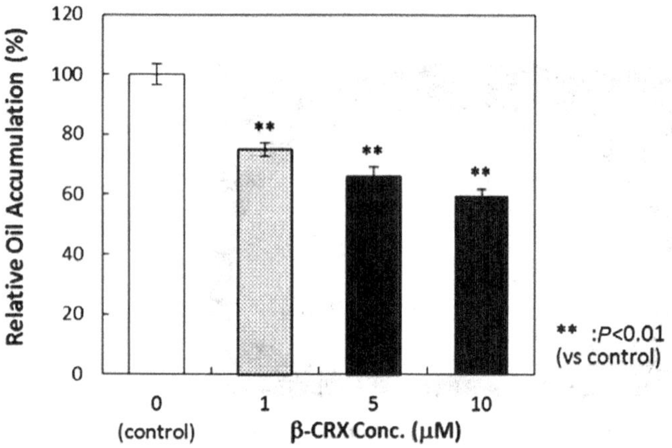

FIGURE 34.14 Inhibition of lipid accumulation in the presence of beta-cryptoxanthin in 3T3-L1 preadipocytes. β-CRX, beta-cryptoxanthin.

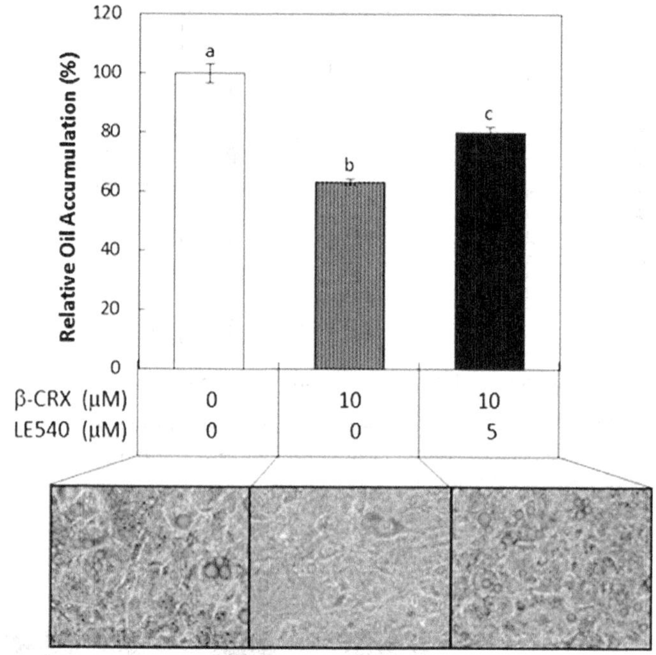

FIGURE 34.15 The effect of LE540 on inhibition of lipid accumulation by beta-cryptoxanthin. Different letters (a, b, and c) indicate statistically significant differences ($P<0.05$) in Oil Red O staining. β-CRX, beta-cryptoxanthin. (See color plate at the back of the book)

All-*trans* retinoic acid (ATRA) suppresses adipocyte differentiation together with RARs.

Several other nuclear receptors are also reported to be related to adipocyte differentiation [54], especially PPAR-γ and retinoic acid receptor RXR-alpha (RXRα). As mentioned in the previous section, PPAR-γ is the master regulator of adipocyte differentiation, which controls adipocyte-specific gene expression [55]. RXRα/PPAR-γ heterodimer formation is required for early-stage differentiation of adipocytes [56]. These reports indicate that nuclear receptors are strongly involved in adipocyte differentiation and subsequent lipid accumulation.

To identify the functional contribution of these nuclear receptors to adipocyte differentiation via the ligand activity of β-CRX, we performed an in vitro nuclear receptor-binding assay. Nuclear receptor-binding assays were performed using an RCAS kit (Enbiotech Laboratories, Tokyo, Japan) to assess PPAR-γ and RXRα ligand activity. Nu ligand kits (Mycrosystems, Kyoto, Japan) were used to assess RARα and RARγ ligand activity. All results were normalized to positive controls: troglitazone for PPAR-γ, tributyltin chloride for RXRα, and ATRA for RARs.

As shown in Fig. 34.16A and B, no binding of β-CRX to PPAR-γ and RXRα was observed. Together with other results indicating that β-CRX does not affect PPAR-γ activation by troglitazone (data not shown), we concluded that β-CRX does not act as an antagonist to PPAR-γ. In contrast, Fig. 34.16C and D demonstrate that β-CRX can efficiently bind to RARα and RARγ, indicating that β-CRX can act as a ligand for RARα and RARγ.

Fig. 34.17 shows the chemical structure of LE540. LE540, 4-(13H-10,11,12,13-tetrahydro-10,10,13,13,15-pentamethyldinaphtho[2,3-b][1,2-e]diazepin-7-yl) benzoic acid, is a diazepinylbenzoic acid derivative that can act as a pan-agonist for RAR [57]. To investigate the involvement of β-CRX in 3T3-L1 differentiation via RARα and RARγ activation, 3T3-L1 preadipocytes were differentiated in the presence of β-CRX and LE540. 3T3-L1 cells were cultured and differentiated to adipocytes in normal (no supplement), β-CRX-supplemented, and β-CRX- and LE540-supplemented differentiation media. The resulting lipid accumulation in each adipocyte was assayed by Oil Red O staining. As shown in Fig. 34.15, β-CRX inhibited lipid accumulation at a concentration of 10 μM; inhibition

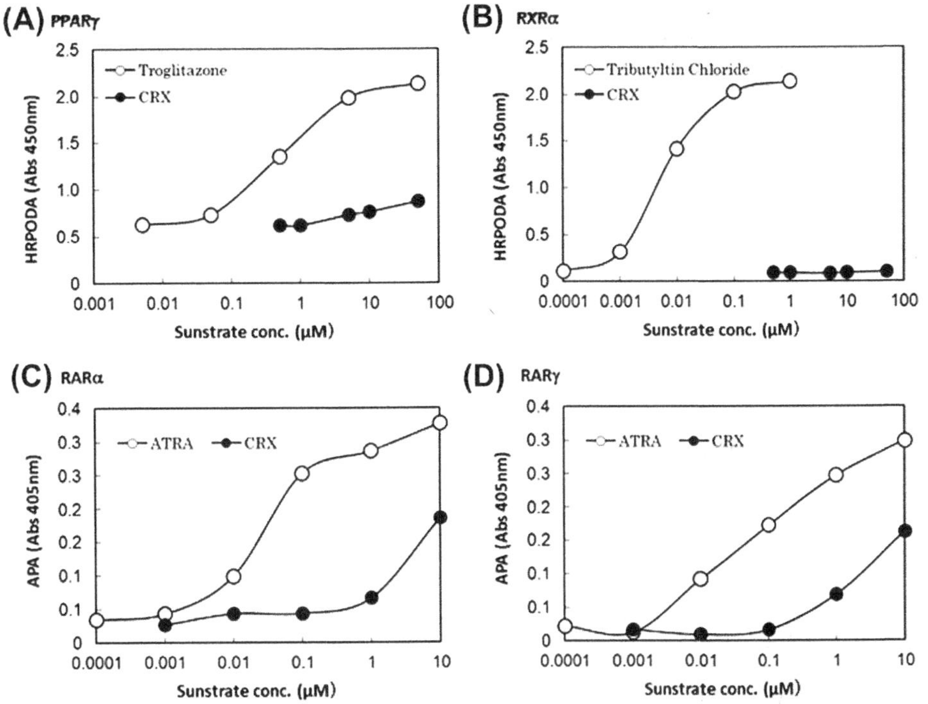

FIGURE 34.16 **In vitro nuclear receptor-binding assays.** Nuclear-binding activities were determined as horseradish peroxidase activity (HRPOSA; A and B) or alkaline phosphatase activity (APA; C) and D). Closed circles indicate beta-cryptoxanthin (CRX), while open circles indicate positive controls. ATRA, all-*trans* retinoic acid.

was blocked in the presence of 5μM LE540. Because no cytotoxic effect of the β-CRX and LE540 treatments was observed, these results indicate that β-CRX inhibits 3T3-L1 adipogenesis via RARα and RARγ activation.

To gain further insight into the role of β-CRX inhibition in 3T3-L1 cell lipid accumulation, real-time RT-PCR analysis was performed (Table 34.8 provides a list of target gene and the primer sequences used) [58–62]. Total RNA was isolated with Isogen (Nippon Gene, Tokyo, Japan) from 3T3-L1 differentiated cell lysates at 48 and 192h after initiation according to the manufacturer's protocol. For RT-PCR analysis, cDNA was synthesized from total RNA using a PrimeScript RT reagent kit (TaKaRa Bio, Shiga, Japan). Real-time quantitative RT-PCR analysis was performed using Sybr Premix Ex Taq (TaKaRa Bio, Shiga, Japan) and automated sequence detection systems (StepOne; Applied Biosystems Japan Ltd, Tokyo, Japan). Cycling conditions were 40 cycles of 95°C for 15s followed by 60°C for 1min.

As shown in Fig. 34.18, β-CRX decreased *Pparg* mRNA levels (encoding PPAR-γ) but not *Cebpb* [encoding CCAAT/enhancer-binding protein beta (C/EBPβ)] at concentrations of 1 and 10μM. This inhibition was reversed in the presence of 5μM LE540. Together with the in vitro-binding assays, these data demonstrate that β-CRX activates cellular retinoic acid-binding protein 2 (CRABP-II) and RARγ2 in response to RAR activation [61,62]. From these results, we conclude that β-CRX affects 3T3-L1 differentiation via downregulating PPAR-γ expression through RAR activation.

Results from our human and animal trials suggest that β-CRX has a practical antiobesity effect through targeting adipocytes. 3T3-L1 preadipocyte and in vitro nuclear receptor-binding assays were performed in order to identify the mechanism.

Several nuclear receptors have been reported to have an effect on adipocyte differentiation [54]; among them, PPAR-γ, RXRα, RARα, and RARγ are important for adipocyte differentiation and proliferation (as previously discussed). We found that β-CRX suppresses 3T3-L1 adipogenesis in a dose-dependent manner (Fig. 34.14). At first, we suspected that this was due to PPAR-γ antagonist

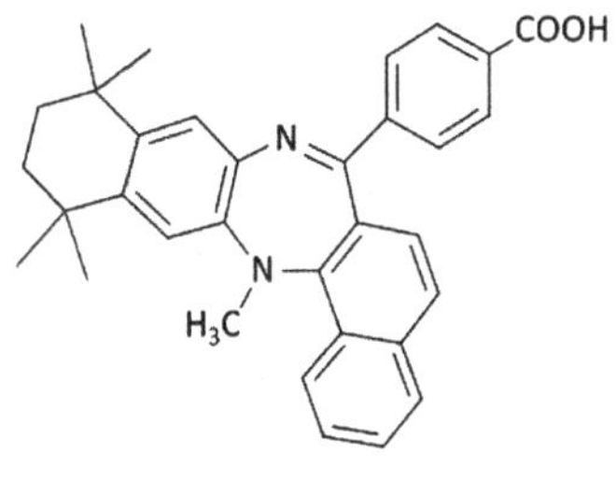

FIGURE 34.17 Chemical structure of LE540.

TABLE 34.8 RT-PCR Target Genes and Primer Sequences

Gene	Sense	Antisense	Reference
Pparg	5′-GATGCACTGCCTATGAGCACTT-3′	5′-AGAGGTCCACAGAGCTGATTCC-3′	[58]
Cebpb	5′-GCAAGAGCCGCGACAAG-3′	5′-GGCTCGGGCAGCTGCTT-3′	[59]
Fabp4	5′-CAGAAGTGGGATGGAAAGTCG-3′	5′-CGACTGACTATTGTAGTGTTTGA-3′	[60]
Rarg	5′-TGGTGTTCTAGCACCCAGTT-3′	5′-AAACGATTCCATGCAGTCGT-3′	[61]
Crabp2	5′-CCTGGAGCCGAGAACTGACCAA-3′	5′-TGGGAGGGAGGTTTGTGTCCTGTA-3	[62]

RT-PCR, reverse transcription polymerase chain reaction.

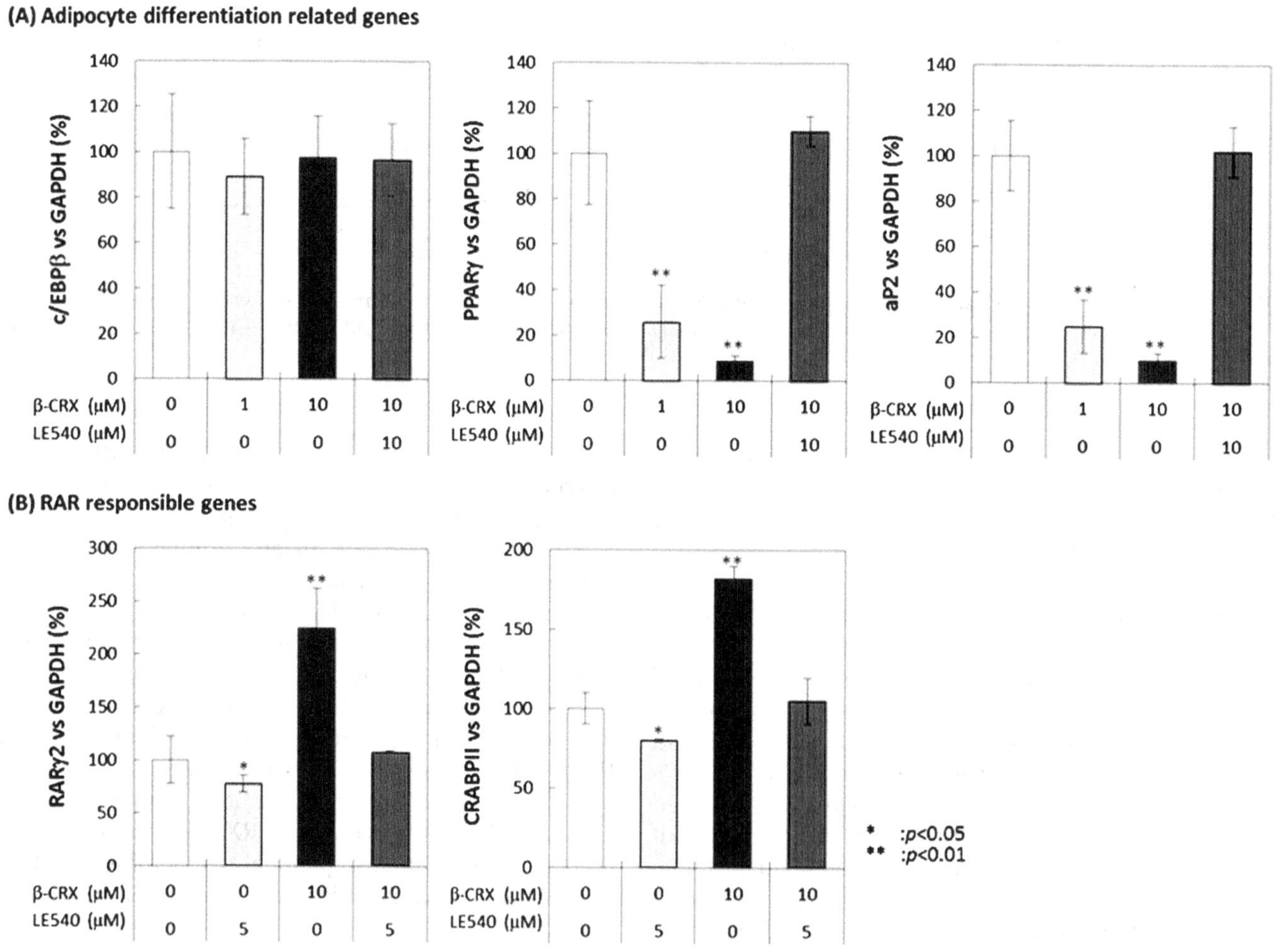

FIGURE 34.18 Gene expression analysis following beta-cryptoxanthin and LE540 treatment. (A) and (B) represent gene expression in the presence or absence of beta-cryptoxanthin (β-CRX) and/or LE540. Each value was normalized to GAPDH expression.

activity because PPAR-γ upregulates adipocyte differentiation and lipid accumulation. However, we found β-CRX to have no binding affinity for PPAR-γ in an in vitro-binding assay, indicating that β-CRX does not act as either an agonist or an antagonist. Instead, we revealed that β-CRX can act as a ligand for RARα and RARγ. Moreover, we showed that this effect could be blocked by LE540, an RAR antagonist. Real-time RT-PCR analysis showed that β-CRX downregulates *Pparg* mRNA expression, which regulates differentiation via C/EBPβ. These results strongly indicate that β-CRX inhibits 3T3-L1 adipogenesis via downregulating of PPAR-γ transcription through RAR activation.

Like β-CRX, ATRA (an in vivo RAR ligand) affects cellular differentiation. ATRA has been widely used as a medicine for specific types of blood cancer; however, serious side effects following its application have been reported [63].

As shown in Figs 34.16 and 34.18, the RAR ligand activity of β-CRX appeared too low to reach the potency of ATRA. However, serum concentrations of β-CRX are higher than those of ATRA: it reached 1–2 μM after the oral intake of a drink containing β-CRX for 8 weeks [22], which was enough to activate RARs. β-CRX was also more stable in serum and showed longer RAR ligand activity than ATRA without any side effects. These results highlight the attractive possibility that β-CRX can substitute for ATRA therapy. This should be reviewed in the near future.

A working model linking RAR activation and adipocyte differentiation has previously been reported. Studies have indicated that RAR binds to CCAAT (a c/EBP-binding element) in specific gene promoters, where it prevents transcription [64]. Other reports have demonstrated that Smad3 (which binds to c/EBPβ and inhibits its transcriptional activation) is upregulated by ATRA [65], while ATRA downregulation of PPAR-γ has been previously reported [53]. Taken together, these studies indicate that RAR, when activated by β-CRX, either binds to the C/EBP response element in the PPAR-γ promoter or inhibits PPAR-γ transcription by an indirect mechanism.

Some reports indicate that some food compounds, e.g. neoxanthin [66], catechin, genistein, and capsaicin [67], can suppress 3T3-L1 differentiation in a different way. For example, neoxanthin downregulates *Pparg* transcription, while catechin, genistein and capsaicin activate AMP-activated protein kinase to suppress 3T3-L1 differentiation. Each compound has different modes of action and differs from that of β-CRX, thus demonstrating the complexity of adipocyte differentiation. These data also suggest that the combined intake of foods containing these compounds may have a synergistic effect.

CONCLUSION

β-CRX is a carotenoid found in the blood of humans. Although it was discovered nearly a century ago, its effects on human health have not yet been fully explored. The reason for this may be the low serum levels of β-CRX, together with the low oral intake in Western countries. It is surprising that several cohort studies suggest a correlation between β-CRX serum levels and the risk of developing diseases such as lung cancer. This finding suggests that there is a strong potential for β-CRX to promote health in humans.

Satsuma mandarin is a unique citrus species found in Japan: approximately 1,000,000 tons of this fruit are produced annually. Since it is particularly rich in β-CRX, satsuma mandarin may be the best β-CRX source in the world.

β-CRX is the only carotenoid among the six carotenoids found in human blood that has not been commercialized. Sugiura et al. showed that satsuma mandarin consumption reflects serum β-CRX levels [4,5]. They also reported that high serum β-CRX levels reduce the risk of diabetic hepatic dysfunction, arteriosclerosis, and postmenopausal osteoporosis, in addition to HOMA-IR improvement.

We have shown that oral intake of satsuma mandarin-derived β-CRX can reduce visceral fat, body weight, and waist circumference in mildly obese men. We also found that these effects are due to the downregulation of PPAR-γ expression via RAR agonist activity, resulting in the repression of adipocyte hypertrophy and lipid accumulation. An important point is that these benefits are obtained without any undesirable side effects or damage to health.

Japanese people have consumed satsuma mandarins for over four centuries and they know empirically that the satsuma mandarin is good for their health. We have now scientifically demonstrated one of its beneficial effects by showing that β-CRX prevents obesity and promotes visceral fat reduction. Other benefits are also under investigation; once we verify these results, we may be able to convince populations worldwide of the benefits of β-CRX and of satsuma mandarin consumption.

References

[1] Smith TA. Carotenoids and cancer: prevention and potential therapy. Br J Biomed Sci 1998;55:268–75.

[2] Young AJ, Lowe GM. Antioxidant and prooxidant properties of carotenoids. Arch Biochem Biophys 2001;385:20–7.

[3] Mangels AR, Holden J, Beecher M, Beecher GR, Forman MR, Lanza E. Carotenoid content of fruits and vegetables: an evaluation of analytic data. J Am Diet Assoc 1993;93:284–96.

[4] Sugiura M, Kato M, Matsumoto H, Nagao A, Yano M. Serum concentration of β-cryptoxanthin in Japan reflects the frequency of Satsuma mandarin (Citrus unshiu Marc.) consumption. J Health Sci 2002;48:350–3.

[5] Sugiura M, Matsumoto H, Kato M, Ikoma Y, Yano M, Nagao A. Multiple linear regression analysis of the seasonal changes in the serum concentration of β-cryptoxanthin. J Nutr Sci Vitaminol 2004;50:196–202.

[6] Bramlev PV. Is lycopene beneficial to human health? Phytochemistry 2000;54:233–6.

[7] Cooney RV, Bertram JS, Hankin JH, Kolonel LN, Miyake A, Billings K, et al. Relationship between dietary, serum, and tissue levels of carotenoids. Cancer Lett 1991;61:81–7.

[8] Glise D, Riondel J, Favier A. Comparative distribution of b-carotene and lycopene after intraperitoneal administration in mice. In Vivo 1998;12:447–54.

[9] Kaplan LA, Lau JM, Stein EA. Carotenoid composition, concentration, and relationships in various human organs. Clin Physiol Biochem 1990;8:1–10.

[10] Nair PP, Lohani A, Norkus EP, Feagins H, Bhagavan HN. Uptake and distribution of carotenoids, retinal, and tocopherols in human colonic epithelial cells in vivo. Cancer Epidemiol Biomarkers Prev 1996;5:913–6.

[11] Sugiura M, Nakamura M, Ikoma Y, Yano M, Ogawa K, Matsumoto H, et al. High serum carotenoids are inversely associated with serum γ-glutamyltransferase in alcohol drinkers within normal liver function. J Epidemiol 2005;15:180–6.
[12] Sugiura M, Nakamura M, Ikoma Y, Yano M, Ogawa K, Matsumoto H, et al. Serum carotenoid concentrations are inversely associated with serum aminotransferases in hyperglycemic subjects. Diabetes Res Clin Pract 2006;71:82–91.
[13] Nishino H, Tokuda H, Murakoshi M, Satomi Y, Masuda M, Onozuka M, et al. Cancer prevention by natural carotenoids. Biofactors 2000;13:89–94.
[14] Rauscher R, Edenharfer R, Platt KL. In vitro antimutagenic and in vivo anticlasogenic effects of carotenoids and solvent extracts from fruits and vegetables rich in carotenoids. Mutat Res 1998;413:129–42.
[15] Tanaka T, Kohno H, Murakami M, Shimada R, Kagami S, Sumida T, et al. Suppression of azoxymethane-induced colon carcinogenesis in male F344 rats my mandarin juices rich in β-cryptoxanthin and hesperidin. Int J Cancer 2000;88:146–50.
[16] Uchiyama S, Yamaguchi M. Oral administration of β-cryptoxanthin prevents bone loss in ovariectomized rats. Int J Mol Med 2006;17:15–20.
[17] Sugiura M, Nakamura M, Ogawa K, Ikoma Y, Ando F, Yano M. Bone mineral density in post-menopausal female subjects is associated with serum antioxidant carotenoids. Osteoporos Int 2008;19:211–9.
[18] Sugiura M, Nakamura M, Ogawa K, Ikoma Y, Ando F, Shimokata H, et al. Dietary patterns of antioxidant vitamin and carotenoid intake associated with bone mineral density: findings from post-menopausal Japanese female subjects. Osteoporos Int 2011;22:143–52.
[19] Sugiura M, Nakamura M, Ikoma Y, Yano M, Ogawa K, Matsumoto H, et al. The homeostasis model assessment-insulin resistance index is inversely associated with serum carotenoids in non-diabetic subjects. J Epidemiol 2006;16:71–8.
[20] Sugiura M, Ogawa K, Yano M. Effect of chronic administration of fruit extract (Citrus unshiu Marc.) on glucose tolerance in GK rats, a model of type 2 diabetes. Biosci Biotechnol Biochem 2006;70:293–5.
[21] Sugiura M, Matsumoto H, Kato M, Ikoma Y, Yano M, Nagao A. Seasonal changes in the relationship between serum concentration of β-cryptoxanthin and serum lipid levels. J Nutr Sci Vitaminol (Tokyo) 2004;50:410–5.
[22] Tsuchida T, Minagawa K, Mukai K, Mizuno Y, Mashiko K, Minagawa K. The comparative study of β-cryptoxanthin derived from Satsuma mandarin for fat of human body. Jpn Pharmacol Ther 2008;36:247–53.
[23] Hirayama I, Yi Z, Izumi S, Arai I, Suzuki W, Nagamachi Y, et al. Genetic analysis of obese diabetes in the TSOD mouse. Diabetes 1999;48:1183–91.
[24] Suzuki W, Iizuka S, Tabuchi M, Funo S, Yanagisawa T, Kimura M, et al. A new mouse model of spontaneous diabetes derived from ddY strain. Exp Anim 1999;48:181–9.
[25] Wahlqvist ML, Wattanapenpaiboon N, Macrae FA, Lambert JR, MacLennan R, Hsu-Hage BH. Changes in serum carotenoids in subjects with colorectal adenomas after 24 mo of 6-carotene supplementation. Am J Clin Nutr 1994;60:936–43.
[26] Michaud DS, Giovannucci EL, Ascherio A, Rimm EB, Forman MR, Sampson L, et al. Associations of plasma carotenoid concentrations and dietary intake of specific carotenoids in samples of two prospective cohort studies using a new carotenoid database. Cancer Epidemiol Biomarker Prev 1998;7:283–90.
[27] Jenkins DJ, Popovich DG, Kendall CW, Vidgen E, Tariq N, Ransom TP, et al. Effect of a diet high in vegetables, fruit, and nuts on serum lipids. Metabolism 1997;46:530–7.
[28] Feldman EB. Fruits and vegetables and the risk of stroke. Nutr Rev 2001;59:24–7.
[29] Ford ES, Mokdad AH. Fruit and vegetable consumption and diabetes mellitus incidence among U.S. adults. Prev Med 2001;32:33–9.
[30] Terry P, Terry JB, Wolk A. Fruit and vegetable consumption in the prevention of cancer: an update. J Intern Med 2001;250:280–90.
[31] Campbell DR, Gross MD, Martini MC, Grandits GA, Stavin JL, Potter JD. Plasma carotenoids as biomarkers of vegetable and fruit intake. Cancer Epidemiol Biomarkers Prev 1994;3:493–500.
[32] Drewnowski A, Rock CL, Henderson SA, Shore AB, Fischler C, Galan P, et al. Serum b-carotene and vitamin C as biomarkers of vegetable and fruit intakes in a community-based sample of French adults. Am J Clin Nutr 1997;65:1796–802.
[33] Tucker KL, Chen H, Vogel S, Wilson PW, Schaefer EJ, Lammi-Keefe CJ. Carotenoid intakes, assessed by dietary questionnaire, are associated with plasma carotenoid concentrations in an elderly population. J Nutr 1999;129:438–45.
[34] van Kappel AL, Steghens JP, Zeleniuch-Jacquotte A, Chajes V, Toniolo P, Riboli E. Serum carotenoids as biomarkers of fruit and vegetable consumption in the New York Women's Health Study. Public Health Nutr 2001;4:829–35.
[35] Papas A, Stacewicz-Sapuntzakis M, Lagiou P, Bamia C, Chloptsios Y, Trichopoulou A. Plasma retinol and tocopherol levels in relation to demographic, lifestyle and nutritional factors of plant origin in Greece. Br J Nutr 2003;89:83–7.
[36] Nakamura M, Sugiura M, Aoki N. High beta-carotene and beta-cryptoxanthin are associated with low pulse wave velocity. Atherosclerosis 2006;184:363–9.
[37] Montonen J, Knekt P, Järvinen R, Reunanen A. Dietary antioxidant intake and risk of type 2 diabetes. Diabetes Care 2004;27:362–6.
[38] Suzuki K, Ito Y, Ochiai J, Kusuhara Y, Hashimoto S, Tokudome S, et al. Relationship between obesity and serum markers of oxidative stress and inflammation in Japanese. Asian Pac J Cancer Prev 2003;4:259–66.
[39] Takaishi N, Satsu H, Takayanagi K, Mukai K, shimizu M. In vivo and in vitro studies on the absorption characteristics of b-cryptoxanthin in the intestine. Biosci Biotechnol Biochem 2012;76:120511–120515.
[40] Huang DW, Sherman BT, Lempicki RA. Systematic and integrative analysis of large gene lists using DAVID bioinformatics resources. Nat Protoc 2009;4:44–57.
[41] Kanehisa M, Goto S, Furumichi M, Tanabe M, Hirakawa M. KEGG for representation and analysis of molecular networks involving diseases and drugs. Nucleic Acids Res 2010;38:D355–60.
[42] Hertzel AV, Smith LA, Berg AH, Cline GW, Shulman GI, Scherer PE, et al. Lipid metabolism and adipokine levels in fatty acid-binding protein null and transgenic mice. Am J Physiol Endocrinol Metab 2006;290:814–23.
[43] Choi BH, Kim YH, Ahn IS, Ha JH, Byun JM, Do MS. The inhibition of inflammatory molecule expression on 3. T3–L1 adipocytes by berberine is not mediated by leptin signaling. Nutr Res Pract 2009;3:84–8.
[44] Ajuwon KM, Spurlock ME. Adiponectin inhibits LPS-induced NF-κB activation and IL-6 production and increases PPARγ2 expression in adipocytes. Am J Physiol Regul Integr Comp Physiol 2005;288:1220–5.
[45] Iizuka S, Suzuki W, Tabuchi M, Nagata M, Imamura S, Kobayashi Y, et al. Diabetic complications in a new animal model (TSOD mouse) of spontaneous NIDDM with obesity. Exp Anim 2005;54:71–83.
[46] Kawada T, Miyata S, Shimada T, Sanzen Y, Ito M, Hemmi C, et al. A study of cardiovascular function in Tsumura Suzuki obese diabetes, a new model mouse of type 2 diabetes. Biol Pharm Bull 2010;33:998–1003.

[47] Rabe K, Lehrke M, Parhofer KG, Broedl UC. Adipokines and insulin resistance. Mol Med 2008;14:741–51.
[48] Mourier A, Gautier JF, De Kerviler E, Bigard AX, Villette JM, Garnier JP, et al. Mobilization of visceral adipose tissue related to the improvement in insulin sensitivity in response to physical training in NIDDM: effects of branched-chain amino acid supplements. Diabetes Care 1997;20:385–91.
[49] Issemann I, Green S. Activation of a member of the steroid hormone receptor superfamily by peroxisome proliferators. Nature 1990;347:645–50.
[50] Matsumoto A, Mizukami H, Mizuno S, Umegaki K, Nishikawa J, Shudo K, et al. β-Cryptoxanthin, a novel natural RAR ligand, induces ATP-binding cassette transporters in macrophages. Biochem Pharmacol 2007;74:256–64.
[51] Chawla A, Schwarz EJ, Dimaculangan DD, Lazar MA. Peroxisome proliferator-activated receptor (PPAR) γ: adipose-predominant expression and induction early in adipocyte differentiation. Endocrinology 1994;135:798–800.
[52] Yoon M. The role of PPARγ in lipid metabolism and obesity: focusing on the effect of estrogen on PPARα actions. Pharmacol Res 2009;60:151–9.
[53] Schwarz EJ, Reginato MJ, Shao D, Krakow SL, Lazar MA. Retinoic acid blocks adipogenesis by inhibiting C/EBPβ-mediated transcription. Mol Cell Biol 1997;17:1552–61.
[54] Fu M, Sun T, Bookout AL, Downes M, Yu RT, Evans RM. A nuclear receptor atlas: 3T3–L1 adipogenesis. Mol Endocrinol 2005;19:2437–50.
[55] Sandouk T, Reda D, Hofmann C. Antidiabetic agent pioglitazone enhances adipocyte differentiation of 3T3–F442A cells. Am J Physiol 1993;264:C1600–8.
[56] Noon LA, Clark AJ, King PJ. A peroxisome proliferator-response element in the murine mc2-r promoter regulates its transcriptional activation during differentiation of 3T3–L1 adipocytes. J Biol Chem 2004;279:22803–8.
[57] Saito A, Sugawara A, Uruno A, Kudo M, Kagechika H, Sato Y, et al. All-trans retinoic acid induces in vitro angiogenesis via retinoic acid receptor: possible involvement of paracrine effects of endogenous vascular endothelial growth factor signaling. Endocrinology 2007;148:1412–23.
[58] Saito T, Abe D, Sekiya K. Nobiletin enhances differentiation and lipolysis of 3T3–L1 adipocytes. Biochem Biophys Res Commun 2007;357:371–6.
[59] Karamanlidis G, Karamitri A, Docherty K, Hazlerigg DG, Lomax MA. C/EBPβ reprograms white 3T3–L1 preadipocytes to a Brown adipocyte pattern of gene expression. J Biol Chem 2007;282:24660–9.
[60] Hertzel AV, Smith LA, Berg AH, Cline GW, Shulman GI, Scherer PE, Bernlohr DA. Lipid metabolism and adipokine levels in fatty acid-binding protein null and transgenic mice. Am J Physiol Endocrinol Metab 2006;290:E814–23.
[61] Bour G, Plassat JL, Bauer A, Lalevée S, Rochette-Egly C. Vinexin beta interacts with the non-phosphorylated AF-1 domain of retinoid receptor γ (RAR γ) and represses RARγ-mediated transcription. J Biol Chem 2005;280:17027–37.
[62] Bry K, Lappalainen U. Pathogenesis of bronchopulmonary dysplasia: the role of interleukin 1β in the regulation of inflammation-mediated pulmonary retinoic acid pathways in transgenic mice. Semin Perinatol 2006;30:121–8.
[63] Yarali N, Tavil B, Kara A, Ozkasap S, Tunç B. Acute renal failure during ATRA treatment. Pediatr Hematol Oncol 2008;25:115–8.
[64] Kirfel J, Kelter M, Cancela LM, Price PA, Schüle R. Identification of a novel negative retinoic acid responsive element in the promoter of the human matrix Gla protein gene. Proc Natl Acad Sci USA 1997;94:2227–32.
[65] Marchildon F, St-Louis C, Akter R, Roodman V, Wiper-Bergeron NL. Transcription factor Smad3 is required for the inhibition of adipogenesis by retinoic acid. J Biol Chem 2010;285:13274–84.
[66] Okada T, Nakai M, Maeda H, Hosokawa M, Sashima T, Miyashita K. Suppressive effect of neoxanthin on the differentiation of 3T3–L1 adipose cells. J Oleo Sci 2008;56:345–51.
[67] Hwang JT, Park IJ, Shin JI, Lee YK, Lee SK, Baik HW, et al. Genistein, EGCG, and capsaicin inhibit adipocyte differentiation process via activating AMP-activated protein kinase. Biochem Biophys Res Commun 2005;338:694–9.

CHAPTER

35

A Diet with Carbohydrates Eaten Primarily at Dinner: an Innovative, Nutritional Approach to End the Vicious Cycle of Abdominal Obesity

Sigal Sofer[a], Aliza Stark[a], Gershon Fink[b], and Zecharia Madar[b]

aInstitute of Biochemistry, Food Science and Nutrition, The Robert H. Smith Faculty of Agriculture, Food and Environment, The Hebrew University of Jerusalem, Jerusalem, Israel, [b]Kaplan Medical Center, Rehovot, Israel

THE VICIOUS CYCLE OF ABDOMINAL OBESITY AND THE METABOLIC SYNDROME

Without a doubt, obesity is the epidemic of the millennium and a worldwide public health challenge. Abdominal obesity is particularly problematic and is associated with higher levels of hunger and low rates of satiety, which leads to continuous overeating and abdominal adipose tissue accumulation. This viscous cycle makes weight loss almost impossible and accelerates the development of insulin resistance, inducing the metabolic syndrome and inflammation, which increases the probability of developing diabetes mellitus and coronary heart disease. Weight reduction is the most widespread method of treatment [1,2], yet the majority of obese subjects trapped in "obesity's vicious cycle" fail to maintain long-term diets and regain body weight over and over again [3,4]. Weight loss diets with differing compositions of fat, protein, and carbohydrates have not demonstrated significant differences in levels of weight loss, percentage weight regain, waist circumference reductions, hunger-satiety scores (H-SSc), and dietary adherence. Changes in body composition, abdominal fat, or hepatic fat were also not significantly altered among diets with varying macronutrient compositions [5]. All of these diets led to modest improvements of risk factors for diabetes and cardiovascular diseases [6].

The manipulation of physiological pathways to reduce symptoms of severe abdominal obesity and the metabolic syndrome is, and should be, a major focus of nutritional research worldwide. Patients suffering from severe or morbid obesity and the nutritionist community are urgently looking for evidence-based alternatives and detailed guidelines.

FAT TISSUE AS AN ENDOCRINE ORGAN AND ITS INFLUENCE ON FOOD INTAKE AND THE METABOLIC SYNDROME

The fact that a large number of obese individuals fail to maintain long-term diets, regain body weight, develop metabolic complications, and in time become diabetic and/or cardiac patients can be explained, at least in part, by our increased understanding of the metabolic role of the adipose tissue.

Adipose tissue is no longer considered exclusively an energy storage site for the body. Today, it is referred to as an endocrine organ that synthesizes and secretes hormones. Some of these hormones regulate hunger/satiety and food intake and others impact the development of insulin resistance, the metabolic syndrome, and inflammation [7].

Leptin is often called *the satiety hormone*. In the long term, it provides the brain with information about the status of the adipose tissue and helps to stabilize body weight. It is secreted from adipose tissue and its level, which correlates with body fat mass, limits weight loss and prevents underweight or weight gain, thus

Nutrition in the Prevention and Treatment of Abdominal Obesity
http://dx.doi.org/10.1016/B978-0-12-407869-7.00035-0

preventing obesity. In the short term, it regulates hunger, satiety, and food intake [7–9]. Several studies have described typical diurnal patterns of serum leptin concentrations and indicate that levels fall during the day, from 0800 to 1600 hours, reaching a nadir at 1300 and increasing from 1600, with a zenith at 0100 [10,11] It is rather ironic that this crucial hormone, responsible for satiety, is at its highest levels when we are sleeping.

Ghrelin, known as the *hunger hormone*, is produced in the stomach, not in adipose tissue, and is involved in regulating food consumption [12]. Ghrelin's long-term functions are negatively associated with energy balance and, similar to leptin, it is important for maintaining a constant body weight. In the short term, ghrelin serum concentrations rise in the preprandial period, stimulating meal initiation [8,13,14]. Studies describing typical circadian patterns for serum ghrelin indicate that ghrelin levels are reciprocal to leptin. This pattern is also somewhat problematic, as high values are maintained throughout the day with a zenith after 1300 hours and low values at night, with a nadir at 0400 [11,12].

Adiponectin, which is secreted by adipose tissue, is considered to be "the link between obesity, insulin resistance and the metabolic syndrome" [15–17]. Adiponectin plays a role in energy regulation as well as in lipid and carbohydrate metabolism, by reducing serum glucose and lipids, inducing insulin sensitization, and acting as an anti-inflammatory agent [18]. Adiponectin's serum diurnal pattern has been described in the literature. In obese individuals including those with abdominal obesity, secretion levels are low, with little fluctuation throughout the day. In normal-weight subjects or following a weight-loss process, overall higher serum adiponectin concentrations are detected, as well as a rise in the diurnal pattern during the daytime, with zeniths at 1100 and 0100 hours and a decline at night, reaching a nadir at 0400 [11,19].

Leptin, Ghrelin, and Neural Control Mechanisms of Food Intake and Body Weight

Understanding the molecular and neural factors that control body weight homeostasis and food intake may help establish innovative nutritional approaches for morbidly obese patients. Several hypothalamic cell groups express leptin and/or ghrelin receptors and appear to be crucial sites of integration for leptin and ghrelin pathways. Two distinct leptin- and ghrelin-responsive cell groups exist within the arcuate nucleus (ARC). The first is identified by the coexpression of proopiomelanocortin (POMC) and cocaine- and amphetamine-regulated transcript protein (CART) and is an anorexigenic neuron population. The second distinct population of neurons is orexigenic and coexpresses neuropeptide Y (NPY) and agouti-related gene product (AgRP) [20]. It has been reported that in the fed state, serum leptin rises, crosses the blood–brain barrier (BBB), and activates POMC neurons causing secretion of POMC. POMC is fractured to smaller segments including alpha melanocyte-stimulating hormone (αMSH) that activates melanocortin receptors (MC4, MC3) in the lateral hypothalamus (LH). Activation of these receptors is known to delay melanin-concentrating hormone and orexin secretion, leading to lower wakefulness and decreased food-seeking behavior, thus reducing food consumption. Simultaneously, leptin inhibits NPY/AgRP neurons and prevents release of the potent orexigenic neuropeptides NPY and AgRP that would otherwise inhibit POMC by competition of AgRP with αMSH on the MC4 receptor. Ghrelin also crosses the BBB and causes activation of AgRP/NPY neurons through growth hormone secretagog receptor (GHSR). NPY attaches to receptor Y and stimulates MCH and orexin secretion from the LH [20].

Adiponectin, Insulin Resistance, and Metabolic and Inflammatory Status

Abdominal obesity can develop to morbid obesity within a short period of time. Severe abdominal obesity is accompanied by hyperinsulinemia that commonly leads to insulin resistance, metabolic syndrome, inflammation, and eventually to diabetes mellitus and coronary heart disease. A better understanding of the factors and metabolites responsible for the development of metabolic diseases and ways to prevent life-threatening outcomes are needed. It is known that adiponectin activates 5′-AMP-activated protein kinase (AMPK), which is an energy regulator in the body [21,22]. Activated (i.e. phosphorylated) AMPK increases glucose uptake in the liver and muscle and reduces levels of the gluconeogenetic enzymes phosphoenolpyruvate carboxykinase (PEPCK) and glucose-6-phosphatase (G6Pase) in the liver, leading to lower glucose output. In general, serum glucose levels decrease and insulin secretion is lowered. AMPK activation by adiponectin deactivates, by phosphorylation, acetyl-coenzyme A carboxylase (ACC) in muscle cells, promoting fatty acid oxidation and decreasing serum triglycerides, which also improves insulin sensitivity [21]. In addition, it is well established that adiponectin activates the peroxisome proliferator-activated receptor alpha (PPAR-α) transcription factor that causes changes in lipid profiles, and stimulates usage of fatty acids, thus decreasing triglyceride levels in muscle and liver tissue and again improving insulin sensitivity [21]. It is also recognized that obesity increases inflammation induced by macrophage infiltration of adipose tissue and secretion of proinflammatory cytokines such as C-reactive protein (CRP), interleukin-6 (IL-6), and tumor necrosis factor (TNF-α) [23,24]. PPAR-α can reduce macrophage infiltration of fat tissue, thus reducing inflammation and insulin resistance [23,25]. In addition, adiponectin has inhibitory effects on atherosclerotic cellular changes. Physiological concentrations of adiponectin have been found to inhibit the expression of adhesion molecules and nuclear factor-kappa-B (NF-κB) activation, thereby decreasing monocyte adhesion to endothelial cells. Adiponectin also decreased oxidized low-density lipoprotein (LDL) uptake by macrophages, reducing foam cell formation and inhibiting the proliferation and migration of smooth muscle cells by competitive binding that decreases the action of growth factors [26].

STUDIES IN MUSLIM POPULATIONS DURING RAMADAN

Innovative dietary regimens that can modify hormonal secretion patterns along with neural and metabolic pathways may be beneficial for people suffering from severe or morbid abdominal obesity. Manipulating leptin and ghrelin secretion patterns may influence the hunger and satiety balance during waking hours and modifying the adiponectin diurnal curve might improve metabolic status. The idea of studying the effect of a low-calorie diet with carbohydrates eaten primarily at dinner on hormonal diurnal secretion patterns was inspired by studies carried out in Muslim populations during Ramadan (i.e. fasting during the day and consuming a carbohydrate-rich meal after sundown). These studies found that the diurnal pattern of leptin secretion changed during the month-long Ramadan fast. In 2004, Kassab et al. [27] recognized that the Ramadan month is a unique metabolic model. Kassab and his associates conducted a study in 46 healthy Muslim females (22 ± 2 years, BMI 25.3 ± 0.7 kg/m^2). Serum levels of leptin were measured at baseline and on days 14 and 28 of the month of Ramadan and 2 weeks after Ramadan. Blood samples were taken at 1300–1400 hours (normally a nadir point for leptin levels under regular conditions) on each of the test days. The results demonstrated a 41% rise in leptin levels after the month of Ramadan (day 28). A second study conducted by Bogdan et al. [28] in 10 healthy Muslim males (34 ± 3.7 years) measured leptin levels around the clock at 4-h intervals from 0815 hours. The data included 24-h leptin curves a week before Ramadan and a second curve demonstrating leptin levels after 23 days of daytime fasting. A shift in the circadian pattern of leptin concentrations was observed. The standard pre-Ramadan curve of a midday nadir and a zenith at night was replaced on day 23 by a curve with high leptin levels during the daytime. In addition to these findings, euglycemic hyperinsulinemic clamp studies have demonstrated elevated serum leptin concentrations 6–8 h after insulin infusions [10]. To the best of our knowledge, no data is available regarding the diurnal secretion patterns of ghrelin and adiponectin during the Ramadan fast. Furthermore, sufficient data on hunger/satiety levels and the biochemical and inflammation status in individuals under similar conditions are not available. Considering these points, we decided to investigate the effect of a low-calorie diet with carbohydrates eaten primarily at dinner on average daily concentrations and diurnal secretion patterns of adiponectin, ghrelin, and leptin in human subjects. Effects on hunger and satiety, anthropometric outcomes, and biochemical and inflammatory profiles of our study participants were also evaluated. We hypothesized that consumption of carbohydrates mostly in the evening would modify the typical diurnal pattern of leptin secretion, as observed in Muslim populations during Ramadan. Since the experimental diet diminishes insulin secretion during the day, causing a single maximal insulin secretion in the evening, we assumed that, similar to the euglycemic hyperinsulinemic clamp trials, the diet would lead to higher relative concentrations of leptin starting in the morning and increasing throughout the day. We thought that this might lead to enhanced satiety during daylight hours and improve adherence to the weight loss diet.

Since the secretory pattern of the hunger hormone ghrelin is reciprocal to that of leptin [29], it was hypothesized that ghrelin's diurnal pattern might also be inverted, leading to the initiation of hunger sensations later in the day.

Studies have shown that there is a negative correlation between insulin and adiponectin levels [30]. Our experimental diet allowed virtually no carbohydrate consumption during the daytime, which theoretically should lead to a reduction in insulin secretion. Thus, we hypothesized that an increase in adiponectin concentrations would be observed throughout the day, thus improving insulin resistance, diminishing symptoms of the metabolic syndrome, and downregulating inflammation.

THE EFFECT OF A DIET WITH CARBOHYDRATES EATEN PRIMARILY AT DINNER ON ABDOMINAL OBESITY, INSULIN RESISTANCE, AND THE METABOLIC SYNDROME: BASIC RESEARCH

Our clinical study objectives were to test the effectiveness of a low-calorie diet with carbohydrates eaten primarily at dinner as a possible nutritional approach to treat patients with severe abdominal obesity, insulin resistance, and metabolic syndrome [31,32]. Specifically, we aimed to demonstrate that changes in the hormonal profiles of leptin and ghrelin caused by the timing of daily carbohydrate consumption might increase satiety and lead to improved adherence to long-term dietary regimens, with better anthropometric outcomes in comparison to standard weight loss diets. We also wanted to provide evidence supporting the hypothesis that changes in adiponectin profiles following the experimental diet could lead to improved biochemical and inflammatory parameters compared to standard diet regimens.

One hundred police officers (men and women, aged 25–55 years, BMI > 30) from the Israeli Police Force, Tel Aviv District, were enrolled in our study in May 2006. Individuals with cardiovascular diseases, hypertension, diabetes mellitus, or other primary diseases, individuals that followed any type of diet regime within 1 year prior to the study, and pregnant individuals were excluded from the study. Seventy-eight individuals met study criteria and 63 subjects finished the study protocol. On the first day (day 0), the police officers participated in a day-long event (24-h period) at a vacation resort run by the Israeli Police. A meeting with the study dietitian took place, personal questionnaires were filled out, and anthropometric measurements (height, weight, abdominal circumference, and percentage body fat) were taken. Randomization was done and each participant was assigned to either the experimental or the control group and received a diet according to the experimental protocol: a standard low-calorie diet (20% protein, 30–35% fat, 45–50% carbohydrates, 1300–1500 kcal) providing carbohydrates only at dinner (experimental diet) or a standard low-calorie diet (20% protein, 30–35% fat, 45–50% carbohydrates, 1300–1500 kcal) providing carbohydrates throughout the day (control diet; Table 35.1). Fasting (12-h) blood samples were taken at 0800 hours and then at 4-h intervals (at 1200, 1600, and 2000 hours). Participants filled out hunger/satiety questionnaires every 4 h, while waiting for blood tests. The hunger/satiety questionnaires were originally developed by Paul E. Garfinkel [33]; questions were slightly modified and translated into Hebrew. The final questionnaire dealt with hunger, satiety, and related issues. Participants were asked to select one answer to each question that best described how they were feeling at each time point. The day was filled with lectures, workshops, and leisure and entertainment activities. Blood samples and hunger/satiety questionnaires (as on day 0) were taken again after 1 week (day 7), 3 months (day 90), and 6 months (day 180). The study dietitian met all participants personally at each of the four day-long events in order to perform a comprehensive inquiry and estimate adherence to the dietary regime. In addition, participants had one-on-one meetings with the dietitian at 1–3-week intervals at Tel Aviv Police district headquarters throughout the entire study period. Body weight, abdominal circumference, and percentage body fat were measured regularly. Participants that did not attend meetings with the dietitian were excluded from the study. Blood samples collected at each of the four full-day events were centrifuged and serum was collected and stored at −80°C for future analysis. Analysis of levels of leptin, ghrelin (total), and adiponectin (high molecular weight) were later performed in our laboratories using sandwich enzyme-linked immunosorbent assay (ELISA) kits. Insulin was analyzed using Microparticle Enzyme Immunoassay test kits; glucose was analyzed enzymatic ultraviolet test kits, cholesterol, high-density lipoprotein (HDL) cholesterol, LDL cholesterol, and triglycerides was analyzed by enzymatic color test kits; and CRP was analyzed using immunoturbidimetric test kits. Insulin resistance was evaluated using homeostasis model assessment of insulin resistance (HOMA-IR); IL-6 and TNF-α were measured using high-sensitivity sandwich ELISA kits.

Anthropometric Measurements

As expected, significant weight loss and reductions in abdominal circumference, BMI, and percentage body fat were found in both experimental and control groups. A significantly greater average weight loss was observed in the experimental group compared with the control group at the end of the study (11.6 ± 0.84 vs. 9.06 ± 0.84 kg, $P = 0.024$). Trends of a greater average absolute BMI reduction (3.99 ± 0.24 vs. 3.16 ± 0.27) and superior average abdominal circumference reduction (11.7 ± 0.66 vs. 9.39 ± 0.98 cm) were observed in the experimental group. A trend toward a greater average reduction in absolute percentage body fat (6.98% ± 0.95% vs. 5.13% ± 0.59%) was also observed at the end of the study in the experimental diet group, compared to controls.

Hunger/Satiety and Thoughts About Food

High H-SSc indicate that subjects were less hungry and more satiated. The H-SSc was 13.7% higher after 180 days on the experimental diet compared to the first week of the diet ($P < 0.05$; Fig. 35.1A). In contrast, the control group reported a 5.9% lower H-SSc compared to baseline. It was found that control group participants felt significantly hungrier at noon on days 90 and 180 compared to the first week (19.3% and 22.4% lower H-SSc, respectively, $P < 0.05$; Fig. 35.1B). It was also found that the experimental group felt less hungry in the afternoon on days 90 and 180 compared to the first week (27.7% and 25.1% higher H-SSc, respectively, $P < 0.05$). The experimental group also felt less hungry in the evening of day 180 compared to the first week (28.0% higher H-SSc, $P < 0.05$). A significant difference between the groups in the H-SSc change from baseline was found on day 180 in the evening (28.0% increase vs. 6.6% decrease in H-SSc respectively, $P = 0.03$).

TABLE 35.1 Experimental and Control Diets

Experimental Diet	
Breakfast	Coffee/tea + artificial sweetener + 1/5 cup of low-fat milk + 7 walnut halves/7 almonds
Morning snack (10:00)	Plain low-fat yogurt/white cheese (1/2 cup) + vegetable
Lunch	Meat/fish dish (without breading, excluding ground meat)
	+ boiled vegetables/vegetable soup
	+ vegetable salad + 1 teaspoon of oil/tablespoon of dressing (from the permitted list)
Afternoon snack (16:00)	Coffee/tea + artificial sweetener + 1/5 cup of low-fat milk + 7 walnut halves/7 almonds
Dinner	Coffee/tea + artificial sweetener + 1/5 cup of low-fat milk + alternative A or B
	Alternative A:
	2–4 pieces of bread/4–6 pieces of reduced calorie bread
	+1/2 cup of white cheese/1 slice of yellow cheese/2 tablespoons of humus/an egg/1/2 can of tuna fish/4 slices of pastrami
	+vegetable salad
	+1 teaspoon of oil/tablespoon of tahini/1/4 avocado/1 tablespoon of dressing
	+fruit/fruit yogurt/diet ice cream/2 biscuits/1 cookie
	Alternative B:
	1–2 cups of cooked rice/pasta/puree/corn/legumes/1 potato/1 sweet potato
	+1 tablespoon of gravy
	+boiled vegetables/vegetables salad
	+1 teaspoon of oil/tablespoon of tahini/1/4 avocado/1 tablespoon of dressing
	+fruit yogurt/diet ice cream/2 biscuits/1 cookie
Night-time snack (if needed)	Coffee/tea + artificial sweetener + 1/5 cup of low-fat milk
	+7 walnut halves/7 almonds
	+plain yogurt/white cheese (1/2 cup)
Beverages	Water/no-calorie diet drinks
Control diet	
Breakfast	Coffee/tea + artificial sweetener + low-fat milk
	+1–2 pieces of bread/2 pieces of reduced calorie bread/2 crackers/ 2 biscuits
	+white cheese
Morning snack (10:00)	Plain yogurt/fruit yogurt + 7 walnut halves/7 almonds
Lunch	Meat/fish dish
	+boiled vegetables/vegetable soup
	+vegetable salad + 1 teaspoon of oil/tablespoon of dressing
	+1/2 cup of cooked rice/pasta/puree/corn/legumes/1/2 potato/1/2 sweet potato
Afternoon snack (16:00)	Coffee/tea + artificial sweetener + low-fat milk
	+2 biscuits/fruit + 7 walnut halves/7 almonds
Dinner	Coffee/tea + artificial sweetener + low-fat milk
	+1–2 pieces of bread/2 pieces of light bread/2 crackers
	+1/2 cup of white cheese/1 slice of yellow cheese/2 tablespoons of humus/egg/1/2 can of tuna fish/4 slices of sliced turkey breast
	+vegetable salad
	+1 teaspoon of oil/ tablespoon of tahini/1/4 avocado/ tablespoon of dressing
Night-time snack (if needed)	Coffee/tea + artificial sweetener + low-fat milk
	+7 walnut halves/7 almonds + plain yogurt/fruit yogurt/diet ice cream
Beverages	Water/no-calorie diet drinks

Source: Sofer et al. [31].

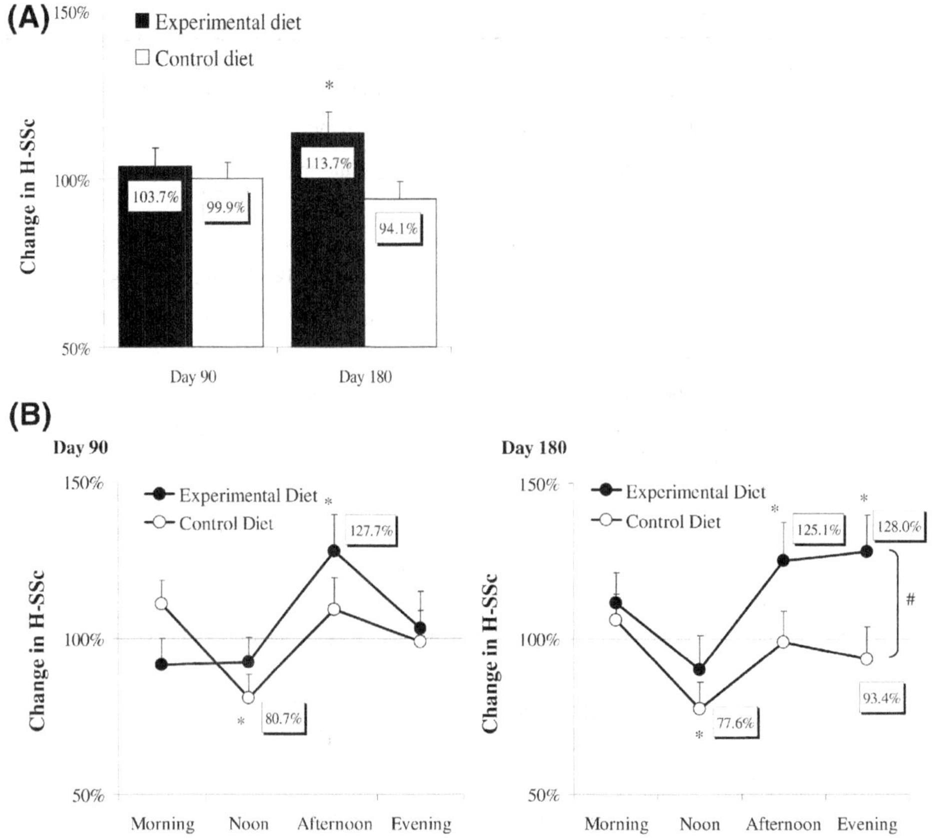

FIGURE 35.1 (A) Least square mean ± SE hunger-satiety scores (H-SSc) on day 90 and day 180 as a percentage of baseline (average of daily satiety on days 0 and 7) in the experimental ($n=18$) and control ($n=21$) groups. Comparison of groups by repeated measures ANOVA. $^{*}P<0.05$ for difference from baseline. (B) Mean ± SE percentage of H-SSc at day 90 and at day 180 compared to scores at the same time points on the first week of the diet (average of days 0 and day 7) *, $P<0.05$ as compared to the same time points in the first week. $^{\#}$, $P=0.030$, comparing control and experimental groups by contrast t-test following repeated measures ANOVA at day 180. *Source: Sofer et al. [31].*

Analysis of the question related to "the urge to eat," revealed significant differences between the groups on day 180 in the afternoon. In the experimental diet group, 67% of participants had a reduced urge to eat (median difference 0.5 on a 1–4 scale), compared to the first week (average of days 0 and 7 at the same time), whereas only 19% of control group participants had a lower urge to eat (median difference 0) compared to the first week [$P<0.05$ by the chi-squared (χ^2) test and the Wilcoxon rank sum test]. When the question related to "preoccupation with thoughts about food" was analyzed, differences between groups were observed on day 180 in the afternoon. In the experimental group, none of the participants had an enhanced preoccupation with thoughts about food (median difference 0.5 on a 1–4 scale) compared to the first week (average of days 0 and 7 at the same time), whereas 33% of control group participants had a higher preoccupation with food (median difference 0) compared to the first week [borderline significant by the Wilcoxon rank sum test ($P=0.067$) and χ^2test ($P=0.052$)].

Biochemical Parameters

Biochemical parameters are summarized in Table 35.2. After 180 days on the experimental diet, significantly lower daily insulin concentrations were observed compared to baseline measurements (68.0%, $P<0.05$). In contrast, after 180 days, the control group had insulin levels higher than those measured at baseline. When comparing the two dietary regimens, insulin concentrations as percentage baseline values were significantly lower for the experimental diet in comparison to control group (68.0% of baseline vs. of 122.6% from baseline, $P=0.006$). The experimental diet led to a significant decrease (20%, $P<0.01$) in fasting glucose concentrations after 180 days compared to baseline, while the control diet did not significantly reduce fasting glucose (8.3% decrease from baseline). A similar trend was observed on day 90 (11.4% vs. 3.3% decrease respectively). After 90 days on the diet, a 30.9% decrease in HOMA-IR was observed in the experimental group, whereas a 19.7% increase was observed in the control group. The difference between the groups

TABLE 35.2 Biochemical and Inflammatory Parameters and Percentage of Baseline

	Day	Experimental Group ($n=18$)		Control Group ($n=21$)		Comparison of Groups
		Absolute Mean	% of Baseline[a]	Absolute Mean	% of Baseline[a]	
Insulin (mU/L)	0	29.8±5.52	–	23.2±4.48	–	–
	90	16.1±1.93	84.4±13.7	20.0±3.61	102.9±13.1	$P=0.332$
	180	14.9±2.79	68.0±14.3*	16.6±1.63	122.6±12.8	$P=0.006$
Glucose (mM)	0	5.10±0.26	–	4.85±0.25	–	–
	90	4.81±0.15	88.6±8.35	4.77±0.08	96.7±6.84	$P=0.454$
	180	4.71±0.18	80.0±7.53**	4.71±0.16	93.7±6.84	$P=0.184$
HOMA-IR	0	1.68±0.24	–	1.33±0.20	–	–
	90	1.14±0.15	69.1±15.8	1.33±0.16	119.7±12.8	$P=0.015$
	180	1.09±0.12	89.0±15.2	1.20±0.15	121.3±13.2	$P=0.114$
Triglycerides (mM)	0	1.88±0.17	–	2.00±0.17	–	–
	90	1.22±0.09	69.2±7.20***	1.22±0.14	65.8±5.92***	$P=0.717$
	180	1.20±0.13	70.6±6.95***	1.33±0.17	68.7±6.00***	$P=0.834$
Total cholesterol (mM)	0	5.46±0.18	–	5.02±0.15	–	–
	90	4.94±0.17	91.9±2.63**	4.76±0.18	95.7±2.45	$P=0.290$
	180	5.32±0.23	97.6±2.75	4.87±0.18	96.3±2.48	$P=0.733$
LDL cholesterol (mM)	0	3.66±0.18	–	3.14±0.15	–	–
	90	3.29±0.18	89.0±3.52**	3.18±0.15	97.8±3.28	$P=0.073$
	180	3.43±0.22	90.3±3.70*	3.00±0.13	92.43.26*	$P=0.670$
HDL cholesterol (mM)	0	0.78±0.06	–	0.83±0.05	–	–
	90	0.88±0.04	114.3±4.48**	0.91±0.04	110.4±4.18*	$P=0.525$
	180	1.07±0.09	140.8±4.65***	1.05±0.05	126.0±4.16***	$P=0.022$
CRP (mg/L)	0	8.2±2.0	–	3.4±0.6	–	–
	90	5.6±1.6	99.0±19.8adj	2.5±0.4	98.3±19.1 adj	$P=0.979$
	180	3.9±1.1	72.2±20.8 adj	2.2±0.4	94.2±19.5 adj	$P=0.456$
TNF-α (pg/mL)	0	1.89±0.15	–	1.93±0.24	–	–
	90	1.85±0.18	101.4±8.39	2.14±0.29	117.3±7.80*	$P=0.169$
	180	1.65±0.16	90. 8±8.82	2.12±0.33	116.2±7.78*	$P=0.034$
IL-6 (pg/mL)	0	2.71±0.33	–	2.52±0.26	–	–
	90	2.22±0.33	84.8±13.4	2.06±0.27	91.5±11.9	$P=0.710$
	180	1.61±0.21	63.0±13.4**	1.84±0.20	76.3±12.2	$P=0.465$

*significant difference from baseline ($P<0.05$ respectively). **significant difference from baseline ($P<0.01$ respectively). ***significant difference from baseline ($P<0.0001$ respectively). [a]percentage baseline values were calculated for each subject and averaged; adj, adjusted for baseline differences.*

Least squares mean±SE for absolute values and percent of baseline. Insulin, glucose, homeostasis model assessment of insulin resistance (HOMA-IR), triglycerides C-reactive protein (CRP), tumor necrosis factor (TNF-α) and interleukin-6 (IL-6) were calculated as a percentage of day-0 values. Total cholesterol, low-density lipoprotein (LDL) cholesterol, and high-density lipoprotein (HDL) cholesterol were calculated as percentage of the average day-0 and day-7 values.To convert values for glucose, triglycerides, total cholesterol, LDL cholesterol, and HDL cholesterol to mg/dL, divide by 0.05551, 0.01129, 0.02586, 0.02564, and 0.02564 respectively.

Source: Sofer et al. [31].

was significant ($P=0.015$). A similar trend was found on day 180 (11.0% decrease vs. 21.3% increase respectively). Both the experimental and the control diets led to similar significant reductions in morning fasting triglyceride concentrations when compared to baseline (30.8% and 34.2% on day 90, respectively; 29.4% and 31.3% on day 180, respectively; $P<0.0001$). The experimental diet led to a significant 8.1% decrease in total cholesterol concentrations ($P<0.01$), whereas only a 4.3% decrease was observed in controls on day 90. The effect was not observed on day 180. An earlier and significant decrease of 11.0% in LDL cholesterol concentration was found in the experimental group on day 90 ($P<0.01$), whereas on day 180 a significant decrease in LDL cholesterol was measured for both diets (9.7% and 7.6% decrease, respectively; $P<0.05$). Significant increases in HDL cholesterol concentrations were observed for both diets on days 90 and 180 (14.3%, $P<0.01$ vs. 10.4%, $P<0.05$ on day 90 and 40.8%, $P<0.0001$ vs. 26.0%, $P<0.01$ on day 180). The HDL cholesterol increase in the experimental diet was significantly greater than the control diet increase after 180 days ($P=0.022$).

Inflammatory Parameters

Inflammatory parameters are shown in Table 35.2. A trend toward a greater reduction in serum CRP levels was observed in the experimental group (27.8% vs. 5.8%). Significant differences were not obtained after adjusting for baseline levels. On day 180, subjects on the experimental diet had significantly lower TNF-α concentrations, with a 9.2% average decrease from baseline measurements. In contrast, the control diet led to an average 16.1% increase in TNF-α ($P=0.034$ for the between-group difference). Both diets lowered IL-6 concentrations at days 90 and 180 compared to baseline. On day 180, the experimental diet led to a significant reduction of 37.8% ($P<0.01$), whereas a smaller nonsignificant reduction of 23.7% was measured in control subjects. On day 90, a similar trend was observed (15.8% vs. 10% reduction from baseline, respectively).

Daily Average and Diurnal Curves of Serum Hormonal Levels

Both diets decreased the average 12-h leptin concentrations on days 90 and 180 compared to baseline ($P<0.05$). Overall, a trend toward smaller reductions in leptin levels from baseline was observed in the experimental group (29.3% and 20.6% decreases in the experimental group on days 90 and 180, and 31.4% and 26.2% decreases in the control group). The experimental diet led to changes in the diurnal secretion pattern of leptin (Fig. 35.2). At baseline, both groups demonstrated typical concave diurnal leptin curves, including a fall throughout the hours of 0800–1600, reaching a nadir in the afternoon and a rise from 1600. On day 180, leptin curves were lower compared to baseline in both groups. In the experimental group, the curve became more convex, with a nadir only in the evening and not in the afternoon (Fig. 35.2B). A significant difference was observed within the experimental group between days 0 and 180 in the morning and the evening ($P=0.016$ and $P=0.040$, respectively).

Due to a technical problem with blood collection, data for ghrelin were available only for days 7 and 90. A significant difference in average daily ghrelin concentrations as a percentage change from baseline (day 7) between groups was observed on day 90 (2.6% increase vs 5.5% decrease in the experimental and control group, respectively; $P<0.05$). The trend of ghrelin's diurnal pattern tended to change after the experimental diet (Fig. 35.3). On day 7 (used as baseline), both groups demonstrated convex curves with a typical diurnal pattern, including high values at daytime with a zenith in the afternoon. On day 90, a trend toward modification of the curve from convex to concave was observed in the experimental diet group, with a zenith only in the evening and not in the afternoon (Fig. 35.3B). We observed a significant difference in ghrelin concentrations in the experimental group in the evening compared to the same hour at baseline ($P=0.045$).

The experimental diet led to a significant increase (43.5%, $P<0.05$) in average 12-h adiponectin concentrations, whereas the control diet led to a smaller and nonsignificant (13.9%) increase after 180 days. The same trend was observed on day 90 (15.3% vs. 1.9%, respectively). The experimental diet modified adiponectin's diurnal secretion (Fig. 35.4). At baseline, both groups demonstrated low, flat curves typical of obese individuals. In the experimental group, the curve showed a rise on day 180 compared to day 0 (Fig. 35.4B); in contrast, the control group curve remained low and flat (Fig. 35.4A). Significant differences in adiponectin concentrations at noon and in the afternoon were observed in the experimental group on day 180, compared to baseline ($P=0.040$ and $P=0.051$, respectively).

In summary, we observed better anthropometric outcomes, higher satiety, and a better biochemical and inflammation status after the experimental diet compared to control. Changes in the levels and circadian patterns of the hormones analyzed were as predicted.

The decrease in overall daily leptin concentrations and in leptin curves for both groups was expected. Decreased leptin levels following weight loss diets have been well documented in previous studies [3,4,8,34,35] and may be explained by reduced body fat mass. Reduced leptin serum concentrations during weight loss programs are commonly associated with a decline in satiety levels [3,4,35,36], as observed in our control

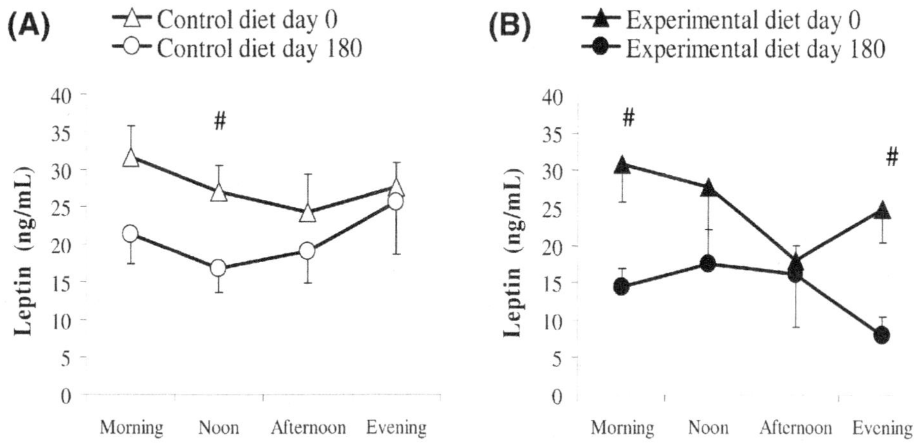

FIGURE 35.2 Effect of diets on leptin's diurnal curves. Mean ± SE on day 0 and on day 180 in the control (A) and experimental (B) groups. #, $P = 0.016$ and $P = 0.040$, comparing day 0 and day 180 for the experimental group ($n = 18$) by t-test in the morning and the afternoon, respectively. *Source: Sofer et al. [32].*

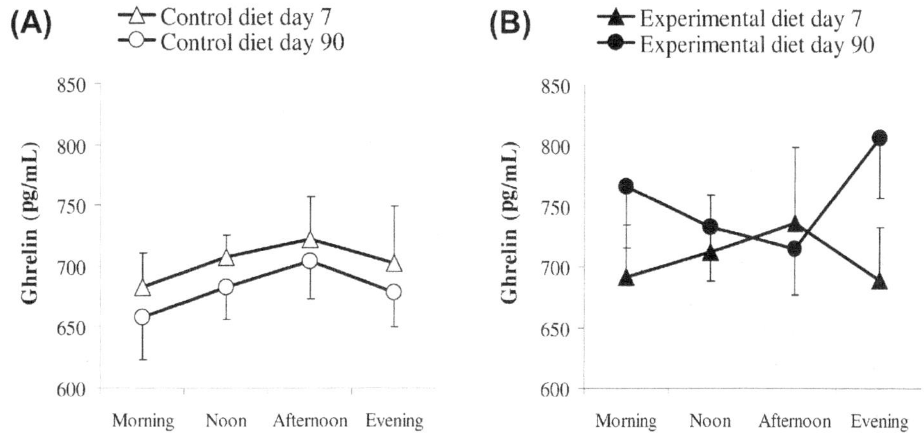

FIGURE 35.3 Effect of diets on ghrelin's diurnal curves. Mean ± SE on day 7 and day 90 in the control (A) and experimental (B) groups. #, $P = 0.045$, comparing day 7 and day 90 for the experimental group ($n = 18$) by t-test in the evening. *Source: Sofer et al. [32].*

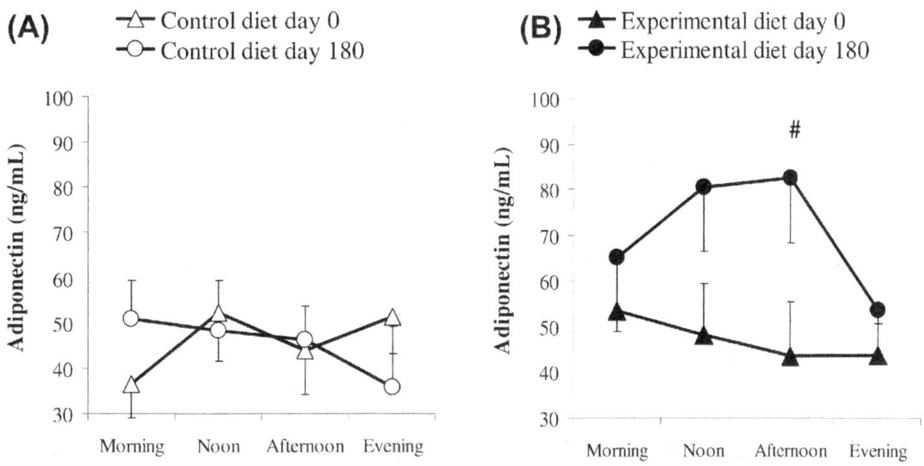

FIGURE 35.4 Effect of diet on adiponectin's diurnal curve. Mean ± SE on day 0 and on day 180 in the control (A) and experimental (B) groups. #, $P = 0.040$ and $P = 0.051$, comparing day 0 and day 180 for the experimental group ($n = 18$) by t-test at noon and in the afternoon, respectively. *Source: Sofer et al. [32].*

group. In the experimental group, this expected satiety reduction did not occur. On the contrary, at the end of the study, the experimental diet group had higher H-SSc in comparison to baseline. Previous studies with different diets reported that, during weight loss, leptin concentrations decreased, satiety levels were reduced, food intake was renewed, and a slow regain of body weight occurred [35–37]. It is obvious that dietary manipulations that maintain higher leptin concentrations through waking hours during weight loss process will be beneficial for dieters. We suggest that a higher relative concentration of leptin at midday and during the afternoon is one of the factors that led to the elevated daytime satiety in our experimental diet group. Decreased levels of leptin in the evening were immediately prior to consumption of the evening meal and therefore did not present a problem with adherence to the dietary regimen. It has been suggested that leptin therapy might negate leptin depletion during the weight loss process and contribute to the ongoing maintenance of dietary regimens [8]. However, Phase III trials of leptin treatment showed low efficacy, and side effects included the formation of antibodies [38]. Dietary manipulations such as our experimental diet that maintain relatively higher daytime leptin concentrations during the weight loss process may make an important contribution to the success rate of the diet.

The rise in ghrelin following consumption of the experimental diet was expected because it is well documented that ghrelin concentrations are upregulated by weight loss (typically after loss of approximately 10% of body weight) [14]. Despite the significant weight loss that was achieved in the control group, the ghrelin curve was not upregulated in this group. A possible explanation is the higher insulin levels that occurred throughout the day in the control group who ate carbohydrates during daylight hours and the reported reciprocal relationship between insulin and ghrelin secretion [14,39–42]. It was expected that ghrelin's overall increase in the experimental group would contribute to hunger sensations as the diet progressed, as has been described previously [8,36,40,43]; however, this was not the case and the experimental group reported higher levels of satiety. We propose that the change in ghrelin's curve to lower relative concentrations in the afternoon may contribute to the enhanced daytime satiety experienced by the experimental diet group. We believe that the alteration in the timing of ghrelin's peak from daylight hours to the evening just before dinner was another cause for the elevated daylight hour satiety, improved persistence in the weight loss process, and better anthropometric outcomes that were measured. Ghrelin's homeostatic mechanism provides an additional explanation for weight regain after dieting. It was shown that ghrelin inhibition can prevent increased food intake in rats and mice [8]. In humans, inhibiting ghrelin as a tool to avoid weight regain after weight loss is under investigation. A decade after its discovery, no ghrelin-based antiobesity therapies are close to reaching the market [8,44]. As for dietary manipulations, it is known that low-fat, high-carbohydrate weight loss diets do not upregulate ghrelin; instead, they decrease leptin concentrations [45]. We suggest that our experimental dietary manipulation might be advantageous because it modifies ghrelin curves to relatively lower concentrations in the afternoon in addition to its beneficial modification of the leptin curve.

Although, no specific nutritional guidance regarding glucose balance, lipids profiles, or inflammation status was given to participants, improvements in these parameters were observed. It is of great interest that for nearly all of these parameters, significantly greater improvements were observed in the experimental diet group, even though both diet groups experienced weight loss accompanied by body fat and abdominal circumference reductions. Studies have reported diverse results, including increased, decreased, or unchanged plasma adiponectin levels after low-calorie diets [39,46–51]. It has been speculated that upregulated adiponectin concentrations during the weight loss process depends on the type of diet administered. It is thought that obesity-related hypoadiponectinemia can only be corrected by a weight reduction process that reverses insulin resistance [52–54]. Our experimental diet led to lower insulin concentrations during daylight hours and improved insulin resistance, as seen in HOMA-IR results. Therefore, eating carbohydrates primarily in the evening lowered insulin levels, which led to an increase in adiponectin concentrations above levels measured in controls and exclusively changed the daily adiponectin curve. Previous studies found that in obesity (primarily abdominal), adiponectin concentrations were low, insulin resistance was high, the risk of type 2 diabetes increased, an atherogenic lipid profile developed, and a high concentration of several inflammatory markers appeared [50,52,55,56]. It is also well established that losing weight, especially from abdominal fat stores, increases adiponectin concentrations and improves all of these parameters because adiponectin is insulin sensitizing, directly reduces metabolic and vascular disorders, and acts as an anti-inflammatory adipokine [52,55,57]. In insulin-resistant mice treated with physiologic concentrations of adiponectin, glucose tolerance improved and insulin resistance was reduced [58]. It was also found that in lean mice injected with adiponectin combined with a high-fat, high-sugar diet, postprandial increases in plasma glucose, free fatty acid, and triacylglycerol concentrations were attenuated [58]. It has been suggested that long-term administration of adiponectin would be effective as an antidiabetic, antiatherogenic agent;

however, large-scale production of the native forms of full-length adiponectin with all post-translational modifications cannot be achieved at commercially viable prices [59]. Thus, dietary manipulations that enhance endogenous adiponectin expression are promising.

Overall, we have demonstrated improved hunger/satiety status, persistence in the weight loss process, better anthropometric outcomes, improved insulin sensitivity, improved metabolic syndrome parameters, reduced inflammation, and hormonal profile changes following simple carbohydrate manipulation. Our results provide an important scientific basis for proposing possible dietary alternatives that may be beneficial for people suffering from severe morbid abdominal obesity, insulin resistance, and the metabolic syndrome who experience difficulties in maintaining a weight loss diet over the long term. Further research into the diurnal profile of the hormones investigated in this study is required to fully establish a causal relationship. The molecular mechanisms by which this diet exerts its effects are currently under investigation in our laboratory.

FUTURE RESEARCH: UNDERSTANDING THE PHYSIOLOGICAL MECHANISMS

In order to understand the mechanisms and characterize the pathways and metabolites underlying the phenomena observed in our clinical studies, additional experiments are being carried out in our laboratory in an animal model. We will examine changes in neural hypothalamic pathways that control body weight and food intake following consumption of the experimental diet. We aim to elucidate the mechanisms that allow our innovative nutritional approach to facilitate maintenance of a long-term weight loss diet. Investigation into changes in the metabolic status of the liver, muscle, and adipose tissue will be also carried out and we intend to assess overall health advantages.

DIETARY ALTERNATIVES TO REPLACE MEDICATIONS: "NUTRITION TARGETING"

The snowball effect of abdominal obesity and its sequence of metabolic complications must be stopped as early as possible to avoid diabetes, coronary heart diseases, and other obesity-related diseases. Several of the factors and metabolites discussed in this chapter are the targets of drugs already prescribed to delay morbidity and reduce mortality associated with abdominal obesity. Three groups of medications, thiazolidinediones (TZDs), biguanides, and fibrates, operate via different metabolic pathways and are commonly used worldwide. Each of these groups of medications is associated with potential adverse effects and possible risks.

Thiazolidinediones

Obesity is defined as increased adipose tissue mass and characterized by hypertrophy of adipocytes. It is well known that large adipocytes size is a significant factor in the pathology of metabolic syndrome. TZDs, also known as *glitazones*, are a family of drugs used in the treatment of diabetes. TZDs bind to PPAR-γ in adipose tissue, leading to cell differentiation that increases the number of small differentiated adipocytes, which secrete more adiponectin and are more insulin sensitive. It has been shown that upregulation of adiponectin expression in white adipose tissue and plasma is one of the main mechanisms of action of TZDs [60]. Higher serum adiponectin levels decrease plasma glucose levels by suppressing hepatic glucose production and decreasing fatty acid concentration through oxidizing fatty acids in the muscle [61]. These pathways work through activation of AMPK, which has an important role in insulin signaling, energy balance, and the metabolism of glucose and fats in tissues [62]. In addition, activation of PPAR-γ and higher serum adiponectin appear to reduce the levels of proinflammatory transcription factors such as NF-κB, and thus decrease transcription of a number of proinflammatory factors, including various interleukins and tumor necrosis factors [63–67]. TZDs increase the synthesis of certain proteins, which reduces the levels of certain types of lipids and circulating free fatty acids. TZDs generally decrease triglycerides and increase HDL cholesterol and LDL cholesterol. Although the increase in LDL is mainly of the larger LDL particles, which may be less atherogenic, the clinical significance of this is currently unknown [65]. The main side effect of TZDs is water retention and weight gain, which can lead to heart failure. In addition, there are an increasing number of reports of hepatitis and potential liver failure associated with this medication [68,69].

Biguanides

Biguanides (mainly Metformin) are widely prescribed antihyperglycemic agents that suppress hepatic glucose production, increase peripheral glucose uptake, and moderately reduce LDL cholesterol and triglyceride levels. Glucose control with the aid of biguanides appears to decrease the risk of diabetes-related complications, and is not associated with weight gain. This medication is reportedly associated with fewer hypoglycemic episodes than other lines of drugs. Biguanides activate AMPK, thus improving insulin signaling, whole-body energy balance, and the metabolism of glucose and fats [62]. Activation of AMPK by biguanides inhibits the expression of the hepatic gluconeogenic genes encoding PEPCK and G6Pase, thereby lowering glucose output [70]. Increased AMPK activity in skeletal muscle by biguanides causes solute carrier family 2, facilitated glucose transporter member 4 (GLUT4) positioning on the plasma membrane, leading to peripheral glucose uptake. Activation of AMPK by biguanides in hepatocytes and muscle cells reduces ACC activity and induces fatty acid oxidation [71]. The most common adverse effect of biguanides is gastrointestinal distress, including diarrhea, cramps, nausea, vomiting, and increased flatulence [72]. Long-term use of biguanides has been associated with decreased absorption of vitamin B12 [73]. The most serious and rare side effect of biguanides use is lactic acidosis, which in most cases appears to be related to comorbidities such as impaired liver or kidney function [74].

Fibrates

The fibrates are a class of hypolipidemic agents that increase HDL levels and decrease triglyceride levels, leading to improved insulin resistance. They are often used in combination therapy with statins.

Fibrates are the best known synthetic ligand for PPARs: they activate PPAR-α and alter lipid metabolism through multiple mechanisms such as stimulation of lipid oxidation and alterations in lipoprotein metabolism. Inhibition of vascular inflammation is also associated with fibrate use [65,75–77]. PPAR-α activation by fibrates increases hepatic uptake and the esterification of free fatty acids. In skeletal muscle and heart, activation of PPAR-α increases mitochondrial free fatty acid uptake and oxidation [65]. The effect of fibrates on the metabolism of triglyceride-rich lipoproteins is due to a PPAR-α-dependent inhibition of apolipoprotein C-III (ApoC-III) expression and stimulation of lipoprotein lipase (LPL) expression in the liver. The increase in plasma HDL cholesterol depends on overexpression of ApoA-I and ApoA-II [69]. PPAR-α is expressed in monocytes and endothelial and smooth muscle cells, and its activation can inhibit nuclear factor-kappa-B (NF-κB), thus reducing inflammatory responses by downregulating inducible nitric oxide synthase (iNOS), IL-6 and other proinflammatory factors [66,69]. Fibrates can cause mild stomach upset and sometimes diarrhea. Since fibrates increase the cholesterol content of bile, they increase the risk for gallstones. The most common side effect of fibrates is myopathy (muscle pain with creatine kinase elevations). In combination with statins, fibrates cause an increased risk of rhabdomyolysis and destruction of muscle tissue, leading to renal failure. In addition, fibrates can irritate the liver; the irritation is usually mild and reversible, but occasionally requires discontinuation of treatment [78,79].

Dietary manipulations that can modify pathways that are treated today by the medications discussed above are less invasive and less expensive, with a low probability of side effects or risks.

We believe that when dealing with abdominal obesity and metabolic syndrome, "nutrition targeting" should be taken into consideration and should attract the attention of scientists, doctors, and dietitians at least as much as, if not more than, traditional drug targeting.

Our past, present, and future work is aimed to establish that our dietary intervention of consuming carbohydrates primarily in the evening might be a method of "nutrition targeting." We believe our diet has the potential to modify the same metabolic pathways as those currently targeted by traditional medications. Natural, dietary alternatives are clearly the preferred treatment choice for reducing risk factors associated with abdominal obesity.

INTERIM CONCLUSIONS

Over the years, scientists have explored ways to stop the "vicious metabolic cycle" of abdominal obesity that leads to morbid obesity, diabetes, and coronary heart disease. Therapeutic approaches studied include diets, medications, and invasive treatments such as bariatric surgery. We believe that our dietary regimen that modifies daily hormonal secretion patterns of leptin, ghrelin, and adiponectin, increases satiety scores, and improves anthropometric biochemical and inflammatory parameters may provide an innovative nutritional approach for ending this cycle. We trust that the results of our studies in human subjects, along with our current and upcoming research in an animal model, will establish specific, evidence-based dietary guidelines for the nutritional treatment of patients with abdominal obesity. We propose that a simple dietary manipulation that can modify hormonal profiles, induce weight loss, and break the vicious metabolic cycle of abdominal obesity has numerous advantages over pharmaceutical and surgical interventions and should be used as a first line of treatment.

References

[1] Orzano AJ, Scott JG. Diagnosis and treatment of obesity in adults: an applied evidence-based review. J Am Board Fam Pract 2004;17(5):359–69.

[2] Nakata Y, Okura T, Matsuo T, Tanaka K. Factors alleviating metabolic syndrome via diet-induced weight loss with or without exercise in overweight Japanese women. Prev Med 2009;48(4):351–6.

[3] Erez G, Tirosh A, Rudich A, Meiner V, Schwarzfuchs D, Sharon N, et al. Phenotypic and genetic variation in leptin as determinants of weight regain. Int J Obes (Lond) 35(6):785–92.

[4] Crujeiras AB, Goyenechea E, Abete I, et al. Weight regain after a diet-induced loss is predicted by higher baseline leptin and lower

ghrelin plasma levels. J Clin Endocrinol Metab 2010;95(11): 5037–44.

[5] de Souza RJ, Bray GA, Carey VJ, et al. Effects of 4 weight-loss diets differing in fat, protein, and carbohydrate on fat mass, lean mass, visceral adipose tissue, and hepatic fat: results from the POUNDS LOST trial. Am J Clin Nutr 2012;95(3):614–25.

[6] Sacks FM, Bray GA, Carey VJ, et al. Comparison of weight-loss diets with different compositions of fat, protein, and carbohydrates. N Engl J Med 2009;360(9):859–73.

[7] Ronti T, Lupattelli G, Mannarino E. The endocrine function of adipose tissue: an update. Clin Endocrinol (Oxf) 2006;64(4):355–65.

[8] Klok MD, Jakobsdottir S, Drent ML. The role of leptin and ghrelin in the regulation of food intake and body weight in humans: a review. Obes Rev 2007;8(1):21–34.

[9] Pico C, Oliver P, Sanchez J, Palou A. Gastric leptin: a putative role in the short-term regulation of food intake. Br J Nutr 2003;90(4):735–41.

[10] Coleman RA, Herrmann TS. Nutritional regulation of leptin in humans. Diabetologia 1999;42(6):639–46.

[11] Yildiz BO, Suchard MA, Wong ML, McCann SM, Licinio J. Alterations in the dynamics of circulating ghrelin, adiponectin, and leptin in human obesity. Proc Natl Acad Sci USA 2004;101(28):10434–9.

[12] Natalucci G, Riedl S, Gleiss A, Zidek T, Frisch H. Spontaneous 24-h ghrelin secretion pattern in fasting subjects: maintenance of a meal-related pattern. Eur J Endocrinol 2005;152(6):845–50.

[13] Ueno H, Yamaguchi H, Kangawa K, Nakazato M. Ghrelin: a gastric peptide that regulates food intake and energy homeostasis. Regul Pept 2005;126(1–2):11–19.

[14] Wells T. Ghrelin—Defender of fat. Prog Lipid Res 2009;48(5): 257–74.

[15] Gil-Campos M, Canete RR, Gil A. Adiponectin, the missing link in insulin resistance and obesity. Clin Nutr 2004;23(5):963–74.

[16] Matsuzawa Y. Establishment of a concept of visceral fat syndrome and discovery of adiponectin. Proc Jpn Acad Ser B Phys Biol Sci 2010;86(2):131–41.

[17] Koh SB, Yoon J, Kim JY, et al. Relationships between Serum Adiponectin with metabolic syndrome and components of metabolic syndrome in non-diabetic Koreans: ARIRANG Study. Yonsei Med J 2011;52(2):234–41.

[18] Chandran M, Phillips SA, Ciaraldi T, Henry RR. Adiponectin: more than just another fat cell hormone? Diabetes Care 2003;26(8):2442–50.

[19] Calvani M, Scarfone A, Granato L, et al. Restoration of adiponectin pulsatility in severely obese subjects after weight loss. Diabetes 2004;53(4):939–47.

[20] Zigman JM, Elmquist JK. Minireview: from anorexia to obesity—the yin and yang of body weight control. Endocrinology 2003;144(9):3749–56.

[21] Kadowaki T, Yamauchi T. Adiponectin and adiponectin receptors. Endocr Rev 2005;26(3):439–51.

[22] Steinberg GR, Macaulay SL, Febbraio MA, Kemp BE. AMP-activated protein kinase—the fat controller of the energy railroad. Can J Physiol Pharmacol 2006;84(7):655–65.

[23] Tsuchida A, Yamauchi T, Takekawa S, et al. Peroxisome proliferator-activated receptor (PPAR)alpha activation increases adiponectin receptors and reduces obesity-related inflammation in adipose tissue: comparison of activation of PPARalpha, PPARgamma, and their combination. Diabetes 2005;54(12):3358–70.

[24] Bouloumie A, Curat CA, Sengenes C, Lolmede K, Miranville A, Busse R. Role of macrophage tissue infiltration in metabolic diseases. Curr Opin Clin Nutr Metab Care 2005;8(4):347–54.

[25] Ye J, Gao Z, Yin J, He Q. Hypoxia is a potential risk factor for chronic inflammation and adiponectin reduction in adipose tissue of *ob/ob* and dietary obese mice. Am J Physiol Endocrinol Metab 2007;293(4):E1118–28.

[26] Matsuzawa Y, Funahashi T, Kihara S, Shimomura I. Adiponectin and metabolic syndrome. Arterioscler Thromb Vasc Biol 2004;24(1):29–33.

[27] Kassab S, Abdul-Ghaffar T, Nagalla DS, Sachdeva U, Nayar U. Interactions between leptin, neuropeptide-Y and insulin with chronic diurnal fasting during Ramadan. Ann Saudi Med 2004;24(5):345–9.

[28] Bogdan A, Bouchareb B, Touitou Y. Response of circulating leptin to Ramadan daytime fasting: a circadian study. Br J Nutr 2005;93(4):515–8.

[29] Kalra SP, Ueno N, Kalra PS. Stimulation of appetite by ghrelin is regulated by leptin restraint: peripheral and central sites of action. J Nutr 2005;135(5):1331–5.

[30] Goropashnaya AV, Herron J, Sexton M, et al. Relationships between plasma adiponectin and body fat distribution, insulin sensitivity, and plasma lipoproteins in Alaskan Yup'ik Eskimos: the Center for Alaska Native Health Research study. Metabolism 2009;58(1):22–9.

[31] Sofer S, Eliraz A, Kaplan S, et al. Greater weight loss and hormonal changes after 6 months diet with carbohydrates eaten mostly at dinner. Obesity (Silver Spring) 2011;19(10):2006–14.

[32] Sofer S, Eliraz A, Kaplan S, et al. Changes in daily leptin, ghrelin and adiponectin profiles following a diet with carbohydrates eaten at dinner in obese subjects. Nutr Metab Cardiovasc Dis 2012;23(8):744–50.

[33] Garfinkel P. In: Corcoran K, Fischer J, editors. Hunger satiety scales. Measures for clinical practice: a sourcebook. Third ed. New York: Free Press; 2000. p. 343–6.

[34] Elloumi M, Ben Ounis O, Makni E, Van Praagh E, Tabka Z, Lac G. Effect of individualized weight-loss programmes on adiponectin, leptin and resistin levels in obese adolescent boys. Acta Paediatr 2009;98(9):1487–93.

[35] Mars M, de Graaf C, de Groot LC, Kok FJ. Decreases in fasting leptin and insulin concentrations after acute energy restriction and subsequent compensation in food intake. Am J Clin Nutr 2005;81(3):570–7.

[36] Beck B, Richy S. Dietary modulation of ghrelin and leptin and gorging behavior after weight loss in the obese Zucker rat. J Endocrinol 2009;202(1):29–34.

[37] Ahima RS. Revisiting leptin's role in obesity and weight loss. J Clin Invest 2008;118(7):2380–3.

[38] Cawthorne MA. Opportunities and challenges for the development of pharmacological therapies for obesity treatment. Obes Rev 2007;8(Suppl. 1):131–6.

[39] Montecucco F, Mach F. Update on therapeutic strategies to increase adiponectin function and secretion in metabolic syndrome. Diabetes Obes Metab 2009;11(5):445–54.

[40] Blom WA, Stafleu A, de Graaf C, Kok FJ, Schaafsma G, Hendriks HF. Ghrelin response to carbohydrate-enriched breakfast is related to insulin. Am J Clin Nutr 2005;81(2):367–75.

[41] Robertson MD, Henderson RA, Vist GE, Rumsey RD. Plasma ghrelin response following a period of acute overfeeding in normal weight men. Int J Obes Relat Metab Disord 2004;28(6):727–33.

[42] Greenman Y, Golani N, Gilad S, Yaron M, Limor R, Stern N. Ghrelin secretion is modulated in a nutrient- and gender-specific manner. Clin Endocrinol (Oxf) 2004;60(3):382–8.

[43] Leidy HJ, Gardner JK, Frye BR, et al. Circulating ghrelin is sensitive to changes in body weight during a diet and exercise program in normal-weight young women. J Clin Endocrinol Metab 2004;89(6):2659–64.

[44] Patterson M, Bloom SR, Gardiner JV. Ghrelin and appetite control in humans—potential application in the treatment of obesity. Peptides 2011;32(11):2290–4.

[45] Reinehr T, Roth CL, Alexy U, Kersting M, Kiess W, Andler W. Ghrelin levels before and after reduction of overweight due to a

low-fat high-carbohydrate diet in obese children and adolescents. Int J Obes (Lond) 2005;29(4):362–8.
[46] Park TG, Hong HR, Lee J, Kang HS. Lifestyle plus exercise intervention improves metabolic syndrome markers without change in adiponectin in obese girls. Ann Nutr Metab 2007;51(3):197–203.
[47] Keogh JB, Brinkworth GD, CliFTOn PM. Effects of weight loss on a low-carbohydrate diet on flow-mediated dilatation, adhesion molecules and adiponectin. Br J Nutr 2007;98(4):852–9.
[48] Behre CJ, Gummesson A, Jernas M, et al. Dissociation between adipose tissue expression and serum levels of adiponectin during and after diet-induced weight loss in obese subjects with and without the metabolic syndrome. Metabolism 2007;56(8):1022–8.
[49] Monzillo LU, Hamdy O, Horton ES, et al. Effect of lifestyle modification on adipokine levels in obese subjects with insulin resistance. Obes Res 2003;11(9):1048–54.
[50] Kopp HP, Krzyzanowska K, Mohlig M, Spranger J, Pfeiffer AF, Schernthaner G. Effects of marked weight loss on plasma levels of adiponectin, markers of chronic subclinical inflammation and insulin resistance in morbidly obese women. Int J Obes (Lond) 2005;29(7):766–71.
[51] Lammert A, Kratzsch J, Selhorst J, et al. Clinical benefit of a short term dietary oatmeal intervention in patients with type 2 diabetes and severe insulin resistance: a pilot study. Exp Clin Endocrinol Diabetes 2008;116(2):132–4.
[52] Fasshauer M, Paschke R, Stumvoll M. Adiponectin, obesity, and cardiovascular disease. Biochimie 2004;86(11):779–84.
[53] Lu JY, Huang KC, Chang LC, et al. Adiponectin: a biomarker of obesity-induced insulin resistance in adipose tissue and beyond. J Biomed Sci 2008;15(5):565–76.
[54] Kamari Y, Peleg E, Herman MO, Bursztyn M, Grossman E, Sharabi Y. The effect of chronic hyperinsulinemia on plasma adiponectin levels in Sprague-Dawley rats. Horm Metab Res 2009;41(1):46–9.
[55] Ouchi N, Kihara S, Funahashi T, Matsuzawa Y, Walsh K. Obesity, adiponectin and vascular inflammatory disease. Curr Opin Lipidol 2003;14(6):561–6.
[56] Gil-Campos M, Aguilera CM, Ramirez-Tortosa MC, Canete R, Gil A. Fasting and postprandial relationships among plasma leptin, ghrelin, and insulin in prepubertal obese children. Clin Nutr 29(1):54–9.
[57] Ouchi N, Walsh K. A novel role for adiponectin in the regulation of inflammation. Arterioscler Thromb Vasc Biol 2008;28(7):1219–21.
[58] Greenberg AS, Obin MS. Obesity and the role of adipose tissue in inflammation and metabolism. Am J Clin Nutr 2006;83(2): 461S–5S.
[59] Shetty S, Kusminski CM, Scherer PE. Adiponectin in health and disease: evaluation of adiponectin-targeted drug development strategies. Trends Pharmacol Sci 2009;30(5):234–9.
[60] Kubota N, Terauchi Y, Kubota T, et al. Pioglitazone ameliorates insulin resistance and diabetes by both adiponectin-dependent and -independent pathways. J Biol Chem 2006;281(13):8748–55.
[61] Evans RM, Barish GD, Wang YX. PPARs and the complex journey to obesity. Nat Med 2004;10(4):355–61.
[62] Towler MC, Hardie DG. AMP-activated protein kinase in metabolic control and insulin signaling. Circ Res 2007;100(3): 328–41.
[63] Sharabi Y, Oron-Herman M, Kamari Y, et al. Effect of PPAR-gamma agonist on adiponectin levels in the metabolic syndrome: lessons from the high fructose fed rat model. Am J Hypertens 2007;20(2):206–10.
[64] Kubota N, Yano W, Kubota T, et al. Adiponectin stimulates AMP-activated protein kinase in the hypothalamus and increases food intake. Cell Metab 2007;6(1):55–68.
[65] Jay MA, Ren J. Peroxisome proliferator-activated receptor (PPAR) in metabolic syndrome and type 2 diabetes mellitus. Curr Diabetes Rev 2007;3(1):33–9.
[66] Li AC, Glass CK. PPAR- and LXR-dependent pathways controlling lipid metabolism and the development of atherosclerosis. J Lipid Res 2004;45(12):2161–73.
[67] Guri AJ, Hontecillas R, Bassaganya-Riera J. Dietary modulators of peroxisome proliferator-activated receptors: implications for the prevention and treatment of metabolic syndrome. J Nutrigenet Nutrigenomics 2008;1(3):126–35.
[68] Mannucci E, Monami M, Lamanna C, Gensini GF, Marchionni N. Pioglitazone and cardiovascular risk. A comprehensive meta-analysis of randomized clinical trials. Diabetes Obes Metab 2008;10(12):1221–38.
[69] Tobin JF, Freedman LP. Nuclear receptors as drug targets in metabolic diseases: new approaches to therapy. Trends Endocrinol Metab 2006;17(7):284–90.
[70] Kim YD, Park KG, Lee YS, et al. Metformin inhibits hepatic gluconeogenesis through AMP-activated protein kinase-dependent regulation of the orphan nuclear receptor SHP. Diabetes 2008;57(2):306–14.
[71] Zhang BB, Zhou G, Li C. AMPK: an emerging drug target for diabetes and the metabolic syndrome. Cell Metab 2009;9(5):407–16.
[72] Bolen S, Feldman L, Vassy J, et al. Systematic review: comparative effectiveness and safety of oral medications for type 2 diabetes mellitus. Ann Intern Med 2007;147(6):386–99.
[73] Andres E, Noel E, Goichot B. Metformin-associated vitamin B12 deficiency. Arch Intern Med 2002;162(19):2251–2.
[74] Khurana R, Malik IS. Metformin: safety in cardiac patients. Heart 2010;96(2):99–102.
[75] Fruchart JC, Duriez P. Mode of action of fibrates in the regulation of triglyceride and HDL-cholesterol metabolism. Drugs Today (Barc) 2006;42(1):39–64.
[76] Fruchart JC, Duriez P, Staels B. Peroxisome proliferator-activated receptor-alpha activators regulate genes governing lipoprotein metabolism, vascular inflammation and atherosclerosis. Curr Opin Lipidol 1999;10(3):245–57.
[77] Fruchart JC, Staels B, Duriez P. PPARS, metabolic disease and atherosclerosis. Pharmacol Res 2001;44(5):345–52.
[78] McClure DL, Valuck RJ, Glanz M, Murphy JR, Hokanson JE. Statin and statin-fibrate use was significantly associated with increased myositis risk in a managed care population. J Clin Epidemiol 2007;60(8):812–8.
[79] Amend KL, Landon J, Thyagarajan V, Niemcryk S, McAfee A. Incidence of hospitalized rhabdomyolysis with statin and fibrate use in an insured US population. Ann Pharmacother 45(10):1230–9.

PART H

MICROMOLECULES AND NUTRIENTS AS MODULATORS OF VISCERAL FAT

CHAPTER

36

Effects of Different Dietary Fatty Acids on Human Energy Balance, Body Weight, Fat Mass, and Abdominal Fat

Sze Yen Tan

University of South Australia, School of Pharmacy and Medical Sciences, Adelaide, Australia

INTRODUCTION

A shift in energy supply leads to a transition from malnutrition as a major public health concern in the last century to the high prevalence of overweight and obesity in the present. The body mass index (BMI), calculated as weight in kilograms ÷ (height in meters)^2, provides a quick and easy way to classify body weight status [1], but this approached has been criticized because global BMI cutoffs may not be appropriate for certain groups of individuals such as children, older adults, certain ethnic groups, or athletes with a higher lean mass [2–5]. Body fat and its distribution have been proposed to be used in conjunction with BMI as an additional criterion for overweight and obesity diagnosis because these indices also predict obesity-related comorbidities [6]. Specifically, central overweight or obesity, defined as a BMI greater than 25 kg/m^2, plus the accumulation of adipose tissues in the upper body has been shown to be an independent predictor of several metabolic diseases [7]. Weight loss strategies that promote abdominal fat loss are thus the priority of medical nutrition therapy.

While the etiology of overweight and obesity in the population is not known, it has been suggested that the weight problem we face is predominantly caused by an increase in food supply [8] and less so by reduced physical activity over the past few decades [9,10]. In general, excessive body weight is a result of cumulative positive energy balance, a condition in which energy intake exceeds energy expenditure in the body. While this view offers a straightforward strategy for weight management in a clinical setting (e.g. eat less and exercise more to reverse the positive energy balance) [11–13], it oversimplifies the problem by omitting many important aspects of overweight and obesity such as (1) taste, food environment, socioeconomic status, convenience, and food affordability that collectively determine food selection, purchase, and consumption [14]; (2) multiple dietary factors (e.g. rheology, portion size, energy density, and types of foods) that regulate appetite and food intake [15–20]; (3) dietary components that exert differential physiological and metabolic responses in the body [21–27]; and (4) occupational and environmental factors that can influence level of the physical activity [28–30]. This chapter will focus primarily on the roles of dietary fat on human energy balance and discuss how a shift in energy balance by dietary fat alterations can translate into body weight, body composition, and body fat distribution differences. Dietary fat was chosen as the topic of review due to the controversies it has generated in the past, as well as a renewed interest concerning its role in causing obesity [31,32]. Scientific evidence suggests that dietary fat may not necessarily be detrimental; it may even be beneficial if the right amount and types of dietary fat are included in a healthy balanced diet.

DIETARY FAT AND HUMAN ENERGY BALANCE

Humans obtain energy from three macronutrients in the diet: carbohydrates, fats, and proteins. Although alcohol also supplies energy to the body, it is not regarded as a nutrient and the adverse effects of alcohol may outweigh the energy it provides, especially in an environment where excessive energy intake is already a major health concern. One view proposes that dietary fat is the major contributor to the increasing prevalence

Nutrition in the Prevention and Treatment of Abdominal Obesity
http://dx.doi.org/10.1016/B978-0-12-407869-7.00036-2

of overweight and obesity. Furthermore, a lower consumption of dietary fat is often recommended in the context of weight maintenance and weight loss because of its adverse impacts on energy balance. In terms of energy intake, dietary fat has the highest energy density (9 kcal/g) compared to dietary carbohydrate and protein (both 4 kcal/g). Foods higher in fat, either naturally or after processing and cooking, are also reported to be more palatable [33], and highly palatable foods are associated with greater intake [34,35].

At the opposite end of the energy balance equation, dietary fat is the least thermogenic when compared with other macronutrients (in the order of protein > carbohydrate > fat), where the digestion, absorption, metabolism, and excretion of fat is associated with the least loss of energy [36]. This is particularly problematic to the population at risk for or already overweight and obese. Highest per-gram energy content of fat, coupled with its low thermic effect means that most of the energy from fat is available to the body, either as fuel or as storage. Furthermore, there exists a hierarchy of macronutrient oxidation, in which macronutrients with limited storage in the body such as proteins and carbohydrates are preferentially oxidized (so that they are minimally retained in the body), while dietary fat is often the last substrate to be oxidized due to the relatively unlimited storage capacity of adipose tissues [36]. This is particularly the case during positive energy balance because the oxidation of dietary fat is often suppressed due to the prioritization of protein and carbohydrate oxidation and excretion [37,38].

However, a diet very low in fat should not be advocated because dietary fat plays other important roles. To name a few examples, dietary fat is essential in supporting healthy brain/neural cell development, the integrity of cell membranes, the digestion and absorption of fat-soluble vitamins, and maintaining healthy skin and hair [39]. From nutritional and dietary perspectives, it is challenging, if not impossible, to drastically reduce dietary fat because most foods contain fat in various proportions. Furthermore, it should be noted that dietary fat is a collective term, which includes three categories of fatty acids (based on their degrees of saturation) in the diet: saturated fat (SFA), monounsaturated fat (MUFA), and polyunsaturated fat (PUFA). Evidence shows that these three types of fat evoke different physiological responses that may have an impact on energy balance, body weight, and body composition (presented in the following sections). If true, it implies that one should not put efforts into limiting total dietary fat intake alone, but instead emphasize increasing the proportion of dietary subtypes that can preferentially support body weight and fat mass loss. The potential benefits of dietary fat type manipulation are depicted in Fig. 36.1.

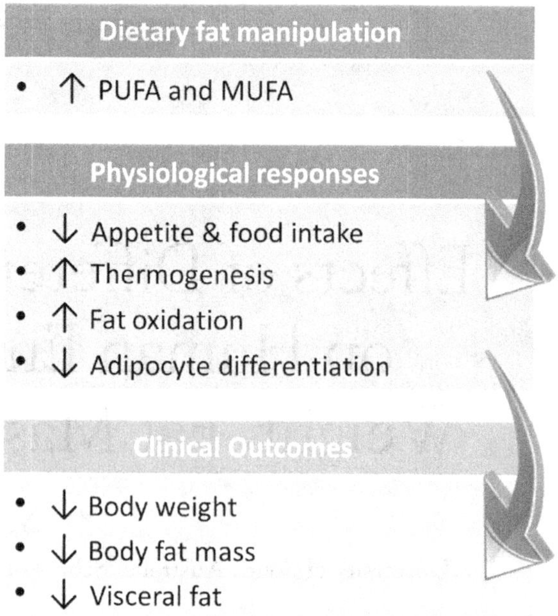

FIGURE 36.1 Dietary fat manipulation and clinical outcomes: a theoretical framework. MUFA, monounsaturated fat; PUFA, polyunsaturated fat. (See color plate at the back of the book.)

PHYSIOLOGICAL EFFECTS OF DIFFERENT DIETARY FAT SUBTYPES

Appetite and Dietary Intake

Appetite is a collective term that describes internal sensations related to feeding behaviors. Appetitive sensations are typically measured in acute studies that use preload designs, in which subjects are provided with a test food and followed by the measurement of appetitive responses using various methods. The appetite of animals is commonly assessed by quantifying their food intake after a preload, but multiple approaches are used to measure human appetite sensations. The most common approach is the subjective assessment of self-reported sensations such as hunger, fullness, desire to eat, and prospective consumption on visual analog scales (VAS) [40,41]. These sensations are representative of different aspects of human appetite, i.e. the hunger sensation initiates food-seeking behaviors and an eating event, satiety (opposite of hunger) prolongs the latency of meals, the fullness sensation determines the amount of food consumed or size of an eating event (also known as satiation), and the desire-to-eat sensation promotes eating either in the presence or absence of hunger. Objective measurements are also used in conjunction with subjective measurements: these measurements include quantification of the amount of challenge meal consumed by participants or meal latency (amount of time elapsed before the initiation of next eating event) after a test preload [42]. Although not widely accepted, the measurements of gut peptides, e.g. anorexic hormones such as cholecystokinin (CCK), glucagon-like-protein-1 (GLP-1), gastric inhibitory polypeptide [glucose-dependent insulinotropic peptide (GIP)], protein YY (PYY), and leptin, and the orexigenic hormone ghrelin, have been used as biomarkers for appetite [43].

A number of studies have reported differential effects of dietary macronutrients on human appetite. Protein was observed to be the most satiating macronutrient, followed by carbohydrate, while fat was the least satiating. However, other studies have failed to observe differential effects on appetite between these macronutrients after controlling for the energy density of test meals [26,44]. This raises an important question of whether the higher satiating effect of protein and carbohydrate compared to fat was confounded by other dietary factors, such as the volume, fiber content, portion size, and food form (solid versus liquid preloads) of the test meals employed in these studies. Palatability and other sensory aspects of the test meals have also been shown to influence human appetite: individuals who were repeatedly provided similar foods or meals reported reducing levels of appetite over time relative to an uneaten food. This phenomenon is referred to as sensory-specific satiety [45–47].

Within the same macronutrient type, fats with different carbon chain length and degree of saturation have been observed to have different effects on human appetite. In one human study, 6g of unsaturated fats (MUFA and PUFA) delivered via a nasoileal catheter, were shown to significantly increase fullness and reduce hunger sensations in 15 healthy adults. These appetitive effects may be mediated by increased CCK secretion. However, these appetitive sensations failed to translate into lower subsequent meal intake 75min after nasoileal fat infusion [48]. Another study further revealed that PUFA, consumed as part of a meal, suppressed appetite more than MUFA or SFA, and resulted in lower consumption of a subsequent meal in 40 healthy adults. However, many other human studies have failed to document the differential effects of fat subtypes on human appetite reported by these two studies [49–54]. The lack of effects of PUFA on food intake was also supported by observations from animal studies [55,56]. Investigation into the effect of supplementation with conjugated linoleic acid [(CLA; a group of PUFA that exists as positional and stereoisomers of octadecadienoic acid (C18:2)] on animal feed intake was also inconclusive (see reviews [57,58]). The beneficial effects of PUFA on human appetite regulation remain inconclusive, and the reasons for the conflicting results between human studies may be a result of the lack of measurement sensitivity, between-individual variability, or subtlety of the true appetitive effects of PUFA [59].

Thermogenesis

Relative to dietary protein and carbohydrate, dietary fat has been reported to have a low thermic effect, and is the last macronutrient to be oxidized in the human body. However, some evidence has shown that these observations may not hold for, or cannot be generalized to, all fat types. In an acute crossover feeding study in which 29 adult participants were fed three isoenergetic diets that were high in SFA from dairy products, high in MUFA from olive oil, or high in PUFA from walnuts, significantly higher postprandial energy expenditure (for 5h) was observed following the consumption of MUFA- and PUFA-rich diets when compared to a SFA-rich diet. The thermic effect of food for PUFA and MUFA diets were reported to be 12.3% and 11.8%, respectively, and only 9.6% in the SFA diet ($P < 0.05$) [53]. In another crossover study, a diet high in MUFA maintained, while an isoenergetic high-SFA diet significantly decreased, total daily energy expenditure after 28days of consumption [60]. The underlying mechanisms of elevated thermic effect by unsaturated fats may be due to an increase in the expression of *UCP2* mRNA (encoding mitochondrial uncoupling protein 2) in the liver and *UCP3* mRNA in skeletal muscle, as previously demonstrated in animal studies [56,61–63]. CLA has also been shown to increase the expression of uncoupling proteins and oxygen consumption (for underlying mechanisms please refer to [57,64,65]). However, it should be noted that other human studies that prescribed higher levels of MUFA and PUFA in the experimental diets failed to document the thermogenic effects of PUFA [66–69], thus raising the question of whether the thermogenic effects of PUFA shown by the first study was amplified by the higher total fat (50% of total energy), PUFA (33% of total energy), or the energy content of the test diet. Nevertheless, one study reported that the thermogenic effect of MUFA was only observed in the overweight but not the lean population [70].

Fat Oxidation

In addition to thermogenesis, the level of dietary fat saturation has been shown to be an important factor in determining fat oxidation rates in the body. A study in which human subjects were fed ^{13}C-labeled fatty acids with similar carbon chain lengths but differing degrees of saturation observed that the highest recovery of ^{13}C from the breath over a 24-h period (indicating higher oxidation rates) followed the consumption of MUFA (oleic acid; C18:1), followed by PUFA (linoleic acid; C18:2n-6), and the least occurred with SFA (stearic acid; C18:0) [71]. Observations from this study were later confirmed by another study, which also found higher oxidation rates of MUFA (oleic acid) and PUFA (α-linolenic acid;

C18:3n-3) [72]. However, in a more recent study, PUFA (linoleic and α-linolenic acids) were observed to be more rapidly oxidized than MUFA (oleic acid), which in turn were oxidized faster than SFA (stearic acid) during a 9-h measurement period [73]. Overall, the postprandial oxidation rates of unsaturated fats appear to be higher than those of SFA.

Besides using a stable isotope method, the oxidation rate of different macronutrients can also be evaluated through gaseous exchange, namely carbon dioxide production (VCO_2) and oxygen consumption (VO_2), measured with an indirect calorimeter, and urinary nitrogen excretion [74,75]. In animals, fat oxidation was significantly increased in broiler chickens fed PUFA (linseed oil and sunflower oil) compared to those fed SFA (beef tallow) [76]. Rats fed a PUFA (safflower oil) diet and CLA also exhibited higher oxygen consumption and fat oxidation than those fed a SFA-rich diet [61,77]. Higher beta-oxidation of fat is partly due to PUFA-induced higher levels of muscle carnitine *O*-palmitoyltransferase 1 (CPT1-M) and mitochondrial hydroxyacyl-coenzyme A dehydrogenase (HCDH) [78], as well as carnitine *O*-palmitoyltransferase 1 (CPT-1) in skeletal muscle [79–81]. Findings from an acute human feeding study showed a similar trend: diets high in PUFA and MUFA increased fat oxidation (albeit not in a statistically significant manner), in contrast to decreased fat oxidation observed with a high-SFA diet [53,70]. In a short-term study, replacing 6g of visible fat with PUFA as fish oil for 3weeks also successfully and significantly increased fat oxidation in humans [68]. The increase in fat oxidation was accompanied by a decrease in carbohydrate oxidation.

Gaseous exchanges can also be used to calculate the respiratory quotient ($RQ = VCO_2 \div VO_2$). The RQs of carbohydrate, protein, and fat are approximately 1.00, 0.80, and 0.67, respectively. A diet comprised of three macronutrients in various proportions will produce an average 24-h RQ of between 0.67 and 1.00. A shift in RQ toward 1.00 indicates an increase in carbohydrate oxidation, while a decrease in RQ indicates enhanced fat oxidation in the body. Using RQ as an indicator of substrate oxidation, animals that were fed PUFA (fish oil and sunflower oil) has significantly lower RQs than those fed SFA (beef tallow) [82]. In a human study, participants who followed a high-MUFA diet for 28days also showed a significant decrease in RQ compared to those who followed a high-SFA diet [60]. In another 6-month study, RQ was also observed to be significantly lower when participants followed a high-MUFA diet [69]. Three weeks of fish oil (PUFA) supplementation (6g/day) also significantly reduces RQ [68]. Together, the findings of these studies suggest that the fat oxidation-enhancing effects of PUFA and MUFA can be maintained over the short and longer terms.

Adipose Tissue Differentiation and Metabolism

Understanding adipose tissue growth and its metabolism is critical for weight management or the prevention of adipose tissue accumulation. Although dietary fat has been shown to be the least oxidized macronutrient (relative to dietary protein and carbohydrate, and hence easily deposited in the adipose tissues), increased PUFA intake suppresses adipose tissue differentiation in animals. Mechanistic studies in animal models also reported downregulation of genes encoding adipocyte fatty acid-binding protein (*Fabp4/aP2*) and complement factor D [adipsin (*Cfd*)] [55]; both these proteins are abundant during adipocyte differentiation [83]. Therefore, the reversal of adipocyte differentiation through the suppression of *aP2* and *Cfd* gene expression may have important implications for obesity treatment. However, PUFA does not have an effect on the size of adipocytes [84]. The inhibition of adipocyte differentiation was also partly achieved through the modulation of lipolysis, lipogenesis, and adipokine and cytokine levels. Specifically, PUFA decreased the levels of mRNA encoding fatty acid synthase (FAS), lipoprotein lipase (LPL), hormone-sensitive lipase (HSL), phosphoenolpyruvate carboxykinase (PEPCK), CCAAT/enhancer-binding protein alpha (C/EBPα), and leptin, predominantly in the visceral, but not the subcutaneous, fat pool [84]. Genes that encode proteins that regulate oxidative metabolism, e.g. peroxisome proliferator-activated receptor alpha (PPAR-α), PPAR-γ coactivator 1 alpha (PGC-1α), and nuclear respiratory factor-1 (NRF1), were also upregulated by increased PUFA intake [85,86]. PUFA in the form of CLA also suppresses adipocyte differentiation, fatty acid transportation, and lipogenesis, and increases proteins that promote fat oxidation in animals and humans [57,65]. CLA has also been shown to promote the apoptosis of preadipocytes and adipocytes, leading to a reduction in adipose cell numbers [87,88].

The effect of PUFA on adipose tissue differentiation and metabolism appears to be specific to visceral adipose tissue because the elevated expression of these genes was found only in the epididymal fat pad of animals fed high-PUFA diets [76,86]. The fact that PUFA preferentially targets visceral fat metabolism may have additional benefits for overweight and obese individuals [89] because visceral adipose tissue is an independent predictor of insulin resistance and other metabolic conditions due to its proximity to organs (e.g. the liver) and its high lipolytic activities [90–95].

Effects of Unsaturated Fats on Body Weight and Fat Mass

Cross-sectional studies have revealed a number of correlations between dietary fat subtype intake, fatty

TABLE 36.1 A Summary of Studies on the Effects of Fat Subtypes on Body Weight, Total Fat Mass, and Abdominal Fat in Humans

Study	Design	Duration	Participants	Intervention	Control	Outcomes		
						Weight	Fat Mass	Abdominal Fat
Walker [101]	Crossover	3 months	16 adults with T2DM	MUFA (olive oil)	CHO	–	N.S.	Lower UF:LF ratio in MUFA
Piers [103]	Crossover	4 weeks	8 overweight / obese men	MUFA (olive oil)	SFA (cream)	Greater weight loss in MUFA	Greater fat mass loss in MUFA	Greater trunk fat loss in MUFA
Paniagua [102]	Crossover	28 days	11 adults with insulin resistance	MUFA (olive oil)	SFA, CHO	N.S.	N.S.	Lower UF in MUFA and SFA than CHO
Luscombe-Marsh [106]	RCT	16 weeks	57 overweight adults	MUFA (various)	Protein	N.S.	N.S.	–
Wien [107]	RCT	24 weeks	65 overweight adults	MUFA (almonds)	CHO	Greater weight loss in MUFA	Greater fat mass loss in MUFA	Greater WC loss in MUFA
Summers [114]	Crossover	5 weeks	17 adults (lean, overweight, T2DM)	PUFA (spread and oil)	SFA	N.S.	N.S.	Lower SAT in females; lower VAT in T2DM
Tapsell [116]	RCT	6 months	58 adults with T2DM	PUFA (walnut)	SFA	N.S.	N.S. (trend of lower fat mass)	–
Tapsell [117]	RCT	12 months	35 adults with T2DM	PUFA (walnut)	SFA	N.S.	N.S.	N.S. (trends of lower SAT and higher VAT)
Tapsell [118]	RCT	12 weeks	150 adults	PUFA (various)	SFA	N.S.	N.S.	N.S. (trends of lower SAT and higher VAT)
Couet [68]	Crossover	3 weeks	6 adults	PUFA (fish oil)	Visible fat	N.S.	Greater fat mass loss in PUFA	–
Thorsdottir [115]	RCT	8 weeks	324 overweight young adults	PUFA (fish oil and fish)	PUFA (sunflower oil)	Greater weight loss in males in fish oil and fish groups	N.S.	Greater WC loss in males in fish oil and fish groups
Krebs [119]	RCT	24 weeks	93 women with insulin resistance	PUFA (fish oil)	Placebo oil	N.S.	N.S.	N.S. in WC and abdominal fat changes
Hill [120]	RCT	12 weeks	65 overweight adults	PUFA (fish oil)	PUFA (sunflower oil)	N.S.	Lower gain in fish oil group	–
Munro [121]	RCT	12 weeks	35 overweight adults	PUFA (fish oil)	MUFA	N.S.	N.S.	–

CHO, carbohydrate; LF, lower body fat; MUFA, monounsaturated fat; PUFA, polyunsaturated fat; RCT, randomized controlled, parallel-arm trial; SAT, subcutaneous adipose tissue; SFA, saturated fat; T2DM, type 2 diabetes; UF, upper body fat; LF, lower body fat; UF, upper body fat; VAT, visceral adipose tissue WC, waist circumference (indicator of upper body fat). N.S., no significant difference between control and intervention groups.

acid composition of adipose tissues, and fat mass distribution. Abdominal fat is positively correlated with habitual SFA intake [96], but negatively associated with dietary MUFA and n-3 PUFA intake [97]. Adherence to a Mediterranean diet (high in unsaturated fat and other healthy dietary components) was also related to a lower waist circumference. Waist circumference is commonly used as a clinical indicator of upper body or abdominal fat accumulation [98]. The analysis of adipose tissue biopsies in cross-sectional studies found that the size of subcutaneous and visceral adipocytes was negatively associated with dietary PUFA intake, while adipocyte cell number negatively correlated with MUFA and positively correlated with SFA intake [99]. The fatty acid content of visceral fat was also higher in SFA and lower in unsaturated fatty acids compared to subcutaneous fat [97,100], suggesting that the visceral fat depot is a major storage site of SFA. Collectively, epidemiological data appear to support a potential protective role for unsaturated fat against body fat mass accumulation, especially in the abdominal region. However, causation cannot be established based on epidemiological studies. In contrast to epidemiological data, a randomized, controlled trial design can demonstrate cause-and-effect relationships between dietary fat subtypes and body fat mass distribution.

Various strategies have been used in randomized controlled trials to achieve target dietary fat levels, ranging from the use of dietary supplements or substitutions (e.g. oil capsules and cooking oil) to the inclusion of foods rich in dietary unsaturated fats (e.g. nuts, olives). The use of a whole-food approach is a double-edge sword: while this approach is more aligned to and compatible with habitual dietary intake, it limits researchers' ability to attribute intervention outcomes to fat subtype effects alone, since many other dietary factors are contributed by the prescribed foods (for example, fiber and protein in nuts). These other dietary components may also dilute the effects of fat manipulation, leading to small or insignificant clinical outcomes, as documented in some of the following studies (Table 36.1).

Monounsaturated Fats

The effects of increased MUFA intake on body weight and body composition were investigated using a within-subject crossover and a randomized controlled experimental design (Table 36.1). In one crossover study, 16 adults with type 2 diabetes mellitus (T2DM) received two test diets, one high in carbohydrate and another high in MUFA (from olive oil), for 3 months per diet (separated by a 1-month washout period). Total body fat mass decreased after the intervention periods but was not significantly different between the two diets. However, there appeared to be a trend of different fat mass loss patterns: participants lost upper body fat with the MUFA diet but gained upper body fat slightly during the high-carbohydrate diet. When examined as a ratio of upper-to-lower body fat mass, the high-carbohydrate diet induced a significantly higher ratio than the high-MUFA diet ($P < 0.01$) [101]. A more recent crossover study that fed 11 insulin-resistant adults high-SFA, high-MUFA, and high-carbohydrate diets in a random order for 28 days each also failed to document additional effects of increased MUFA intake on body weight and fat mass loss. However, the MUFA-rich diet did prevent upper body fat accumulation that was induced by the high-carbohydrate diet. Consequently, the upper-to-lower body fat ratio was significantly higher in that diet group [102]. Similar to the aforementioned studies, one study documented greater upper body fat loss after following a high-MUFA diet (vs. a high-SFA diet) for 4 weeks [103]. This study also recorded significant losses in body weight and total body fat mass, which was not found in the other two studies. Differences in the study populations may explain the contradictory observations regarding total body fat mass loss: studies that included adults with T2DM or insulin resistance reported no additional benefits of MUFA on body weight and fat mass, while studies that recruited healthy male adults did. Impaired fatty acid oxidation has been previously reported in adults with T2DM [104,105].

The randomized controlled, parallel-arm studies that tested the effects of MUFA on body weight and body composition are limited, and were conducted using a weight loss paradigm. In one study, 57 overweight and obese adults were randomly assigned to follow a low-fat, high-protein (30% fat, 35% protein) or a high-fat, standard-protein (45% fat high in MUFA from mixed nuts and canola oil and 18% protein) diet [106]. During the first 12 weeks of this trial, energy restriction was prescribed to promote weight loss; this was followed by an energy balance period of 4 weeks. This study did not find significant differences in body weight and fat mass loss between the two diets. The lack of effects of MUFA in this trial may be due to (1) the simultaneous manipulation of two dietary components (e.g. protein and fat); (2) the absence of a proper control group; (3) subtle acute physiological effects of MUFA that failed to translate into clinical observations; or (4) adaptation of the body to increased dietary MUFA during the study period. However, these possibilities are yet to be evaluated.

Another randomized controlled trial compared the weight- and fat-mass-reducing effects of a high-MUFA (from almonds) vs. a high-carbohydrate energy-restricted diet for 24 weeks [107]. Like the previous study, the two intervention diets differed in more than one aspect: the MUFA diet contained higher total fat and lower carbohydrate (39% fat, 32% carbohydrate) than the high-carbohydrate diet (19% fat, 53% carbohydrate). In this study, greater reductions in weight (−18% vs. −11%), fat mass (−30% vs. 20%), and waist circumference (an indicator of abdominal fat; −14% vs. −9%) were observed in the high-MUFA group, although it should be pointed out that these superior clinical outcomes may not be attributable to MUFA alone. Almonds (the vehicle of MUFA used in this study) influence energy balance by promoting satiety [108,109] and dietary compensation [110–112], and the absorption of dietary fat from almonds is lower than previously thought [113]. In summary, the presence of confounding factors in the intervention studies limits the ability to draw conclusions as to whether MUFA has therapeutic effects on body weight and total fat mass reduction. More longer-term and better-controlled intervention trials are therefore warranted.

Polyunsaturated Fats: Long Chain, Very Long Chain, and Conjugated Linoleic Acid

In a randomized crossover study, body weight, total body fat mass, and abdominal fat mass changes were not significantly different in 17 participants who consumed a diet high in either SFA or PUFA for 5 weeks (Table 36.1) [114]. The effects of PUFA on weight and fat mass were also examined in randomized controlled trials. Except for one clinical trial [115], no additional weight loss was observed with increased PUFA intake [68,116–120]. The prescription of CLA, a subtype of PUFA, also did not promote greater weight loss in most clinical trials, as documented in a systematic review [58]. Two studies that prescribed high-PUFA diets enriched with walnuts [predominantly linoleic acid (C18:2n-6) and α-linolenic acid (C18:3n-3)] to individuals with T2DM observed a trend of decreasing total body fat mass with increasing PUFA in the diet after 6 and 12 months [116,117]. Studies that prescribed fish oil (very-long-chain PUFA) also reported either a greater decrease in fat mass [68] or a prevention of fat mass gain [120]. However, a comparable number of studies failed to reproduce the fat mass-reducing effects of fish oil [115,119,121]. Based on two systematic reviews of randomized controlled trials, CLA supplements also did not promote fat mass loss in most studies [58,122]. Nonetheless, a meta-analysis in humans showed that a minimum dose of 3.2 g/day is required to produce a modest fat mass loss.

In addition to anthropometric measurements, a number of studies also assessed visceral and subcutaneous adipose tissue areas in the abdominal region (at the L4 level) using a magnetic resonance imaging or a computed tomography method. Researchers in a crossover study observed that a PUFA-rich diet preferentially and significantly reduced abdominal subcutaneous fat in females and those who did not have T2DM. PUFA was found to have limited effects on the abdominal visceral fat pool, except for in individuals with diabetes who documented a greater decrease with the high-PUFA diet in the same study [114]. In two randomized controlled, parallel-arm studies, increased PUFA intake was observed to prevent the redistribution of fat into the subcutaneous depot during energy balance and promote greater subcutaneous fat loss during hypoenergetic conditions, but it inhibited visceral fat loss under both energy balance or hypoenergetic conditions (although interaction effects were not statistically significant) [117,118].

Visceral fat forms part of the total body fat mass; it has been demonstrated that visceral fat loss is allometric (proportionate to) total body fat mass loss [123]. Therefore, the independent comparison of visceral fat changes between control and intervention groups in the aforementioned clinical trials may be problematic without considering total fat mass loss. In fact, reanalysis of data from multiple weight loss studies that reported significant visceral fat loss revealed that different types of weight loss strategies (e.g. energy restriction, exercise, or gastric bypass surgery) did not promote additional loss of visceral fat mass after adjusting for total body fat mass loss [124]. Data analysis from our trials also found that PUFA did not preferentially increase visceral fat loss; the observed effects were mainly attributable to energy restriction [125]. The beneficial effects of PUFA on subcutaneous fat reduction appear to be consistent throughout human studies, but the lack of its effect on the abdominal visceral fat pool in human subjects remains unexplained. In contrast, animal studies have consistently reported abdominal visceral fat loss rather than subcutaneous fat loss with increased PUFA intake [55,56,78,82,85,126,127]. Differences between animal and human studies may be caused by (1) inherent physiological differences; (2) differences in visceral fat quantification (e.g. separation of fat from animal carcasses vs. imaging technique used in humans); (3) the dose of PUFA relative to body mass; (4) differences in fat subtypes and methods of delivery; and (5) lack of analysis standardization between animal and human models.

CONCLUSIONS AND RECOMMENDATIONS

Dietary PUFA induces several postprandial physiological responses that modulate appetite, food intake, energy expenditure, adipose tissue metabolism, and fat oxidation. For these reasons, PUFA is a potential candidate to help achieve a negative energy balance, support weight loss, and reduce fat mass, especially in the abdominal region. However, available human data suggest that the acute postingestive effects of PUFA manipulation are not sustained, which results in limited or modest body weight and fat mass loss over a longer period of time. Treatment of obesity should also aim to reduce the abdominal visceral fat depot, which is an independent predictor of metabolic syndrome in overweight and obese individuals. While animal studies may have demonstrated the visceral fat-reducing effects of PUFA, these effects are yet to be replicated in humans. To date, the effects of PUFA on weight loss and fat mass reduction in the abdominal region in humans are modest and may be of little clinical importance. Until there is more evidence for the beneficial effects of PUFA, a solid recommendation for PUFA in abdominal adiposity treatment cannot be made. Nonetheless, an increase in the proportion of PUFA within a low-fat diet may be beneficial in other respects such as reducing blood pressure and inflammation, and improving blood lipids and insulin sensitivity [128–131].

Acknowledgments

The author thanks Richard Mattes for his comments and suggestions.

References

[1] World Health Organization. Obesity: preventing and managing the global epidemic. Geneva, 2000.
[2] McCarthy HD, Cole TJ, Fry T, Jebb S, Prentice AM. Body fat reference curves for children. Int J Obes 2006;30:598–602.
[3] Prentice AM, Jebb S. Beyond body mass index. Obesity Reviews 2001;2:141–7.
[4] Romero-Corral A, Somers VK, Sierra-Johnson J, Thomas RJ, Collazo-Clavell ML, Korinek J, et al. Accuracy of body mass index in diagnosing obesity in the adult general population. Int J Obes Relat Metab Disord 2008;32:959–66.
[5] WHO expert consultation . Appropriate body-mass index for Asian populations and its implication for policy abd intervention strategies. The Lancet 2004;363:157–63.
[6] Burkhauser RV, Cawley J. Beyond BMI: the value of more accurate measures of fatness and obesity in social science research. J Health Econ 2008;27:519–29.
[7] Jensen MD. Role of body fat distribution and the metabolic complications of obesity. Journal of Clinical Endocrinology & Metabolism 2008;93:S57–63.
[8] Swinburn BA, Sacks G, Ravussin E. Increased food energy supply is more than sufficient to explain the US epidemic of obesity. Am J Clin Nutr 2009;90:1453–6.
[9] Westerterp KR, Speakman JR. Physical activity energy expenditure has not declined since the 1980s and matches energy expenditures of wild mammals. Int J Obes 2008;32:1256–63.
[10] Dugas LR, Harders R, Merrill S, Ebersole K, Shoham DA, Rush EC, et al. Energy expenditure in adults living in developing compared with industrialized countries: a meta-analysis of doubly-labeled water studies. Am J Clin Nutr 2011;93:427–41.
[11] Hill JO, Peters JC, Wyatt HR. Using the energy gap to address obesity: a commentary. J Am Diet Assoc 2009;11:1848–53.
[12] Swinburn BA, Sacks G, Lo SK, Westerterp KR, Rush EC, Rosenbaum M, et al. Estimating the changes in energy flux that characterize the rise in obesity prevalence. Am J Clin Nutr 2009;89:1723–8.
[13] Veerman JL, Barendregt JJ, van Beeck EF, Seidell JC, Mackenbach JP. Stemming the obesity epidemic: a tantalizing prospect. Obesity (Silver Spring) 2007;15:2365–70.
[14] Swinburn BA, Sacks G, Hall KD, McPherson K, Finegood DT, Moodie ML, et al. The global obesity pandemic: shaped by global drivers and local environments. The Lancet 2011;378:804–14.
[15] Mattes RD. Food palatability, rheology, and meal patterning. Jpen 2008;32:572–4.
[16] Leidy HJ, Apolzan JW, Mattes RD, Campbell WW. Food form and portion size affect postprandial appetite sensations and hormonal responses in healthy, nonobese, older adults. Obesity 2010;18:293–9.
[17] Levitsky DA, Youn T. The more food young adults are served, the more they overeat. J Nutr 2004;134:2546–9.
[18] Rolls BJ, Morris EL, Roe LS. Portion size of food affects energy intake in normal-weight and over-weight men and women. Am J Clin Nutr 2002;76:1207–13.
[19] Rolls BJ, Roe LS, Meengs JS. The effect of large portion sizes on energy intake is sustained for 11 days. Obesity 2007;15:1535–43.
[20] Mattes RD, Campbell WW. Effects of food form and timing of ingestion on appetite and energy intake in lean young adults and in young adults with obesity. J Am Diet Assoc 2009;109:430–7.
[21] Alfenas RC, Mattes RD. Influence of glycemic index/load on glycemic response, appetite, and food intake in healthy humans. Diabetes Care 2005;28:2123–9.
[22] Hill AJ, Blundell JE. Macronutrients and satiety: the effects of a high-protein or high-carbohydrate meal on subjective motivation to eat and food preferences. Nutrition and Behavior 1986;3:133–44.
[23] Labayen I, Diez N, Parra D, Gonzalez A, Martinez JA. Basal and postprandial substrate oxidation rates in obese women receiving two test meals with different protein content. Clin Nutr 2004;23:571–8.
[24] Ludwig DS, Majzoub JA, Al-Zahrani A, Dallal GE, Blanco I, Roberts SB. High glycemic index foods, overeating, and obesity. Pediatrics 1999;103:E26.
[25] Poppitt SD, McCormack DN, Buffenstein R. Short-term effects of macronutrient preloads on appetite and energy intake in lean women. Physiol Behav 1998;64:279–85.
[26] Raben A, Agerholm-Larsen L, Flint A, Holst JJ, Astrup A. Meals with similar energy densities but rich in protein, fat, carbohydrate, or alcohol have different effects on energy expenditure and substrate metabolism but not on appetite and energy intake. Am J Clin Nutr 2003;77:91–100.
[27] Stubbs J, Whybrow S, Mamat N. Macronutrients, feeding behavior, and weight control in humans. In: Harris R, Mattes RD, editors. Appetite and Food Intake. Boca Raton: CRC; 2009. p. 295–322.
[28] Handy SL, Boarnet MG, Ewing R, Killingsworth RE. How the built environment affects physical activity. Am J Prev Med 2002;23:64–73.
[29] Church TS, Thomas DM, Tudor-Locke C, Katzmarzyk PT, Earnest CP, Rodarte RQ, et al. Trends over 5 decades in U.S. occupation-related physical activity and their associations with obesity. PLoS ONE 2011;6:e19657.
[30] Powell-Wiley TM, Ayers CR, de Lemos JA, Lakoski SG, Vega GL, Grundy S, et al. Relationship between perceptions about neighborhood environment and prevalent obesity: data from the dallas heart study. Obesity 2013;21:E14–21.
[31] Bray GA, Paeratakul S, Popkin BM. Dietary fat and obesity: a review of animal, clinical and epidemiological studies. Physiol Behav 2004;82:549–55.

[32] Drewnowski A. The real contribution of added sugars and fats to obesity. Epidemiol Rev 2007;29:160–71.
[33] Drewnowski A, Greenwood MR. Cream and sugar: human preferences for high-fat foods. Physiol Behav 1983;30:629–33.
[34] de Castro JM, Bellisle F, Dalix A-M, Pearcey SM. Palatability and intake relationships in free-living humans: characterization and independence of incluence in North Americans. Physiol Behav 2000;70:343–50.
[35] Sorensen LB, Moller P, Flint A, Martens M, Raben A. Effect of sensory perception of foods on appetite and food intake: a review of studies on humans. Int J Obes Relat Metab Disord 2003;27:1152–66.
[36] Stubbs J, Raben A, Westerterp-Plantenga MS. Macronutrient metabolism and appetite. In: Westerterp-Plantenga MS, , Steffens AB, Tremblay A, editors. Regulation of foods intake and energy expenditure. Edra: Milan; 1999. p. 59–84.
[37] Horton TJ, Drougas H, Brachey A, Reed GW, Peters JC, Hill JO. Fat and carbohydrate overfeeding in humans: different effects on energy storage. Am J Clin Nutr 1995;62:19–29.
[38] McDevitt RM, Poppitt SD, Murgatroyd PR, Prentice AM. Macronutrient disposal during controlled overfeeding with glucose, fructose, sucrose, or fat in lean and obese women. Am J Clin Nutr 2000;72:369–77.
[39] Dunn C. Nutrition decisions. 1st edn. Burlington, MA: Jones & Barlett Learning; 2013.
[40] Flint A, Raben A, Blundell JE, Astrup A. Reproducibility, power and validity of visual analogue scales in assessment of appetite sensations in single test meal studies. Int J Obes 2000;24:38–48.
[41] Stubbs RJ, Hughes DA, Johnstone AM, Rowley E, Reid C, Elia M, et al. The use of visual analogue scales to assess motivation to eat in human subjects: a review of their reliability and validity with an evaluation of new hand-held computerized systems for temporal tracking of appetite ratings. Br J Nutr 2000;84:405–15.
[42] Marmonier C, Chapelot D, Louis-Sylvestre J. Effects of macronutrient content and energy density of snacks consumed in a satiety state on the onset of the next meal. Appetite 2000;34:161–8.
[43] de Graaf C, Blom WA, Smeets PA, Stafleu A, Hendriks HF. Biomarkers of satiation and satiety. Am J Clin Nutr 2004;79:946–61.
[44] De Graaf C, Hulshof T, Westrate JA, Jas P. Short-term effects of different amounts of protein, fats, and carbohydrates on satiety. Am J Clin Nutr 1992;55:33–8.
[45] Brondel L, Romer M, Van Wymelbeke V, Pineau N, Jiang T, Hanus C, et al. Variety enhances food intake in humans: role of sensory-specific satiety. Physiol Behav 2009;97:44–51.
[46] Inman JJ. The role of sensory-specific satiety in attribute-level variety seeking. J Consum Res 2001;28:105–20.
[47] Rolls BJ. Sensory-Specific Satiety. Nutr Rev 1986;44:93–101.
[48] Maljaars J, Romeyn EA, Haddeman E, Peters HPF, Masclee AAM. Effect of fat saturation on satiety, hormone release, and food intake. Am J Clin Nutr 2009;89:1019–24.
[49] French SJ, Conlon CA, Mutuma ST, Arnold M, Read NW, Meijer G, et al. The effects of intestinal infusion of long-chain fatty acids on food intake in humans. Gastroenterology 2000;119:943–6.
[50] Strik CM, Lithander F, McGill A-T, MacGibbon AK, McArdle BH, Poppitt SD. No evidence of differential effects of SFA, MUFA or PUFA on post-ingestive satiety and energy intake: a randomised trial of fatty acid saturation. Nutrition Journal 2010;9:1–12.
[51] Alfenas RC, Mattes RD. Effect of fat sources on satiety. Obes Res 2003;11:183–7.
[52] Iyer SS, Boateng LA, Sales RL, Coelho SB, Lokko P, Monteiro JB, et al. Effects of peanut oil consumption on appetite and food choice. Int J Obes 2006;30:704–10.
[53] Casas-Agustench P, Lopez-Urirte P, Bullo M, Ros E, Gomez-Flores A, Salas-Salvado J. Acute effects of 3 high-fat meals with different saturation on energy expenditure, substrate oxidation and satiety. Clin Nutr 2009;28:39–45.
[54] MacIntosh CG, Holt SHA, Brand-Miller JC. The degree of fat saturation does not alter glycemic, insulinemic or satiety responses to a starchy staple in healthy men. J Nutr 2003;133:2577–80.
[55] Okuno M, Kajiwara K, Imai S, Kobayashi T, Honma N, Maki T, et al. Perilla oil prevents the excessive growth of visceral adipose tissue in rats by down-regulating adipocyte differentiation. J Nutr 1997;127:1752–7.
[56] Hun CH, Hasegawa K, Kawabata T, Kato M, Shimokawa T, Kagawa Y. Increased uncoupling protein2 mRNA in white adipose tissue, and decrease in leptin, visceral fat, blood glucose, and cholesterol in KK-Ay mice fed with eicosapentaenoic and docosahexaenoic acids in addition to linolenic acid. Biochem Biophys Res Commun 1999;259:85–90.
[57] House RL, Cassady JP, Eisen EJ, McIntosh MK, Odle J. Conjugated linoleic acid evokes de-lipidation through the regulation of genes controlling lipid metabolism in adipose and liver tissue. Obesity Reviews 2005;6:247–58.
[58] Li J-J, Huang CJ, Xie D. Anti-obesity effects of conjugated linoleic acid, docosahexanoic acid, and eicosapentanoic acid. Mol Nutr Food Res 2008;52:631–45.
[59] Mattes RD, Hollis J, Hayes D, Stunkard AJ. Appetite: measurement and manipulation misgivings. J Am Diet Assoc 2005;105:S87–97.
[60] Kien CL, Bunn JY, Ugrasbul F. Increasing dietary palmitic acid decreases fat oxidation and daily energy expenditure. Am J Clin Nutr 2005;82:320–6.
[61] Choi JS, Jung MH, Park HS, Song J. Effects of conjugated lioleic acid isomers on insulin resistance and mRNA levels of gene regulating energy metabolism in high-fat-fed rats. Nutrition (Burbank, Los Angeles County, Calif) 2004;20:1008–17.
[62] Ealey KN, El-Sohemy A, Archer MC. Effects of dietary conjugated linoleic acid on the expression of uncoupling proteins in mice and rats. Lipids 2002;37:853–61.
[63] Tsuboyama-Kasaoka N, Takahashi M, Kim H, Ezaki O. Up-regulation of liver uncoupling protein-2 mRNA by either fish oil feeding or fibrate administration in mice. Biochem Biophys Res Commun 1999;257:879–85.
[64] Park Y, Pariza MW. Mechanisms of body fat modulation by conjugated linoleic acid (CLA). Food Res Int 2007;40:311–23.
[65] Belury MA. Dietary conjugated linoleic acid in health: physiological effects and mechanisms of action. Annu Rev Nutr 2002;22:505–31.
[66] Jones PJH, Ridgen JE, Phang PT, Birmingham CL. Influence of dietary fat polyunsaturated to saturated ratio on energy substrate utilization in obesity. Metabolism 1992;41:396–401.
[67] Jones PJH, Schoeller DA. Polyunsaturated: Saturated ratio of diet fat influences energy substrate utilization in the human. Metabolism 1988;37:145–51.
[68] Couet C, Delarue J, Ritz P, Antoine J-M, Lamisse F. Effect of dietary fish oil on body fat mass and basal fat oxidation in healthy adults. Int J Obes 1997;21:637–43.
[69] Rasmussen LG, Larsen TM, Mortensen PK, Due A, Astrup A. Effect on 24-h energy expenditure of a moderate-fat diet high in monounsaturated fatty acids compared with that of a low-fat, carbohydrate-rich diet: a 6-mo controlled dietary intervention trial. Am J Clin Nutr 2007;85:1014–22.
[70] Soares MJ, Cummings SJ, Mamo JCL, Kenrick M, Piers LS. The acute effects of olive oil v. cream on postprandial thermogenesis and substrate oxidation in postmenopausal women. Br J Nutr 2004;91:245–52.

[71] Jones PJ, Pencharz PB, Clandinin MT. Whole body oxidation of dietary fatty acids: implications for energy utilization. Am J Clin Nutr 1985;42:769–77.
[72] Pan DA, Hulbert AJ, Storlien LH. Dietary fats, membrane phospholipids and obesity. J Nutr 1994;124:1555–65.
[73] DeLany JP, Windhauser MM, Champagne CM, Bray GA. Differential oxidation of individual dietary fatty acids in humans. Am J Clin Nutr 2000;72:905–11.
[74] Elia M, Livesey G. Energy expenditure and fuel selection in biological systems: the theory and practice of calculations based on indirect calorimetry and tracer methods. World Review in Nutrition and Dietetics 1992;70:68–131.
[75] Frayn KN. Calculation of substrate oxidation rates in vivo from gaseous exchange. J Appl Physiol 1983;55:628–34.
[76] Crespo N, Esteve-Garcia E. Dietary linseed oil produces lower abdominal fat deposition but higher de novo fatty acid synthesis in broiler chickens. Poult Sci 2002;81:1555–62.
[77] Shimomura Y, Tamura T, Suzuki M. Less body fat accumulation in rats fed a safflower oil diet than in rats fed a beef tallow diet. J Nutr 1990;120:1291–6.
[78] Sanz M, Lopez-Bote CJ, Menoyo D, Bautista JM. Abdominal fat deposition and fatty acid synthesis are lower and β-oxidation is higher in broiler chickens fed diets containing unsaturated rather than saturated fat. J Nutr 2000;130:3034–7.
[79] Nagao K, Inoue N, Wang YM, Shirouchi B, Yanagita T. Dietary conjugated linoleic acid alleviates momalcoholic fatty liver disease in zucker (fa/fa) rats. J Nutr 2005;135.
[80] Degrace P, Demizieux L, Gresti J, Chardigny JM, Sebedio JL, Clouet P. Hepatic steatosis is not due to impaired fatty acid oxidation capacities in C57BL/6J mice fed the conjugated trans-10, cis-12-isomer of linoleic acid. J Nutr 2004;134:861–7.
[81] Bouthegourd JC, Even PC, Gripois D, Tiffon B, Blouquit MF, Roseau S, et al. A CLA mixture prevents body triglyceride accumulation without affecting energy expenditure in syrian hamster. J Nutr 2002;132.
[82] Newman RE, Bryden WL, Fleck E, Ashes JR, Buttermer WA, Storlien LH, et al. Dietary n-3 and n-6 fatty acids alter avian metabolism: metabolism and abdominal fat deposition. Br J Nutr 2002;88:11–18.
[83] Cook KS, Groves DL, Min HY, Spiegelman BM. A developmentally regulated mRNA from 3T3 adipocytes encodes a novel serine protease homologue. Proceedings of the National Academy of Sciences of the United States 1985;82:6480–4.
[84] Raclot T, Groscolas R, Langin D, Ferre P. Site-specific regulation of gene expression by n-3 polyunsaturated fatty acids in rat white adipose tissues. J Lipid Res 1997;38:1963–72.
[85] Jang IS, Hwang DY, Chae KR, Lee JE, Kim YK, Kang TS, et al. Role of dietary fat type in the development of adiposity from dietary obesity susceptible Sprague-Dawley rats. Br J Nutr 2003;89:429–37.
[86] Flachs P, Horakova O, Brauner P, Rossmeisl M, Pecina P, Franssen-van Hal N, et al. Polyunsaturated fatty acids of marine origin upregulate mitochondrial biogenesis and induce β-oxidation in white fat. Diabetologia 2005;48:2365–75.
[87] Hargrave KM, Meyer BJ, Li C, Azain MJ, Baile CA, Miner JL. Influence of dietary conjugated linoleic acid and fat source on body fat and apoptosis in mice. Obes Res 2004;12:1435–44.
[88] McNeel RL, Mersmann HJ. Effects of isomers of conjugated linoleic acid on procine adipocyte growth and differentiation. Journal of Nutritional Biochemistry 2003;14:266–74.
[89] Zhou Y-T, Wang Z-W, Higa M, Newgard CB, Unger RH. Reversing adipocyte differentiation: implications for treatment od obesity. Proceedings of the National Academy of Sciences of the United States 1999;96:2391–5.
[90] Frayn KN. Visceral fat and insulin resistance - sausative or correlative? Br J Nutr 2000;83:S71–7.
[91] Fox CS, Massaro JM, Hoffmann U, Pou KM, Maurovich-Hovart P, Liu CY, et al. Abdominal visceral and subcutaneous adipose tissue compartments: association with metabolic risk factors in the Framingham Heart Study. Circulation 2007;116:39–48.
[92] Foster MT, Pagliassotti MJ. Metabolic alterations following visceral fat removal and expansion: beyond anatomic location. Adipocyte 2012;1:192–9.
[93] Gastaldelli A, Cusi K, Pettiti M, Hardies J, Miyazaki Y, Berria R, et al. Relationship between hepatic/visceral fat and hepatic insulin resistance in nondiabetic and type 2 diabetic subjects. Gastroenterology 2007;133:496–506.
[94] Bergman RN, Kim SP, Catalano KJ, Hsu IR, Chiu JD, Kabir M, et al. Why visceral fat is bad: mechanisms of the metabolic syndrome. Obesity 2006;14:16S–9S.
[95] Despres J-P, Lemieux I. Abdominal obesity and metabolic syndrome. Nature 2006;444:881–7.
[96] Ward KD, Sparrow D, Vokonas PS, Willett WC, Landsberg L, Weiss ST. The relationships of abdominal obesity, hyperinsulinemia and saturated fat intake to serum lipid levels: the Normative Aging Study. Int J Obes 1994;18:137–44.
[97] Garaulet M, Pérez-Llamas F, Pérez-Ayala M, Martínez P, de Medina FS, Tebar FJ, et al. Site-specific differences in the fatty acid composition of abdominal adipose tissue in an obese population from a Mediterranean area: relation with dietary fatty acids, plasma lipid profile, serum insulin, and central obesity. Am J Clin Nutr 2001;74:585–91.
[98] Romaguera D, Norat T, Mouw T, May AM, Bamia C, Slimani N, et al. Adherence to the Mediterranean diet is associated with lower abdominal adiposity in European men and women. J Nutr 2009;139:1728–37.
[99] Garaulet M, Hernandez-Morante JJ, Lujan J, Tebar FJ, Zamora S. Relationship between fat cell size and number and fatty acid composition in adipose tissue from different fat depots in overweight/obese humans. Int J Obes 2006;30:899–905.
[100] Machann J, Stefan N, Schabel C, Schleicher E, Fritsche A, Würslin C, et al. Fraction of unsaturated fatty acids in visceral adipose tissue (VAT) is lower in subjects with high total VAT volume-a combined 1H MRS and volumetric MRI study in male subjects. NMR Biomed 2013;26:232–6.
[101] Walker KZ, O'Dea K, Johnson L, Sinclair AJ, Piers LS, Nicholson GC, et al. Body fat distribution and non-insulin-dependent diabetes: comparison of a fiber-rich, high-carbohydrate, low-fat (23%) diet and a 35% fat diet high in monounsaturated fat. Am J Clin Nutr 1996;63:254–60.
[102] Paniagua JA, de la Sacristana AG, Romero I, Vidal-Puig A, Latre JM, Sanchez E, et al. Monounsaturated fat-rich diet prevents central body fat distribution and decreases postprandial adiponectin expression induced by a carbohydrate-rich diet in insulin-resistant subjects. Diabetes Care 2007;30:1717–23.
[103] Piers LS, Walker KZ, Stoney RM, Soares MJ, O'Dea K. Substitution of saturated with monounsaturated fat in a 4-week diet affects body weight and composition of overweight and obese men. Br J Nutr 2003;90:717–27.
[104] Kelley DE, He J, Menshikova EV, Ritov VB. Dysfunction of mitochondria in human skeletal muscle in type 2 diabetes. Diabetes Metab 2002;51:2944–50.
[105] Kelley DE, Simoneau JA. Impaired free fatty acid utilization by skeletal muscle in non-insulin-dependent diabetes mellitus. J Clin Invest 1994;94:2349–56.
[106] Luscombe-Marsh ND, Noakes M, Wittert G, Keogh JB, Foster P, Clifton PM. Carbohydrate-restricted diets high in either monounsaturated fat or protein are equally effective at promoting fat

loss and improving blood lipids. Am J Clin Nutr 2005;81:762–72.

[107] Wien MA, Sabate JM, Ikle DN, Cole SE, Kandeel FR. Almonds vs complex carbohydrates in a weight reduction program. Int J Obes 2003;27:1365–72.

[108] Cassady BA, Hollis JH, Fulford AD, Considine RV, Mattes RD. Mastication of almonds: effects of lipid bioaccessibility, appetite, and hormone response. Am J Clin Nutr 2009;89:794–800.

[109] Mori AM, Considine RV, Mattes RD. Acute and second-meal effects of almond form in impaired glucose tolerant adults: a randomized crossover trial. Nutr Metab 2011;8:1–8.

[110] Fraser GE, Bennett HW, Jaceldo KB, Sabate J. Effect on body weight of a free 76 Kilojoule (320 calorie) daily supplement of almonds for six months. J Am Coll Nutr 2002;21:275–83.

[111] Hollis J, Mattes R. Effect of chronic consumption of almonds on body weight in healthy humans. Br J Nutr 2007;98:651–6.

[112] Jenkins DJA, Kendall CWC, Marchie A, Parker TL, Connelly PW, Qian W, et al. Dose response of almonds on coronary heart disease risk factors: blood lipids, oxidized low-density lipoproteins, lipoprotein(a), homocysteine, and pulmonary nitric oxide: a randomized, controlled, crossover trial. Circulation 2002;106:1327–32.

[113] Novotny JA, Gebauer SK, Baer DJ. Discrepancy between the Atwater factor predicted and empirically measured energy values of almonds in human diets. Am J Clin Nutr 2012;96:296–301.

[114] Summers LKM, Fielding BA, Bradshaw HA, Ilic V, Beysen C, Clark ML, et al. Substituting dietary saturated fat with polyunsaturated fat changes abdominal fat distribution and improves insulin sensitivity. Diabetologia 2002;45:369–77.

[115] Thorsdottir I, Tomasson H, Gunnarsdottir I, Gisladottir E, Kiely M, Parra MD, et al. Randomized trial of weight-loss-diets for young adults varying in fish and fish oil content. Int J Obes 2007;31:1560–6.

[116] Tapsell LC, Gillen LJ, Patch CS, Batterham M, Owen A, Bare M, et al. Including walnuts in a low-fat/modified-fat diet improves HDL cholesterol-to-total cholesterol ratios in patients with type 2 diabetes. Diabetes Care 2004;27:2777–83.

[117] Tapsell LC, Batterham MJ, Teuss G, Tan SY, Dalton S, Quick CJ, et al. Long-term effects of increased dietary polyunsaturated fat from walnuts on metabolic parameters in type II diabetes. Eur J Clin Nutr 2009;63:1008–15.

[118] Tapsell LC, Batterham MJ, Huang XF, Tan S-Y, Teuss G, Charlton K, et al. Short term effects of energy restriction and dietary fat sub-type on weight loss and disease risk factors. Nutrition, Metabolism and Cardiovascular Diseases 2010;20:317–25.

[119] Krebs JD, Browning LM, McLean NK, Rothwell JL, Mishra GD, Moore CS, et al. Additive benefits of long-chain n-3 polyunsaturated fatty acids and weight-loss in the management of cardiovascular disease risk in overweight hyperinsulinaemic women. Int J Obes 2006;30:1535–44.

[120] Hill AM, Buckley JD, Murphy KJ, Howe PR. Combining fish-oil supplements with regular aerobic exercise improves body composition and cardiovascular disease risk factors. Am J Clin Nutr 2007;85:1267–74.

[121] Munro IA, Garg ML. Dietary supplementation with long chain omega-3 polyunsaturated fatty acids and weight loss in obese adults. Obes Res Clin Pract 2013. http://dx.doi.org/10.1016/j.orcp.2011.11.001.

[122] Salas-Salvado J, Marquez-Sandoval F, Bullo M. Conjugated linoleic acid intake in humans: a systematic review focusing on its effect on body composition, glucose, and lipid metabolism. Crit Rev Food Sci Nutr 2006;46:479–88.

[123] Smith SR, Zachwieja JJ. Visceral adipose tissue: a critical review of intervention strategies. Int J Obes Relat Metab Disord 1999;23:329–35.

[124] Hallgreen CE, Hall KD. Allometric relationship between changes of visceral fat and total fat mass. Int J Obes 2008;32:845–52.

[125] Tan S-Y, Batterham M, Tapsell L. Increased intake of dietary polyunsaturated fat does not promote whole body or preferential abdominal fat mass loss in overweight adults. Obesity Facts 2011;4:352–7.

[126] Belzung F, Raclot T, Groscolas R. Fish oil n-3 fatty acids selectively limit the hypertrophy of abdominal fat depots in growing rats fed high-fat diets. Am J Physiol 1993;264:R1111–8.

[127] Crespo N, Esteve-Garcia E. Dietary fatty acid profile modifies abdominal fat deposition in broiler chickens. Poult Sci 2001;80:71–8.

[128] Heyden S. Polyunsaturated and monounsaturated fatty acids in the diet to prevent coronary heart disease via cholesterol reduction. Ann Nutr Metab 2008;38:117–22.

[129] Calder PC. Polyunsaturated fatty acids and inflammatory processes: new twists in an old tale. Biochimie 2009.

[130] Iacono JM, Dougherty RM, Puska P. Reduction of blood pressure associated with dietary polyunsaturated fat. Hypertension 1982;4:III-34–III-42.

[131] Ruxton CHS, Reed SC, Simpson MJA, Millington KJ. The health benefits of omega-3 polyunsaturated fatty acids: a review of the evidence. J Hum Nutr Diet 2004;17:449–59.

CHAPTER

37

Conjugated Linoleic Acid in Human Health Effects on Weight Control

Yeonhwa Park

Department of Food Science, University of Massachusetts, Amherst, MA, USA

INTRODUCTION

Health concerns over the consumption of *trans* fatty acids compared to the known health benefits of fish oil clearly illustrate how different dietary fats contribute to our health. The *trans* fatty acids can be further divided into unconjugated and conjugated *trans* fatty acids based on their structural features. Unconjugated *trans* fatty acids found in foods from ruminant sources are referred to as ruminant *trans* fatty acids. Unconjugated *trans* fatty acids derived from partially hydrogenated vegetable oils are referred to as industrial *trans* fatty acids. These industrial *trans* fatty acids are known to be the major dietary source of *trans* fatty acids and are also considered to be a major health concern, particularly for cardiovascular diseases [1,2].

Current regulation by the U.S. Food and Drug Administration for *trans* fat labeling specifically defines "all unsaturated fatty acids that contain one or more isolated double bonds (i.e. non conjugated) in a *trans* configuration" [3]. Based on this definition, the "conjugated" *trans* fatty acids, primarily conjugated linoleic acid (CLA), have been excluded from the current *trans* fat labeling. In addition, with current approval for CLA as generally recognized as safe (GRAS) and a food additive for use in certain types of food in the U.S. since 2008, the consumption of CLA associated with dietary supplements or foods is expected to rise significantly. Thus, it is important to review the current knowledge on CLA, and particularly its human health implications. This chapter will primarily focus on CLA publications involving human studies on body fat and weight control [4,5].

DISCOVERY AND ORIGINS OF CONJUGATED LINOLEIC ACID

As early as 1932, the existence of CLA was reported in a scientific paper, although it was not until much later that its structure was identified and it was given the name "CLA" [6]. The first report of CLA was from milk, in which increased ultraviolet absorption at 230 nm in summer milk compared to winter milk was reported, suggesting the presence of a conjugated double bond in CLA's structure [6]. In the 1980s, Dr Pariza's group at the University of Wisconsin-Madison investigated the relationship between mutagen formation and cooking temperature and time using cooked ground beef to expand on previous observations that eating overcooked meat can cause cancer [7,8]. They found that increased cooking temperature and time potentiated mutagen formation by cooked beef, but interestingly they also identified a beef extract fraction that inhibited mutagenesis [7,8]. The principal compound responsible for this activity was identified as a conjugated isomer of linoleic acid and thus named *conjugated linoleic acid* [7,8].

CLA was discovered in beef and the primary dietary source of CLA is ruminant products. CLA is derived from biohydrogenation of linoleic acid to stearic acid by rumen bacteria [9]. Among a number of potential CLA isomers (please see below for details), the main CLA isomer from biohydrogenation is the *cis*-9,*trans*-11 isomer, a stable intermediate of biohydrogenation [9]. This isomer is also called *rumenic acid*, which implies that it is produced by rumen bacteria [10]. Similarly, *trans*-11 vaccenic acid, the other stable intermediate of biohydrogenation, escapes this process and can be converted to

Nutrition in the Prevention and Treatment of Abdominal Obesity
http://dx.doi.org/10.1016/B978-0-12-407869-7.00037-4

TABLE 37.1 Effects of Conjugated Linoleic Acid on Body Composition in Humans

Reference	CLA Supplementation		*n* (sex)	Results[a]					Other Comments or Conclusions
	Dose (g/day)	Duration		BW	BFM	BMI	LBM	Waist (SAD)	
Berven et al. 2000 [121]	3.4	12 weeks	47 (F/M)	↓[b] 1.1	—	↓[b] 0.4	—	—	–
Blankson et al. 2000 [45]	1.7/3.4/5.1/6.8	6 and 12 weeks	47 (F/M)	—	↓ 0.43–1.73	—	↑[b] 0.54–1.26 at 12 weeks	–	No additional benefits with >3.4 g CLA/day; exercise outcome reported
Zambell et al. 2000 [70]	2.5	9 weeks	17 (F)	—	—	—	—	–	No Δ RMR[a] and respiratory exchange ratio
Mougios et al. 2001 [189]	0.7/1.4	4 weeks each	22 (F/M)	—	↓[b] 0.7 from week 4 to week 8	—	–	–	Skinfolds↓[b]; isoenergetically fed
Riserus et al. 2001 [177]	3.3	4 weeks	24 (M)	—	–	—	–	↓[b] 1.5 (0.6)	Subjects with metabolic syndrome
Smedman and Vessby 2001 [190]	3.2	12 weeks	50 (F/M)	—	↓ 3.84%	—	–	—	–
Thom et al. 2001 [88]	1.8	12 weeks	20 (F/M)	—	↓ ≈3%	—	–	–	Exercise
Kreider et al. 2002 [86]	6.0	4 weeks	23 (M)	—	—	–	—	–	Exercise
Noone et al. 2002 [32]	2.0	8 weeks	51 (F/M)	—	–	—	–	–	–
Riserus et al. 2002 [178]	3.4 as a mixture or t10c12	12 weeks	57 (M)	↓[b] 0.88 by t10c12	↓[b] 0.92–1.02%	↓[b] 0.27 by t10c12	—	↓[b] 1.57 or 0.88 (S) by t10c12	Subjects with metabolic syndrome: greater effects with t10c12 than mixture
Belury et al. 2003 [78]	6.1	8 weeks	21 (F/M)	Inverse correlation	–	–	–	–	Type 2 diabetes; plasma level of CLA inversely linked to leptin
Kamphuis et al. 2003 [48]	1.8/3.6	13 weeks	54 (F/M)	—	↓[b] 1.1–1.4%	—	↑[b] 2.7–3.3%	–	Weight regain; no effect on BW regain; ↑ RMR[a]
Eyjolfson et al. 2004 [191]	3.0	8 weeks	16 (F/M)	—	—	—	–	–	Sedentary
Gaullier et al. 2004 [21]	3.4 or 3.6	1 year	180 (F/M)	↓ 1.1–1.8	↓ 1.7–2.4	↓ 0.4–0.6	↑ 0.6–0.7	–	No difference between free and TG form of CLA; recommended to ↓ intake by approx. 200 kcal/day
Malpuech-Brugere et al. 2004 [33]	1.5/3.0, t10c12	18 weeks	81 (F/M)	—	—	—	—	–	Ns ↓ intake by t10c12

(Continued)

TABLE 37.1 Continued

Reference	CLA Supplementation		n (sex)	Results[a]					Other Comments or Conclusions
	Dose (g/day)	Duration		BW	BFM	BMI	LBM	Waist (SAD)	
Whigham et al. 2004 [82]	6.0	1 year	46 (F/M)	—	—	–	–	–	Weight loss and maintenance; 3 phases of study: low-calorie diet (phase 1), refeed (phase 2), and open label (phase 3)
Gaullier et al. 2005 [52]	3.4 or 3.6 at year 1 and 3.4 at year 2	2 years	125 (F/M)	↓[b] 1.5–2.4	↓[b] 1.8–2.7	↓[b] 0.6–0.9	—	–	↓[b] energy intake; ↓[b] leptin; 1-year extension open study of Gaullier et al. 2004 [21]
Adams et al. 2006 [87]	3.2	4 weeks	28 (M)	—	–	—	–	–	Exercise; no Δ visceral adipose tissue; crossover design (4 weeks CLA + 4 weeks placebo)
Colakoglu et al. 2006 [43]	3.6[d]	6 weeks	44 (F)	↓[b] 0.8%, 1.67% w/exercise	↓[b] 8.1%	↓[b] 0.8%	↑[b] 1.6%	↓[b] 3.4%	Exercise; greater effect of CLA when combined with exercise
Larsen et al. 2006 [104]	3.4	1 year	83 (F/M)	—	—	—	—	—	Weight regain; Hypocaloric diet
Pinkoski et al. 2006 [67]	5.1	7 weeks	76 (F/M)	-	↓[b] 0.8	-	↑[b] 1.3	-	Exercise; no Δ RMR[a]; ↑ Strength; ↓ protein degradation; some subjects crossed over for 7 weeks
Taylor et al. 2006 [99]	4.5	12 weeks	40 (M)	↓[b] 1.1 ($P=0.06$)	—	↓[b] 0.4 ($P=0.07$)	-	—	↓ skinfolds in limbs
Attar-Bashi et al. 2007 [105]	3.2	8 weeks	16 (F/M)	-	—	—	-	—	Cosupplementation with 11 g/day α-linolenic acid
Gaullier et al. 2007 [55]	3.4	6 months	105 (F/M)	—	↓[b] 1.0	↓[b] 0.3–0.5 for BMI > 30	↑[b] 0.5	↓[b] 2.6	Greater effects in women and BMI > 30; ↓ fat mass mostly in arms and legs in women; no Δ cal intake
Lambert et al. 2007 [68]	2.6	12 weeks	62 (F/M)	—	—	-	—	—	Exercise; no Δ RMR; no Δ appetite
Laso et al. 2007 [192]	3	12 weeks	54 (F/M)	-	↓ 0.6 for BMI ≤ 30	—	—	—	↓ trunk fat mass w/BMI ≤ 30
Nazare et al. 2007 [65]	2.8	14 weeks	44 (F/M)	—	—	—	—	-	Exercise; ↑[b] RMR

(Continued)

TABLE 37.1 Continued

	CLA Supplementation			Results[a]					
Reference	**Dose (g/day)**	**Duration**	***n* (sex)**	**BW**	**BFM**	**BMI**	**LBM**	**Waist (SAD)**	**Other Comments or Conclusions**
Steck et al. 2007 [69]	3.2/6.4	12 weeks	48 (F/M)	—	—	—	↑[b] 0.64 in 6.4 CLA	—	no Δ RMR
Syvertsen et al. 2007 [193]	3.4	6 months	41 (F/M)	—	—	—	-	—	-
Tarnopolsky et al. 2007 [90]	5.4	6 months	39 (F/M)	—	↓ 1.9	—	↑ 2.1	-	Cosupplementation with 5 g/day creatine monohydrate; aging; exercise
Thursh et al. 2007 [194]	3.1	12 weeks	9 (F/M)	—	—	—	-	—	No Δ in caloric intake; open study without placebo
Watras et al. 2007 [49]	3.2	6 months	40 (F/M)	↓ 0.6	↓ ≈1.0	↓ 0.2	—	-	Holiday weight gain; ↑[b] RMR; no Δ energy intake
Diaz et al. 2008 [89]	1.8	12 weeks	38 (F)	—	—	-	—	-	Cosupplementation with 400 μg/day chromium picolinate; exercise; premenopausal
Park et al. 2008 [195]	2.4	8 weeks	30 (F/M)	↓[b] 0.8	—	↓[b] 0.2	—	-	↓ hip circumference
Raff et al. 2008 [162]	4.3	5 weeks	38 (M)	—	-	-	-	-	Control group consumed low-CLA butter
Sneddon et al. 2008 [98]	2.3	12 weeks	59 (M)	↑[b] 1.31 in young obese	—	↑[b] 0.42 in young obese	↑ 0.88 in young obese	—	Cosupplementation with 1.5 g/day EPA/DHA[a]; young vs. older; crossover design (12-week washout)
Cornish et al. 2009 [56]	4.3	5 weeks	69 (F/M)	—	—	—	↑ ≈2.5% by CLA and creatine	-	Cosupplementation with 9 g/day creatine monohydrate and 36 g/day whey protein; strength training; no Δ energy intake
Herrmann et al. 2009 [37]	3.4 mixture or t10c12	4 weeks	34 (M)	—	-	—	-	↓ 0.9 by t10c12	-
Norris et al. 2009 [57]	6.4	16 weeks	35 (F)	↓ 0.8–1.3	↓[b] 1.1–1.6	↓ 0.4–0.5	—	—	Type 2 diabetes; postmenopausal; crossover design (4-week washout)
MacRedmond et al. 2010 [196]	4.5 (3.3 as CLA)	12 weeks	26 (F/M)	↓ 2.0	-	↓ 0.5	-	-	Subjects with mild/moderate asthma; improved airway hyperresponsiveness

(*Continued*)

TABLE 37.1 Continued

	CLA Supplementation			Results[a]					
Reference	**Dose (g/day)**	**Duration**	***n*** **(sex)**	**BW**	**BFM**	**BMI**	**LBM**	**Waist (SAD)**	**Other Comments or Conclusions**
Michishita et al. 2010 [91]	1.6	16 weeks	41 (F/M)	—	—	—	–	↓ 3.2	Cosupplementation with 1.52 g/day amino acid mixture; exercise; ↓ 2.5 cm hip circumference
Raff et al. 2009 [38]	5.5	16 weeks	75 (F)	—	↓ 1.0	–	↑ 0.4 for lower body	–	Postmenopausal; greater effects on lower body fat mass
Zhao et al. 2009 [106]	4.5	8 weeks	80 (F/M)	—	↓ 4.8%	—	–	↓ 3.2 ($P=0.06$)	Cosupplementation with 37.5 mg/day ramipril; hypertensive; ↓ hip circumference
Racine et al. 2010 [31]	2.4	7 months	53 (F/M)	↓ 0.5 gain	↓ 1.0 gain	↓ 0.6 gain	↑ 0.5% gain	–	Children; all subjects were growing and gaining weight; ↓ peripheral and abdominal fat; 6–10 year-olds, prepubertial, BMI >85 percentile
Venkatramanan et al. 2010 [41]	1.3	8 weeks	15 (F/M)	—	—	—	–	–	Hyperlipidemic; crossover design
Joseph et al. 2011 [40]	3.5 (2.8 as CLA)	8 weeks	27 (M)	—	—	—	—	–	Crossover design; slightly hyperlipidemic men
Pfeuffer et al. 2011 [124]	4.5 (3.4 as CLA)	4 weeks	81 (M)	↓ 1.13	–	↓ 0.35	–	–	Significant ↓ in diastolic BP
Chen et al. 2012 [197]	3.4	12 weeks	63 (F/M)	↓[b] 0.7	↓[b] 0.5	↓[b] 0.32	—	–	↓ subcutaneous fat mass; ↓ Waist-Hip ratio; greater effects w subjects >27 BMI and Females
Macaluso et al. 2012 [93]	6 (4.8 as CLA)	3 weeks	10 (M)	–	—	–	—	–	Crossover design; physically active subjects; ↑ serum testosterone after exercise
Rubin et al. 2012 [80]	4.25 mixture or t10c12 (3.4 as CLA)	4 weeks	35 (M)	—	–	—	–	–	PPAR-γ polymorphism (Pro-Ala); crossover design: c9t11 and mixture, improve HOMA-IR; t10c12, worsens weight gain and BMI; Pro, no effect; t10c12 decreases waist

[a]*Numbers are kg (BW, BFM, and LBM), kg/m² (BMI), or cm (waist and SAD; SAD in parenthesis), unless indicated as%.* [b]*Significantly different within group.*
–, missing value; —, no change; Δ, change; ↓, decrease; ↑, increase; BFM, body fat mass; BMI, body mass index; BP, blood pressure; BW, body weight; c9t11, *cis*-9,*trans*-11; CLA, conjugated linoleic acid; DHA, docosahexaenoic acid; EPA, eicosapentaenoic acid; F, female; HOMA-IR, homeostatic model assessment of insulin resistance; LBM, lean body mass; M, male; ns, not significant; RMR, resting metabolic rate; t10c12, *trans*-10,*cis*-12; TG, triglyceride; SAD, sagittal abdominal diameter.

the *cis*-9,*trans*-11 isomer by delta-9 desaturase expressed in mammalian tissue [11,12]. This is considered an alternative source of tissue *cis*-9,*trans*-11 CLA [11,12].

Even though foods from ruminant origins are considered to be good sources of CLA, typical concentrations of *cis*-9,*trans*-11 CLA in food are relatively low, less than 10 mg CLA per g fat [13]. CLA intake varies greatly depending on a person's dietary pattern: high CLA intake with high dairy consumption (up to 291 mg/day) versus low-CLA intake with low dairy consumption (approximately 15 mg/day) [14]. It has been estimated that the average intake of CLA from foods is 176–212 mg/day for men and 104–151 mg/day for women in the USA [15–18].

In addition to the *cis*-9,*trans*-11 CLA isomer, a number of other positional and geometric isomers of CLA have been reported from foodstuffs: double bonds at (7,9), (8,10), (9,11), (10,12), and (11,13), with either *cis* or *trans* configurations [19]. The most noteworthy is the *trans*-10,*cis*-12 CLA isomer. This isomer is found at very low levels in food; however, when CLA is prepared chemically from linoleic acid this isomer is present in significant amounts [13]. Most CLA preparations made using this method typically consist of about 35–45% *trans*-10,*cis*-12 isomer along with similar amounts of the *cis*-9,*trans*-11 isomer, often referred to as *CLA mixture* or *50:50 mix*. The current knowledge on the biological activities of CLA is derived mainly from research using CLA mixture, with limited studies using the two individual isomers. This does not necessarily suggest that other CLA isomers have no biological activities; rather, there is relatively limited knowledge regarding the activities of other isomers [4].

Due to the nature of CLA preparation, synthetically prepared CLA contains the free fatty acid form of CLA [13], while the natural form of fat, including CLA in foodstuffs, is present as triglycerides (TG). Thus, there was concern that there may be differences in the bioavailability and/or bioactivity of the free fatty acid vs. the TG form of CLA. However, both forms of CLA were equally effective in modulating body composition in animal models as well as in human trials [20,21]. This chapter will focus on these two major isomers of CLA and will not necessarily distinguish the form of CLA.

ANTIOBESITY EFFECTS OF CONJUGATED LINOLEIC ACID

It is estimated that currently about two-thirds of the U.S. population is classified as either overweight or obese [22,23]. As obesity is one of the major risk factors for other chronic diseases, such as type 2 diabetes and metabolic syndrome, the incidences of these diseases are simultaneously on the rise [24,25]. Along with efforts to control obesity via modifications to activity and dietary habits, there are various attempts to control the obesity epidemic using diet or dietary supplements, one of which is CLA.

Since the original discovery of CLA's effects in preventing cancer development, a number of other beneficial effects of CLA have been reported. One of the most interesting aspects of CLA is its ability to modulate body composition by reducing body fat and improving lean body mass [18,20,26–28]. The first report used mouse models, in which CLA reduced body fat significantly by 60% compared to respective controls [29]. This has been consistently observed in a number of other animal models [20,27,28].

Overview of Human Studies on Conjugated Linoleic Acid

Currently about 100 human trials have been conducted and published worldwide: these have investigated not only the effects of CLA on body fat regulation but also other health benefits as well as potential adverse effects [18,30]. Table 37.1 summarizes human studies involving CLA: of particular interest are publications in which markers of body composition were reported, such as body weight (BW), body fat mass (BFM), body mass index (BMI), lean body mass (LBM), and waist circumference or sagittal abdominal diameter (SAD). The 50 studies are included in this table, which used either CLA mixture or *trans*-10,*cis*-12 isomers for periods as short as 4 weeks and up to 2 years. All but one used adults and the majority used overweight subjects, although normal and/or obese subjects were often included. Racine et al. [31] published the only study of young growing children.

About 10 studies used the *cis*-9,*trans*-11 CLA isomer preparation to determine its effects on body composition [32–41]. Some studies used the *cis*-9,*trans*-11 as a part of the study, along with CLA mixture and the *trans*-10,*cis*-12 isomer. Others used this isomer only, either from synthetic preparation or from enriched food products. Consistent with observations from animal studies that the *trans*-10,*cis*-12 CLA isomer is positively associated with body fat reduction [42], human studies using the *cis*-9,*trans*-11 CLA isomer showed no significant differences in any of the markers summarized in Table 37.1, and were thus excluded from the table. These data clearly also support an independent role for the *trans*-10,*cis*-12 CLA isomer in the modulation of body composition in humans.

A number of human trials reported the benefits of taking CLA supplementation to reduce BW and BFM, as well as to improve LBM, BMI, and waist measurement or SAD. However, the results varied and were not dramatic, with only marginal effects on BW (less than 2 kg) or BFM (best outcome was 8% reduction with exercise) [43], while others reported no benefits of supplementing CLA (Table 37.1). The meta-analysis by Whigham et al. [44] reported the significance of dose and duration for CLA's efficacy in weight control. They reported that the CLA dose negatively correlated with its effect on BFM, and that 3.2 g CLA/day was enough to cause a significant reduction in BFM. This was consistent with Blankson et al. [45], who reported no additional benefits of CLA doses greater than 3.4 g/day on BFM reduction. Whigham et al. [44] also reported that the effects of CLA on BFM were linear up to 6 months, then slowed and plateaued at about 2 years. Similarly, Onakpoya et al. [46] performed a meta-analysis of long-term CLA supplementation studies and concluded that CLA supplementation results in statistically significant loss in both BW and BFM compared to placebo. However, they specifically stated that this was "a small difference" (−0.70 weight or −1.33 kg BFM) [46].

The meta-analysis by Schoeller et al. [47] reported the effect of CLA on LBM (or fat-free mass). This study concluded that CLA had a relatively rapid and significant, but small, effect on improving LBM. This effect was not correlated with the length of supplementation or the dose of CLA used. The gain in LBM may be perceived as weight gain; however, this change in body composition would be considered beneficial beyond simple weight reduction. This is particularly important during the weight gain/regain period: Kamphuis et al. [48] reported the benefits of CLA supplementation during weight regain periods and found no significant difference in overall BW; however, CLA significantly improved LBM gain while reducing BFM gain. Similarly, Watras et al. [49] provided CLA during holiday periods and observed that CLA supplementation significantly reduced holiday weight gain and fat mass gain compared to the placebo group.

Mechanisms of Body Fat Regulation by Conjugated Linoleic Acid

Multiple mechanisms of action for CLA on body fat regulation have been suggested from animal and human studies: these include changes in food intake, energy expenditure, fatty acid beta-oxidation, and/or lipid/adipocyte metabolism [4,20].

Earlier studies of CLA in animal models reported significant reductions in food intake, although these were inconsistent [29,42,50]. Since reduced food intake would impact an animal's weight and body fat, the study by Park et al. [51] determined the role of reduced food intake by CLA on body fat reduction by using pair feeding. From this study, it was clear that CLA-induced reductions in body fat were independent of its effects on food intake [51]. In human studies, there were reports that subjects had reduced caloric intake [33,52]. However, others failed to observe an impact of CLA on caloric intake [49,53–58]. Thus, it is very unlikely that CLA controls body composition by influencing overall caloric intake.

Second, it was reported that CLA supplementation increased energy expenditure in animal models [59–64]. Several clinical studies reported that CLA supplementation increased resting metabolic rate (RMR) [48,49,65,66]; however, others failed to observe an influence of CLA on RMR, even when reduced BW or fat deposition was observed [67–70]. With minimal effects of CLA on BW or BFM in human studies, it may not be easy to observe any significant difference in energy expenditure, unlike in animal models.

As part of CLA's biochemical mechanisms leading to reduced body fat, increased fatty acid beta-oxidation in skeletal muscle was suggested by animal models, as observed by enhanced activity and expression of carnitine *O*-palmitoyltransferase 1 (CPT-1) [29,42,71–75]. This was not due to oxidative changes in CLA itself, as Malpuech-Brugere et al. [76] reported that the oxidation rate of the *trans*-10,*cis*-12 isomer (the active isomer for body fat reduction) was not significantly different from that of oleic acid. The only human study involving CLA's effects on fat oxidation was done by Close et al. [66]: 6 months of CLA supplementation resulted in increased fat oxidation during sleep, along with a reduced percentage of energy obtained from protein during the same time period.

There are many publications reporting CLA's mechanisms of action on lipid and adipocyte metabolism, including cytokine- or adipokine-associated mechanisms using in vitro and animal models [20,27]. However, there are limited studies on these aspects of CLA in humans. In tissue culture or animal studies, CLA has been shown to (1) inhibit lipoprotein lipase in adipocytes; (2) inhibit stearoyl-CoA desaturase; (3) enhance apoptosis in preadipocytes and adipocytes; (4) modulate lipolysis by adipocytes; (5) inhibit adipocyte differentiation via peroxisome proliferator-activated receptor gamma (PPAR-γ)- and nuclear factor-kappa-B (NF-κB)-dependent mechanisms; and (6) modulate tumor necrosis factor (TNF-α) or other cytokines/adipokines. Medina et al. [77] reported that a CLA supplementation of 3 g/day in healthy women could produce a temporary decline in leptin levels, which was consistent with reports from animal models [50,78,79]. It is also interesting to point out that Rubin et al. [80] recently reported that a PPAR-γ_2 polymorphism may play a significant role in CLA's effects on BW and insulin levels in middle-aged subjects, which supports the potential involvement of PPAR-γ in CLA's activity.

Lastly, Kamphuis et al. [81] reported a favorable effect of CLA on appetite (i.e. hunger satiety, and fullness). Similarly, CLA supplementation alleviated clinical symptoms associated with a hypocaloric diet, such as appetite, stress, sleep, depression, and irritability [45,82]. However, other reports failed to observe any effects of CLA on appetite, fullness, or satiety [68,77]. Although it is difficult to draw any conclusions from these limited studies, their observations are certainly very intriguing and may have great potential future implications.

Exercise and Conjugated Linoleic Acid Supplementation

A proper supply of energy during exercise, particularly via mitochondrial fatty acid beta-oxidation, is critical to increase endurance capacity [83]. Based on the observation that CLA increased skeletal muscle fatty acid beta-oxidation, it may be hypothesized that CLA enhances exercise performance. In fact, Mizunoya et al. [84] reported that CLA supplementation enhanced maximum swimming capacity by increasing fat oxidation in mice. In addition, Kim et al. [85] reported that CLA increased maximum running time and distance in trained mice, and was specifically associated with the *trans*-10,*cis*-12 isomer. It is also interesting that CLA not only improved endurance exercise performance but also increased voluntary movements in a mouse model [60].

Currently, 11 clinical trials have tested CLA along with exercise in the study design: four of them included cosupplementation with creatine monohydrate, chromium picolinate, or an amino acid mixture [43,56,65,67,68,86–91]. The overall outcomes of these studies were inconsistent: six reported positive effects on at least one of the parameters (BW, BFM, BMI, LBM, or waist circumference) compared to control [43,56,67,88,90,91], while others showed no effects [65,68,86,87,89].

Six of the aforementioned studies also reported exercise outcomes [43,45,56,67,86,90]. Four of these reported a significant improvement in exercise performance following CLA supplementation, such as increased training hours, improved bench-press strength, and improved muscular endurance [45,56,67,90]. These include two studies that involved cosupplementation with creatine monohydrate [56,90], as this is a popular dietary supplement used by athletes to improve exercise-related outcomes [92]. In addition, Macaluso et al. [93] reported that CLA supplementation significantly increased serum testosterone levels after resistance exercise. Although it was a relatively short supplementation period (3 weeks), it may have contributed to CLA's effect on exercise outcome. Along with animal studies of CLA on improved endurance performance, these reports suggest a potential role for CLA in maintaining proper muscle mass [84,85].

Importantly, Tarnopolsky et al. [90] reported improved exercise outcomes in older subjects (>65 years) after cosupplementation of CLA and creatine monohydrate. Therefore, CLA may have great (although limited) potential to elderly people who are at a great risk of developing sarcopenia, i.e. the age-dependent gradual loss of skeletal muscle mass resulting in decreased muscle strength. Sarcopenia is prevalent in approximately 15% of those under 70 years or greater than 50% of those over 80 years of age [94–97]. Further clinical trials of CLA with exercise regimes, particularly in the elderly, are therefore needed before a general conclusion can be made.

Subject Age and Conjugated Linoleic Acid Supplementation

Racine et al. [31] reported the only CLA trial that included young children, aged 6–10 years: all subjects (overweight or obese children) gained BW during the 7-month study period. In this study, CLA attenuated the increase in BW gain, BFM gain, and BMI gain, and was associated with improved LBM gain. These results show a potential use for CLA in growing children who are at risk of developing obesity later in life.

Sneddon et al. [98] compared the effects of 3 g CLA and 3 g/day ω-3 fatty acids for 12 weeks on young and old subjects. They reported significant increases in BW, BMI, and LBM with CLA supplements in young obese subjects, while no differences were observed in older subjects. However, it was unclear whether the significant effects were due to CLA or to ω-3 fatty acids in this study.

Similarly, Tarnopolsky et al. [90] conducted a placebo-controlled, double-blind study in older subjects (between 65 and 85 years) using cosupplementation of 6 g/day CLA and 5 g/day creatine monohydrate for 6 months, with a particular focus on strength performance. Cosupplementation resulted in a significant reduction in BFM (1.9 kg) with enhanced LBM (2.1 kg) without changes in BW. Again, it was unclear whether CLA supplementation alone would have had similar results in older subjects.

Two studies have involved postmenopausal women [38,57]. Subjects in the Norris et al. [57] study were an average of 60 years old and received 6.4 g/day CLA supplementation for 16 weeks. The authors reported significant reductions in BW, BFM, and BMI without significant changes in LBM and waist circumference. Raff et al. [38] also reported that 5.5 g/day CLA for 16 weeks in postmenopausal women (≈ 60 years old) decreased BFM and improved lower LBM. In these limited studies, it is difficult to draw any concrete conclusion; however, they suggest that CLA administration to certain populations may lead to health benefits, including regulation of body composition as well as other benefits described in a later section.

Conjugated Linoleic Acid: Other Considerations

Data on the effects of CLA on body compositional modulation in humans are clearly weaker than those observed in animal models [4,28,44,99–102]. This difference may derive from differences in experimental design, dose administered, relative feeding duration (short period vs. life span), or species-dependent variation in metabolic rate [4,20,100,103].

Most animal studies (with a few exceptions) investigated the role of CLA during a positive energy balance period (rapid growth period with ad libitum dietary regimes) and reported that CLA showed dramatic effects on body composition [20]. Five clinical trials have focused on potential weight gain with CLA [31,48,49,82,104]. Among them, three reported that CLA supplementation had a positive impact on weight gain, such as reduced BFM gain, reduced BW gain, or reduced BMI gain [31,48,49]. The other two studies failed to show any positive outcome following CLA supplementation [82,104]. Along with an animal study showing no beneficial effects of CLA on body fat under dietary restriction [51], this suggests that CLA may be more effective at reducing fat mass "gain" during a positive energy balance period [48,49,54,81,82,104].

The CLA doses used in human studies were about 3g/day (range 0.7–6.8g/day; Table 37.1). In contrast, the doses of CLA used in mice were typically 0.5% (w/w) of diet, which is equivalent to ≈56g CLA/day/70kg BW, which is much higher than the doses used in human studies [33]. Second, considering the relative life spans, the study duration in animals was much longer than those used in humans (4weeks to 2years). It is noteworthy that all human CLA studies with a supplementation period shorter than 4-weeks did not report any significant difference in body composition [4], whereas studies with CLA supplementation periods longer than 6months reported better outcomes (shown in Table 37.2). Third, metabolic differences between species may have significantly contributed to the greater efficacy in mice compared to other species, including humans [103]. Lastly, several studies have used CLA with other dietary supplements or drugs, such as creatine monohydrate, fish oil, chromium picolinate, whey protein, or antihypertensive drug, which may help to potentiate CLA's efficacy [56,89,90,98,105,106]. All of these factors may help explain the wide variations observed in CLA studies and indicate that further studies are required to evaluate the specific conditions under which CLA may have the most health benefits.

OTHER HEALTH BENEFITS OF CONJUGATED LINOLEIC ACID

Cancer Prevention and Conjugated Linoleic Acid

As stated earlier, the original discovery of CLA was based on its anticancer effect; however, only a small number of human studies involve CLA effects on cancer. All of these have investigated the link between naturally occurring CLA (thus, mainly the *cis*-9,*trans*-11 isomer) and cancer incidence [107–114]. Knekt et al. [107] made the first report of the inverse correlation between breast cancer incidence and milk consumption, which has since been confirmed by others [108,110]. However, four other studies have reported no association between either CLA intake or CLA levels in tissue and breast cancer incidence [109,111–113]. Larsson et al. [114] was the only group to report the effects of CLA on colorectal cancer: they found a significant negative association between colorectal cancer incidence and the consumption of high fat dairy and CLA.

Since CLA has been associated with reduced food intake in certain studies, there has been concern over its antiappetite effects in cancer patients [115]. However, earlier work with CLA using immune stimulation showed a positive influence on food intake by CLA in animal models [116,117]. Future controlled trials are therefore needed to determine the potential benefits of CLA on specific types of cancer, along with its effects on food intake, particularly in cancer patients.

Cardiovascular Disease and Conjugated Linoleic Acid

One of the earlier reports of CLA demonstrated its preventive effects on the development of atherosclerosis in rabbits [118]. As cardiovascular diseases are the leading cause of death in USA, the potential use of CLA for preventing cardiovascular diseases is of great interest. A significant number of clinical trials involving CLA have measured blood markers for lipids, such as total cholesterol, low-density lipoprotein (LDL) cholesterol, high-density lipoprotein (HDL) cholesterol, and TG [18,30,119,120]. Overall, most studies reported that CLA did not have any effects on those markers; others reported either increased LDL or decreased HDL cholesterol, although values were all in the normal range. CLA effects on other markers of cardiovascular disease were also reported; however, all

TABLE 37.2 Summary of Long-Term Conjugated Linoleic Acid Clinical Trials

Reference	CLA Supplementation		Key Notes	Results[a]								Other observations
	Dose (g/day)	Duration		BW[a]	BFM[a]	BMI[a]	LBM[a]	Waist	Glucose	Insulin	Insulin sensitivity	
Gaullier et al. 2007 [55]	3.4	6 months	No difference in caloric intake	—	↓[b] 1.0	↓[b] 0.3–0.5 for BMI >30	↑[b] 0.5	↓[b] 2.6	↓[b]	—	–	Greater effects in women and BMI >30; ↓fat mass mostly in arms and legs in women
Syvertsen et al. 2007 [193]	3.4		–	—	—	—	–	—	—	—	—	–
Tarnopolsky et al. 2007 [90]	5.4		Cosupplementation with 5 g/day creatine monohydrate; older subjects; with exercise	—	↓ 1.9	—	↑ 2.1	–	—	–	—	Cosupplementation with 5 g/day creatine monohydrate; aging; exercise
Watras et al. 2007 [49]	3.2		Holiday weight gain	↓ 0.6	↓ ≈1.0	↓0.2	—	–	—	—	—	↑[b] RMR; no Δ energy intake
Racine et al. 2010 [31]	2.4	7 months	Children (6–10 years)	↓ 0.5 gain	↓ 1.0 gain	↓ 0.6 gain	↑ 0.5% gain	–	—	—	—	↓ Peripheral and abdominal fat
Gaullier et al. 2004 [21]	3.4 or 3.6	1 year	Decreased caloric intake (200 kcal)	↓ 1.1–1.8	↓ 1.7–2.4	↓ 0.4–0.6	↑ 0.6–0.7	–	—	–	–	–
Whigham et al. 2004 [82]	6.0		Weight loss and maintenance	—	—	–	–	–	↑ at week 2 only	—	—	–
Larsen et al. 2006 [104]	3.4		Weight regain; hypocaloric diet	—	—	—	—	—	—	—	—	–
Gaullier et al. 2005 [52]	3.4 or 3.6 at year 1 and 3.4 at year 2	2 years	1-year extension open study of Gaullier et al. 2004 [21]	↓[b] 1.5–2.4	↓[b] 1.8–2.7	↓[b] 0.6–0.9	—	–	—	↑ with TG, CLA	–	↓[b] energy intake; ↓[b] leptin

[a]*Numbers are kg (BW, BFM, and LBM), kg/m² (BMI), or cm (waist), unless indicated as%.* [b]*Significantly different within group only.*
–, missing value; —, no change; Δ, change; ↓, decrease; ↑, increase; BFM, body fat mass; BMI, body mass index; BW, body weight; CLA, conjugated linoleic acid; EPA, eicosapentaenoic acid; LBM, lean body mass; RMR, resting metabolic rate.

were inconsistent except for C-reactive protein (CRP), which was increased by CLA supplementation [18,30]. Increased CRP levels due to CLA will be discussed in the section entitled "Immune and Inflammatory Responses and Conjugated Linoleic Acid."

Six studies have reported antihypertensive effects of CLA [53,106,121–124]. Among them, two reports by Herrera et al. [122,123] found that CLA supplementation significantly reduced pregnancy-induced hypertension. Zhao et al. [106] reported the cosupplementation of CLA and ramipril, an antihypertensive drug, enhanced the effects of ramipril on reducing blood pressure in hypertensive patients: the decrease of 18 mmHg systolic and 19 mmHg diastolic pressures were significantly greater than the decrease of 7 mmHg systolic and 11 mmHg diastolic pressure observed with ramipril treatment alone. These effects were associated with decreased serum angiotensinogen levels without altering angiotensin-converting enzyme (ACE) activity [106]. As reducing blood pressure alone can reduce the risk of developing cardiovascular diseases, the hypotensive effects of CLA may be highly significant. In addition, Smit et al. [125] reported an association between adipose tissue *cis*-9,*trans*-11 CLA and a lowered risk of myocardial infarction among Costa Rican subjects. This suggests that the benefits of CLA on reducing cardiovascular diseases is not limited to its effects as a cosupplement; rather, naturally occurring CLA may also have significant effects on reducing cardiovascular diseases [125]. This, along with CLA's hypotensive effects, warrants further investigation.

Bone Health and Conjugated Linoleic Acid

Unlike the consistent effects of CLA on body fat reduction reported in animal studies, the effects of CLA on bone health are inconsistent [126–138]. Nine studies have investigated the effects of CLA on bone markers in humans [21,31,52,55,86,90,122,139,140], and most have reported no significant effects of CLA on bone mineral content, bone mineral mass, or bone mineral density [21,52]. The only positive outcome was reported by Brownbill et al. [139], who observed a positive association between food rich in CLA, thus mainly the *cis*-9,*trans*-11 isomer, and bone mineral density in postmenopausal women taking calcium supplements. This suggests a potential interaction between CLA and calcium in bone formation, as well as in calcium absorption, as previously suggested [140–144]. In addition, it has been suggested CLA's role in bone adiposity may involve effects on bone formation [145–148].

Immune and Inflammatory Responses and Conjugated Linoleic Acid

Most human studies did not report any significant changes in immune and inflammatory markers after CLA supplementation [18,30,120,149,150]. Stickford et al. [151] reported that 8-week CLA supplementation did not improve exercise-induced bronchoconstriction in asthma patients, although others reported promising results such as reduced allergic symptoms, improved antibody production after hepatitis B vaccination, reduced total symptom scores after rhinovirus infection, and reduced atopic dermatitis [152–155]. Although it was unclear whether a particular CLA isomer contributed to these activities, improved allergic symptoms and reduced atopic dermatitis were reported to be associated with the *cis*-9,*trans*-11 isomer [152,154,155].

Some studies indicate that serum CRP levels are increased after CLA supplementation [49,55,69,86,156–158], while others report no significant changes in CRP by CLA [35,39,90,149,150,154,159–162]. CRP is a serum inflammatory marker used to indicate increased risk of cardiovascular disease [163]. However, the risks of cardiovascular disease are often accompanied with increased levels of other inflammatory markers, such as TNF-α and interleukin 1β, 2, 6, and 10 [18,30,120]. Increased CRP alone, as seen with CLA supplementation, without changes to other markers is not indicative of an increased risk of cardiovascular disease.

Health Concerns Associated with Conjugated Linoleic Acid Consumption

Safety is of the utmost concern for any dietary supplement. The approval of CLA as a food additive in the USA was based on an extensive evaluation of its potential health impact, particularly the adverse effects associated with CLA [30,46]. The currently approved preparation of CLA as a food additive is the CLA mixture, containing approximately 60–90% of the two biologically active isomers: *cis*-9,*trans*-11 and *trans*-10,*cis*-12 CLA. There have been three clinical trials with CLA lasting longer than 1 year, one of which continued for another full year as an open study [52]. All reports from these trials indicate no major concerns with CLA supplementation. Thus, it may be considered that the consumption of CLA in the range of $\geq$6 g/day for 1 year and $\geq$3.4 g/day for up to 2 years has no adverse effects [21,52,82,104]. However, based on animal and human studies, four effects of CLA supplementation still need to be addressed in detail: (1) oxidative stress; (2) insulin sensitivity; (3) maternal milk fat; and (4) liver functions [4,156,164–168].

Oxidative Stress

Oxidative stress is a condition caused by an imbalance between oxygen-derived free radicals and antioxidative mechanisms, and increased oxidative stress is linked to development of chronic diseases. There are consistent reports that CLA supplementation increases oxidative markers in human studies, which are associated with both cis-9,trans-11 and trans-10,cis-12 isomers [34,56,65,99,124,150,154,156,169–171]. These include increased serum or urine isoprostanes, 8-iso-prostaglandin F2α (8-iso-PGF2α; a nonenzymatic oxidative marker) and/or 15-ketodihydro-PGF2α (an enzymatic oxidative marker) [34,56,99,124,150,154,156,169–171]. However, no other biomarkers of oxidative stress have been linked to CLA, suggesting that the increases of these markers may not indicate oxidative stress; rather, they reflect an interaction of CLA with isoprostane metabolism. This is supported by previous reports that CLA is metabolized by beta-oxidation to generate shorter carbon conjugated fatty acids [172,173]. It is also suggested that CLA-originated isoprostanes or similar metabolites may not be distinguishable by typical methods to determine isoprostanes, such as immune-based assays [174,175].

Pfeuffer et al. [124] provided further evidence that CLA supplementation does not change the levels of oxidized LDL, which is related to oxidative stress. In addition, Kim et al. [176] reported that CLA supplementation for 8 weeks did not alter serum lipid peroxidation or lipid antioxidant concentrations, thus confirming there may be no need for concern regarding CLA-associated oxidative stress.

Glucose Metabolism

CLA's effects on glucose metabolism in animal studies have been inconsistent: different responses were observed between normal and obese/diabetic models [20,28]. CLA's effects on glucose metabolism in humans were also inconsistent. The majority of human CLA studies reported no changes of glucose or insulin levels following CLA supplementation; however, some reports indicate that CLA adversely influences one or the other [53,159,177]. It is also important to note here that the *trans*-10,*cis*-12 CLA isomer, but not the *cis*-9,*trans*-11, has been associated with insulin resistance, which was not seen when CLA mixture was used in the same study [156,178]. This suggests that the *cis*-9,*trans*-11 isomer may antagonize the adverse effects of the *trans*-10,*cis*-12 isomer on insulin resistance.

Effects of CLA (longer than 6-month supplementation) on glucose and insulin levels are summarized in Table 37.2. Whigham et al. [82] reported the temporal increase in glucose levels after 2-week CLA supplementation that disappeared after that period. In addition, Gaullier et al. [52] reported increased insulin levels after 2-year CLA supplementation (only with the TG form of CLA). However, in the same report, insulin C-peptide levels (a better indicator of active insulin) were not altered in the CLA group. In conclusion, there is no significant concern over the use of CLA with regard to glucose metabolism, particularly when CLA mixture is used.

Milk Fat Depression

CLA supplementation has resulted in not only decreased body fat but also reduced milk fat in animal studies, particularly cows [179,180]. This raised concerns over the use of CLA in lactating women. Four publications have determined the role of CLA on milk fat in humans [181–184]. These studies were relatively short (5 days), except for Rizenthaler et al. [184], who used an 8-week CLA supplementation period. Two publications reported no influence of CLA on milk fat content [181,182]; in contrast, Masters et al. [183] reported a significant reduction in milk fat after CLA supplementation, although the milk fat content values were all within the normal range. Rizenthaler et al. [184] reported no effects on milk fat content with the longer supplementation period. However, they used naturally occurring *cis*-9,*trans*-11 CLA, which is not the active isomer for fat reduction. The primary source of milk fat is de novo fatty acid synthesis in ruminants, while it is diet and stored dietary fat in humans [179,180,185]. Thus, the inhibitory effects of CLA on de novo fatty acid synthesis may have greater impact in cows than in humans. However, three human studies used a short study period of 5 days, and it is important to determine the long-term effects of maternal CLA supplementation on milk fat.

Liver Function

In animal studies, CLA feeding resulted in altered liver functions, particularly in fatty liver [79,165,186,187]. Several human studies reported either no change or increased levels of liver function markers following CLA supplementation, although all were within the normal range [30,46,58]. Others reported no significant changes in liver structure or morphology or in signs of lipodystrophy after an 18-week CLA supplementation, except for a single case of CLA-induced acute hepatitis [33,188]. Wanders et al. [58] reported that short-term supplementation of high-dose CLA (19.3 g/day: 14.6 g *cis*-9,*trans*-11 and 4.7 g *trans*-10,*cis*-12) for 3 weeks had no adverse effect on liver function in healthy subjects. Thus, it is likely that CLA-induced alterations in liver function are specific to rodents. With the doses and treatment periods of CLA used in clinical trials, it is unlikely that CLA will cause liver dysfunction; however, it is important to follow up the serum markers to ensure the safety of CLA supplementation, particularly for long-term use.

CONCLUSION

Dietary factors affect a number of chronic diseases in both negative and positive ways. An ongoing primary effort to improve overall human health is to modify our dietary patterns, where CLA can serve as a beneficial component. However, it is apparent that CLA itself may not dramatically reduce body fat in humans, as has been seen in animal models. This does not exclude the applicability of CLA to the current effort to control obesity as well as other chronic diseases, including cancer. Close monitoring of efficacy as well as safety issues associated with CLA consumption will help to strengthen the future of CLA.

Acknowledgments

The author thanks Ms Jayne M. Storkson for help in preparing this manuscript. The author is one of the inventors of the CLA use patents assigned to the Wisconsin Alumni Research Foundation.

References

[1] Willett WC, Stampfer MJ, Manson JE, Colditz GA, Speizer FE, Rosner BA, et al. Intake of trans fatty acids and risk of coronary heart disease among women. Lancet 1993;341(8845):581–5.

[2] Lichtenstein AH, Ausman LM, Jalbert SM, Schaefer EJ. Effects of different forms of dietary hydrogenated fats on serum lipoprotein cholesterol levels. N.Engl. J. Med. 1999;340(25):1933–40.

[3] U.S. Food and Drug Administration. Nutrition labeling: trans fat labeling, <http://www.fda.gov/Food/Guidance Regulation/GuidanceDocumentsRegulatoryInformation/Labeling Nutrition/ucm064904.htm#transfatl>; 2013 [accessed 26.03.13].

[4] Park Y. Conjugated linoleic acid (CLA): Good or bad *trans* fat? J. Food Comp. Anal. 2009;22S:S4–S12.

[5] Park Y, Pariza MW. Bioactivities and potential mechanisms of action for conjugated fatty acids. Food Sci. Biotech. 2009;18(3):586–93.

[6] Parodi PW. Conjugated Linoleic Acid: The Early Years. In: Yurawecz MP, , Mossoba MM, , Kramer JKG, , Pariza MW, Nelson GJ, editors. Advances in Conjugated Linoleic Acid Resear, Vol. 1. Champaign, IL: AOCS Press; 1999. p. 1–11.

[7] Pariza MW, Hargraves WA. A beef-derived mutagenesis modulator inhibits initiation of mouse epidermal tumors by 7,12-dimethylbenz[a]anthracene. Carcinogenesis 1985;6(4):591–3.

[8] Ha YL, Grimm NK, Pariza MW. Anticarcinogens from fried ground beef: heat-altered derivatives of linoleic acid. Carcinogenesis 1987;8(12):1881–7.

[9] Kepler CR, Hirons KP, McNeill JJ, Tove SB. Intermediates and products of the biohydrogenation of linoleic acid by Butyrinvibrio fibrisolvens. J. Biol. Chem. 1966;241(6):1350–4.

[10] Kramer JK, Parodi PW, Jensen RG, Mossoba MM, Yurawecz MP, Adlof RO. Rumenic acid: a proposed common name for the major conjugated linoleic acid isomer found in natural products. Lipids 1998;33(8):835.

[11] Kay JK, Mackle TR, Auldist MJ, Thomson NA, Bauman DE. Endogenous synthesis of cis-9, trans-11 conjugated linoleic acid in dairy cows fed fresh pasture. J. Dairy Sci. 2004;87(2):369–78.

[12] Corl BA, Barbano DM, Bauman DE, Ip C. Cis-9, trans-11 CLA derived endogenously from trans-11 18:1 reduces cancer risk in rats. J. Nutr. 2003;133(9):2893–900.

[13] Chin SF, Storkson JM, Ha YL, Pariza MW. Dietary sources of conjugated dienoic isomers of linoleic acid. J. Food Comp. Anal. 1992;5:185–97.

[14] Park Y, McGuire MK, Behr R, McGuire MA, Evans MA, Shultz TD. High-fat dairy product consumption increases delta 9c,11t-18:2 (rumenic acid) and total lipid concentrations of human milk. Lipids 1999;34(6):543–9.

[15] Mushtaq S. Heather Mangiapane E, Hunter KA. Estimation of cis-9, trans-11 conjugated linoleic acid content in UK foods and assessment of dietary intake in a cohort of healthy adults. Br. J. Nutr. 2010;8(103):1366–74.

[16] Ritzenthaler KL, McGuire MK, Falen R, Shultz TD, Dasgupta N, McGuire MA. Estimation of conjugated linoleic acid intake by written dietary assessment methodologies underestimates actual intake evaluated by food duplicate methodology. J. Nutr. 2001;131(5):1548–54.

[17] Herbel BK, McGuire MK, McGuire MA, Shultz TD. Safflower oil consumption does not increase plasma conjugated linoleic acid concentrations in humans. Am. J. Clin. Nutr. 1998;67(2):332–7.

[18] McCrorie TA, Keaveney EM, Wallace JM, Binns N, Livingstone MB. Human health effects of conjugated linoleic acid from milk and supplements. Nutr. Res. Rev. 2011;24(2):206–27.

[19] Kramer JK, Sehat N, Dugan ME, Mossoba MM, Yurawecz MP, Roach JA, et al. Distributions of conjugated linoleic acid (CLA) isomers in tissue lipid classes of pigs fed a commercial CLA mixture determined by gas chromatography and silver ion-high-performance liquid chromatography. Lipids 1998;33(6):549–58.

[20] Park Y, Pariza MW. Mechanisms of body fat modulation by conjugated linoleic acid (CLA). Food Res. Int. 2007;40:311–23.

[21] Gaullier JM, Halse J, Hoye K, Kristiansen K, Fagertun H, Vik H, et al. Conjugated linoleic acid supplementation for 1 y reduces body fat mass in healthy overweight humans. Am. J. Clin. Nutr. 2004;79(6):1118–25.

[22] Kelly T, Yang W, Chen CS, Reynolds K, He J. Global burden of obesity in 2005 and projections to 2030. Int. J. Obes. (Lond) 2008;32(9):1431–7.

[23] Wang Y, Lobstein T. Worldwide trends in childhood overweight and obesity. Int. J. Pediatr. Obes. 2006;1(1):11–25.

[24] Biro FM, Wien M. Childhood obesity and adult morbidities. Am. J. Clin. Nutr. 2010;91(5):1499S–505S.

[25] Wang Y, Beydoun MA, Liang L, Caballero B, Kumanyika SK. Will all Americans become overweight or obese? estimating the progression and cost of the US obesity epidemic. Obesity (Silver Spring) 2008;16(10):2323–30.

[26] Pariza MW, Park Y, Cook ME. The biologically active isomers of conjugated linoleic acid. Prog. Lipid Res. 2001;40(4):283–98.

[27] Bhattacharya A, Banu J, Rahman M, Causey J, Fernandes G. Biological effects of conjugated linoleic acids in health and disease. J. Nutr. Biochem. 2006;17(12):789–810.

[28] Kennedy A, Martinez K, Schmidt S, Mandrup S, LaPoint K, McIntosh M. Antiobesity mechanisms of action of conjugated linoleic acid. J. Nutr. Biochem. 2010;21(3):171–9.

[29] Park Y, Albright KJ, Liu W, Storkson JM, Cook ME, Pariza MW. Effect of conjugated linoleic acid on body composition in mice. Lipids 1997;32(8):853–8.

[30] Dilzer A, Park Y. Implication of Conjugated Linoleic Acid (CLA) in Human Health. Crit. Rev. Food Sci. Nutr. 2012;52:488–513.

[31] Racine NM, Watras AC, Carrel AL, Allen DB, McVean JJ, Clark RR, et al. Effect of conjugated linoleic acid on body fat accretion in overweight or obese children. Am. J. Clin. Nutr. 2010;3(91):1157–64.

[32] Noone EJ, Roche HM, Nugent AP, Gibney MJ. The effect of dietary supplementation using isomeric blends of conjugated linoleic acid on lipid metabolism in healthy human subjects. Br. J. Nutr. 2002;88(3):243–51.

[33] Malpuech-Brugere C, Verboeket-van de Venne WP, Mensink RP, Arnal MA, Morio B, Brandolini M, et al. Effects of two conjugated linoleic Acid isomers on body fat mass in overweight humans. Obes. Res. 2004;12(4):591–8.

[34] Riserus U, Vessby B, Arnlov J, Basu S. Effects of cis-9, trans-11 conjugated linoleic acid supplementation on insulin sensitivity, lipid peroxidation, and proinflammatory markers in obese men. Am. J. Clin. Nutr. 2004;80(2):279–83.

[35] Desroches S, Chouinard PY, Galibois I, Corneau L, Delisle J, Lamarche B, et al. Lack of effect of dietary conjugated linoleic acids naturally incorporated into butter on the lipid profile and body composition of overweight and obese men. Am. J. Clin. Nutr. 2005;82(2):309–19.

[36] Tricon S, Burdge GC, Jones EL, Russell JJ, El-Khazen S, Moretti E, et al. Effects of dairy products naturally enriched with cis-9, trans-11 conjugated linoleic acid on the blood lipid profile in healthy middle-aged men. Am. J. Clin. Nutr. 2006;83(4):744–53.

[37] Herrmann J, Rubin D, Hasler R, Helwig U, Pfeuffer M, Auinger A, et al. Isomer-specific effects of CLA on gene expression in human adipose tissue depending on PPARgamma2 P12A polymorphism: a double blind, randomized, controlled cross-over study. Lipids Health. Dis. 2009;18(8):35.

[38] Raff M, Tholstrup T, Toubro S, Bruun JM, Lund P, Straarup EM, et al. Conjugated linoleic acids reduce body fat in healthy postmenopausal women. J. Nutr. 2009;139(7):1347–52.

[39] Sluijs I, Plantinga Y, de Roos B, Mennen LI, Bots ML. Dietary supplementation with cis-9, trans-11 conjugated linoleic acid

and aortic stiffness in overweight and obese adults. Am. J. Clin. Nutr. 2010;91(1):175–83.

[40] Joseph SV, Jacques H, Plourde M, Mitchell PL, McLeod RS, Jones PJ. Conjugated linoleic acid supplementation for 8 weeks does not affect body composition, lipid profile, or safety biomarkers in overweight, hyperlipidemic men. J. Nutr. 2011;141(7):1286–91.

[41] Venkatramanan S, Joseph SV, Chouinard PY, Jacques H, Farnworth ER, Jones PJ. Milk enriched with conjugated linoleic acid fails to alter blood lipids or body composition in moderately overweight, borderline hyperlipidemic individuals. J. Am. Coll. Nutr. 2010;29(2):152–9.

[42] Park Y, Storkson JM, Albright KJ, Liu W, Pariza MW. Evidence that the trans-10, cis-12 isomer of conjugated linoleic acid induces body composition changes in mice. Lipids 1999;34(3):235–41.

[43] Colakoglu S, Colakoglu M, Taneli F, Cetinoz F, Turkmen M. Cumulative effects of conjugated linoleic acid and exercise on endurance development, body composition, serum leptin and insulin levels. J. Sports Med. Phys. Fitness 2006;46(4):570–7.

[44] Whigham LD, Watras AC, Schoeller DA. Efficacy of conjugated linoleic acid for reducing fat mass: a meta-analysis in humans. Am. J. Clin. Nutr. 2007;85(5):1203–11.

[45] Blankson H, Stakkestad JA, Fagertun H, Thom E, Wadstein J, Gudmundsen O. Conjugated linoleic acid reduces body fat mass in overweight and obese humans. J. Nutr. 2000;130(12):2943–8.

[46] Onakpoya IJ, Posadzki PP, Watson LK, Davies LA, Ernst E. The efficacy of long-term conjugated linoleic acid (CLA) supplementation on body composition in overweight and obese individuals: a systematic review and meta-analysis of randomized clinical trials. Eur. J. Nutr. 2012;51(2):127–34.

[47] Schoeller DA, Watras AC, Whigham LD. A meta-analysis of the effects of conjugated linoleic acid on fat-free mass in humans. Appl. Physiol. Nutr. Metab. 2009;34(5):975–8.

[48] Kamphuis MM, Lejeune MP, Saris WH, Westerterp-Plantenga MS. The effect of conjugated linoleic acid supplementation after weight loss on body weight regain, body composition, and resting metabolic rate in overweight subjects. Int. J. Obes. Relat. Metab. Disord. 2003;27(7):840–7.

[49] Watras AC, Buchholz AC, Close RN, Zhang Z, Schoeller DA. The role of conjugated linoleic acid in reducing body fat and preventing holiday weight gain. Int. J. Obes. (Lond) 2007;31(3):481–7.

[50] DeLany JP, Blohm F, Truett AA, Scimeca JA, West DB. Conjugated linoleic acid rapidly reduces body fat content in mice without affecting energy intake. Am. J. Physiol. 1999;276(4 Pt 2):R1172–9.

[51] Park Y, Albright KJ, Storkson JM, Liu W, Pariza MW. Conjugated Linoleic Acid (CLA) Prevents Body Fat Accumulation and Weight Gain in an Animal Model. J. Food Sci. 2007;72(8):S612–7.

[52] Gaullier JM, Halse J, Hoye K, Kristiansen K, Fagertun H, Vik H, et al. Supplementation with conjugated linoleic acid for 24 months is well tolerated by and reduces body fat mass in healthy, overweight humans. J. Nutr. 2005;135(4):778–84.

[53] Iwata T, Kamegai T, Yamauchi-Sato Y, Ogawa A, Kasai M, Aoyama T, et al. Safety of dietary conjugated linoleic acid (CLA) in a 12-weeks trial in healthy overweight Japanese male volunteers. J. Oleo Sci. 2007;56(10):517–25.

[54] Atkinson RL. Conjugated linoleic acid for altering body composition and treating obesity. In: Yurawecz MP, , Mossoba MM, , Kramer JKG, , Pariza MW, Nelson GJ, editors. Advances in conjugated linoleic acid research, Vol. 1. Champaign, IL: AOCS Press; 1999. p. 348–53.

[55] Gaullier JM, Halse J, Hoivik HO, Hoye K, Syvertsen C, Nurminiemi M, et al. Six months supplementation with conjugated linoleic acid induces regional-specific fat mass decreases in overweight and obese. Br. J. Nutr. 2007;97(3):550–60.

[56] Cornish SM, Candow DG, Jantz NT, Chilibeck PD, Little JP, Forbes S, et al. Conjugated linoleic acid combined with creatine monohydrate and whey protein supplementation during strength training. Int. J. Sport Nutr. Exerc. Metab. 2009;19(1):79–96.

[57] Norris LE, Collene AL, Asp ML, Hsu JC, Liu LF, Richardson JR, et al. Comparison of dietary conjugated linoleic acid with safflower oil on body composition in obese postmenopausal women with type 2 diabetes mellitus. Am. J. Clin. Nutr. 2009;90(3):468–76.

[58] Wanders AJ, Leder L, Banga JD, Katan MB, Brouwer IA. A high intake of conjugated linoleic acid does not affect liver and kidney function tests in healthy human subjects. Food Chem. Toxicol. 2010;22(48):587–90.

[59] West DB, Delany JP, Camet PM, Blohm F, Truett AA, Scimeca J. Effects of conjugated linoleic acid on body fat and energy metabolism in the mouse. Am. J. Physiol. 1998;275(3 Pt 2):R667–72.

[60] Park Y, Park Y. Conjugated fatty acids increase energy expenditure in part by increasing voluntary movement in mice. Food Chem. 2012;133:400–9.

[61] Nagao K, Inoue N, Wang YM, Hirata J, Shimada Y, Nagao T, et al. The 10trans,12cis isomer of conjugated linoleic acid suppresses the development of hypertension in Otsuka Long-Evans Tokushima fatty rats. Biochem. Biophys. Res. Commun. 2003;306(1):134–8.

[62] Ohnuki K, Haramizu S, Oki K, Ishihara K, Fushiki T. A single oral administration of conjugated linoleic acid enhanced energy metabolism in mice. Lipids 2001;36(6):583–7.

[63] Ohnuki K, Haramizu S, Ishihara K, Fushiki T. Increased energy metabolism and suppressed body fat accumulation in mice by a low concentration of conjugated linoleic acid. Biosci. Biotechnol. Biochem. 2001;65(10):2200–4.

[64] Terpstra AH, Beynen AC, Everts H, Kocsis S, Katan MB, Zock PL. The decrease in body fat in mice fed conjugated linoleic acid is due to increases in energy expenditure and energy loss in the excreta. J. Nutr. 2002;132(5):940–5.

[65] Nazare JA, de la Perriere AB, Bonnet F, Desage M, Peyrat J, Maitrepierre C, et al. Daily intake of conjugated linoleic acid-enriched yoghurts: effects on energy metabolism and adipose tissue gene expression in healthy subjects. Br. J. Nutr. 2007;97(2):273–80.

[66] Close RN, Schoeller DA, Watras AC, Nora EH. Conjugated linoleic acid supplementation alters the 6-mo change in fat oxidation during sleep. Am. J. Clin. Nutr. 2007;86(3):797–804.

[67] Pinkoski C, Chilibeck PD, Candow DG, Esliger D, Ewaschuk JB, Facci M, et al. The effects of conjugated linoleic acid supplementation during resistance training. Med. Sci. Sports Exerc. 2006;38(2):339–48.

[68] Lambert EV, Goedecke JH, Bluett K, Heggie K, Claassen A, Rae DE, et al. Conjugated linoleic acid versus high-oleic acid sunflower oil: effects on energy metabolism, glucose tolerance, blood lipids, appetite and body composition in regularly exercising individuals. Br. J. Nutr. 2007;97(5):1001–11.

[69] Steck SE, Chalecki AM, Miller P, Conway J, Austin GL, Hardin JW, et al. Conjugated linoleic acid supplementation for twelve weeks increases lean body mass in obese humans. J. Nutr. 2007;137(5):1188–93.

[70] Zambell KL, Keim NL, Van Loan MD, Gale B, Benito P, Kelley DS, et al. Conjugated linoleic acid supplementation in humans: effects on body composition and energy expenditure. Lipids 2000;35(7):777–82.

[71] Bouthegourd JC, Even PC, Gripois D, Tiffon B, Blouquit MF, Roseau S, et al. A CLA mixture prevents body triglyceride accumulation without affecting energy expenditure in Syrian hamsters. J. Nutr. 2002;132(9):2682–9.

[72] Degrace P, Demizieux L, Gresti J, Chardigny JM, Sebedio JL, Clouet P. Hepatic steatosis is not due to impaired fatty acid oxidation capacities in C57BL/6J mice fed the conjugated trans-10, cis-12-isomer of linoleic acid. J. Nutr. 2004;134(4):861–7.

[73] Nagao K, Inoue N, Wang YM, Shirouchi B, Yanagita T. Dietary conjugated linoleic acid alleviates nonalcoholic fatty liver disease in Zucker (fa/fa) rats. J. Nutr. 2005;135(1):9–13.

[74] Peters JM, Park Y, Gonzalez FJ, Pariza MW. Influence of conjugated linoleic acid on body composition and target gene expression in peroxisome proliferator-activated receptor alpha-null mice. Biochim. Biophys. Acta 2001;1533(3):233–42.

[75] Ribot J, Portillo MP, Pico C, Macarulla MT, Palou A. Effects of trans-10, cis-12 conjugated linoleic acid on the expression of uncoupling proteins in hamsters fed an atherogenic diet. Br. J. Nutr. 2007;97(6):1074–82.

[76] Malpuech-Brugere C, Mensink RP, Loreau O, Maret A, Fernie CE, Lassel TS, et al. Comparison of postprandial oleic acid, 9c,11t CLA and 10t,12c CLA oxidation in healthy moderately overweight subjects. Lipids 2010;45(11):1047–51.

[77] Medina EA, Horn WF, Keim NL, Havel PJ, Benito P, Kelley DS, et al. Conjugated linoleic acid supplementation in humans: effects on circulating leptin concentrations and appetite. Lipids 2000;35(7):783–8.

[78] Belury MA, Mahon A, Banni S. The conjugated linoleic acid (CLA) isomer, t10c12-CLA, is inversely associated with changes in body weight and serum leptin in subjects with type 2 diabetes mellitus. J. Nutr. 2003;133(1):257S–60S.

[79] Tsuboyama-Kasaoka N, Takahashi M, Tanemura K, Kim HJ, Tange T, Okuyama H, et al. Conjugated linoleic acid supplementation reduces adipose tissue by apoptosis and develops lipodystrophy in mice. Diabetes 2000;49(9):1534–42.

[80] Rubin D, Herrmann J, Much D, Pfeuffer M, Laue C, Winkler P, et al. Influence of different CLA isomers on insulin resistance and adipocytokines in pre-diabetic, middle-aged men with PPARgamma2 Pro12Ala polymorphism. Genes Nutr. 2012;7(4):499–509.

[81] Kamphuis MM, Lejeune MP, Saris WH, Westerterp-Plantenga MS. Effect of conjugated linoleic acid supplementation after weight loss on appetite and food intake in overweight subjects. Eur. J. Clin. Nutr. 2003;57(10):1268–74.

[82] Whigham LD, O'Shea M, Mohede IC, Walaski HP, Atkinson RL. Safety profile of conjugated linoleic acid in a 12-month trial in obese humans. Food Chem. Toxicol. 2004;42(10):1701–9.

[83] Fushiki T, Matsumoto K, Inoue K, Kawada T, Sugimoto E. Swimming endurance capacity of mice is increased by chronic consumption of medium-chain triglycerides. J. Nutr. 1995;125(3):531–9.

[84] Mizunoya W, Haramizu S, Shibakusa T, Okabe Y, Fushiki T. Dietary conjugated linoleic acid increases endurance capacity and fat oxidation in mice during exercise. Lipids 2005;40(3):265–71.

[85] Kim JH, Kim J, Park Y. Trans-10, cis-12 CLA enhances endurance capacity by increasing fatty acid oxidation and reducing glycogen utilization in mice. Lipids 2012;47:855–63.

[86] Kreider RB, Ferreira MP, Greenwood M, Wilson M, Almada AL. Effects of conjugated linoleic acid supplementation during resistance training on body composition, bone density, strength, and selected hematological markers. J. Strength Cond. Res. 2002;16(3):325–34.

[87] Adams RE, Hsueh A, Alford B, King C, Mo H, Wildman R. Conjugated linoleic Acid supplementation does not reduce visceral adipose tissue in middle-aged men engaged in a resistance-training program. J. Int. Soc. Sports Nutr. 2006;13(3):28–36.

[88] Thom E, Wadstein J, Gudmundsen O. Conjugated linoleic acid reduces body fat in healthy exercising humans. J. Int. Med. Res. 2001;29(5):392–6.

[89] Diaz ML, Watkins BA, Li Y, Anderson RA, Campbell WW. Chromium picolinate and conjugated linoleic acid do not synergistically influence diet- and exercise-induced changes in body composition and health indexes in overweight women. J. Nutr. Biochem. 2008;19(1):61–8.

[90] Tarnopolsky M, Zimmer A, Paikin J, Safdar A, Aboud A, Pearce E, et al. Creatine monohydrate and conjugated linoleic acid improve strength and body composition following resistance exercise in older adults. PLoS ONE 2007;2(10):e991.

[91] Michishita T, Kobayashi S, Katsuya T, Ogihara T, Kawabuchi K. Evaluation of the antiobesity effects of an amino acid mixture and conjugated linoleic acid on exercising healthy overweight humans: a randomized, double-blind, placebo-controlled trial. J. Int. Med. Res. 2010;38(3):844–59.

[92] Brosnan JT, Brosnan ME. Creatine: endogenous metabolite, dietary, and therapeutic supplement. Annu. Rev. Nutr. 2007;27:241–61.

[93] Macaluso F, Morici G, Catanese P, Ardizzone NM, Marino Gammazza A, Bonsignore G, et al. Effect of conjugated linoleic acid on testosterone levels in vitro and in vivo after an acute bout of resistance exercise. J. Strength Cond Res. 2012;26(6):1667–74.

[94] Glass D, Roubenoff R. Recent advances in the biology and therapy of muscle wasting. Ann.N.Y.Acad.Sci. 2010;1211:25–36.

[95] Narici MV, Maffulli N. Sarcopenia: characteristics, mechanisms and functional significance. Br. Med. Bull. 2010;95:139–59.

[96] Houston DK, Nicklas BJ, Zizza CA. Weighty concerns: the growing prevalence of obesity among older adults. J. Am. Diet. Assoc. 2009;109(11):1886–95.

[97] Zamboni M, Mazzali G, Fantin F, Rossi A, Di Francesco V. Sarcopenic obesity: a new category of obesity in the elderly. Nutr. Metab. Cardiovasc. Dis. 2008;18(5):388–95.

[98] Sneddon AA, Tsofliou F, Fyfe CL, Matheson I, Jackson DM, Horgan G, et al. Effect of a conjugated linoleic acid and omega-3 fatty acid mixture on body composition and adiponectin. Obesity (Silver Spring) 2008;16(5):1019–24.

[99] Taylor JS, Williams SR, Rhys R, James P, Frenneaux MP. Conjugated linoleic acid impairs endothelial function. Arterioscler. Thromb. Vasc. Biol. 2006;26(2):307–12.

[100] Li JJ, Huang CJ, Xie D. Anti-obesity effects of conjugated linoleic acid, docosahexaenoic acid, and eicosapentaenoic acid. Mol. Nutr. Food Res. 2008;52(6):631–45.

[101] Wang Y, Jones PJ. Dietary conjugated linoleic acid and body composition. Am. J. Clin. Nutr. 2004;79(6 Suppl):1153S–8S.

[102] Terpstra AH. Effect of conjugated linoleic acid on body composition and plasma lipids in humans: an overview of the literature. Am. J. Clin. Nutr. 2004;79(3):352–61.

[103] Terpstra AH. Differences between humans and mice in efficacy of the body fat lowering effect of conjugated linoleic acid: role of metabolic rate. J. Nutr. 2001;131(7):2067–8.

[104] Larsen TM, Toubro S, Gudmundsen O, Astrup A. Conjugated linoleic acid supplementation for 1 y does not prevent weight or body fat regain. Am. J. Clin. Nutr. 2006;83(3):606–12.

[105] Attar-Bashi NM, Weisinger RS, Begg DP, Li D, Sinclair AJ. Failure of conjugated linoleic acid supplementation to enhance biosynthesis of docosahexaenoic acid from alpha-linolenic acid in healthy human volunteers. Prostaglandins Leukot. Essent. Fatty Acids 2007;76(3):121–30.

[106] Zhao WS, Zhai JJ, Wang YH, Xie PS, Yin XJ, Li LX, et al. Conjugated linoleic acid supplementation enhances

antihypertensive effect of ramipril in Chinese patients with obesity-related hypertension. Am. J. Hypertens. 2009;22(6):680–6.
[107] Knekt P, Jarvinen R, Seppanen R, Pukkala E, Aromaa A. Intake of dairy products and the risk of breast cancer. Br. J. Cancer 1996;73(5):687–91.
[108] Aro A, Mannisto S, Salminen I, Ovaskainen ML, Kataja V, Uusitupa M. Inverse association between dietary and serum conjugated linoleic acid and risk of breast cancer in postmenopausal women. Nutr. Cancer 2000;38(2):151–7.
[109] Chajes V, Lavillonniere F, Ferrari P, Jourdan ML, Pinault M, Maillard V, et al. Conjugated linoleic acid content in breast adipose tissue is not associated with the relative risk of breast cancer in a population of French patients. Cancer Epidemiol. Biomarkers Prev. 2002;11(7):672–3.
[110] Voorrips LE, Brants HA, Kardinaal AF, Hiddink GJ, van den Brandt PA, Goldbohm RA. Intake of conjugated linoleic acid, fat, and other fatty acids in relation to postmenopausal breast cancer: the Netherlands Cohort Study on Diet and Cancer. Am. J. Clin. Nutr. 2002;76(4):873–82.
[111] Chajes V, Lavillonniere F, Maillard V, Giraudeau B, Jourdan ML, Sebedio JL, et al. Conjugated linoleic acid content in breast adipose tissue of breast cancer patients and the risk of metastasis. Nutr. Cancer 2003;45(1):17–23.
[112] Rissanen H, Knekt P, Jarvinen R, Salminen I, Hakulinen T. Serum fatty acids and breast cancer incidence. Nutr. Cancer 2003;45(2):168–75.
[113] McCann SE, Ip C, Ip MM, McGuire MK, Muti P, Edge SB, et al. Dietary intake of conjugated linoleic acids and risk of premenopausal and postmenopausal breast cancer, Western New York Exposures and Breast Cancer Study (WEB Study). Cancer Epidemiol. Biomarkers Prev. 2004;13(9):1480–4.
[114] Larsson SC, Bergkvist L, Wolk A. High-fat dairy food and conjugated linoleic acid intakes in relation to colorectal cancer incidence in the Swedish Mammography Cohort. Am. J. Clin. Nutr. 2005;82(4):894–900.
[115] Rastmanesh R. An urgent need to include risk-benefit analysis in clinical trials investigating conjugated linoleic acid supplements in cancer patients. Contemp. Clin. Trials 2011;32(1):69–73.
[116] Cook ME, Miller CC, Park Y, Pariza M. Immune Modulation by Altered Nutrient Metabolism - Nutritional Control of Immune-Induced Growth Depression. Poult. Sci. 1993;72(7):1301–5.
[117] Miller CC, Park Y, Pariza MW, Cook ME. Feeding conjugated linoleic acid to animals partially overcomes catabolic responses due to endotoxin injection. Biochem. Biophys. Res. Commun. 1994;198(3):1107–12.
[118] Lee KN, Kritchevsky D, Pariza MW. Conjugated linoleic acid and atherosclerosis in rabbits. Atherosclerosis 1994;108(1):19–25.
[119] Wanders AJ, Brouwer IA, Siebelink E, Katan MB. Effect of a high intake of conjugated linoleic acid on lipoprotein levels in healthy human subjects. PLoS One 2010;5(2):e9000.
[120] Sofi F, Buccioni A, Cesari F, Gori AM, Minieri S, Mannini L, et al. Effects of a dairy product (pecorino cheese) naturally rich in cis-9, trans-11 conjugated linoleic acid on lipid, inflammatory and haemorheological variables: A dietary intervention study. Nutr. Metab. Cardiovasc. Dis. 2010;20(2):117–24.
[121] Berven G, Bye A, Hals O, Blankson H, Fagertun H, Thom E, et al. Safety of conjugated linoleic acid (CLA) in overweight or obese human volunteers. Eur. J. Lipid Sci. Tech. 2000;102(7):455–62.
[122] Herrera JA, Arevalo-Herrera M, Shahabuddin AK, Ersheng G, Herrera S, Garcia RG, et al. Calcium and conjugated linoleic acid reduces pregnancy-induced hypertension and decreases intracellular calcium in lymphocytes. Am. J. Hypertens. 2006;19(4):381–7.
[123] Herrera JA, Shahabuddin AK, Ersheng G, Wei Y, Garcia RG, Lopez-Jaramillo P. Calcium plus linoleic acid therapy for pregnancy-induced hypertension. Int. J. Gynaecol. Obstet. 2005;91(3):221–7.
[124] Pfeuffer M, Fielitz K, Laue C, Winkler P, Rubin D, Helwig U, et al. CLA does not impair endothelial function and decreases body weight as compared with safflower oil in overweight and obese male subjects. J. Am. Coll. Nutr. 2011;30(1):19–28.
[125] Smit LA, Baylin A, Campos H. Conjugated linoleic acid in adipose tissue and risk of myocardial infarction. Am. J. Clin. Nutr. 2010;92(1):34–40.
[126] Watkins BA, Shen CL, McMurtry JP, Xu H, Bain SD, Allen KG, et al. Dietary lipids modulate bone prostaglandin E2 production, insulin-like growth factor-I concentration and formation rate in chicks. J. Nutr. 1997;127(6):1084–91.
[127] Li Y, Watkins BA. Conjugated linoleic acids alter bone fatty acid composition and reduce ex vivo prostaglandin E2 biosynthesis in rats fed n-6 or n-3 fatty acids. Lipids 1998;33(4):417–25.
[128] Turek JJ, Li Y, Schoenlein IA, Allen KGD, Watkins BA. Modulation of macrophage cytokine production by conjugated linoleic acids is influenced by the dietary n-6: n-3 fatty acid ratio. J. Nutr. Biochem. 1998;9(5):258–66.
[129] Li Y, Seifert MF, Ney DM, Grahn M, Grant AL, Allen KG, et al. Dietary conjugated linoleic acids alter serum IGF-I and IGF binding protein concentrations and reduce bone formation in rats fed (n-6) or (n-3) fatty acids. J. Bone Miner. Res. 1999;14(7):1153–62.
[130] Thiel-Cooper RL, Parrish Jr FC, Sparks JC, Wiegand BR, Ewan RC. Conjugated linoleic acid changes swine performance and carcass composition. J. Anim. Sci. 2001;79(7):1821–8.
[131] Demaree SR, Gilbert CD, Mersmann HJ, Smith SB. Conjugated linoleic acid differentially modifies fatty acid composition in subcellular fractions of muscle and adipose tissue but not adiposity of postweaning pigs. J. Nutr. 2002;132(11):3272–9.
[132] Kelly O, Cusack S, Cashman KD. The effect of bovine whey protein on ectopic bone formation in young growing rats. Br. J. Nutr. 2003;90(3):557–64.
[133] Ostrowska E, Suster D, Muralitharan M, Cross RF, Leury BJ, Bauman DE, et al. Conjugated linoleic acid decreases fat accretion in pigs: evaluation by dual-energy X-ray absorptiometry. Br. J. Nutr. 2003;89(2):219–29.
[134] Berge GM, Ruyter B, Asgard T. Conjugated linoleic acid in diets for juvenile Atlantic salmon (Salmo salar); effects on fish performance, proximate composition, fatty acid and mineral content. Aquaculture 2004;237(1–4):365–80.
[135] Banu J, Bhattacharya A, Rahman M, O'Shea M, Fernandes G. Effects of conjugated linoleic acid and exercise on bone mass in young male Balb/C mice. Lipids Health. Dis. 2006;23(5):7.
[136] Burr LL, Taylor CG, Weiler HA. Dietary conjugated linoleic acid does not adversely affect bone mass in obese fa/fa or lean Zucker rats. Exp. Biol. Med. (Maywood) 2006;231(10):1602–9.
[137] Weiler H, Austin S, Fitzpatrick-Wong S, Nitschmann E, Bankovic-Calic N, Mollard R, et al. Conjugated linoleic acid reduces parathyroid hormone in health and in polycystic kidney disease in rats. Am. J. Clin. Nutr. 2004;79(6 Suppl):1186S–9S.
[138] Kelly O, Cashman KD. The effect of conjugated linoleic acid on calcium absorption and bone metabolism and composition in adult ovariectomised rats. Prostaglandins Leukot. Essent. Fatty Acids 2004;71(5):295–301.
[139] Brownbill RA, Petrosian M, Ilich JZ. Association between dietary conjugated linoleic acid and bone mineral density in postmenopausal women. J. Am. Coll. Nutr. 2005;24(3):177–81.
[140] Doyle L, Jewell C, Mullen A, Nugent AP, Roche HM, Cashman KD. Effect of dietary supplementation with conjugated linoleic acid on markers of calcium and bone metabolism in healthy adult men. Eur. J. Clin. Nutr. 2005;59(3):432–40.
[141] Park Y, Terk M, Park Y. Interaction between dietary conjugated linoleic acid and calcium supplementation affecting bone and fat mass. J. Bone Miner. Metab. 2011;10(29):268–78.

[142] Park Y, Park YH, Rhee S, Park GK. Effect of interaction between dietary conjugated linoleic acid (CLA) and calcium on body composition. FASEB J. 2006;20:A570.

[143] Murphy EF, Hooiveld GJ, Muller M, Calogero RA, Cashman KD. The effect of trans-10, cis-12 conjugated linoleic acid on gene expression profiles related to lipid metabolism in human intestinal-like Caco-2 cells. Genes Nutr. 2009;4(2):103–12.

[144] Murphy EF, Jewell C, Hooiveld GJ, Muller M, Cashman KD. Conjugated linoleic acid enhances transepithelial calcium transport in human intestinal-like Caco-2 cells: an insight into molecular changes. Prostaglandins Leukot. Essent. Fatty Acids 2006;74(5):295–301.

[145] Ing SW, Belury MA. Impact of conjugated linoleic acid on bone physiology: proposed mechanism involving inhibition of adipogenesis. Nutr. Rev. 2011;69(3):123–31.

[146] Halade GV, Rahman MM, Williams PJ, Fernandes G. Combination of conjugated linoleic acid with fish oil prevents age-associated bone marrow adiposity in C57Bl/6J mice. J. Nutr. Biochem. 2011;22(5):459–69.

[147] Rahman MM, Halade GV, Williams PJ, Fernandes G. t10c12-CLA maintains higher bone mineral density during aging by modulating osteoclastogenesis and bone marrow adiposity. J. Cell. Physiol. 2011;226(9):2406–14.

[148] Kim J, Park Y, Lee SH, Park Y. Trans-10, cis-12 Conjugated linoleic acid promotes bone formation by inhibiting adipogenesis by peroxisome proliferator activated receptor-gamma-dependent mechanisms and by directly enhancing osteoblastogenesis from bone marrow mesenchymal stem cells. J. Nutr. Biochem. 2013;24(4):672–9.

[149] Asp ML, Collene AL, Norris LE, Cole RM, Stout MB, Tang SY, et al. Time-dependent effects of safflower oil to improve glycemia, inflammation and blood lipids in obese, post-menopausal women with type 2 diabetes: a randomized, double-masked, crossover study. Clin. Nutr. 2011;30(4):443–9.

[150] Smit LA, Katan MB, Wanders AJ, Basu S, Brouwer IA. A high intake of trans fatty acids has little effect on markers of inflammation and oxidative stress in humans. J. Nutr. 2011;141(9):1673–8.

[151] Stickford JL, Mickleborough TD, Fly AD, Stager JM. Conjugated linoleic acid's lack of attenuation of hyperpnea-induced bronchoconstriction in asthmatic individuals in the short term. Int. J. Sport Nutr. Exerc. Metab. 2011;21(1):40–7.

[152] Albers R, van der Wielen RP, Brink EJ, Hendriks HF, Dorovska-Taran VN, Mohede IC. Effects of cis-9, trans-11 and trans-10, cis-12 conjugated linoleic acid (CLA) isomers on immune function in healthy men. Eur. J. Clin. Nutr. 2003;57(4):595–603.

[153] Peterson KM, O'Shea M, Stam W, Mohede IC, Patrie JT, Hayden FG. Effects of dietary supplementation with conjugated linoleic acid on experimental human rhinovirus infection and illness. Antivir. Ther. 2009;14(1):33–43.

[154] Turpeinen AM, Ylonen N, von Willebrand E, Basu S, Aro A. Immunological and metabolic effects of cis-9, trans-11-conjugated linoleic acid in subjects with birch pollen allergy. Br. J. Nutr. 2008;100(1):112–9.

[155] Thijs C, Muller A, Rist L, Kummeling I, Snijders BE, Huber M, et al. Fatty acids in breast milk and development of atopic eczema and allergic sensitisation in infancy. Allergy 2011;66(1):58–67.

[156] Riserus U, Basu S, Jovinge S, Fredrikson GN, Arnlov J, Vessby B. Supplementation with conjugated linoleic acid causes isomer-dependent oxidative stress and elevated C-reactive protein: a potential link to fatty acid-induced insulin resistance. Circulation 2002;106(15):1925–9.

[157] Riserus U, Vessby B, Arner P, Zethelius B. Supplementation with trans10cis12-conjugated linoleic acid induces hyperproinsulinaemia in obese men: close association with impaired insulin sensitivity. Diabetologia 2004;47(6):1016–9.

[158] Smedman A, Basu S, Jovinge S, Fredrikson GN, Vessby B. Conjugated linoleic acid increased C-reactive protein in human subjects. Br. J. Nutr. 2005;94(5):791–5.

[159] Moloney F, Yeow TP, Mullen A, Nolan JJ, Roche HM. Conjugated linoleic acid supplementation, insulin sensitivity, and lipoprotein metabolism in patients with type 2 diabetes mellitus. Am. J. Clin. Nutr. 2004;80(4):887–95.

[160] Tricon S, Burdge GC, Kew S, Banerjee T, Russell JJ, Grimble RF, et al. Effects of cis-9, trans-11 and trans-10, cis-12 conjugated linoleic acid on immune cell function in healthy humans. Am. J. Clin. Nutr. 2004;80(6):1626–33.

[161] Ramakers JD, Plat J, Sebedio JL, Mensink RP. Effects of the individual isomers cis-9, trans-11 vs. trans-10, cis-12 of conjugated linoleic acid (CLA) on inflammation parameters in moderately overweight subjects with LDL-phenotype B. Lipids 2005;40(9):909–18.

[162] Raff M, Tholstrup T, Basu S, Nonboe P, Sorensen MT, Straarup EM. A diet rich in conjugated linoleic acid and butter increases lipid peroxidation but does not affect atherosclerotic, inflammatory, or diabetic risk markers in healthy young men. J. Nutr. 2008;138(3):509–14.

[163] Madjid M, Willerson JT. Inflammatory markers in coronary heart disease. Br. Med. Bull. 2011;100:23–38.

[164] Kelley DS, Erickson KL. Modulation of body composition and immune cell functions by conjugated linoleic acid in humans and animal models: benefits vs. risks. Lipids 2003;38(4):377–86.

[165] Larsen TM, Toubro S, Astrup A. Efficacy and safety of dietary supplements containing CLA for the treatment of obesity: evidence from animal and human studies. J. Lipid Res. 2003;44(12):2234–41.

[166] Tricon S, Yaqoob P. Conjugated linoleic acid and human health: a critical evaluation of the evidence. Curr. Opin. Clin. Nutr. Metab. Care 2006;9(2):105–10.

[167] Pariza MW. Perspective on the safety and effectiveness of conjugated linoleic acid. Am. J. Clin. Nutr. 2004;79(6 Suppl):1132S–6S.

[168] Clement L, Poirier H, Niot I, Bocher V, Guerre-Millo M, Krief S, et al. Dietary trans-10, cis-12 conjugated linoleic acid induces hyperinsulinemia and fatty liver in the mouse. J. Lipid Res. 2002;43(9):1400–9.

[169] Basu S, Riserus U, Turpeinen A, Vessby B. Conjugated linoleic acid induces lipid peroxidation in men with abdominal obesity. Clin. Sci. (Lond) 2000;99(6):511–6.

[170] Basu S, Smedman A, Vessby B. Conjugated linoleic acid induces lipid peroxidation in humans. FEBS Lett. 2000;468(1):33–6.

[171] Smedman A, Vessby B, Basu S. Isomer-specific effects of conjugated linoleic acid on lipid peroxidation in humans: regulation by alpha-tocopherol and cyclo-oxygenase-2 inhibitor. Clin. Sci. (Lond) 2004;106(1):67–73.

[172] Iannone A, Petroni A, Murru E, Cordeddu L, Carta G, Melis MP, et al. Impairment of 8-iso-PGF(2ALPHA) isoprostane metabolism by dietary conjugated linoleic acid (CLA). Prostaglandins Leukot Essent Fatty Acids 2009;80(5–6):279–87.

[173] Park Y, Storkson JM, Albright KJ, Liu W, Pariza MW. Biological activities of conjugated fatty acids: conjugated eicosadienoic (conj. 20:2delta(c11, t13/t12, c14)), eicosatrienoic (conj. 20:3delta(c8, t12, c14)), and heneicosadienoic (conj. 21:2delta(c12, t14/c13, t15)) acids and other metabolites of conjugated linoleic acid. Biochim. Biophys. Acta 2005;1687(1–3):120–9.

[174] Banni S, Petroni A, Blasevich M, Carta G, Cordeddu L, Murru E, et al. Conjugated linoleic acids (CLA) as precursors of a distinct family of PUFA. Lipids 2004;39(11):1143–6.

[175] Sebedio JL, Angioni E, Chardigny JM, Gregoire S, Juaneda P, Berdeaux O. The effect of conjugated linoleic acid isomers on fatty acid profiles of liver and adipose tissues and their conversion to isomers of 16:2 and 18:3 conjugated fatty acids in rats. Lipids 2001;36(6):575–82.

[176] Kim J, Paik HD, Shin MJ, Park E. Eight weeks of conjugated linoleic acid supplementation has no effect on antioxidant status in healthy overweight/obese Korean individuals. Eur. J. Nutr. 2012;51(2):135–41.

[177] Riserus U, Berglund L, Vessby B. Conjugated linoleic acid (CLA) reduced abdominal adipose tissue in obese middle-aged men with signs of the metabolic syndrome: a randomised controlled trial. Int. J. Obes. Relat. Metab. Disord. 2001;25(8):1129–35.

[178] Riserus U, Arner P, Brismar K, Vessby B. Treatment with dietary trans10cis12 conjugated linoleic acid causes isomer-specific insulin resistance in obese men with the metabolic syndrome. Diabetes Care 2002;25(9):1516–21.

[179] Bernard L, Leroux C, Chilliard Y. Expression and nutritional regulation of lipogenic genes in the ruminant lactating mammary gland. Adv. Exp. Med. Biol. 2008;606:67–108.

[180] Bauman DE, Griinari JM. Nutritional regulation of milk fat synthesis. Annu. Rev. Nutr. 2003;23:203–27.

[181] Hasin A, Griinari JM, Williams JE, Shahin AM, McGuire MA, McGuire MK. Consumption of c9, t11–18:2 or t10, c12–18:2 enriched dietary supplements does not influence milk macronutrients in healthy, lactating women. Lipids 2007;42(9):835–43.

[182] Mosley SA, Shahin AM, Williams J, McGuire MA, McGuire MK. Supplemental conjugated linoleic acid consumption does not influence milk macronutrient contents in all healthy lactating women. Lipids 2007;42(8):723–9.

[183] Masters N, McGuire MA, Beerman KA, Dasgupta N, McGuire MK. Maternal supplementation with CLA decreases milk fat in humans. Lipids 2002;37(2):133–8.

[184] Ritzenthaler KL, McGuire MK, McGuire MA, Shultz TD, Koepp AE, Luedecke LO, et al. Consumption of conjugated linoleic acid (CLA) from CLA-enriched cheese does not alter milk fat or immunity in lactating women. J. Nutr. 2005;135(3):422–30.

[185] Hachey DL, Silber GH, Wong WW, Garza C. Human lactation. II: Endogenous fatty acid synthesis by the mammary gland. Pediatr. Res. 1989;25(1):63–8.

[186] Belury MA, Kempa-Steczko A. Conjugated linoleic acid modulates hepatic lipid composition in mice. Lipids 1997;32(2):199–204.

[187] Jaudszus A, Moeckel P, Hamelmann E, Jahreis G. Trans-10, cis-12-CLA-caused lipodystrophy is associated with profound changes of fatty acid profiles of liver, white adipose tissue and erythrocytes in mice: possible link to tissue-specific alterations of fatty acid desaturation. Ann. Nutr. Metab. 2010;57(2):103–11.

[188] Ramos R, Mascarenhas J, Duarte P, Vicente C, Casteleiro C. Conjugated Linoleic Acid-Induced Toxic Hepatitis: First Case Report. Dig. Dis. Sci. 2009;23(54):1141–3.

[189] Mougios V, Matsakas A, Petridou A, Ring S, Sagredos A, Melissopoulou A, et al. Effect of supplementation with conjugated linoleic acid on human serum lipids and body fat. J. Nutr. Biochem. 2001;12(10):585–94.

[190] Smedman A, Vessby B. Conjugated linoleic acid supplementation in humans–metabolic effects. Lipids 2001;36(8):773–81.

[191] Eyjolfson V, Spriet LL, Dyck DJ. Conjugated linoleic acid improves insulin sensitivity in young, sedentary humans. Med. Sci. Sports Exerc. 2004;36(5):814–20.

[192] Laso N, Brugue E, Vidal J, Ros E, Arnaiz JA, Carne X, et al. Effects of milk supplementation with conjugated linoleic acid (isomers cis-9, trans-11 and trans-10, cis-12) on body composition and metabolic syndrome components. Br. J. Nutr. 2007;98(4):860–7.

[193] Syvertsen C, Halse J, Hoivik HO, Gaullier JM, Nurminiemi M, Kristiansen K, et al. The effect of 6 months supplementation with conjugated linoleic acid on insulin resistance in overweight and obese. Int. J. Obes. (Lond) 2007;31(7):1148–54.

[194] Thrush AB, Chabowski A, Heigenhauser GJ, McBride BW, Or-Rashid M, Dyck DJ. Conjugated linoleic acid increases skeletal muscle ceramide content and decreases insulin sensitivity in overweight, non-diabetic humans. Appl. Physiol. Nutr. Metab. 2007;32(3):372–82.

[195] Park E, Kim J, Kim K, Paik H. Conjugated Linoleic Acid (CLA) Supplementation for 8 Weeks Reduces Body Weight in Healthy Overweight/Obese Korean Subjects. Food Science and Biotechnology 2008;17(6):1261–4.

[196] MacRedmond R, Singhera G, Attridge S, Bahzad M, Fava C, Lai Y, et al. Conjugated linoleic acid improves airway hyper-reactivity in overweight mild asthmatics. Clin. Exp. Allergy 2010;40(7):1071–8.

[197] Chen SC, Lin YH, Huang HP, Hsu WL, Houng JY, Huang CK. Effect of conjugated linoleic acid supplementation on weight loss and body fat composition in a Chinese population. Nutrition 2012;28(5):559–65.

CHAPTER

38

Essential Amino Acid Supplementation for the Prevention and Treatment of Obesity

Giuseppe D'Antona

Department of Molecular Medicine and the Laboratory for the Study of Motor Activities in Rare Diseases, University of Pavia, Voghera, Italy

MACRONUTRIENTS AND OBESITY

Obesity, which arises when the dietary intake of energy exceeds whole-body energy expenditure and fat is accumulated in white adipose tissue, is a growing concern for health professionals due to the concomitant high prevalence (about 32.2% of adult men and 35.5% of adult women in the United States [1]) and a strict correlation with the development of chronic diseases.

There is unchallenged evidence that obesity is a major risk factor for coronary heart disease and is associated with higher risk of hypertension, type 2 diabetes mellitus (T2DM), dyslipidemia [elevated total cholesterol and low-density lipoprotein (LDL) cholesterol, and reduced levels of high-density lipoprotein cholesterol], stroke, osteoarthritis, sleep apnea, and breast, prostate, and colon cancer [2–4].

Inadequate lifestyle factors such as reduced physical activity and poor nutrition are considered the leading behavioral risk factors for the development of obesity; therefore, adequate exercise load and nutrition strategies can help to prevent and/or reduce abdominal adipose tissue accumulation and cardiovascular risk. With this aim, and based on the assumption that physical activity has been shown to result in an improved health risk profile in individuals even in presence of overweight or obesity [5], regular exercise programs have been developed and practiced since the 1990s, with variable compliance and success. In parallel, to aid the goal of weight loss and/or improved body composition, dieting strategies and nutritional supplementations have been adopted to combat obesity and promote health [6].

From the beginning of the twentieth century until the 1950s, a high-fat diet was recommended by the medical profession as a suitable diet for health maintenance and the treatment of diabetes. The first recommendation to reduce dietary fat content was introduced in the 1970s as a means of lowering serum cholesterol and preventing heart disease [7].

Nowadays, although controversy still exists over whether fat consumption is the major determinant of body fat mass [8], the generally accepted paradigm is that low-fat/high-carbohydrate diets promote weight loss and/or prevent weight gain. This kind of diet can particularly promote weight loss if the carbohydrate-rich foods are vegetables and whole grains of a low glycemic index, but it has been linked to unfavorable effects because it may promote the insulin resistance [9–12] or determine the transformation of large LDLs into the more atherogenic, small LDLs [13]. Recently, low-carbohydrate diets (including the so-called Atkins diet with low carbohydrate, high protein, and high fat) have been the focus of several studies [14–18] and there is evidence that they have advantages over low-energy, high-carbohydrate diets (i.e. so-called conventional diets: low calorie, high carbohydrate, low fat) in terms of improvements to lipid profile elements [14–17] and insulin sensitivity [15,16], and a greater and more rapid weight loss that was observed following energy restriction and low fat [15–17]. Importantly, after several months (12 months) following a low-carbohydrate diet, significant improvements in weight loss have been observed in comparison with a conventional diet, suggesting that the rapid weight loss induced by this kind of diet is regained faster than with a conventional low-fat diet [17].

Nutrition in the Prevention and Treatment of Abdominal Obesity
http://dx.doi.org/10.1016/B978-0-12-407869-7.00038-6

Thus, the weight-reducing properties of low-carbohydrate diets appear similar to those of conventional diets; this effect may be mainly due to the decreased energy intake and higher satiety induced by proteins in comparison with carbohydrates [19,20]. In fact, important findings in mammals have shown decreased food intake immediately followed by a reduction in body weight [21,22] when a high-protein diet is fed ad libitum; this was demonstrated in humans by Skov and colleagues by increasing the relative dietary protein content from normal (10–15%) to a higher level (20–40%) [19]. This capacity has been also described in additional studies demonstrating that short- and long-term nutritional interventions with high-protein diets appear to offer advantages over conventional weight loss regimens for weight loss maintenance after the initial body weight loss [22,23]; mechanisms include (apart from increased and sustained satiety despite a negative energy balance) increased thermogenesis and basal energy expenditure, and a significant sparing of lean body mass [24]. Lean body mass is a major determinant of the resting metabolic rate during weight reduction, and is particularly important in sarcopenic obesity [25]. Several mechanisms may contribute to the metabolic improvements related to high-protein intake, at least in the short term, finally leading to increased energy expenditure and increased satiety [26]. Specific amino acids disproportionately contribute to these effects.

Although low-carbohydrate/high-protein diets have been shown to promote weight loss in obese subjects, and particularly in short-term intervention studies [16,27,28], long-term intervention studies have had mixed results [17,29–33]. In particular, observational studies have recently shown a positive correlation between an increased proportion of proteins in the diet and weight gain [34–37]. In these studies, the risk of becoming overweight has been positively linked with increased energy disposal from animal (in contrast to vegetable) proteins [38] and this hyperconsumption has been associated with higher mortality [39]. In particular, a significantly higher risk of becoming overweight was found when the average percentage energy derived from protein exceeded the amount currently recommended by the World Health Organization (10–15%) [40], being significantly higher starting from 18% of energy from protein in normal-weight subjects and from 20% of energy from protein in overweight subjects [34,41]. Interestingly, following protein excess, a higher weight gain was observed when the proportion of protein was increased at the expense of good-quality carbohydrates (rich in fiber) compared to low-quality carbohydrates (low in fiber) [34]. Importantly, the mechanisms underlying the long-term effects of protein excess on overweight are not currently known. Intriguingly, the decreased food intake associated with protein-enriched diets may be counterbalanced by the hypothalamic melanocortin system, which seems to play a central role in the control of food intake through adjustments that evolved to defend the body against variations in food intake and body weight changes [42]. Nevertheless, limitations of the aforementioned studies (mainly related to the complexity in controlling variables), highlight the need for future studies involving large cohorts of subjects to investigate the mechanisms by which a sustained high proportion of dietary protein may lead to long-term weight gain in humans.

Overall, a possible correlation between protein excess and body weight is in apparent contrast with results from high-quality studies such as the population-based International Study of Macro- and Micronutrients and Blood Pressure (INTERMAP) [43], which demonstrates that a higher intake of essential amino acids (EAAs), and in particular branched-chain amino acids (BCAAs), is associated with a lower prevalence of overweight or obesity in middle-aged individuals from East Asian and Western countries. This evidence appears to strengthen the hypothesis that EAAs, unlike non-EAAs, may exert unique obesity-related effects [44] because effects on obesity have been related to increased fat leptin secretion [45], decreased food intake and body weight via serine/threonine-protein kinase mTOR signaling [46], and improved muscle glucose uptake and whole-body glucose metabolism [47]; thus, their supplementation is a potential strategy for the prevention and treatment of obesity, in addition to changing macronutrients regimes.

ESSENTIAL AMINO ACIDS AND THE CONTROL OF SATIETY

The satiating efficacies of macronutrients have a strict correspondence with the timing of their metabolism, with protein generally being the most satiating and fat the least [48], although this hierarchy is not always observed in rats [49] or humans [50,51].

Protein-induced satiety has been observed following acute high-protein intake in a dose-dependent fashion [48,52] and following prolonged high-protein diets [53], thus contributing to weight regain limitations after weight loss. Diverse mechanisms (both peripheral and central) may contribute to the satiating effect of dietary amino acids. In fact, amino acid consumption is detected by several pre- and postabsorptive signals originating from visceral and metabolic sources and subsequently recorded by the central nervous system (CNS). Satiation feedback signals originate in the stomach and result from volumetric signals produced by mechanoreceptors that detect increased gastric secretion and water intake [54]. Next, dietary proteins and amino acids are detected within the lumen of the duodenum [55] and by hepatic portal vein vagal afferents [56].

The process of amino acid detection at the level of the upper intestine appears to be linked to di- and tripeptide absorption by enterocytes, mediated by solute carrier family 15 member 1 [peptide transporter 1 (PepT1)], a member of the peptide transporter family found in all species from bacteria to humans [57] This protein is expressed on the apical membrane of enterocytes and on cholecystokinin (CCK)-endocrine cells [58–61] and its expression is regulated by its substrate [59]. Alternatively, amino acids may be detected by nutrient-specific receptors on the apical side of enterocytes and enteroendocrine cells [56,62,63]. Ultimately, amino acid and oligopeptide detection in the intestinal wall is dependent upon the release of CCK by enteroendocrine cells, followed by the activation of C-C motif chemokine 28 (CCK1) receptors and an increase in the firing rate of afferent vagal nerve terminals located close to the brush border. This conveys information to the nuclei of the solitary tract (NTS; the main entry point of the vagus nerve into the CNS) in the brainstem [64]. Interestingly, a role for PepT1 has also been determined in the secretion of CCK [65], but the underlying mechanisms remain unclear [66].

Importantly, another mechanism consisting of the inhibition of proximal gastrointestinal motility and secretion by a means of local feedback arising in the lower intestine may exert a direct or indirect impact on eating behavior and satiety (the so-called *ileal brake* [55]). Ileal infusion with proteins activates the ileal brake by the long-lasting release of peptide YY (PYY) by L intestine cells [67,68]. In fact, a high-protein diet, unlike other diets, increases total plasma PYY and integrated PYY levels in normal and obese subjects, followed by hunger reduction. Interestingly, in mice, PYY knockout abolishes the satiating and weight-reducing effects of proteins and produces obesity that appears to be reversed by exogenous PYY treatment [69].

Mediators other than CCK and PYY may also play a role in the regulation of protein intake. In particular, these include proteins that appear to be strong stimulators of glucagon-like peptide 1 (GLP-1; which acts on vagal afferent terminals in close vicinity to the enteroendocrine L cells [68]) release by the small intestine [70] and inhibitors of the orexigenic blood-borne peptide ghrelin [71]. As suggested by several authors, a complex cooperative interplay might occur between anorexigenic hormones, resulting in potential synergistic effects [72]. Once generated, anorexigenic signals may act on the CNS, first via the vagus nerve at the gastrointestinal tract to the brainstem within the NTS, and secondly via a direct effect on the hypothalamus [mainly the arcuate nucleus of the hypothalamus (ARC)] and brainstem via the bloodstream. As intracerebroventricular or dietary administration of leucine is sufficient to suppress food intake in rats and mice [46], it has been suggested that changes in blood amino acids may act directly on brain regions. The first evidence in rats suggested that the protein-induced suppression of the feeling of hunger arises from signals (mainly vagus mediated) directed to the NTS and the hypothalamus [73]. It is currently accepted that high-protein diets trigger the activation of noradrenergic and adrenergic neurons in the NTS and melanocortin neurons in the ARC and inhibit the activation of opioid and GABAergic neurons in the nucleus accumbens, thus restraining food intake by reducing the hedonic response to food. Considering that the intracerebroventricular injection of leucine has been found to exert the same depressive effects on satiety as a leucine-containing amino acid mixture [74], until now the central effects of high-protein diets have been exclusively attributed to leucine, mainly through neural mechanisms involving mTOR and 5′-AMP-activated protein kinase (AMPK) [75]. AMPK is activated by an increased adenosine monophosphate:adenosine triphosphate (AMP:ATP) ratio, and phosphorylates acetyl-CoA carboxylase (ACC), thus switching on energy-producing pathways in the cell.

It has been shown in the rat ARC and paraventricular nuclei of the hypothalamus that leucine suppresses AMPK and ACC phosphorylation, concomitant with a decreased AMP:ATP ratio, and activates mTOR, which is known to be sensitive to nutrients such as amino acids and growth factors [74,75]. The activation of mTOR and suppression of AMPK-dependent phosphorylation seem to modulate hypothalamic neuropeptides, including decreasing neuropeptide Y (NPY) and agouti-related peptide (Agrp; both orexigenic neuropeptides) and increasing proopiomelanocortin (POMC; which is anorexigenic).

Interestingly, recent results suggest that direct central effects on satiety cannot be exclusively attributed to leucine. In fact, an equimolar substitution of leucine by alanine seems to exert the same effect as leucine on body fat accumulation in male mice fed ad libitum with high-fat diets, thus suggesting that changes in energy and substrate metabolism induced by high-protein diets are only partially related to the specific effects of single amino acids such as leucine; instead, increased protein, i.e. nitrogen, consumption [76] may have a general impact on satiety. Notwithstanding the possibility that different amino acids may contribute to the direct central satiating effect of proteins, to date there is not enough evidence that amino acid precursors of neurotransmitters can explain the decreased food intake induced by proteins. For example, no effects on hunger have been found following the addition of free tryptophan (the precursor of serotonin, which is known to inhibit appetite [77]) to gelatin (a protein that does not contain tryptophan) to the same level as that of α-lactalbumin, which is high in tryptophan [78]. Similarly, no effects on satiety have been obtained by tyrosine (a precursor of dopamine) supplementation in the diet of rats [79]. Finally, contradictory results have been obtained in rats supplemented with histidine (a precursor of histamine) by different research teams adding the same amount of the amino acid to the diet [79,80].

Another intriguing aspect of central satiety regulation by amino acids is how the time course of changing circulating amino acid levels may contribute to the overall satiating power of proteins of different origins. In fact, the higher peak of circulating amino acids following whey protein ingestion in comparison with casein may explain the lower satiating power of the latter [81]. Thus, both the composition and the time course of amino acid absorption and plasma appearance may affect the overall satiating effect of ingested proteins. Importantly, an additional limiting factor in the overall satiating effect of proteins consists of the habitual protein-intake level [82] because the beneficial effect of high protein on satiety may be attenuated by habituation to an increased protein intake [34].

AMINO ACIDS AND THE PRESERVATION OR AUGMENTATION OF LEAN BODY MASS IN OBESE INDIVIDUALS

From the second to the eighth decade of life, lean body mass decreases by about 18% in sedentary men and by 27% in sedentary women [83]. This change is associated with a concomitant increase in fat body mass, as described by increased body mass index (BMI), waist circumference (WC), or waist-hip ratio. This trend of change has been confirmed in the 10 years between the ages of 60 and 70 years, in which a continuous small increase of the BMI occurs, especially in women (Scottish Health Survey) [84]. During the same period, a disproportionate increase in WC with a smaller increase in BMI suggests the presence of a simultaneous gain in visceral fat mass and loss of lean tissues. The loss of lean body mass in aged skeletal muscles is known as *sarcopenia*; it is associated with progressive skeletal muscle weakening due to a reduction in mass and concomitant changes in phenotype, including the selective loss of fast (type II) fibers [85]. Recently, the importance of excess of fat (as a percentage of body weight) associated with reduced lean mass has been highlighted [86]. This condition, known as *sarcopenic obesity* [87], has been clearly linked with a greater decrease in physical function than either obesity or sarcopenia alone [88], and an increased incidence of noninsulin-dependent diabetes [89]. Importantly, some correlation has been found between mortality and increased adiposity (measured by BMI) after adjustment for individual lifestyle characteristics, whereas a strict inverse correlation exists between muscle mass and reduced central fat [90,91]. These findings highlight the importance of lean mass in preserving or promoting health and identify sarcopenia as an important cause of frailty among the obese elderly [92]. Furthermore, wasting of lean tissue is a probable negative event that should be taken seriously when applying strategies for weight loss in obesity.

Several factors may contribute to sarcopenia of aging, including a reduced protein and caloric intake and an altered turnover of myofibrillar proteins as a result of reduced synthesis and/or increased catabolism [93]. Of importance, a general [94] or selective [95] reduction in muscle protein synthesis (MPS) has been observed in the aged muscle, thus indicating that the efficiency of protein turnover and its responsiveness to specific stimuli, including mechanical stress, electrical stimulation, anabolic hormones (i.e. insulin), and amino acids (i.e. EAAs) may be gradually and partially lost during this period of life. Studies in humans have shown that the age-dependent reduction in MPS can be attributed, at least in part, to altered efficiency of the mTOR signaling pathway [96], which is now recognized to be a key regulator of cell growth and a pivotal sensor of nutritional status throughout the life span by regulating messenger RNA translation [93]. mTOR was first discovered as a target of the potent immunosuppressant, rapamycin. Next, a single gene encoding mTOR (*MTOR*) was identified in the eukaryote genome [97,98]. mTOR belongs to a group of kinases known as the phosphatidylinositol kinase-related kinases (or PIKKs). In cells, mTOR forms two distinct complexes known as mTORC1 and mTORC2: when bound to regulatory associated protein of mTOR (raptor), mTOR forms mTORC1 [99], which regulates cell growth and protein synthesis through phosphorylating downstream translation regulators such as ribosomal protein S6 kinase beta-1 (S6K1) and eukaryotic translation initiation factor 4E-binding protein 1 (4E-BP1) [100]. In particular, mTOR-mediated activation of 4E-BP1 releases inhibition of the eukaryotic factors complex (eIF4F) and is thus responsible for translation initiation [101], whereas the activation (by threonine-389 phosphorylation) of S6K1 by mTORC1 regulates the activity of eukaryotic elongation factor 2 kinase (eEF-2k) [93].

In aging, although the basal levels of activation of mTORC1 and downstream target kinases S6K1 and 4E-BP1 appear almost normal, the physiological increase in MPS induced by mechanical and nutritional stimuli is attenuated [102]. This bias is particularly evident in fast twitch muscles [103]. In agreement with these results, other studies have shown that in the elderly an altered change in MPS to mechanical load is associated with a significantly delayed and partially reduced activation response of the mTOR/S6K1 pathway [104]. These data strongly suggest that sarcopenia and the observed reduction of muscle growth induced by mechanical stimuli in the aged muscle may be in part due to a failure in the activation of signals involved in the control of translation. Several in vitro and in vivo studies have shown that EAAs, unlike non-EAAs [105], are fundamental regulators of MPS through the regulation of translation initiation, mitochondrial biogenesis and reactive oxygen species production [106], and ameliorated lipid profile [107], both in the young [108] and in the elderly [109]. These effects identify supplementation with EAAs as a useful strategy to counteract the skeletal muscle loss associated with sarcopenic obesity [93,110]. Among the EAAs, BCAAs (leucine, isoleucine, and valine) play a very important role as nutrient signals that regulate MPS [111,112]. In particular, available data suggest that at least part of the postprandial translational activation is attributable to BCAAs (leucine) through activation of mTOR and its downstream signaling molecules (elF4G, S6K1, and 4E-BP1). The acute BCAA-induced stimulation of MPS is not maintained for prolonged periods, despite continued activation of mTOR signaling, because levels of circulating amino acids fall as they are utilized for protein synthesis. However, when circulating amino acid levels are maintained, leucine-induced stimulation of MPS is maintained for prolonged periods. Thus, adequate protein intake, especially of leucine-enriched balanced amino acids, may enhance MPS and preserve muscle mass and strength. Indeed, several studies have highlighted the fact that high-protein diets [113], and in particular leucine supplementation [114], may minimize lean tissue loss in obese subjects who are fasting to obtain weight reduction. In particular, weigh loss trials with an isocaloric hyperprotein diet that provides an extra dose of leucine (10 g/day) were associated with a greater loss of body fat and an attenuated loss of lean tissue in comparison with subjects consuming a high-carbohydrate diet [115,116]. In accordance, diets with a total protein intake of greater than 1.5 g/kg/day and a reduced amount of carbohydrates (<150 g/day) were associated with attenuated loss of lean tissue [24,117,118].

Overall, the effects of BCAAs on protein synthesis are independent of changes in anabolic hormone concentration [119,120], although insulin availability is required for the effects on translation [121]. In fact, a transient spike of circulating insulin is observed within minutes following BCAA administration and may facilitate the stimulatory effect on MPS [122]. On the other hand, amino acids are necessary for insulin-induced activation of mTOR signaling and translation [123], which also occurs in the presence of insulin resistance [124]. As a matter of fact, a postprandial rise in BCAAs and insulin independently stimulates MPS in the elderly [125,126]. Importantly BCAA-mediated effects on MPS and mitochondrial biogenesis appear to be considerably enhanced by combined exercise training in both aged rodents [106] and humans [127,128], and is strongly attenuated in endothelial nitric oxide synthase-null mice ($eNOS^{-/-}$) or after rapamycin treatment [106]. In fact, an increased protein anabolic response has been detected when amino acids and carbohydrates ingestion followed exercise, due to increased protein synthesis and a minor reduction in protein catabolism independent of circulating insulin. Thus, although initiated at different levels, BCAAs and mechanical load seem to have a common target in the mTOR pathway; thus, they control MPS through interactive mechanisms that are not well defined. For example, it has recently been demonstrated that eccentric exercise can activate S6K1 through changing the level of phosphatidic acid (PA), followed by activation of phospholipase D, which plays an important role in mediating MPS [129]. In fact, blocking the synthesis of PA with l-butanol, an inhibitor of phospholipase D, completely abolishes the increased activation of S6K1 by eccentric exercise, thus inhibiting MPS [130]. The existence of a common endpoint may also help to explain the appearance of a considerably enhanced effect when nutrient supplementation is combined with exercise training in the elderly. For instance, a resistance exercise session is followed by a significant increase in MPS lasting for ≥2 days [128], and postexercise protein intake may potentiate the rise of MPS up to levels that exceed the amount of protein degraded, resulting in a clearly positive protein balance and consequent protein accretion [108]. This effect seems to be the consequence of the synergic action of EAAs and contraction on downstream targets of the mTOR/S6K1 pathway, as was demonstrated in the isolated soleus of aged rats (D'Antona unpublished observations).

As controversy remains about the effects of BCAAs on insulin sensitivity [93], cross talk between insulin and BCAAs at the level of mTOR signaling may represent a crucial limiting factor in the physiological anabolic response to BCAAs in obesity and sarcopenic obesity because increased body fat/abdominal obesity are key factors in the increasing incidence of noninsulin-dependent diabetes mellitus (NIDDM) among the elderly [25]. Importantly, when the risk of metabolic syndrome is calculated from regression models controlled for several variables, including age and sex, sarcopenic obesity is associated with a higher risk in comparison with nonsarcopenic obesity, which manifests a higher risk in comparison with the control group [131].

The current understanding of the regulation of insulin signaling mediated by mTOR is focused on the function of insulin receptor substrate 1 (IRS-1), which is directly involved in transmission of the insulin signal by serving as a docking site for many effector proteins that contain a Src homology 2 (SH2) phosphotyrosine-binding domain [132]. Phosphorylation of IRS-1 on different serine residues (serines 636 and 639) [132] enhances or blocks insulin signaling, while phosphorylation on different tyrosine residues activates the insulin response [133]. A large number of kinases phosphorylate serine residues of IRS-1; these include S6K1, the acute activation of which promotes insulin resistance [134] through a negative feedback mechanism. This loop may contribute to extinction of the insulin signal [135]. In fact, the function of IRS-1 is negatively regulated by degradation through the ubiquitin-proteasome pathway [136–138] and inhibition by suppressor of cytokine signaling (SOCS) proteins [139]. After prolonged insulin stimulation, IRS-1 serine phosphorylation causes its dissociation from the insulin receptor (IR) and association with an E3 ubiquitin-protein ligase (Mdm2) that can ubiquitinate IRS-1. This sequence of events induces its degradation by the 26S proteasome [138,140]. Importantly, IRS-1 phosphorylation through S6K1 activation can also be directly triggered by acute infusion with EAAs, and this effect appears to be reversed by rapamycin. In fact, in humans, amino acid infusion increases IRS-1 phosphorylation at serine-312 and serines 636/639 [141]; this effect may prevent redundancy of the stimulus on the signal transduction pathway. Although acute resistance to insulin may arise from BCAA stimulation of the mTOR/S6K1 pathway, the role of BCAAs in mediating IRS-1 phosphorylation in the setting of chronic nutrient supplementation is only partially understood, as contradictory results have been reported. In particular, improved glucose metabolism was observed following long-term dietary supplementation with leucine in mice maintained on a high-fat diet [142] or in the presence of an elevated EAA:non-EAA ratio with no change in dietary carbohydrate and fat content [143]. Indeed, oral administration of a BCAA-enriched mixture and high glucose improved glucose tolerance in comparison with unsupplemented rats [144]. This result was confirmed in elderly rodents following prolonged supplementation with a BCAA-enriched mixture; their basal level of IRS-1 serine-636 phosphorylation appeared to be unchanged [123]. In contrast, leucine deprivation was observed to increase whole-body insulin sensitivity by decreasing mTOR/S6K1 signaling and activating AMPK signaling in the liver [145]. In humans, prolonged administration of a BCAA-enriched mixture resulted in increased insulin sensitivity, even in presence of NIDDM [146,147]. In this randomized trial involving 41 subjects with sarcopenia of aging, intake of the BCAA-enriched mixture increased muscle mass, reduced tumor necrosis factor (TNF-α), and improved insulin sensitivity. This observation may be related to increased expression and autophosphorylation of the IR, as observed in experimental and clinical T2DM [148]. In line with this observation, BCAA supplementation has been linked to reduced insulin resistance in patients with chronic viral liver disease [149,150] and in patients with nonalcoholic steatohepatitis-related liver cirrhosis [151]. Interestingly, beneficial effects of BCAA supplementation have been also observed in animal models of insulin-dependent diabetes mellitus, such as the streptozotocin rat model [152–154], suggesting a possible metabolic amelioration in the presence of normal insulin sensitivity and loss of insulin activation.

An intriguing aspect of the overall effect of EAA supplementation on insulin resistance is the apparent contrast between the observed beneficial effects of supplementation and the correlation between insulin resistance and an identified cluster of obesity-related changes in specific circulating amino acids. By metabolic profiling, Newgard et al. [155] studied subjects that become obese on a typical Western diet. In these subjects, circulating levels of BCAAs were higher in obese than in lean subjects [155]. Obesity was also associated with decreased availability of insulin-like growth factor I (IGF-I), thus suggesting that overnutrition and low IGF-I levels are associated with increased circulating BCAA and that the subsequent overload of BCAA catabolism contributes to insulin resistance in obese subjects. More recently, the Framingham Offspring Study investigated whether metabolite profiles could predict the development of NIDDM [156]. Fasting concentrations of BCAAs and of two aromatic amino acids (phenylalanine and tyrosine) were found to be elevated up to 12 years before the onset of diabetes, as compared to control subjects. The strongest risk of future diabetes was associated with a combination of three amino acids (isoleucine, phenylalanine, and tyrosine). In a more heterogeneous study sample, obtained by looking at a random set of controls from the Framingham cohort, the relative risk associated with elevated amino acids, although still significant, was attenuated [156]. Interestingly, in the presence of insulin resistance or the diabetic state circulating patterns of only a limited number of amino acids (BCAAs and the sulfur-containing amino acids, phenylalanine and tyrosine) appeared to be altered.

As the circulating signature of BCAAs depends on their catabolism, loss of catabolic capacity has been identified as a potential contributor to the obesity-related rise in circulating BCAAs [157].

The first step in BCAA breakdown is the reversible transfer of the α-amino group to α-ketoglutarate to form glutamate and the respective branched-chain α-keto acids in a reaction catalyzed by branched-chain aminotransferase (BCAT) isozymes. The next irreversible step in BCAA catabolism is oxidative decarboxylation of the branched-chain α-keto acid products of the transamination reaction. This step is catalyzed by the mitochondrial branched-chain α-keto acid dehydrogenase multienzyme complex (BCKD) [158]. BCKD expression and activity is rather ubiquitous in humans, whereas BCAT activity is negligible in hepatocytes. Thus, the liver is a poor consumer of BCAAs but an active site of branched-chain α-keto acid utilization [159,160]. This process ultimately forms intramitochondrial acetyl-CoA (leucine) or anaplerotic metabolite succinyl-CoA via propionyl-CoA (valine and isoleucine). As the rate-limiting enzyme in BCAA catabolism, BCKD is a major player in terms of regulating the complete combustion of BCAAs, significant reductions in its activity in metabolically active tissues is predicted to result in increased tissue and circulating BCAA levels.

A number of reports have demonstrated that BCKD expression and activity are significantly reduced in obesity or insulin resistance compared to lean controls [47,161–163]. In particular, She et al. found tissue specific alterations in BCAA catabolic enzymes involving a reduction in the BCKDH E1α subunit in liver and adipose tissue, but not in skeletal muscle. Thus, it is reasonable to consider that raised blood BCAA and branched-chain α-keto acid concentrations in obesity, the insulin-resistant state, or NIDDM are a direct consequence of reduced BCKD activity in the liver and adipose tissue, but not in muscle.

Importantly, BCAAs are also known to modulate the function of the BCKD complex. In particular, leucine is known to increase the concentration of α-ketoisocaproate [164], a potent inhibitor of the BCKD kinase that is responsible for phosphorylation and inactivation of the BCKD. Inhibition of the BCKD kinase results in dephosphorylation and activation of the BCKD, and its activation stimulates decarboxylation of BCAAs, thus committing them to oxidation. At the same time, the increase in leucine concentration also inhibits pyruvate dehydrogenase, thus limiting pyruvate oxidation. This process spares pyruvate carbon as alanine through transamination and stimulates glucose utilization as a glycolytic fuel [165].

Overall, the observed beneficial effects of BCAA supplementation on insulin sensitivity and of an increased circulating BCAA signature in the presence of increased insulin resistance seem to suggest that BCAAs may be metabolic markers (rather than effectors) of insulin resistance, and their supplementation may ameliorate overall metabolic control in obesity. Nevertheless, further studies are needed to clarify this issue.

CONCLUSIONS

Dietary supplementation is a particularly attractive approach to combat obesity, as it may contribute to weight loss and attenuate some related risks, even without changes in macronutrient consumption. In this regard, BCAA supplementation may play a major role. In fact, accumulating experimental evidence demonstrates that BCAAs may be effective in promoting fat loss, preserving lean mass, and improving metabolic control.

In any case, many questions still await answers, including the significance of specific BCAA signatures that have been correlated with obesity, diabetes, and insulin resistance. In particular, whether their roles are causative or descriptive, and the consequence of overlapping amino acid fluctuations due to dietary supplementation should be analyzed in the near future.

CONFLICT OF INTEREST STATEMENT

The authors have no conflict of interest to declare in relation to this manuscript.

References

[1] Flegal KM, Carroll MD, Ogden CL, Curtin LR. Prevalence and trends in obesity among US adults, 1999–2008. JAMA 2010;303(3):235–41.
[2] Campos P, Saguy A, Ernsberger P, Oliver E, Gaesser G. The epidemiology of overweight and obesity: public health crisis or moral panic? Int J Epidemiol 2006;35(1):55–60.
[3] Goldenberg I, Benderly M, Sidi R, Boyko V, Tenenbaum A, Tanne D, et al. Relation of clinical benefit of raising high-density lipoprotein cholesterol to serum levels of low-density lipoprotein cholesterol in patients with coronary heart disease (from the Bezafibrate Infarction Prevention Trial). Am J Cardiol 2009;103(1):41–5.
[4] Barter P, Gotto AM, LaRosa JC, Maroni J, Szarek M, Grundy SM, et al. HDL cholesterol, very low levels of LDL cholesterol, and cardiovascular events. N Engl J Med 2007;357(13):1301–10.
[5] Kullo IJ, Khaleghi M, Hensrud DD. Markers of inflammation are inversely associated with V02 max in asymptomatic men. J Appl Physiol 2007;102(4):1374–9.
[6] Nesheim MC. What is the research base for the use of dietary supplements? Public Health Nutr 1999;2(1):35–8.
[7] Stamler J. Diet and coronary heart disease. Biometrics 1982;38 (Suppl.):95–118.
[8] Willett WC. Is dietary fat a major determinant of body fat? Am J Clin Nutr 1998;67(3 Suppl.):556S–62S.
[9] Abbasi F, McLaughlin T, Lamendola C, Kim HS, Tanaka A, Wang T, et al. High carbohydrate diets, triglyceride-rich lipoproteins, and coronary heart disease risk. Am J Cardiol 2000;85(1):45–8.
[10] Jeppesen J, Hein HO, Suadicani P, Gyntelberg F. Relation of high TG-low HDL cholesterol and LDL cholesterol to the incidence of ischemic heart disease. An 8-year follow-up in the Copenhagen Male Study. Arterioscler Thromb Vasc Biol 1997;17(6):1114–20.
[11] Jeppesen J, Schaaf P, Jones C, Zhou MY, Chen YD, Reaven GM. Effects of low-fat, high-carbohydrate diets on risk factors for ischemic heart disease in postmenopausal women. Am J Clin Nutr 1997;65(4):1027–33.
[12] Garg A, Grundy SM, Unger RH. Comparison of effects of high and low carbohydrate diets on plasma lipoproteins and insulin sensitivity in patients with mild NIDDM. Diabetes 1992;41(10):1278–85.
[13] Krauss RM. Dietary and genetic effects on low-density lipoprotein heterogeneity. Annu Rev Nutr 2001;21:283–95.
[14] Westman EC, Yancy WS, Edman JS, Tomlin KF, Perkins CE. Effect of 6-month adherence to a very low carbohydrate diet program. Am J Med 2002;113(1):30–6.

[15] Brehm BJ, Seeley RJ, Daniels SR, D'Alessio DA. A randomized trial comparing a very low carbohydrate diet and a calorie-restricted low fat diet on body weight and cardiovascular risk factors in healthy women. J Clin Endocrinol Metab 2003;88(4):1617–23.
[16] Samaha FF, Iqbal N, Seshadri P, Chicano KL, Daily DA, McGrory J, et al. A low-carbohydrate as compared with a low-fat diet in severe obesity. N Engl J Med 2003;348(21):2074–81.
[17] Foster GD, Wyatt HR, Hill JO, McGuckin BG, Brill C, Mohammed BS, et al. A randomized trial of a low-carbohydrate diet for obesity. N Engl J Med 2003;348(21):2082–90.
[18] Astrup A, Meinert Larsen T, Harper A. Atkins and other low-carbohydrate diets: hoax or an effective tool for weight loss? Lancet 2004;364(9437):897–9.
[19] Skov AR, Toubro S, Ronn B, Holm L, Astrup A. Randomized trial on protein vs carbohydrate in ad libitum fat reduced diet for the treatment of obesity. Int J Obes Relat Metab Disord 1999;23(5):528–36.
[20] Veldhorst MA, Nieuwenhuizen AG, Hochstenbach-Waelen A, Westerterp KR, Engelen MP, Brummer RJ, et al. Effects of high and normal soyprotein breakfasts on satiety and subsequent energy intake, including amino acid and 'satiety' hormone responses. Eur J Nutr 2009;48(2):92–100.
[21] Potier M, Darcel N, Tome D. Protein, amino acids and the control of food intake. Curr Opin Clin Nutr Metab Care 2009;12(1):54–8.
[22] Westerterp-Plantenga MS, Nieuwenhuizen A, Tome D, Soenen S, Westerterp KR. Dietary protein, weight loss, and weight maintenance. Annu Rev Nutr 2009;29:21–41.
[23] Pi-Sunyer FX. Medical hazards of obesity. Ann Intern Med 1993;119(7 Pt 2):655–60.
[24] Piatti PM, Monti F, Fermo I, Baruffaldi L, Nasser R, Santambrogio G, et al. Hypocaloric high-protein diet improves glucose oxidation and spares lean body mass: comparison to hypocaloric high-carbohydrate diet. Metabolism 1994;43(12):1481–7.
[25] Li Z, Heber D. Sarcopenic obesity in the elderly and strategies for weight management. Nutr Rev 2011;70(1):57–64.
[26] Hochstenbach-Waelen A, Westerterp-Plantenga MS, Veldhorst MA, Westerterp KR. Single-protein casein and gelatin diets affect energy expenditure similarly but substrate balance and appetite differently in adults. J Nutr 2009;139(12):2285–92.
[27] Yancy Jr WS, Olsen MK, Guyton JR, Bakst RP, Westman EC. A low-carbohydrate, ketogenic diet versus a low-fat diet to treat obesity and hyperlipidemia: a randomized, controlled trial. Ann Intern Med 2004;140(10):769–77.
[28] Layman DK, Evans EM, Erickson D, Seyler J, Weber J, Bagshaw D, et al. A moderate-protein diet produces sustained weight loss and long-term changes in body composition and blood lipids in obese adults. J Nutr 2009;139(3):514–21.
[29] Dansinger ML, Gleason JA, Griffith JL, Selker HP, Schaefer EJ. Comparison of the Atkins, Ornish, Weight Watchers, and Zone diets for weight loss and heart disease risk reduction: a randomized trial. JAMA 2005;293(1):43–53.
[30] Due A, Toubro S, Skov AR, Astrup A. Effect of normal-fat diets, either medium or high in protein, on body weight in overweight subjects: a randomised 1-year trial. Int J Obes Relat Metab Disord 2004;28(10):1283–90.
[31] Gardner CD, Kiazand A, Alhassan S, Kim S, Stafford RS, Balise RR, et al. Comparison of the Atkins, Zone, Ornish, and LEARN diets for change in weight and related risk factors among overweight premenopausal women: the A TO Z Weight Loss Study: a randomized trial. JAMA 2007;297(9):969–77.
[32] Sacks FM, Bray GA, Carey VJ, Smith SR, Ryan DH, Anton SD, et al. Comparison of weight-loss diets with different compositions of fat, protein, and carbohydrates. N Engl J Med 2009;360(9):859–73.
[33] Shai I, Schwarzfuchs D, Henkin Y, Shahar DR, Witkow S, Greenberg I, et al. Weight loss with a low-carbohydrate, Mediterranean, or low-fat diet. N Engl J Med 2008;359(3):229–41.
[34] Vergnaud AC, Norat T, Mouw T, Romaguera D, May AM, Bueno-de-Mesquita HB, et al. Macronutrient composition of the diet and prospective weight change in participants of the EPIC-PANACEA study. PloS One 2013;8(3):e57300.
[35] Halkjaer J, Olsen A, Bjerregaard LJ, Deharveng G, Tjonneland A, Welch AA, et al. Intake of total, animal and plant proteins, and their food sources in 10 countries in the European Prospective Investigation into Cancer and Nutrition. Eur J Clin Nutr 2009;63(Suppl. 4):S16–36.
[36] Halkjaer J, Olsen A, Overvad K, Jakobsen MU, Boeing H, Buijsse B, et al. Intake of total, animal and plant protein and subsequent changes in weight or waist circumference in European men and women: the Diogenes project. Int J Obes 2011;35(8):1104–13.
[37] Vergnaud AC, Norat T, Romaguera D, Mouw T, May AM, Travier N, et al. Meat consumption and prospective weight change in participants of the EPIC-PANACEA study. Am J Clin Nutr 2010;92(2):398–407.
[38] Bujnowski D, Xun P, Daviglus ML, Van Horn L, He K, Stamler J. Longitudinal association between animal and vegetable protein intake and obesity among men in the United States: the Chicago Western Electric Study. J Am Diet Assoc 2011;111(8):1150–5.
[39] Fung TT, van Dam RM, Hankinson SE, Stampfer M, Willett WC, Hu FB. Low-carbohydrate diets and all-cause and cause-specific mortality: two cohort studies. Ann Intern Med 2010;153(5):289–98.
[40] World Health Organization. Diet, nutrition and the prevention of chronic diseases. World Health Organization technical report series; 2003. p. 916, i–viii, 1–149, back cover.
[41] Elmadfa I, Meyer A, Nowak V, Hasenegger V, Putz P, Verstraeten R, et al. European nutrition and health report 2009. Ann Nutr Metab 2009;55(Suppl. 2):1–40.
[42] Pillot B, Duraffourd C, Begeot M, Joly A, Luquet S, Houberdon I, et al. Role of hypothalamic melanocortin system in adaptation of food intake to food protein increase in mice. PloS One 2011;6(4):e19107.
[43] Qin LQ, Xun P, Bujnowski D, Daviglus ML, Van Horn L, Stamler J, et al. Higher branched-chain amino acid intake is associated with a lower prevalence of being overweight or obese in middle-aged East Asian and Western adults. J Nutr 2011;141(2):249–54.
[44] Valerio A, D'Antona G, Nisoli E. Branched-chain amino acids, mitochondrial biogenesis, and healthspan: an evolutionary perspective. Aging 2010;3(5):464–78.
[45] Lynch CJ, Gern B, Lloyd C, Hutson SM, Eicher R, Vary TC. Leucine in food mediates some of the postprandial rise in plasma leptin concentrations. Am J Physiol 2006;291(3):E621–30.
[46] Cota D, Proulx K, Smith KA, Kozma SC, Thomas G, Woods SC, et al. Hypothalamic mTOR signaling regulates food intake. Science 2006;312(5775):927–30.
[47] She P, Van Horn C, Reid T, Hutson SM, Cooney RN, Lynch CJ. Obesity-related elevations in plasma leucine are associated with alterations in enzymes involved in branched-chain amino acid metabolism. Am J Physiol 2007;293(6):E1552–63.
[48] Veldhorst M, Smeets A, Soenen S, Hochstenbach-Waelen A, Hursel R, Diepvens K, et al. Protein-induced satiety: effects and mechanisms of different proteins. Physiol Behav 2008;94(2):300–7.
[49] Geliebter A, Liang JT, Van Itallie TB. Effects of repeated isocaloric macronutrient loads on daily food intake of rats. Am J Physiol 1984;247(2 Pt 2):R387–92.
[50] Marmonier C, Chapelot D, Fantino M, Louis-Sylvestre J. Snacks consumed in a nonhungry state have poor satiating efficiency:

influence of snack composition on substrate utilization and hunger. Am J Clin Nutr 2002;76(3):518–28.

[51] Raben A, Agerholm-Larsen L, Flint A, Holst JJ, Astrup A. Meals with similar energy densities but rich in protein, fat, carbohydrate, or alcohol have different effects on energy expenditure and substrate metabolism but not on appetite and energy intake. Am J Clin Nutr 2003;77(1):91–100.

[52] Smeets AJ, Soenen S, Luscombe-Marsh ND, Ueland O, Westerterp-Plantenga MS. Energy expenditure, satiety, and plasma ghrelin, glucagon-like peptide 1, and peptide tyrosine-tyrosine concentrations following a single high-protein lunch. J Nutr 2008;138(4):698–702.

[53] Lejeune MP, Kovacs EM, Westerterp-Plantenga MS. Additional protein intake limits weight regain after weight loss in humans. Br J Nutr 2005;93(2):281–9.

[54] Powley TL, Phillips RJ. Gastric satiation is volumetric, intestinal satiation is nutritive. Physiol Behav 2004;82(1):69–74.

[55] Fromentin G, Darcel N, Chaumontet C, Marsset-Baglieri A, Nadkarni N, Tome D. Peripheral and central mechanisms involved in the control of food intake by dietary amino acids and proteins. Nutr Res Rev 2012;25(1):29–39.

[56] Darcel NP, Liou AP, Tome D, Raybould HE. Activation of vagal afferents in the rat duodenum by protein digests requires PepT1. J Nutr 2005;135(6):1491–5.

[57] Adibi SA. The oligopeptide transporter (Pept-1) in human intestine: biology and function. Gastroenterology 1997;113(1):332–40.

[58] Raybould HE, Glatzle J, Freeman SL, Whited K, Darcel N, Liou A, et al. Detection of macronutrients in the intestinal wall. Auton Neurosci 2006;125(1–2):28–33.

[59] Adibi SA. Regulation of expression of the intestinal oligopeptide transporter (Pept-1) in health and disease. Am J Physiol Gastrointest Liver Physiol 2003;285(5):G779–88.

[60] Hussain I, Zanic-Grubisic T, Kudo Y, Boyd CA. Functional and molecular characterization of a peptide transporter in the rat PC12 neuroendocrine cell line. FEBS Lett 2001;508(3):350–4.

[61] Ogihara H, Saito H, Shin BC, Terado T, Takenoshita S, Nagamachi Y, et al. Immuno-localization of H+/peptide cotransporter in rat digestive tract. Biochem Biophys Res Commun 1996;220(3):848–52.

[62] Lindemann B. Receptors and transduction in taste. Nature 2001;413(6852):219–25.

[63] Liou AP, Chavez DI, Espero E, Hao S, Wank SA, Raybould HE. Protein hydrolysate-induced cholecystokinin secretion from enteroendocrine cells is indirectly mediated by the intestinal oligopeptide transporter PepT1. Am J Physiol Gastrointest Liver Physiol 2011;300(5):G895–902.

[64] Eastwood C, Maubach K, Kirkup AJ, Grundy D. The role of endogenous cholecystokinin in the sensory transduction of luminal nutrient signals in the rat jejunum. Neurosci Lett 1998;254(3):145–8.

[65] Cordier-Bussat M, Bernard C, Haouche S, Roche C, Abello J, Chayvialle JA, et al. Peptones stimulate cholecystokinin secretion and gene transcription in the intestinal cell line STC-1. Endocrinology 1997;138(3):1137–44.

[66] Buchan AM. Nutrient tasting and signaling mechanisms in the Gut III. Endocrine cell recognition of luminal nutrients. Am J Physiol 1999;277(6 Pt 1):G1103–7.

[67] Meyer JH, Hlinka M, Tabrizi Y, DiMaso N, Raybould HE. Chemical specificities and intestinal distributions of nutrient-driven satiety. Am J Physiol 1998;275(4 Pt 2):R1293–307.

[68] Moran TH, Dailey MJ. Intestinal feedback signaling and satiety. Physiol Behav 2011;105(1):77–81.

[69] Batterham RL, Heffron H, Kapoor S, Chivers JE, Chandarana K, Herzog H, et al. Critical role for peptide YY in protein-mediated satiation and body-weight regulation. Cell Metab 2006;4(3):223–33.

[70] Bowen J, Noakes M, Clifton PM. Appetite regulatory hormone responses to various dietary proteins differ by body mass index status despite similar reductions in ad libitum energy intake. J Clin Endocrinol Metab 2006;91(8):2913–9.

[71] Blom WA, Lluch A, Stafleu A, Vinoy S, Holst JJ, Schaafsma G, et al. Effect of a high-protein breakfast on the postprandial ghrelin response. Am J Clin Nutr 2006;83(2):211–20.

[72] Rehfeld JF. Incretin physiology beyond glucagon-like peptide 1 and glucose-dependent insulinotropic polypeptide: cholecystokinin and gastrin peptides. Acta Physiol (Oxford, England) 2011;201(4):405–11.

[73] Faipoux R, Tome D, Gougis S, Darcel N, Fromentin G. Proteins activate satiety-related neuronal pathways in the brainstem and hypothalamus of rats. J Nutr 2008;138(6):1172–8.

[74] Morrison CD, Xi X, White CL, Ye J, Martin RJ. Amino acids inhibit Agrp gene expression via an mTOR-dependent mechanism. Am J Physiol 2007;293(1):E165–71.

[75] Ropelle ER, Pauli JR, Fernandes MF, Rocco SA, Marin RM, Morari J, et al. A central role for neuronal AMP-activated protein kinase (AMPK) and mammalian target of rapamycin (mTOR) in high-protein diet-induced weight loss. Diabetes 2008;57(3):594–605.

[76] Freudenberg A, Petzke KJ, Klaus S. Dietary L-leucine and L-alanine supplementation have similar acute effects in the prevention of high-fat diet-induced obesity. Amino Acids 2013;44(2):519–28.

[77] Blundell JE, Latham CJ. Serotonergic influences on food intake: effect of 5-hydroxytryptophan on parameters of feeding behaviour in deprived and free-feeding rats. Pharmacol Biochem Behav 1979;11(4):431–7.

[78] Veldhorst MA, Nieuwenhuizen AG, Hochstenbach-Waelen A, Westerterp KR, Engelen MP, Brummer RJ, et al. A breakfast with alpha-lactalbumin, gelatin, or gelatin + TRP lowers energy intake at lunch compared with a breakfast with casein, soy, whey, or whey-GMP. Clin Nutr (Edinburgh, Scotland) 2009;28(2):147–55.

[79] Bassil MS, Hwalla N, Obeid OA. Meal pattern of male rats maintained on histidine-, leucine-, or tyrosine-supplemented diet. Obesity 2007;15(3):616–23.

[80] Kasaoka S, Tsuboyama-Kasaoka N, Kawahara Y, Inoue S, Tsuji M, Ezaki O, et al. Histidine supplementation suppresses food intake and fat accumulation in rats. Nutrition 2004;20(11–12):991–6.

[81] Mellinkoff SM, Frankland M, Boyle D, Greipel M. Relationship between serum amino acid concentration and fluctuations in appetite. J Appl Physiol 1956;8(5):535–8.

[82] Long SJ, Jeffcoat AR, Millward DJ. Effect of habitual dietary-protein intake on appetite and satiety. Appetite 2000;35(1):79–88.

[83] Evans WJ, Cyr-Campbell D. Nutrition, exercise, and healthy aging. J Am Diet Assoc 1997;97(6):632–8.

[84] Han TS, Tajar A, Lean ME. Obesity and weight management in the elderly. Br Med Bull 2011;97:169–96.

[85] D'Antona G, Pellegrino MA, Adami R, Rossi R, Carlizzi CN, Canepari M, et al. The effect of ageing and immobilization on structure and function of human skeletal muscle fibres. J Physiol 2003;552(Pt 2):499–511.

[86] Newman AB, Kupelian V, Visser M, Simonsick E, Goodpaster B, Nevitt M, et al. Sarcopenia: alternative definitions and associations with lower extremity function. J Am Geriatr Soc 2003;51(11):1602–9.

[87] Heber D, Ingles S, Ashley JM, Maxwell MH, Lyons RF, Elashoff RM. Clinical detection of sarcopenic obesity by bioelectrical impedance analysis. Am J Clin Nutr 1996;64(3 Suppl):472S–7S.

[88] Baumgartner RN. Body composition in healthy aging. Ann N Y Acad Sci 2000;904:437–48.

[89] Kim TN, Park MS, Yang SJ, Yoo HJ, Kang HJ, Song W, et al. Prevalence and determinant factors of sarcopenia in patients with type 2 diabetes: the Korean Sarcopenic Obesity Study (KSOS). Diabetes Care 2010;33(7):1497–9.

[90] Zamboni M, Mazzali G, Zoico E, Harris TB, Meigs JB, Di Francesco V, et al. Health consequences of obesity in the elderly: a review of four unresolved questions. Int J Obes 2005;29(9):1011–29.

[91] Wannamethee SG, Shaper AG, Lennon L, Whincup PH. Decreased muscle mass and increased central adiposity are independently related to mortality in older men. Am J Clin Nutr 2007;86(5):1339–46.

[92] Narici MV, Maffulli N. Sarcopenia: characteristics, mechanisms and functional significance. Br Med Bull 2010;95:139–59.

[93] D'Antona G, Nisoli E. MTOR signaling as a target of amino acid treatment of the age-related sarcopenia. Interdiscip Top Gerontol 2010;37:115–41.

[94] Balagopal P, Rooyackers OE, Adey DB, Ades PA, Nair KS. Effects of aging on in vivo synthesis of skeletal muscle myosin heavy-chain and sarcoplasmic protein in humans. Am J Physiol 1997;273(4 Pt 1):E790–800.

[95] Welle S, Bhatt K, Thornton C. Polyadenylated RNA, actin mRNA, and myosin heavy chain mRNA in young and old human skeletal muscle. Am J Physiol 1996;270(2 Pt 1):E224–9.

[96] Guillet C, Prod'homme M, Balage M, Gachon P, Giraudet C, Morin L, et al. Impaired anabolic response of muscle protein synthesis is associated with S6K1 dysregulation in elderly humans. FASEB J 2004;18(13):1586–7.

[97] Crespo JL, Powers T, Fowler B, Hall MN. The TOR-controlled transcription activators GLN3, RTG1, and RTG3 are regulated in response to intracellular levels of glutamine. Proc Natl Acad Sci USA 2002;99(10):6784–9.

[98] Crespo JL, Diaz-Troya S, Florencio FJ. Inhibition of target of rapamycin signaling by rapamycin in the unicellular green alga Chlamydomonas reinhardtii. Plant Physiol 2005;139(4):1736–49.

[99] Wullschleger S, Loewith R, Hall MN. TOR signaling in growth and metabolism. Cell 2006;124(3):471–84.

[100] Kozma SC, Thomas G. P70s6k/p85s6k: mechanism of activation and role in mitogenesis. Semin Cancer Biol 1994;5(4):255–60.

[101] Flati V, Pasini E, D'Antona G, Speca S, Toniato E, Martinotti S. Intracellular mechanisms of metabolism regulation: the role of signaling via the mammalian target of rapamycin pathway and other routes. Am J Cardiol 2008;101(11A):16E–21E.

[102] Cuthbertson D, Smith K, Babraj J, Leese G, Waddell T, Atherton P, et al. Anabolic signaling deficits underlie amino acid resistance of wasting, aging muscle. FASEB J 2005;19(3):422–4.

[103] Tamaki T, Uchiyama S, Uchiyama Y, Akatsuka A, Yoshimura S, Roy RR, et al. Limited myogenic response to a single bout of weight-lifting exercise in old rats. Am J Physiol Cell Physiol 2000;278(6):C1143–52.

[104] Dreyer HC, Fujita S, Cadenas JG, Chinkes DL, Volpi E, Rasmussen BB. Resistance exercise increases AMPK activity and reduces 4E-BP1 phosphorylation and protein synthesis in human skeletal muscle. J Physiol 2006;576(Pt 2):613–24.

[105] Smith K, Reynolds N, Downie S, Patel A, Rennie MJ. Effects of flooding amino acids on incorporation of labeled amino acids into human muscle protein. Am J Physiol 1998;275(1 Pt 1):E73–8.

[106] D'Antona G, Ragni M, Cardile A, Tedesco L, Dossena M, Bruttini F, et al. Branched-chain amino acid supplementation promotes survival and supports cardiac and skeletal muscle mitochondrial biogenesis in middle-aged mice. Cell Metab 2010;12(4):362–72.

[107] Brocca L, Mascaro A, D'Antona G. Proteomic analysis of plasma after branched chain enriched mixture supplementation in mice. J Int Soc Sports Nutr 2013;10(1):19.

[108] Biolo G, Tipton KD, Klein S, Wolfe RR. An abundant supply of amino acids enhances the metabolic effect of exercise on muscle protein. Am J Physiol 1997;273(1 Pt 1):E122–9.

[109] Volpi E, Ferrando AA, Yeckel CW, Tipton KD, Wolfe RR. Exogenous amino acids stimulate net muscle protein synthesis in the elderly. J Clin Invest 1998;101(9):2000–7.

[110] Dillon EL, Sheffield-Moore M, Paddon-Jones D, Gilkison C, Sanford AP, Casperson SL, et al. Amino acid supplementation increases lean body mass, basal muscle protein synthesis, and insulin-like growth factor-I expression in older women. J Clin Endocrinol Metab 2009;94(5):1630–7.

[111] Lynch CJ, Halle B, Fujii H, Vary TC, Wallin R, Damuni Z, et al. Potential role of leucine metabolism in the leucine-signaling pathway involving mTOR. Am J Physiol 2003;285(4):E854–63.

[112] Lynch CJ, Hutson SM, Patson BJ, Vaval A, Vary TC. Tissue-specific effects of chronic dietary leucine and norleucine supplementation on protein synthesis in rats. Am J Physiol 2002;283(4):E824–35.

[113] Bistrian DR, Winterer J, Blackburn GL, Young V, Sherman M. Effect of a protein-sparing diet and brief fast on nitrogen metabolism in mildly obese subjects. J Lab Clin Med 1977;89(5):1030–5.

[114] Sherwin RS. Effect of starvation on the turnover and metabolic response to leucine. J Clin Invest 1978;61(6):1471–81.

[115] Layman DK, Evans E, Baum JI, Seyler J, Erickson DJ, Boileau RA. Dietary protein and exercise have additive effects on body composition during weight loss in adult women. J Nutr 2005;135(8):1903–10.

[116] Layman DK, Boileau RA, Erickson DJ, Painter JE, Shiue H, Sather C, et al. A reduced ratio of dietary carbohydrate to protein improves body composition and blood lipid profiles during weight loss in adult women. J Nutr 2003;133(2):411–7.

[117] Parker B, Noakes M, Luscombe N, Clifton P. Effect of a high-protein, high-monounsaturated fat weight loss diet on glycemic control and lipid levels in type 2 diabetes. Diabetes Care 2002;25(3):425–30.

[118] Farnsworth E, Luscombe ND, Noakes M, Wittert G, Argyiou E, Clifton PM. Effect of a high-protein, energy-restricted diet on body composition, glycemic control, and lipid concentrations in overweight and obese hyperinsulinemic men and women. Am J Clin Nutr 2003;78(1):31–9.

[119] Svanberg E, Zachrisson H, Ohlsson C, Iresjo BM, Lundholm KG. Role of insulin and IGF-I in activation of muscle protein synthesis after oral feeding. Am J Physiol 1996;270(4 Pt 1):E614–20.

[120] Svanberg E, Moller-Loswick AC, Matthews DE, Korner U, Andersson M, Lundholm K. Effects of amino acids on synthesis and degradation of skeletal muscle proteins in humans. Am J Physiol 1996;271(4 Pt 1):E718–24.

[121] Preedy VR, Garlick PJ. The response of muscle protein synthesis to nutrient intake in postabsorptive rats: the role of insulin and amino acids. Biosci Rep 1986;6(2):177–83.

[122] Anthony JC, Anthony TG, Kimball SR, Jefferson LS. Signaling pathways involved in translational control of protein synthesis in skeletal muscle by leucine. J Nutr 2001;131(3):856S–60S.

[123] Flati V, Caliaro F, Speca S, Corsetti G, Cardile A, Nisoli E, et al. Essential amino acids improve insulin activation of AKT/MTOR signaling in soleus muscle of aged rats. Int J Immunopathol Pharmacol 2010;23(1):81–9.

[124] Drummond MJ, Dreyer HC, Pennings B, Fry CS, Dhanani S, Dillon EL, et al. Skeletal muscle protein anabolic response to resistance exercise and essential amino acids is delayed with aging. J Appl Physiol 2008;104(5):1452–61.

[125] Volpi E, Kobayashi H, Sheffield-Moore M, Mittendorfer B, Wolfe RR. Essential amino acids are primarily responsible for the amino acid stimulation of muscle protein anabolism in healthy elderly adults. Am J Clin Nutr 2003;78(2):250–8.

[126] Rennie MJ, Bohe J, Wolfe RR. Latency, duration and dose response relationships of amino acid effects on human muscle protein synthesis. J Nutr 2002;132(10):3225S–7S.

[127] Murphy C, Miller BF. Protein consumption following aerobic exercise increases whole-body protein turnover in older adults. Appl Physiol Nutr Metab (Physiologie appliquee, nutrition et metabolisme) 2010;35(5):583–90.

[128] Phillips SM, Tipton KD, Aarsland A, Wolf SE, Wolfe RR. Mixed muscle protein synthesis and breakdown after resistance exercise in humans. Am J Physiol 1997;273(1 Pt 1):E99–E107.

[129] O'Neil TK, Duffy LR, Frey JW, Hornberger TA. The role of phosphoinositide 3-kinase and phosphatidic acid in the regulation of mammalian target of rapamycin following eccentric contractions. J Physiol 2009;587(Pt 14):3691–701.

[130] Wang X, Devaiah SP, Zhang W, Welti R. Signaling functions of phosphatidic acid. Prog Lipid Res 2006;45(3):250–78.

[131] Lim S, Kim JH, Yoon JW, Kang SM, Choi SH, Park YJ, et al. Sarcopenic obesity: prevalence and association with metabolic syndrome in the Korean Longitudinal Study on Health and Aging (KLoSHA). Diabetes Care 2010;33(7):1652–4.

[132] Sun XJ, Rothenberg P, Kahn CR, Backer JM, Araki E, Wilden PA, et al. Structure of the insulin receptor substrate IRS-1 defines a unique signal transduction protein. Nature 1991;352(6330):73–7.

[133] Gual P, Le Marchand-Brustel Y, Tanti JF. Positive and negative regulation of insulin signaling through IRS-1 phosphorylation. Biochimie 2005;87(1):99–109.

[134] Um SH, Frigerio F, Watanabe M, Picard F, Joaquin M, Sticker M, et al. Absence of S6K1 protects against age- and diet-induced obesity while enhancing insulin sensitivity. Nature 2004;431(7005):200–5.

[135] Tremblay F, Marette A. Amino acid and insulin signaling via the mTOR/p70 S6 kinase pathway. A negative feedback mechanism leading to insulin resistance in skeletal muscle cells. J Biol Chem 2001;276(41):38052–60.

[136] Smith LK, Rice KM, Garner CW. The insulin-induced down-regulation of IRS-1 in 3T3-L1 adipocytes is mediated by a calcium-dependent thiol protease. Mol Cell Endocrinol 1996;122(1):81–92.

[137] Sun XJ, Goldberg JL, Qiao LY, Mitchell JJ. Insulin-induced insulin receptor substrate-1 degradation is mediated by the proteasome degradation pathway. Diabetes 1999;48(7):1359–64.

[138] Pederson TM, Kramer DL, Rondinone CM. Serine/threonine phosphorylation of IRS-1 triggers its degradation: possible regulation by tyrosine phosphorylation. Diabetes 2001;50(1): 24–31.

[139] Ueki K, Kondo T, Kahn CR. Suppressor of cytokine signaling 1 (SOCS-1) and SOCS-3 cause insulin resistance through inhibition of tyrosine phosphorylation of insulin receptor substrate proteins by discrete mechanisms. Mol Cell Biol 2004;24(12):5434–46.

[140] Usui I, Imamura T, Huang J, Satoh H, Shenoy SK, Lefkowitz RJ, et al. Beta-arrestin-1 competitively inhibits insulin-induced ubiquitination and degradation of insulin receptor substrate 1. Mol Cell Biol 2004;24(20):8929–37.

[141] Tremblay F, Jacques H, Marette A. Modulation of insulin action by dietary proteins and amino acids: role of the mammalian target of rapamycin nutrient sensing pathway. Curr Opin Clin Nutr Metab Care 2005;8(4):457–62.

[142] Zhang Y, Guo K, LeBlanc RE, Loh D, Schwartz GJ, Yu YH. Increasing dietary leucine intake reduces diet-induced obesity and improves glucose and cholesterol metabolism in mice via multimechanisms. Diabetes 2007;56(6):1647–54.

[143] Noguchi Y, Nishikata N, Shikata N, Kimura Y, Aleman JO, Young JD, et al. Ketogenic essential amino acids modulate lipid synthetic pathways and prevent hepatic steatosis in mice. PloS One 2010;5(8):e12057.

[144] Bernard JR, Liao YH, Hara D, Ding Z, Chen CY, Nelson JL, et al. An amino acid mixture improves glucose tolerance and insulin signaling in Sprague-Dawley rats. Am J Physiol 2011;300(4):E752–60.

[145] Xiao F, Huang Z, Li H, Yu J, Wang C, Chen S, et al. Leucine deprivation increases hepatic insulin sensitivity via GCN2/mTOR/S6K1 and AMPK pathways. Diabetes 2011;60(3):746–56.

[146] Solerte SB, Fioravanti M, Locatelli E, Bonacasa R, Zamboni M, Basso C, et al. Improvement of blood glucose control and insulin sensitivity during a long-term (60 weeks) randomized study with amino acid dietary supplements in elderly subjects with type 2 diabetes mellitus. Am J Cardiol 2008;101(11A):82E–8E.

[147] Solerte SB, Gazzaruso C, Bonacasa R, Rondanelli M, Zamboni M, Basso C, et al. Nutritional supplements with oral amino acid mixtures increases whole-body lean mass and insulin sensitivity in elderly subjects with sarcopenia. Am J Cardiol 2008;101(11A):69E–77E.

[148] Iritani N, Sugimoto T, Fukuda H, Komiya M, Ikeda H. Dietary soybean protein increases insulin receptor gene expression in Wistar fatty rats when dietary polyunsaturated fatty acid level is low. J Nutr 1997;127(6):1077–83.

[149] Kawaguchi T, Taniguchi E, Itou M, Sumie S, Oriishi T, Matsuoka H, et al. Branched-chain amino acids improve insulin resistance in patients with hepatitis C virus-related liver disease: report of two cases. Liver Int 2007;27(9):1287–92.

[150] Kawaguchi T, Nagao Y, Matsuoka H, Ide T, Sata M. Branched-chain amino acid-enriched supplementation improves insulin resistance in patients with chronic liver disease. Int J Mol Med 2008;22(1):105–12.

[151] Miyake T, Abe M, Furukawa S, Tokumoto Y, Toshimitsu K, Ueda T, et al. Long-term branched-chain amino acid supplementation improves glucose tolerance in patients with nonalcoholic steatohepatitis-related cirrhosis. Intern Med 2012;51(16):2151–5.

[152] Pellegrino MA, Patrini C, Pasini E, Brocca L, Flati V, Corsetti G, et al. Amino acid supplementation counteracts metabolic and functional damage in the diabetic rat heart. Am J Cardiol 2008;101(11A):49E–56E.

[153] Brocca L, D'Antona G, Bachi A, Pellegrino MA. Amino acid supplements improve native antioxidant enzyme expression in the skeletal muscle of diabetic mice. Am J Cardiol 2008;101(11A):57E–62E.

[154] Eizirik DL, Germano CM, Migliorini RH. Dietetic supplementation with branched chain amino acids attenuates the severity of streptozotocin-induced diabetes in rats. Acta Diabetol 1988;25(2):117–26.

[155] Newgard CB, An J, Bain JR, Muehlbauer MJ, Stevens RD, Lien LF, et al. A branched-chain amino acid-related metabolic signature that differentiates obese and lean humans and contributes to insulin resistance. Cell Metab 2009;9(4):311–26.

[156] Wang TJ, Larson MG, Vasan RS, Cheng S, Rhee EP, McCabe E, et al. Metabolite profiles and the risk of developing diabetes. Nat Med 2011;17(4):448–53.

[157] Adams SH. Emerging perspectives on essential amino acid metabolism in obesity and the insulin-resistant state. Adv Nutr 2011;2(6):445–56.

[158] Brodan V, Kuhn E, Pechar J, Tomkova D. Changes of free amino acids in plasma of healthy subjects induced by physical exercise. Eur J Appl Physiol 1976;35(1):69–77.

[159] Suryawan A, Hawes JW, Harris RA, Shimomura Y, Jenkins AE, Hutson SM. A molecular model of human branched-chain amino acid metabolism. Am J Clin Nutr 1998;68(1):72–81.

[160] Sweatt AJ, Wood M, Suryawan A, Wallin R, Willingham MC, Hutson SM. Branched-chain amino acid catabolism: unique segregation of pathway enzymes in organ systems and peripheral nerves. Am J Physiol 2004;286(1):E64–76.

[161] Kuzuya T, Katano Y, Nakano I, Hirooka Y, Itoh A, Ishigami M, et al. Regulation of branched-chain amino acid catabolism in rat

models for spontaneous type 2 diabetes mellitus. Biochem Biophys Res Commun 2008;373(1):94–8.
[162] Bajotto G, Murakami T, Nagasaki M, Sato Y, Shimomura Y. Decreased enzyme activity and contents of hepatic branched-chain alpha-keto acid dehydrogenase complex subunits in a rat model for type 2 diabetes mellitus. Metabolism 2009;58(10):1489–95.
[163] Doisaki M, Katano Y, Nakano I, Hirooka Y, Itoh A, Ishigami M, et al. Regulation of hepatic branched-chain alpha-keto acid dehydrogenase kinase in a rat model for type 2 diabetes mellitus at different stages of the disease. Biochem Biophys Res Commun 2010;393(2):303–7.
[164] Layman DK, Walker DA. Potential importance of leucine in treatment of obesity and the metabolic syndrome. J Nutr 2006;136(1 Suppl.):319S–23S.
[165] Chang TW, Goldberg AL. Leucine inhibits oxidation of glucose and pyruvate in skeletal muscles during fasting. J Biol Chem 1978;253(10):3696–701.

PART I

ACTIVITY OF ADIPOCYTES: ROLE IN GROWTH AND ACCUMULATION OF FAT

CHAPTER

39

Fibroblast Growth Factor 21 is a Regulator of Energy Metabolism in the Liver and Adipose Tissue

Niina Matikainen

Department of Endocrinology and Cardiovascular Research Unit, Heart and Lung Center, Helsinki University Central Hospital, University of Helsinki, Helsinki, Finland

Abbreviations

BMI, body mass index; CNS, central nervous system; CVD, cardiovascular disease; FGF, fibroblast growth factor; FGFR, fibroblast growth factor receptor; NAFLD, nonalcoholic fatty liver disease

BACKGROUND

The fibroblast growth factor (FGF) family of signaling proteins comprises several members that are mostly involved in mediating autocrine or paracrine metabolic signaling. The twenty-first of the documented FGFs was described in 2000 and was named FGF-21. Of these FGFs, only three, namely FGF-15/19, FGF-21, and FGF-23, also act through systemic circulation, are unable to bind heparin, and thus possess classical hormonal functions i.e. they are secreted proteins that mediate their biological responses by binding to and activating cell-surface FGF receptors (FGFRs) [1]. The actions of FGF-21 are two-fold: besides its hormone-like properties, it also possesses paracrine/autocrine protein or adipokine-like properties. FGF-21 is recognized as a central player in the control of adaptation to nutritional status, along with having profound effects on lipid and carbohydrate metabolism [2]. FGF-21 gained wide scientific attention after the publication of a paper showing both in vitro and in vivo FGF-21-stimulated glucose uptake into fat cells by the induction of glucose transporter synthesis [2].

While pharmacological FGF-21 treatment alleviates hyperglycemia, improves the lipid profile, and reduces ectopic fat (including hepatic triglycerides) and body weight in animal models, FGF-21 has appeared as an interesting regulator of metabolic pathways in humans and a candidate target for the treatment of metabolic diseases associated with dysregulation of body fat depots such as the metabolic syndrome and type 2 diabetes mellitus (T2DM) [2,3]. The need for an enhanced understanding of the pathways underlying metabolic diseases and a search for novel therapies to tackle these diseases is obvious. The modern obesity epidemic has led to a dramatic rise in deaths related to metabolic diseases, mainly due to cardiovascular disease (CVD), in particular stroke and myocardial infarction. The median survival time of morbidly obese people with a body mass index (BMI) of 40–45 kg/m^2 is 8–10 years less than those with normal BMI [4]. The key pathological mediator that link obesity to excess CVD and mortality is inflammation and dysfunction of adipose tissue [5]. In obesity, the limited ability to store fat in subcutaneous fat depots leads to accumulation of hepatic and visceral fat. This is associated with overproduction of proinflammatory adipokines, de novo triglyceride (TG) production, hyperglycemia, and insulin resistance. On the other hand, the biological action of protective adipokines such as adiponectin, leptin, and FGF-21 is decreased [6,7].

FGF-21 STRUCTURE, EXPRESSION, AND RECEPTOR BINDING

FGF-21 is a secreted protein consisting of 210 amino acids with a hydrophobic amino terminus. Its closest structural resemblance is to FGF-19 and FGF-23, the two other hormone-like FGFs [8]. It is predominantly, but not exclusively, expressed in the liver. Other tissues that

Nutrition in the Prevention and Treatment of Abdominal Obesity
http://dx.doi.org/10.1016/B978-0-12-407869-7.00039-8

produce FGF-21 are white and brown adipose tissue, skeletal muscle, and pancreatic beta cells, which are all involved in the control of carbohydrate and lipid metabolism [9–11].

FGF-21 acts through a subset of cell-surface FGFRs. FGFRs known to bind FGF-21 include FGFR-1, FGFR-2, FGFR-3, and FGFR-4, but the relative affinity of FGF-21 binding to the various FGFRs is unknown [12]. These FGFRs are tyrosine kinases that require a coreceptor, beta-klotho, to form a FGF-21-beta-klotho-FGFR active complex [13,14]. FGFR activation leads to induction of the classical receptor tyrosine kinase signaling pathway, with stimulation of extracellular signal-regulated kinases (ERK) 1 and 2, MAPK 3/ERK-1, and protein kinase B (Akt). Whether physiologically relevant FGF-21 activation can also occur independently of beta-klotho is still under debate. However, some actions of FGF-21 are detected in beta-klotho knockout mice [15]. The presence of both FGFR and beta-klotho determine tissue responsiveness to FGF-21.

PARACRINE/AUTOCRINE, ENDOCRINE, AND PHARMACOLOGICAL ROLES OF FGF-21

In healthy animals and also in humans, liver is the major source of circulating, hormone-like FGF-21, which mostly operates in the fasting state. In contrast, adipose tissue is the main site of FGF-21 local actions that occur without changes in plasma FGF-21 concentrations (outlined in Fig. 39.1). Local paracrine/autocrine actions of FGF-21 control a wide range of metabolic functions in adipose tissue that are considered to operate in the fed state [16,17].

The dual roles of FGF-21 as a paracrine/autocrine adipokine and a circulating hormone-like molecule may partly overlap so as to increase both hepatic and adipose tissue fatty acid oxidation. However, tissue-specific actions may have opposing metabolic effects, e.g. stimulation of gluconeogenesis in the liver and increased glucose uptake in adipose tissue (Fig. 39.1). The actions of FGF-21 may occur in various tissues depending on

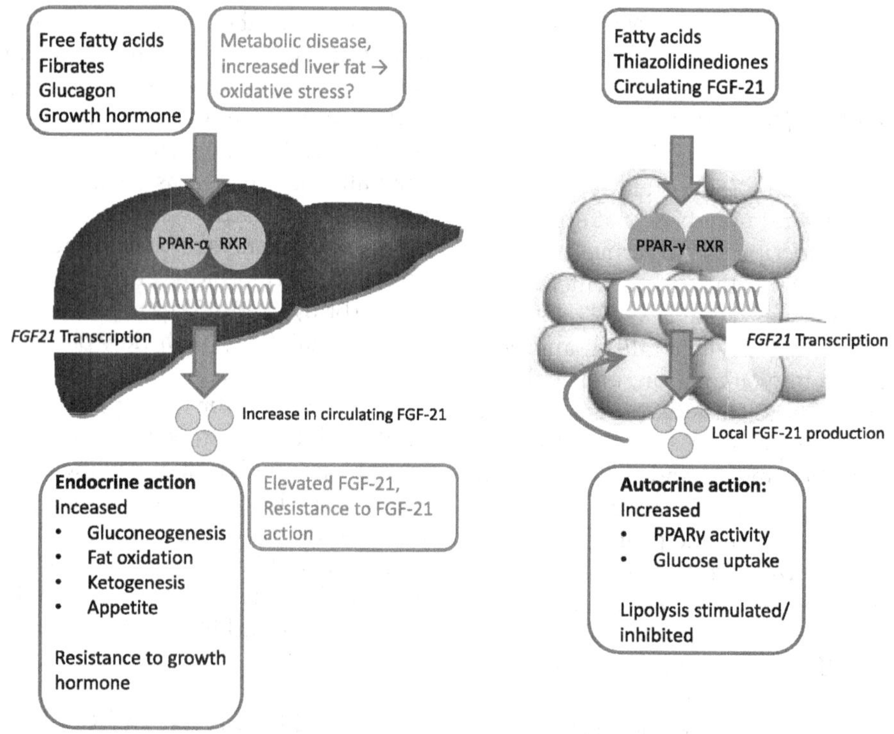

FIGURE 39.1 The physiological regulation of endocrine (hormone-like) and paracrine/autocrine synthesis of FGF21 is tissue-specific. In the liver (left panel) the transcription of FGF21 is stimulated by fasting or fibrate drugs. Also, thyroid hormones, lactation and heavy exercise may regulate FGF21 expression. Under physiological conditions indicated in left panel, rise in plasma FGF21 induces ketogenegis, increase in glucose concentration, and utilization of fat as energy source, and resistance to growth hormone action. In conditions associated with high liver fat or obesity, oxidative stress induces hepatic overexpression of FGF21 (middle panel). The plasma levels of FGF21 increase but do not lead to alleviation of hyperglycemia, triglyceride metabolism or liver fat content due to resistance to FGF21 action. The paracrine/autocrine actions of FGf21 take place in the adipose tissue (right panel), where the FGF21 expression is regulated by PPARγ agonists (thiazolinediones), by circulating FGF21 and also by free fatty acids. The current concept suggests that this pathway is activated mainly in the fed state. This metabolic loop increases local FGF21 concentrations and activates PPARγ transcription, which lead to increased glucose uptake and altered lipolysis. (See color plate at the back of the book.)

physiological status i.e. fasting vs. fed, or normal vs. cold temperatures. Therefore, it is vital to consider separately the physiological settings in which tissue-specific or systemic FGF-21 action takes place [16]. Circulating FGF-21 mainly comes from the liver. The hormone-like functions of FGF-21 are mediated through FGFRs in metabolic tissues that express beta-klotho [13]. It has been proposed that tissue-specific expression of beta-klotho in combination with local expression of specific FGFR type(s) may determine the responsiveness and actions of FGF-21 within a target tissue. FGF-21 target tissues include liver, adipose tissue, pancreas, and also the central nervous system (CNS) [12,18]. FGF-21 appears to be able to cross the blood-brain barrier and, importantly, beta-klotho is expressed in the hypothalamus (at least), thus enabling FGF-21 effects to occur in the CNS [19].

In addition to hormone-like and autocrine/paracrine physiological functions, administered FGF-21 analogs may reach pharmacological plasma concentrations that produce effects different from those seen at physiological concentrations. So far, the many FGF-21 roles across species are insufficiently described, with most data deriving from rodent and primate studies [7].

EXPRESSION AND REGULATION OF FGF-21

In Vitro and Animal Studies

Plasma concentrations and hepatic *FGF21* mRNA expression increase during fasting and starvation, whereas in the fed state FGF-21 expression and plasma levels are low in rodents as well as in healthy human subjects [20,21]. The main stimuli that induce hepatic FGF-21 expression during fasting are free fatty acids (FFAs). FFAs bind to hepatic peroxisome proliferator-activated receptor alpha (PPAR-α) and enhance signaling, which upregulates hepatic *FGF21* transcription [22–24]. The factors that increase plasma FFAs and subsequently activate PPAR-α such as fibrates, glucagon, somatotropin/growth hormone (GH) therapy, intensive physical activity, and lactation can all induce FGF-21 expression in the liver and increase plasma concentrations of FGF-21, as outlined in Fig. 39.1 [7,25–27]. Thus, PPAR-α is the key regulator of hepatic FGF-21 expression and mediates the hormone-like actions of FGF-21.

Recently, it was shown that glucagon modulates FGF-21 expression [28]. Glucagon exerts a regulatory role in FGF-21 secretion independent of the prevailing insulin concentrations; however, like FFA, this pathway also is PPAR-α dependent [25,28,29]. In addition, thyroid hormones may be involved in the hepatic activation of FGF-21 expression. This was shown by Adams et al., who treated mice with triiodothyronine and found a dose-dependent enhancement in hepatic FGF-21 expression [30]. This study added thyroid receptor beta to the factors that can induce FGF-21 expression. Further research is required to demonstrate whether FGF-21 links the thyroid hormone balance to lipid, glucose, and energy metabolism.

FGF-21 is suggested to operate during feeding, mostly through tissue-level effects. In the fed state, an abundance of circulating FFAs stimulates local FGF-21 expression in adipose tissue, which increases glucose uptake and alters lipolysis. For example, the glucose-lowering and antilipolytic effects of rosiglitazone, a PPAR-γ agonist, may be partly explained by FGF-21 induction in adipose tissue [31]. The mechanism of action of FGF-21 in adipose tissue is thus PPAR-γ dependent (Fig. 39.1).

Food intake suppresses FGF-21 expression, but repressors of FGF-21 are not well known. Expression of FGF-21 in the liver is downregulated by a cholesterol-enriched diet in mice through a pathway involving oxysterols receptor LXR-alpha (LXRα) and LXRβ, ligand-activated transcription factors belonging to the nuclear receptor superfamily [32]. Further proof for an involvement of this pathway comes from a study showing that LXR agonist treatment results in repression of FGF-21 levels induced by fasting. The decrease in FGF-21 expression may explain why LXR agonists increase hepatic steatosis in mice [33].

Human Studies

Relatively little is known about the regulation of FGF-21 in humans, as compared to in vitro or experimental animal data. Genetic factors contribute only moderately to plasma FGF-21 levels, with a heritability of 40% in healthy human subjects [34]. The unresolved question is whether FGF-21 is a critical regulator of either fasting or feeding, or a surrogate marker of energy metabolism in humans. However, it is clear from human studies under fasting conditions that FGF-21 is not a simple nutritional switch in humans, and that the FGF-21 regulatory pathways described in rodents are not directly applicable to humans; instead, that more complex metabolic interactions are involved.

The role of FGF-21 in the fasting state is poorly understood. Human *FGF21* gene expression studies in mouse hepatocytes reveal that the paradoxical expression of FGF-21 in both the fasting and fed states also apply in humans. Two fasting signals [PPAR-α and glucagon-protein kinase A (PKA)] and two feeding signals (glucose and xylitol) can increase FGF-21 expression in vitro. The human *FGF21* gene contains a carbohydrate-response element in addition to a PPAR-response element. Furthermore, (over) feeding of glucose results in a dose-dependent increase in FGF-21 expression in cell lines. In addition, basal FGF-21 expression has been shown in humans to be independent of known stimuli, including PPAR-α, glucagon, glucose, and xylitol [35]. Previous fasting studies show no effect of 2 days of food deprivation on FGF-21 levels and an increase in plasma concentrations only after 1 week of unphysiological food deprivation or after infusion of supraphysiological FFA concentrations [20,36]. Together, these findings suggest that in humans FGF-21 may be a signal of ultimate crisis in energy metabolism, with high levels in appearing in plasma under both starvation and overfeeding conditions; however, the regulatory pathways and sources of FGF-21 in these opposite nutritional states are poorly characterized [35].

The effects of physiological concentrations of insulin on FGF-21 concentrations are under debate. In theory, Akt contributes to FGF-21 expression, and slight increases in plasma FGF-21 were observed during a hyperinsulinemic clamp study, supporting a role for high insulin concentrations in FGF-21 regulation [10,37]. The role of glucagon in FGF-21 regulation may be independent of insulin and contribute to lipolytic activity [29]. However, PPAR-α and FFAs appear to be the most important regulators of FGF-21 under physiological energy balance in humans as well [20,37,38]. In addition, PPAR-α ligands such as fenofibrate can increase hepatocyte *FGF21* expression and plasma FGF-21 concentrations [20,23,39]. These findings in humans may reflect the tissue-specific regulation of FGF-21 in the background of varying physiological energy balance; thus, future studies into the tissue-specific regulation of FGF-21 expression in humans are warranted.

PHYSIOLOGICAL ROLE OF FGF-21

Fasting and Fed Conditions

In rodents, FGF-21 represents a nutritional switch in the adaptation to starvation and is thought to act as an endocrine feedback signal regulating energy balance. In vitro and animal data demonstrate that during food deprivation or a ketogenic diet an increase in FGF-21 levels mediates a shift in energy balance in hepatocytes, adipocytes, pancreatic islet beta cells, and possibly the CNS, with an associated increase in gluconeogenesis, lipid oxidation, and ketogenesis [40]. This fasting response is mediated by PPAR-α activation in the liver, which increases hepatic FGF-21 expression and, subsequently, plasma FGF-21 levels. In the liver, FGF-21 activates the master regulator of mitochondrial biogenesis, PPAR-γ coactivator 1 alpha (PGC-1α), which negatively regulates FGF-21 expression [24]. The downstream signaling of FGF-21 in adipocytes operates through 5′-AMP-activated protein kinase (AMPK), NAD-dependent protein deacetylase sirtuin-1 (SIRT1), and PGC-1α to enhance mitochondrial function and oxidative capacity. This leads to the activation of multiple metabolic pathways that turn on oxygen consumption and citrate synthase activity and induce the expression of key metabolic genes [41,42]. Hepatic activation of FGF-21 expression changes energy handling in the liver itself, and circulating FGF-21 signals the nutritional balance to other tissues involved in energy regulation; however, the balance between FGF-21 local production and systemic effects are not well understood.

The importance of FGF-21 in rodent fasting-feeding adaptation is well recognized. FGF-21 mediates the increase in gluconeogenesis, fatty acid oxidation, and hunger signaling under fasting conditions. FGF-21 knockout mice cannot adapt to food deprivation by exploiting their fat tissue as the source of energy. While wild-type mice lose weight during a ketogenic diet, FGF-21 knockout mice gain weight, develop hepatosteatosis, and show a marked impairment in ketogenesis and glucose control [43]. FGF-21 controls glycemia via both regulating hepatic glucose flux and improving insulin sensitivity. In the liver, FGF-21 induces gluconeogenesis through the PGC-1α pathway and thus increases the availability of carbohydrates. However, it does not contribute to increased glycogenolysis in the fasting state [24]. In addition, increased FGF-21 expression augments hepatic fatty acid oxidation, thus enabling the use of fat stores as an energy source [44].

The well-known effects of starvation on growth retardation are at least partly explained by FGF-21 effects. In the fasting state, FGF-21 in the liver inhibits the GH-activated tyrosine-protein kinase JAK2-signal transducer and activator of transcription 5 (STAT5) signaling, causing resistance to GH action that helps conserve energy [45]. On the other hand, impaired GH signaling leads to activation of de novo hepatic lipogenesis, leading to an increase in liver fat content and the possible development of nonalcoholic fatty liver disease (NAFLD). Thus, liver fat accumulation in GH-resistant states may be partly due to the relative suppression of hepatic FGF-21 expression or activity that permits the activation of lipogenic enzymes sterol regulatory element-binding proteins (SREBPs) 1 and 2 and enhanced lipid synthesis [46].

In adipose tissue, both circulating and locally produced FGF-21 regulate fat tissue energy metabolism both in vitro and in vivo through stimulating glucose uptake into fat cells by inducing solute carrier family 2 facilitated glucose transporter member 1 (GLUT1), as first described by Kharitonenkov [2]. This pathway is distinct from that of insulin, which activates GLUT4 translocation. In addition, FGF-21 can stimulate lipolysis in adipocytes [22,29]; however, inhibitory effects on lipolysis have also been demonstrated [47]. These studies suggest that local FGF-21 mostly inhibits lipolysis during feeding and that systemic FGF-21 mostly stimulates it during fasting. In adipocytes, FGF-21 enhances mitochondrial oxidative capacity through PGC-1α, which promotes the utilization of fat [48]. Most data on the local autocrine/paracrine function of FGF-21 in adipose tissue suggest that it is important in the fed state.

FGF-21 Augments Adaptation to Cold Temperatures and Controls Thermogenesis

Energy homeostasis is closely linked to the adaptation to cold temperatures, which is critical for the survival for all endothermic species but is also an important determinant of the basal metabolic rate in humans. Adaptation mechanisms for coping in cold temperatures involve important FGF-21-dependent paracrine/autocrine actions. In pharmacological doses, FGF-21 can induce thermogenic responses in both brown adipose tissue and thermogenically competent white adipose tissue depots. Recent studies show that the thermogenic properties of FGF-21 are linked to increased expression of thermogenic genes, such as *UCP1* [encoding mitochondrial brown fat uncoupling protein 1 (UCP 1)] and *CIDEA* (encoding cell death activator CIDE-A), in brown adipose tissue and primary brown adipocytes by the induction of PGC-1α protein [49,50]. Besides the paracrine/autocrine nature of this metabolic pathway, changes in levels of circulating FGF-21 upon cold exposure are also detected [50]. Interestingly, FGF-21 may activate thermogenic gene expression in specific thermogenically competent white adipose tissue depots even more profoundly than in brown adipose tissue [51]. Therefore, FGF-21 may operate differently in the various types of adipose tissue.

In rodents, FGF-21 also reduces physical activity and induces a short-term hibernation-like state of regulated hypothermia that conserves energy, called *torpor* [22]. Of note, pharmacological doses of FGF-21 may even increase activity levels. FGF-21 also possesses other functions linked to cold adaptation and survival: a study by Hondoras et al. found that FGF-21 can increase the expression of thermogenic genes, such as *Ucp1* and *Ppargc1a* (encoding PGC-1α) in brown adipose tissue and through increasing oxidation can raise the body temperature of neonate mice. They proposed the novel theory that when placental glucose during fetal period is changed to milk enriched with FFAs at birth, the change in nutritional composition serves as a signal to induce *Fgf21* expression. Therefore, FGF-21 may represent the key sensor in the change of nutritional status and mediate the activation of brown adipose tissue thermogenesis that is critical for survival during the fetal to neonate transition [52].

FGF-21 Controls Glucose and Lipid Metabolism and Body Weight

FGF-21 regulates the energy balance through both the CNS control of food intake and adaptation of hepatic, adipose tissue, and possibly pancreatic metabolism to fasting-feeding periods. Importantly, the effects of FGF-21 on metabolism are dependent on the physiological state and also the source of FGF-21. If FGF-21 expression is stimulated under fasting conditions, it induces hepatic gluconeogenesis to raise plasma glucose concentration in order to secure the supply of energy to the tissues. In contrast, at pharmacological concentrations FGF-21 treatment reduces plasma glucose concentrations, although the mechanisms for this action are not well understood. After feeding, FGF-21 levels fall in healthy animals. Raised plasma insulin concentration after macronutrient intake may be an important regulator of this fall in FGF-21. In mice, the postprandial decrease in FGF-21 is associated with repression of the transcriptional repressor, nuclear factor interleukin-3-regulated protein/E4 promoter-binding protein 4 (E4BP4). In mouse hepatocytes, insulin acts directly through Akt to induce E4BP4, thus providing an interesting link from feeding to FGF-21 suppression by insulin [53].

FGF-21 has an impact on pancreatic alpha and beta cell function, and possibly on pancreatic autoimmune processes. In pancreatic islets isolated from diabetic rodents, FGF-21 treatment increases islet insulin content and glucose-induced insulin secretion, as well as inhibiting glucagon secretion [54]. Whether FGF-21 has a positive effect on beta cell survival and prevents islet cell from glucolipotoxicity is under debate [54]. The pancreatic effects of FGF-21 may be of importance in type 1 and latent autoimmune diabetes, in which FGF-21 levels correlate positively with C-peptide levels but inversely with titers of islet autoantibodies [55]. Furthermore, FGF-21 knockout mice are prone to develop insulitis, but FGF-21 transgenic mice are more resistant to it [56].

Studies in rodents suggest that FGF-21 increases food intake and may therefore be added to the list of orexigenic hormones. FGF-21 activates FGFR-1 and thereby initiates a pathway that is important for appetite regulation. Inhibition of FGFR-1 in primates and rodents induces hypophagia and results in weight loss [57]. Again, physiological effects of FGF-21 during starvation may differ from those seen with pharmacological concentrations. In a hamster model of seasonal obesity, pharmacological FGF-21 treatment produced an 18% loss of body weight associated with a reduction in food intake and decreased respiratory exchange ratio, indicating increased fat oxidation. These findings applied only during long-day but not short-day conditions. It can be speculated that day length-induced changes in FGF-21 sensitivity are related to the seasonal variations in adipose tissue mass that are typical for rodents [58]. Whether this model of seasonal weight variation also operates in humans remains to be studied.

Obesity is linked to altered FGF-21 metabolism, termed *FGF-21-resistance*, especially affecting white adipose tissue that serves as energy depot and also controls energy homeostasis. Dysregulation of fat tissue metabolism also involves a number of other adipokines, and plasma concentrations of TNF-α, adipocyte fatty acid-binding protein (AFABP), neutrophil gelatinase-associated lipocalin (NGAL)/lipocalin-2, plasminogen activator inhibitor-1 (PAI-1), C-C motif chemokine 2 [monocyte chemotactic protein 1 (MCP-1)], and resistin are increased. Protective adipokines such as adiponectin may be downregulated and circulate in low concentrations [6]. Despite high plasma concentrations, the action of FGF-21 and insulin are impaired. Of these factors, FGF-21-based therapy has the widest effects on metabolic diseases associated with obesity and adipose tissue dysregulation. PPAR-γ activation in concert with local FGF-21 effects has been shown to promote glucose uptake and adipocyte differentiation, which may promote obesity [59]. In a mouse model of obesity, an increased contribution of fat tissue to circulating FGF-21 levels has been noted [60]. In addition, FGF-21 knockout mice show defects in PPAR-γ signaling, decreased body adiposity, and resistance to the actions of rosiglitazone, a PPAR-γ agonist. PPAR-γ transcription is also reduced in FGF-21 knockout mice. These findings suggest that in adipose tissue, FGF-21 pathway is fundamentally important for both insulin sensitization and the weight gain and edema-predisposing effects of PPAR-γ agonists, and that FGF-21 paracrine/autocrine actions can promote adipogenesis in white adipose tissue [31]. It is not known whether FGF-21 is causally linked to obesity. However, in a mouse model of diet-induced obesity, treatment with exendin-4 decreased both glucose and liver fat and also elevated FGF-21 protein levels [61].

FGF-21 and Human Metabolism

In humans, the physiological functions of FGF-21 in energy metabolism remain under debate; Table 39.1 summarizes the data accumulated from animal and human studies. The FGF-21 concentration oscillates with a frequency of 6–12 times/day [62]. FGF-21 levels are highly variable after an overnight fast but show little intraindividual or fasting-feeding variation during a 25-h period in healthy subjects. A 48-h ketogenic diet does not change FGF-21 levels despite a 40-fold increase in beta-hydroxybutyrate concentrations that signals highly activated lipid oxidation during fasting. However, FGF-21 concentrations are induced after 7 days of unphysiological food deprivation that increase beta-hydroxybutyrate by 70-fold and reduces body weight by 7%. Despite profound ketosis, the FGF-21 concentration increases by only 74% [20]. It can be concluded that, in analogy to experimental animals, a rise in adipose tissue lipolysis and consequently in FFA concentration during fasting can induce FGF-21 expression in healthy subjects, but that this phenomenon requires an extended period of fasting for several days; thus, FGF-21 is not a major player in the adaptation to physiological fasting periods in humans [44]. Therefore, in contrast to findings in rodents, FGF-21 is not considered a vital hormonal switch of nutritional fasting vs. feeding status in humans [20,63].

TABLE 39.1 Physiological Roles of FGF-21 in Experimental Animals and Humans

Function	Animals	Humans	Reference(s)
Stimulation of fasting lipolysis	+	(+)	[29,47]
Adaptation to ketosis	+	−	[2,20]
Adaptation to prolonged fasting	+	−	[2,20]
Hibernation	+	−	[22]
Adaptation to cold	+	(+)	[49,66]
Resistance to growth hormone	+	(+)	[45,84]
Food intake	+	(+)	[83,86]

+, Positive effects; −, negative effects. Less well characterized or controversial roles for FGF-21 in humans are shown in brackets.

Food intake clearly decreases plasma FGF-21 levels from fasting levels in healthy subjects. Ingestion of a mixed meal consisting of fat, carbohydrates, and protein suppresses FGF-21 concentrations 4-h postprandially in metabolically healthy subjects [21]. After an oral glucose tolerance test, the FGF-21 nadir is reached after 60 min and the fasting values, as well as the post-glucose decline, correlates inversely with glucose and insulin levels [64]. During the day-long sequential ingestion of standardized meals, FGF-21 levels peak in the early morning after an overnight fast and oscillate in parallel to the changes in FFA and cortisol concentrations, but in the opposite directions to glucose and insulin concentrations [65].

Although pharmacological concentrations of FGF-21 have a major impact on lipid metabolism in rodents and primates, the significance of FGF-21 in human lipid metabolism is less clear. In healthy, normal-weight adults, low-density (LDL) and high-density lipoprotein cholesterol concentrations are not related to FGF-21 levels, although this may be different in subjects with metabolic diseases. Instead, plasma TG levels correlate with FGF-21 levels in most but not all studies [20,34]. In addition, the postprandial decrease in FGF-21 is closely inversely related to postprandial intestinal and hepatic TG-rich lipoproteins and their degradation products termed remnant lipoproteins in healthy subjects. Surprisingly, postprandial plasma FFAs are not clearly related to FGF-21 concentration in humans [21], despite the fact that FFAs are potent regulators of fasting FGF-21 expression [44]. Together, these findings indicate that fasting, but not postprandial, FFAs are closely linked to FGF-21 concentrations.

FGF-21 may also be important in the adaptation to temperature variations in humans because a change in environmental temperature affects the circadian rhythm of FGF-21. In calorimetry studies performed at various temperatures in healthy adults, a diminished diurnal reduction in FGF-21 was noted at 19 °C as compared to 24 °C during daytime, together with a 37% increase in overall diurnal FGF-21 levels. Concomitantly, glycerol release from adipose tissue was increased, suggesting an increase in cold-induced thermogenesis occurs via FGF-21 signaling [66]. Thus, minor changes in environmental temperature are sufficient to modulate FGF-21 diurnal levels in humans and may mediate cold-induced metabolic changes similar to those reported in rodents. However, whether FGF-21 controls the expression of thermogenic genes such as *UCP1* and the basic metabolic rate in humans is unknown. It may be speculated that variations in FGF-21 expression also contribute to the lean phenotype in humans [67].

THE ROLE OF FGF-21 IN HUMAN METABOLIC DISEASES

In healthy subjects, fasting plasma levels of FGF-21 are low, but high levels of FGF-21 are commonly found in diseases characterized by the accumulation of ectopic fat in the liver and dysregulation of adipose tissue metabolism (Table 39.2). However, the role of FGF-21 in these metabolic diseases is not straightforward. It is unknown whether adipose tissue FGF-21 autocrine/paracrine signaling pathway is disturbed in addition to increased systemic, secreted FGF-21 levels. The observed high circulating plasma FGF-21 concentrations presumably represent FGF-21 resistance, similar to the insulin and leptin resistance typically observed in obesity, NAFLD, insulin resistance, and T2DM [39,60,63,68–70]. As well as the liver, adipose tissue also contributes to excessive levels of circulating FGF-21 in obesity, in which increased *FGF21* mRNA expression in adipose tissue may represent an imbalance between hepatic vs. other tissue-derived FGF-21 in obesity [39,60].

Other conditions linked to increased levels of FGF-21 and FGF-21 resistance include dysmetabolic conditions such as dyslipidemia and coronary heart disease [71]. Lately, high FGF-21 levels have been described in subjects with hypertension and end-stage renal disease [72,73]. In addition, patients with human immunodeficiency virus infection and Cushing disease show similar patterns of FGF-21 resistance [74–76]. These studies all demonstrate elevated fasting FGF-21 levels in metabolic conditions that are closely linked to increased liver fat and NAFLD [63,77]. In healthy human subjects, fasting and postprandial FGF-21 levels correlate with liver fat and visceral fat, as measured with magnetic resonance imaging spectroscopy, indicating that the relationship also exists in normal-weight to mildly obese healthy individuals [21]. Compared to healthy controls, subjects with impaired glucose tolerance and T2DM show a gradual impairment in the suppression of postprandial FGF-21 levels in an oral glucose tolerance test [64]. These findings suggest that FGF-21 resistance develops simultaneously with metabolic syndrome, but whether FGF-21 dysregulation precedes the onset of metabolic disease or vice versa remains unknown.

In Asian populations, FGF-21 has been shown to predict the development of metabolic syndrome and T2DM [60,78]. In another epidemiological follow-up study of Caucasian individuals, FGF-21 levels independently predicted the incidence of metabolic syndrome, progression to impaired glucose metabolism, and T2DM [79]. In any case, elevated plasma FGF-21 levels are a uniform finding

TABLE 39.2 FGF-21 Concentrations in Metabolic Diseases that are Associated with Obesity, Increased Liver Fat, and Dysregulation of Fat Depots

Disease	Insulin Signaling	FGF-21 Concentration	Risk of Vascular Disease
Hypertension	Resistance	Increased	Increased
Obesity	Resistance	Increased	Increased
Nonalcoholic fatty liver disease	Resistance	Increased	Increased
Type 2 diabetes mellitus	Resistance	Increased	Increased
Cushing syndrome	Resistance	Increased	Increased
Lipodystrophy by HIV-1	Resistance	Increased	Increased
End-stage renal disease	Resistance	Increased	Increased

The association between FGF-21 resistance and increased cardiovascular morbidity and mortality is remains to be elucidated. HIV-1, human immunodeficiency virus type 1.

in diseases linked to obesity and high liver fat. In line with these cross-sectional and follow-up data, *FGF21* single nucleotide polymorphisms are associated with obesity, metabolic syndrome, and T2DM phenotypes [80].

How are obesity and FGF-21 linked? Obesity is characterized by chronic oxidative stress that promotes the expression of nuclear factor erythroid 2-related factor 2 (Nrf2), a transcription factor that controls a set of antioxidant and detoxification genes under both basal and stress conditions. In a mouse model of long-term high-fat diet-induced obesity, Nrf2 knockout mice were partially protected from obesity and the insulin-resistant phenotype. Interestingly, this phenomenon was related to higher plasma FGF-21 levels and higher hepatic and white adipose tissue *Fgf21* mRNA levels than in wild-type mice. Overexpression of Nrf2 in cultured cell has consistently resulted in decreased *FGF21* mRNA levels, as well as in suppressed *FGF21* promoter activity. Nrf2 may downregulate hepatic FGF-21 under conditions of increased oxidative stress, but this finding must be considered preliminary and does not explain FGF-21 resistance [81]. The role of increased cellular stress as the cause of elevated FGF-21 levels in patients with NAFLD was supported by a study showing that hepatoma cells and rat hepatocytes overproduce FGF-21 in the presence of intracellular stress induced by either nutrient (amino acid deprivation) or oxidative (arsenite) stress [82]. These data provide a biological link between metabolic defects of the liver and FGF-21 overexpression. However, the mechanisms of FGF-21 resistance that function at the tissue level are not known.

It is unknown whether FGF-21 represents an important regulator of human weight and a satiety signal to ingested nutrients in humans. Recently, the *FGF21* gene variant rs838133 was found to affect dietary macronutrient intake in a population-based genome-wide meta-analysis [83]. Interestingly, obesity-associated human metabolic diseases are characterized by impaired satiety and FGF-21 resistance [39]. In anorexia nervosa, the other extreme of food intake and weight, reduced FGF-21 levels are reported and provide further proof that FGF-21 is an important hormone involved in signaling between adipose tissue metabolism and central regulation of food intake, although the causality remains unexplored [44]. In addition, FGF-21 is thought to mediate the characteristic resistance to GH action in anorexia nervosa, in analogy to famine [84].

FGF-21-TARGETED THERAPY

Animal and In Vitro Models of Therapeutic FGF-21 Intervention

Hopes for FGF-21-based therapy are based on the multiple metabolic benefits observed in rodent and primate models, in which exogenous FGF-21 at pharmacological concentrations induces the potent lowering of blood glucose, improves insulin sensitivity, and enhances pancreatic beta cell function and mass (Table 39.3). Furthermore, pharmacological effects of FGF-21 include the reversal of hepatosteatosis, lowering of plasma TGs, and reductions in body weight and adipose tissue mass. All of these changes point toward a reduction in CVD risk markers with FGF-21-based therapy [12]. Transgenic mice overexpressing FGF-21 provide an interesting rodent model for studying the biological actions of FGF-21. These mice consistently demonstrate 5-10 times higher FGF-21 plasma levels than wild-type mice throughout their life span. FGF-21 transgenic mice have a 30–40% longer life span without caloric restriction, slightly increased energy intake, lower body weight without change in fat vs. lean body mass, and marked improvement both in glucose and lipid metabolism compared to wild-type mice on a standard diet. Female FGF-21 transgenic mice extend their life span even further than the males; about a third of female FGF-21 transgenic mice were still alive after 44 months, compared to an average life span of 28 months in wild-type mice [85].

Administration of FGF-21 to leptin-deficient rodents decreases serum glucose and TG concentrations and enhances insulin sensitivity and glucose clearance [2]. Mice overexpressing FGF-21 in the liver are resistant to diet-induced weight gain [2]. In diabetic rhesus monkeys, pharmacological doses of FGF-21 reduce glucose, insulin, and, importantly, atherogenic lipoproteins, LDL cholesterol and very-low-density lipoprotein subfractions. These monkeys also demonstrate a small but significant weight loss [86]. Chronic FGF-21 administration also improves insulin sensitivity and fasting hyperglycemia in genetically obese mice [3]. In *ob/ob* mice, FGF-21 treatment for 2 weeks induces fat oxidation and reduced weight by 20%, despite minor increases in energy intake. In addition, glucose levels are improved and hepatic TG content decreases through the reduced

TABLE 39.3 Effects of Pharmacological Administration of Recombinant FGF-21 or Long-Acting FGF-21 Analogs in Rodents and Primates

FGF-21-Based Pharmacological Therapy
Weight loss
Minor change in appetite and caloric intake
Increased activity
Improved glycemic control
Increase in insulin sensitivity
Improvement of dyslipidemia
Decrease in liver fat
Decrease in bone mass

activity of key lipogenic enzymes [41]. In rats, hepatic *Fgf21* gene expression is inversely related to hepatic TG concentration [25]. In B6.V-*Lep*^{ob}/J leptin-deficient mice, pharmacological administration of recombinant FGF-21 protein improves glucose parameters but not TG or cholesterol levels. This contrasts with many reports showing significant improvements in hyperlipidemia after chronic treatment with FGF-21 in high-fat diet models [87].

The use of wild-type native FGF-21 as therapeutic agent is complicated by its short half-life and susceptibility to proteolytic degradation. Long-acting FGF-21 analogs are under development and have demonstrated comparable efficacy to that reported for native FGF-21 [88,89]. Possible concerns associated with FGF-21-based therapies include reduced bone mass. Studies in young and older FGF-21 transgenic mice demonstrate that bone mass decreases, partly due to increased differentiation of marrow adipocytes and a corresponding decrease in osteoblast differentiation [85,90]. Other mechanisms such as inhibition of GH action at the growth plate and further changes in the GH-insulin-like growth factor I (IGF-I) axis may also apply [91,92]. It is unknown whether FGF-21 causes bone loss in humans. The observed changes in bone metabolism resemble those seen with thiazolidinedione treatment. Taking into account that FGF-21 is essential for both the wanted and unwanted effects of rosiglitazone, it is important to consider the typical side effects of thiazolidinediones if FGF-21-based therapies are to be used in humans [31].

FGF-21 and the Treatment of Human Metabolic Diseases

In humans, the pharmacological actions of FGF-21 are unknown. Lifestyle modification is the first-line therapy for all metabolic diseases, including metabolic syndrome, T2DM, NAFLD, and obesity. Therefore, it is relevant to ask whether weight loss, diet, or exercise interventions decrease elevated FGF-21 levels or alleviate FGF-21 resistance in human metabolic diseases. During ketogenic diet and 9% weight loss, FGF-21 levels decreased [38]. In a study of 40 obese women, a 3-month combined aerobic and resistance exercise program decreased both plasma FGF-21 levels and arterial stiffness [93]. In addition, weight loss in obese children decreased FGF-21 levels [69]. In contrast, a modest weight loss from a BMI of 37.4–32.8 kg/m^2 by a hypocaloric diet and exercise or significant postbariatric surgery weight loss did not affect FGF-21 levels, despite a significant improvement in the metabolic profile [36,94]. Taken together, these studies are inconclusive about whether improvements in FGF-21 metabolism are linked to beneficial changes in metabolic profile after weight loss.

If T2DM is treated with pioglitazone, no changes in plasma FGF-21 ensue, despite a reduction in liver fat. However, whether local FGF-21 metabolism in fat tissue is affected remains an open question. Instead, pioglitazone in combination with exenatide reduces FGF-21 levels [61]. Of the lipid-lowering drugs, fibrates are activators of hepatic PPAR-α and therefore of special interest. In subjects with T2DM, a 5-year treatment with fenofibrate increased plasma FGF-21 concentration by 85%, and similar findings are reported with short-term fibrate treatment [20,39,95]. However, whether these changes in FGF-21 during pharmacological therapy cause improved outcomes is unknown. Until now, one study [96] has reported improvement in the metabolic profile and decrease of body weight with a FGF-21 analog treatment.

So far, multiple roles of FGF-21 as a paracrine/autocrine and hormonal regulator of hepatic and adipose tissue metabolism have been unraveled, suggesting that many FGF-21 functions remain to be discovered in future studies. The clinical entities characterized by ectopic fat accumulation in the liver represent proatherogenic states that are linked to dysregulated FGF-21 metabolism and FGF-21 resistance both in animal models and in humans. Preliminary animal and in vitro data exists for FGF-21 or FGF-21 analog therapy, but whether FGF-21-based therapies represent a treatment option for metabolic diseases and weight loss in humans remains to be explored.

CONFLICT OF INTEREST STATEMENT

The author has no conflict of interest to declare.

References

[1] Tacer KF, Bookout AL, Ding X, Kurosu H, John GB, Wang L, et al. Research resource: comprehensive expression atlas of the fibroblast growth factor system in adult mouse. Mol Endocrinol 2010;24(10):2050–64.

[2] Kharitonenkov A, Shiyanova TL, Koester A, Ford AM, Micanovic R, Galbreath EJ, et al. FGF-21 as a novel metabolic regulator. J Clin Invest 2005;115(6):1627–35.

[3] Berglund ED, Li CY, Bina HA, Lynes SE, Michael MD, Shanafelt AB, et al. Fibroblast growth factor 21 controls glycemia via regulation of hepatic glucose flux and insulin sensitivity. Endocrinology 2009;150(9):4084–93.

[4] Whitlock G, Lewington S, Sherliker P, Clarke R, Emberson J, Halsey J, et al. Body-mass index and cause-specific mortality in 900 000 adults: collaborative analyses of 57 prospective studies. Lancet 2009;373(9669):1083–96.

[5] Boren J, Taskinen MR, Olofsson SO, Levin M. Ectopic lipid storage and insulin resistance: a harmful relationship. J Intern Med 2013;274(1):25–40.

[6] Hui X, Lam KS, Vanhoutte PM, Xu A. Adiponectin and cardiovascular health: an update. Br J Pharmacol 2012;165(3):574–90.

[7] Cuevas-Ramos D, Aguilar-Salinas CA, Gomez-Perez FJ. Metabolic actions of fibroblast growth factor 21. Curr Opin Pediatr 2012;24(4):523–9.

[8] Itoh N. Hormone-like (endocrine) Fgfs: their evolutionary history and roles in development, metabolism, and disease. Cell Tissue Res 2010;342(1):1–11.
[9] Nishimura T, Nakatake Y, Konishi M, Itoh N. Identification of a novel FGF, FGF-21, preferentially expressed in the liver. Biochim Biophys Acta 2000;1492(1):203–6.
[10] Izumiya Y, Bina HA, Ouchi N, Akasaki Y, Kharitonenkov A, Walsh K. FGF21 is an Akt-regulated myokine. FEBS Lett 2008;582(27):3805–10.
[11] Kliewer SA, Mangelsdorf DJ. Fibroblast growth factor 21: from pharmacology to physiology. Am J Clin Nutr 2010;91(1):254S–7S.
[12] Kharitonenkov A, Larsen P. FGF21 reloaded: challenges of a rapidly growing field. Trends Endocrinol Metab 2011;22(3):81–6.
[13] Ogawa Y, Kurosu H, Yamamoto M, Nandi A, Rosenblatt KP, Goetz R, et al. BetaKlotho is required for metabolic activity of fibroblast growth factor 21. Proc Natl Acad Sci U S A 2007;104(18):7432–7.
[14] Yie J, Hecht R, Patel J, Stevens J, Wang W, Hawkins N, et al. FGF21 N- and C-termini play different roles in receptor interaction and activation. FEBS Lett 2009;583(1):19–24.
[15] Tomiyama K, Maeda R, Urakawa I, Yamazaki Y, Tanaka T, Ito S, et al. Relevant use of Klotho in FGF19 subfamily signaling system in vivo. Proc Natl Acad Sci U S A 2010;107(4):1666–71.
[16] Potthoff MJ, Kliewer SA, Mangelsdorf DJ. Endocrine fibroblast growth factors 15/19 and 21: from feast to famine. Genes Dev 2012;26(4):312–24.
[17] Woo YC, Xu A, Wang Y, Lam KS. Fibroblast growth factor 21 as an emerging metabolic regulator: clinical perspectives. Clin Endocrinol (Oxf) 2013;78(4):489–96.
[18] Ito S, Kinoshita S, Shiraishi N, Nakagawa S, Sekine S, Fujimori T, et al. Molecular cloning and expression analyses of mouse betaklotho, which encodes a novel Klotho family protein. Mech Dev 2000;98(1–2):115–9.
[19] Hsuchou H, Pan W, Kastin AJ. The fasting polypeptide FGF21 can enter brain from blood. Peptides 2007;28(12):2382–6.
[20] Galman C, Lundasen T, Kharitonenkov A, Bina HA, Eriksson M, Hafstrom I, et al. The circulating metabolic regulator FGF21 is induced by prolonged fasting and PPARalpha activation in man. Cell Metab 2008;8(2):169–74.
[21] Matikainen N, Taskinen MR, Stennabb S, Lundbom N, Hakkarainen A, Vaaralahti K, et al. Decrease in circulating fibroblast growth factor 21 after an oral fat load is related to postprandial triglyceride-rich lipoproteins and liver fat. Eur J Endocrinol 2012;166(3):487–92.
[22] Inagaki T, Dutchak P, Zhao G, Ding X, Gautron L, Parameswara V, et al. Endocrine regulation of the fasting response by PPARα-mediated induction of fibroblast growth factor 21. Cell Metab 2007;5(6):415–25.
[23] Badman MK, Pissios P, Kennedy AR, Koukos G, Flier JS, Maratos-Flier E. Hepatic fibroblast growth factor 21 is regulated by PPARalpha and is a key mediator of hepatic lipid metabolism in ketotic states. Cell Metab 2007;5(6):426–37.
[24] Potthoff MJ, Inagaki T, Satapati S, Ding X, He T, Goetz R, et al. FGF21 induces PGC-1α and regulates carbohydrate and fatty acid metabolism during the adaptive starvation response. Proc Natl Acad Sci U S A 2009;106(26):10853–8.
[25] Uebanso T, Taketani Y, Fukaya M, Sato K, Takei Y, Sato T, et al. Hypocaloric high-protein diet improves fatty liver and hypertriglyceridemia in sucrose-fed obese rats via two pathways. Am J Physiol Endocrinol Metab 2009;297(1):E76–84.
[26] Chen W, Hoo RL, Konishi M, Itoh N, Lee PC, Ye HY, et al. Growth hormone induces hepatic production of fibroblast growth factor 21 through a mechanism dependent on lipolysis in adipocytes. J Biol Chem 2011;286(40):34559–66.
[27] Schoenberg KM, Giesy SL, Harvatine KJ, Waldron MR, Cheng C, Kharitonenkov A, et al. Plasma FGF21 is elevated by the intense lipid mobilization of lactation. Endocrinology 2011;152(12):4652–61.
[28] Berglund ED, Kang L, Lee-Young RS, Hasenour CM, Lustig DG, Lynes SE, et al. Glucagon and lipid interactions in the regulation of hepatic AMPK signaling and expression of PPARα and FGF21 transcripts in vivo. Am J Physiol Endocrinol Metab 2010;299(4):E607–14.
[29] Arafat AM, Kaczmarek P, Skrzypski M, Pruszynska-Oszmalek E, Kolodziejski P, Szczepankiewicz D, et al. Glucagon increases circulating fibroblast growth factor 21 independently of endogenous insulin levels: a novel mechanism of glucagon-stimulated lipolysis? Diabetologia 2013;56(3):588–97.
[30] Adams AC, Astapova I, Fisher FM, Badman MK, Kurgansky KE, Flier JS, et al. Thyroid hormone regulates hepatic expression of fibroblast growth factor 21 in a PPARalpha-dependent manner. J Biol Chem 2010;285(19):14078–82.
[31] Dutchak PA, Katafuchi T, Bookout AL, Choi JH, Yu RT, Mangelsdorf DJ, et al. Fibroblast growth factor-21 regulates PPARγ activity and the antidiabetic actions of thiazolidinediones. Cell 2012;148(3):556–67.
[32] Uebanso T, Taketani Y, Yamamoto H, Amo K, Tanaka S, Arai H, et al. Liver X receptor negatively regulates fibroblast growth factor 21 in the fatty liver induced by cholesterol-enriched diet. J Nutr Biochem 2012;23(7):785–90.
[33] Archer A, Venteclef N, Mode A, Pedrelli M, Gabbi C, Clement K, et al. Fasting-induced FGF21 is repressed by LXR activation via recruitment of an HDAC3 corepressor complex in mice. Mol Endocrinol 2012;26(12):1980–90.
[34] Tyynismaa H, Raivio T, Hakkarainen A, Ortega-Alonso A, Lundbom N, Kaprio J, et al. Liver fat but not other adiposity measures influence circulating FGF21 levels in healthy young adult twins. J Clin Endocrinol Metab 2011;96(2):E351–5.
[35] Uebanso T, Taketani Y, Yamamoto H, Amo K, Ominami H, Arai H, et al. Paradoxical regulation of human FGF21 by both fasting and feeding signals: is FGF21 a nutritional adaptation factor? PLoS ONE 2011;6(8):e22976.
[36] Mai K, Schwarz F, Bobbert T, Andres J, Assmann A, Pfeiffer AFH, et al. Relation between fibroblast growth factor-21, adiposity, metabolism, and weight reduction. Metab Clin Exp 2011;60(2):306–11.
[37] Mai K, Andres J, Biedasek K, Andres J, Assmann A, Pfeiffer AFH, et al. Free fatty acids link metabolism and regulation of the insulin-sensitizing fibroblast growth factor-21. Diabetes 2009;58(7):1532–8.
[38] Christodoulides C, Dyson P, Sprecher D, Tsintzas K, Karpe F. Circulating fibroblast growth factor 21 is induced by peroxisome proliferator-activated receptor agonists but not ketosis in man. J Clin Endocrinol Metab 2009;94(9):3594–601.
[39] Mraz M, Bartlova M, Lacinova Z, Michalsky D, Kasalicky M, Haluzikova D, et al. Serum concentrations and tissue expression of a novel endocrine regulator fibroblast growth factor-21 in patients with type 2 diabetes and obesity. Clin Endocrinol (Oxf) 2009;71(3):369–75.
[40] Kralisch S, Fasshauer M. Fibroblast growth factor 21: effects on carbohydrate and lipid metabolism in health and disease. Curr Opin Clin Nutr Metab Care; 2011.
[41] Coskun T, Bina HA, Schneider MA, Dunbar JD, Hu CC, Chen Y, et al. Fibroblast growth factor 21 corrects obesity in mice. Endocrinology 2008;149(12):6018–27.
[42] Chau MDL, Gao J, Yang Q, Wu Z, Gromada J. Fibroblast growth factor 21 regulates energy metabolism by activating the AMPK-SIRT1-PGC-1α pathway. Proc Natl Acad Sci U S A 2010;107(28):12553–8.
[43] Badman MK, Koester A, Flier JS, Kharitonenkov A, Maratos-Flier E. Fibroblast growth factor 21-deficient mice demonstrate impaired adaptation to ketosis. Endocrinology 2009;150(11):4931–40.

[44] Domouzoglou EM, Maratos-Flier E. Fibroblast growth factor 21 is a metabolic regulator that plays a role in the adaptation to ketosis. Am J Clin Nutr 2011;93(4):901S–5S.

[45] Inagaki T, Lin VY, Goetz R, Mohammadi M, Mangelsdorf DJ, Kliewer SA. Inhibition of growth hormone signaling by the fasting-induced hormone FGF21. Cell Metab 2008;8(1):77–83.

[46] Barclay JL, Nelson CN, Ishikawa M, Murray LA, Kerr LM, McPhee TR, et al. GH-dependent STAT5 signaling plays an important role in hepatic lipid metabolism. Endocrinology 2011;152(1):181–92.

[47] Hotta Y, Nakamura H, Konishi M, Murata Y, Takagi H, Matsumura S, et al. Fibroblast growth factor 21 regulates lipolysis in white adipose tissue but is not required for ketogenesis and triglyceride clearance in liver. Endocrinology 2009;150(10):4625–33.

[48] Long YC, Kharitonenkov A. Hormone-like fibroblast growth factors and metabolic regulation. Biochim Bioph Acta Mol Basis Dis 2011;1812(7):791–5.

[49] Chartoumpekis DV, Habeos IG, Ziros PG, Psyrogiannis AI, Kyriazopoulou VE, Papavassiliou AG. Brown adipose tissue responds to cold and adrenergic stimulation by induction of FGF21. Mol Med 2011;17(7–8):736–40.

[50] Hondares E, Iglesias R, Giralt A, Gonzalez FJ, Giralt M, Mampel T, et al. Thermogenic activation induces FGF21 expression and release in brown adipose tissue. J Biol Chem 2011;286(15): 12983–90.

[51] Fisher FM, Kleiner S, Douris N, Fox EC, Mepani RJ, Verdeguer F, et al. FGF21 regulates PGC-1α and browning of white adipose tissues in adaptive thermogenesis. Genes Dev 2012;26(3):271–81.

[52] Hondares E, Rosell M, Gonzalez FJ, Giralt M, Iglesias R, Villarroya F. Hepatic FGF21 expression is induced at birth via PPARα in response to milk intake and contributes to thermogenic activation of neonatal brown fat. Cell Metab 2010;11(3):206–12.

[53] Tong X, Muchnik M, Chen Z, Patel M, Wu N, Joshi S, et al. Transcriptional repressor E4-binding protein 4 (E4BP4) regulates metabolic hormone fibroblast growth factor 21 (FGF21) during circadian cycles and feeding. J Biol Chem 2010;285(47):36401–9.

[54] Wente W, Efanov AM, Brenner M, Kharitonenkov A, Koster A, Sandusky GE, et al. Fibroblast growth factor-21 improves pancreatic beta-cell function and survival by activation of extracellular signal-regulated kinase 1/2 and Akt signaling pathways. Diabetes 2006;55(9):2470–8.

[55] Xiao Y, Xu A, Law LSC, Chen C, Li H, Li X, et al. Distinct changes in serum fibroblast growth factor 21 levels in different subtypes of diabetes. J Clin Endocrinol Metab 2012;97(1):E54–8.

[56] Johnson CL, Weston JY, Chadi SA, Fazio EN, Huff MW, Kharitonenkov A, et al. Fibroblast growth factor 21 reduces the severity of cerulein-induced pancreatitis in mice. Gastroenterology 2009;137(5):1795–804.

[57] Sun HD, Malabunga M, Tonra JR, DiRenzo R, Carrick FE, Zheng H, et al. Monoclonal antibody antagonists of hypothalamic FGFR1 cause potent but reversible hypophagia and weight loss in rodents and monkeys. Am J Physiol Endocrinol Metabol 2007;292(3):E964–76.

[58] Murphy M, Samms R, Warner A, Bolborea M, Barrett P, Fowler MJ, et al. Increased responses to the actions of fibroblast growth factor 21 on energy balance and body weight in a seasonal model of adiposity. J Neuroendocrinol 2013;25(2):180–9.

[59] Moyers JS, Shiyanova TL, Mehrbod F, Dunbar JD, Noblitt TW, Otto KA, et al. Molecular determinants of FGF-21 activity-synergy and cross-talk with PPARgamma signaling. J Cell Physiol 2007;210(1):1–6.

[60] Zhang X, Yeung DC, Karpisek M, Stejskal D, Zhou ZG, Liu F, et al. Serum FGF21 levels are increased in obesity and are independently associated with the metabolic syndrome in humans. Diabetes 2008;57(5):1246–53.

[61] Samson SL, Sathyanarayana P, Jogi M, Gonzalez EV, Gutierrez A, Krishnamurthy R, et al. Exenatide decreases hepatic fibroblast growth factor 21 resistance in non-alcoholic fatty liver disease in a mouse model of obesity and in a randomised controlled trial. Diabetologia 2011;54(12):3093–100.

[62] Lee SA, Jeong E, Kim EH, Shin MS, Hwang JY, Koh EH, et al. Various oscillation patterns of serum fibroblast growth factor 21 concentrations in healthy volunteers. Diab Metab J 2012;36(1):29–36.

[63] Dushay J, Chui PC, Gopalakrishnan GS, Varela-Rey M, Crawley M, Fisher FM, et al. Increased fibroblast growth factor 21 in obesity and nonalcoholic fatty liver disease. Gastroenterology 2010;139(2):456–63.

[64] Lin Z, Gong Q, Wu C, Yu J, Lu T, Pan X, et al. Dynamic change of serum FGF21 levels in response to glucose challenge in human. J Clin Endocrinol Metab 2012;97(7):E1224–8.

[65] Yu H, Xia F, Lam KSL, et al. Circadian rhythm of circulating fibroblast growth factor 21 is related to diurnal changes in fatty acids in humans. Clin Chem 2011;57(5):691–700.

[66] Lee P, Brychta RJ, Linderman J, Smith S, Chen KY, Celi FS. Mild cold exposure modulates fibroblast growth factor 21 (FGF21) diurnal rhythm in humans: relationship between FGF21 levels, lipolysis, and cold-induced thermogenesis. J Clin Endocrinol Metab 2013;98(1):E98–E102.

[67] Flachs P, Rossmeisl M, Kuda O, Kopecky J. Stimulation of mitochondrial oxidative capacity in white fat independent of UCP1: A key to lean phenotype. Biochim Bioph Acta Mol Cell Biol, Lipids 2013;1831(5):986–1003.

[68] Chavez AO, Molina-Carrion M, Abdul-Ghani MA, Folli F, Defronzo RA, Tripathy D. Circulating fibroblast growth factor-21 is elevated in impaired glucose tolerance and type 2 diabetes and correlates with muscle and hepatic insulin resistance. Diabetes Care 2009;32(8):1542–6.

[69] Reinehr T, Woelfle J, Wunsch R, Roth CL. Fibroblast growth factor 21 (FGF-21) and its relation to obesity, metabolic syndrome, and nonalcoholic fatty liver in children: a longitudinal analysis. J Clin Endocrinol Metab 2012;97(6):2143–50.

[70] Flier JS. Hormone resistance in diabetes and obesity: insulin, leptin, and FGF21. Yale J Biol Med 2012;85(3):405–14.

[71] Lin Z, Wu Z, Yin X, Liu Y, Yan X, Lin S, et al. Serum levels of FGF-21 are increased in coronary heart disease patients and are independently associated with adverse lipid profile. PLoS ONE 2010;5(12):e15534.

[72] Semba RD, Sun K, Egan JM, Crasto C, Carlson OD, Ferrucci L. Relationship of serum fibroblast growth factor 21 with abnormal glucose metabolism and insulin resistance: the Baltimore Longitudinal Study of Aging. J Clin Endocrinol Metab 2012;97(4):1375–82.

[73] Han SH, Choi SH, Cho BJ, Lee Y, Lim S, Park YJ, et al. Serum fibroblast growth factor-21 concentration is associated with residual renal function and insulin resistance in end-stage renal disease patients receiving long-term peritoneal dialysis. Metab Clin Exp 2010;59(11):1656–62.

[74] Domingo P, Gallego-Escuredo JM, Domingo JC, Gutierrez Mdel M, Mateo MG, Fernandez I, et al. Serum FGF21 levels are elevated in association with lipodystrophy, insulin resistance and biomarkers of liver injury in HIV-1-infected patients. AIDS 2010;24(17):2629–37.

[75] Lindegaard B, Hvid T, Grondahl T, Frosig C, Gerstoft J, Hojman P, et al. Expression of fibroblast growth factor-21 in muscle is associated with lipodystrophy, insulin resistance and lipid disturbances in patients with HIV. PLoS ONE 2013;8(3):e55632.

[76] Ďurovcová V, Marek J, Hána V, Matoulek M, Zikán V, Haluzíková D, et al. Plasma concentrations of fibroblast growth factors 21 and 19 in patients with Cushing's syndrome. Physiol Res 2010;59(3):415–22.

[77] Li H, Fang Q, Gao F, Fan J, Zhou J, Wang X, et al. Fibroblast growth factor 21 levels are increased in nonalcoholic fatty liver disease patients and are correlated with hepatic triglyceride. J Hepatol 2010;53(5):934–40.
[78] Chen C, Cheung BM, Tso AW, Wang Y, Law LS, Ong KL, et al. High plasma level of fibroblast growth factor 21 is an Independent predictor of type 2 diabetes: a 5.4-year population-based prospective study in Chinese subjects. Diabetes Care 2011;34(9):2113–5.
[79] Bobbert T, Schwarz F, Fischer-Rosinsky A, Pfeiffer AF, Mohlig M, Mai K, et al. Fibroblast growth factor 21 predicts the metabolic syndrome and type 2 diabetes in Caucasians. Diabetes Care 2013;36(1):145–9.
[80] Zhang M, Zeng L, Wang YJ, An ZM, Ying BW. Associations of fibroblast growth factor 21 gene 3′ untranslated region single-nucleotide polymorphisms with metabolic syndrome, obesity, and diabetes in a Han Chinese population. DNA Cell Biol 2012;31(4):547–52.
[81] Chartoumpekis DV, Ziros PG, Psyrogiannis AI, Papavassiliou AG, Kyriazopoulou VE, Sykiotis GP, et al. Nrf2 represses FGF21 during long-term high-fat diet-induced obesity in mice. Diabetes 2011;60(10):2465–73.
[82] Schaap FG, Kremer AE, Lamers WH, Jansen PLM, Gaemers IC. Fibroblast growth factor 21 is induced by endoplasmic reticulum stress. Biochimie 2013;95(4):692–9.
[83] Chu AY, Workalemahu T, Paynter NP, Rose LM, Giulianini F, Tanaka T, et al. Novel locus including FGF21 is associated with dietary macronutrient intake. Hum Mol Genet 2013;22(9):1895–902.
[84] Fazeli PK, Misra M, Goldstein M, Miller KK, Klibanski A. Fibroblast growth factor-21 may mediate growth hormone resistance in anorexia nervosa. J Clin Endocrinol Metab 2010;95(1):369–74.
[85] Zhang Y, Xie Y, Berglund ED, Coate KC, He TT, Katafuchi T, et al. The starvation hormone, fibroblast growth factor-21, extends lifespan in mice. eLife 2012;1:e00065.
[86] Kharitonenkov A, Wroblewski VJ, Koester A, Chen YF, Clutinger CK, Tigno XT, et al. The metabolic state of diabetic monkeys is regulated by fibroblast growth factor-21. Endocrinology 2007;148(2):774–81.
[87] Wu X, Ge H, Baribault H, Gupte J, Weiszmann J, Lemon B, et al. Dual actions of fibroblast growth factor 19 on lipid metabolism. J Lipid Res 2013;54(2):325–32.
[88] Hecht R, Li YS, Sun J, Belouski E, Hall M, Hager T, et al. Rationale-based engineering of a potent long-acting FGF21 analog for the treatment of type 2 diabetes. PLoS ONE 2012;7(11):e49345.
[89] Kharitonenkov A, Beals JM, Micanovic R, Strifler BA, Rathnachalam R, Wroblewski VJ, et al. Rational design of a fibroblast growth factor 21-based clinical candidate, LY2405319. PLoS ONE 2013;8(3):e58575.
[90] Wei W, Dutchak PA, Wang X, Ding X, Wang X, Bookout AL, et al. Fibroblast growth factor 21 promotes bone loss by potentiating the effects of peroxisome proliferator-activated receptor. Proc Natl Acad Sci U S A 2012;109(8):3143–8.
[91] Wu S, Levenson A, Kharitonenkov A, De Luca F. Fibroblast growth factor 21 (FGF21) inhibits chondrocyte function and growth hormone action directly at the growth plate. J Biol Chem 2012;287(31):26060–7.
[92] Wan Y. Bone marrow mesenchymal stem cells: fat on and blast off by FGF21. Int J Biochem Cell Biol 2013;45(3):546–9.
[93] Yang SJ, Hong HC, Choi HY, Yoo HJ, Cho GJ, Hwang TG, et al. Effects of a three-month combined exercise programme on fibroblast growth factor 21 and fetuin-A levels and arterial stiffness in obese women. Clin Endocrinol (Oxf) 2011;75(4):464–9.
[94] Woelnerhanssen B, Peterli R, Steinert RE, Peters T, Borbely Y, Beglinger C. Effects of postbariatric surgery weight loss on adipokines and metabolic parameters: comparison of laparoscopic Roux-en-Y gastric bypass and laparoscopic sleeve gastrectomy—a prospective randomized trial. Surg Obes Rel Dis 2011;7(5):561–8.
[95] Ong KL, Rye KA, O'Connell R, et al. Long-term fenofibrate therapy increases fibroblast growth factor 21 and retinol-binding protein 4 in subjects with type 2 diabetes. J Clin Endocrinol Metab 2012;97(12):4701–8.
[96] Gaich G, Chien JY, Fu H, Glass LC, Deeg MA, Holland WL, et al. The effect of LY2405319, an FGF21 analog, in obese human subjects with type 2 diabetes. Cell Metabolism 2013;18(3):333–40.

CHAPTER

40

Genetics of Abdominal Obesity

Min Xu[a,b] and Lu Qi[a,c]

[a]Department of Nutrition, Harvard School of Public Health, Boston, MA, USA; [b]Shanghai Clinical Center for Endocrine and Metabolic Diseases, Shanghai Institute of Endocrine and Metabolic Diseases, Ruijin Hospital Affiliated to Shanghai Jiao Tong University School of Medicine, Shanghai, China; [c]Channing Division of Network Medicine, Department of Medicine, Brigham and Women's Hospital and Harvard Medical School, Boston, MA, USA

INTRODUCTION

Obesity is a heterogeneous phenotype associated with metabolic disturbances affecting not only the overall amount of body fat but also the distribution of body fat. In epidemiological studies, altered regional adiposity has been related to various metabolic disorders such as dyslipidemia, insulin resistance, diabetes, and cardiovascular disease, independent of overall adiposity. Among the various depots of body fat, those that accumulate in abdominal regions are particularly detrimental.

Terms such as *abdominal obesity* and *central obesity* are used to describe excess intra-abdominal adipose tissue accumulation. In population studies, waist circumference (WC) and waist-hip ratio (WHR) are most widely used to indicate the severity of abdominal obesity. Definitions of abdominal obesity vary across different agencies. For example, the World Health Organization defines abdominal obesity as a WHR of >0.9 for men and >0.85 for women, while the National Health and Nutrition Examination Survey (NHANES III) defines abdominal obesity as a WC of >102 cm (40 inches) in men and >88 cm (35 inches) in women). More precise measures of abdominal adipose tissue using dual-energy X-ray absorptiometry (DEXA), computed tomography, and magnetic resonance imaging (MRI) are less frequently employed in large population settings.

It has been known for a long time that environmental factors such as diet and lifestyle play key roles in determining obesity, including abdominal obesity. Classical genetic analyses in families, adoptees, and twins have also clearly shown the genetic contribution to abdominal obesity. It is now widely accepted that abdominal obesity has a genetic basis but requires environmental influences to be revealed. This chapter will summarize major efforts made over the past few decades in genetic research on abdominal obesity, recent advances in the detection of the genetic markers, and published empirical evidence for interactions between genetic components and environmental factors, especially lifestyle and diet.

HERITABILITY

Obesity, especially abdominal obesity, is among several conditions that show the most widespread ethnic variations, even among people who live in analogous environments. This suggests that ethnic-specific genetic makeup may account for at least part of the distinction. The heritable nature is also supported by the observation of a high concordance of abdominal obesity among genetically related individuals. In classic genetic research, heritability (i.e. the proportion of the phenotypic variance accounted for by genetic factors) is usually estimated from twin studies or family studies.

Twin studies have advantages in the study of heritability: they provide a unique method for disentangling nature and nurture by taking advantage of the fact that monozygotic twins share all of their genes, whereas dizygotic twins on average share half of their segregating genes [1]. The classical twin model is based upon the key assumption that both prenatal and postnatal environmental covariance are the same for monozygotic and dizygotic twin pairs. If genetics contribute to phenotype variance, concordance in the phenotype would be higher in monozygotic twins than in dizygotic twins. Heritability estimates for overall adiposity [(most commonly measured by body mass index (BMI)] in adults range from 55% to 85% [2–5]. It is believed that certain genetic

Nutrition in the Prevention and Treatment of Abdominal Obesity
http://dx.doi.org/10.1016/B978-0-12-407869-7.00040-4

components contribute to both overall adiposity and abdominal adiposity, while phenotype-specific genetic effects may also exist. In a large-scale twin study including 1813 monozygotic (845 males and 968 females) and 3279 dizygotic (818 males and 840 females; and n = 1621 opposite-sex) subjects with an average age of 9.9 years (range 8.3-11.6), BMI and WC showed a high correlation ($r = 0.77$). Even so, it was found that 40% of the heritability of WC is independent of the genetic influence on BMI [6]. Of note, estimates of measures for abdominal obesity vary considerably across studies. For example, heritability estimates for WC [7–9] ranged from 37% in an old order Amish community to 81% in nondiabetic Native American Pima people, from 6% to 30% in Taiwan Chinese for WHR [10–12], and from 35% to 63% in a Taiwan Chinese population for percentage body fat [12–15]. A twin study and the Health, Risk Factors, Exercise Training, and Genetics (HERITAGE) family study reported a similar heritability of 63% and 62%, respectively [13,14]. In an Indian population, >90% heritability has been reported for abdominal fat accumulation [16].

Many reasons may explain the high variation in heritability estimates. For example, the influence of shared environment on the estimate of heritability may vary across studies. In addition, the participants in different studies varied significantly in age, sex, BMI, and other characteristics related to abdominal obesity. Moreover, a small study sample size may generate unstable estimates of heritability.

MONOGENIC OBESITY

More direct evidence supporting the genetic contribution to obesity-related traits was obtained from the identification of a monogenic form of obesity. Monogenic obesity is a kind of Mendelian disorder that is caused by mutations in genes that encode proteins mainly involved in energy intake or expenditure, such as appetite regulation. The known monogenic forms of obesity can be divided into three broad categories. The first category is obesity caused by mutations in genes that have a physiologic role in the hypothalamic leptin-melanocortin system of energy balance, such as mutations in human genes encoding for leptin (*LEP*) [17], leptin receptor (*LEPR*) [18], proopiomelanocortin (*POMC*) [19], melanocortin receptor 4 (*MC4R*) [20] and neuroendocrine convertases 1-3/prohormone convertases 1-3 [proprotein convertase subtilisin/kexin type 1 (*PCSK1*)] [21], most of which have been associated with juvenile-onset morbid obesity. Mutations in the gene that encodes MC4R account for the frequent autosomal dominant forms of obesity [20,22]. MC4R deficiency represents the most common monogenic obesity disorder that has been identified so far, and occurs in 1-6% of obese individuals from different ethnic groups [23]. The second category is obesity resulting from mutations in the three genes necessary for development of the hypothalamus: single-minded homolog 1 (*SIM1*), brain-derived neurotrophic factor (*BDNF*), and neurotrophic tyrosine kinase, receptor, type 1 (*NTRK*) [24]. These genes have important roles in hypothalamic development and lead to severe obesity when mutated. The third category is obesity presenting as part of a complex syndrome caused by mutations in genes whose functional relationship to obesity is unclear. Most of these obesity syndromes are distinguished by the presence of mental retardation. There are about 30 Mendelian disorders in which obesity or abdominal obesity is a clinical feature, often associated with mental retardation, dysmorphic features, and organ-specific developmental abnormalities, such as Bardet-Biedl syndrome, Albright hereditary osteodystrophy, and fragile X syndrome [25].

GENOME-WIDE LINKAGE STUDY

Genetic linkage analysis is one of the principal approaches used to identify genomic regions that contain genes predisposing to disease. Linkage analysis is often performed as the first stage in the genetic investigation of a trait, since it can be used to identify broad genomic regions that might contain a disease gene, even in the absence of previous biologically driven hypotheses [1].

A logarithm of the odds (LOD) score is usually used to indicate the significance level of the linkage: LOD ≥ 3 is widely accepted as the cutoff point for genome-wide significance. This score was first proposed by Morton in 1955 [26]. It is a function of the recombination fraction (θ) or chromosomal position, measured in centimorgans. Large positive scores are evidence of linkage (or cosegregation), and negative scores are evidence against linkage [1]. A genome region identified from linkage analysis is termed a *quantitative trait locus* (QTL). As of October 2005, 253 QTLs for obesity-related phenotypes have been reported from 61 genome-wide linkage scans (Fig. 40.1). A total of 52 genomic regions harbor QTLs supported by two or more studies [24]. However, the vast majority of these linkage analyses focused on overall adiposity, and a few of the studies found evidence of linkage with measures related to abdominal obesity, such as WC or WHR [27–30]. For instance, QTL 1q21-q25 in the Hong Kong Family Diabetes Study and QTL 6q23-25 in the Framingham Heart Study were found to be in linkage with WC [27,30]. Suggestive linkage was found in European Americans and African-Americans, both with LOD scores of 2.7 at the Xp21.3 and Xp11.3 regions [28]. Some studies have reported regions in linkage with percentage body fat [31–35], including two

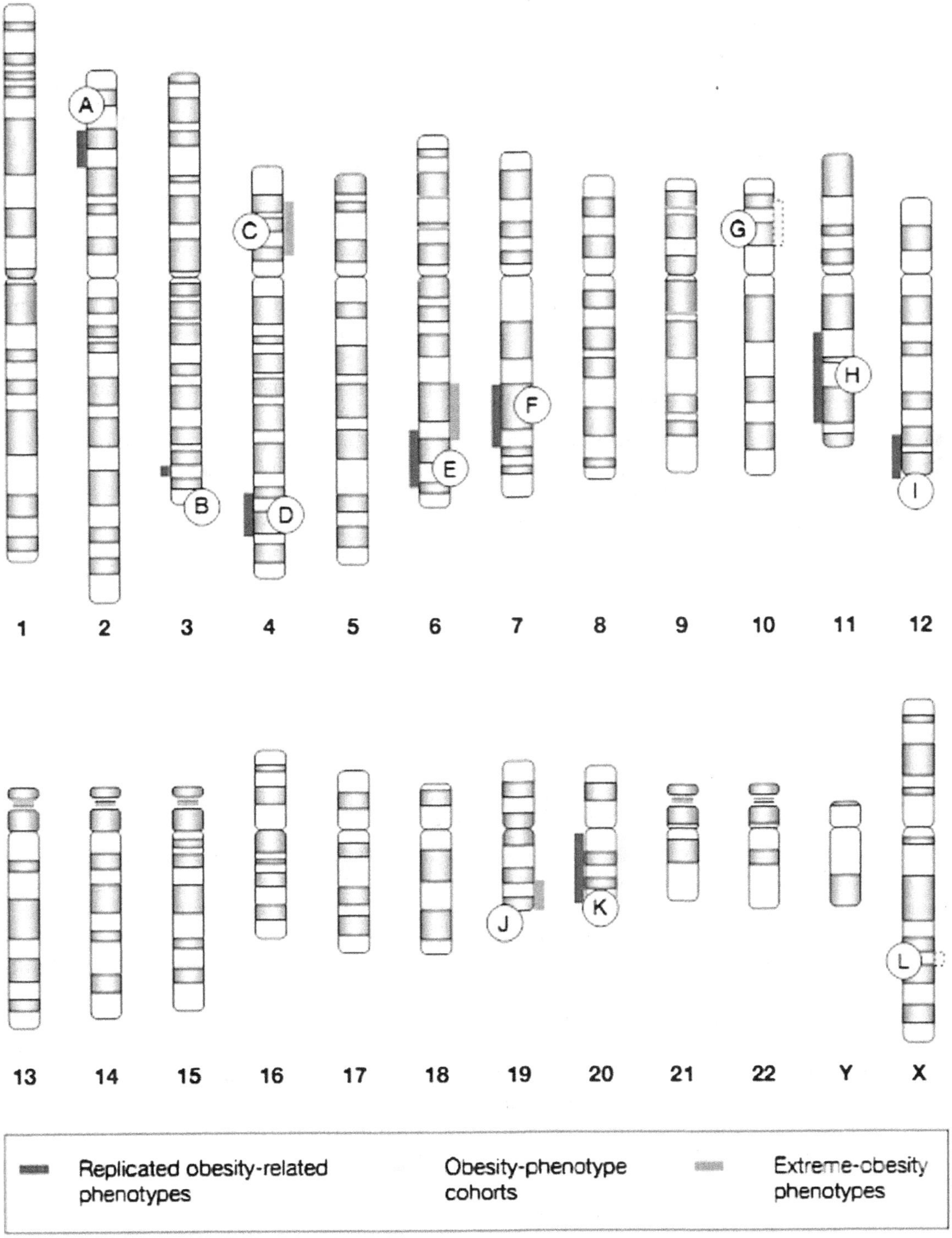

FIGURE 40.1 Genetic linkage map for obesity. Loci found to be linked with obesity. Blue bars indicate regions that have been replicated in several studies. Yellow bars represent loci that were found in cohorts selected specifically for obesity, and dotted lines around these bars indicate replication in other obesity cohorts. Red bars indicate regions identified in groups with extreme obesity phenotypes. A, 2p21-p23; B, 3q27; C, 4p15-p14; D, 4q31-q32; E, 6q22.31-q23.2; F, 7q31-q32; G, 10p11-p12; H, 11q14-q24; I, 12q23-q24; J, 19q13.33-q13.43; K, 20q11-q13; L, Xq24. *Source: Bell et al.* [36]. (See color plate at the back of the book.)

studies performed in non-Hispanic whites and European-American families: both observed a LOD score of 3.8 in chromosome 12q24 [33,34].

Several limitations of linkage studies of obesity-related phenotypes should be acknowledged. First, the relatively small study sample size may limit the power of genome scans to detect relatively moderate genetic effects. Second, multiple tests performed in each study increased type 1 error, and correction for multiple testing is necessary to claim significant levels. Third, the heterogeneity of the study populations makes it difficult to detect true linkages that can be validated across studies. The lack of replication of the findings from genome-wide linkage study has been a major concern.

CANDIDATE GENE ASSOCIATION STUDY

Before the genome-wide association approach was first introduced to the field, candidate gene association study was a predominant method to detect genetic variants for complex disorders including abdominal obesity. The design of the candidate gene association study is simple: it includes the identification of genes relevant to the outcome phenotype of interest; selection of polymorphic markers within the candidate genes; and analyses of associations between the genetic markers, with the outcomes in a suitable set of subjects. Identification of potential candidate genes is the main stumbling block. Two major types of candidate genes are generally considered: functional and positional [36]. Functional candidates are genes with products that are in some way involved in the pathogenesis of the disease. Clearly, this is highly dependent on the current state of knowledge about a disease. In the case of obesity or abdominal obesity, there is confirmed evidence that genes influencing energy homeostasis and thermogenesis, adipogenesis, leptin-insulin signaling transduction, and hormonal signaling peptides play critical roles [37]. Positional candidates are genes identified by linkage or association studies, or by the detection of chromosomal translocations that disrupt the gene. The number of studies reporting associations between DNA sequence variation in specific genes and obesity phenotypes has increased considerably, with 426 findings of positive associations in 127 candidate genes by October 2005. A promising observation is that 22 genes are each supported by at least five positive studies [24].

Most candidate genes are found to be associated with overall obesity. It is worth mentioning that several candidate genes have shown biological effects underlying the genetically association. In addition to peroxisome proliferative activated receptor gamma (*PPARG*; encoding a nuclear receptor) [38–40], *POMC* [41] and *MC4R* [42] were demonstrated to associate with common obesity. The beta 2 and beta 3 adrenoceptor (*ADRB2* and *ADRB3*) [43,44], uncoupling protein 1 and 3 gene (*UCP1* and *UCP3*) [45], adrenoceptor alpha 2A gene (*ADRA2A*) [46], angiotensin I converting enzyme gene (*ACE*) [47], apolipoprotein A-II gene (*APOA2*) [48], fatty acid binding protein 2 gene (*FABP2*) [49], lymphotoxin alpha gene (*LTA*) [50], microsomal triglyceride transfer protein gene (*MTTP*) [51], perlipin gene (*PLIN*) [52], *PPARG* [53] and acyl-CoA dehydrogenase gene (*ACDC*) [54] genes have been linked to WC, WHR, or abdominal fat. The *ADRB3* gene is predominantly expressed in adipose tissue and regulates lipid metabolism and thermogenesis [55], and genetic variants at *ADRB3* locus have been associated with body weight across diverse populations. A meta-analysis including 31 studies with more than 9000 individuals demonstrated a significant association of the Trp64Arg polymorphism of the *ADRB3* gene with BMI [56]. The *ADRB3* genotype has also been related to WC, a measure of abdominal obesity. The beta-2 adrenergic receptor is expressed in visceral fat in humans [57] and is responsible for increased lipolysis and the delivery of free fatty acid into the portal vein. In one study of 335 subjects from western Finland of 207 nondiabetic subjects and 128 patients affected by noninsulin-dependent diabetes mellitus (NIDDM), the Trp64Arg allele of *ADRB3* gene was found to be associated with abdominal obesity [44].

Many studies have suggested relations between UCP family genes and both obesity and fat distribution. The major function of UCPs is to uncouple oxidative phosphorylation of adenosine diphosphate (ADP) to adenosine triphosphate (ATP), leading to the generation of heat [58]. The UCP family includes three different proteins: UCP 1 expressed in brown adipose tissue, UCP 2 expressed in most tissues, including white adipose tissue), and UCP 3 expressed in skeletal muscle. *UCP2* and *UCP3* genes are located adjacent to each another on chromosome 11q13 [59]. The G866A polymorphism of the *UCP2* gene has been related in Chinese and Indian men [60] and Finnish overweight individuals [61] to increased risk of central obesity and overall obesity [62,63]. However, the association was not consistently observed [64].

The neuropeptide Y gene (*NPY*), containing four exons, is located on chromosome 7p15.1 and encodes a 36-amino acid peptide that is secreted by neurons in the hypothalamus [65]. The neuropeptide has orexigenic effects, affecting appetite and food intake in animals. Injection of this peptide directly into the central nervous system of animals leads to obesity through increased feeding [66]. In addition, a maternal low-protein diet upregulates the neuropeptide system in visceral fat and leads to abdominal obesity and glucose intolerance in a sex- and time-specific manner [67].

Although candidate gene association studies have suggested that genetic variants in several biologically relevant genes might be related to abdominal obesity, it is also notable that most of the findings are not reproducible. In fact, no loci have been convincingly confirmed to be associated with abdominal obesity to date. Of note, most of the candidate gene association studies are relatively small in size and were performed without replications [68]. In addition, candidate gene association studies usually focus on limited variants in the studied regions, thus failing to capture the overall genetic variance [69]. Moreover, selection of candidate genes relies on current knowledge of their biological relevance, thus seriously limiting the power for detection of novel genetic variations affecting the outcomes of interest.

GENOME-WIDE ASSOCIATION STUDY

Genetic research into complex diseases has achieved a remarkable leap since the first application of a genome-wide association approach in 2006 [70]. Such revolutionary progress in the field is largely due to the completion of Human Genome Project and breakthroughs in high-throughput, genome-wide genotyping technology. During the past few years, genome-wide association studies (GWAS) have been extensively employed in the detection of genetic determinants for various diseases (e.g. diabetes, obesity, cancers, cardiovascular diseases, dyslipidemia, neuropsychiatric diseases, autoimmune diseases, and infectious diseases) and metabolic quantitative traits (e.g. body height, blood glucose, BMI, and WC/WHR). Thus far, these studies have identified hundreds of susceptibility loci associated with complex diseases and metabolic traits (see http://www.genome.gov/gwastudies/), including measures of abdominal obesity (Fig. 40.2) [71].

Unlike candidate gene association studies, GWAS are conducted without a prior hypothesis. The widely used genome-wide scan platforms cover up to several million genetic variants—single nucleotide polymorphisms (SNPs) or structural variants such as copy number variants—over the human genome. Another significant improvement in study design is that all GWAS have a replication mechanism and typically include a large sample size. The number of susceptibility loci for obesity has grown dramatically. It has now been demonstrated that 36 susceptibility loci are associated with BMI and/or obesity [72–74] and 14 loci associated with WHR adjusted for BMI (Table 40.1) [75,76]. Given the high correlation between BMI and WHR/WC, the GWAS for indicators of abdominal obesity, WHR, or WC, should consider independent genetic determinants after adjusting for BMI.

Two rounds of GWAS have been performed to detect novel genetic loci for abdominal obesity. The first round of study was performed by using a meta-analysis of 16 GWAS ($n=38{,}580$) informative for adult WC and WHR. The investigators then selected 26 SNPs for follow-up, for which the evidence of association with measures of abdominal adiposity (WC and/or WHR) was strong and disproportionate to that for overall adiposity or height. Follow-up studies in a maximum of 70,689 individuals identified two loci strongly associated with measures of abdominal adiposity: *TFAP2B* (WC, $P=1.9\times10^{-11}$) and *MSRA* (WC, $P=8.9\times10^{-9}$). Another locus, near *LYPLAL1*, was associated with WHR in women only ($P=2.6\times10^{-8}$). Variants near *TFAP2B* appear to influence abdominal adiposity through an effect on overall obesity/fat mass, whereas *LYPLAL1* displays a strong female-only association with fat distribution. The study provided proof of principle for the genetic control of body fat distribution distinct from that of overall adiposity. The second round of GWAS was performed within the Genetic Investigation of Anthropometric Traits (GIANT) consortium. The authors performed a large-scale meta-analysis of GWAS informative for WHR using adjustment for BMI to focus discovery to genetic loci associated with body fat distribution rather than overall adiposity [75]. In first stage of the meta-analysis of 32 GWAS for WHR adjusted for BMI (including up to 77,167 European ascent participants and 2,850,269 imputed and genotyped SNPs), the top 16 independent (defined as being located >1 Mb apart) regions of association (discovery $P<1.4\times10^{-6}$) were selected and evaluated in an additional 29 studies (comprising up to 113,636 subjects). Joint analysis of the discovery and follow-up results revealed genome-wide significant associations for 14 signals (with *P* values between 1.9×10^{-9} and 1.8×10^{-40}), 13 of which are new loci (in or near *RSP03, VEGFA, TBX15-WARS2, NFE2L3, GRB14, DNM3-PIGC, ITPR2-SSPN, LY86, HOXC13, ADAMTS9, ZNRF3-KREMEN1, NISCH-STAB1,* and *CPEB4* ($P=1.9\times10^{-9}$ to 1.8×10^{-40}) and one known signal at *LYPLAL1*. Sex-specific analysis revealed that seven of these loci (those near *RSP03, VEGFA, GRB14, LYPLAL1, HOXC13, ITPR2-SSPN,* and *ADAMTS9*) exhibited marked sexual dimorphism, all with a stronger effect on WHR in women than men (*P* for sex difference $=1.9\times10^{-3}$ to 1.2×10^{-13}). These findings provide evidence for multiple loci that modulate body fat distribution independent of overall adiposity and reveal strong gene-sex interactions.

Although many genetic loci have been found to be related to complex diseases or traits, including overall obesity and abdominal obesity, the established loci for complex traits only account for a small proportion of trait heritability [77]. One potential way for increasing new genetic discoveries is to exploit the extremes of trait distribution, where there may be less locus heterogeneity, greater genetic contributions, and enrichment for highly

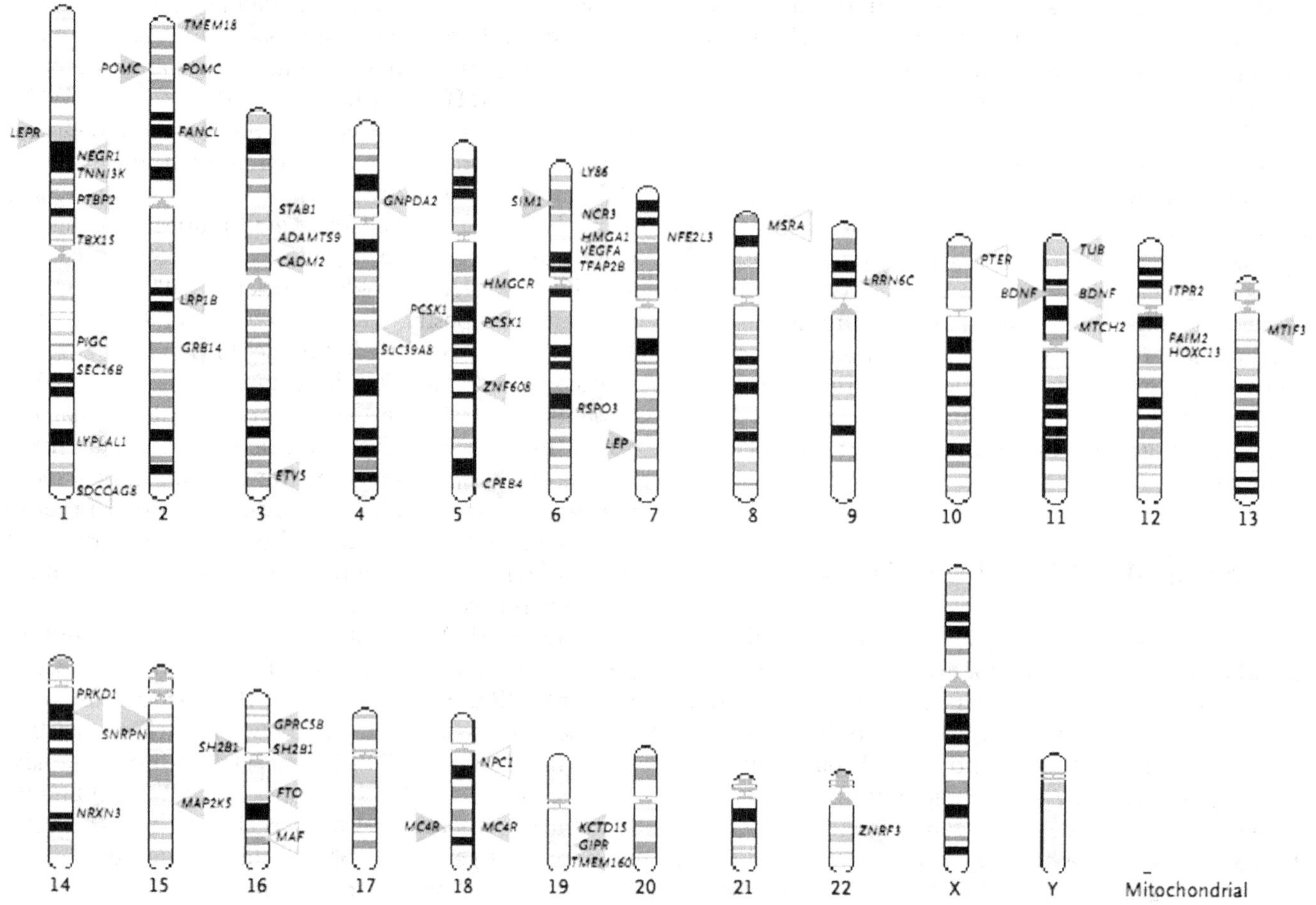

FIGURE 40.2 **Genomic locations of proven signals of body mass index, obesity, and related phenotypes.** Signals are shown according to their location on each chromosome. Genes that cause monogenic and selected syndromic forms of obesity (red triangles) are shown on the left. Common variants that have significant genome-wide associations with body mass index (BMI) or multifactorial obesity are shown on the right: loci implicated in BMI or weight variation at the population level (solid blue triangles), additional loci identified in case-control analyses of extreme obesity (open blue triangles), and variants identified primarily because of their association with waist circumference or waist-hip ratio (solid green triangles). For the variants shown on the right, genes named within the triangles are indicative of signal position, but in most instances formal proof that these are the specific genes responsible for the association is lacking. *Source: McCarthy et al.* [71]. (See color plate at the back of the book.)

penetrant variants. The use of population extremes has also been proposed to improve cost efficiency because effect sizes may be larger, fewer subjects may be needed for genotyping, and a smaller proportion of the variance may be attributable to environmental factors. Where there is heterogeneity, analyzing extremes by case-control design may offer superior power [78]. A updated meta-GWAS analysis for anthropometric traits aimed to use and compare different distribution cutoff points for the identification of genetic loci for anthropometric traits was conducted and identified another 11 new loci for anthropometric traits, including clinical obesity (*HNF4G, RPTOR, GNAT2, MRPS33P4, ADCY9, HS6ST3,* and *ZZZ3*) [79]. Four SNPs that reached genome-wide significance ($P<5\times10^{-8}$) have previously been identified as WHR-associated loci in the general population [75]. The authors concluded that a large overlap was found in genetic structure and the distribution of variants between traits based on extremes and the general population, with little etiological heterogeneity between obesity subgroups [79].

GENE-ENVIRONMENT INTERACTIONS

Although GWAS have shown tremendous success in identifying genetic variants for abdominal obesity, it is notable that the established genetic markers only account for a small proportion of the variance (<5%) in phenotype, leaving considerable "missing heritability" unexplained. Several reasons have been proposed to explain why missing heritability may exist. For example, current GWAS only focus on common variants and not

TABLE 40.1 Genetic Loci Associated with Waist Circumference/Waist-Hip Ratio at the Genome-Wide Significance Level (5.0×10^{8}) By 28 April 2013

Year	Reported Gene(s)	Strongest SNP Risk Allele	Region	Population	Risk Allele Frequency	*P* Value	Traits/ Phenotypes	Beta	95% CI	Reference
2008	*MC4R*	rs12970134-A	18q21.32	Asian Indian and European ancestry	0.36	2.00×10^{9}	Waist circumference	0.88	0.59-1.17 cm increase	[110]
2009	*TFAP2B*	rs987237-G	6p12	European ancestry	NR	1.87×10^{11}	Waist circumference	NR	NR	[76]
	MSRA	rs7826222-G	8p23.1	–	NR	8.89×10^{9}		NR	NR	
	LYPLAL1	rs2605100	1q41	–	NR	2.55×10^{8}	waist-hip ratio	NR	NR	
2009	*FTO*	rs1558902-?	16q12.2	European ancestry	NR	5.00×10^{19}	Waist circumference	NR	NR	[111]
	NRXN3	rs10146997-G	14q31.1	–	NR	5.00×10^{8}		0.65	[NR] cm increase	
2010	*ZNRF3-KREMEN1*	rs4823006-A	22q12.1	European ancestry	0.57	1.10×10^{11}	Waist-hip ratio	0.02	[NR] unit increase	[75]
	LYPLAL1	rs4846567-G	1q41	–	0.28	6.89×10^{21}		0.03	[NR] unit increase	
	GRB14	rs10195252-T	2q24.3	–	0.6	2.09×10^{24}		0.03	[NR] unit increase	
	RSP03	rs9491696-G	6q22.33	–	0.52	1.84×10^{40}		0.04	[NR] unit increase	
	DNM3-PIGC	rs1011731-G	1q24.3	–	0.57	9.51×10^{18}		0.03	[NR] unit increase	
	TBX15-WARS2	rs984222-G	1p12	–	0.37	8.69×10^{25}		0.03	[NR] unit increase	
	NISCH-STAB1	rs6784615-T	3p21.1	–	0.94	3.84×10^{10}		0.04	[NR] unit increase	
	ADAMTS9	rs6795735-C	3p14.1	–	0.41	9.79×10^{14}		0.03	[NR] unit increase	
	HOXC13	rs1443512-A	12q13.13	–	0.24	6.38×10^{17}		0.03	[NR] unit increase	
	NFE2L3	rs1055144-T	7p15.2	–	0.21	9.97×10^{25}		0.04	[NR] unit increase	
	ITPR2-SSPN	rs718314-G	12p12.1	–	0.74	1.14×10^{17}		0.03	[NR] unit increase	
	VEGFA	rs6905288-A	6p21.1	–	0.56	5.88×10^{25}		0.04	[NR] unit increase	
	CPEB4	rs6861681-A	5q35.2	–	0.34	1.91×10^{9}		0.02	[NR] unit increase	
	LY86	rs1294421-G	6p25.1	–	0.39	1.75×10^{17}		0.03	[NR] unit increase	
2011	*CCDC121*	rs3749147-C	2p23.3	European ancestry	NR	1.00×10^{9}	Waist circumfer-ence-triglycer-ides	0.18	0.12-0.24 unit decrease	[112]
	ZNF259	rs2075290-C	11q23.3	–	NR	1.00×10^{16}		0.41	0.31-0.51 unit increase	
	GCKR	rs780093-A	2p23.3	–	NR	2.00×10^{12}		0.19	[0.13-0.25] unit increase	
	C20rf16	rs1919128-A	2p23.3	–	NR	2.00×10^{9}		0.18	[0.12-0.24] unit decrease	
	BUD13	rs10790162-A	11q23.3	–	NR	7.00×10^{16}		0.39	[0.29-0.49] unit increase	
	ZNF512	rs13022873-A	2p23.3	–	NR	5.00×10^{9}		0.17	[0.11-0.23] unit decrease	
	APOA5	rs2266788-A	11q23.3	–	NR	2.00×10^{16}		0.41	[0.31-0.51] unit increase	

CI, confidence interval; NR, not reported; SNP, single nucleotide polymorphism.

variants with low frequency; structural variants are not extensively examined; and the sample sizes are still too small to discover more moderate genetic effects. In addition, it has been acknowledged that for most complex diseases, including obesity, both genetic and environmental factors are involved in the pathogenesis processes. However, the previous GWAS did not consider the potential interactions between genetic variants and environmental factors. Gene-environment interaction analysis is now becoming one of the new frontiers for genetic discovery.

Diet and physical activity are among the most important environmental factors affecting obesity. The *FTO* gene shows the strongest association with both overall adiposity and abdominal obesity. A recent meta-analysis reported that the obesogenic effect of the *FTO* rs9939609 minor allele is substantially diminished by physical activity [80]. The analysis comprised up to 218,166 adults and 19,268 children or adolescents and provided strong statistical evidence supporting this interaction. In the studies included in the meta-analysis, the physical activity data were standardized using categorical data. The adults were defined as being "inactive" when they had a sedentary occupation and if they reported less than 1h of moderate-to-vigorous leisure-time or commuting physical activity per week. With regard to the continuous data on physical activity, adults were defined as being "inactive" when their level of physical activity was in the lowest sex-specific 20% of the study population concerned. All other individuals were defined as "physically active." For children and adolescents, a more stringent cutoff for "inactivity" was chosen than for adults because of the high average physical activity levels in younger children and the known weaker association between physical activity and childhood BMI. Thus, children and adolescents were defined as being "inactive" when their level of physical activity was in the lowest sex- and age-specific 10% of the study population. Overall, 25% of adults and 13% of children were categorized as inactive. In adults, the minor (A) allele of rs9939609 increased the odds of obesity by 1.23-fold/allele [95% confidence interval (CI)1.20-1.26], but physical activity attenuated this effect ($P_{\text{interaction}} = 0.001$). More specifically, the minor allele of rs9939609 increased the odds of obesity less in the physically active group [odds ratio (OR) 1.22/allele, 95% CI 1.19-1.25] than in the inactive group (OR 1.30/allele, 95% CI 1.24-1.36). However, no such interaction was found in children and adolescents. Lifestyle intervention trials generally support the beneficial effects of physical activity on overall adiposity measures, regardless of *FTO* genotype [81,82]. Sedentary behavior as indicated by television (TV) watching was also found as a modification factor influencing the genetic effect on obesity. In two large prospective cohorts from the Nurses' Health Study and the Health Professionals Follow-up Study, investigators analyzed interactions between TV watching, leisure-time physical activity, and genetic predisposition in relation to BMI in 7740 women and 4564 men [83]. They used 32 established BMI-associated variants to calculate a weighted obesity genetic risk score. The genetic risk score has been related to measures of abdominal obesity such as WHR. To lower the risk of reverse causation, physical activity and TV watching were collected 2 years before the assessment of BMI. In both women and men, genetic associations with BMI strengthened with increased hours of TV watching. An increment of the weighted genetic risk score (each 10 points) was associated with 0.8, 0.8, 1.4, 1.5, and 3.4 kg/m^2 higher BMI across the five categories of TV watching (0-1, 2-5, 6-20, 21-40, and >40 h/week; $P_{\text{interaction}} = 0.001$), while the genetic association with BMI weakened with increased levels of physical activity (each 10 points associated with 1.5, 1.3, 1.2, 1.2, and 0.8 kg/m^2 higher BMI across the quintiles of physical activity). The interactions of TV watching and physical activity with genetic predisposition in relation to BMI were independent of each other. Although the study did not specifically examine measures of abdominal obesity, given the high correlation between overall adiposity and abdominal adiposity and the fact that obesity genes are also related to abdominal measures, it is expected that physical activity and TV watching may both modify abdominal obesity in similar manner.

Several recent studies also observed significant interactions between dietary factors and genetic variants in relation to obesity. Gene-diet interaction occurs when the dietary effect on a person's health is conditional on a specific genotype [84–86]. Although the topic of gene-diet interaction has been extensively discussed, detection of such interaction in human studies was not fruitful because most of the findings were not reproducible [84,87], mainly because of relatively small sample size and cross-sectional design. Although GWAS have demonstrated the validity of studies with cross-sectional design in identifying disease-predisposing variants, which are less likely to correlate with the potential confounders and are free of reverse causation, the inherent bias of cross-sectional analysis become paramount in testing for gene-diet interactions [88]. In addition, lack of replication is another serious limitation. An epidemiological framework for evaluating gene-diet interactions has yet to be well established. However, several recent large-scale studies with prospective design and replication have emerged and may shed light on the ways to plug the gap in this fast-moving area.

Temporal patterns in the increasing consumption of sugar-sweetened beverages have paralleled the rise in the prevalence of obesity in the United States, with both more than doubling since the late 1970s [89]. Compelling evidence supports a positive link between the consumption of sugar-sweetened beverages and the risk of obesity [90–92]. However, there is scare evidence concerning whether the risk of obesity is modified by the genetic background. Qi et al. analyzed the interaction between genetic predisposition and the intake of sugar-sweetened beverages in relation to BMI and obesity risk in 6934 women from the Nurses' Health Study, 4423 men from the Health Professionals Follow-up Study, and a replication cohort of 21,740 women from the Women's Genome Health Study. The genetic association with adiposity, a long-term BMI increase, and the risk of incident obesity appeared to be more pronounced with a greater intake of sugar-sweetened beverages. When the three cohorts were combined, the pooled relative risk of obesity incidence for each increment of 10 risk alleles were 1.35 (95% CI 1.18-1.54), 1.59 (95% CI 1.33-1.91), 1.56 (95% CI 1.26-1.92), and 3.35 (95% CI 2.22-5.05) across the four categories of intake ($P_{interaction} < 0.001$; Fig. 40.3) [93].

In addition to observational studies, gene-diet interactions have been also reported in randomized diet intervention trials. A unique strength of diet intervention trials in testing for gene-diet interactions is that such studies may provide more direct evidence to instruct genetic-targeted diet interventions in future public health practices. However, as most of existing diet intervention trials are relatively small in sample size, the power of detection of moderate gene-diet interactions would be a major concern [88]. The Preventing Overweight Using Novel Dietary Strategies (POUNDS LOST) trial is a clinical trial including a total of 811 overweight (BMI $\geq$ 25 kg/m^2) and obese (BMI $\geq$ 30 kg/m^2) adult men and women who were randomly assigned to one of four weight loss diets varying in macronutrient contents (dietary fat, protein, and carbohydrates) for 2 years [94]. An analysis based on the POUNDS LOST trial showed that *FTO* variant rs1558902 had significant modifying effects on interventions varying in dietary protein in 2-year changes in fat-free mass, whole-body total percentage of fat mass, total adipose tissue mass, visceral adipose tissue mass, and superficial adipose tissue mass in 742 obese adults [95]. Interestingly, the authors indicated that carriers of the risk allele (A allele) had a greater reduction in weight, body composition, and fat distribution in response to a high-protein diet, whereas an opposite genetic effect was observed on changes in fat distribution in response to a low-protein diet during 2 years of follow-up. The data suggest that a high-protein diet may be beneficial for weight loss and improvement to body composition and fat distribution in individuals with the risk allele of the *FTO* variant

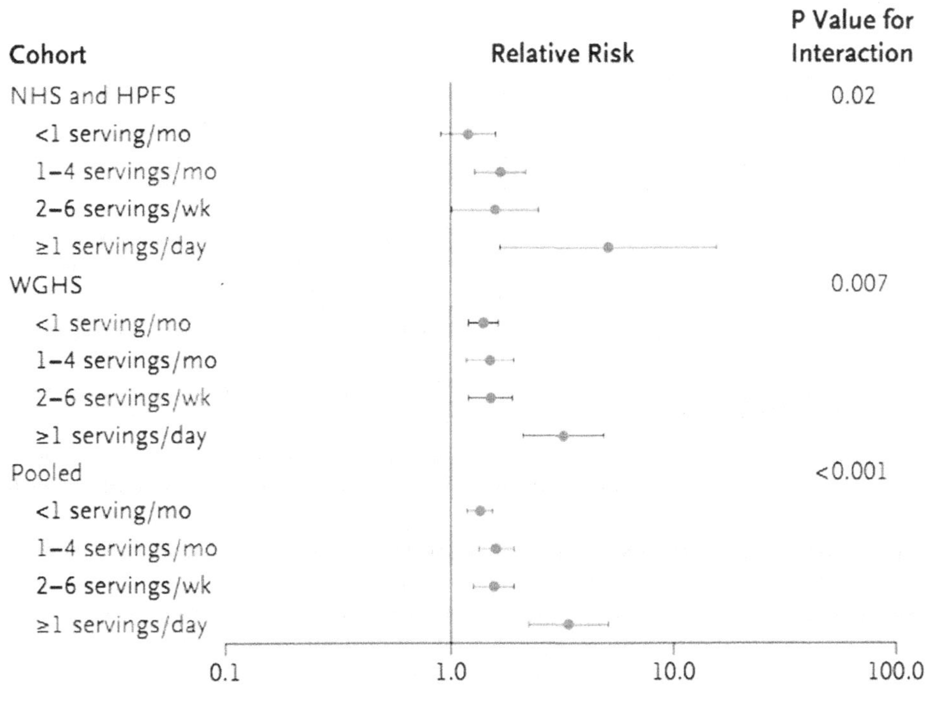

FIGURE 40.3 Relative risk of the development of obesity per increment of 10 risk alleles, according to intake of sugar-sweetened beverages. The data were from Nurses' Health Study (NHS) and Health Professionals Follow-up Study (HPFS) cohorts; analyses were based on 18 years of follow-up for 6402 initially nonobese women with 1107 incident cases of obesity, 12 years of follow-up for 3889 initially nonobese men with 297 incident cases of obesity, and a median of 6 years of follow-up for 18,127 initially nonobese women with 2280 incident cases of obesity from the Women's Genome Health Study (WGHS) cohort. Shown are the relative risks of incident obesity, with adjustment for age, geographic region, eigenvectors, level of physical activity, and status with respect to current smoking, alcohol intake, and total energy intake. Horizontal bars indicate 95% confidence intervals. *Source: Qi et al.* [93].

rs1558902. Previous studies have shown associations between branched amino acids (BCAAs) or aromatic amino acids (AAAs) with obesity, insulin sensitivity, and incident type 2 diabetes mellitus (T2DM) [96–98] and weight loss induced by gastric bypass surgery or behavioral/dietary intervention [99,100]. In the POUNDS LOST trial, investigators found a significant interaction between the amino acid metabolite-related genotype rs1440581 (*PPM1K*) [101] and dietary fat on weight loss and changes in insulin resistance [102]. In the energy restricted high-fat diet group, the C allele was related to less weight loss (adjusted means: TT, −6.7 kg; CT, −5.8 kg; and CC, −4.1 kg, respectively; $P = 0.001$ in an additive pattern), whereas no significant genetic effect was observed in the low-fat diet group ($P = 0.53$) after 6 months of intervention. Participants carrying the C allele had smaller decreases in serum insulin and homeostatic model assessment of insulin resistance (known as HOMA-IR) values than those without this allele in the high-fat diet group (both $P = 0.02$), while an opposite effect was observed in participants assigned to the low-fat diet group ($P = 0.02$ and 0.04, respectively). In the Diabetes Prevention Program (DPP), in which 908 measures of adiposity derived from computed tomography were available, it was found that in the insulin-induced gene 2 (*INSIG2*) rs7566605 genotype the minor C allele was associated with more subcutaneous adiposity at baseline. In an additive model, there were significant gene-lifestyle interactions on weight change and subcutaneous and visceral adipose areas [81]. The common G allele was associated with less reduction in subcutaneous and visceral adipose areas following treatment with a lifestyle intervention, whereas the change in adipose area in those assigned to the placebo group was similar across genotypes. These findings provide novel information on effective dietary intervention strategies based on genetic background for use in preventing or curing diseases related to central obesity.

SEXUAL DIMORPHISM

There is a sex difference in regional fat distribution: women have more subcutaneous fat, whereas men have more visceral fat. Therefore, obesity-related metabolic disorders are much lower in premenopausal women than in men. On the one hand, differences in cardiovascular disease may be under the influence of sex hormones either directly in the brain or through their influence on body fat distribution. On the other hand, a genetic predisposition may cause this sex-specific fat distribution. A previous study demonstrated that genetic variance is significantly higher in women for the waist, hip, and thigh circumference and WHR, implying that genes account for more variance in fat distribution in women than in men [103]. In addition, by examining morbidly obese U.S. subjects in "affected clusters" (i.e. groups of three or more closely related individuals with $BMI \geq 40$), Stone et al. identified a female-only predisposition locus at chromosome 4p15-p14, although the authors did not claim that this was a genuine sex-specific effect [104]. In a genome-wide linkage study performed in non-Hispanic whites and African-Americans (the HyperGEN study), sex-specific linkage was observed for human fatness [33]. Lewis et al. found a QTL influencing percentage body fat in women on chromosome12q (12q24.3-12q24.32; maximum empirical LOD score = 3.8); a QTL influencing this phenotype in men was found on chromosome 15q (15q25.3; maximum empirical LOD score = 3.0). These QTLs were detected in both African-American and white women (12q) and men (15q). In the largest meta-GWAS of WHR to date, 14 loci were identified as being related to WHR at a genome-wide significant level. Among them, seven loci (RSP03, *VEGFA*, *GRB14*, *LYPLAL1*, *HOXC13*, *ITPR2-SSPN*, and *ADAMTS9*) exhibited marked sexual dimorphism, with a stronger effect in women than in men. These findings provide evidence for multiple loci that modulate body fat distribution independent of overall adiposity and reveal strong gene-sex interactions. These 14 loci explain 1.34% of the variance in WHR (after adjustment for BMI and age) in women but only 0.46% of the WHR variance in men. The sex-specific genetic loci for association with WC are summarized in Fig. 40.4.

EPIGENETICS

Epigenetics literally means "on top of genetics," and is defined as the heritable changes that affect gene expression through mechanisms not associated with concomitant alterations in the DNA sequence; these include DNA methylation and histone modifications. Epigenetics research has increased exponentially during the last few years. Gene-specific epigenetic marks have been associated with disease—and also obesity—and related conditions. The vast majority of studies have focused on methylation of CpG islands (CpG-rich sites).

The study of the epigenetics of obesity and related metabolic disorders is only just beginning. To date, relatively few studies have explored the epigenetic characterization of humans at risk of obesity (Table 40.2), and most have focused on characterizing the methylation status of selected CpG sites in candidate genes [105]. They have provided novel ideals about the pathogenesis of obesity. Similar to the genetic association studies based on the candidate genes, there are several limitations of these studies. First, the poorly powered sample size and lack of replication have been major concerns. Usually, the measurement of epigenetic markers is very

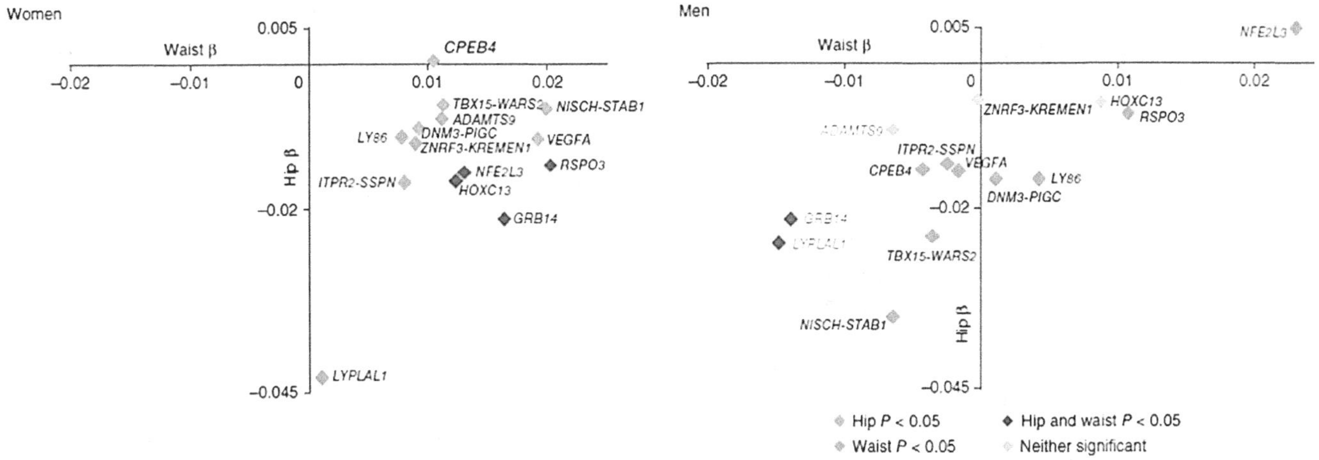

FIGURE 40.4 Sex-specific genetic loci for association with waist circumference. Association of the 14 waist-hip ratio (WHR) loci with waist and hip circumference. β, coefficients for waist circumference (WC; *x* axis) and hip circumference (HIP; *y* axis) in women and men derived from the joint discovery and follow-up analysis. *P* values for WC and HIP are represented by colors. In men, gray gene labels refer to those single nucleotide polymorphisms that were not significant in the male-specific WHR analysis. *Source: Heid et al.* [75]. (See color plate at the back of the book.)

TABLE 40.2 DNA Methylation Candidate Gene and Epigenome-Wide Association Studies for Obesity

Candidate Genes/ EWAS	Phenotypes	Case Control/ Quantitative Traits	Sample Size	Tissue	Replication	References
ALOX12, ALPL, BCL2A1, CASP10, CAV1, CCL3, CD9, CDKN1C, DSC2, EPHA1, EVI2A, HLA, IRF5, KRT1, LCN2, MLLT4, MMP9, MPL, NID1, NKX31, PMP22, S100A12, TAL1, VIM	BMI, fat mass and lean mass	Quantitative traits	178 individuals	Umbilical cord blood	–	[113]
GNAS, GRB10, H19, IGF2, KCNQ10T1, MEST, SNRPN	Discordant BMI in twins	Case control	16 twins	Saliva	–	[114]
MCHR1	BMI	Quantitative analysis	49 individuals	Whole blood	–	[115]
POMC	Childhood obesity	Case control	71 obese and 36 normal-weight subjects	Whole blood	100 obese and 54 normal-weight subjects	[116]
IL8, NOS3, PIK3CD, RXRA, SOD1	Fat mass and percentage fat mass	Quantitative analysis	78 individuals	Umbilical cord blood	–	[117]
SLC6A4	BMI, weight, and waist circumference	Quantitative analysis	168 individuals	Peripheral blood leukocytes	–	[118]
TACSTD2	Fat mass	Quantitative analysis	94 individuals	Whole blood	161 individuals	[119]
EWAS	BMI	Quantitative analysis	74 individuals	Leukocyte DNA	–	[120]
EWAS	Obesity	Case control	7 obese and 7 lean subjects	Leukocyte DNA	46 obese and 46 lean subjects	[121]
EWAS	Obesity	Case control	23 obese and 24 control subjects	Whole blood	–	[108]

BMI, body mass index; EWAS, epigenome-wide association study.

expensive (compared with genotyping), thus making it difficult to conduct in large populations. In addition, epigenetic variations differ among various tissues. Therefore, methylation profiles measured in accessible samples (e.g. peripheral blood) may not be representative of those occurring in more obesity-relevant, but largely inaccessible, tissues, such as adipose tissue or the hypothalamus [105]. Given these limitations, previous studies have led to largely inconclusive results.

The largest epigenome-wide association study for T2DM conducted in a sample of ≈1150 cases and controls from Israel [106]. The best-studied and most promising region was the obesity-associated gene *FTO*, in which methylation levels at a CpG site within the first intron of the *FTO* gene were correlated with genotype at nearby BMI-associated SNPs. Associations between the *FTO* risk allele with hypermethylation have now been demonstrated and replicated in several studies [107,108], but it remains unclear whether methylation is the causal link between the *FTO* risk allele and T2DM [106].

The big challenge for epigenome-wide studies is that, unlike DNA genotypes, epigenetic marks can change over time, and apparent associations with disease are prone to confounding and reverse causation due to the disease of interest or its treatment [109].

Although there is ample evidence that epigenetic effects are likely to play a role in the pathogenesis of obesity and to contribute to the observed familial aggregation, experimental studies that conclusively define key loci responsible in disease-relevant tissues have yet to be performed (Table 40.2). It is also worth noting that existing studies have focused almost exclusively on DNA methylation, leaving other components of the epigenetic machinery (such as chromatin state) largely unexplored. Given the limited access to disease-relevant human tissues, progress will almost certainly depend on centralized community efforts such as the International Human Epigenome Consortium, which is generating reference epigenomes (including detailed methylome maps) for a panel of human tissues and cell types [109]. This epigenetic counterpart of the Human HapMap effort will provide tissue-specific maps of methylation correlation structures, document the positions of variably methylated sites, and empower future epigenome-wide association study efforts [105].

CONCLUSIONS

Obesity has become an epidemic in the United States and worldwide since the early 1980s, and is one of the greatest challenges in public health care and research today. In epidemiological studies, abdominal obesity and overall adiposity have been independently associated with a variety of metabolic disorders, such as T2DM and cardiovascular diseases, and even all-cause mortality. Evidence from genetic research, especially those collected from GWAS over the past few years, has clearly indicated the importance of the human genome in determining susceptibility to obesity including abdominal obesity. However, our current knowledge of the genomic basis for abdominal obesity is still limited.

An unhealthy diet, physical inactivity, and a sedentary lifestyle have been identified among the primary contributors for the increase of obesity. Recently emerged data on gene-environment interaction suggest that these factors may not affect obesity on themselves, but they can upon interaction with an individual's genomic makeup. Although the supporting evidence is still weak at this time, available studies have indicated considerable diversity in levels of obesity may exist at individual levels in response to obesogenic risk factors.

Individual risk-based, or "personalized," diet and lifestyle interventions have long been proposed as attractive targets in future prevention efforts tailored to the reduction of obesity. A thorough understanding of the genetic basis of gene-environment interactions underlying obesity may foster more efficient intervention strategies and thus may assist in improving the quality of life for affected individuals. Advances in high-throughput genotyping technology are facilitating the offer of direct-to-consumer genetic testing services, and have raised great hope and expectations that genetic testing will pave the way to personalized prevention. In the light of such a trend, debates about how to establish preventive genomics based genetic testing in a medically and socially responsible way have just begun.

References

[1] Hopper JL, Bishop DT, Easton DF. Population-based family studies in genetic epidemiology. Lancet 2005;366:1397–406.
[2] Schousboe K, Willemsen G, Kyvik KO, Mortensen J, Boomsma DI, Cornes BK, et al. Sex differences in heritability of BMI: a comparative study of results from twin studies in eight countries. Twin Res 2003;6:409–21.
[3] Malis C, Rasmussen EL, Poulsen P, Petersen I, Christensen K, Beck-Nielsen H, et al. Total and regional fat distribution is strongly influenced by genetic factors in young and elderly twins. Obes Res 2005;13(12):2139–45.
[4] Bulik CM, Sullivan PF, Kendler KS. Genetic and environmental contributions to obesity and binge eating. Int J Eat Disord 2003;33:293–8.
[5] Romeis JC, Grant JD, Knopik VS, Pedersen NL, Heath AC. The genetics of middle-age spread in middle-class males. Twin Res 2004;7:596–602.
[6] Wardle J, Carnell S, Haworth CM, Plomin R. Evidence for a strong genetic influence on childhood adiposity despite the force of the obesogenic environment. Am J Clin Nutr 2008;87(2):398–404.
[7] Hunt KJ, Duggirala R, Göring HH, Williams JT, Almasy L, Blangero J, et al. Genetic basis of variation in carotid artery

plaque in the San Antonio Family Heart Study. Stroke 2002;33(12):2775–80.

[8] Hsueh WC, Mitchell BD, Aburomia R, Pollin T, Sakul H, Gelder Ehm M, et al. Diabetes in the Old Order Amish: characterization and heritability analysis of the Amish Family Diabetes Study. Diabetes Care 2000;23(5):595–601.

[9] Sakul H, Pratley R, Cardon L, Ravussin E, Mott D, Bogardus C. Familiality of physical and metabolic characteristics that predict the development of non-insulin-dependent diabetes mellitus in Pima Indians. Am J Hum Genet 1997;60(3):651–6.

[10] Freeman MS, Mansfield MW, Barrett JH, Grant PJ. Heritability of features of the insulin resistance syndrome in a community-based study of healthy families. Diabet Med 2002;19(12):994–9.

[11] Poulsen P, Vaag A, Kyvik K, Beck-Nielsen H. Genetic versus environmental aetiology of the metabolic syndrome among male and female twins. Diabetologia 2001;44(5):537–43.

[12] Wu DM, Hong Y, Sun CA, Sung PK, Rao DC, Chu NF. Familial resemblance of adiposity-related parameters: results from a health check-up population in Taiwan. Eur J Epidemiol 2003;18(3):221–6.

[13] Rice T, Daw EW, Gagnon J, Bouchard C, Leon AS, Skinner JS, et al. Familial resemblance for body composition measures: the HERITAGE Family Study. Obes Res 1997;5(6):557–62.

[14] Luke A, Guo X, Adeyemo AA, Wilks R, Forrester T, Lowe Jr W, et al. Heritability of obesity-related traits among Nigerians, Jamaicans and US black people. Int J Obes Relat Metab Disord 2001;25(7):1034–41.

[15] Schousboe K, Visscher PM, Erbas B, Kyvik KO, Hopper JL, Henriksen JE, et al. Twin study of genetic and environmental influences on adult body size, shape, and composition. Int J Obes Relat Metab Disord 2004;28(1):39–48.

[16] Davey G, Ramachandran A, Snehalatha C, Hitman GA, McKeigue PM. Familial aggregation of central obesity in Southern Indians. Int J Obes Relat Metab Disord 2000;24(11):1523–7.

[17] Montague CT, Farooqi IS, Whitehead JP, Soos MA, Rau H, Wareham NJ, et al. Congenital leptin deficiency is associated with severe early-onset obesity in humans. Nature 1997;387(6636):903–8.

[18] Clément K, Vaisse C, Lahlou N, Cabrol S, Pelloux V, Cassuto D, et al. A mutation in the human leptin receptor gene causes obesity and pituitary dysfunction. Nature 1998;392(6674):398–401.

[19] Krude H, Biebermann H, Luck W, Horn R, Brabant G, Grüters A. Severe early-onset obesity, adrenal insufficiency and red hair pigmentation caused by POMC mutations in humans. Nat Genet 1998;19(2):155–7.

[20] Vaisse C, Clement K, Guy-Grand B, Froguel P. A frameshift mutation in human MC4R is associated with a dominant form of obesity. Nat Genet 1998;20(2):113–4.

[21] Jackson RS, Creemers JW, Ohagi S, Raffin-Sanson ML, Sanders L, Montague CT, et al. Obesity and impaired prohormone processing associated with mutations in the human prohormone convertase 1 gene. Nat Genet 1997;16(3):303–6.

[22] Yeo GS, Farooqi IS, Aminian S, Halsall DJ, Stanhope RG, O'Rahilly S. A frameshift mutation in MC4R associated with dominantly inherited human obesity. Nat Genet 1998;20(2):111–2.

[23] Lubrano-Berthelier C, Durand E, Dubern B, Shapiro A, Dazin P, Weill J, et al. Intracellular retention is a common characteristic of childhood obesity-associated MC4R mutations. Hum Mol Genet 2003;12(2):145–53.

[24] Rankinen T, Zuberi A, Chagnon YC, Weisnagel SJ, Argyropoulos G, Walts B, et al. The human obesity gene map: the 2005 update. Obesity (Silver Spring) 2006;14(4):529–644.

[25] Farooqi IS, O'Rahilly S. Monogenic obesity in humans. Annu Rev Med 2005;56:443–58.

[26] Morton N. Sequential tests for the detection of linkage. Am J Hum Genet 1955;7:277–318.

[27] Ng MC, So WY, Lam VK, Cockram CS, Bell GI, Cox NJ, et al. Genome-wide scan for metabolic syndrome and related quantitative traits in Hong Kong Chinese and confirmation of a susceptibility locus on chromosome 1q21-q25. Diabetes 2004;53(10):2676–83.

[28] Price RA, Kilker R, Li WD. An X-chromosome scan reveals a locus for fat distribution in chromosome region Xp21-22. Diabetes 2002;51:1989–91.

[29] Hsueh WC, Mitchell BD, Schneider JL, St Jean PL, Pollin TI, Ehm MG, et al. Genome-wide scan of obesity in the Old Order Amish. J Clin Endocrinol Metab 2001;86(3):1199–205.

[30] Fox CS, Heard-Costa NL, Wilson PW, Levy D, St D'Agostino RB, Atwood LD. Genome-wide linkage to chromosome 6 for waist circumference in the Framingham Heart Study. Diabetes 2004;53(5):1399–402.

[31] Li WD, Dong C, Li D, Zhao H, Price RA. An obesity-related locus in chromosome region 12q23-24. Diabetes 2004;53(3):812–20.

[32] Guo YF, Shen H, Liu YJ, Wang W, Xiong DH, Xiao P, et al. Assessment of genetic linkage and parent-of-origin effects on obesity. J Clin Endocrinol Metab 2006;91(10):4001–5.

[33] Lewis CE, North KE, Arnett D, Borecki IB, Coon H, Ellison RC, et al. Sex-specific findings from a genome-wide linkage analysis of human fatness in non-Hispanic whites and African Americans: the HyperGEN study. Int J Obes (Lond) 2005;29(6):639–49.

[34] Dong C, Li WD, Li D, Price RA. Interaction between obesity-susceptibility loci in chromosome regions 2p25-p24 and 13q13-q21. Eur J Hum Genet 2005;13(1):102–8.

[35] Chagnon YC, Rice T, Pérusse L, Borecki IB, Ho-Kim MA, Lacaille M, et al. Genomic scan for genes affecting body composition before and after training in Caucasians from HERITAGE. J Appl Physiol 2001;90(5):1777–87.

[36] Bell CG, Walley AJ, Froguel P. The genetics of human obesity. Nat Rev Genet 2005;6(3):221–34.

[37] Loktionov A. Common gene polymorphisms and nutrition: emerging links with pathogenesis of multifactorial chronic diseases. J Nutr Biochem 2003;14:426–51.

[38] Deeb SS, Fajas L, Nemoto M, Pihlajamäki J, Mykkänen L, Kuusisto J, et al. A Pro12Ala substitution in PPARgamma2 associated with decreased receptor activity, lower body mass index and improved insulin sensitivity. Nat Genet 1998;20(3):284–7.

[39] Ek J, Urhammer SA, Sørensen TI, Andersen T, Auwerx J, Pedersen O. Homozygosity of the Pr012Ala variant of the peroxisome proliferation-activated receptor-gamma2 (PPAR-gamma2): divergent modulating effects on body mass index in obese and lean Caucasian men. Diabetologia 1999;42(7):892–5.

[40] Vidal-Puig AJ, Considine RV, Jimenez-Liñan M, Werman A, Pories WJ, Caro JF. Peroxisome proliferator-activated receptor gene expression in human tissues. Effects of obesity, weight loss, and regulation by insulin and glucocorticoids. J Clin Invest 1997;99(10):2416–22.

[41] Challis BG, Pritchard LE, Creemers JW, Delplanque J, Keogh JM, Luan J, et al. A missense mutation disrupting a dibasic prohormone processing site in pro-opiomelanocortin (POMC) increases susceptibility to early-onset obesity through a novel molecular mechanism. Hum Mol Genet 2002;11(17):1997–2004.

[42] Geller F, Reichwald K, Dempfle A, Illig T, Vollmert C, Herpertz S, et al. Melanocortin-4 receptor gene variant I103 is negatively associated with obesity. Am J Hum Genet 2004;74(3):572–81.

[43] Large V, Hellström L, Reynisdottir S, Lönnqvist F, Eriksson P, Lannfelt L, et al. Human beta-2 adrenoceptor gene polymorphisms are highly frequent in obesity and associate with altered adipocyte beta-2 adrenoceptor function. J Clin Invest 1997;100(12):3005–13.

[44] Widén E, Lehto M, Kanninen T, Walston J, Shuldiner AR, Groop LC. Association of a polymorphism in the beta

3-adrenergic-receptor gene with features of the insulin resistance syndrome in Finns. N Engl J Med 1995;333(6):348–51.

[45] Herrmann SM, Wang JG, Staessen JA, Kertmen E, Schmidt-Petersen K, Zidek W, et al. Uncoupling protein 1 and 3 polymorphisms are associated with waist-to-hip ratio. J Mol Med (Berl) 2003;81(5):327–32.

[46] Garenc C, Pérusse L, Chagnon YC, Rankinen T, Gagnon J, Borecki IB, et al. The alpha 2-adrenergic receptor gene and body fat content and distribution: the HERITAGE Family Study. Mol Med 2002;8(2):88–94.

[47] Katzov H, Bennet AM, Kehoe P, Wiman B, Gatz M, Blennow K, et al. A cladistic model of ACE sequence variation with implications for myocardial infarction, Alzheimer disease and obesity. Hum Mol Genet 2004;13(21):2647–57.

[48] Lara-Castro C, Hunter GR, Lovejoy JC, Gower BA, Fernández JR. Apolipoprotein A-II polymorphism and visceral adiposity in African-American and white women. Obes Res 2005;13(3):507–12.

[49] Lara-Castro C, Hunter GR, Lovejoy JC, Gower BA, Fernández JR. Association of the intestinal fatty acid-binding protein Ala54Thr polymorphism and abdominal adipose tissue in African-American and Caucasian women. J Clin Endocrinol Metab 2005;90(2):1196–201.

[50] Hamid YHUS, Glümer C, Borch-Johnsen K, Jørgensen T, Hansen T, Pedersen O. The common T60N polymorphism of the lymphotoxin-alpha gene is associated with type 2 diabetes and other phenotypes of the metabolic syndrome. Diabetologia 2005;48(3):445–51.

[51] Berthier MT, Houde A, Paradis AM, Couture P, Gaudet D, Després JP, et al. Molecular screening of the microsomal triglyceride transfer protein: association between polymorphisms and both abdominal obesity and plasma apolipoprotein B concentration. J Hum Genet 2004;49(12):684–90.

[52] Qi L, Shen H, Larson I, Schaefer EJ, Greenberg AS, Tregouet DA, et al. Gender-specific association of a perilipin gene haplotype with obesity risk in a white population. Obes Res 2004;12(11):1758–65.

[53] Kim KS, Choi SM, Shin SU, Yang HS, Yoon Y. Effects of peroxisome proliferator-activated receptor-gamma 2 Pro12Ala polymorphism on body fat distribution in female Korean subjects. Metabolism 2004;53(12):1538–43.

[54] Menzaghi C, Ercolino T, Di Paola R, Berg AH, Warram JH, Scherer PE, et al. A haplotype at the adiponectin locus is associated with obesity and other features of the insulin resistance syndrome. Diabetes 2002;51(7):2306–12.

[55] Emorine L, Blin N, Strosberg AD. The human b3-adrenergic receptor: the search for a physiological function. Trends Pharmacol Sci 1994;5:3–7.

[56] Fujisawa T, Ikegami H, Kawaguchi Y, Ogihara T. Meta-analysis of the association of Trp64Arg polymorphism of beta 3-adrenergic receptor gene with body mass index. J Clin Endocrinol Metab 1998;83(7):2441–4.

[57] Krief S, Lönnqvist F, Raimbault S, Baude B, Van Spronsen A, Arner P, et al. Tissue distribution of b3-adrenergic receptor mRNA in man. J Clin Invest 1993;91:344–9.

[58] Flier JS, Lowell BB. Obesity research springs a proton leak. Nat Genet 1997;15:223–4.

[59] Fleury C, Neverova M, Collins S, Raimbault S, Champigny O, Levi-Meyrueis C, et al. Uncoupling protein-2: a novel gene linked to obesity and hyperinsulinemia. Nat Genet 1997;15:269–72.

[60] Shen H, Qi L, Tai ES, Chew SK, Tan CE, Ordovas JM. Uncoupling protein 2 promoter polymorphism -866G/A, central adiposity, and metabolic syndrome in Asians. Obesity (Silver Spring) 2006;14(4):656–61.

[61] Salopuro T, Pulkkinen L, Lindström J, Kolehmainen M, Tolppanen AM, Eriksson JG, et al. Variation in the UCP2 and UCP3 genes associates with abdominal obesity and serum lipids: the Finnish Diabetes Prevention Study. BMC Med Genet 2009;10:94.

[62] Dalgaard L. Genetic variance in uncoupling protein 2 in relation to obesity, type 2 diabetes, and related metabolic traits: focus on the functional-866G>A promoter variant (rs659366). J Obes 2011;2011:340241.

[63] Warden C. Genetics of uncoupling proteins in humans. Int J Obes Relat Metab Disord 1999(Suppl. 6):S46–8.

[64] Kovacs P, Ma L, Hanson RL, Franks P, Stumvoll M, Bogardus C, et al. Genetic variation in UCP2 (uncoupling protein-2) is associated with energy metabolism in Pima Indians. Diabetologia 2005;48(11):2292–5.

[65] Ding B, Kull B, Liu Z, Mottagui-Tabar S, Thonberg H, Gu HF, et al. Human neuropeptide Y signal peptide gain-of-function polymorphism is associated with increased body mass index: possible mode of function. Regul Pept 2005;127:45–53.

[66] Patel HR, Qi Y, Hawkins EJ, Hileman SM, Elmquist JK, Imai Y, et al. Neuropeptide Y deficiency attenuates responses to fasting and high-fat diet in obesity-prone mice. Diabetes 2006;55(11):3091–8.

[67] Han R, Li A, Li L, Kitlinska JB, Zukowska Z. Maternal low-protein diet up-regulates the neuropeptide Y system in visceral fat and leads to abdominal obesity and glucose intolerance in a sex- and time-specific manner. FASEB J 2012;26(8):3528–36.

[68] Lohmueller KE, Pearce CL, Pike M, Lander ES, Hirschhorn JN. Meta-analysis of genetic association studies supports a contribution of common variants to susceptibility to common disease. Nat Genet 2003;33(2):177–82.

[69] Clayton DG, Walker NM, Smyth DJ, Pask R, Cooper JD, Maier LM, et al. Population structure, differential bias and genomic control in a large-scale, case-control association study. Nat Genet 2005;37(11):1243–6.

[70] Klein RJ, Zeiss C, Chew EY, Tsai JY, Sackler RS, Haynes C, et al. Complement factor H polymorphism in age-related macular degeneration. Science 2005;308(5720):385–9.

[71] McCarthy M. Genomics, type 2 diabetes, and obesity. N Engl J Med 2010;363(24):2339–50.

[72] Speliotes EK, Willer CJ, Berndt SI, Monda KL, Thorleifsson G, Jackson AU, et al. Association analyses of 249,796 individuals reveal 18 new loci associated with body mass index. Nat Genet 2010;42(11):937–48.

[73] Okada Y, Kubo M, Ohmiya H, Takahashi A, Kumasaka N, Hosono N, et al. Common variants at CDKAL1 and KLF9 are associated with body mass index in east Asian populations. Nat Genet 2012;44(3):302–6.

[74] Wen W, Cho YS, Zheng W, Dorajoo R, Kato N, Qi L, et al. Meta-analysis identifies common variants associated with body mass index in East Asians. Nat Genet 2012;44(3):307–11.

[75] Heid IM, Jackson AU, Randall JC, Winkler TW, Qi L, Steinthorsdottir V, et al. Meta-analysis identifies 13 new loci associated with waist-hip ratio and reveals sexual dimorphism in the genetic basis of fat distribution. Nat Genet 2010;42(11):949–60.

[76] Lindgren CM, Heid IM, Randall JC, Lamina C, Steinthorsdottir V, Qi L, et al. Genome-wide association scan meta-analysis identifies three Loci influencing adiposity and fat distribution. PLoS Genet 2009;5(6):e1000508.

[77] Lee SH, Wray NR, Goddard ME, Visscher PM. Estimating missing heritability for disease from genome-wide association studies. Am J Hum Genet 2011;88(3):294–305.

[78] Pütter C, Pechlivanis S, Nöthen MM, Jöckel KH, Wichmann HE, Scherag A. Missing heritability in the tails of quantitative traits? A simulation study on the impact of slightly altered true genetic models. Hum Hered 2011;72(3):173–81.

[79] Berndt SI, Gustafsson S, Mägi R, Ganna A, Wheeler E, Feitosa MF, et al. Genome-wide meta-analysis identifies 11 new loci for

anthropometric traits and provides insights into genetic architecture. Nat Genet 2013;45(5):501–12.

[80] Kilpeläinen TO, Qi L, Brage S, Sharp SJ, Sonestedt E, Demerath E, et al. Physical activity attenuates the influence of *FTO* variants on obesity risk: a meta-analysis of 218,166 adults and 19,268 children. PLoS Med 2011;8(11):e1001116.

[81] Franks PW, Jablonski KA, Delahanty LM, McAteer JB, Kahn SE, Knowler WC. Assessing gene-treatment interactions at the *FTO* and INSIG2 loci on obesity-related traits in the Diabetes Prevention Program. Diabetologia 2008;51(12):2214–23.

[82] Dlouhá D, Suchánek P, Lánská V, Hubáček JA. Body mass index change in females after short-time life style intervention is not dependent on the *FTO* polymorphisms. Physiol Res 2011;60(1):199–202.

[83] Qi Q, Li Y, Chomistek AK, Kang JH, Curhan GC, Pasquale LR, et al. Television watching, leisure time physical activity, and the genetic predisposition in relation to body mass index in women and men. Circulation 2012;126(15):1821–7.

[84] Qi L, Cho YA. Gene-environment interaction and obesity. Nutr Rev 2008;66(12):684–94.

[85] Qi L, Hu FB, Hu G. Genes, environment, and interactions in prevention of type 2 diabetes: a focus on physical activity and lifestyle changes. Curr Mol Med 2008;8:519–32.

[86] Qi L, Liang J. Interactions between genetic factors that predict diabetes and dietary factors that ultimately impact on risk of diabetes. Curr Opin Lipidol 2010;21:31–7.

[87] Perusse L, Bouchard C. Gene-diet interactions in obesity. Am J Clin Nutr 2000;72:1285S–90S.

[88] Qi L. Gene-diet interactions in complex disease: current findings and relevance for public health. Curr Nutr Rep 2012;1(4):222–7.

[89] Popkin B. Patterns of beverage use across the lifecycle. Physiol Behav 2010;100(1):4–9.

[90] Mozaffarian D, Hao T, Rimm EB, Willett WC, Hu FB. Changes in diet and lifestyle and long-term weight gain in women and men. N Engl J Med 2011;364(25):2392–404.

[91] Malik VS, Popkin BM, Bray GA, Després JP, Hu FB. Sugar-sweetened beverages, obesity, type 2 diabetes mellitus, and cardiovascular disease risk. Circulation 2010;121(11):1356–64.

[92] Schulze MB, Manson JE, Ludwig DS, Colditz GA, Stampfer MJ, Willett WC, et al. Sugar-sweetened beverages, weight gain, and incidence of type 2 diabetes in young and middle-aged women. JAMA 2004;292(8):927–34.

[93] Qi Q, Chu AY, Kang JH, Jensen MK, Curhan GC, Pasquale LR, et al. Sugar-sweetened beverages and genetic risk of obesity. N Engl J Med 2012;367(15):1387–96.

[94] Sacks FM, Bray GA, Carey VJ, Smith SR, Ryan DH, Anton SD, et al. Comparison of weight-loss diets with different compositions of fat, protein, and carbohydrates. N Engl J Med 2009;360(9):859–73.

[95] Zhang X, Qi Q, Zhang C, Smith SR, Hu FB, Sacks FM, et al. *FTO* genotype and 2-year change in body composition and fat distribution in response to weight-loss diets: the POUNDS LOST Trial. Diabetes 2012;61(11):3005–11.

[96] Huffman KM, Shah SH, Stevens RD, Bain JR, Muehlbauer M, Slentz CA, et al. Relationships between circulating metabolic intermediates and insulin action in overweight to obese, inactive men and women. Diabetes Care 2009;32:1678–83.

[97] Newgard CB, An J, Bain JR, Muehlbauer MJ, Stevens RD, Lien LF, et al. A branched-chain amino acid-related metabolic signature that differentiates obese and lean humans and contributes to insulin resistance. Cell Metab 2009;9:311–26.

[98] Wang TJ, Larson MG, Vasan RS, Cheng S, Rhee EP, McCabe E, et al. Metabolite profiles and the risk of developing diabetes. Nat Med 2011;17:448–53.

[99] Laferrere B, Reilly D, Arias S, Swerdlow N, Gorroochurn P, Bawa B, et al. Differential metabolic impact of gastric bypass surgery versus dietary intervention in obese diabetic subjects despite identical weight loss. Sci Transl Med 2011;3:80re2.

[100] Shah SH, Crosslin DR, Haynes CS, Nelson S, Turer CB, Stevens RD, et al. Branched-chain amino acid levels are associated with improvement in insulin resistance with weight loss. Diabetologia 2012;55:321–30.

[101] Kettunen J, Tukiainen T, Sarin AP, Ortega-Alonso A, Tikkanen E, Lyytikäinen LP, et al. Genome-wide association study identifies multiple loci influencing human serum metabolite levels. Nat Genet 2012;44:269–76.

[102] Xu M, Qi Q, Liang J, Bray GA, Hu FB, Sacks FM, et al. Genetic determinant for amino acid metabolites and changes in body weight and insulin resistance in response to weight-loss diets: the preventing overweight using novel dietary strategies (POUNDS LOST) trial. Circulation 2013;127(12):1283–9.

[103] Zillikens MC, Yazdanpanah M, Pardo LM, Rivadeneira F, Aulchenko YS, Oostra BA, et al. Sex-specific genetic effects influence variation in body composition. Diabetologia 2008;51(12):2233–41.

[104] Stone S, Abkevich V, Hunt SC, Gutin A, Russell DL, Neff CD, et al. A major predisposition locus for severe obesity, at 4p15-p14. Am J Hum Genet 2002;70(6):1459–68.

[105] Drong AW, Lindgren CM, McCarthy MI. The genetic and epigenetic basis of type 2 diabetes and obesity. Clin Pharmacol Ther 2012;92(6):707–15.

[106] Toperoff G, Aran D, Kark JD, Rosenberg M, Dubnikov T, Nissan B, et al. Genome-wide survey reveals predisposing diabetes type 2-related DNA methylation variations in human peripheral blood. Hum Mol Genet 2012;21(2):371–83.

[107] Bell CG, Finer S, Lindgren CM, Wilson GA, Rakyan VK, Teschendorff AE, et al. Integrated genetic and epigenetic analysis identifies haplotype-specific methylation in the *FTO* type 2 diabetes and obesity susceptibility locus. PLoS One 2010;5(11):e14040.

[108] Almén MS, Jacobsson JA, Moschonis G, Benedict C, Chrousos GP, Fredriksson R, et al. Genome wide analysis reveals association of a *FTO* gene variant with epigenetic changes. Genomics 2012;99(3):132–7.

[109] Rakyan VK, Down TA, Balding DJ, Beck S. Epigenome-wide association studies for common human diseases. Nat Rev Genet 2011;12(8):529–41.

[110] Chambers JC, Elliott P, Zabaneh D, Zhang W, Li Y, Froguel P, et al. Common genetic variation near MC4R is associated with waist circumference and insulin resistance. Nat Genet 2008;40(6):716–8.

[111] Heard-Costa NL, Zillikens MC, Monda KL, Johansson A, Harris TB, Fu M, et al. NRXN3 is a novel locus for waist circumference: a genome-wide association study from the CHARGE Consortium. PLoS Genet 2009;5(6):e1000539.

[112] Kraja AT, Vaidya D, Pankow JS, Goodarzi MO, Assimes TL, Kullo IJ, et al. A bivariate genome-wide approach to metabolic syndrome: STAMPEED consortium. Diabetes 2011;60(4):1329–39.

[113] Relton CL, Groom A, St Pourcain B, Sayers AE, Swan DC, Embleton ND, et al. DNA methylation patterns in cord blood DNA and body size in childhood. PLoS One 2012;7(3):e31821.

[114] Souren NY, Tierling S, Fryns JP, Derom C, Walter J, Zeegers MP. DNA methylation variability at growth-related imprints does not contribute to overweight in monozygotic twins discordant for BMI. Obesity (Silver Spring) 2011;19(7):1519–22.

[115] Stepanow S, Reichwald K, Huse K, Gausmann U, Nebel A, Rosenstiel P, et al. Allele-specific, age-dependent and BMI-associated DNA methylation of human MCHR1. PLoS One 2011;6(5):e17711.

[116] Kuehnen P, Mischke M, Wiegand S, Sers C, Horsthemke B, Lau S, et al. An Alu element-associated hypermethylation variant of

the POMC gene is associated with childhood obesity. PLoS Genet 2012;8(3):e1002543.

[117] Godfrey KM, Sheppard A, Gluckman PD, Lillycrop KA, Burdge GC, McLean C, et al. Epigenetic gene promoter methylation at birth is associated with child's later adiposity. Diabetes 2011;60(5):1528–34.

[118] Zhao J, Goldberg J, Vaccarino V. Promoter methylation of serotonin transporter gene is associated with obesity measures: a monozygotic twin study. Int J Obes (Lond) 2013;37(1):140–5.

[119] Groom A, Potter C, Swan DC, Fatemifar G, Evans DM, Ring SM, et al. Postnatal growth and DNA methylation are associated with differential gene expression of the TACSTD2 gene and childhood fat mass. Diabetes 2012;61(2):391–400.

[120] Feinberg AP, Irizarry RA, Fradin D, Aryee MJ, Murakami P, Aspelund T, et al. Personalized epigenomic signatures that are stable over time and covary with body mass index. Sci Transl Med 2010;2(49):49ra67.

[121] Wang X, Zhu H, Snieder H, Su S, Munn D, Harshfield G, et al. Obesity related methylation changes in DNA of peripheral blood leukocytes. BMC Med 2010;8:87.

CHAPTER

41

The Role of Site-Specific Adipose Tissue Fatty Acid Composition in Obesity

Fátima Pérez de Heredia[a] *and Marta Garaulet*[b]

[a]School of Natural Sciences and Psychology, Liverpool John Moores University, Liverpool, United Kingdom; [b]Dept. Physiology, Faculty of Biology, University of Murcia, Murcia, Spain

Research since the late twentieth century has greatly changed our perception of adipose tissue. The passive fuel storage view has given way to a complex picture of metabolic, genetic, endocrine, and immune cross talk. Nevertheless, energy storage in the form of triglycerides remains adipose tissue's main function, and maintaining energy homeostasis forms the basis of its amazing plethora of interconnected functions. Lipids accumulated within adipocytes experience a slow yet constant turnover, with continuous flux between the adipose and plasma compartments. Adipose tissue is the most important source of fatty acids for lipid synthesis throughout the organism [1].

The fatty acid composition of adipose tissue, together with the degree of lipid mobilization, varies significantly between different depots. These differences will define the relative contributions of adipose regions to the plasma lipid profile and, consequently, concomitant metabolic alterations. In addition, the composition of fatty acids will also influence the endocrine and metabolic properties of adipose tissue itself, and the relative impact of the different regions on adipose-associated alterations, such as obesity, metabolic syndrome, and chronic inflammation.

FATTY ACID COMPOSITION OF ADIPOSE TISSUE

Triglycerides are incessantly being synthesized, stored, and mobilized within the adipocyte. The fatty acid profile of adipose tissue is a result of the continuous fluxes in and out of triglycerides [2]. The main sources of fatty acids into the adipocyte are the exogenous input of dietary fatty acids circulating in plasma and the endogenous synthesis and/or transformation of these fatty acids: the balance between these two sources will determine adipose tissue fatty acid profile.

Despite the great importance of adipose tissue as the organismal fatty acid reservoir, its composition in humans was not well studied until well into the twentieth century. The first data available date from 1925; however, the first relevant study on the topic was conducted in 1943, when Cramer and Brown performed a comprehensive chemical analysis of body fat using fractional distillation of fatty acid methyl esters combined with their new low-temperature crystallization technique. These researchers were the first to describe the presence of monounsaturated fatty acids (MUFAs) consisting of 14 and 16 carbon atoms, and of 18-carbon isomers of MUFAs and polyunsaturated fatty acids (PUFAs) [3]. After the 1960s, the study of adipose tissue fatty acid composition gained interest, and a series of studies showed that more than 40 different fatty acids are present in body fat, although only six of these comprise up to 90-97% of the total fatty acids: myristic (C14:0), palmitic (C16:0), palmitoleic (C16:1*n*-7), stearic (C18:0), oleic (C18:1*n*-9), and linoleic (C18:2*n*-6) acids [4–7]. Later, lauric (C12:0), γ-linoleic (18:3*n*-6), and vaccenic (18:1*n*-7) acids were also considered major fatty acids in human body fat (Table 41.1) [8–13]. The main fatty acid families, their chemical structures, and the synthetic reactions to form new fatty acids from their precursors are summarized in Fig. 41.1.

Fig. 41.2 shows the relative proportions of the major fatty acids in human adipose tissue in a Mediterranean (Spanish) population [14]. Oleic acid was the most abundant fatty acid, amounting to almost half of the total fat (47%), and its proportion was negatively associated with those of myristic, palmitic, linoleic, and vaccenic acids. The second most abundant was palmitic acid (21.5%),

Nutrition in the Prevention and Treatment of Abdominal Obesity
http://dx.doi.org/10.1016/B978-0-12-407869-7.00041-6

TABLE 41.1 Most Abundant Fatty Acids in Human Adipose Tissue

Trivial Name	Systematic Name	Structure	Type
Lauric	Dodecanoic	12:0	SFA
Miristic	Tetradecanoic	14:0	SFA
Palmitic	Hexadecanoic	16:0	SFA
Stearic	Octodecanoic	18:0	SFA
Palmitoleic	9-Hexadecenoic	16:1*n*-7	*n*-7 MUFA
Vaccenic	11-Octadecenoic	18:1*n*-7	*n*-7 MUFA
Oleic	9-Octadecenoic	18:1*n*-9	*n*-9 MUFA
Linoleic	9,12-Octadecadienoic	18:2*n*-6	*n*-6 PUFA
γ-Linolenic	6,9,12-Octadecatrienoic	18:3*n*-6	*n*-6 PUFA

MUFA, monounsaturated fatty acid; PUFA, polyunsaturated fatty acid; SFA, saturated fatty acid.

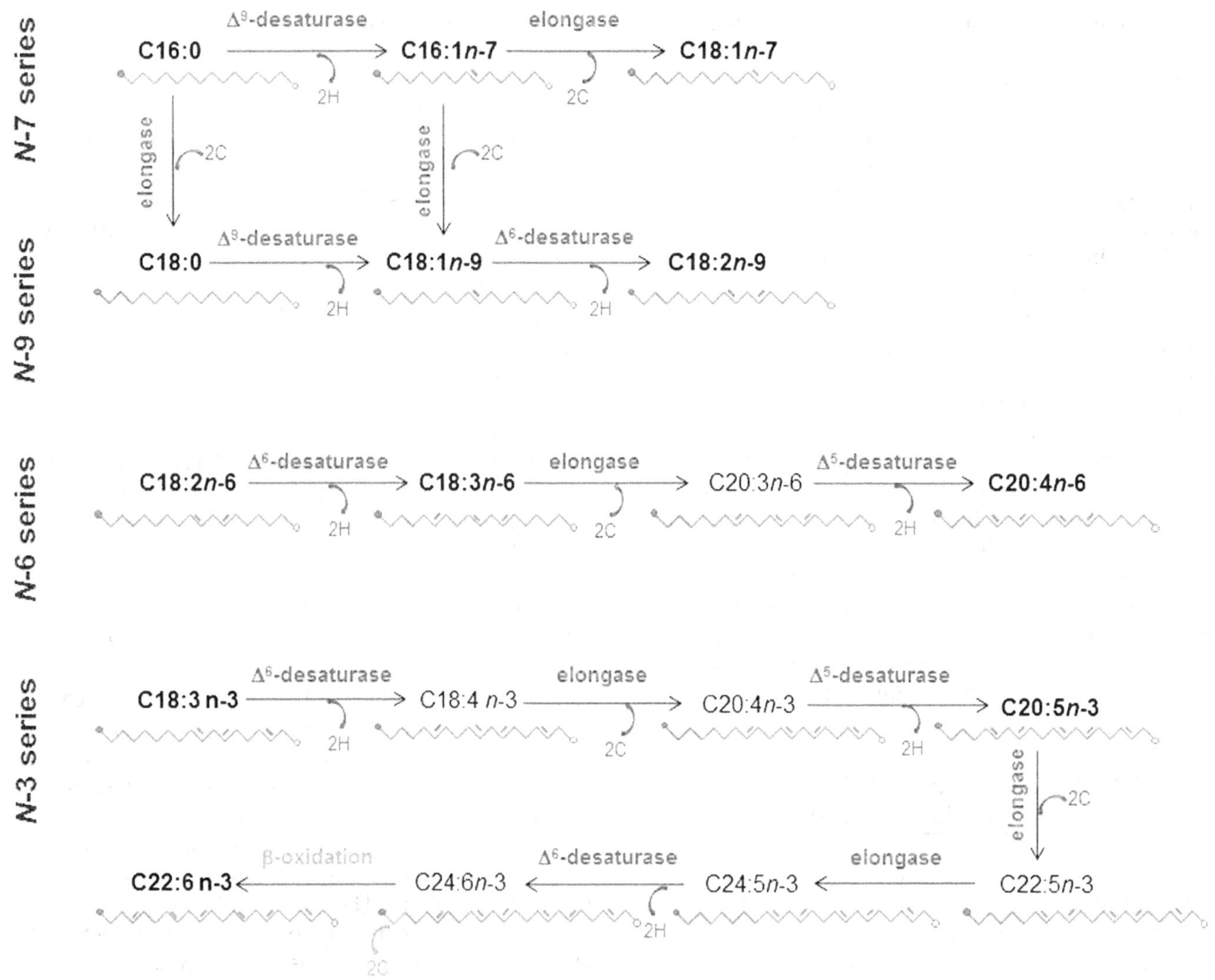

FIGURE 41.1 The main representatives of the different fatty acid families and their metabolic interconversions. Δ^5, delta-5; Δ^6, delta-6; Δ^9, delta-9. (See color plate at the back of the book.)

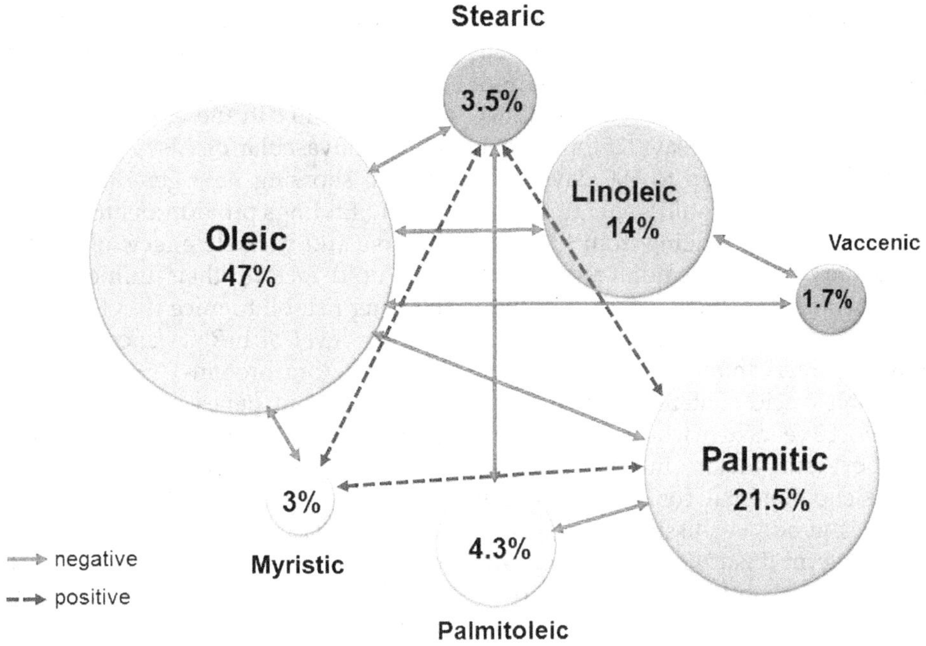

FIGURE 41.2 Relative proportions of the major fatty acids in human adipose tissue.

the proportion of which positively correlated with the other saturated fatty acids (SFAs) myristic and stearic, and negatively with oleic and palmitoleic. Linoleic acid was the third most abundant, showing an inverse association with vaccenic and oleic acids. Palmitoleic and stearic acids normally occurred in similar proportions, and were inversely correlated. Finally, myristic and vaccenic acids were the least abundant of the seven major fatty acids. The associations represented in the figure reflect how changes in the amount of one particular fatty acid will affect those of others, due to competition for transport, uptake and binding to mono- and diacylglycerides, or elongation and unsaturation/desaturation reactions. The adipose tissue profile shown in Fig. 41.2 is similar but not identical to those described in other countries and populations, such as Americans or Japanese [15], thus providing evidence for the greater influence of dietary contribution over endogenous metabolism on the fatty acid composition of adipose tissue.

WHICH FACTORS DETERMINE ADIPOSE TISSUE FATTY ACID PROFILE?

Diet and Adipose Tissue Fatty Acid Composition

In Europe, fat intake accounts for approximately 34% of the total caloric intake in women and 36% in men for most countries [16], representing a great diversity in its origin and chemical nature. Except for the Greek, Spanish, and Italian centers, the average MUFA intake has been shown to range between 10% and 13% of total energy, with a high proportion derived from animal sources. SFA intake is lowest in the Greek, Spanish, Italian, and UK cohorts, and highest in the Swedish centers. The mean PUFA intake is in the range of 4-8% total energy.

Changing the source of dietary lipids means changing which fatty acids are available within the organism, and therefore the composition and metabolic function of adipose tissue, as evidenced by studies with animal models. For instance, experiments with rats [17], mice [18,19], broiler chickens [20], and guinea pigs [21] demonstrate that the linoleic acid content of body fat increases along with its presence in the diet. Similarly, diets with a higher content in *trans* fatty acid-rich sources alter adipose tissue lipid composition [22]. The discovery of the beneficial effects of *n*-3 PUFAs in relation to cardiovascular health led to considerable interest in studying their presence in adipose tissue and its relationship with dietary intake; a strong positive correlation between their concentration in the diet and in adipose tissue was found in animal models [23]. The dietary content of SFAs and MUFAs can also influence adipose tissue composition, although the relationship is not as strong as that observed with PUFAs [21,24].

Regarding humans, regulation of the fatty acid composition of adipose tissue is still a matter for research. However, factors like age or gender do not seem to be significant modulators of fatty acid profile, whereas dietary intake appears to be the determining factor. The relationship between diet and adipose tissue composition has been analyzed using two main approaches:

observational studies on habitual diets, and interventional studies that manipulate the source of dietary fat. For the latter, adipose tissue turnover must be taken into account to establish the duration of interventions. This was generally considered to be 350–375 days [25], although some authors produced figures of up to 680 days [26]. Isotope-labeling studies observed different turnover rates in different adipose regions, ranging from 134 days in the abdominal depot to 305 in the femoral region and 326 in the gluteal subcutaneous pads. These findings indicate that changes in adipose tissue composition require long-term dietary interventions. For example, an attempt to alter the linoleic acid content in human adipose tissue needed almost 3 years to reach a new set-point [27]. Consequently, short-term dietary interventions do not provide adequate experimental conditions to produce significant changes in adipose tissue composition. On the other hand, long-term dietary manipulations are often nonviable, due to ethical and methodological concerns. Therefore, the most frequent scientific approach takes the form of cross-sectional and observational studies on the habitual diets of individuals, comparing them with their adipose tissue compositions.

Types of Diet and Adipose Tissue Composition

An analysis of fatty acid composition in the adipose tissue of Spanish and Greek populations found high percentages of oleic acid. These populations are well known for the high consumption of olive oil in their diets [14–28]. In other populations, it has been demonstrated that the consumption of coconut oil increases the adipose tissue content of lauric and myristic acids, both SFAs [29], and adipose tissue samples from Japanese populations presented elevated proportions of PUFAs of the *n*-3 family such as eicosapentaenoic (EPA; C20:5*n*-3) and docosahexaenoic (DHA; C22:6*n*-3) acids, which were associated with high fish intake [15]. When vegetarians and nonvegetarians were compared, the former had higher proportions of linoleic acid in their adipose tissues, and were also believed to have higher PUFA intakes [30]. In addition, a five-year intervention study showed that manipulating the diet in order to significantly increase the PUFA content resulted in 22% greater linoleic acid in the adipose tissue of the participants [26].

The observation that Greenland Eskimos, who consume animal fats of marine origin with high *n*-3 PUFA contents, have a very low incidence of cardiovascular diseases attracted scientific interest in these fatty acids [31]. Nowadays, the diminished cardiovascular risk associated with *n*-3 PUFA consumption is a well-known fact [32]. Indeed, fish oil consumption may help normalize the prethrombotic state and reduce arterial disease. This antithrombotic potential of *n*-3 PUFA-rich fish oil has been attributed to a reduction in platelet activation, a lowering of plasma triglycerides and vitamin K-dependent coagulation factors, and a decrease in vascular tone. However, there is considerable between-subject variability in the effects of *n*-3 PUFA consumption on cardiovascular diseases, and new nutrigenetics studies are showing new gene × environment interactions. Recent findings provide an attractive explanation for the diverse and variable effects of *n*-3 PUFA on hemostatic and lipid factors: their influence on gene expression. Feeding fish oil to mice was found to downregulate the hepatic level of mRNA encoding sterol regulatory element-binding protein-1 (SREPB-1), which controls several lipogenic genes [33]. Also in mice, *n*-3 PUFAs suppress the expression of endogenous peroxisome proliferator-activated receptor alpha (PPAR-α), a ligand-activated transcription factor [34], whereas oxidized *n*-3 PUFAs activate PPAR- α [35]. In addition, genetic polymorphisms in genes encoding hemostatic factors may be associated with the variable, subject-dependent response to PUFAs of genes encoding apolipoproteins [36].

On the other hand, research has long suggested that the consumption of certain *trans* isomers of fatty acids has detrimental health effects, such as impairing platelet aggregation, inhibition of elongation, and desaturation of essential fatty acids (and thus a reduction in the availability of long-chain PUFAs) [37]. Several studies have shown that consumption of these *trans* fatty acids is linked to their storage in adipose tissue, and how a chronic intake can alter lipid metabolism leading to decreased fat storage in adipose tissue, an effect probably linked to diminished insulin sensitivity [38]. Moreover, the mechanism by which *trans* fatty acids induce insulin resistance differs from that by which diets enriched with saturated fats achieve this outcome [39,40].

Relationship Between Diet and Adipose Tissue Composition: Beynen's Mathematical Model

In 1980, Beynen and colleagues developed a mathematical model that explained the relationship between fatty acid composition of adipose tissue of individuals and their usual diets [41]. They observed that the strongest correlations were found with the relative proportions of PUFAs. PUFA are essential dietary components; although some can be obtained by enzymatic modification (i.e. elongation and desaturation) of other fatty acids, the initial *n*-3 and *n*-6 structures cannot be synthesized by human cells and must therefore be ingested with food. Consequently, the content of these fatty acids in adipose tissue provides useful information about their presence in the diet.

In contrast, for both SFAs (myristic, palmitic, and stearic) and MUFAs (palmitoleic, oleic, and vaccenic), studies showed a weaker relationship between the percentages of these fatty acids in the diet and in adipose tissue. SFAs and MUFAs are the most abundant fatty acids in adipose tissue and are also present in high proportions in most habitual diets. In addition, any excess carbohydrate or protein intake, as well as alcohol intake, will eventually find its way to the form of fatty acids to be stored in the fat depots, mainly in the form of saturated fats. Endogenous interconversion among fatty acids of these families can also determine their concentrations in adipose tissue. However, as mentioned earlier, in populations with a high intake of MUFAs (e.g. Mediterranean populations), a stronger relationship can be found between intake and adipose tissue content [14].

According to Beynen and colleagues, certain fatty acids appear in either smaller or greater percentages in adipose tissue than in the diet [41]. For example, the presence of lauric, myristic, stearic, and linoleic acids in the diet normally exceeds that in adipose tissue; in contrast, palmitoleic and oleic acids are more abundant in tissue than in the diet [15]. In addition, if PUFA consumption exceeds 30% of total dietary fat, this will not be translated into adipose tissue fatty acid profile, indicating that the diet has a limited ability to affect adipose tissue composition [41].

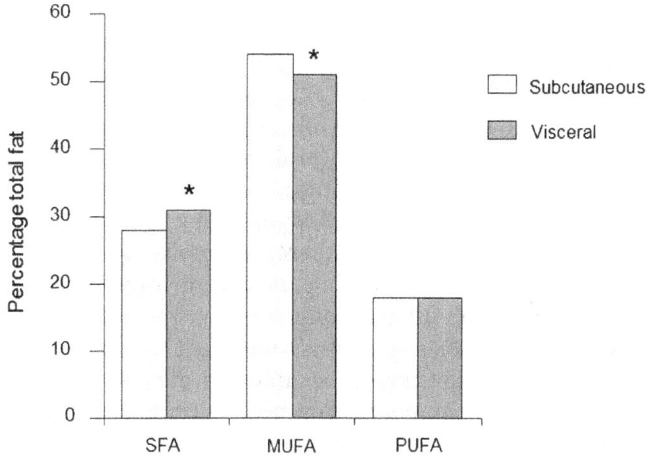

FIGURE 41.3 Differences in fat composition between subcutaneous and visceral fat in a Mediterranean Spanish population. MUFA, monounsaturated fatty acid; PUFA, polyunsaturated fatty acid; SFA, saturated fatty acid. *, $P < 0.05$ for differences in fatty acid percentages between adipose depots. (See color plate at the back of the book.) *Source: Garaulet et al. [14].*

Site-Related Differences in Adipose Tissue Composition

The study of animal fat showed over a century ago that *superficial* (i.e. subcutaneous) fat is softer than *deep* (i.e. visceral) fat depots. The greater exposure of superficial fat to lower ambient temperatures requires higher concentrations of unsaturated fatty acids to maintain optimal fluidity and function [42]. In relation to humans, some authors have reported that the fatty acid profile of deep fat is similar to that of the subcutaneous fat [43]. However, we and others claimed that, like in animals, human visceral fat is more saturated than subcutaneous fat, with a higher proportion of stearic acid and lower proportions of palmitoleic and oleic acids [5,11,14]. Fig. 41.3 illustrates the differences in fatty acid composition between subcutaneous and visceral adipose depots in a Mediterranean population [14]. As shown in the figure, fatty acid composition is related to adipose tissue distribution. More specifically, central obesity is positively associated with *n*-6 PUFAs and inversely with MUFAs and *n*-3 PUFAs in adipose tissue [14]. These data are in agreement with previous studies by Phinney and colleagues, performed in 1994 [12]. Moreover, similar recently published results show a negative correlation between MUFAs and central obesity [44].

Subcutaneous Adipose Tissue

The subcutaneous depot is the biggest fat storage compartment in the body and, consequently, the major energy reservoir. Thanks to the development of simple suction techniques [25,45], it has become relatively easy to conduct analyses on human subcutaneous fat. Several studies have compared the fatty acid profiles of different subcutaneous fat depots and, although some authors reported no site-specific variance [46], others did find changes in the content of SFAs and MUFAs between abdominal and gluteal-femoral subcutaneous fat, with the former being richer in SFA [27,47]. Thus, site-related differences in adipose tissue composition may not only be linked to how deep the fat depot is located but also to a more specific regional distribution. This indicates that several factors other than diet can affect adipose tissue fatty acid composition; we will discuss these next.

Temperature

The melting temperature of the major fatty acids varies in the different adipose depots: subcutaneous fat's melting point is approximately 41°C, while visceral fat's is 49°C. Visceral fat is normally exposed to physiological temperatures (37°C), and therefore it needs a higher melting point to maintain its physicochemical properties in a semisolid, semifluid state. On the other hand, subcutaneous fat needs to have a lower melting point as it is also exposed to lower temperatures, and consequently contains a greater proportion of unsaturated lipids to maintain its optimal physiological state.

Malcolm and colleagues, however, suggested that the mechanisms underlying fatty acid profile in adipose tissue should be more complex than simply consisting of a response to surrounding and environmental temperatures [47].

Function

Differences in function between the different fat depots may determine fatty acid content. It was initially believed that subcutaneous fat is mainly responsible for thermal isolation, while visceral tissue exerts a preeminently mechanical role, acting as a cushion for the inner organs. This function would require fat in this region to be harder and more solid (therefore, more highly saturated). Nowadays, following the recent huge increase in knowledge about the complex metabolic functions of visceral fat, this hypothesis may seem too simplistic; however, we must remember that the mechanical role of this fat depot in conferring protection for our inner organs remains an important part of our physiology.

Rate and Degree of Adaptation to Dietary Changes

It has been suggested that the correlations between fatty acids in the diet and in adipose tissue described by the Beynen model vary according to the localization of the fat depots. Field and colleagues stated that regional diversity in adipose tissue composition is due to different rates of dietary adaptation [48].

Experiments in animals have shown site-specific differences in the sensitivity of adipose tissue to dietary changes. For example, in rats given a diet enriched with fish oil, *n*-3 PUFA uptake into adipose tissue was greater in the subcutaneous and mesenteric fat depots than in the retroperitoneal and omental ones [49]. In humans, Katan and coworkers made similar findings. By supplying fish oil in varying amounts to 58 men for 12 months, they found that *n*-3 PUFA incorporation occurred at different speeds in the different fat depots: after 6 months of treatment, it had reached 67% in the gluteal depot and 75% in the subcutaneous abdominal depot [50].

In the case of subcutaneous fat, this difference is consistent with the need for a greater degree of unsaturation due to exposure to lower temperatures, as mentioned above. It has also been suggested that intra-abdominal adipose tissue has a reduced capacity to take up exogenous free fatty acids when compared to subcutaneous [50]. As for mesenteric fat, it can be hypothesized that its close association with the intestine turns it into the first storage site and that it thus somehow acts as a retention filter. However, interscapular fat has been shown to adapt to dietary changes faster than subcutaneous and even mesenteric tissues [51].

Beta-Oxidation

Another factor that influences the composition of adipose tissue is the types of fatty acids that are mobilized for oxidation. If we consider that the average person consumes between 5 and 10 times the equivalent of their body energy content per year, we can appreciate that there is an excess of substrates from which to choose which should be stored and which should be oxidized. In this context, SFAs are the preferred oxidation substrates because unsaturated fatty acid catabolism requires more complex enzymatic machinery and is less efficient in terms of net energy yield.

Different Enzyme Affinities

The enzymes involved in the synthesis of glycerolipids selectively influence fatty acid uptake. For instance, several studies have shown that enzymes responsible for de novo synthesis usually place a SFA in the first position of the triglyceride (R1; see Fig. 41.4). This implies that half of the fatty acids in diacylglycerides and one-third in triglycerides are saturated. Unsaturated fatty acids are esterified in the second position (R2), and highly unsaturated fatty acids (20-22 carbon atoms long) are unsaturated in the third position (R3) [52]. Triglyceride stereochemistry is not only important for the acylation process but it also determines lipolytic and lipogenic reactions. Hormone-sensitive lipase (HSL), the enzyme responsible for fatty acid release from adipose tissue, has a preference for fatty acids unsaturated in the R3 position in particular, and for PUFAs in general.

Site-dependent distribution of enzymatic activities and affinities will therefore result in a site-dependent diacylglyceride and triglyceride composition. Indeed, research has shown that the different adipose regions present distinct lipase, lipoprotein lipase (LPL), and HSL activities. The positions on which these lipases act in each fat depot will determine the selective release and uptake of fatty acids in the adipocytes, and consequently adipose tissue composition.

Influence of Sex Hormones

Some authors defend the idea that the regional differences in fatty acid storage are related more to sex

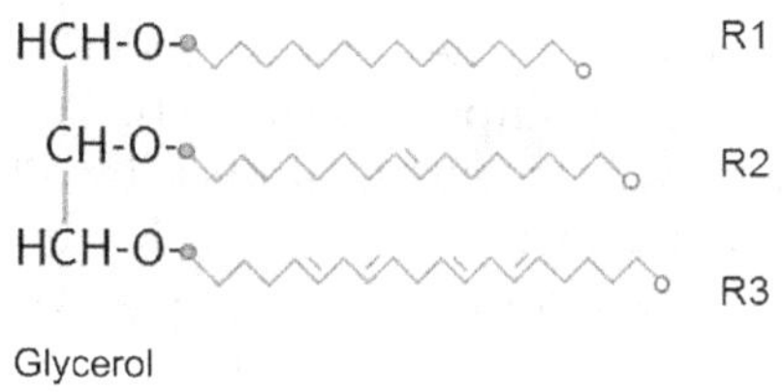

FIGURE 41.4 Structure of a trygliceride, showing the glycerol molecule esterified to different fatty acids.Most commonly, the first position (R1) is occupied by a saturated acid, the second (R2) by an unsaturated acid, and third (R3) position usually by a long-chain highly unsaturated fatty acid. (See color plate at the back of the book.)

differences in body fat distribution rather than to the patterns of dietary fatty acid storage. This is not only the case for experimental animals [53], but also for humans [54]. To illustrate this, storage rates of palmitic acid were measured in omental and abdominal subcutaneous fat in both men and women, along with enzymes involved in fatty acid storage. Researchers found that direct fatty acid storage rates were significantly greater in omental than in abdominal subcutaneous tissue for both sexes, and greater in women than in men for both depots. They also found that the proportion of fatty acids stored in subcutaneous adipose tissue (and their and rates of storage) via direct reuptake were greater in women than in men [54].

Site-specific concentrations and activities of sex hormones are factors that can also influence differences in fatty acid composition within the different adipose tissue depots and its association with sex. A good example is provided by data showing the effects of dehydroepiandrosterone (DHEA) and its sulfate on experimental animals and humans [55–57]. The level of this particular hormone, a precursor of most androgens and estrogens, is strongly related to body fat distribution and also with fatty acid profiles of adipose tissue and plasma.

In vitro experiments showed that 3T3-L1 adipocytes treated with DHEA had a shift toward higher proportions of oleic (C18:1) and stearic (C18:0) acids, and lower proportions of palmitic (C16:0) acid [55]. In our laboratory, we observed that rats receiving DHEA orally for 13 weeks reproduced some of the changes observed in 3T3-L1 cells. Besides having a significantly lower percentage body fat, DHEA-treated rats had higher proportions of stearic and oleic acids and a lower proportion of palmitoleic acid in their adipose depots [56]. Total *n*-6 PUFAs were also decreased, while *n*-3 PUFAs were increased, leading to significant reductions in *n*-6:*n*-3 PUFA ratios. We later confirmed these results in vitro in human subcutaneous and visceral adipose tissue samples treated with DHEA sulfate (DHEAS): there was a reduction in palmitic acid, total SFAs, total *n*-6 PUFAs, and *n*-6:*n*-3 PUFA ratios after DHEAS treatment, whereas MUFAs were increased [57]. Additionally, markers of delta-6 desaturase activity were significantly increased by DHEA and DHEAS in both rats and humans [56,57].

In rats, the effect of DHEA on adipose tissue fatty acid profile was more marked in the subcutaneous than in visceral depots; even more, DHEA was shown to increase the proportion of *n*-3 PUFAs, particularly in interscapular brown adipose tissue [56]. In contrast, the effects of DHEAS on the fatty acid profile seemed to be similar in the two human depots [57]. Nevertheless, human adipose tissues did vary in their lipolytic response to DHEAS stimulation, and this effect was shown to be sex specific: in men, the hormone stimulated lipolysis to a higher extent in the visceral depot, whereas in women this response was more evident in the subcutaneous depot [57].

The Influence of Adipose Tissue Clock Genes

In mammals, a network of circadian clock genes regulates 24-h rhythms of behavior and physiology. Different studies developed by our group and others have consistently demonstrated associations between different clock genetic variants and fatty acid composition from the diet or from erythrocyte membranes [58,59]. We have also shown that adipose tissue expresses its own clock genes that regulate different aspects of the adipose tissue metabolism [60]. Our studies also pointed out that the epigenetic imprint of several clock genes is related to MUFA and PUFA intake [58]. However, the site-specific influence of clock genes on adipose tissue fatty acid composition has not yet been demonstrated, and further investigations in this area are required. Of note, it has recently been shown that diurnal variations in lipolysis rates correlate with the rhythmic regulation of two adipocyte clocks [61], and also that circadian clock disruption promotes the accumulation of triglycerides in adipose tissue, leading to increased adiposity and adipocyte hypertrophy. These results demonstrate that circadian modulation of lipolysis rates regulates the availability of lipid-derived energy during the day, thus suggesting a role for white adipose tissue clocks in the regulation of energy homeostasis [61].

ADIPOSE TISSUE FATTY ACIDS AND OBESITY

Fatty Acid Profile and Degree of Obesity

Previous studies in rats showed that obesity was characterized by significant modifications in fatty acid composition in the subcutaneous and mesenteric adipose tissue, and these changes were not reversed upon feeding a low-calorie diet. In addition, the changes differed among the adipose depots [62]. However, it is important to note that the lipogenic capacity of human adipose tissue is lower than that of rats. This diminished lipogenic activity in humans does not seem to be related to differences in diet, but it is instead partly due to a lower concentration of fatty acid synthase (FAS) and a lower abundance of sterol regulatory element-binding protein 1c (SREBP-1c) [63].

It appears that certain enzymes of lipid metabolism, in particular the delta-9 and delta-6 desaturases, alter their activity in both the liver and adipose tissue depending on the degree of obesity [64]. Indeed, in humans, an association between delta-9 desaturase (also known as stearoyl-CoA desaturase) activity and both adiposity and plasma lipid profile was suggested in a group of healthy adolescent women, supporting the assumption that delta-9 activity is independently linked to higher body mass index (BMI) and higher circulatory triglyceride levels [65]. Some authors reported that palmitoleic acid content is higher in adipose tissue of obese individuals when compared to normal-weight individuals, and suggested that the increase in due to higher delta-9 desaturase activity [64]. These results were later replicated by other authors, who found palmitoleic acid levels in adipose tissue triglycerides to be correlated with multiple measures of adiposity and adipose tissue distribution [66]. This work revealed that the percentage palmitoleic acid in serum and adipose tissue were highly similar between monozygotic twins, independent of dietary fat intake, both before and after a weight loss intervention followed by 1-year weight maintenance. This result suggests that palmitoleic acid is a metabolic indicator of endogenous lipogenesis under genetic control [66]. In experimental studies, palmitoleic acid was suggested as a possible *lipokine* that allows adipose tissue to communicate with distant organs [67]. However, this lipokine function was not confirmed by other authors, who showed that adipose tissue levels of palmitoleic acid correspond to endogenous lipogenesis [68].

Obesity is also associated with a defect in the oxidation of long-chain triglycerides [62] that is probably linked to an excessive input of these fatty acids in the diet. In contrast, oxidation of mid-chain triglycerides does not seem to be affected by obesity. Other studies have found negative correlations between body weight and the proportions of lauric, myristic, and stearic fatty acids, while *n*-6 PUFA content, and in particular that of linoleic acid, is increased in obese subjects when compared to those of normal weight [6]. Linoleic acid is an essential nutrient and can therefore only be obtained from the diet; this has led to suggest that its relative increase in obesity is due to higher overall fat intake, which is commonly seen in obese subjects [69]. In relation to *n*-3 PUFAs, there seems to be a tendency toward lower proportions with increasing obesity, especially abdominal obesity [14]; this could contribute to the greater cardiovascular risk in obese individuals. In addition, *n*-3 PUFAs are known ligands of uncoupling protein 2 (UCP 2; responsible for nonshivering thermogenesis), and their levels in adipose tissue have been positively associated with UCP 2 activity [70] and negatively with adipocyte size [71,72], implying a thermogenic, antilipogenic action for these fatty acids. However, in populations with a usual high consumption of fish, such as Japanese or Eskimos, obesity is associated with elevated *n*-3 PUFA content in adipose tissue [73]. These apparently contradictory results may be related to the fact that in those specific populations, unlike in Western or Mediterranean ones, the adipose tissue *n*-3 PUFA content may be an accurate marker of total fat intake. Therefore, in these particular populations, the high proportions of *n*-3 PUFAs seen in obesity should not be considered an indicator of a potential obesogenic role for this type of fatty acid.

The relationships observed between adipocyte size and fatty acids deserve further attention. In the beginning of the twenty-first century, several authors proposed that enlarged fat cells exhibit biochemical features that could be involved in the metabolic complications of obesity at the systemic level [74,75]. In other words, that cell hypertrophy per se could lead to the hormonal and metabolic alterations occurring in obesity as part of an adaptive mechanism linked to the status of energy stores in adipose tissue. Thus, understanding the effects of fatty acids on factors such as adipocyte size, number, and function is of great interest in the prevention and treatment of obesity.

Adipose Tissue Fatty Acid Composition and Metabolic Syndrome

Abdominal obesity is one of the critical factors in the definition of the metabolic syndrome [76,77]. It still remains to be unraveled whether the association between these two alterations is a causal relationship (i.e. visceral fat accumulation leads to metabolic risk) or whether they are both the consequences of a third factor. The quest to elucidate mechanisms responsible for the strong association between central fat accumulation and metabolic disturbances has been the origin of multiple epidemiological, clinical, and molecular studies worldwide. Different explanations have been proposed during the years.

It was initially suggested that the positive correlation between metabolic syndrome and body fat distribution was due to the greater lipolytic activity of abdominal fat. Fatty acids released from this depot would arrive to the liver directly through the portal vein [78], and their deposition in the liver would impair insulin signaling, eventually leading to systemic insulin resistance and hyperinsulinemia. At the same time, this influx of free fatty acids would induce hepatic glucose synthesis by stimulating gluconeogenesis, thus contributing to hyperglycemia and consequently further hyperinsulinemia. Arguments against this hypothesis were raised, however; it was claimed that there was no evidence of increased portal free fatty acid influx in visceral obesity [79].

Adipose Tissue Fatty Acid Composition and Cardiovascular Risk

Adipose tissue composition may still play an important role in the development of insulin resistance and cardiovascular damage associated with metabolic syndrome. In relation to cardiovascular risk, there seems to be a connection between adipose tissue fatty acid profile and atheromatosis. Triglycerides from this tissue constitute the most important source of fatty acids for the synthesis of complex lipids and energy production; different studies have shown that adipose tissue fatty acids are in a state of constant mobilization, regardless of whether the individual is losing or gaining weight. Phinney and colleagues demonstrated back in 1990 that the rate of fatty acid mobilization is higher than that of oxidation; net oxidation would thus result from the difference between lipolysis and reesterification of fatty acids [80]. This continuous mobilization has an influence on plasma fatty acid composition and, therefore, on cardiovascular diseases.

Despite this obvious influence, little information was available on the relationship between adipose tissue composition and cardiovascular disease until relatively recently. Some studies found weak associations between certain fatty acids in subcutaneous fat and various factors of cardiovascular risk (age, BMI, blood pressure, and levels of cholesterol and lipoproteins) [81]. Since the early 2000s, our own group has conducted research showing that subcutaneous and visceral abdominal fat depots differ significantly not only in their fatty acid composition but also in the way this is associated with plasma lipid profile, with visceral adipose tissue having a greater number of significant associations [14]. In particular, adipose tissue levels of oleic acid (C18:1*n*-9) and *n*-3 PUFAs negatively correlate with plasma triglyceride and apolipoprotein B (ApoB) levels. For their part, stearic (C18:0) and eicosapentaenoic (C20:5*n*-3) acids positively correlate with high-density lipoprotein cholesterol and ApoA levels; consequently, these fatty acids appear to be cardioprotective. In contrast, myristic acid (C14:0) is associated with lower ApoA levels and therefore appears potentially atherogenic.

Adipose Tissue Fatty Acids and Insulin Resistance

Excess fatty acid release from adipose tissue into the circulation may end up accumulating in nonfatty tissues, mainly the liver and skeletal muscle. This leads to impaired insulin signaling in these organs and, consequently, decreased peripheral insulin sensitivity, a phenomenon that Russell came to call *lipotoxicity* [82]. Back in the 1960s, Randle and colleagues proposed that the decrease in insulin sensitivity had its origin in elevated levels of circulating free fatty acids, which would result in an imbalance between the oxidation of fatty acids and that of glucose [83]. Decades later, Roden and coworkers refined this hypothesis by showing that plasma fatty acids inhibited glucose transport and oxidation [84].

The relationship between fatty acids and insulin function is, however, more complex than this (for a more extensive review on this particular topic, see [85]). It is not merely the total amount of circulating free fatty acids, but their particular chemical nature, that modulates insulin sensitivity in target tissues. Already in the twenty-first century, it was proposed that SFAs, and particularly palmitic acid, are converted into ceramides, and that it is these compounds that are responsible for impaired insulin signaling [86,87]. More recently, a euglycemic clamp study conducted in an elderly population showed that adipose tissue enriched with palmitic acid and depleted of essential PUFAs was associated with insulin resistance [88]. Indeed, levels of palmitic acid (C16:0), the major SFA in the diet and in adipose tissue, negatively correlated with insulin sensitivity, while DHA (C22:6*n*-3) positively correlated with this outcome. Moreover, studies have demonstrated that endothelial dysfunction in type 2 diabetics is also related to fatty acid composition and in the same direction: SFAs were positively related to endothelial dysfunction, while PUFAs showed protective effects [89].

A mechanism proposed for PUFA modulation of insulin sensitivity involves the regulation of genes involved in adipogenesis, in particular *PPARG*, which encodes the transcription factor PPAR-γ. This factor acts to promote adipocyte differentiation, lipid storage, and, consequently, sensitivity to insulin. Natural ligands of this transcription factor are linoleic (C18:2*n*-6), γ -linolenic (C18:3*n*-6), arachidonic (C20:4*n*-6), and EPA (C20:5*n*-3) acids [90].

Less clear seem to be the effects of MUFAs on insulin sensitivity, or the mechanisms by which these fatty acids operate, but epidemiological evidence indicates that olive oil and MUFAs can enhance systemic insulin sensitivity [85].

When we analyzed the relationship between adipose tissue fatty acid composition and markers of insulin resistance, our data showed that visceral fat composition was significantly associated with circulating insulin levels. This association was positive with adipose tissue SFAs and negative with MUFAs, especially with oleic acid. This provides more evidence in favor of a protective nature for this fatty acid, and consequently of olive oil and the Mediterranean diet [91]. No significant associations were found between insulin levels and subcutaneous tissue fatty acid composition. In agreement with our previous comments related to the continuous mobilization of fatty acids, the composition of intra-abdominal adipose tissue seems to be more relevant than that of subcutaneous adipose tissue concerning the metabolic syndrome. As a result, the existing differences between subcutaneous and visceral adipose tissue fatty acid compositions and mobilization rates lead to differences in their atherogenic capacity.

Fatty Acids as Modulators of Adipocyte Function

Apart from exerting a detrimental effect when ectopically deposited in nonadipose tissues and organs, fatty acids have been shown to also have an impact within adipose tissue itself. We have previously seen that the specificity of enzymes involved in lipid metabolism can determine fatty acid composition in adipose tissue. But this is not a one direction relationship; instead, fatty acids have also been shown to act upon these enzymes. Particular fatty acids or the fatty acid profile as a whole can alter essential metabolic processes like fat accumulation, synthesis (lipogenesis), and oxidation (lipolysis). The capacity of *n*-6 and, especially, *n*-3 PUFAs to limit lipid storage and, consequently, adipocyte size and hypertrophy of adipose tissue has been well documented in experimental animals [49,92–94], and it was suggested that oils containing these fatty acids suppressed the growth of fat tissues [95]. We have already mentioned that in our population of overweight and obese subjects, a significant inverse correlation was found between the adipose tissue content of *n*-3 PUFAs and fat cell size [71]. *N*-3 PUFAs can suppress fatty acid synthesis, increase their oxidation [96], and reduce triacylglycerol synthesis [97]. EPA (C20:5*n*-3) and DHA (C22:6*n*-3), in particular, are closely associated with the expression of genes encoding enzymes involved in lipogenesis (such as FAS and LPL), lipolysis (HSL), or gluconeogenesis [phosphoenolpyruvate carboxykinase (PEPCK)], and also with genes expressing transcription factors [like CCAAT/enhancer binding protein alpha (C/EBPα) and leptin] [49]. All these proteins control fat accumulation and, consequently, adipocyte size.

Furthermore, the influence of fatty acids on adipocyte function extends beyond lipid metabolism. Fatty acids have been recognized as modulators of gene expression in both adipocytes and preadipocytes by acting as ligands of transcription factors, in a similar way to hormones. In this sense, they influence the mechanisms of proliferation and differentiation of fat cells (adipogenesis; reviewed in Azain 2004 [98]). Despite their roles as natural ligands for the adipogenic factor PPAR-γ, we have mentioned throughout this chapter that PUFAs are associated with decreased adipocyte size and lower body fat content. It has been suggested that *n*-6 PUFAs are more efficient than *n*-3 PUFAs in inhibiting adipocyte differentiation and fatty acid synthesis [99]. However, a recent report showed that changes in adipocyte fatty acid profile were accompanied by changes in adipogenesis. 3T3-L1 cells were transfected with the *Caenorhabditis .elegans fat-1* gene and a reduction in the *n*-6:*n*-3 ratio was observed, together with impaired preadipocyte differentiation, as revealed by lower expression of key genes including those encoding PPAR- γ, adipocyte fatty acid-binding protein/aP2, and UCP 2 [100]. The interpretation of these and other seemingly contradictory results in relation to PUFAs and adipogenesis has now become one of the main challenges in understanding the role of fatty acids in adipose tissue metabolism, so it is necessary to investigate how to reconcile an inhibitory effect on fat cell proliferation with an insulin-sensitizing action. The key to unravel these questions will probably lie in the *n*-6:*n*-3 PUFA ratios, or even in the balance between all of the different fatty acid types (in other words, in the fatty acid profile of the tissues), rather than the absolute levels of particular fatty acids.

Finally, it is necessary to mention the effect of fatty acids on the expression, synthesis, and secretion of adipokines, with leptin and adiponectin being the most widely researched. In either case, a distinct pattern of association is still lacking. In the case of leptin, for instance, *n*-6 PUFAs have been shown to downregulate its production in rodent brown adipocytes [101]; in contrast, EPA has been reported to stimulate leptin release from primary cultures of rat adipocytes [102], but diets with a high *n*-3 PUFA content have also been associated with decreased circulating leptin levels [101].

Especial attention should be paid to the interaction between fatty acids and adiponectin, an adipokine involved in insulin sensitivity and cardiovascular health. Experiments using 3T3-L1 adipocytes found a reduction in adiponectin expression after treatment with palmitic acid, linoleic acid, EPA, and DHA [103]. Results obtained by our group in rats showed significant negative correlations between *Adipoq* gene (encoding adiponectin) expression and the tissue content of lauric, myristic, and palmitoleic acids in visceral fat depots, and positive ones with stearic acid in the periovarian depot and linoleic acid in the subcutaneous. We also found a significant negative association between adipokine gene expression levels and the subcutaneous adipose tissue content of *n*-3 PUFAs [104]. In human samples of visceral adipose tissue, we again found negative associations between SFAs and adiponectin expression, while oleic acid content was positively correlated with the expression of this cardioprotective and insulin-sensitizing adipokine [105].

Similar to our discussion in relation to fatty acids and insulin sensitivity, the meaning of the interactions between fatty acids and adipokines deserves thorough consideration, as we are probably facing a highly complex metabolic cross talk. As an example, we also recently observed that the effect of fatty acids on adipocyte function will vary depending on the status of adipose tissue. In adipocytes cultured under standard conditions, no significant effects were observed on the expression of genes encoding adipokines involved in angiogenesis (like angiopoietin-related protein 4) or inflammation [e.g. interleukin-6 (IL-6) and IL-1β]. However, when cells were cultured under hypoxia in order to replicate the proinflammatory conditions seen in obesity, stimulation with fatty acids had a synergistic upregulatory effect on gene expression [106].

ADIPOSE TISSUE FATTY ACID COMPOSITION AS A PREDICTOR OF WEIGHT LOSS

One of the most important questions related to adipose tissue is whether fatty acid composition changes with weight loss. Most importantly, several authors have been interested in assessing the predictive role of adipose triglyceride fatty acids in weight loss and long-term weight loss maintenance after dietary intervention. In this regard, a relatively recent study has demonstrated that weight change after the maintenance phase correlated positively with baseline levels of adipose tissue palmitoleic, myristoleic and *trans* palmitoleic acids [44]. This outcome is in agreement with previously described findings suggesting that palmitoleic acid levels in adipose tissue reflect endogenous lipogenesis [68]. Also myristoleic acid (a product of myristic acid desaturation in humans), a minor fatty acid in adipose tissue, seems to be an indicator of endogenous lipogenesis [1]. Of note, lower initial oleic acid predicts lower weight decrease [44]. These results suggest a specific role for adipose tissue MUFA content in weight management and as a weight change predictor that may contribute to the protective role of the Mediterranean diet against obesity [107].

SUMMARY

We could take the popular statement "we are what we eat" and give it an extra twist: we are what *remains* of what we ate. It is true that diet exerts a great influence on adipose tissue fatty acid composition, but it is no less certain that diverse aspects of lipid metabolism operate to maintain as stable a body fat composition as possible to minimize the effect of fortuitous changes in our daily diet.

Adipose tissue fatty acid composition links diet, obesity, and metabolic syndrome. Differences in composition between visceral and subcutaneous depots, along with the higher lipolytic activity of the former and its strong association with plasma lipids and insulin levels, may help to explain the processes leading to the development of metabolic syndrome.

References

[1] Lands WE. Long term fat intake and biomarkers. Am J Clin Nutr 1995;61(Suppl):72S–5S.
[2] Lands WE, Morris A, Libelt B. Quantitative effects of dietary polyunsaturated fats on the composition of fatty acids in rat tissues. Lipids 1990;25:505–16.
[3] Cramer DL, Brown JB. The component fatty acids of human depot fat. J Biol Chem 1943;151:427–39.
[4] Hegsted DM, Jacx CW, Stare FJ. The composition of human adipose tissue from several parts of the world. Am J Clin Nutr 1962;10:11–18.
[5] McLaren DS, Ajans ZA, Awdeh Z. Composition of human adipose tissue, with special reference to site and age differences. Am J Clin Nutr 1965;17:171–6.
[6] Insull W, Barch GE. Fatty acid composition of human adipose tissue related to age, sex and race. Am J Clin Nutr 1967;20:13–23.
[7] Konatnur MG, Oalmann MC, Johnson WD, Malcom GT, Strong JP. Fatty acid composition of human adipose tissue from two anatomical sites in a biracial community. Am J Clin Nutr 1979;32:2198–205.
[8] McLaren DS, Read WWC. Fatty acid composition of adipose tissue: a study in three races in East Africa. Clin Sci 1962;23:247–50.
[9] Hefferman GA. The fatty acid composition of human adipose tissue. Clin Sci 1963;25:423–9.
[10] Hefferman GA. Fatty acid composition of adipose tissue in normal and abnormal subjects. Am J Clin Nutr 1964;15:5–10.
[11] Calder PC, Harvey DJ, Pond CM, Newsholme EA. Site-specific differences in the fatty acid composition of human adipose tissue. Lipids 1992;27:716–20.
[12] Phinney SD, Stern JS, Burke KE, Tang AB, Miller G, Holman RT. Human subcutaneous adipose tissue shows site-specific differences in fatty acid composition. Am J Clin Nutr 1994;60:725–9.
[13] Schoen RE, Evans KW, Sankey SS, Weissfeld JL, Kuller L. Does visceral adipose tissue differ from subcutaneous adipose tissue in fatty acid content? Int J Obes 1996;20(4):346–52.
[14] Garaulet M, Pérez-Llamas F, Pérez-Ayala M, Martínez P, de Medina FS, Tebar FJ, et al. Site-specific differences in the fatty acid composition of abdominal adipose tissue in an obese population from a Mediterranean area (South-east Spain): relationship with dietary fatty acids, plasma lipid profile and central obesity. Am J Clin Nutr 2001;74:585–91.
[15] Insull W, Lang PD, Hsi BP, Yoshimura S. Studies of atherosclerosis in Japanese and American men. J Clin Invest 1969;48:1313–27.
[16] Linseisen J, Welch AA, Ocké M, Amiano P, Agnoli C, Ferrari P, et al. Dietary fat intake in the European Prospective Investigation into Cancer and Nutrition: results from the 24-h dietary recalls. Eur J Clin Nutr 2009;63(Suppl 4):S61–80.
[17] Awad AB. Effect of dietary lipids on composition and glucose utilization by rat adipose tissue. J Nutr 1981;111:34–9.
[18] Tove SB, Smith FH. Kinetics of the depletion of linoleic acid in mice. Arch Biochem Biophys 1959;85:325–65.
[19] Tove SB, Smith FH. Changes in the fatty acid composition of the depot fat of mice induced by feeding oleate and linoleate. J Nutr 1960;71:264–72.
[20] Bartov I. Nutritional factors affecting quantity and quality of carcass fat in chickens. Fed Proc 1979;38:2627–30.

[21] Gurr MI, Robinson MP, Kirtland J, Widdowson EM. Body lipids of guinea pigs exposed to different dietary fats from mid-gestation to 3 months of age III. Fatty acid composition of the lipids of plasma, adipose tissue, liver and muscle at months of age. Nutr Metab 1975;20:364–7.

[22] Schrock CG, Connor WE. Incorporation of the dietary trans fatty acid (c18:1) into the serum lipids, the serum lipoproteins and adipose tissue. Am J Clin Nutr 1975;28:1020–7.

[23] Leray C, Raclot T, Groscolas R. Positional distribution of n-3 fatty acids in triacilglycerols from rat adipose tissue during fish oil feeding. Lipids 1993;4:279–83.

[24] Ostwald R, Okey R, Shannon A, Tinoco J. Changes in tissue lipids in response to diet. I. Fatty acids of subcutaneous, mesenteric and interscapular fat. J Nutr 1962;76:341–52.

[25] Hirsch J, Gallian E. Methods for the determination of adipose cell size in man and animals. J Lipid Res 1968;9:110–9.

[26] Dayton S, Hashimoto S, Dixon W, Pearce ML. Composition of lipids in human serum and adipose tissue during prolonged feedings of a diet high in unsaturated fat. J Lipid Res 1966;7:103–11.

[27] Christakis GJ, Rinzler SH, Archer M, Hashim SA, Van Itallie TB. Effect of serum cholesterol-lowering diet on composition of depot fat in man. Am J Clin Nutr 1965;16:243–51.

[28] Fordyce MK, Christakis G, Kafatos A, Duncan R, Cassadi J. Adipose tissue fatty acid composition of adolescents in a US-Greece cross-cultural study of coronary heart disease risk factors. J Chronic Dis 1983;36:481–6.

[29] Shortland FB, Czochanska Z, Prior IAM. Studies on fatty acid composition of adipose tissue and blood lipids of Polynesians. Am J Clin Nutr 1969;22:594–605.

[30] Sanders TAB, Ellis FR, Path RFC, Dickerson JWT, Biol FI. Studies of vegans: the fatty acid composition of plasma choline phosphoglycerides, eythrocytes, adipose tissue and breast milk, and some indicators of susceptibility to ischemic heart disease in vegans and omnivore controls. Am J Clin Nutr 1978;31:805–13.

[31] Bang HO, Dyerberg J, Hyone N. The composition on food consumed by Greenlandic Eskimos. Acta Med Scand 1976;220:69–73.

[32] Vanschoonbeek K, de Maat MP, Heemskerk JW. Fish oil consumption and reduction of arterial disease. J Nutr 2003;133(3):657–60.

[33] Kim HJ, Takahashi M, Ezaki O. Fish oil feeding decreases mature sterol regulatory element-binding protein 1 (SREBP-1) by down-regulation of SREBP-1c mRNA in mouse liver. J Biol Chem 1999;274:25892–8.

[34] Tsutsumi S, Aburatani H, Ezaki O. Fish oil feeding alters liver gene expressions to defend against PPARα activation and ROS production. Am J Physiol 2002;282:G338–48.

[35] Sethi S, Ziouzenkova O, Ni H, Wagner DD, Plutzky J, Mayadas TN. Oxidized ω-3 fatty acids in fish oil inhibit leukocyte-endothelial interactions through activation of PPARα. Blood 2002;100:1340–6.

[36] Wallace AJ, Humphries SE, Fisher RM, Mann JI, Chisholm A, Sutherland WHF. Genetic factors associated with response of LDL subfractions to change in the nature of dietary fat. Atherosclerosis 2000;149(2):387–94.

[37] Simopoulos AP, Koletzko B, Anderson RE, Hornstra G, Mensink RP, Weksler BB, et al. The 1st congress of the International Society for the Study of Fatty Acids and Lipids (ISSFAL): fatty acids and lipids from cell biology to human disease. J Lipid Res 1994;35:169–73.

[38] Machado RM, Stefano JT, Oliveira CP, Mello ES, Ferreira FD, Nunes VS, et al. Intake of trans fatty acids causes non-alcoholic steatohepatitis and reduces adipose tissue fat content. J Nutr 2010;140(6):1127–32.

[39] Lottenberg AM, Afonso Mda S, Lavrador MS, Machado RM, Nakandakare ER. The role of dietary fatty acids in the pathology of metabolic syndrome. J Nutr Biochem 2012;23(9):1027–40.

[40] Dorfman SE, Laurent D, Gounarides JS, Li X, Mullarkey TL, Rocheford EC, et al. Metabolic implications of dietary trans-fatty acids. Obesity (Silver Spring) 2009;17(6):1200–7. Erratum in: Obesity (Silver Spring) 2009; 17(7):1474

[41] Beynen AC, Hermus RJJ, Hautrast JGAJ. A mathematical relationship between the fatty acid composition of the diet and that of the adipose tissue in man. Am J Clin Nutr 1980;33:81–5.

[42] Hilditch TP. The chemical constitution of natural fats. London: Champman Hall, Ltd; 1949. pp. 65–113.

[43] Brook CGD. Composition of human adipose tissue from deep and subcutaneous sites. Br J Nutr 1970;25:377–80.

[44] Kunešová M, Hlavatý P, Tvrzická E, Staňková B, Kalousková P, Viguerie N, et al. Fatty acid composition of adipose tissue triglycerides after weight loss and weight maintenance: the DIOGENES study. Physiol Res 2012;61(6):597–607.

[45] Kolacynski JW, Morales LM, Moore JH, Considine RV, Pietrzkowski Z, Noto PF, et al. A new technique for biopsy of human abdominal fat under local anaesthesia with lidocaine. Int J Obes 1994;18:161–6.

[46] Kingsbury KJ, Paul S, Crossley A, Morgan DM. The fatty acid composition of human depot fat. Biochem J 1961;78:541.

[47] Malcom GT, Bhattacaryya AK, Vélez-Durán M, Guzmán MA, Oalmann MC, Strong JP. Fatty acid composition of adipose tissue in humans: differences between subcutaneous sites. Am J Clin Nutr 1989;52:486–90.

[48] Field CJ, Ángel A, Clandini MT. Relationship of diet to the fatty acid composition of human adipose tissue storage and structural lipids. Am J Clin Nutr 1985;42:1206–20.

[49] Raclot T, Groscolas R, Langin D, Ferre P. Site-specific regulation of gene expression by n-3 polyunsaturated fatty acids in rat white adipose tissues. J Lipid Res 1997;38:1963–72.

[50] Katan MB, Deslypere JP, Van-Birgelen AP, Penders M, Zegwaard M. Kinetics of the incorporation of dietary fatty acids into serum cholesteryl esters, erythrocyte membranes, and adipose tissue: an 18-month controlled study. J Lipid Res 1997;38:2012–22.

[51] Raclot T, Groscolas R. Individual fish-oil n-3 polyunsaturated fatty acid deposition and mobilization rates for adipose tissue of rats in a nutritional steady state. Am J Clin Nutr 1994;60(1):72–8.

[52] Raclot T, Groscolas R, Leray C. Composition and structure of triacylglycerols in brown adipose tissue of rats fed fish oil. Lipids 1994;29:759–64.

[53] Estrany ME, Proenza AM, Lladó I, Gianotti M. Isocaloric intake of a high-fat diet modifies adiposity and lipid handling in a sex dependent manner in rats. Lipids Health Dis 2011;10:52.

[54] Ali AH, Koutsari C, Mundi M, Heimbach JK, Taler SJ, Nygren J, et al. Free fatty acid storage in human visceral and subcutaneous adipose tissue: role of adipocyte proteins. Diabetes 2011;60(9):2300–7.

[55] Gómez EF, Miyazaki M, Kim YC, Marwah P, Lardy HA, Ntambi JM, et al. Molecular differences caused by differentiation of 3T3-L1 preadipocytes in the presence of either dehydroepiandrosterone (DHEA) or 7-oxo-DHEA. Biochemistry 2002;41:5473–82.

[56] Pérez de Heredia F, Larqué E, Zamora S, Garaulet M. DHEA modifies rat fatty acid composition of serum and different adipose tissue depots towards an insulin-sensitizing profile. J Endocrinol 2009;201:67–74.

[57] Hernandez-Morante JJ, Cerezo D, Cruz RM, Larque E, Zamora S, Garaulet M. Dehydroepiandrosterone-sulfate modifies human fatty acid composition of different adipose tissue depots. Obes Surg 2011;21(1):102–11.

[58] Milagro FI, Gómez-Abellán P, Campión J, Martínez JA, Ordovás JM, Garaulet M. CLOCK, PER2 and BMAL1 DNA methylation: association with obesity and metabolicsyndrome characteristics and monounsaturated fat intake. Chronobiol Int 2012;29(9):1180–94.

[59] Garaulet M, Lee YC, Shen J, Parnell LD, Arnett DK, Tsai MY, et al. CLOCK genetic variation and metabolic syndrome risk:

modulation by monounsaturated fatty acids. Am J Clin Nutr 2009;90(6):1466–75.
[60] Garaulet M, Ordovás JM, Gómez-Abellán P, Martínez JA, Madrid JA. An approximation to the temporal order in endogenous circadian rhythms of genes implicated in human adipose tissue metabolism. J Cell Physiol 2011;226(8):2075–80.
[61] Shostak A, Meyer-Kovac J, Oster H. Circadian regulation of lipid mobilization in white adipose tissues. Diabetes 2013;62(7):2195–203.
[62] Portillo MP, Cantoral R, Torres MI, De-Diego MA, Macarulla MT. Fatty acid profiles in subcutaneous and mesenteric adipose tissues from Zucker rats after energy restriction. Influence of dietary fat. Rev Esp Fisiol 1997;53:317–25.
[63] Letexier D, Pinteur C, Large V, Fréring V, Beylot M. Comparison of the expression and activity of the lipogenic pathway in human and rat adipose tissue. J Lipid Res 2003;44(11):2127–34.
[64] Jones BH, Maher MA, Banz WJ, Zemel MB, Whelan J, Smith PJ, et al. Adipose tissue stearoyl-CoA desaturase mRNA is increased by obesity and decreased by polyunsaturated fatty acids. Am J Physiol 1996;271:E44–9.
[65] Zhou YE, Egeland GM, Meltzer SJ, Kubow S. The association of desaturase 9 and plasma fatty acid composition with insulin resistance-associated factors in female adolescents. Metabolism 2009;58:158–66.
[66] Kunešová M, Phinney S, Hainer V, Tvrzická E, Stich V, Parízková J, et al. The responses of serum and adipose fatty acids to a one-year weight reduction regimen in female obese monozygotic twins. Ann N Y Acad Sci 2002;967:311–23.
[67] Cao H, Gerhold K, Mayers JR, Wiest MM, Watkins SM, Hotamisligil GS. Identification of a lipokine, a lipid hormone linking adipose tissue to systemic metabolism. Cell 2008;134:933–44.
[68] Gong J, Campos H, McGarvey S, Wu Z, Goldberg R, Baylin A. Adipose tissue palmitoleic acid and obesity in humans: does it behave as a lipokine? Am J Clin Nutr 2011;93:186–91.
[69] Garaulet M, Pérez-Llamas F, Tebar FJ, Zamora S. Endocrine, metabolic and nutritional factors in obesity and their relative significance as revealed by factor analysis. Int J Obes 2001;25:243–51.
[70] Hun CS, Hasegawa K, Kawabata T, Kato M, Shimokawa T, Kagawa Y. Increased uncoupling protein 2 mRNA in white adipose tissue, and decrease in leptin, visceral fat, blood glucose, and cholesterol in KK-Ay mice fed with eicosapentaenoic and docosahexaenoic acids in addition to linolenic acid. Biochem Biophys Res Commun 1999;27:85–90.
[71] Garaulet M, Hernández-Morante JJ, Luján J, Tebar FJ, Zamora S. Relationship between fat cell size and number and fatty acid composition in adipose tissue from different fat depots in overweight/obese humans. Int J Obes 2006;30:899–905.
[72] Pérez de Heredia F, Larque E, del Puy Portillo M, Canteras M, Zamora S, Garaulet M. Age-related changes in fatty acids from different adipose depots in rat and their association with adiposity and insulin. Nutrition 2008;24:1013–22.
[73] Bjerregaard P, Jorgensen ME, Andersen S, Mulvad G, Borch-Johnsen K. The Greenland population study. Decreasing overweight and central fat pattering with Westernization among the Inuit in Greenland and Inuit migrants. Int J Obes 2002;26:1503–10.
[74] Le Lay S, Krief S, Farnier C, Lefrère I, Le Liepvre X, Bazin R, et al. Cholesterol, a cell-size dependent signal that regulates glucose metabolism and gene expression in adipocytes. J Biol Chem 2001;276:16904–10.
[75] Trayhurn P, Wood IS. Adipokines: inflammation and the pleiotropic role of white adipose tissue. Br J Nutr 2004;92:347–55.
[76] Alberti KGMM, Zimmet P, Shaw J. The metabolic syndrome—a new worldwide definition. Lancet 2005;366:1059–62. for the IDF Epidemiology Task Force Consensus Group.
[77] Zimmet P, Alberti KGMM, Serrano Ríos M. A new International Diabetes Federation (IDF) worldwide definition of the metabolic syndrome: the rationale and the results. Rev Esp Cardiol 2005;58(12):1371–6.
[78] Kaplan NM. The deadly quartet upper-body obesity, glucose intolerance, hypertriglyceridemia and hypertension. Arch Inter Med 1989;149:1514–20.
[79] Frayn K. Visceral fat in relation to health: is it a major culprit or simply an innocent bystander? Int J Obes 1997;21:1191–2.
[80] Phinney SD, Tang AB, Johnson SB, Holman RT. Reduced adipose 18:3 omega 3 with weight loss by very low calorie dieting. Lipids 1990;25(12):798–806.
[81] Hudgins LC, Hirsch J, Emken EA. Correlation of isomeric fatty acids in human adipose tissue with clinical risk factors for cardiovascular disease. Am J Clin Nutr 1991;53:474–82.
[82] Russell AP. Lipotoxicity: the obese and endurance-trained paradox. Int J Obes Relat Metab Disord 2004;28(Suppl 4):S66–71.
[83] Randle PJ, Garland PB, Hales CN, Newsholme EA. The glucose fatty-acid cycle. Its role in insulin sensitivity and the metabolic disturbances of diabetes mellitus. Lancet 1963;1:785–9.
[84] Roden M, Price TB, Perseghin G, Petersen KF, Rothman DL, Cline GW, et al. Mechanism of free fatty acid-induced insulin resistance in humans. J Clin Invest 1996;97:2859–65.
[85] Tierney AC, Roche HM. The potential role of olive oil-derived MUFA in insulin sensitivity. Mol Nutr Food Res 2007;51:1235–48.
[86] Chavez JA, Summers SA. Characterizing the effects of saturated fatty acids on insulin signaling and ceramide and diacylglycerol accumulation in 3T3-L1 adipocytes and C2C12 myotubes. Arch Biochem Biophys 2003;419(2):101–9.
[87] Sabin MA, Stewart CE, Crowne EC, Turner SJ, Hunt LP, Welsh GI, et al. Fatty acid-induced defects in insulin signalling, in myotubes derived from children, are related to ceramide production from palmitate rather than the accumulation of intramyocellular lipid. J Cell Physiol 2007;211(1):244–52.
[88] Iggman D, Arnlöv J, Vessby B, Cederholm T, Sjögren P, Risérus U. Adipose tissue fatty acids and insulin sensitivity in elderly men. Diabetologia 2010;53(5):850–7.
[89] Perassolo MS, Almeida JC, Steemburgo T, Dall'Alba V, de Mello VD, Zelmanovitz T, et al. Endothelial dysfunction and serum fatty acid composition in patients with type 2 diabetes mellitus. Metabolism 2008;57:1167–72.
[90] Daynes RA, Jones DC. Emerging roles of PPARs in inflammation and immunity. Nat Rev Immunol 2002;2:748–59.
[91] Garaulet M, Pérez-Llamas F, Zamora S, Sánchez de Medina F, Pérez-Ayala M, Martínez P, et al. Adipose tissue and obesity. Reply to HS Kahn and R Valdez. Am J Clin Nutr 2002;75:1124.
[92] Belzung F, Raclot T, Groscolas R. Fish oil n-3 fatty acids selectively limit the hypertrophy of abdominal fat depots in growing rats fed high-fat diets. Am J Physiol 1993;264:R1111–8.
[93] Okuno M, Kajiwara K, Imai S, Kobayashi T, Honma N, Maki T, et al. Perilla oil prevents the excessive growth of visceral adipose tissue in rats by down-regulating adipocyte differentiation. J Nutr 1997;127:1752–7.
[94] Fickova M, Hubert P, Cremel G, Leray C. Dietary (n-3) and (n-6) polyunsaturated fatty acids rapidly modify fatty acid composition and insulin effects in rat adipocytes. J Nutr 1998;128:512–9.
[95] Sessler AM, Ntambi JM. Polyunsaturated fatty acid regulation of gene expression. J Nutr 1998;128:923–6.
[96] Willumsen N, Skorve J, Hexeberg S, Rustan AC, Berge RK. The hypotriglyceridemic effect of eicosapentaenoic acid in rats is reflected in increased mitochondrial fatty acid oxidation followed by diminished lipogenesis. Lipids 1993;28:683–90.
[97] Surette ME, Whelan J, Broughton KS, Kinsella JE. Evidence for mechanisms of hypotriglyceridemic effect of n-3 polyunsaturated fatty acids. Biochim Biophys Acta 1992;1126:199–205.

[98] Azain MJ. Role of fatty acids in adipocyte growth and development. J Anim Sci 2004;82(3):916–24.
[99] Madsen L, Petersen RK, Kristiansen K. Regulation of adipocyte differentiation and function by polyunsaturated fatty acids. Biochim Biophys Acta 2005;1740(2):266–86.
[100] An L, Pang YW, Gao HM, Tao L, Miao K, Wu ZH, et al. Heterologous expression of C. elegans fat-1 decreases the n-6/n-3 fatty acid ratio and inhibits adipogenesis in 3T3-L1 cells. Biochem Biophys Res Commun 2012;428(3):405–10.
[101] Wilding JP. Leptin and the control of obesity. Curr Opin Pharmacol 2001;1:656–61.
[102] Perez-Matute P, Marti A, Martinez JA, Fernández-Otero MP, Stanhope KL, Havel PJ, et al. Eicosapentaenoic fatty acid increases leptin secretion from primary cultured rat adipocytes: role of glucose metabolism. Am J Physiol Regul Integr Comp Physiol 2005;288:R1682–8.
[103] Bueno A, Oyama L, de Oliveira C, Pisani LP, Ribeiro EB, Silveira VL, et al. Effects of different fatty acids and dietary lipids on adiponectin gene expression in 3T3-L1 cells and C57BL/6J mice adipose tissue. Pflügers Archiv—Eur. J Physiol 2008;455:701–9.
[104] Pérez de Heredia F, Sánchez J, Priego T, Larqué E, Portillo MP, Palou A, et al. Adiponectin is associated with serum and adipose tissue fatty acid composition in rats. J Endocrinol Invest 2009;32:659–65.
[105] Hernandez-Morante JJ, Milagro FI, Larque E, Lujan J, Martinez JA, Zamora S, et al. Relationship among adiponectin, adiponectin gene expression and fatty acids composition in morbidly obese patients. Obes Surg 2007;17(4):516–24.
[106] González-Muniesa P, de Oliveira C, Pérez de Heredia F, Thompson MP, Trayhurn P. Fatty acids and hypoxia stimulate the expression and secretion of the adipokine Angpt14 (angiopoietin-like protein 4/fasting-induced adipose factor) from human adipocytes. J Nutrigenet Nutrigenomics 2011;4(3):146–53.
[107] Garaulet M, Pérez de Heredia F. Behavioural therapy in the treatment of obesity (II): role of the Mediterranean diet. Nutr Hosp 2010;25:9–17.

PART J

FIBER AND VISCERAL OBESITY

CHAPTER

42

Using Psyllium to Prevent and Treat Obesity Comorbidities

Sebely Pal, Simone Radavelli-Bagatini, Suleen Ho, Jenny-Lee McKay, and Monica Jane

School of Public Health, Curtin Health Innovation Research Institute, Curtin University of Technology, Perth, Western Australia, Australia

INTRODUCTION

Overweight and obesity are some of today's most visible public health problems; there is an escalating global epidemic [1], with approximately 1.5 billion adults being overweight [2] and 300 million being obese [3]. In recent years, obesity has superseded malnutrition in becoming the predominant public health issue [4]. Being obese significantly increases the risk of developing metabolic syndrome (MS), which is associated with increased cardiovascular morbidity and mortality, and has been implicated in the development of atherosclerosis [5].

MS consists of a combination of different abnormalities [6], such as glucose intolerance, insulin resistance, abdominal obesity, atherogenic dyslipidemia, impaired endothelial function, hypertension, and inflammation [7]. The prevalence of MS is quoted as 34% according to National Health and Nutrition Examination Survey (NHANES) 2003–2006 figures; however, the prevalence of MS is approaching 50% worldwide [8]. The risk of having a heart attack or stroke is three times more likely and the risk of developing type 2 diabetes mellitus (T2DM) is five times more likely with MS compared to those without MS [9].

Epidemiological and cohort studies have consistently revealed that higher fiber intakes produce health benefits and a consequent risk reduction for MS, cardiovascular disease (CVD), and type 2 diabetes mellitus (T2DM) resulting from a lower body weight, lower body mass index (BMI), lower waist circumference [10,11], improved plasma lipid profiles [12–21], and improved glycemia and insulinemia [22]. Current dietary fiber recommendations for adults in Australia, Canada, the United States, and Europe are 25–30 g/day; to be achieved by consuming fiber-rich foods such as fruit, vegetables, legumes, and whole grains [23]. However, it is estimated that the intake of fiber in the United States and many other developed countries is around 15 g/day [24], only half the amount recommended by the American Heart Association [23]. Although the benefits of fiber are well known, most find it difficult to eat the required amounts of fiber by increasing fruit and vegetable intake, as shown by the Continuing Survey of Food Intakes by Individuals 1994–96, 1998 [25,26]. Therefore, fiber supplements may provide a cost-effective and easy alternative for increasing the fiber content of a diet, without the need for other major dietary modifications.

Psyllium seed husk is a viscous, water-soluble fiber supplement [27]. It is one of the most widely used fiber supplements in the world, because it is reasonably cheap, available in several flavors, and sold as powdered drink mixes, capsules, or wafers. Psyllium is better tolerated than other fiber supplements because it causes less abdominal bloating; thus, it has advantages over other types of soluble fiber [27]. Psyllium has been shown to be an effective adjunct to dietary intervention in the control of body weight, body composition, cholesterol, glucose, insulin, and triglyceride (TG) levels both in animal [28–30] and human studies [31–36]. Therefore, the aim of this chapter is to review the benefits of psyllium fiber on several components of MS, such as body weight, body composition, satiety, glucose and insulin homeostasis, lipids and lipoproteins, blood pressure, and vascular function.

Nutrition in the Prevention and Treatment of Abdominal Obesity
http://dx.doi.org/10.1016/B978-0-12-407869-7.00032-5

PSYLLIUM AND HEALTH

Dietary fiber is an edible component of all plants that is defined as being resistant to digestion and absorption in the small intestine; it usually undergoes partial or complete fermentation in the large intestine [37,38].

Psyllium is a well-established blood cholesterol-lowering agent and bowel regulator [39,40]. These physiological benefits are thought to be due to its composition: it is a soluble gel-forming mucilage from the *Plantago ovata* plant, the bioactive fraction of which is a fiber composed of highly branched arabinoxylan [27], in which xylose forms the backbone, and arabinose and xylose form the side chains. Psyllium causes less flatulence and abdominal distending because it is less readily fermented than other fiber types [27]. Interestingly, a study in rats showed that arabinose undergoes less fermentation in comparison to xylose [41]. Arabinose digestibility was also found to be lower than xylose digestibility in human studies of psyllium [42,43]. Thus, it seems that the linear chain of psyllium is fermented until an atypical branch point (that is unavailable to microbial activity) is reached [42]; this explains why it is less completely fermented than other fibers, thus causing less gastrointestinal issues.

BODY COMPOSITION AND APPETITE

Improvements in body weight have been linked to psyllium in animal studies [28]; however, this issue is still controversial in humans [35,36,44–48]. Galisteo et al. observed that Zucker rats (a model for T2DM) fed a psyllium-supplemented diet for 25 weeks had a significantly reduced body weight gain compared with those fed a standard diet [28]. Results of a parallel-design study by Pal et al. are in agreement with these data [35]. Investigators compared the effects of four different diets in obese adults with an average BMI of 34 kg/m^2: a control diet (with placebo), a control diet supplemented with 21 g of psyllium (FIB), a healthy diet plus placebo (HLT), and a healthy diet supplemented with 21 g of psyllium (HLT-FIB) [35]. They found that both diets containing psyllium (FIB and HLT-FIB) significantly reduced body weight (−2.1 kg, $P=0.007$ and −2.6 kg, $P<0.001$, respectively), and percentage total body fat (−2.3%, $P=0.002$ and −2.7%, $P<0.001$, respectively) compared to the control diet after 12 weeks [35].

In contrast, a study of 83 normal-weight subjects randomized to receive placebo or 16.5 g Minolest (containing 16% guar gum and 62% psyllium as the principal active ingredients,) per day for 3 months found no differences in body weight and BMI between the two treatments [47]. The lack of weight loss in the latter four studies may be related to the fact that the participants were in the healthy weight range or only slightly overweight. However, another study found some improvements in BMI after 6 months of 10.5 g/day of either psyllium or guar fiber supplementation compared with a standard diet in hypertensive, slightly overweight individuals [33]. In the psyllium-treated patients, the BMI decrease was statistically significant after 4 months of supplementation (−0.8 ± 0.2), and continued up to 6 months (−2.0 ± 0.3) [33]. In the guar-treated patients, the BMI decrease was already statistically significant after the first 2 months of supplementation (−0.9 ± 0.2) and it progressively continued up to 6 months (−1.8 ± 0.3) [33]. In addition, a randomized crossover design study for 3 weeks separated by a 2-week washout period compared the effects of low-viscosity wheat bran at 10.8 g/day, medium-viscosity psyllium at 9 g/day, and a high-viscosity fiber blend at 5.1 g/day in 23 healthy-weight participants with an average BMI of 23.8 ± 4.6 kg/m^2 [48]. This study found no differences among the treatments in the amount of food consumed, total dietary fiber intake, reported physical activity, and body weight [48]. A double-blind placebo-controlled study, which included 125 normal-weight and overweight patients with T2DM, showed no significant changes in body weight in either the low-fat diet plus 15 g/day psyllium or the low-fat diet plus placebo after a 6-week period [46]. Another study showed no significant changes in BMI in slightly overweight type 2 diabetics with an average BMI of 26.7 kg/m^2 following the consumption for 8 weeks of 10.2 g/day of psyllium compared to placebo [36].

The role of psyllium in appetite control has been investigated but the findings are inconsistent [49,50]. Dietary protein is thought to be the most satiating macronutrient compared with others such as fat or carbohydrate [51–54]; however, psyllium fiber may also possess satiating qualities. Female subjects were randomized to one of three treatment groups: psyllium (20 g granules with 200 mL water), placebo (20 g granules with 200 mL water), or plain water (200 mL), 3 h before meals and the same dose immediately after meals [50]. Psyllium consumption significantly increased fullness (measured using visual analog scales) 1 h postmeal compared to both placebo and water groups ($P<0.05$). The authors concluded that psyllium may be a useful supplement in weight control diets because it affects fat intake and may affect subjective feelings of fullness [50].

Fiber-enriched meals have also been shown to significantly decrease ghrelin and peptide YY (PYY) appetite hormone responses in healthy subjects compared to protein-enriched meals [49]. Interestingly, a study showed postprandial ratings of appetite to be similar after meals supplemented with either psyllium fiber or protein [49]. Psyllium has been shown to produce a greater suppression of snack intake compared with wheat bran in a study that compared the effects on short-term (24-h) appetite of three isocaloric breakfasts containing high-insoluble fiber cereal (22 g total: 4.4 g psyllium and 17.6 g wheat bran), high-soluble fiber cereal (22 g total: 17.6 g psyllium and 4.4 g wheat bran), or a low-fiber cereal (3 g; 1.5 g of both soluble and insoluble fiber) in healthy, normal-weight males after an overnight fast [55]. However, there was no significant effect of breakfast type on total daily energy intake [55]; although appetite seems to decrease after the consumption of psyllium, this effect does not appear to differ from those of other sources of fiber [50,55].

The mechanisms through which dietary fiber, including psyllium, can affect weight loss, appetite, and energy intake include its effects on gastric emptying [56], satiety [57], and gut hormones such as cholecystokinin [58], as well as alterations to glycemic index or insulin response [59]. The act of chewing takes longer when consuming fiber-rich foods, which may increase sensory satiety and diminish meal size [60–62]. Dietary fiber reduces the energy density of foods, which may directly moderate energy intake and indirectly decrease appetite [63]. Another mechanism to explain the satiating power of psyllium includes the role of fiber in decreasing intestinal passage rates, which leads to prolonged nutrient absorption and, consequently, increased satiety [64]. Soluble fiber ferments in the large intestine, thus increasing the concentration of short-chain fatty acids that may enhance satiety [65]. In addition, fiber has also been suggested to decrease energy absorption by lowering the bioavailability of fatty acids and proteins [66]. The effects of fiber-rich diets on appetite control, energy intake, and body weight may be related to the chemical structure of the fiber and its physicochemical properties such as solubility, viscosity, water-holding capacity, and fermentability, rather than on the amount of fiber ingested [61,67].

While psyllium fiber seems to improve body weight in animals [28], the lack of a significant change in body weight in many of the human studies may be due to the fact that most of the participants had a healthy starting weight; however, weight loss has been observed in studies with obese participants. In addition, the controls in many of these studies varied, including a standard or low-fat diet plus placebo, placebo only, or even antidiabetic drugs, thus making it difficult to unravel the true effect of psyllium on body weight alone due to confounding effects of the background diet. In addition, a variety of studies designs have been used. Further, no trials have examined the additional effects of psyllium supplementation and a weight loss diet on body composition. The duration of consumption also varied greatly in the studies described above, from 3 weeks to 6 months [33,36,46–48], which may be related to the differing outcomes. The amount of psyllium supplementation also needs to be considered because many of the highlighted studies report no change in body weight with doses below 15 g/day psyllium supplementation.

Therefore, future weight loss studies with psyllium need to consider the starting weight or BMI of individuals because this may be a limiting factor on the magnitude of weight loss. Again, future studies could consider including psyllium supplementation with and without a hypocaloric diet. In addition, doses higher than 15 g/day need to be considered in future trials. Out of all the papers cited in this section, the work published by Pal seems to be the strongest overall in terms of research design, duration, and number of cases, thus strengthening our suggestion that psyllium supplement could improve body composition in overweight and obese people [35].

BLOOD SUGAR LEVELS AND INSULIN REGULATION

Psyllium intake has been shown to improve glucose and insulin responses in animal [28,30] and human studies [35,36,50,68]. The effects of psyllium supplementation on peripheral insulin sensitivity and skeletal muscle solute carrier family 2, facilitated glucose transporter member 4 (GLUT4) protein expression were studied in male, stroke-prone, spontaneously hypertensive rats fed a hypercaloric diet from 5 to 9 weeks of age. An oral glucose tolerance test showed that fasting plasma glucose was significantly reduced in the psyllium-supplemented group compared to the cellulose-supplemented group.

A study in individuals with T2DM included three phases: phase 1 (1 week, subjects followed a diet designed for diabetes and received the diabetes medication, sulfonylurea); phase 2 (6 weeks, patients continued with both the diet and sulfonylurea and also received 14 g/day psyllium fiber); and phase 3 (4 weeks, subjects followed the diet for diabetes and received sulfonylurea) [68]. A clinical evaluation was performed at the end of each phase after the ingestion of a test breakfast of 436 kcal (1824 kJ). Psyllium supplementation significantly decreased postprandial blood glucose by 12.2% and 11.9% in phase 2, compared to the results at the end of phases 1 and 3, respectively [68]. However, this reduction was not associated with a change in insulin levels (5%) [68]. Psyllium supplementation at 10.2 g/day for 8 weeks significantly improved glucose and glycated hemoglobin (HbA1c) in individuals with T2DM, compared to a placebo [36]. Human studies support the results of animal studies. In one study, 16 healthy, nonobese participants were randomized to one of the following five isocaloric test meals: (1) low in protein (2.8 g) and fiber (7.6 g); (2) low in protein (2.6 g) and high in soluble fiber (23 g psyllium); (3) high in protein (19.7 g soy) and low in fiber (6.2 g); (4) high in protein (18.4 g) and soluble fiber (23 g psyllium); and (5) white wheat bread [49]. Psyllium fiber-enriched meals significantly decreased glucose and insulin compared to non-fiber-enriched meals [49]. A study by Pal et al. showed that insulin levels were significantly decreased in a group of overweight subjects consuming a healthy diet with a daily addition of 21 g psyllium compared to a control group after 6 and 12 weeks of intervention [35]. However, glucose levels were not significantly different between the groups [35]. Another study showed that the oral ingestion of 10.5 g/day psyllium or guar gum powder for 6 months significantly improved glucose and insulin concentrations, as well as the homeostatic model assessment of insulin resistance (HOMA-IR) index in hypertensive overweight adults [33], suggesting that longer time frames may be required to see improvements.

The glucose-reducing action of psyllium is proposed to result from the formation of a viscous gel in aqueous solution. This gel may hinder the access of glucose to the absorptive epithelium of the small intestine, thereby blunting postprandial glucose peaks [69]. In addition, soluble fiber may delay gastric emptying, thus slowing carbohydrate uptake [70]. Another mechanism that may contribute to the postprandial effect of psyllium is the sequestration of carbohydrates ingested with the meal, thus retarding their access to digestive enzymes [71].

The trials cited above included overweight and obese individuals, subjects with hypertension or T2DM, and even healthy adults. In addition, many of these studies have used a great variety of control groups, including placebo, placebo in combination with antidiabetic drugs, or a standard diet (not specified) [33,35,36,68]. The trial periods ranged from 6 weeks to 6 months [33,35,36,68]. A dose of 10–14 g/day psyllium reduced glucose levels over a period of 6–8 weeks [36,68]. Interestingly, reductions in plasma insulin levels seemed to require a greater dose of around 21–23 g/day, as seen in studies with test meals [49], or an intervention of at least 12 weeks at this dose [35]. One 6-month study suggested that a longer period of psyllium supplementation may be necessary to improve both glucose and insulin levels at a lower dose of 10 g/day [33].

Overall, psyllium seems to improve glucose levels and the insulin response in most animal and human studies reported so far. The mechanisms responsible for these effects may be related to the prevention of glucose peaks, delay of gastric emptying, and delayed carbohydrate access to digestive enzymes.

BLOOD LIPIDS

Recently, human and animal models have indicated that psyllium fiber may provide cardiovascular benefits [28,33,35,36,47,55]. Increasing dietary fiber intake may elicit favorable changes in circulating lipid and lipoprotein levels, including reductions in low-density lipoprotein (LDL), serum TG, and total serum cholesterol levels, as well as an increase in high-density lipoprotein (HDL) concentrations, all of which are independent risk factors for CVD.

An animal study showed that a psyllium-supplemented diet for 25 weeks significantly reduced plasma concentrations of TG, total cholesterol, and free fatty acids in Zucker rats compared with those fed the standard diet [28]. A meta-analysis conducted to determine the effect of consuming psyllium-enriched cereal products (the amount of psyllium soluble fiber ranged from 3–12 g/day) for a period of 14–56 days (mean, 42 days) on lipid and lipoprotein levels in 404 adults with mild-to-moderate hypercholesterolemia, who consumed a low-fat diet included eight published and four unpublished studies conducted in four countries [72]. It showed that subjects who consumed psyllium cereal had lower total cholesterol and LDL concentrations than did subjects who consumed the control cereal; however, LDL concentrations were unaffected [72]. The authors concluded that consuming psyllium-enriched cereal as part of a low-fat diet improves the blood lipid profile of hypercholesterolemic adults over that which can be achieved with a low-fat diet alone [72]. A study of overweight and obese men evaluated the postprandial effects of consuming a low-fiber meal containing 3 g of psyllium versus a high-fiber meal containing 15 g of psyllium, and observed a significantly lower TG concentration after consumption of the high-fiber meal during a 6-h postprandial period, compared with the low-fiber meal [34]. The plasma concentration of apolipoprotein B48 (ApoB48; a marker for TG-rich chylomicrons) was significantly lower after the consumption of a high-fiber meal after the first hour of the postprandial period [34]. The authors suggest that a single acute dose of dietary fiber in the form of a psyllium supplement can decrease arterial exposure to TG and modify chylomicron responses in the postprandial period [34]. According to the U.S. Food and Drug Administration (FDA), the consumption of a 1.78-g serving of psyllium four times a day can improve lipid levels, thereby reducing cardiovascular risk factors [73]. Jenkins et al. assessed the efficacy of this dose of fiber in reducing serum lipid risk factors for CVD in 68 hyperlipidemic adults, who consumed a test diet (4 servings of high-fiber foods per day: 1.8–2.5 g psyllium or 0.75 g β-glucan per serving, which delivered 8 g/day more soluble fiber than the control diet) and a control low-fat, low-cholesterol diet for 1 month each in a randomized crossover study [74]. Compared with the control diet, the psyllium-enriched diet reduced total cholesterol, total cholesterol:HDL ratio, LDL:HDL ratio, and ApoB:ApoA-I ratio, thus confirming a reduction of cardiovascular risk of 4.2% ± 1.4% by the Framingham equation [74]. The investigators concluded that the reduction in serum lipid risk factors for CVD supports the FDA's approval of a health claim for a dietary fiber intake of 4 servings/day [74]. At the end of a 6-week study which included the consumption of 14 g/day of psyllium by individuals with T2DM, total cholesterol and LDL levels significantly decreased (by 7.7% and 9.2%, respectively) [68]. Another study found that a 10.2-g psyllium treatment over 8 weeks significantly increased HDL levels and decreased the LDL:HDL ratio in individuals with T2DM [36]. A double-blind, placebo-controlled parallel study of 26 men with mild-to-moderate hypercholesterolemia that involved following their usual diets with 3.4 g of psyllium or cellulose placebo at mealtimes (three times a day) for 8 weeks found that psyllium reduced total serum cholesterol levels by 14.8%, LDL levels by 20.2%, and LDL:HDL ratio by 14.8% relative to baseline values [31]. Pal et al. demonstrated that adding psyllium fiber supplementation (21 g/day) to a normal diet was sufficient to see improvements in total cholesterol and LDL cholesterol in overweight and obese individuals, compared with control, after 12 weeks [35]. Cholesterol levels in the fiber only, healthy diet, and healthy diet plus psyllium groups were lower by 21%, 19%, and 20%, respectively, at week 12 compared with the control group; however, there were no significant differences between groups. The LDL level was lower after the 12-week intervention in the three groups by 29%, 24%, and 28%, respectively, compared with the control group. Thus, a high-fiber diet consisting of a psyllium supplement plus the fiber present in a healthy diet provided the greatest improvements in MS risk factors. A randomized, placebo-controlled, double-blind, parallel-group study assessed the effect of Minolest on the lipid profile and obesity [47]: 83 subjects were randomized to receive placebo or 16.5 g/day of Minolest for 3 months. Minolest produced a 3.24% decrease in total cholesterol and a 5.45% decrease in LDL but no significant difference in serum TG compared to the placebo group [47]. Psyllium supplementation at 10.5 g/day for 6 months led to a significant improvement in plasma TG concentration (of 13.3%) but did not affect LDL levels (compared to guar gum supplementation) in hypertensive overweight adults [33]. Another meta-analysis of eight studies looked at the effects of psyllium in an attempt to more precisely define the hypolipidemic effects and safety of psyllium when used as an adjunct to a low-fat diet in men and women with hypercholesterolemia [39]. All studies evaluated the hypocholesterolemic effects of 10.2 g/day psyllium as adjunctive to a low-fat diet in individuals with mild-to-moderate hypercholesterolemia for ≥8 weeks. The meta-analysis found that the consumption of 10.2 g/day of psyllium lowered total serum cholesterol by 4%, LDL by 7%, and the ApoB:ApoA-I ratio by 6% relative to a placebo, but had no effect on serum LDL or TG concentrations [39].

Three major hypotheses have frequently been postulated to explain the cholesterol-lowering action of soluble dietary fiber, including psyllium [39,75,76]. First, the digestion of macronutrients is delayed by viscous soluble fiber, which slows gastric emptying, thus decreasing the transport and mixing of digestive enzymes, and increasing the resistance of the unstirred water layer lining the mucosa to intestinal absorption [77]. This can lead to a reduced glycemic response due to a reduction in glucose absorption [78] and a subsequent decrease in postprandial glucose levels, which is accompanied by a reduction in insulin levels [79]. Decreased insulin levels can then result in the inhibition of 3-hydroxy-3-methylglutaryl-coenzyme A reductase (HMG-CoA reductase) and a subsequent reduction in hepatic cholesterol synthesis [80]. Second, the presence of soluble fiber in the small intestine may physically prevent bile salt reabsorption into the enterohepatic circulation, resulting in increased fecal bile salt excretion [81,82]. This may deplete bile salt in the liver, causing cholesterol to be rapidly catabolized in hepatocytes to replenish the bile salt pool via activation of cholesterol 7-alpha-monooxygenase. In addition, there is increased production of LDL surface membrane receptors, thus enhancing LDL uptake from the bloodstream and consequently lowering cholesterol levels [83]. Third, fiber reduces hepatic cholesterol synthesis that is modulated by fermentation products, such as propionate, leading to decreased cholesterol absorption and bile acid reabsorption by physically disrupting the intraluminal formation of micelles [44,84]. It is well known that soluble dietary fibers are not digested or absorbed in the small intestine, but instead undergo anaerobic bacterial fermentation in the cecum and colon to produce short-chain fatty acids [85]. Short-chain fatty acids, particularly propionate, seem to deplete plasma cholesterol by inhibiting hepatic cholesterol metabolism via mechanisms that include reducing HMG-CoA receptor activity [45] and inhibiting of acetyl-CoA reductase, which catalyzes the synthesis of acetyl-CoA from acetate.

Overall, psyllium seems to improve the lipid profile of both animals and humans, thereby reducing cardiovascular risk factors. Psyllium seems to improve lipids and lipoproteins regardless of the dose and period of the studies (i.e. 10–20 g/day psyllium for 6 weeks to 6 months). Subjects in the studies discussed were overweight or obese, or had T2DM, hypertension, hypercholesterolemia, or hyperlipidemia. However, these health conditions did not seem to affect the results of the studies. Additionally, although a range of control diets was used, study outcomes consistently showed improved lipid profiles following psyllium consumption. Although the mechanism responsible for effects of fiber on lipids and lipoproteins is still being studied, it seems to be mainly mediated by excess bile salt secretion, which reduces plasma cholesterol.

VASCULAR FUNCTION

The augmentation index (AI) is an indicator of arterial stiffness that has been shown to be higher in those with hypercholesterolemia [86]. It has been suggested that an increase in arterial stiffness is associated with increased systolic (SBP) and diastolic blood pressure (DBP) [87–89]. Arterial stiffness is one of the major risk factors of CVD [90], presenting an independent risk factor for this condition [90,91]. Arterial stiffness is an age-related phenomenon [88,92] and its progression is faster in patients exhibiting MS criteria [92–94], luminal enlargement resulting from wall thickening (remodeling), and a loss of flexibility (stiffening) at the level of the large elastic arteries, namely *arteriosclerosis* [95]. Individuals with MS [96], hypertension [97], or diabetes [98] exhibit increased carotid wall thickness and stiffness; this "accelerated" arterial aging is a well-established risk factor for CVD [99].

An inverse relationship exists between healthy eating and arterial stiffness [98]. However, the specific role of dietary fiber in preventing and improving arterial stiffness in both the short and long term has yet to be fully elucidated. Endothelial function has an important role in regulating blood pressure and vascular resistance [99]. The hypotensive effect of psyllium has been attributed, at least in part, to its ability to inhibit intestinal sodium absorption and improve endothelial function by improving hyperlipidemia and decreasing inflammatory markers [29]. Only one study so far, by Pal et al., has measured the effect of psyllium on arterial stiffness [89]. In this study, the psyllium-supplemented group did present with a lower AI compared with the control group, but this result did not persist until the end of the study at week 12 [89]. Mechanisms that involve lipid lowering may explain the effects of fiber on blood pressure and vascular function.

Collectively, the studies mentioned above, which included hypertensive, non-hypertensive, hyperlipidemic or hypercholesterolemic adults, reported no change in blood pressure compared to the control groups. In these studies, the control groups had a standard diet, a low-fat diet, or placebo. The amount of psyllium in these studies ranged from 7 to 21 g/day and interventions were from 8 to 12 weeks. Only one study found a reduction in both SBP and DBP in hypertensive adults after supplementation with 10.5 g/day psyllium. Overall, increasing psyllium intake may promote a reduction in blood pressure and vascular function; however, this is still unconfirmed. The effect of psyllium might depend on the dose and duration of the treatment, as well as the baseline blood pressure of individuals. Therefore, future studies examining the effect of psyllium supplementation on hypertension should use high doses (21 g/day) in hypertensive individuals consuming their usual diet to reduce the confounding effects of background diets.

Animal [28,29] and human [32,33] studies have demonstrated that dietary fiber intake may be inversely related to blood pressure levels, and may therefore decrease the risk of hypertension. Accordingly, the World Health Organization has recommended an increase in dietary fiber as a safe and practical approach to CVD risk reduction in the hypertensive population [100].

Animal studies suggest that psyllium [28,29] and high-fiber diets [101] decrease blood pressure in hypertensive and obese rats. Consumption of a fiber-supplemented diet containing 3.5% psyllium for 25 weeks improved SBP and endothelial function in obese Zucker rats [28]. Salt-accelerated hypertension was also observed to be significantly attenuated in stroke-prone, spontaneously hypertensive rats supplemented with 3% and 10% psyllium for 30 days [29].

In a 6-month study, psyllium fiber supplementation at 10.5 g/day appeared to significantly reduce both SBP and DBP in overweight, hypertensive subjects [33]. This effect was not observed with guar gum fiber or a standard diet. Another study showed that dietary protein (soy) and soluble fiber (15 g/day psyllium) supplementation for 8 weeks additively lowered blood pressure in hypertensive individuals [32], but there was no difference between the interventions. This result is consistent with another study of hyperlipidemic adults, which observed a slight reduction in both SBP and DBP after high-fiber diet (7.2 g of psyllium and 0.75 g/day of β-glucan) and a control low-fat diet after 1 month. However, the results were not significantly different between groups [74]. Interestingly, a randomized parallel-design study by Pal et al. did not find any improvements in blood pressure or vascular function in nonhypertensive overweight and obese individuals with psyllium fiber supplementation of 21 g/day for 12 weeks [102]. A randomized placebo-controlled, double-blind, parallel-group study with 83 subjects with mild hypercholesterolemia found no significant difference in blood pressure after a 3-month intervention with 16.5 g/day Minolest compared to a placebo group [47]. These differing outcomes indicate that further research in hypertensive individuals may be necessary to elucidate whether psyllium supplementation reduces blood pressure and improves vascular function.

The precise mechanism by which psyllium consumption may regulate blood pressure is currently unclear. It has been shown that high serum cholesterol impairs endothelium-dependent dilation [103] via blood pressure regulation [104]. Interestingly, many hypertensive patients also appear to have increased serum cholesterol levels [105]. However, whether this is only a correlation or whether it represents a pathophysiological link is still under discussion [104]. Hypercholesterolemia is associated with a loss of nitric oxide-induced vasodilation [106] and a subsequent increase in blood pressure [107].

Evidence suggests that cholesterol induces endothelial dysfunction even at normal or high-to-normal ranges by reducing the bioavailability of endothelium-derived nitric oxide [103,106]. Higher cholesterol levels may also be associated with increased numbers of atherosclerotic vessels through an increase in intima media thickness, not only in the carotid circulation but also in other arteries [104]. In addition, water-soluble fiber seems to reduce insulin resistance [108,109], which is thought to be involved in the development of hypertension [110].

Other mechanisms have been hypothesized to account for the effects of dietary fiber intake on blood pressure. Dietary fiber can lower the glycemic index of foods through its effects on the digestion and absorption of foods, thereby altering the insulin response. Insulin plays a role in blood pressure regulation, and dietary fiber can modify insulin levels and vascular endothelial function [111]. Insulin resistance and its concomitant compensatory hyperinsulinemia are suggested to be major underlying pathogenic mechanisms for the development of hypertension [112]. In this way, the effectiveness of both soluble and insoluble fiber in reducing insulin levels, as well as insulin resistance, in both diabetic and healthy persons [113,114] could contribute to the treatment or prevention of hypertension.

CONCLUSION

Research to date supports the notion that the consumption of psyllium may provide benefits to many components of MS. Psyllium supplementation improves glucose levels and the insulin response as well as the lipid profile in both animals and humans, thereby reducing metabolic risk factors. Increasing psyllium intake may also promote a reduction in blood pressure and vascular function; however, this could depend on the dose and duration of the treatment as well as the baseline blood pressure of individuals. Appetite has been reported to decrease after the consumption of psyllium but this effect seems to be similar to that of other sources of fiber [49,50,55]. Psyllium fiber seems to improve body weight in animals [28], but human studies are still inconsistent on this issue, with most studies showing no improvement in body weight and body composition after psyllium consumption [36,46–48]. However, this may be either a dose-related issue or related to the fact that most studies have been conducted in normal-weight or slightly overweight individuals.

CONFLICT OF INTEREST STATEMENT

The authors have no conflict of interest to declare in relation to this manuscript.

Acknowledgments

Dr Pal participated in the conception, design, writing, and critical revision of this chapter. Dr Radavelli-Bagatini participated in the writing and revision of this chapter. Dr Ho, Mrs McKay, Dr Hagger and Ms Jane participated in the revision of this chapter.

References

[1] World Health Organization, WHO. Nutrition: Controlling the global obesity epidemic. <http://www.who.int/nutrition/topics/obesity/en/>; 2002 [accessed 1.10.13].
[2] WHO. Obesity: preventing and managing the global epidemic. Report of a WHO consultation. World Health Organ Tech Rep Ser 2000;894(i–xii):1–253.
[3] Wilborn C, Beckham J, Campbell B, et al. Obesity: prevalence, theories, medical consequences, management, and research directions. J Int Soc Sports Nutr 2005;2:4–31.
[4] Mokdad AH, Ford ES, Bowman BA, et al. Prevalence of obesity, diabetes, and obesity-related health risk factors, 2001. Jama 2003;289:76–9.
[5] Cook S, Hugli O, Egli M, et al. Clustering of cardiovascular risk factors mimicking the human metabolic syndrome X in eNOS null mice. Swiss Med Weekly 2003;133:360–3.
[6] Isomaa B, Almgren P, Tuomi T, et al. Cardiovascular morbidity and mortality associated with the metabolic syndrome. Diabetes care 2001;24:683–9.
[7] Grundy SM. Obesity, metabolic syndrome, and cardiovascular disease. J Clin Endocrinol Metab 2004;89:2595–600.
[8] Kones R. Primary prevention of coronary heart disease: integration of new data, evolving views, revised goals, and role of rosuvastatin in management. A comprehensive survey. Drug Des Devel Ther 2011;5:325–80.
[9] Alberti KG, Zimmet P, Shaw J. Metabolic syndrome—a new world-wide definition. A consensus statement from the international diabetes federation. Diabet Med 2006;23:469–80.
[10] Du H, van der AD, Boshuizen HC, et al. Dietary fiber and subsequent changes in body weight and waist circumference in European men and women. Am J Clin Nutr 2010;91:329–36.
[11] Newby PK, Maras J, Bakun P, Muller D, Ferrucci L, Tucker KL. Intake of whole grains, refined grains, and cereal fiber measured with 7-d diet records and associations with risk factors for chronic disease. Am J Clin Nutr 2007;86:1745–53.
[12] NHMRC. Dietary guidelines for Australian adults. National Health and Medical Research Council; Canberra: Commonwealth of Australia 2003.
[13] Wu H, Dwyer KM, Fan Z, Shircore A, Fan J, Dwyer JH. Dietary fiber and progression of atherosclerosis: the los angeles atherosclerosis study. Am J Clin Nutr 2003;78:1085–91.
[14] Lairon D. Macronutrient intake and modulation on chylomicron production and clearance. Atheroscler Suppl 2008;9:45–8.
[15] Kan H, Stevens J, Heiss G, Klein R, Rose KM, London SJ. Dietary fiber intake and retinal vascular caliber in the atherosclerosis risk in communities study. Am J Clin Nutr 2007;86:1626–32.
[16] Lairon D, Arnault N, Bertrais S, et al. Dietary fiber intake and risk factors for cardiovascular disease in French adults. Am J Clin Nutr 2005;82:1185–94.
[17] Venn BJ, Mann JI. Cereal grains, legumes and diabetes. Eur J Clin Nutr 2004;58:1443–61.
[18] Weickert MO, Pfeiffer AF. Metabolic effects of dietary fiber consumption and prevention of diabetes. J Nutr 2008;138:439–42.
[19] McKeown NM, Meigs JB, Liu S, Wilson PW, Jacques PF. Wholegrain intake is favorably associated with metabolic risk factors for type 2 diabetes and cardiovascular disease in the framingham offspring study. Am J Clin Nutr 2002;76:390–8.

[20] Brown L, Rosner B, Willett WW, Sacks FM. Cholesterol-lowering effects of dietary fiber: a meta-analysis. Am J Clin Nutr 1999;69:30–42.
[21] Pittler MH, Ernst E. Guar gum for body weight reduction: meta-analysis of randomized trials. Am J Med 2001;110:724–30.
[22] Ludwig DS, Pereira MA, Kroenke CH, et al. Dietary fiber, weight gain, and cardiovascular disease risk factors in young adults. Jama 1999;282:1539–46.
[23] Marlett JA, McBurney MI, Slavin JL. Position of the American dietetic association: health implications of dietary fiber. J Am Diet Assoc 2002;102:993–1000.
[24] Alaimo K, McDowell MA, Briefel RR, et al. Dietary intake of vitamins, minerals, and fiber of persons ages 2 months and over in the United States: third national health and nutrition examination survey, Phase 1, 1988–91. Adv Data 1994:1–28.
[25] CSFII. Continuing survey of food intakes by individuals (CSFII) 1994–96, 98. Agricultural Research Services, US Department of Agriculture. <http://sodapop.pop.psu.edu/data-collections/csfii>; 2000 [accessed 22.10.13].
[26] IOM . Dietary, functional, and total fiber. DRI: dietary reference intakes for energy, carbohydrate, fiber, fat, fatty acids, cholesterol, protein, and amino acids food and nutrition board 2005:339–421.
[27] Blackwood AD, Salter J, Dettmar PW, Chaplin MF. Dietary fiber, physicochemical properties and their relationship to health. J R Soc Promot Health 2000;120:242–7.
[28] Galisteo M, Sanchez M, Vera R, et al. A diet supplemented with husks of *Plantago ovata* reduces the development of endothelial dysfunction, hypertension, and obesity by affecting adiponectin and TNF-α in obese Zucker rats. J Nutr 2005;135:2399–404.
[29] Obata K, Ikeda K, Yamasaki M, Yamori Y. Dietary fiber, psyllium, attenuates salt-accelerated hypertension in stroke-prone spontaneously hypertensive rats. J Hypertens 1998;16:1959–64.
[30] Song YJ, Sawamura M, Ikeda K, Igawa S, Yamori Y. Soluble dietary fiber improves insulin sensitivity by increasing muscle GLUT-4 content in stroke-prone spontaneously hypertensive rats. Clin Exp Pharmacol Physiol 2000;27:41–5.
[31] Anderson JW, Zettwoch N, Feldman T, Tietyen-Clark J, Oeltgen P, Bishop CW. Cholesterol-lowering effects of psyllium hydrophilic mucilloid for hypercholesterolemic men. Arch Intern Med 1988;148:292–6.
[32] Burke V, Hodgson JM, Beilin LJ, Giangiulioi N, Rogers P, Puddey IB. Dietary protein and soluble fiber reduce ambulatory blood pressure in treated hypertensives. Hypertension 2001;38:821–6.
[33] Cicero AF, Derosa G, Manca M, Bove M, Borghi C, Gaddi AV. Different effect of psyllium and guar dietary supplementation on blood pressure control in hypertensive overweight patients: a six-month, randomized clinical trial. Clin Exp Hypertens 2007;29:383–94.
[34] Khossousi A, Binns CW, Dhaliwal SS, Pal S. The acute effects of psyllium on postprandial lipaemia and thermogenesis in overweight and obese men. Br J Nutr 2008;99:1068–75.
[35] Pal S, Khossousi A, Binns C, Dhaliwal S, Ellis V. The effect of a fiber supplement compared to a healthy diet on body composition, lipids, glucose, insulin and other metabolic syndrome risk factors in overweight and obese individuals. Br J Nutr 2011;105: 90–100.
[36] Ziai SA, Larijani B, Akhoondzadeh S, et al. Psyllium decreased serum glucose and glycosylated hemoglobin significantly in diabetic outpatients. J Ethnopharmacol 2005;102:202–7.
[37] National Health and Medical Research Council . Nutrient reference values for Australia and New ZealandNHaMR Council, editors. National health and medical research council 2005.
[38] AHA. Fiber. American Heart Association, <http://www.americanheart.org/presenter.jhtml?identifier=4574>; 2009 [accessed 2 October 2009].
[39] Anderson JW, Allgood LD, Lawrence A, et al. Cholesterol-lowering effects of psyllium intake adjunctive to diet therapy in men and women with hypercholesterolemia: meta-analysis of 8 controlled trials. Am J Clin Nutr 2000;71:472–9.
[40] Cummings JH. Fermentation in the human large intestine: evidence and implications for health. Lancet 1983;1:1206–9.
[41] Marlett JA, Fischer MH. A poorly fermented gel from psyllium seed husk increases excreta moisture and bile acid excretion in rats. J Nutr 2002;132:2638–43.
[42] Marlett JA, Fischer MH. The active fraction of psyllium seed husk. Proc Nutr Soc 2003;62:207–9.
[43] Marlett JA, Kajs TM, Fischer MH. An unfermented gel component of psyllium seed husk promotes laxation as a lubricant in humans. Am J Clin Nutr 2000;72:784–9.
[44] Anderson JW, Riddell-Mason S, Gustafson NJ, Smith SF, Mackey M. Cholesterol-lowering effects of psyllium-enriched cereal as an adjunct to a prudent diet in the treatment of mild to moderate hypercholesterolemia. Am J Clin Nutr 1992;56:93–8.
[45] Levrat MA, Favier ML, Moundras C, Remesy C, Demigne C, Morand C. Role of dietary propionic acid and bile acid excretion in the hypocholesterolemic effects of oligosaccharides in rats. J Nutr 1994;124:531–8.
[46] Rodriguez-Moran M, Guerrero-Romero F, Lazcano-Burciaga G. Lipid- and glucose-lowering efficacy of *Plantago psyllium* in type II diabetes. J Diabetes Complications 1998;12:273–8.
[47] Tai ES, Fok AC, Chu R, Tan CE. A study to assess the effect of dietary supplementation with soluble fiber (Minolest) on lipid levels in normal subjects with hypercholesterolaemia. Ann Acad Med Singapore 1999;28:209–13.
[48] Vuksan V, Jenkins AL, Rogovik AL, Fairgrieve CD, Jovanovski E, Leiter LA. Viscosity rather than quantity of dietary fiber predicts cholesterol-lowering effect in healthy individuals. Br J Nutr 2011;106:1349–52.
[49] Karhunen LJ, Juvonen KR, Flander SM, et al. A psyllium fiber-enriched meal strongly attenuates postprandial gastrointestinal peptide release in healthy young adults. J Nutr 2010;140:737–44.
[50] Turnbull WH, Thomas HG. The effect of a *Plantago ovata* seed containing preparation on appetite variables, nutrient and energy intake. Int J Obes Relat Metab Disord 1995;19:338–42.
[51] Jequier E. Pathways to obesity. Int J Obes Relat Metab Disord 2002;26(Suppl 2):S12–17.
[52] Paddon-Jones D, Westman E, Mattes RD, Wolfe RR, Astrup A, Westerterp-Plantenga M. Protein, weight management, and satiety. Am J Clin Nutr 2008;87:1558S–61S.
[53] Anderson GH, Moore SE. Dietary proteins in the regulation of food intake and body weight in humans. J Nutr 2004;134:974S–9S.
[54] Weigle DS, Breen PA, Matthys CC, et al. A high-protein diet induces sustained reductions in appetite, ad libitum caloric intake, and body weight despite compensatory changes in diurnal plasma leptin and ghrelin concentrations. Am J Clin Nutr 2005;82:41–8.
[55] Delargy HJ, O'Sullivan KR, Fletcher RJ, Blundell JE. Effects of amount and type of dietary fiber (soluble and insoluble) on short-term control of appetite. Int J Food Sci Nutr 1997;48:67–77.
[56] Yao M, Roberts SB. Dietary energy density and weight regulation. Nutr Rev 2001;59:247–58.
[57] Holt S, Brand J, Soveny C, Hansky J. Relationship of satiety to postprandial glycaemic, insulin and cholecystokinin responses. Appetite 1992;18:129–41.
[58] Burton-Freeman B, Davis PA, Schneeman BO. Plasma cholecystokinin is associated with subjective measures of satiety in women. Am J Clin Nutr 2002;76:659–67.
[59] Anderson JW, Randles KM, Kendall CWC, Jenkins DJA. Carbohydrate and fiber recommendations for individuals with

diabetes: a quantitative assessment and meta-analysis of the evidence. J Am Coll Nutr 2004;23:5–17.
[60] Pereira MA, Ludwig DS. Dietary fiber and body-weight regulation. Observations and mechanisms. Pediatr Clin North Am 2001;48:969–80.
[61] Zijlstra N, de Wijk RA, Mars M, Stafleu A, de Graaf C. Effect of bite size and oral processing time of a semisolid food on satiation. Am J Clin Nutr 2009;90:269–75.
[62] Zijlstra N, Mars M, de Wijk RA, Westerterp-Plantenga MS, de Graaf C. The effect of viscosity on ad libitum food intake. Int J Obes (Lond) 2008;32:676–83.
[63] Drewnowski A. Energy density, palatability, and satiety: implications for weight control. Nutr Rev 1998;56:347–53.
[64] Dikeman CL, Murphy MR, Fahey Jr GC. Dietary fibers affect viscosity of solutions and simulated human gastric and small intestinal digesta. J Nutr 2006;136:913–9.
[65] Sleeth ML, Thompson EL, Ford HE, Zac-Varghese SE, Frost G. Free fatty acid receptor 2 and nutrient sensing: a proposed role for fiber, fermentable carbohydrates and short-chain fatty acids in appetite regulation. Nutr Res Rev 2010;23:135–45.
[66] Baer DJ, Rumpler WV, Miles CW, Fahey Jr GC. Dietary fiber decreases the metabolizable energy content and nutrient digestibility of mixed diets fed to humans. J Nutr 1997;127:579–86.
[67] Blackwood AD, Salter J, Dettmar PW, Chaplin MF. Dietary fiber, physicochemical properties and their relationship to health. J R Soc. Promot Health 2000;120:242–7.
[68] Sierra M, Garcia JJ, Fernandez N, Diez MJ, Calle AP. Therapeutic effects of psyllium in type 2 diabetic patients. Eur J Clin Nutr 2002;56:830–42.
[69] Moreno LA, Tresaco B, Bueno G, et al. Psyllium fiber and the metabolic control of obese children and adolescents. J Physiol Biochem 2003;59:235–42.
[70] Gropper SS, Acosta PB. The therapeutic effect of fiber in treating obesity. J Am Coll Nutr 1987;6:533–5.
[71] Dunaif G, Schneeman BO. The effect of dietary fiber on human pancreatic enzyme activity in vitro. Am J Clin Nutr 1981;34:1034–5.
[72] Olson BH, Anderson SM, Becker MP, et al. Psyllium-enriched cereals lower blood total cholesterol and LDL cholesterol, but not HDL cholesterol, in hypercholesterolemic adults: results of a meta-analysis. J Nutr 1997;127:1973–80.
[73] FDA . Control of health claims in foods. Lancet 1998;351:609.
[74] Jenkins DJ, Kendall CW, Vuksan V, et al. Soluble fiber intake at a dose approved by the US food and drug administration for a claim of health benefits: serum lipid risk factors for cardiovascular disease assessed in a randomized controlled crossover trial. Am J Clin Nutr 2002;75:834–9.
[75] Cornfine C, Hasenkopf K, Eisner P, Schweiggert U. Influence of chemical and physical modification on the bile acid binding capacity of dietary fiber from lupins (*Lupinus angustifolius* L.). Food Chem 2010;122:638–44.
[76] Anderson JW, Allgood LD, Turner J, Oeltgen PR, Daggy BP. Effects of psyllium on glucose and serum lipid responses in men with type 2 diabetes and hypercholesterolemia. Am J Clin Nutr 1999;70:466–73.
[77] Lairon D, Play B, Jourdheuil-Rahmani D. Digestible and indigestible carbohydrates: interactions with postprandial lipid metabolism. J Nutr Biochem 2007;18:217–27.
[78] Bourdon I, Yokoyama W, Davis P, et al. Postprandial lipid, glucose, insulin, and cholecystokinin responses in men fed barley pasta enriched with beta-glucan. Am J Clin Nutr 1999;69:55–63.
[79] Potter JG, Coffman KP, Reid RL, Krall JM, Albrink MJ. Effect of test meals of varying dietary fiber content on plasma insulin and glucose response. Am J Clin Nutr 1981;34:328–34.
[80] Lundin EA, Zhang JX, Lairon D, et al. Effects of meal frequency and high-fiber rye-bread diet on glucose and lipid metabolism and ileal excretion of energy and sterols in ileostomy subjects. Eur J Clin Nutr 2004;58:1410–9.
[81] Marlett JA, Fischer MH. A poorly fermented gel from psyllium seed husk increases excreta moisture and bile acid excretion in rats. J Nutr 2002;132:2638–43.
[82] Ellegard L, Andersson H. Oat bran rapidly increases bile acid excretion and bile acid synthesis: an ileostomy study. Eur J Clin Nutr 2007;61:938–45.
[83] Brown MS, Goldstein JL. A receptor-mediated pathway for cholesterol homeostasis. Science 1986;232:34–47.
[84] Anderson JW, Davidson MH, Blonde L, et al. Long-term cholesterol-lowering effects of psyllium as an adjunct to diet therapy in the treatment of hypercholesterolemia. Am J Clin Nutr 2000;71:1433–8.
[85] Gunness P, Gidley MJ. Mechanisms underlying the cholesterol-lowering properties of soluble dietary fiber polysaccharides. Food Funct 2010;1:149–55.
[86] Wilkinson IB, Prasad K, Hall IR, et al. Increased central pulse pressure and augmentation index in subjects with hypercholesterolemia. J Am Coll Cardiol 2002;39:1005–11.
[87] Blacher J, Safar ME. Large-artery stiffness, hypertension and cardiovascular risk in older patients. Nat Clin Pract 2005;2:450–5.
[88] Safar ME. Systolic blood pressure, pulse pressure and arterial stiffness as cardiovascular risk factors. Curr Opin Nephrol Hypertens 2001;10:257–61.
[89] Tomiyama H, Hashimoto H, Hirayama Y, et al. Synergistic acceleration of arterial stiffening in the presence of raised blood pressure and raised plasma glucose. Hypertension 2006;47:180–8.
[90] Greenwald SE. Ageing of the conduit arteries. J Pathol 2007;211:157–72.
[91] McEniery CM, Cockcroft JR. Does arterial stiffness predict atherosclerotic coronary events? Adv Cardiol 2007;44:160–72.
[92] Ostmark E, Harrisson S, Wooley KL, Malmstrom EE. Comb polymers prepared by ATRP from hydroxypropyl cellulose. Biomacromolecules 2007;8:1138–48.
[93] Izzo Jr JL, Shykoff BE. Arterial stiffness: clinical relevance, measurement, and treatment. Rev Cardiovas Med 2001;2(29–34):37–40.
[94] Scuteri A, Najjar SS, Muller DC, et al. Metabolic syndrome amplifies the age-associated increases in vascular thickness and stiffness. J Am Coll Cardiol 2004;43:1388–95.
[95] Arnett DK, Tyroler HA, Burke G, Hutchinson R, Howard G, Heiss G. Hypertension and subclinical carotid artery atherosclerosis in blacks and whites. Arch Int Med 1996;156:1983–9.
[96] Amar J, Ruidavets JB, Chamontin B, Drouet L, Ferrieres J. Arterial stiffness and cardiovascular risk factors in a population-based study. J Hypertens 2001;19:381–7.
[97] Benetos A, Waeber B, Izzo J, et al. Influence of age, risk factors, and cardiovascular and renal disease on arterial stiffness: clinical applications. Am J Hypertens 2002;15:1101–8.
[98] Seals DR, Moreau KL, Gates PE, Eskurza I. Modulatory influences on ageing of the vasculature in healthy humans. Exp Gerontol 2006;41:501–7.
[99] Wilkinson IB, Qasem A, McEniery CM, Webb DJ, Avolio AP, Cockcroft JR. Nitric oxide regulates local arterial distensibility in vivo. Circulation 2002;105:213–7.
[100] WHO. Diet, nutrition and the prevention of chronic diseases. World health organization and FAO: Report of the joint WHO/FAO expert consultation. WHO technical report series, No 916 (TRS 916) <http://www.who.int/dietphysicalactivity/publications/trs916/en/>; 2003 [accessed 1.10.13].
[101] Li J, Wang J, Kaneko T, Qin LQ, Sato A. Effects of fiber intake on the blood pressure, lipids, and heart rate in Goto Kakizaki rats. Nutrition 2004;20:1003–7.

[102] Pal S, Khossousi A, Binns C, Dhaliwal S, Radavelli-Bagatini S. The effects of 12-week psyllium fibre supplementation or healthy diet on blood pressure and arterial stiffness in overweight and obese individuals. Br J Nutr 2012;107(5): 725–34.
[103] Creager MA, Cooke JP, Mendelsohn ME, et al. Impaired vasodilation of forearm resistance vessels in hypercholesterolemic humans. J Clin Invest 1990;86:228–34.
[104] Ferrara LA, Guida L, Iannuzzi R, Celentano A, Lionello F. Serum cholesterol affects blood pressure regulation. J Hum Hypertens 2002;16:337–43.
[105] Laurenzi M, Mancini M, Menotti A, et al. Multiple risk factors in hypertension: results from the Gubbio study. J Hypertens Suppl 1990;8:S7–12.
[106] Hayakawa H, Raij L. Relationship between hypercholesterolaemia, endothelial dysfunction and hypertension. J Hypertens 1999;17:611–9.
[107] Vallance P, Collier J, Moncada S. Effects of endothelium-derived nitric oxide on peripheral arteriolar tone in man. Lancet 1989;2:997–1000.
[108] Anderson JW, Zeigler JA, Deakins DA, et al. Metabolic effects of high-carbohydrate, high-fiber diets for insulin-dependent diabetic individuals. Am J Clin Nutr 1991;54:936–43.
[109] Fukagawa NK, Anderson JW, Hageman G, Young VR, Minaker KL. High-carbohydrate, high-fiber diets increase peripheral insulin sensitivity in healthy young and old adults. Am J Clin Nutr 1990;52:524–8.
[110] Ferrannini E, Buzzigoli G, Bonadonna R, et al. Insulin resistance in essential hypertension. N Engl J Med 1987;317:350–7.
[111] Bessesen D. The role of carbohydrates in insulin resistance. J Nutr 2001;131:2782S–6S.
[112] Ferrannini E, Haffner SM, Mitchell BD, Stern MP. Hyperinsulinaemia: the key feature of a cardiovascular and metabolic syndrome. Diabetologia 1991;34:416–22.
[113] King DE, Mainous AG, Egan BM, Woolson RF, Geesey ME. Fiber and C-reactive protein in diabetes, hypertension, and obesity. Diabetes care 2005;28:1487–9.
[114] Qi L, Rimm E, Liu S, Rifai N, Hu FB. Dietary glycemic index, glycemic load, cereal fiber, and plasma adiponectin concentration in diabetic men. Diabetes care 2005;28:1022–8.

CHAPTER

43

Whole Grains in the Prevention and Treatment of Abdominal Obesity

J. Philip Karl and Nicola M. McKeown

Jean Mayer USDA Human Nutrition Research Center on Aging, Tufts University, Boson, MA, USA

INTRODUCTION

Cereal grains have been included in human diets for millennia as important sources of macronutrients, fiber, vitamins, minerals, and a diverse array of phytochemicals [1]. Anatomically, cereal grains are composed of three primary components (Fig. 43.1): the inner germ, which contains the embryo or seed; the outer bran, which acts as a multilayered protective barrier for the grain; and the starchy endosperm, which comprises the majority of the grain and supplies the energy needed for seed maturation [2,3]. The distinct roles of the germ, bran, and endosperm in the growth and maturation of the grain result in a distinctive distribution of nutrients within the grain. Starch and storage proteins, but relatively few additional nutrients, are concentrated in the endosperm. In contrast, the germ and bran contain most of the fiber, vitamins (niacin, pantothenic acid, riboflavin, thiamin, vitamin B6, and vitamin E), minerals (calcium, iron, magnesium, phosphorous, potassium, sodium, and zinc), lipids, and other phytochemicals including lignans, phenolic acids, phytates, and polyphenols within the grain [2,4].

For dietary purposes, the term *whole grain* is defined by the American Association of Cereal Chemists (AACC) and the U.S. Food and Drug Administration as the "intact, ground, cracked or flaked fruit of the grain whose principal components—the starchy endosperm, germ and bran—are present in the same relative proportions as they exist in the intact grain" [5]. In other words, whole-grain ingredients are either intact grains or grains that have been processed and reconstituted with the same relative proportion of bran, germ, and endosperm as are found in the intact grain. In contrast to whole grains, refined grains consist primarily of endosperm retained after separation and removal of the bran and germ. Nutrients are often added to refined grain food products by enrichment and fortification; however, much of the nutritive value of the whole grain is lost in the refining process (Fig. 43.2).

In developed countries, the most commonly consumed grains include wheat, rye, oats, barley, corn, and rice with other grains such as triticale, teff, millets, sorghum, and Job's tears consumed in lesser amounts, and the predominant grains consumed varying by region [2]. Although all cereal grains have similar chemical compositions, the proportions of nutrients vary within different grains (Table 43.1). For example, whole-grain varieties of wheat, rye, and oat contain three times the amount of fiber as brown rice, and the proportions of different types of fiber vary, with oats and barley being rich in β-glucans and rye being rich in arabinoxylan and fructans [6].

The ways in which whole grains are incorporated into foods and into individual diets also varies. Whole grains can be either consumed as a stand-alone food product (e.g. whole oats) or consumed following incorporation as ingredients into grain-based food products (e.g. whole-wheat flour used for bread making). When incorporated into food products, the proportion of grain ingredients that are whole grain can range from almost 0% to 100%. In the United States, the predominant food sources of whole grains include ready-to-eat breakfast cereals, yeast breads, hot cereals, popcorn, crackers, and grain-based desserts [7]. Many of these foods often contain a mixture of both whole and refined grains. Grain-based foods that contain relatively small amounts of whole grain, such as some ready-to-eat breakfast cereals, can make a substantial contribution to the total whole-grain intake in certain subpopulations (e.g. American children [8]), despite containing mostly refined grains in addition to less healthy ingredients such as added sugars and solid fats [9]. Moreover, whole-grain ingredients in both partial whole-grain foods and 100% whole-grain foods are often processed prior to consumption, with the final structure of the grain ingredient existing along a

Nutrition in the Prevention and Treatment of Abdominal Obesity
http://dx.doi.org/10.1016/B978-0-12-407869-7.00043-X

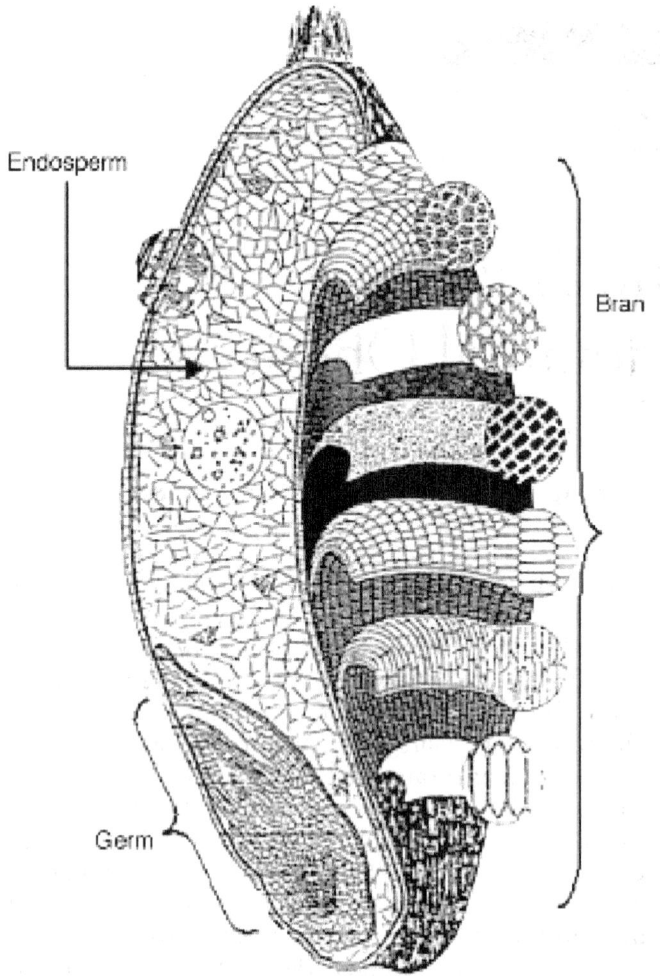

FIGURE 43.1 Anatomy of a whole grain. Reproduced with permission from Ref. [3].

continuum of fully intact to finely milled. Consequently, most whole grains are currently consumed in a processed, rather than a fully or partially intact form and, although the nutrient composition differs from refined grain, the structure does not.

Unless a food is 100% whole grain, the exact proportion of grains that are whole grain is proprietary to the manufacturer and often not disclosed. However, some food-labeling initiatives help provide an indication of whole-grain content. For example, foods in the United States can carry the whole-grain health claim stating that "diets rich in whole grain foods and other plant foods and low in total fat, saturated fat, and cholesterol may help reduce the risk of heart disease and certain cancers" if the food product contains at least 51% whole grains by wet weight [10]. The whole grains stamp is an international food-labeling program developed by the Whole Grains Council, which allows food manufacturers to place a unique icon on food products containing ≥8 g whole grains per serving [11]. Food manufacturers using this program often use the icon to state the per-serving whole-grain content of the food. In addition, AACC International recently defined a whole-grain food product as one containing 8 g or more of whole grain per 30 g of product [11]. This definition is intended to help consumers identify and select whole-grain food products meeting requirements outlined in the Dietary Guidelines for Americans.

The 2010 Dietary Guidelines for Americans recommend consuming at least half of all grains as whole grains, which translates into a recommendation to consume ≥48 g whole grains/2000 kcal/day or, equivalently, ≥3 servings whole grains/2000 kcal/day [12]. One serving (i.e. 16 g) of whole grains can be obtained by eating 1 oz (i.e. 1 slice) of 100% whole-grain bread, 2 slices of 50% whole-grain bread, or half a cup of 100% whole-grain pasta or cereal, for example. Higher daily consumption is recommended in a number of European countries [6,13], where habitual whole-grain intakes tend to be higher than in the United States. However, whole-grain intake remains well below recommended levels for many adults and children [14], especially in the United States [15,16], and public health campaigns worldwide continue to focus on increasing population-level whole-grain consumption. The rationale underpinning these efforts is the superior nutritive value of whole grains relative to refined grains, and associations of increased whole-grain intake with reduced chronic disease risk, including a reduced risk of obesity [17,18].

Multiple bioactive components within whole grains as well as the properties of less-processed whole grains have been shown to favorably modulate appetite, glucose metabolism, insulin sensitivity, and, more recently, the composition of the gut microbiota [2,19]. When packaged in a whole grain, these effects may act synergistically to deter body fat accumulation [3,4]. Consequently, substituting whole grains for refined grains in the diet may be one component of effective strategies for mitigating undesirable weight gain, body fat accumulation, and related sequelae. In this chapter, we discuss evidence for a role of whole grains in the prevention and treatment of abdominal adiposity.

BIOLOGICAL PLAUSIBILITY OF WHOLE GRAIN-MEDIATED EFFECTS ON ADIPOSITY

The 2010 Dietary Guidelines for Americans and various international dietary guidelines recommend increasing whole-grain intake by replacing refined grains with whole grains [6,12,20–24]. If adopting this recommendation is to favorably affect abdominal adiposity, then replacing refined grains with whole grains must, in theory, deter weight gain, promote weight loss, and/or

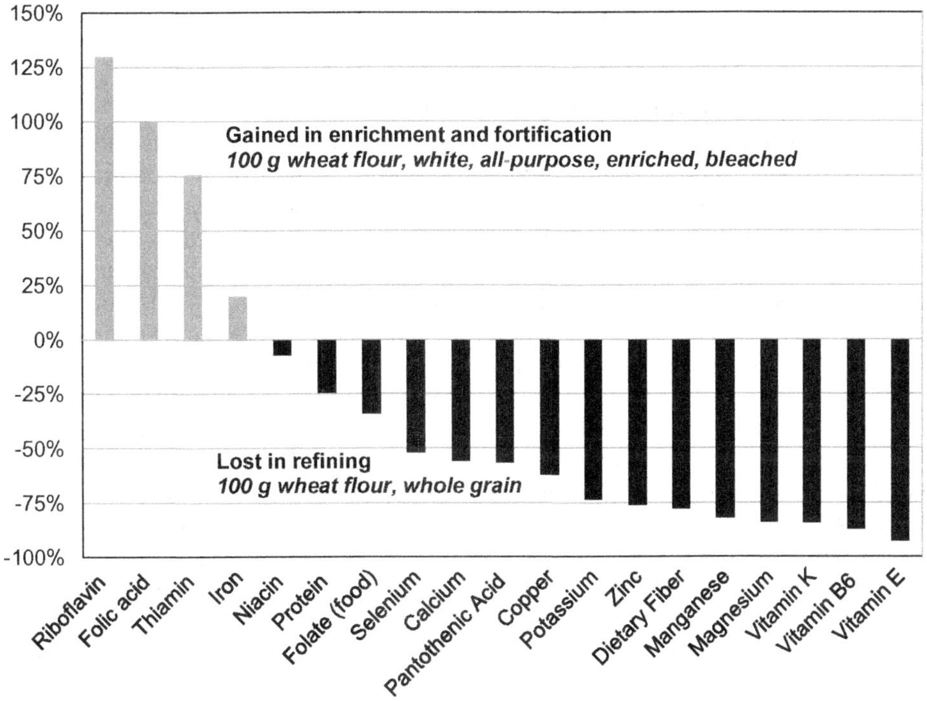

FIGURE 43.2 Percentage of nutrients lost or gained in the refining of wheat. Reprinted from McKeown et al. [62]. *Data source: U.S. Department of Agriculture [117].*

TABLE 43.1 Approximate Concentration of Selected Nutrients in One Serving (16 g) of Commonly Consumed Whole Grains

	Wheat	Rye	Oat	Barley, Hulled	Corn, yellow	Rice, Long-Grain Brown
Carbohydrate (g)	11.9	12.1	10.6	11.8	12.3	12.4
Fat (g)	0.3	0.3	1.1	0.4	0.6	0.5
Protein (g)	1.5	1.6	2.7	2.0	1.1	1.3
Total fiber (g)	2.1	2.4	1.7	2.8	1.2	0.6
Total fiber (% dry matter)	13.5	19.9	10.2	15.2	–	–
Arabinoxylan (% dry matter)	5.6	8.9	2.0	5.2	–	–
Cellulose (% dry matter)	2.5	2.9	1.3	1.9	–	–
β-glucan (% dry matter)	0.8	1.5	5.0	4.6	–	–
Fructan (% dry matter)	1.3	4.1	4.1	1.6	–	–
Thiamin (mg)	0.05	0.1	0.1	0.1	0.04	0.1
Riboflavin (mg)	0.03	0.04	0.02	0.05	0.01	0.01
Niacin (mg)	0.9	0.7	0.2	0.7	0.3	0.8
Vitamin B6 (mg)	0.03	0.05	0.02	0.1	0.1	0.1
Vitamin E (mg)	0.1	0.1	0.1	0.1	0.1	0.2
Magnesium (mg)	19	18	28	21	15	23
Iron (mg)	0.6	0.4	0.8	0.6	0.4	0.2

Sources: Frolich et al. [6] and U.S. Department of Agriculture, Agricultural Research Service [117].

preferentially spare or build lean body mass. As will be discussed below, some of these effects are biologically plausible, and a number of feasible mechanisms have been proposed. These mechanisms include appetite suppression and weight loss, reduced dietary glycemic load, improved insulin sensitivity, and, more recently, modulation of the gut microbiota [2,3,19]. The capacity of whole grains to mediate these mechanisms is attributed to the independent and synergistic physiologic effects of nutrients within whole grains, many of which are lost during refining, and the physical properties of whole grains (e.g. structural intactness and integrity, as well as particle size) [2–4,19].

Fiber is the component of whole grains that is most likely to influence physiologic effects relevant to the regulation of body weight and adiposity. The relationship between fiber and adiposity is mediated by the physicochemical properties of different fibers, which include viscosity, water-binding capacity, and fermentability [25]. Viscous fibers (e.g. arabinoxylans and β-glucans) form gels when mixed with digesta. This slows gastric emptying and nutrient absorption, thereby promoting satiety, reducing energy intake, and attenuating postprandial glycemic responses [26]. The high water-binding capacity and low energy density (i.e. metabolizable energy per unit mass) of fiber also promotes satiety and reduces energy intake by adding bulk and volume without additional energy to the diet [27]. Fermentable fibers (e.g. wheat dextrin, fructans, resistant starches, and β-glucans) have less effect on energy density because they are fermented by bacteria in the colon. The fermentation process produces energy from an otherwise unavailable energy source in the form of short-chain fatty acids (SCFAs) [28]. Although SCFA production increases the metabolizable energy content of fiber, it also influences body weight and composition by directly mediating hepatic and peripheral glucose and lipid oxidation, and stimulating secretion of the gut hormones peptide YY (PYY) and glucagon-like peptide 1 (GLP-1) [29]. The actions of these hormones include appetite suppression, slowed gastrointestinal transit rate, and modulation of glucose metabolism [30]. SCFAs also lower colonic pH and, in combination with the proliferation of bacteria stimulated by fermentable fiber, alter the composition of the microbiota in the colon. Altering gut microbiota composition may have relevant effects on adiposity, given the emerging recognition of gut microbes as important mediators of human metabolism, as well as associations between gut microbiota composition and human obesity [31].

The superior nutrient content of whole grains relative to refined grains may also mediate the effects of whole grains on adiposity. Relative to refined grains, whole grains are higher in magnesium and antioxidants, nutrients that have been associated with lower fasting glucose and insulin levels, and improved insulin sensitivity [32,33]. Moreover, whole grains are rich sources of polyphenols [4]. Polyphenols are metabolized by gut microbes, have antimicrobial properties, and may alter the composition of the gut microbiota [34].

Perhaps the primary determinant of the physiologic effects of whole grains is grain structure. Preserving the grain structure decreases the accessibility of nutrients within the grain to pancreatic amylases. Consequently, intact and less-processed whole grains produce lower postprandial glycemic responses compared to both processed whole grains and refined grains [35]. In support of this, Holt et al. [36] demonstrated progressive increases in postprandial glycemic and insulinemic responses as the particle size of the whole grains consumed progressively decreased from an intact to a finely ground form. Similar findings have been reported for other grains [37–40]. Appetite may also be affected by grain processing because higher satiety ratings following consumption of intact relative to ground grain have been reported [36,41], which may be attributable in part to greater stomach distension with increasing particle size [41]. When available for hydrolysis, the proportion of different starches within the grain also influences postprandial physiology because high-amylose grains attenuate postprandial glycemia and insulinemia owing to the slower rate of hydrolysis of amylose relative to amylopectin [35]. In less-processed whole grains, the decreased availability of starch to amylases results in higher amounts of starch reaching the colon in an undigested state [42]; it can then be readily fermented by gut microbes, resulting in increased SCFA production and possible alterations in gut microbiota composition.

ASSOCIATIONS BETWEEN WHOLE-GRAIN INTAKE AND ADIPOSITY IN OBSERVATIONAL STUDIES

Several cross-sectional studies have observed that higher whole-grain intakes are associated with lower body weight and abdominal adiposity in adults [16,43–49]. In a 2008 meta-analysis of 15 observational studies examining associations between whole-grain intake and body composition [50], 12 studies (80%) documented a significant inverse association between whole-grain intake and body mass index (BMI), and six out of seven studies examining whole-grain intake and either waist circumference (WC) or waist-hip ratio (WHR) reported a significant inverse association. To summarize the data on the physiological effects of whole-grain intake, those adults consuming, on average, ≥3 daily servings of whole grains had a 0.6 kg/m^2 lower BMI, a 2.7 cm lower WC, and a 0.023 lower WHR compared with those consuming <0.5 whole-grain servings/day [50]. A number of subsequent cross-sectional studies have since confirmed these findings [16,44,47].

In observational studies into associations between excess adiposity and chronic disease, BMI and WC are often employed as surrogate markers of total adiposity and abdominal adiposity, respectively, [51]. The increased availability of methods offering more precise measures of adiposity such as dual-energy X-ray absorptiometry (DEXA) and computed tomography (CT) have recently been used to advance observational nutrition research, including investigations into the relationship between whole-grain intake and abdominal adiposity [46,52]. For example, using DEXA, McKeown et al. [46] observed that consuming approximately 3 servings of whole grains/day relative to consuming <0.2 servings of whole grains/day was associated with 2.4% lower total body fat and 3.6% lower trunk fat in adults over the age of 60. In addition, among Framingham Heart Study participants, McKeown and colleagues [52] observed that visceral adipose tissue volume (as measured by CT) was 10% lower in middle-aged adults consuming $\geq$3 servings of whole grains/day compared with those consuming <0.2 servings of whole grains/day. These observations suggest that higher intakes of whole grains may be differentially linked to body fat deposition.

Despite multiple studies observing a cross-sectional association between whole-grain consumption and BMI or abdominal adiposity, the extent to which higher whole-grain intake prevents or reduces long-term (i.e. >1 year) weight gain and body fat accretion has received less attention. However, prospective evidence linking higher whole-grain intake to attenuated increases in body weight or total adiposity as measured by BMI has been demonstrated in several large cohorts of American health professionals [53–55]. In these studies, estimates of whole-grain intake obtained from food frequency questionnaires administered every few years were linked to changes in self-reported body weight or BMI. Using the Nurses' Health Study cohort, Liu et al. [54] reported a 0.1 kg/m^2 lower increase in BMI every 2-4 years in women who increased their whole-grain intake by $\approx$1 serving/1000 kcal/day relative to those who decreased their whole-grain intake by 0.6 servings/1000 kcal/day. Similarly, a 0.5 kg lower weight gain over 8 years was observed in men participating in the Health Professionals Follow-up Study who increased their whole-grain intake by 1.5 servings/day compared to those who reduced their intake by 0.9 servings/day [53]. In a subsequent meta-analysis in which data from these cohorts were combined with additional data from the Nurses' Health Study II cohort, Mozaffarian et al. [55] estimated an annual weight loss of 0.04 kg for every 1 serving/day increase in whole-grain intake. Collectively, these studies provide evidence that higher whole-grain intakes may modestly attenuate weight gain or even promote weight loss in well-educated American adults after controlling for other lifestyle and dietary factors.

Evidence specifically linking higher whole-grain consumption to long-term changes in abdominal adiposity is limited by the lack of prospective cohort studies employing more direct indicators of adiposity than BMI, such as WC or percentage body fat. The few cohort studies that have attempted to explore this relationship have not quantified total whole-grain intake but have instead limited estimates of whole-grain intake to individual food groups or possible surrogate markers of whole-grain intake such as cereal fiber. For example, Du et al. [56] observed that each 10 g/day intake of cereal fiber was associated with a decrease in WC of 0.10 cm/year in one large, multinational European cohort. In contrast, increases in whole-grain bread intake have not been significantly associated with changes in WC [57,58], although a trend toward a reduction in WC over 6 years was observed in women within one study [57].

To put the findings of these observational studies into perspective, each 5 kg/m^2 increase in BMI on a population level has been associated with 30% greater overall mortality [59]. Although effects of whole grains on BMI appear considerably smaller, both the avoidance of weight gain as well as relatively small reductions in body weight are thought to significantly reduce chronic disease risk in the significant proportion of the population that is overweight or obese [60].

Although epidemiological evidence is suggestive and largely consistent, observational studies cannot causally link higher whole-grain intake to reduced abdominal adiposity. Moreover, relatively few studies [53–55] have directly assessed total whole-grain intake in relation to long-term changes in adiposity within large cohorts followed prospectively over years. Although the few available cohort studies suggest marginal benefits of whole-grain consumption on adiposity, definitive conclusions are precluded by the relative lack of relevant trials employing accurate measures of adiposity.

Interpretation of observational studies is also complicated by the methodological difficulty of accurately quantifying whole-grain intake [61,62]. Dietary assessment questionnaires assessing whole-grain intake often only consider breakfast cereals containing $\geq$25% whole grains, dark bread, brown rice, popcorn, oatmeal, and a few additional foods such as wild rice, bran muffins, and whole-wheat crackers as whole grain foods [61]. Furthermore, until recently, estimates of whole-grain intake generally included "added bran" and bran-containing cereals. Thus, the definition applied in the research setting is not consistent with the AACC definition of a whole grain, nor does it align with the U.S. Food and Drug Administration requirement that a food should comprise $\geq$51% whole grain by weight to be eligible for the whole-grain health claim. Further, given the increased availability of whole-grain products in the food supply chain [63], traditional dietary assessment methods and definitions of whole grains may not adequately capture the variety and increasing abundance of dietary sources of whole grains. Coupled with the aforementioned limitations, these methods also fail to account for the considerable variability of whole-grain content among grain-based foods in which whole grains can comprise 0-100% of the total grain content. In order to overcome these limitations, a more quantitative estimate of whole-grain intake is needed. Some studies [43,47,53,64] have applied whole-grain databases that include manufacturer information on the whole-grain content of specific food products. The use of these quantitative estimates of whole-grain intake has led to higher estimates of population-level whole-grain intakes within the same cohort, although study conclusions were not affected [53]. Nonetheless, in combination with the established limitations of dietary recall methods and the difficulties that individuals have in identifying whole-grain foods [65], improvements in the whole-grain databases used in research are necessary to reduce measurement error in observational studies.

Independent biomarkers of food or nutrient intakes are of value in epidemiological studies for confirming observations based on self-reported dietary exposure. To date, plasma [66,67] and urinary [68] concentrations of alkylresorcinols (ARs) and their metabolites have emerged as potentially promising biomarkers of whole-grain intake. ARs are a group of phenolic lipids found in the outer bran of wheat, rye, barley, and triticale [69]. Recently, Ma and colleagues [70] used plasma AR concentrations to confirm a previous observation from their group that whole-grain intake is inversely correlated with BMI and percentage body fat in older adults [70]. However, ARs are only present in wheat, rye, barley, and triticale, and may not be a suitable biomarker in populations where consumption of other grains contributes substantially to total whole-grain intake. Moreover, AR concentrations demonstrate large interindividual variation [67,71], reflect a short half-life [72], and do not demonstrate linear increases at high levels of intake [73], which may limit their use as long-term biomarkers of whole-grain intake [74].

Residual confounding is also of concern when interpreting associations between whole-grain intake and adiposity observed in epidemiological studies. Whole-grain consumers are consistently observed to be more physically active, smoke less, and consume more fruit, vegetables, and dietary fiber than low whole-grain consumers [45,47,52,75]. Similarly, analyses of dietary patterns frequently link whole-grain consumption with greater intakes of fruits, vegetables, and other foods associated with desirable health behaviors [76,77]. Although statistical adjustment for these factors is common, to what extent the associations between high whole-grain intake and lower adiposity reported in epidemiological studies simply reflect the healthier lifestyles of whole-grain consumers remains unclear.

EVIDENCE FROM CLINICAL TRIALS OF WHOLE GRAIN-MEDIATED EFFECTS ON ADIPOSITY

A number of randomized controlled trials have examined the effects of whole grains on adiposity by assessing whether dietary substitution of whole grains for refined grains leads to a spontaneous reduction in energy intake that consequently results in body weight and body fat loss [78–84] or promotes greater body weight and body fat loss when adopting a hypoenergetic weight loss diet (Table 43.2) [85–89]. Taken together, these studies indicate that dietary substitution of whole grains for refined grains does not appear to have a meaningful impact on appetite or body weight [19]. However, some evidence supporting a favorable effect of whole grains on abdominal adiposity independent of effects on body weight has been reported [85–87].

The absence of whole grain-mediated effects on body weight was quantified in a meta-analysis of nine randomized trials published from 1966 to 2012 [17]. The authors calculated a nonsignificant 0.18 kg [95% confidence interval (CI)−0.54-0.18 kg] greater weighted mean weight loss over 6 weeks to 16 weeks in individuals randomized to whole grain relative to refined grain interventions [17]. Recent narrative reviews that include studies not selected for the meta-analysis have likewise concluded that current evidence from clinical trials regarding whole grain-mediated effects on body weight is equivocal [19,62]. Significant heterogeneity in study durations, baseline intake of whole grains, the varieties and quantities of whole grains consumed by participants, assessment of dietary compliance, level of dietary control by study investigators, and the metabolic health of the populations studied has been noted [17,19,62]. In particular, many of the trials have been 12 weeks or less in duration, and longer study durations may be needed to observe differences in body weight resulting from increasing whole-grain intake. One reason for this deficiency is that many of the trials reporting body weight include the measure as a secondary outcome. In these studies, body weight maintenance is desirable in order to minimize the confounding of primary outcomes that may be attributed to differences in body weight change between study groups. The whole-grain sources used in different studies have also been widely variable (Table 43.2), having been derived either from single foods (e.g. bread or breakfast cereal) or grains (e.g. wheat or rye) or

TABLE 43.2 Clinical Trials Comparing Whole Grains to Refined Grains and Reporting Effects on Body Weight and Adiposity

Reference	Design and Population	Intervention	Weight Change (kg)	Change in Adiposity
Energy intake not restricted				
Andersson et al. [80]	6 weeks CO; $n = 30$ Ovwt and Ob M/F, 35–70 years	WG, 112 g WG/day[a]	BMI (kg/m^2):	Not measured
		C, 112 g RG/day	WG, + 0.3**	
			C, + 0.2	
Brownlee et al. [78]	16 weeks RCT; $n = 266$ Ovwt and Ob M/F, 18–65 years	WG1, 60 g WG/day for 8 weeks + 120 g WG/day for 8 weeks[a]	WG1, + 0.2	Total BF:
				WG1, + 0.3%
		WG2, 60 g WG/day for 16 weeks[a]	WG2, + 0.7	WG2, + 1.0%
		C, no intervention	C, 0	C, + 0.3%
				WC: ND
Giacco et al. [81]	3 weeks CO, $n = 15$ Nmwt, Ovwt and Ob M/F, 55 years	WG, WG-containing diet	WG, −0.1	Not measured
		C, RG-containing diet	C, −0.2	
Leinonen et al. [82]	4 weeks CO, $n = 40$ Nmwt, Ovwt and Ob M/F, 43 years	WG, 20% of total energy intake from WG rye bread	WG, −0.4	Not measured
		C, 20% of total energy intake from RG wheat bread	C, 0	
Pinn et al. [83]	12 weeks RCT, $n = 88$ Nmwt, Ovwt and Ob M/F, 33–67 years	WG, 137 g/day WG oat cereals	WG, + 0.5	Not measured
		RG, 146 g/day RG wheat cereals	RG, −0.3	
Ross et al. [79]	2 weeks CO; $n = 17$ Nmwt M/F, 20–50 years	WG, 150 g WG/day[a]	WG, −0.5	Not measured
		C, RG foods	C, 0	
Tucker et al. [84]	6 weeks CO; $n = 28$ Nmwt or Ob hyperglycemic M/F, 43–70 years	WG, 6-7 s/day WG wheat bread	WG, −0.5	WC: ND
		RG, 4-5 s/day RG wheat bread	RG, −0.3	Total BF: ND
Energy intake restricted				
Katcher et al. [85]	12 weeks RCT; $n = 47$ Ob M/F with MS, 20–65 years	WG, 4-7 oz-eq WG foods/day[a]	WG, −3.7	Total BF:
		C, avoid WG foods	C, −5.3	WG, −1.2%
		All, 500 kcal/day energy deficit + diet/activity counselling		C, −1.0%
				Ab BF:
				WG, −2.2%**
				C, −0.9%
				WC:
				WG, −2.5 cm
				C, −4.7 cm

(Continued)

TABLE 43.2 Continued

Reference	Design and Population	Intervention	Weight Change (kg)	Change in Adiposity
Kristensen et al. [86]	12 weeks RCT; $n = 72$ Ovwt and Ob postmenopausal F, 45–70 years	WG, 105 g WG/day[a]	WG, −3.6	Total FM:
		C, RG foods	C, −2.7	WG, −3.0%**,b
		All, 300 kcal/day energy deficit		C, −2.1%
				Central FM:
				WG, −3.8%*,b
				C, −2.7%
				WC:
				WG, −4.1 cm
				C, −4.1 cm
Maki et al. [87]	12 weeks RCT; $n = 144$ Ovwt and Ob M/F, 20–65 years	WG, 3 cups/day oat cereal	WG, −2.2	WC:
		C, low-fiber foods	C, −1.7	WG, −3.3 cm**
		All, 500 kcal/day energy deficit		C, −1.9 cm
Melanson et al. [89]	24 weeks RCT; $n = 92$ Ovwt and Ob M/F, 18–70 years	WG, 40-80 g/day WG breakfast cereal	WG, −4.7	Not measured
		C, avoid breakfast cereals	C, −5.0	
		All, 500 kcal/day energy deficit from diet and exercise		
Saltzman et al. [88]	6 weeks RCT; $n = 41$ Nmwt, Ovwt and Ob M/F, 18–78 years	WG, 45 g/1000 kcal/day oats	WG, −4.4	Total FM:
		C, 45 g/1000 kcal/day RG wheat	C, −4.3	WG, −2.6 kg C, −3.0 kg
		All, 1000 kcal/day energy deficit		

Source: adapted from Karl et al. [19].

$^*P \leq 0.1$ compared to control; $^{**}P < 0.05$ compared to control. [a]Various sources of whole grains consumed. [b]Percentage change.

Ab, abdominal; BF, percentage body fat; C, control; CO, crossover; F, female; FM, fat mass; M, male; MS, metabolic syndrome; ND, no difference (actual values not reported); Nmwt, normal-weight (18.5 kg/m^2 ≤ BMI < 25 kg/m^2); Ob, obese (BMI ≥ 30 kg/m^2); Ovwt, overweight (25 kg/m^2 ≤ BMI < 30 kg/m^2); oz-eq, ounce-equivalents; RCT, randomized controlled trial; RG, refined grain; s/day, servings per day; WC, waist circumference; WG, whole grain.

from a variety of whole-grain sources (e.g. commercially available whole-grain products, including cookies and snack bars). The use of commercial products, in particular, may attenuate beneficial physiologic effects of whole-grain consumption because these products can often include highly processed whole-grain ingredients, as well as less healthy ingredients such as added sugar and solid fats [9].

An additional reason for an absence of whole grain-mediated reductions in body weight may be that, contrary to expectations, when incorporated into diets whole grains do not appear to promote reductions in energy intake. Few clinical studies have controlled all aspects of participant diets by providing complete study diets to participants [79,88,90]. Instead, most studies have provided 3-5 servings/day of whole grain or refined grain foods for incorporation into habitual diets. In some intervention studies, this has led to participants randomized to the whole-grain intervention adding, rather than substituting, the intervention foods to their habitual diets, thereby increasing their energy intake [78,85]. Interestingly, when unintended between-group differences in dietary intake are avoided by providing all foods to participants, evidence of a satiety-enhancing effect of whole grains has been documented [88,90]. However, it could not be determined whether this translates into reduced energy intake because energy intake was strictly controlled. In one study, in which all food was provided but intake was ad libitum, participants did not reduce energy intake despite consuming 150 g whole grain/day, although a trend for weight loss after 2 weeks was reported [79].

Relatively few randomized whole-grain interventions have quantified changes in adiposity using direct, sensitive techniques such as DEXA or hydrostatic weighing. Katcher et al. [85] randomized 50 obese adults with metabolic syndrome to one of two groups receiving dietary advice to obtain all recommended daily grain servings from either whole grain or refined grain sources while reducing habitual energy intake by 500 kcal/day: the whole grain-advice group increased whole-grain intake to an average of 5 servings whole grains/day, whereas the refined grain-advice group consumed <0.25 servings whole grains/day. Foods were not provided by investigators, and the primary whole-grain sources consumed were commercially available breads and rolls, ready-to-eat breakfast cereals, brown rice, oatmeal, pasta, salty snacks (e.g. chips, crackers), and snack bars. Similar reductions in body weight, WC, and total body fat (as measured by DEXA), along with similar improvements in glucose tolerance and insulin sensitivity, were observed in both groups after 12 weeks. However, percentage body fat loss from the abdominal region was 1.3% greater in the whole grain-advice group [85].

Similar findings were reported by Kristensen et al. [86] in a study in which overweight and obese postmenopausal women were randomized into one of two groups instructed to reduce energy intake by 300 kcal/day while including 475 kcal/day of either provided whole grain or refined grain foods to their diets. All of the provided foods were made from wheat and included breads made specifically for the study and commercially available pastas. Changes in glycemic control and insulin sensitivity as measured by hemoglobin A1c, and the homeostatic model assessment of insulin resistance (HOMA-IR) did not differ between groups. Total body and central fat mass (measured by DEXA) and WC were reduced in both groups after 12 weeks. However, a 1.1% greater decrease in total percentage body fat, primarily attributable to fat loss in the abdominal region, was documented in the whole-grain group [86].

Interestingly, neither of these two studies detected between-group differences in changes in WC during the intervention [85,86]. In contrast, Maki et al. [87] reported a 1.2 cm greater decrease in WC over 12 weeks in overweight and obese adults randomized to consume a hypoenergetic diet containing 3 cups/day of a whole-grain oat breakfast cereal compared to a hypoenergetic diet in which low-fiber breakfast foods were included. No significant between-group difference in weight loss was observed [87]. Taken together these three studies suggest that overweight and obese adults substituting whole grains for refined grains on the background of hypoenergetic diets for weight loss may experience modestly greater reductions in adiposity, primarily from the abdominal region, despite no significant weight loss benefit beyond energy restriction alone [85–87].

In contrast, whole-grain foods have not been shown to promote body fat loss in randomized trials that include normal-weight adults (BMI <25 kg/m^2) or that do not include an energy restriction recommendation for weight loss. In the largest randomized trial reporting effects of whole grains on adiposity conducted to date, Brownlee et al. [78] randomized 316 free-living overweight and obese adults who were not habitual consumers of whole grains to one of three different diet arms: control with no dietary change; 60 g whole grains/day for 16 weeks; or 60 g whole grains/day for 8 weeks followed by 120 g whole grains/day for an additional 8 weeks. Whole-grain foods were provided and included a variety of whole grains (i.e. wheat, rice, and oats) and commercially available food products (e.g. breads, ready-to-eat breakfast cereals, chips, and snacks bars). Although participants were instructed to substitute these whole-grain foods for refined grain foods in their normal diets, findings were complicated by the fact that participants appeared to add rather than substitute the whole-grain foods into their diets. Consequently, higher energy intakes were observed in the whole-grain groups compared to the control group, yet no significant between-group differences in BMI, percentage body fat, WC, or insulin sensitivity were observed.

Saltzman et al. [88] randomized healthy adults with BMIs of 18-38 kg/m^2 to hypoenergetic diets containing either 45 g whole-grain rolled oats/1000 kcal/day or the same amount of refined grain wheat. The prescribed energy deficit of 1000 kcal/day was met by providing all food to participants, and body fat was measured by hydrostatic weighing. After 6 weeks, neither body weight nor body fat loss differed between groups [88]. Interestingly, a trend for greater improvement in insulin sensitivity, as measured by oral glucose tolerance test and HOMA-IR, was reported in the oats group [91]. The favorable effects on insulin sensitivity are consistent with another whole-grain intervention in which dietary intake was strictly controlled by providing all food to participants [90]. In that crossover trial, 11 hyperinsulinemic adults consumed isoenergetic weight-maintaining diets that varied only in whether grains were derived from whole-grain or refined grain sources for 6 weeks. Insulin sensitivity, as measured by the euglycemic-hyperinsulinemic clamp, was significantly higher after individuals consumed the whole-grain diet, despite no significant changes in body weight during either diet period [90].

Taken together, these studies suggest that dietary substitution of whole grains for refined grains may preserve lean mass and facilitate greater body fat loss, predominantly from the abdominal region, in overweight and obese adults adopting hypoenergetic diets for weight loss. However, replication of these findings is required in a larger study because the observed effect sizes are relatively small and within the measurement error of the methods used to assess fat mass [92–94]. In addition, the observed effects are not always consistent with changes in WC [85,86]. Moreover, underlying mechanisms remain unclear because studies reporting positive effects on adiposity have not observed concomitant improvements in glycemic control and insulin sensitivity.

A potential mediator, and relatively unexplored mechanism in these studies, is the effect of whole grains on the composition of the gut microbiota. Gut microbiota composition has been linked to human obesity [95–101] and is sensitive to multiple dietary factors [97,102–105]. The gut microbiota plays an essential role in the metabolism of fiber within whole grains [34,106], and metabolic by-products of this metabolism, particularly SCFAs, influence glucose and lipid utilization and storage [29]. Whole grains may, therefore, influence adiposity through a combination of altering gut microbiota composition and providing metabolic substrates for gut microbes.

The first studies to demonstrate whole grain-mediated effects on the gut microbiota separately reported increased fecal *Bifidobacterium* spp. abundance following consumption of 48 g/day of whole-grain maize or wheat breakfast cereal for 2 weeks [107,108]. These interventions were too short to infer effects on adiposity; however, one recent meta-analysis concluded that *Bifidobacterium* is depleted in the gut microbiota of obese relative to lean individuals [109]. Thus, longer interventions resulting in a sustained increase in *Bifidobacterium* abundance may have resulted in favorable effects on adiposity. Martinez et al. [110] recently documented increased bacterial diversity in the gut microbiota of individuals incorporating 60 g/day of whole-grain barley and brown rice into their diets over 4 weeks. Although body composition was not assessed in the study, greater bacterial diversity has been associated with leanness [100]. In addition, shifts in microbiota composition were correlated with decreased glucose and insulin responses to an oral glucose tolerance test [110]. In contrast, incorporating 75 g/day of whole-grain rye bread into habitual diets for 12 weeks had little effect on bacterial populations in another study [111]. The inconsistency with previous studies may reflect differences in the source of whole grains used for the intervention because in vitro models have demonstrated that the type, amount, and structure of whole grains differentially influence bacterial growth [112–114]. In addition, the study was conducted in a population with high habitual whole-grain rye intakes, and reductions in rye intake within the control group resulted in significant decreases in multiple bacterial populations [111]. These changes were not significantly different from those of the whole-grain group but do provide some additional support for whole grain-mediated effects on gut microbiota composition. Unfortunately, while this study was of sufficient duration to detect changes in adiposity, body composition was not reported [111]. As such, to what extent whole grain-mediated effects on the gut microbiota are relevant to the regulation of body fat storage and utilization remains undetermined.

CONCLUSION

All whole grains share nutrients and physicochemical properties thought to benefit body weight and adiposity. Dietary fiber, in particular, has been linked to appetite suppression, improved glycemic control and insulin sensitivity, and weight loss, and is the preferred substrate of gut bacteria. Antimicrobial properties of polyphenols in whole grains are also postulated to alter gut microbiota composition, while magnesium and antioxidants within whole grains have been linked to improved insulin sensitivity. Intact, relative to processed, whole grains attenuate postprandial glycemic responses and may promote satiety. However, diversity in the chemical composition and quantities of indigestible carbohydrates within different whole grains, the degree to which grains are processed prior to consumption, and interactions with the food matrix all influence the physiologic effects of whole grains. Moreover, variations in nutrient composition, the types of foods in which whole-grain ingredients are used, and the structural integrity of different whole grains can be considerable. As such, not all whole-grain and whole grain-containing foods elicit the same physiologic effects, and not all whole-grain foods should be considered healthy or likely to be efficacious in preventing and treating abdominal adiposity.

Although epidemiological evidence consistently demonstrates inverse associations between whole-grain intake and adiposity, findings of controlled clinical trials are inconclusive. Inconsistencies may be attributable to the nature of whole-grain interventions employed because the <10 g/day differences in dietary fiber intake achieved by substituting whole grains for refined grains in many clinical trials [79,80,84–89] is less than the amount reported to induce even modest weight loss [115,116]. In addition, the common use of processed whole-grain products may have mitigated whole grain-mediated effects on physiologic regulators of adiposity.

Insufficient evidence exists to definitively conclude that whole grains are efficacious for preventing and treating abdominal adiposity. Randomized trials of adequate duration to detect sustained effects on body weight and adiposity (i.e. ideally a year or longer) and utilizing whole-grain products likely to optimize effects on body composition (i.e. high fiber and intact grains) are needed.

Nonetheless, whole grains are nutritionally superior to refined grains, and observational evidence consistently links higher whole-grain intakes to lower chronic disease risk, BMI, and adiposity. In the interim, whole-grain consumption should continue to be encouraged as part of a health-promoting diet, with an emphasis placed on consuming whole-grain foods that are minimally processed, high in fiber, and low in added sugar.

References

[1] Spiller GA. Whole grain, whole wheat, and white flours in history. In: Marquat L, , Slavin JL, Fulcher RG, editors. Whole-grain foods in health and disease. St. Paul, MN: Eagan Press; 2002.

[2] Fardet A. New hypotheses for the health-protective mechanisms of whole-grain cereals: what is beyond fibre? Nutr Res Rev 2010;23(1):65–134.

[3] Slavin J. Whole grains and human health. Nutr Res Rev 2004;17(1):99–110.

[4] Okarter N, Liu RH. Health benefits of whole grain phytochemicals. Crit Rev Food Sci Nutr 2010;50(3):193–208.

[5] American association of cereal chemists international . Whole-grain definition. Cereal Foods World 1996;45:79.

[6] Frolich W, Aman P, Tetens I. Whole grain foods and health—a Scandinavian perspective. Food Nutr Res 2013;57:18503.

[7] Bachman JL, Reedy J, Subar AF, Krebs-Smith SM. Sources of food group intakes among the US population, 2001–2002. J Am Diet Assoc 2008;108(5):804–14.

[8] Harnack L, Walters SA, Jacobs Jr DR. Dietary intake and food sources of whole grains among US children and adolescents: data from the 1994–1996 continuing survey of food intakes by individuals. J Am Diet Assoc 2003;103(8):1015–9.

[9] Mozaffarian RS, Andry A, Lee RM, Wiecha JL, Gortmaker SL. Price and healthfulness of snacks in 32 YMCA after-school programs in 4 US metropolitan areas, 2006–2008. Prev Chronic Dis 2012;9:E38.

[10] U.S. Department of Health and Human Services. U.S. FDA. Health claim notification for whole grain foods, <http://www.fda.gov/Food/IngredientsPackagingLabeling/LabelingNutrition/ucm073639.htm>; 2013 [accessed 19.06.2013].

[11] American Association of Cereal Chemists International. AACCI's whole grains working group unveils new whole grain products characterization, <http://www.aaccnet.org/about/newsreleases/Pages/WholegrainProductCharacterization.aspx>; 2013 [accessed 19.06.13].

[12] U.S. Department of Agriculture U.S. Department of Health and Human Services . Dietary Guidelines for Americans, 2010. 7th ed. Washington, DC: U.S. Government Printing Office; December 2010.

[13] McKeown NM, Jacques PF, Seal CJ, de Vries J, Jonnalagadda SS, Clemens R, et al. Whole grains and health: from theory to practice—highlights of the grains for health foundation's whole grains summit 2012. J Nutr 2013;143(5):744S–58S.

[14] Lang R, Jebb SA. Who consumes whole grains, and how much? Proc Nutr Soc 2003;62(1):123–7.

[15] Burgess-Champoux TL, Larson NI, Neumark-Sztainer DR, Hannan PJ, Story MT. Longitudinal and secular trends in adolescent whole-grain consumption, 1999–2004. Am J Clin Nutr 2010;91(1):154–9.

[16] O'Neil CE, Nicklas TA, Zanovec M, Cho S. Whole-grain consumption is associated with diet quality and nutrient intake in adults: the National Health and Nutrition Examination Survey, 1999–2004. J Am Diet Assoc 2010;110(10):1461–8.

[17] Ye EQ, Chacko SA, Chou EL, Kugizaki M, Liu S. Greater whole-grain intake is associated with lower risk of type 2 diabetes, cardiovascular disease, and weight gain. J Nutr 2012;142(7):1304–13.

[18] Aune D, Chan DS, Lau R, Vieira R, Greenwood DC, Kampman E, et al. Dietary fibre, whole grains, and risk of colorectal cancer: systematic review and dose-response meta-analysis of prospective studies. BMJ 2011;343:d6617.

[19] Karl JP, Saltzman E. The role of whole grains in body weight regulation. Adv Nutr 2012;3(5):697–707.

[20] The food pyramid for Germany, Austria, and Switzerland, <http://www.dge.de/modules.php?name=News&file=article&sid=481>: 2013 [accessed 19.06.13].

[21] UK food standards agency healthy eating nutrition essentials, <http://www.eatwell.gov.uk/healthydiet/nutritionessentials>; 2013 [accessed 19.06.13].

[22] Ministry of Health and Welfare SSHC . Dietary guidelines for adults in Greece. Arch Hellenic Med 1999;16(5):516–24.

[23] World Health Organization . Food based dietary guidelines in the WHO European region. Copenhagen, Denmark: WHO Regional, Office; 2003.

[24] Walter P, Infanger E, Muhlemann P. Food pyramid of the swiss society for nutrition. Ann Nutr Metab 2007;51(S2):15–20.

[25] Cui SW, Nie S, Roberts KT. Functional properties of dietary fiber. Comprehensive Biotech 2011;4:517–25.

[26] Dikeman CL, Fahey GC. Viscosity as related to dietary fiber: a review. Crit Rev Food Sci Nutr 2006;46(8):649–63.

[27] Slavin J, Green H. Dietary fibre and satiety. Nutr Bull 2007;32(S1):32–42.

[28] Macfarlane S, Macfarlane GT. Regulation of short-chain fatty acid production. Proc Nutr Soc 2003;62(1):67–72.

[29] Macfarlane GT, Macfarlane S. Bacteria, colonic fermentation, and gastrointestinal health. J AOAC Int 2012;95(1):50–60.

[30] Sleeth ML, Thompson EL, Ford HE, Zac-Varghese SE, Frost G. Free fatty acid receptor 2 and nutrient sensing: a proposed role for fibre, fermentable carbohydrates and short-chain fatty acids in appetite regulation. Nutr Res Rev 2010;23(1):135–45.

[31] Delzenne NM, Cani PD. Interaction between obesity and the gut microbiota: relevance in nutrition. Ann Rev Nutr 2011;31:15–31.

[32] Dong JY, Xun P, He K, Qin LQ. Magnesium intake and risk of type 2 diabetes: meta-analysis of prospective cohort studies. Diabetes Care 2011;34(9):2116–22.

[33] Hamer M, Chida Y. Intake of fruit, vegetables, and antioxidants and risk of type 2 diabetes: systematic review and meta-analysis. J Hypertens 2007;25(12):2361–9.

[34] Tuohy KM, Conterno L, Gasperotti M, Viola R. Up-regulating the human intestinal microbiome using whole plant foods, polyphenols, and/or fiber. J Agric Food Chem 2012;60(36):8776–82.

[35] Hallfrisch J, Behall KM. Mechanisms of the effects of grains on insulin and glucose responses. J Am Coll Nutr 2000;19(3 Suppl):320S–5S.

[36] Holt SH, Miller JB. Particle size, satiety and the glycaemic response. Eur J Clin Nutr 1994;48(7):496–502.

[37] Heaton KW, Marcus SN, Emmett PM, Bolton CH. Particle size of wheat, maize, and oat test meals: effects on plasma glucose and insulin responses and on the rate of starch digestion in vitro. Am J Clin Nutr 1988;47(4):675–82.

[38] Jenkins DJ, Wesson V, Wolever TM, Jenkins AL, Kalmusky J, Guidici S, et al. Wholemeal versus wholegrain breads: proportion of whole or cracked grain and the glycaemic response. BMJ 1988;297(6654):958–60.

[39] Liljeberg H, Granfeldt Y, Bjorck I. Metabolic responses to starch in bread containing intact kernels versus milled flour. Eur J Clin Nutr 1992;46(8):561–75.

[40] O'Dea K, Nestel PJ, Antonoff L. Physical factors influencing postprandial glucose and insulin responses to starch. Am J Clin Nutr 1980;33(4):760–5.

[41] Hlebowicz J, Jonsson JM, Lindstedt S, Bjorgell O, Darwich G, Almer LO. Effect of commercial rye whole-meal bread on postprandial blood glucose and gastric emptying in healthy subjects. Nutr J 2009;8:26.
[42] Englyst KN, Englyst HN. Carbohydrate bioavailability. Br J Nutr 2005;94(1):1–11.
[43] Esmaillzadeh A, Mirmiran P, Azizi F. Whole-grain consumption and the metabolic syndrome: a favorable association in Tehranian adults. Eur J Clin Nutr 2005;59(3):353–62.
[44] Good CK, Holschuh N, Albertson AM, Eldridge AL. Whole grain consumption and body mass index in adult women: an analysis of NHANES 1999–2000 and the USDA pyramid servings database. J Am Coll Nutr 2008;27(1):80–7.
[45] Lutsey PL, Jacobs Jr DR, Kori S, Mayer-Davis E, Shea S, Steffen LM, et al. Whole grain intake and its cross-sectional association with obesity, insulin resistance, inflammation, diabetes and subclinical CVD: The MESA Study. Br J Nutr 2007;98(2):397–405.
[46] McKeown NM, Yoshida M, Shea MK, Jacques PF, Lichtenstein AH, Rogers G, et al. Whole-grain intake and cereal fiber are associated with lower abdominal adiposity in older adults. J Nutr 2009;139(10):1950–5.
[47] Newby PK, Maras J, Bakun P, Muller D, Ferrucci L, Tucker KL. Intake of whole grains, refined grains, and cereal fiber measured with 7-d diet records and associations with risk factors for chronic disease. Am J Clin Nutr 2007;86(6):1745–53.
[48] van de Vijver LP, van den Bosch LM, van den Brandt PA, Goldbohm RA. Whole-grain consumption, dietary fibre intake and body mass index in the Netherlands cohort study. Eur J Clin Nutr 2009;63(1):31–8.
[49] Jacobs Jr DR, Meyer KA, Kushi LH, Folsom AR. Whole-grain intake may reduce the risk of ischemic heart disease death in postmenopausal women: the Iowa women's health study. Am J Clin Nutr 1998;68(2):248–57.
[50] Harland JI, Garton LE. Whole-grain intake as a marker of healthy body weight and adiposity. Public Health Nutr 2008;11(6):554–63.
[51] Grundy SM, Cleeman JI, Daniels SR, Donato KA, Eckel RH, Franklin BA, et al. Diagnosis and management of the metabolic syndrome. An american heart association/National heart, lung, and blood institute scientific statement. Executive summary. Cardiol Rev 2005;13(6):322–7.
[52] McKeown NM, Troy LM, Jacques PF, Hoffmann U, O'Donnell CJ, Fox CS. Whole- and refined-grain intakes are differentially associated with abdominal visceral and subcutaneous adiposity in healthy adults: the Framingham heart study. Am J Clin Nutr 2010;92(5):1165–71.
[53] Koh-Banerjee P, Franz M, Sampson L, Liu S, Jacobs Jr DR, Spiegelman D, et al. Changes in whole-grain, bran, and cereal fiber consumption in relation to 8-y weight gain among men. Am J Clin Nutr 2004;80(5):1237–45.
[54] Liu S, Willett WC, Manson JE, Hu FB, Rosner B, Colditz G. Relation between changes in intakes of dietary fiber and grain products and changes in weight and development of obesity among middle-aged women. Am J Clin Nutr 2003;78(5):920–7.
[55] Mozaffarian D, Hao T, Rimm EB, Willett WC, Hu FB. Changes in diet and lifestyle and long-term weight gain in women and men. N Engl J Med 2011;364(25):2392–404.
[56] Du H, van der AD, Boshuizen HC, Forouhi NG, Wareham NJ, Halkjaer J, et al. Dietary fiber and subsequent changes in body weight and waist circumference in European men and women. Am J Clin Nutr 2010;91(2):329–36.
[57] Halkjaer J, Sorensen TI, Tjonneland A, Togo P, Holst C, Heitmann BL. Food and drinking patterns as predictors of 6-year BMI-adjusted changes in waist circumference. Br J Nutr 2004;92(4):735–48.
[58] Bautista-Castano I, Sanchez-Villegas A, Estruch R, Martinez-Gonzalez MA, Corella D, Salas-Salvado J, et al. Changes in bread consumption and 4-year changes in adiposity in Spanish subjects at high cardiovascular risk. Br J Nutr 2012;110(2):337–46.
[59] Whitlock G, Lewington S, Sherliker P, Clarke R, Emberson J, Halsey J, et al. Body-mass index and cause-specific mortality in 900,000 adults: collaborative analyses of 57 prospective studies. Lancet 2009;373(9669):1083–96.
[60] Clinical Guidelines on the Identification . Evaluation, and Treatment of Overweight and Obesity in Adults—The Evidence Report. National Institutes of Health. Obes Res 1998;6(Suppl 2):51S–209S.
[61] Jonnalagadda SS, Harnack L, Liu RH, McKeown N, Seal C, Liu S, et al. Putting the whole grain puzzle together: health benefits associated with whole grains—summary of American society for nutrition 2010 satellite symposium. J Nutr 2011;141(5):1011S–22S.
[62] McKeown NM, Hruby A, Saltzman E, Choumenkovitch SF, Jacques PF. Weighing in on whole grains: a review of evidence linking whole grains to body weight. Cereal Foods World 2012;57(1):20–7.
[63] Mancino L, Kuchler F, Leibtag E. Getting consumers to eat more whole-grains: the role of policy, information, and food manufacturers. Food Policy 2008;33:489–96.
[64] Thane CW, Stephen AM, Jebb SA. Whole grains and adiposity: little association among British adults. Eur J Clin Nutr 2009;63(2):229–37.
[65] Clemens R, Kranz S, Mobley AR, Nicklas TA, Raimondi MP, Rodriguez JC, et al. Filling America's fiber intake gap: summary of a roundtable to probe realistic solutions with a focus on grain-based foods. J Nutr 2012;142(7):1390S–401S.
[66] Landberg R, Kamal-Eldin A, Andersson A, Vessby B, Aman P. Alkylresorcinols as biomarkers of whole-grain wheat and rye intake: plasma concentration and intake estimated from dietary records. Am J Clin Nutr 2008;87(4):832–8.
[67] Ross AB, Bourgeois A, Macharia HN, Kochhar S, Jebb SA, Brownlee IA, et al. Plasma alkylresorcinols as a biomarker of whole-grain food consumption in a large population: results from the WHOLEheart Intervention Study. Am J Clin Nutr 2012;95(1):204–11.
[68] Landberg R, Townsend MK, Neelakantan N, Sun Q, Sampson L, Spiegelman D, et al. Alkylresorcinol metabolite concentrations in spot urine samples correlated with whole grain and cereal fiber intake but showed low to modest reproducibility over one to three years in U.S. women. J Nutr 2012;142(5):872–7.
[69] Ross AB, Kamal-Eldin A, Aman P. Dietary alkylresorcinols: absorption, bioactivities, and possible use as biomarkers of whole-grain wheat- and rye-rich foods. Nutr Rev 2004;62(3):81–95.
[70] Ma J, Ross AB, Shea MK, Bruce SJ, Jacques PF, Saltzman E, et al. Plasma alkylresorcinols, biomarkers of whole-grain intake, are related to lower BMI in older adults. J Nutr 2012;142(10):1859–64.
[71] Montonen J, Landberg R, Kamal-Eldin A, Aman P, Knueppel S, Boeing H, et al. Reliability of fasting plasma alkylresorcinol concentrations measured 4 months apart. Eur J Clin Nutr 2010;64(7):698–703.
[72] Landberg R, Linko AM, Kamal-Eldin A, Vessby B, Adlercreutz H, Aman P. Human plasma kinetics and relative bioavailability of alkylresorcinols after intake of rye bran. J Nutr 2006;136(11):2760–5.
[73] Landberg R, Aman P, Friberg LE, Vessby B, Adlercreutz H, Kamal-Eldin A. Dose response of whole-grain biomarkers: alkylresorcinols in human plasma and their metabolites in urine in relation to intake. Am J Clin Nutr 2009;89(1):290–6.

[74] Ross AB. Present status and perspectives on the use of alkylresorcinols as biomarkers of wholegrain wheat and rye intake. J Nutr Metab 2012;2012:462967.

[75] Liu E, McKeown NM, Newby PK, Meigs JB, Vasan RS, Quatromoni PA, et al. Cross-sectional association of dietary patterns with insulin-resistant phenotypes among adults without diabetes in the Framingham Offspring Study. Br J Nutr 2009;102(4):576–83.

[76] Kant AK. Dietary patterns and health outcomes. J Am Diet Assoc 2004;104(4):615–35.

[77] Newby PK, Tucker KL. Empirically derived eating patterns using factor or cluster analysis: a review. Nutr Rev 2004;62(5):177–203.

[78] Brownlee IA, Moore C, Chatfield M, Richardson DP, Ashby P, Kuznesof SA, et al. Markers of cardiovascular risk are not changed by increased whole-grain intake: the WHOLEheart study, a randomised, controlled dietary intervention. Br J Nutr 2010;104(1):125–34.

[79] Ross AB, Bruce SJ, Blondel-Lubrano A, Oguey-Araymon S, Beaumont M, Bourgeois A, et al. A whole-grain cereal-rich diet increases plasma betaine, and tends to decrease total and LDL-cholesterol compared with a refined-grain diet in healthy subjects. Br J Nutr 2011;105(10):1492–502.

[80] Andersson A, Tengblad S, Karlstrom B, Kamal-Eldin A, Landberg R, Basu S, et al. Whole-grain foods do not affect insulin sensitivity or markers of lipid peroxidation and inflammation in healthy, moderately overweight subjects. J Nutr 2007;137(6):1401–7.

[81] Giacco R, Clemente G, Cipriano D, Luongo D, Viscovo D, Patti L, et al. Effects of the regular consumption of wholemeal wheat foods on cardiovascular risk factors in healthy people. Nutr Metab Cardiovasc Dis 2010;20(3):186–94.

[82] Leinonen KS, Poutanen KS, Mykkanen HM. Rye bread decreases serum total and LDL cholesterol in men with moderately elevated serum cholesterol. J Nutr 2000;130(2):164–70.

[83] Pins JJ, Geleva D, Keenan JM, Frazel C, O'Connor PJ, Cherney LM. Do whole-grain oat cereals reduce the need for antihypertensive medications and improve blood pressure control? J Fam Pract 2002;51(4):353–9.

[84] Tucker AJ, Mackay KA, Robinson LE, Graham TE, Bakovic M, Duncan AM. The effect of whole grain wheat sourdough bread consumption on serum lipids in healthy normoglycemic/ normoinsulinemic and hyperglycemic/hyperinsulinemic adults depends on presence of the APOE E3/E3 genotype: a randomized controlled trial. Nutr Metab 2010;7:37.

[85] Katcher HI, Legro RS, Kunselman AR, Gillies PJ, Demers LM, Bagshaw DM, et al. The effects of a whole grain-enriched hypocaloric diet on cardiovascular disease risk factors in men and women with metabolic syndrome. Am J Clin Nutr 2008;87(1):79–90.

[86] Kristensen M, Toubro S, Jensen MG, Ross AB, Riboldi G, Petronio M, et al. Whole grain compared with refined wheat decreases the percentage of body fat following a 12-week, energy-restricted dietary intervention in postmenopausal women. J Nutr 2012;142(4):710–6.

[87] Maki KC, Beiseigel JM, Jonnalagadda SS, Gugger CK, Reeves MS, Farmer MV, et al. Whole-grain ready-to-eat oat cereal, as part of a dietary program for weight loss, reduces low-density lipoprotein cholesterol in adults with overweight and obesity more than a dietary program including low-fiber control foods. J Am Diet Assoc 2010;110(2):205–14.

[88] Saltzman E, Moriguti JC, Das SK, Corrales A, Fuss P, Greenberg AS, et al. Effects of a cereal rich in soluble fiber on body composition and dietary compliance during consumption of a hypocaloric diet. J Am Coll Nutr 2001;20(1):50–7.

[89] Melanson KJ, Angelopoulos TJ, Nguyen VT, Martini M, Zukley L, Lowndes J, et al. Consumption of whole-grain cereals during weight loss: effects on dietary quality, dietary fiber, magnesium, vitamin B-6, and obesity. J Am Diet Assoc 2006;106(9):1380–8.

[90] Pereira MA, Jacobs Jr DR, Pins JJ, Raatz SK, Gross MD, Slavin JL, et al. Effect of whole grains on insulin sensitivity in overweight hyperinsulinemic adults. Am J Clin Nutr 2002;75(5):848–55.

[91] Saltzman E, Das SK, Lichtenstein AH, Dallal GE, Corrales A, Schaefer EJ, et al. An oat-containing hypocaloric diet reduces systolic blood pressure and improves lipid profile beyond effects of weight loss in men and women. J Nutr 2001;131(5):1465–70.

[92] Gibson RS. Principles of nutrition assessment. 2nd ed. New York, NY: Oxford University Press; 2005.

[93] Lee RD. Nutritional assessment. 3rd ed. New York, NY: McGraw-Hill; 2000.

[94] Lohman TG, Harris M, Teixeira PJ, Weiss L. Assessing body composition and changes in body composition. Another look at dual-energy X-ray absorptiometry. Ann N Y Acad Sci 2000;904:45–54.

[95] Armougom F, Henry M, Vialettes B, Raccah D, Raoult D. Monitoring bacterial community of human gut microbiota reveals an increase in Lactobacillus in obese patients and methanogens in anorexic patients. PLoS One 2009;4(9):e7125.

[96] Kalliomaki M, Collado MC, Salminen S, Isolauri E. Early differences in fecal microbiota composition in children may predict overweight. Am J Clin Nutr 2008;87(3):534–8.

[97] Ley RE, Turnbaugh PJ, Klein S, Gordon JI. Microbial ecology: human gut microbes associated with obesity. Nature 2006;444(7122):1022–3.

[98] Million M, Maraninchi M, Henry M, Armougom F, Richet H, Carrieri P, et al. Obesity-associated gut microbiota is enriched in Lactobacillus reuteri and depleted in Bifidobacterium animalis and Methanobrevibacter smithii. Int J Obes 2012;36(6):817–25.

[99] Nadal I, Santacruz A, Marcos A, Warnberg J, Garagorri M, Moreno LA, et al. Shifts in clostridia, bacteroides and immunoglobulin-coating fecal bacteria associated with weight loss in obese adolescents. Int J Obes 2009;33(7):758–67.

[100] Turnbaugh PJ, Hamady M, Yatsunenko T, Cantarel BL, Duncan A, Ley RE, et al. A core gut microbiome in obese and lean twins. Nature 2009;457(7228):480–4.

[101] Zhang H, DiBaise JK, Zuccolo A, Kudrna D, Braidotti M, Yu Y, et al. Human gut microbiota in obesity and after gastric bypass. Proc Natl Acad Sci U S A 2009;106(7):2365–70.

[102] Duncan SH, Lobley GE, Holtrop G, Ince J, Johnstone AM, Louis P, et al. Human colonic microbiota associated with diet, obesity and weight loss. Int J Obes 2008;32(11):1720–4.

[103] Fava F, Gitau R, Griffin BA, Gibson GR, Tuohy KM, Lovegrove JA. The type and quantity of dietary fat and carbohydrate alter faecal microbiome and short-chain fatty acid excretion in a metabolic syndrome 'at-risk' population. Int J Obes 2013;37(2):216–23.

[104] Jumpertz R, Le DS, Turnbaugh PJ, Trinidad C, Bogardus C, Gordon JI, et al. Energy-balance studies reveal associations between gut microbes, caloric load, and nutrient absorption in humans. Am J Clin Nutr 2011;94(1):58–65.

[105] Wu GD, Chen J, Hoffmann C, Bittinger K, Chen YY, Keilbaugh SA, et al. Linking long-term dietary patterns with gut microbial enterotypes. Science 2011;334(6052):105–8.

[106] Scott KP, Duncan SH, Flint HJ. Dietary fibre and the gut microbiota. Nutr Bulletin 2008;33:201–11.

[107] Carvalho-Wells AL, Helmolz K, Nodet C, Molzer C, Leonard C, McKevith B, et al. Determination of the in vivo prebiotic potential of a maize-based whole grain breakfast cereal: a human feeding study. Br J Nutr 2010;104(9):1353–6.

[108] Costabile A, Klinder A, Fava F, Napolitano A, Fogliano V, Leonard C, et al. Whole-grain wheat breakfast cereal has a prebiotic effect on the human gut microbiota: a double-blind, placebo-controlled, crossover study. Br J Nutr 2008;99(1):110–20.

[109] Angelakis E, Armougom F, Million M, Raoult D. The relationship between gut microbiota and weight gain in humans. Future Microbiol 2012;7(1):91–109.

[110] Martinez I, Lattimer JM, Hubach KL, Case JA, Yang J, Weber CG, et al. Gut microbiome composition is linked to whole grain-induced immunological improvements. ISME J 2013;7(2):269–80.

[111] Lappi J, Salojarvi J, Kolehmainen M, Mykkanen H, Poutanen K, de Vos WM, et al. Intake of whole-grain and fiber-rich rye bread versus refined wheat bread does not differentiate intestinal microbiota composition in Finnish adults with metabolic syndrome. J Nutr 2013;143(5):648–55.

[112] Connolly ML, Lovegrove JA, Tuohy KM. In vitro fermentation characteristics of whole grain wheat flakes and the effect of toasting on prebiotic potential. J Med Food 2012;15(1):33–43.

[113] Connolly ML, Tuohy KM, Lovegrove JA. Wholegrain oat-based cereals have prebiotic potential and low glycaemic index. Br J Nutr 2012;108(12):2198–206.

[114] Connolly ML, Lovegrove JA, Tuohy KM. In vitro evaluation of the microbiota modulation abilities of different sized whole oat grain flakes. Anaerobe 2010;16(5):483–8.

[115] Howarth NC, Saltzman E, Roberts SB. Dietary fiber and weight regulation. Nutr Rev 2001;59(5):129–39.

[116] Wanders AJ, van den Borne JJ, de Graaf C, Hulshof T, Jonathan MC, Kristensen M, et al. Effects of dietary fibre on subjective appetite, energy intake and body weight: a systematic review of randomized controlled trials. Obes Rev 2011;12(9):724–39.

[117] U.S. Department of Agriculture, Agricultural Research Service. National Nutrient Database for Standard Reference, Release 25, 2012, <http://www.ars.usda.gov/ba/bhnrc/ndl>; 2013 [accessed 19.06.13].

Index

D

T

Color Plates

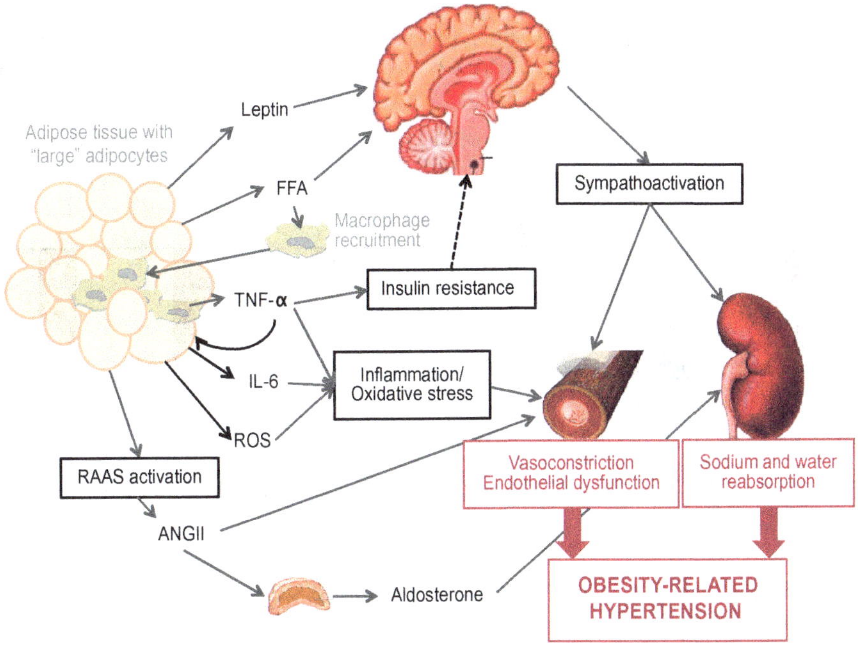

FIGURE 9.2 Simplified scheme of "mechanistic" pathways leading from increased adiposity to elevated blood pressure. ANGII, angiotensin II; FFA, free fatty acids; IL-6, interleukin-6; RAAS, renin-angiotensin-aldosterone system; ROS, reactive oxygen species; TNF-α, tumor necrosis factor.

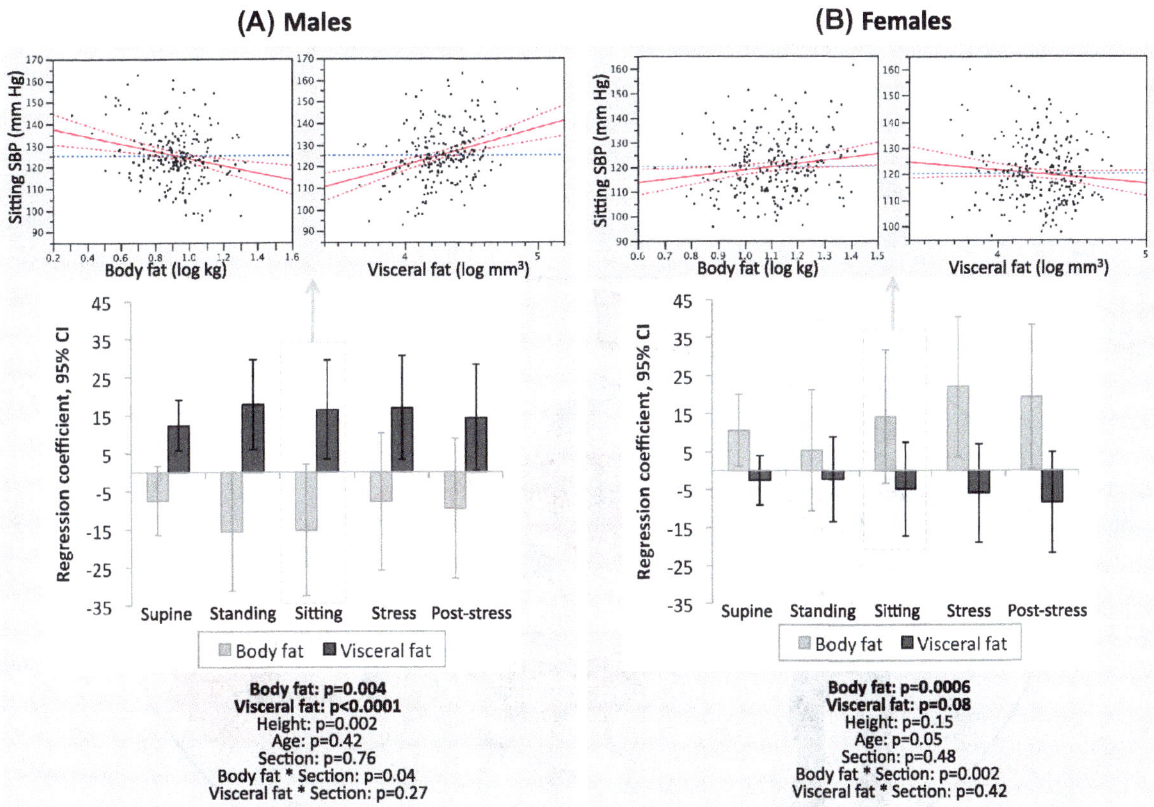

FIGURE 9.4 Multivariable relationships of systolic blood pressure with total body fat and visceral fat in males and females. A multivariable mixed linear model was used to estimate the relative contribution (model coefficient with 95% confidence interval) of each total body fat and visceral fat to systolic blood pressure (SBP) in males (*A*) and females (*B*), while adjusting for interindividual differences in height. SBP means of five consecutive sections of a 52-min cardiovascular protocol (i.e. supine, standing, sitting, stress, and poststress) were included in these analyses as repeated measures. Representative scatter plots of the multivariate associations of SBP with visceral fat and total body fat are also shown; for this purpose, the sitting section of the protocol was chosen. Source: reference [26] with permission.

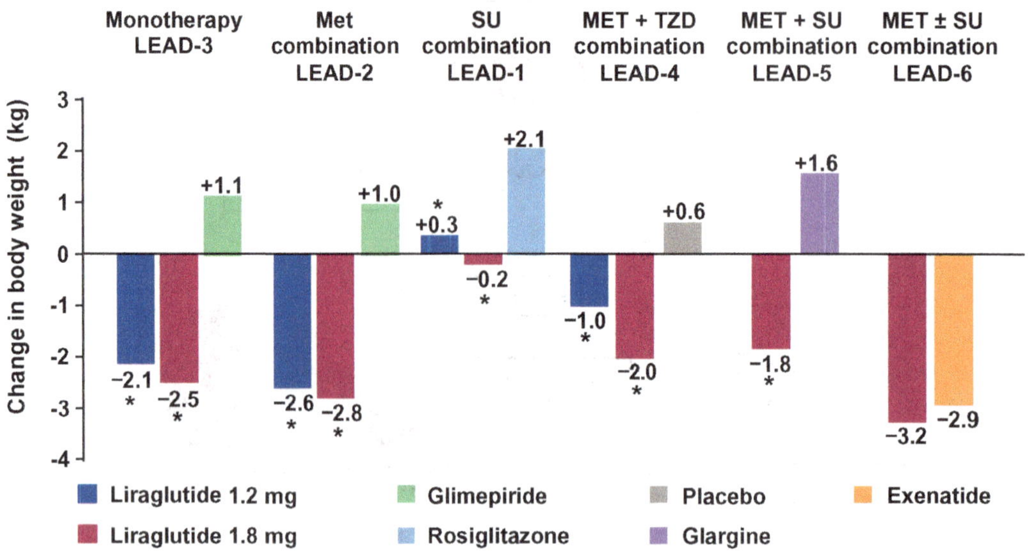

FIGURE 15.1 Changes in body weight from baseline observed in the LEAD trials [55,56,58]. *, statistical significance compared to a trial comparator. LEAD, Liraglutide Effect and Action in Diabetes; Met, metformin; SU, sulfonylurea; TZD, thiazolidinediones.

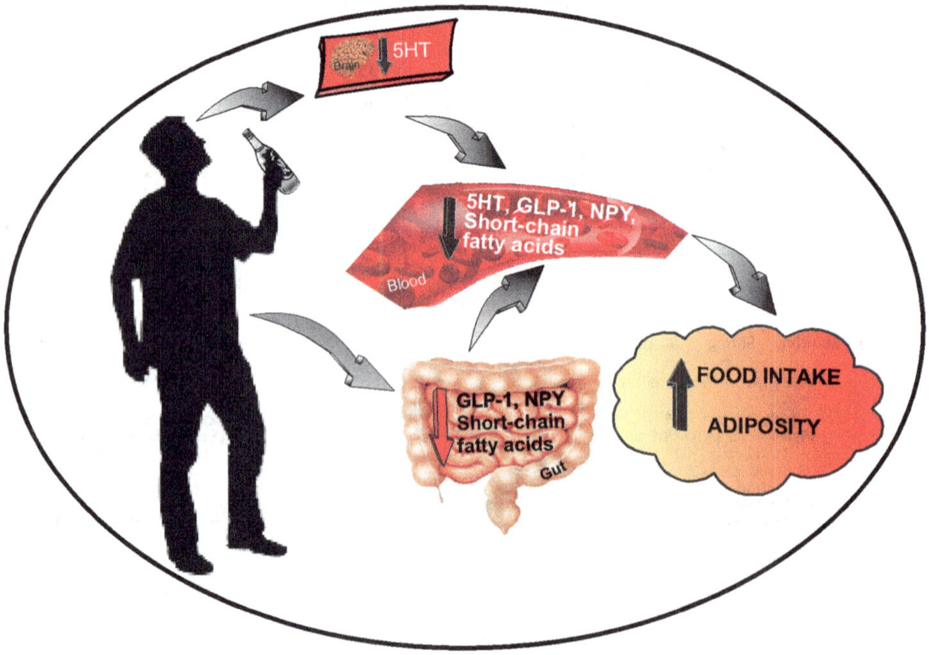

FIGURE 23.1 Schematic diagram showing the effects of ethanol on serotonin [5-hydroxytryptamine (5-HT)], anorexigenic and orexigenic hormones, and short-chain fatty acids, and thus on adiposity and food intake.

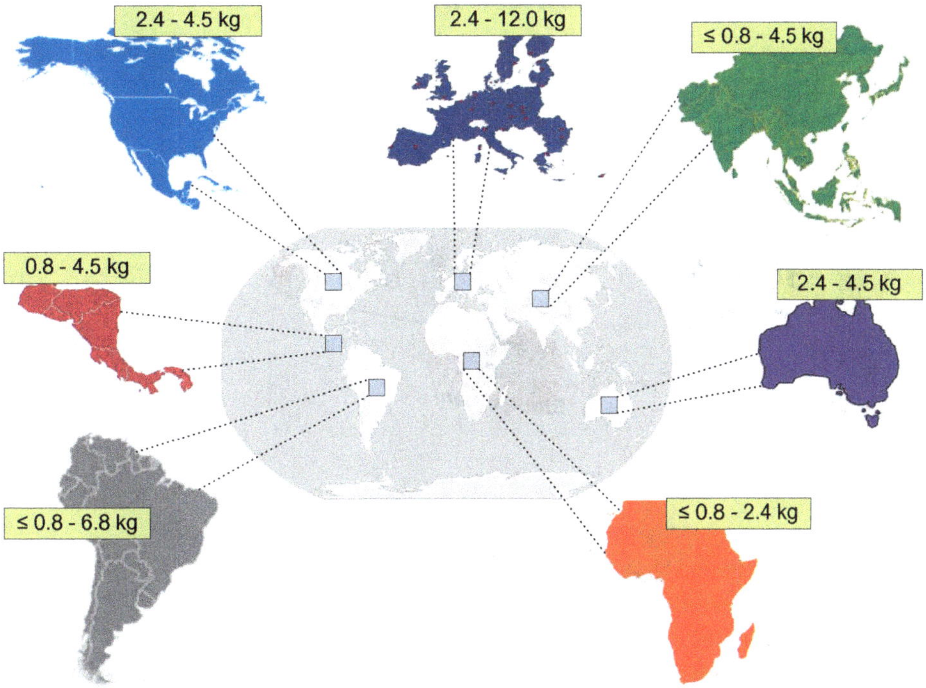

FIGURE 24.1 Current annual coffee consumption per capita per year throughout the world. Gray, South America; red, Central America; blue, North America; dark blue, Europe; green, Asia; purple, Oceania; orange, Africa.

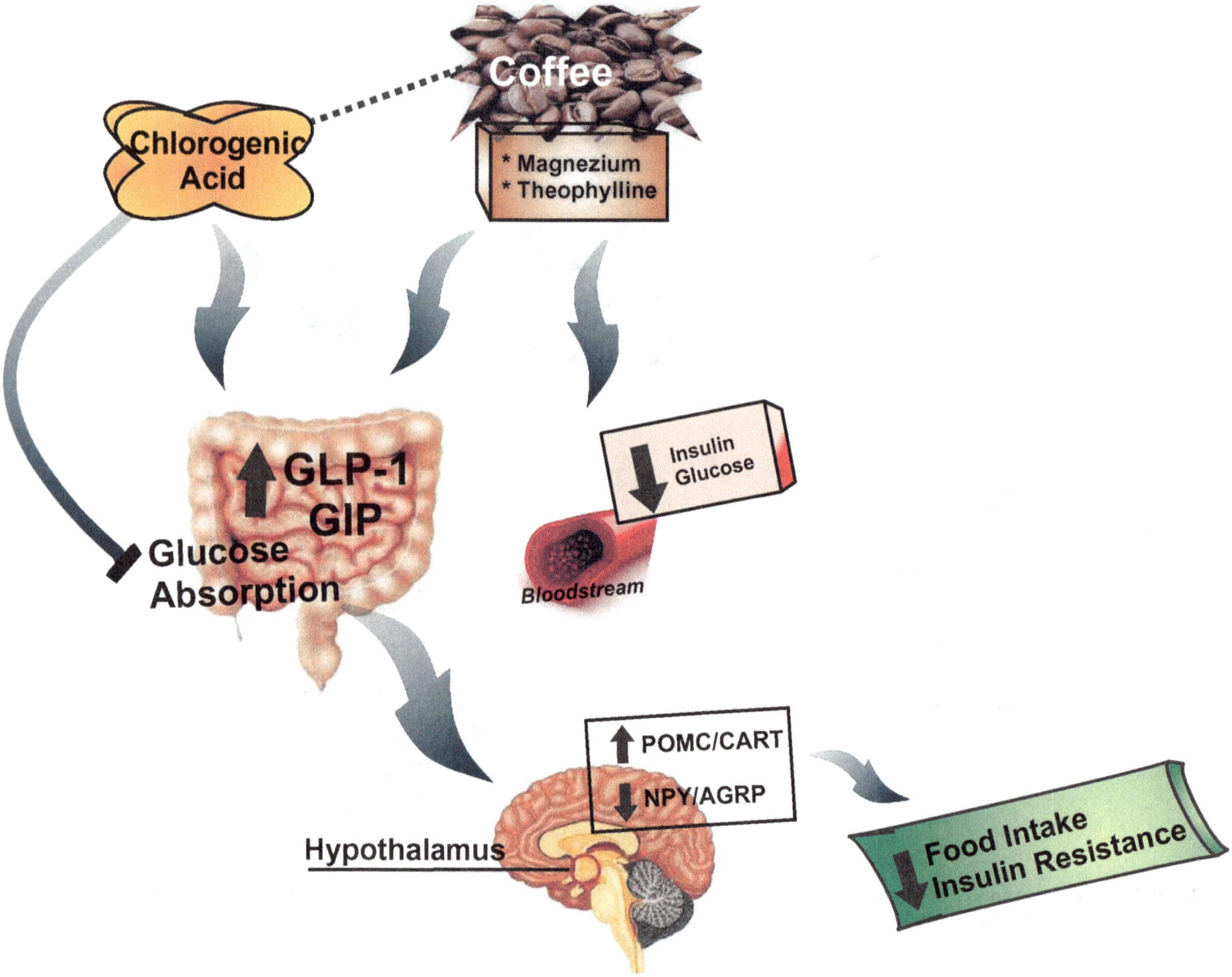

FIGURE 24.2 Schematic diagram showing the effects of coffee and its compounds on reducing food intake and improving insulin resistance. The consumption of coffee, theophylline, and chlorogenic acid has several beneficial actions: it (1) increases serum glucagon-like peptide 1 (GLP-1) and gastric inhibitory polypeptide (GIP) levels; (2) reduces beta cell damage; (3) increases C-peptide levels; (4) inhibits glucose absorption; and (5) reduces blood insulin and glucose concentrations. These effects may activate the neuropeptides proopiomelanocortin (POMC)/cocaine- and amphetamine-regulated transcript (CART) and reduce neuropeptide Y/agouti-related protein (NPY/AgRP), hence decreasing food intake and insulin resistance.

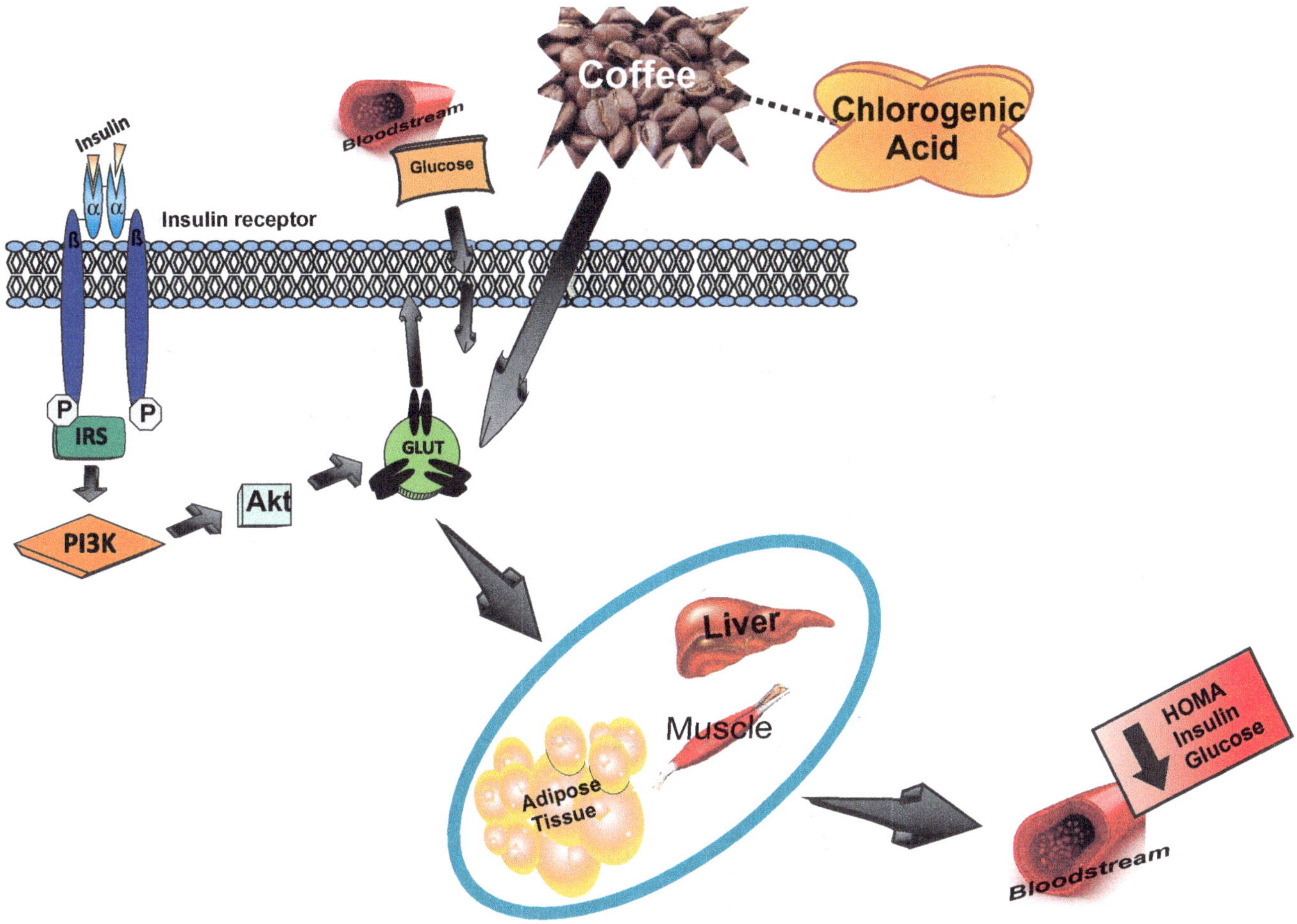

FIGURE 24.3 Diagram showing the effects of coffee and its compounds on glucose metabolism and insulin signaling. In healthy subjects, insulin binds to it receptors, which phosphorylates tyrosine residues in its substrates [insulin receptor substrate (IRS) 1 and 2], which activate phosphoinositide 3-kinase (PI3K), leading to Akt serine phosphorylation, which increases glucose transporters to the plasmatic membrane, which in turn favors the uptake of glucose by liver cells, muscle, and adipose tissue for use as an energy source. Glucose uptake can also be enhanced via 5′-AMP-activated protein kinase (AMPK). However, insulin signaling is blocked or impaired and AMPK is inactivated in obese individuals. Thus, coffee consumption (≥ 3 cups of 150 mL/day) or chlorogenic acid can activate GLUT proteins and induce AMPK phosphorylation, mainly in adipose tissue, the liver, and skeletal muscle.

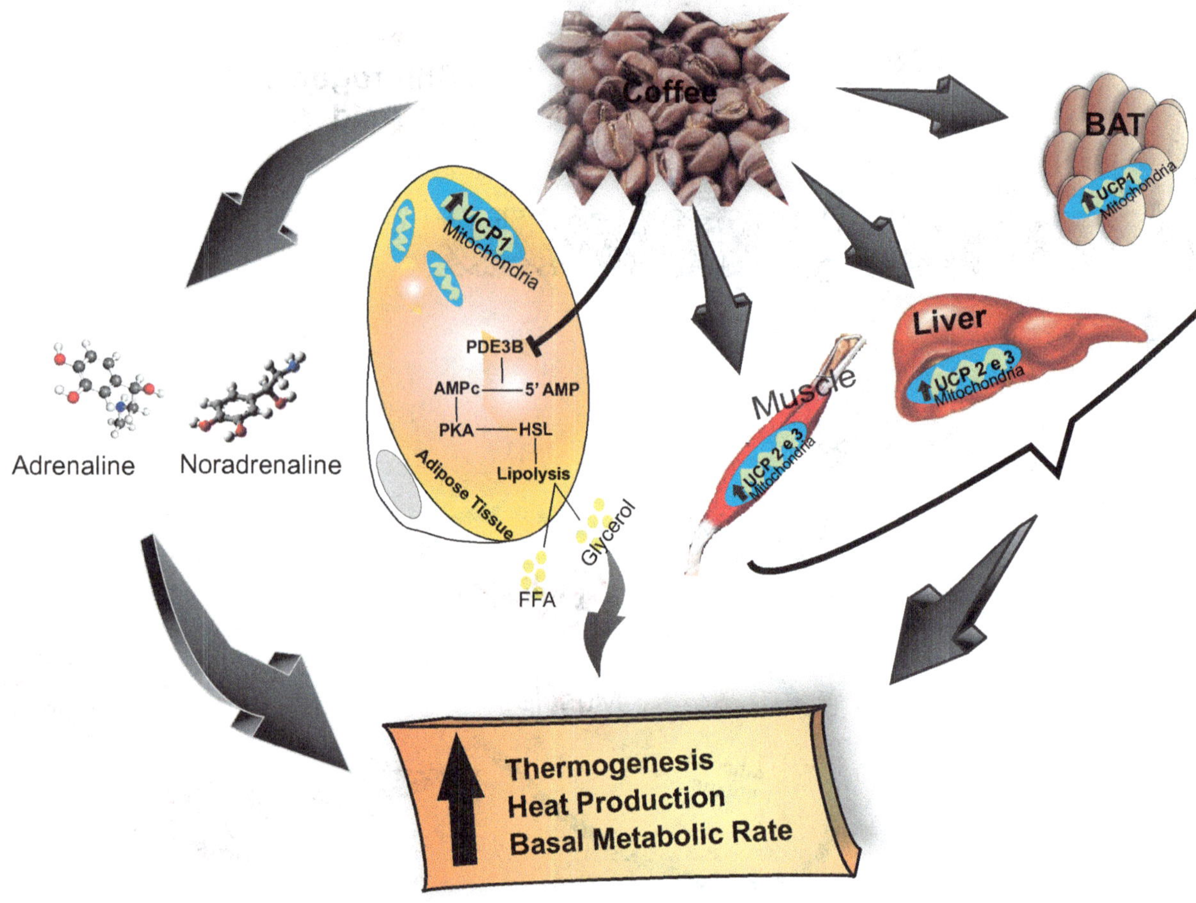

FIGURE 24.4 Main mechanisms of action of coffee and caffeine in increasing thermogenesis. Coffee and caffeine consumption may increase thermogenesis by (1) activating uncoupling proteins (UCPs 1, 2, and 3) in brown adipose tissue (BAT), liver, or skeletal muscle; (2) releasing noradrenaline and adrenaline and increasing lipolysis; and (3) inhibiting phosphodiesterase-induced degradation of intracellular cyclic AMP (cAMP). cAMP activates lipolysis pathway proteins such as protein kinase A (PKA), which phosphorylates hormone-sensitive lipase (HSL) and perilipin, releasing free fatty acids and glycerol to stimulate adrenoceptors, leading to thermogenesis.

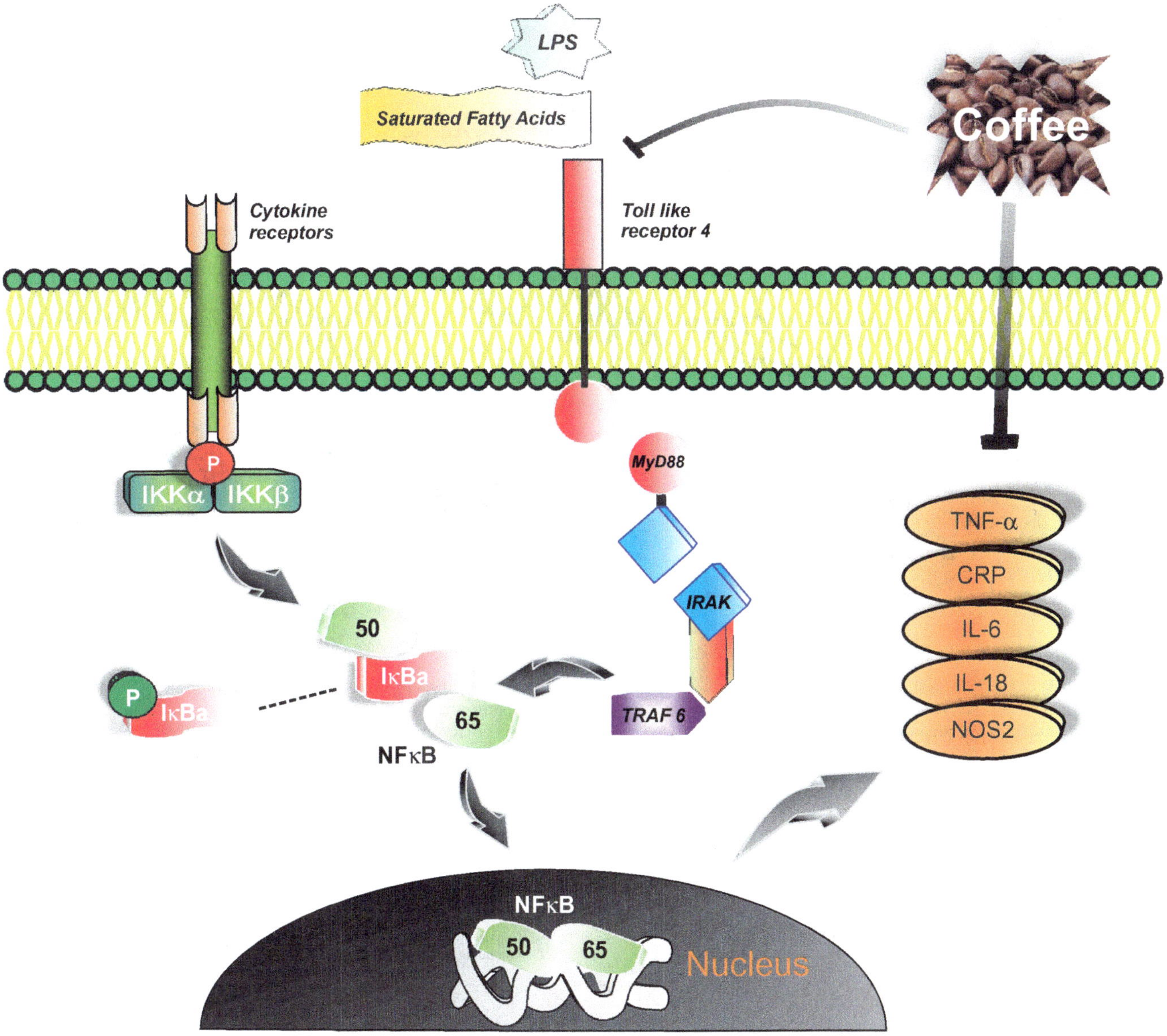

FIGURE 24.5 Schematic diagram showing the effects of coffee on the levels of proinflammatory molecules. In obese patients, inflammatory signaling is activated. A high intake of *trans* or saturated fatty acids, as well as a high lipopolysaccharide (LPS) content in the blood, has been demonstrated to induce proinflammatory cytokine production through the nuclear factor-kappa-B (NFκB) pathway after activation of the toll-like receptor 4 (TLR4). Activation of TLR4 initiates the myeloid differentiation primary response protein (MyD88)-dependent signaling pathway. MyD88 binding to the cytoplasmic domain of TLR4 activates TNF receptor-associated factor 6 (TRAF6), which is recruited by interleukin-1 receptor-associated kinase 1 (IRAK-1). Following IRAK-1 phosphorylation, the TRAF6 complex dissociates from the TLRs and TRAF6 interacts with various proteins to form a large complex that activates of transforming growth factor-beta-activated kinase 1 (TAK1). TAK1 phosphorylates the inhibitor of nuclear factor kappa-B (IκB) kinase (IKK) complex, and phosphorylated IκB is targeted for proteasomal degradation. Thus, the p65 subunit of NFκB is activated and translocates to the nucleus, where it binds to its target genes to produce proinflammatory cytokines, such as tumor necrosis factor (TNF-α), interleukin-6 (IL-6), interleukin-1β (IL-1β), interleukin-13 (IL-13), inducible nitric oxide synthase (iNOS/NOS2) and C-reactive protein (CRP). On the other hand, coffee and chlorogenic acid consumption can reduce proinflammatory cytokines in the blood, brain, and peripheral tissues and inhibit TLR4 expression, thus reducing inflammation and obesity.

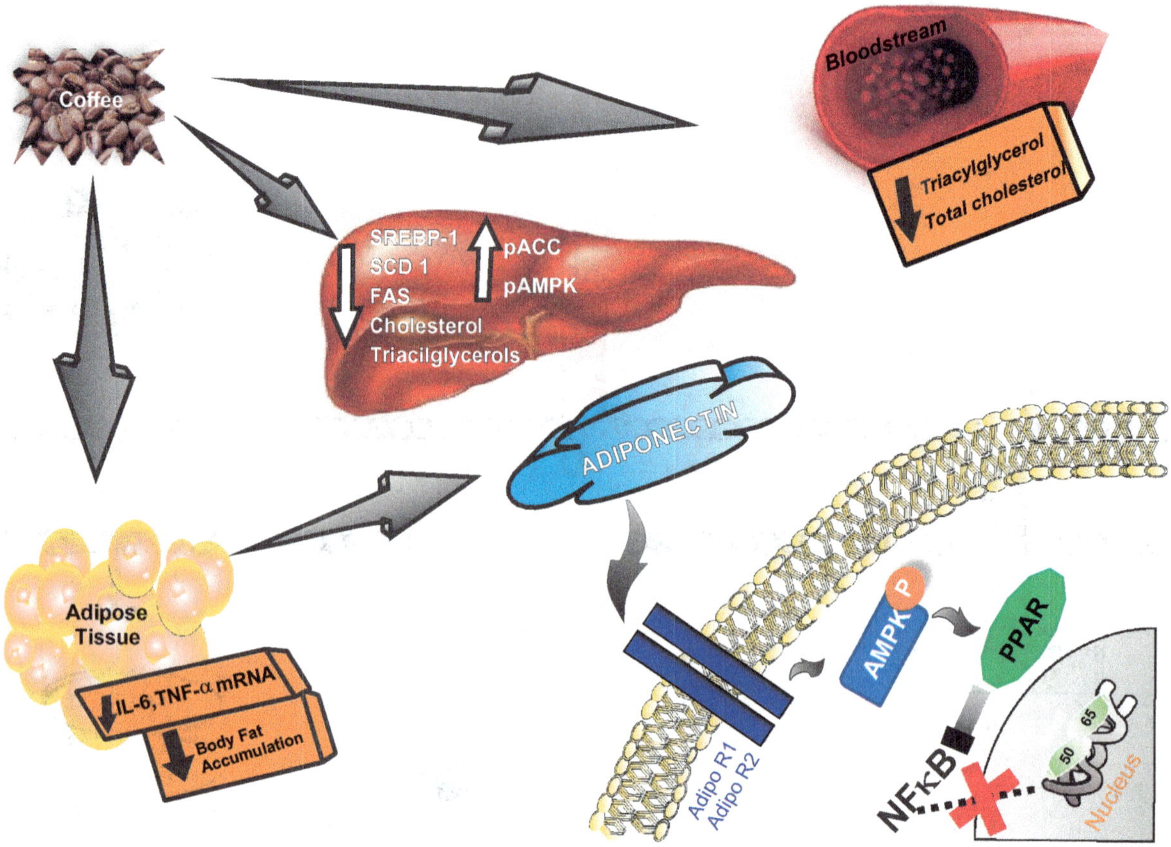

FIGURE 24.6 Schematic diagram showing the effects of coffee on cardiovascular disease indicators and inflammatory parameters in the bloodstream, liver, and white adipose tissue. Obese patients frequently have large amounts of adipose tissue and hepatic steatosis, accompanied by increased proinflammatory protein expression. Thus, coffee intake reduces adiposity and steatosis, as well as inflammation, by inhibiting tumor necrosis factor (TNF-α), interleukin-6 (IL-6), interleukin-1β (IL-1β), total cholesterol, triacylglycerols, glycemia, and insulin, and increasing blood adiponectin levels. Adiponectin binding to its receptors (Adipo R1 and Adipo R2) leads to 5′-AMP-activated protein kinase (AMPK) phosphorylation at threonine-172, which activates peroxisome proliferator-activated receptor gamma (PPAR-γ). This blocks the translocation of nuclear factor-kappa-B (NFκB) into the nucleus and thus reduces levels of inflammatory cytokines.

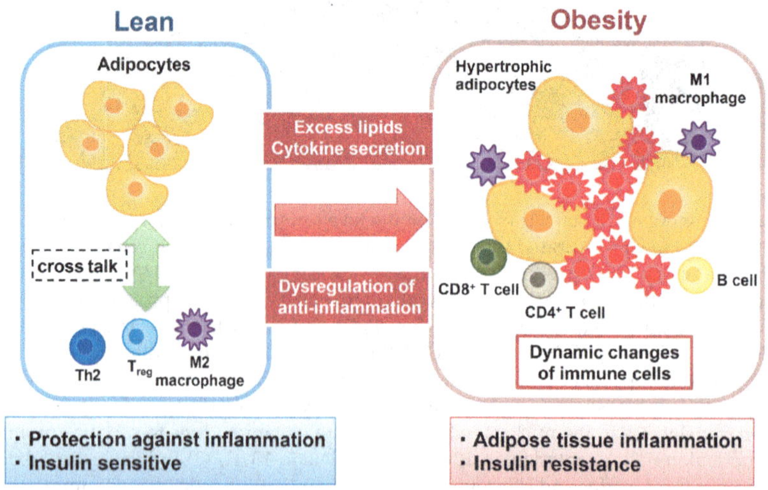

FIGURE 26.1 Functional interactions between adipocytes and immune cells in the lean or obese state. In the lean state, Th2 cells, Treg cells, and M2 macrophages are prominent in adipose tissue. These cells contribute to the suppression of inflammation in adipose tissue. As obesity progresses, excess lipids and proinflammatory cytokines are released and anti-inflammatory regulation by the immune system is impaired. In obese adipose tissue, adipocytes are hypertrophic and infiltrated M1 macrophages, $CD8^+$ T cells, $CD4^+$ T cells, and B cells contribute to induce chronic adipose tissue inflammation and insulin resistance.

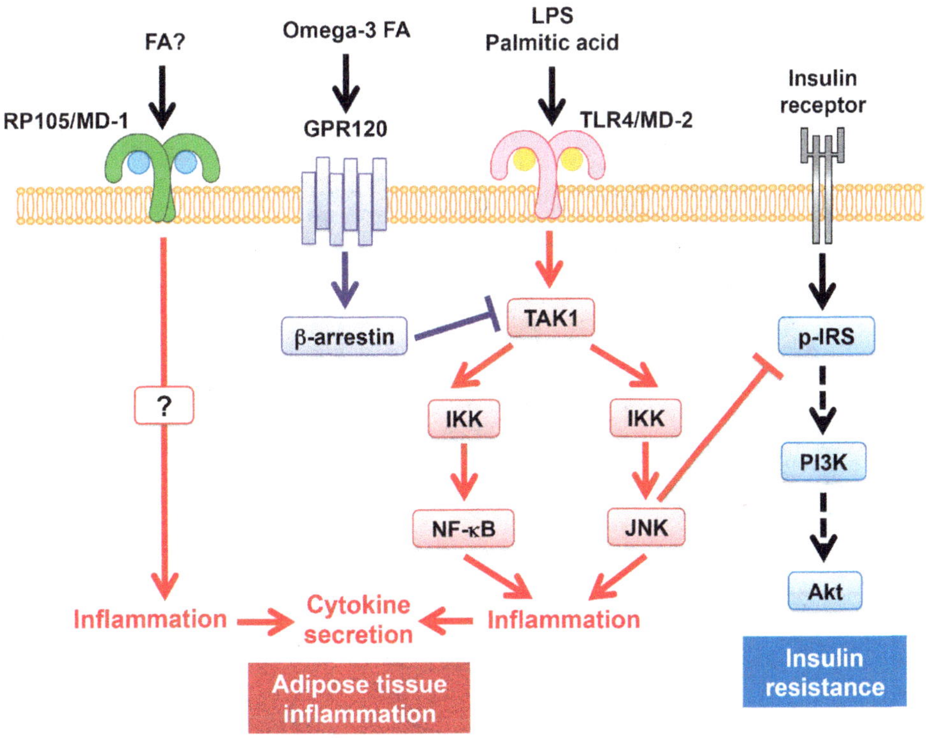

FIGURE 26.2 Inflammatory signaling pathways involved in the development of mechanisms controlling adipose tissue inflammation and insulin resistance. Lipopolysaccharides (LPS) or palmitic acid can signal via TLR4/MD-2 to induce inflammatory responses and inhibit IRS phosphorylation of insulin receptor signaling. Omega-3 fatty acids (FA) signal via GPR120 and inhibit TLR4 signaling via sequestration of TAK1. Signal via RP105/MD-1 may induce inflammatory responses, but the nature of RP105-mediated signaling in adipose tissue inflammation remains unclear.

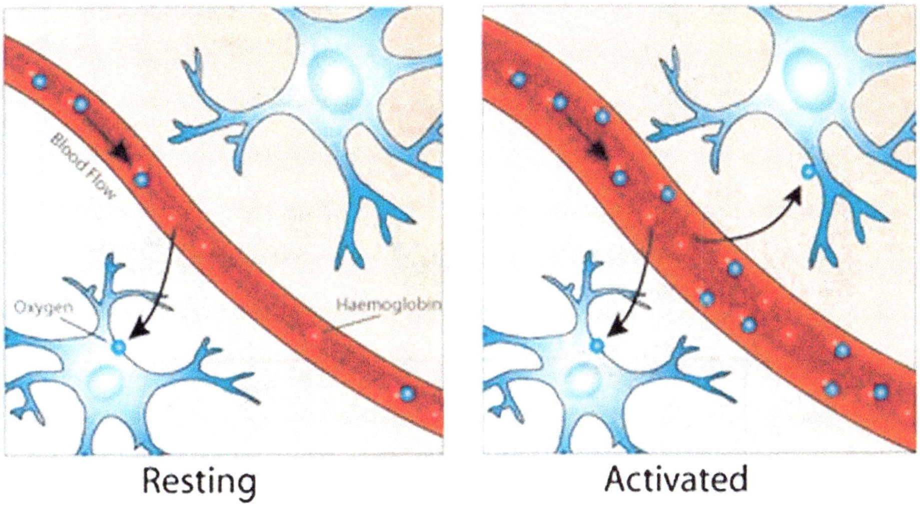

FIGURE 28.3 ***BOLD fMRI Signal.*** When blood hemoglobin is oxygenated, it contains no unpaired electrons and is thus not attracted to a magnetic field. However, it becomes paramagnetic (has unpaired electrons) when deoxygenated. This difference in magnetic properties makes it possible to detect small differences in the magnetic resonance signal of blood. Thus, the changes in oxygenation reflect levels of neural activity. This form of functional magnetic resonance imaging fMRI is known as blood oxygenation level dependent (BOLD) fMRI.

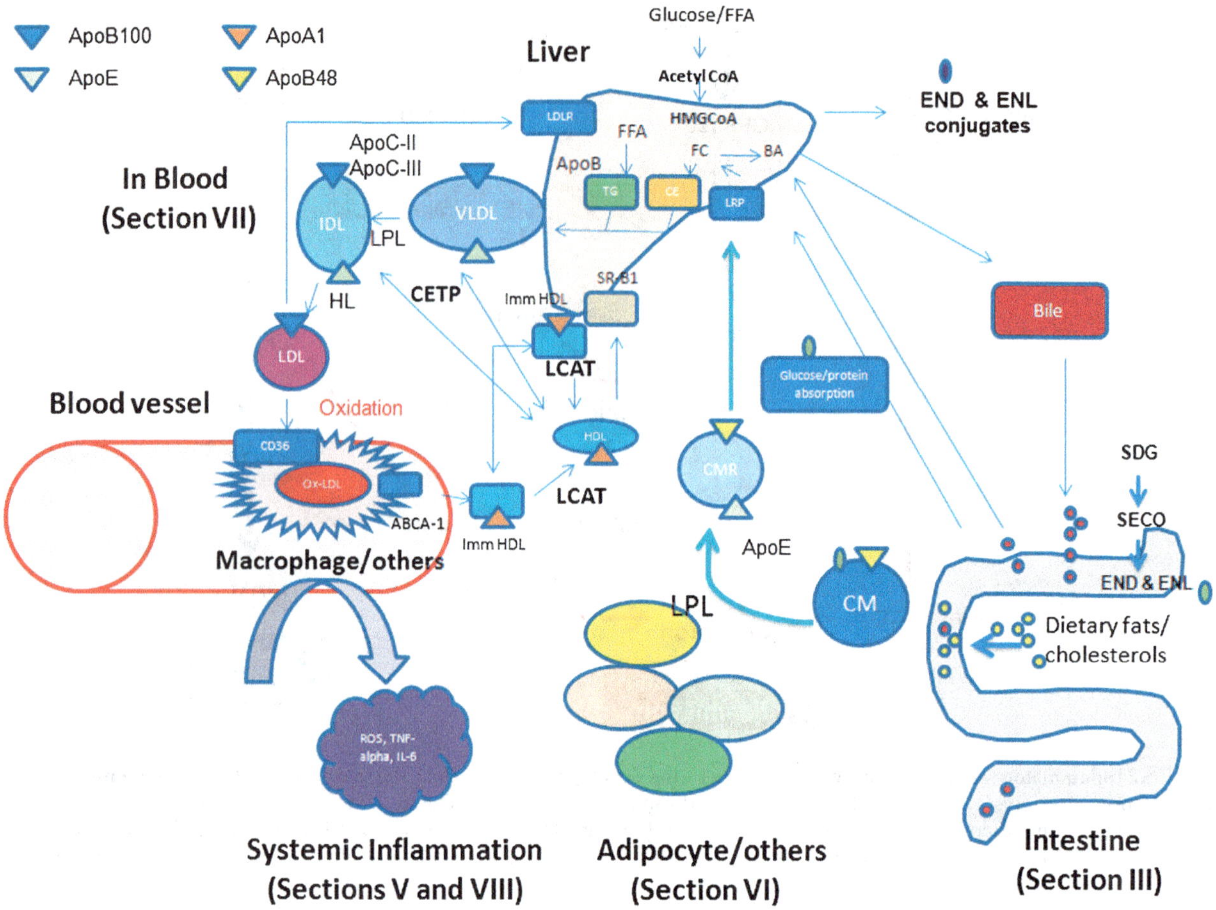

FIGURE 29.2 Diagram of lignan, cholesterol, and lipid absorption, cholesterol metabolism, and systemic inflammation. BA, bile acids; CETP, cholesteryl ester transfer protein; CM, chylomicrons; CMR, chylomicron remnants; END, enterodiol; ENL, enterolactone; FFA, free fatty acids; FC, free cholesterol; HDL, high-density lipoprotein; HL, hepatic lipase; Imm, inner mitochondrial membrane; LCAT, lecithin cholesterol acyl transferase; LPL, lipoprotein lipase; LRP, lipoprotein receptor-related proteins; Ox-LDL, oxidized low-density lipoprotein; SDG, secoisolariciresinol diglucoside; SECO, secoisolariciresinol.

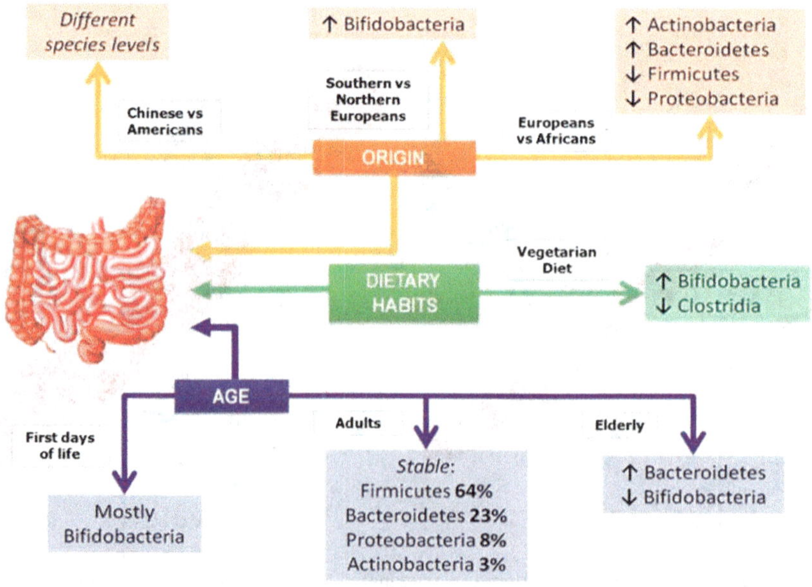

FIGURE 33.4 Factors that influence the gut microbiota. The main factors determining the intestinal microbiota are geographical and ethnic origins, dietary habits, and age.

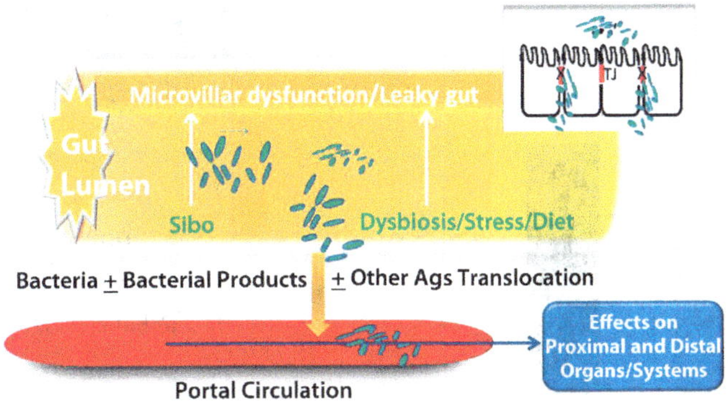

FIGURE 33.5 Events leading to bacterial and bacterial product translocation from the gut lumen to the portal circulation in the presence of microvillar dysfunction/leaky gut, small intestinal bacterial overgrowth (SIBO), gut dysbiosis, stress, or a high-fat diet. Note that tight junction (TJ) malfunction is a critical event. AGs, antigens. *Source: Vajro et al. [51].*

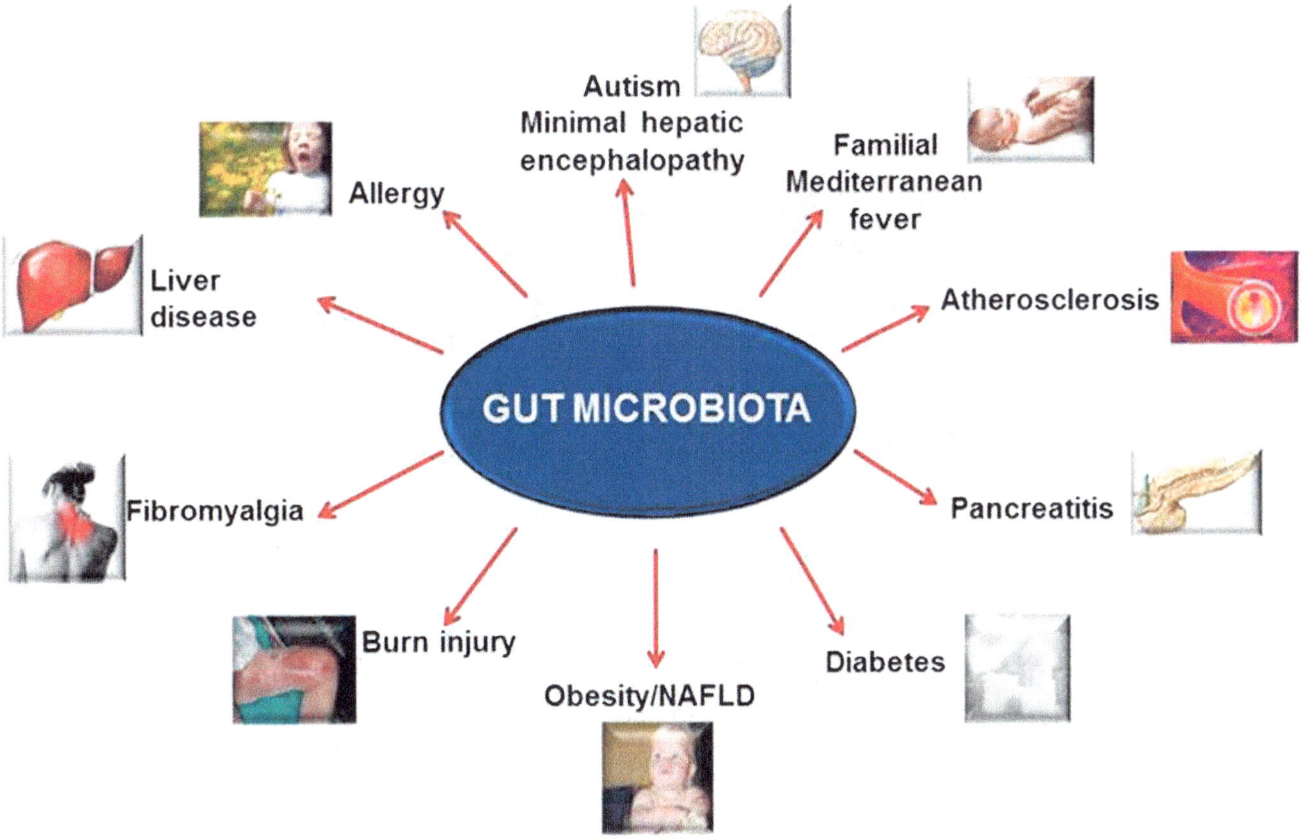

FIGURE 33.6 Proximal and distal organ diseases in which the intestinal microbiota is involved. NAFLD, nonalcoholic fatty liver disease. *Source: Vajro et al. [51].*

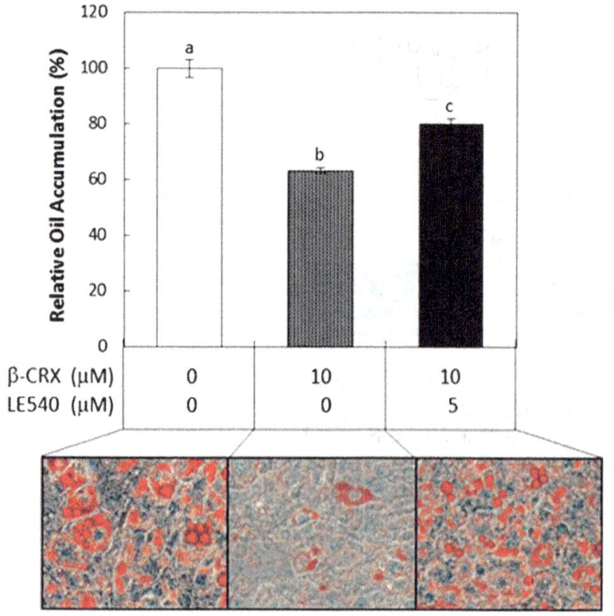

FIGURE 34.15 The effect of LE540 on inhibition of lipid accumulation by beta-cryptoxanthin. Different letters (a, b, and c) indicate statistically significant differences ($P<0.05$) in Oil Red O staining. β-CRX, beta-cryptoxanthin.

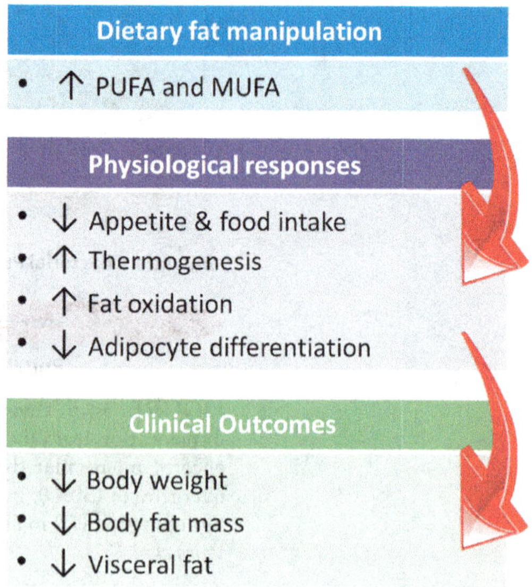

FIGURE 36.1 Dietary fat manipulation and clinical outcomes: a theoretical framework. MUFA, monounsaturated fat; PUFA, polyunsaturated fat.

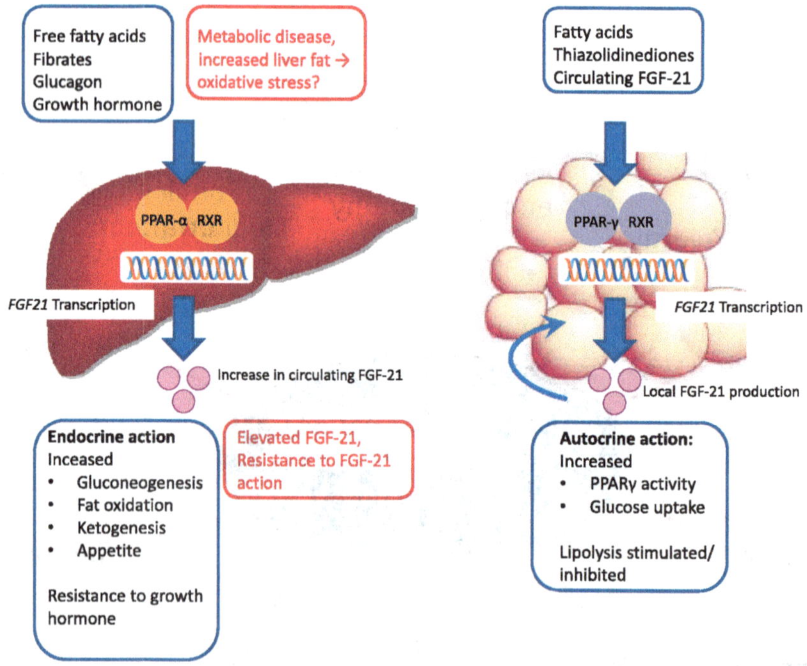

FIGURE 39.1 The physiological regulation of endocrine (hormone-like) and paracrine/autocrine synthesis of FGF21 is tissue-specific. In the liver (left panel) the transcription of FGF21 is stimulated by fasting or fibrate drugs. Also, thyroid hormones, lactation and heavy exercise may regulate FGF21 expression. Under physiological conditions indicated in left panel, rise in plasma FGF21 induces ketogenegis, increase in glucose concentration, and utilization of fat as energy source, and resistance to growth hormone action. In conditions associated with high liver fat or obesity, oxidative stress induces hepatic overexpression of FGF21 (middle panel). The plasma levels of FGF21 increase but do not lead to alleviation of hyperglycemia, triglyceride metabolism or liver fat content due to resistance to FGF21 action. The paracrine/autocrine actions of FGf21 take place in the adipose tissue (right panel), where the FGF21 expression is regulated by PPARγ agonists (thiazolinediones), by circulating FGF21 and also by free fatty acids. The current concept suggests that this pathway is activated mainly in the fed state. This metabolic loop increases local FGF21 concentrations and activates PPARγ transcription, which lead to increased glucose uptake and altered lipolysis.

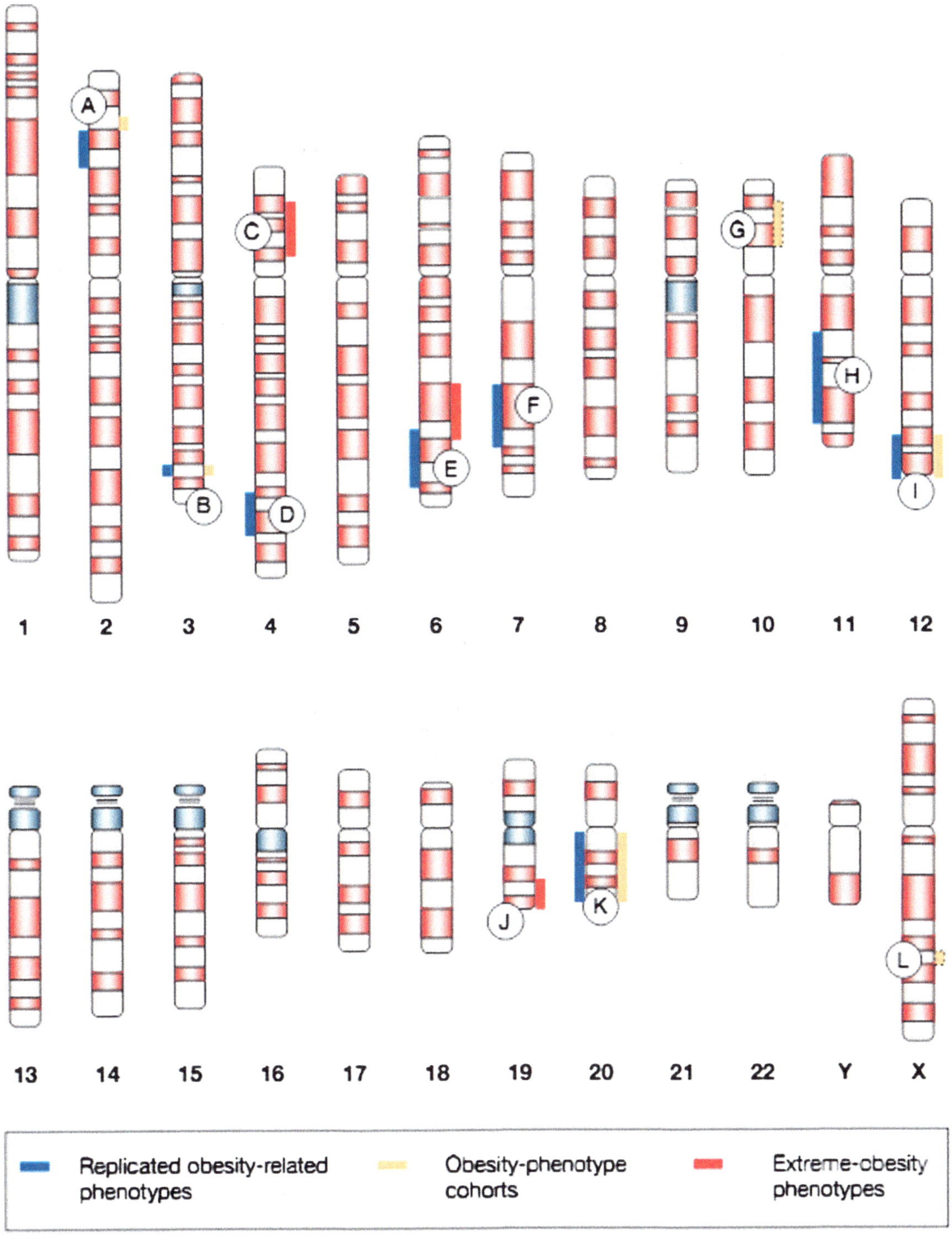

FIGURE 40.1 **Genetic linkage map for obesity**. Loci found to be linked with obesity. Blue bars indicate regions that have been replicated in several studies. Yellow bars represent loci that were found in cohorts selected specifically for obesity, and dotted lines around these bars indicate replication in other obesity cohorts. Red bars indicate regions identified in groups with extreme obesity phenotypes. A, 2p21-p23; B, 3q27; C, 4p15-p14; D, 4q31-q32; E, 6q22.31-q23.2; F, 7q31-q32; G, 10p11-p12; H, 11q14-q24; I, 12q23-q24; J, 19q13.33-q13.43; K, 20q11-q13; L, Xq24. *Source: Bell et al.* [36].

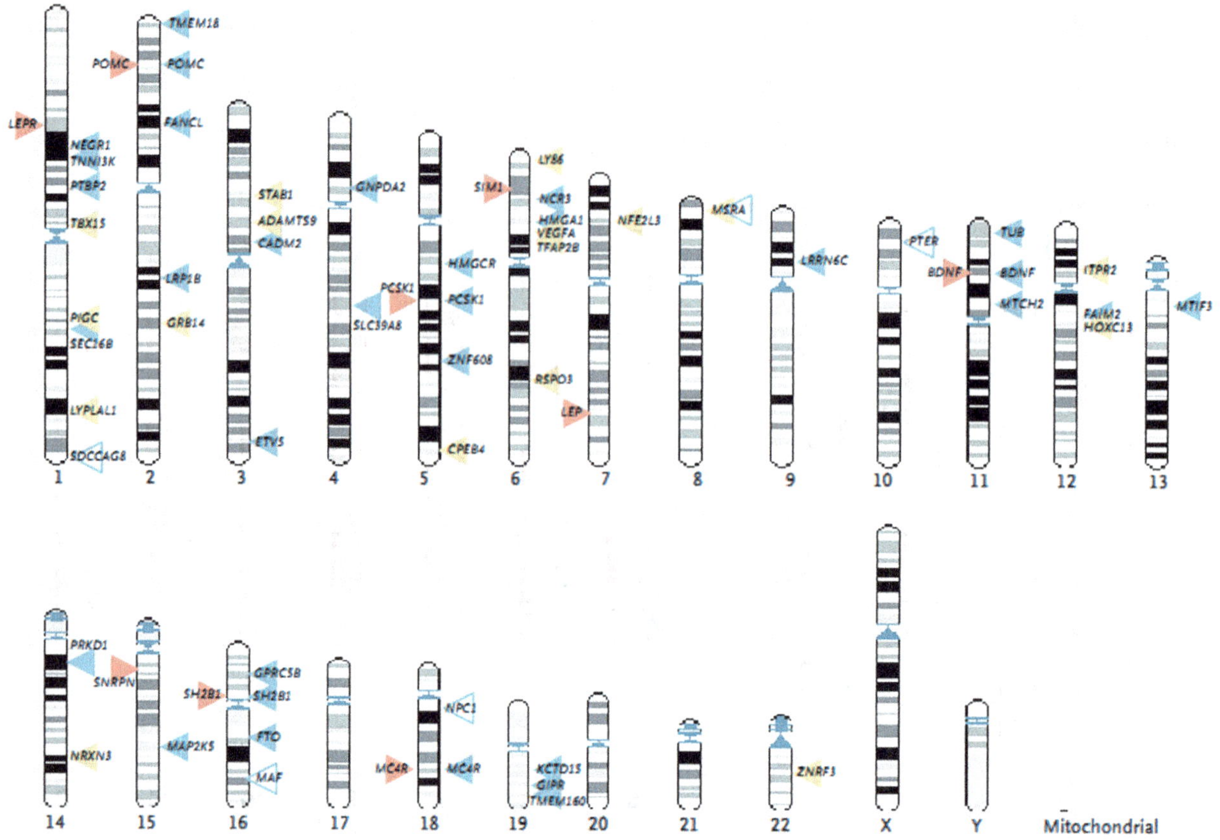

FIGURE 40.2 **Genomic locations of proven signals of body mass index, obesity, and related phenotypes.** Signals are shown according to their location on each chromosome. Genes that cause monogenic and selected syndromic forms of obesity (red triangles) are shown on the left. Common variants that have significant genome-wide associations with body mass index (BMI) or multifactorial obesity are shown on the right: loci implicated in BMI or weight variation at the population level (solid blue triangles), additional loci identified in case-control analyses of extreme obesity (open blue triangles), and variants identified primarily because of their association with waist circumference or waist-hip ratio (solid green triangles). For the variants shown on the right, genes named within the triangles are indicative of signal position, but in most instances formal proof that these are the specific genes responsible for the association is lacking. *Source: McCarthy et al.* [71].

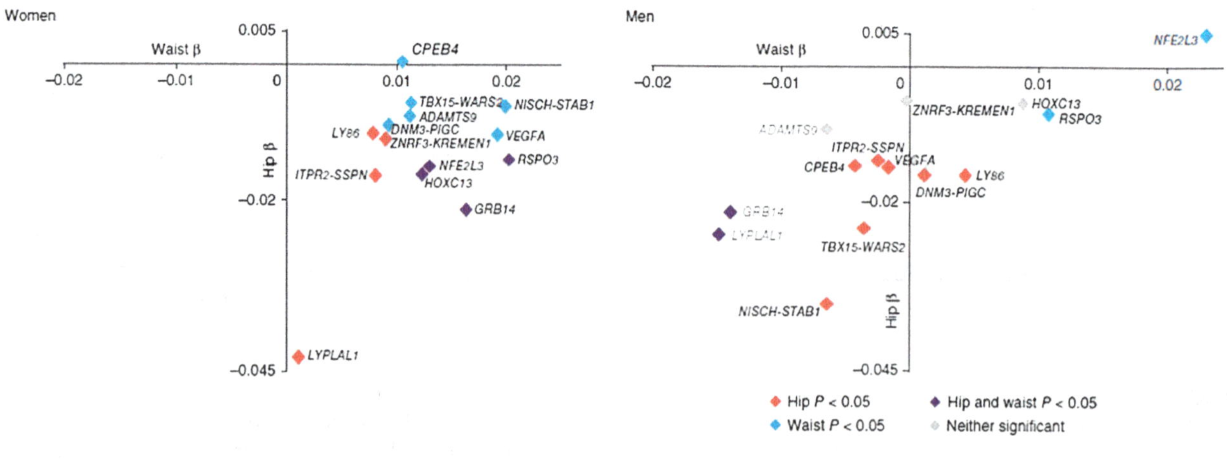

FIGURE 40.4 **Sex-specific genetic loci for association with waist circumference.** Association of the 14 waist-hip ratio (WHR) loci with waist and hip circumference. β, coefficients for waist circumference (WC; *x* axis) and hip circumference (HIP; *y* axis) in women and men derived from the joint discovery and follow-up analysis. *P* values for WC and HIP are represented by colors. In men, gray gene labels refer to those single nucleotide polymorphisms that were not significant in the male-specific WHR analysis. *Source: Heid et al.* [75].

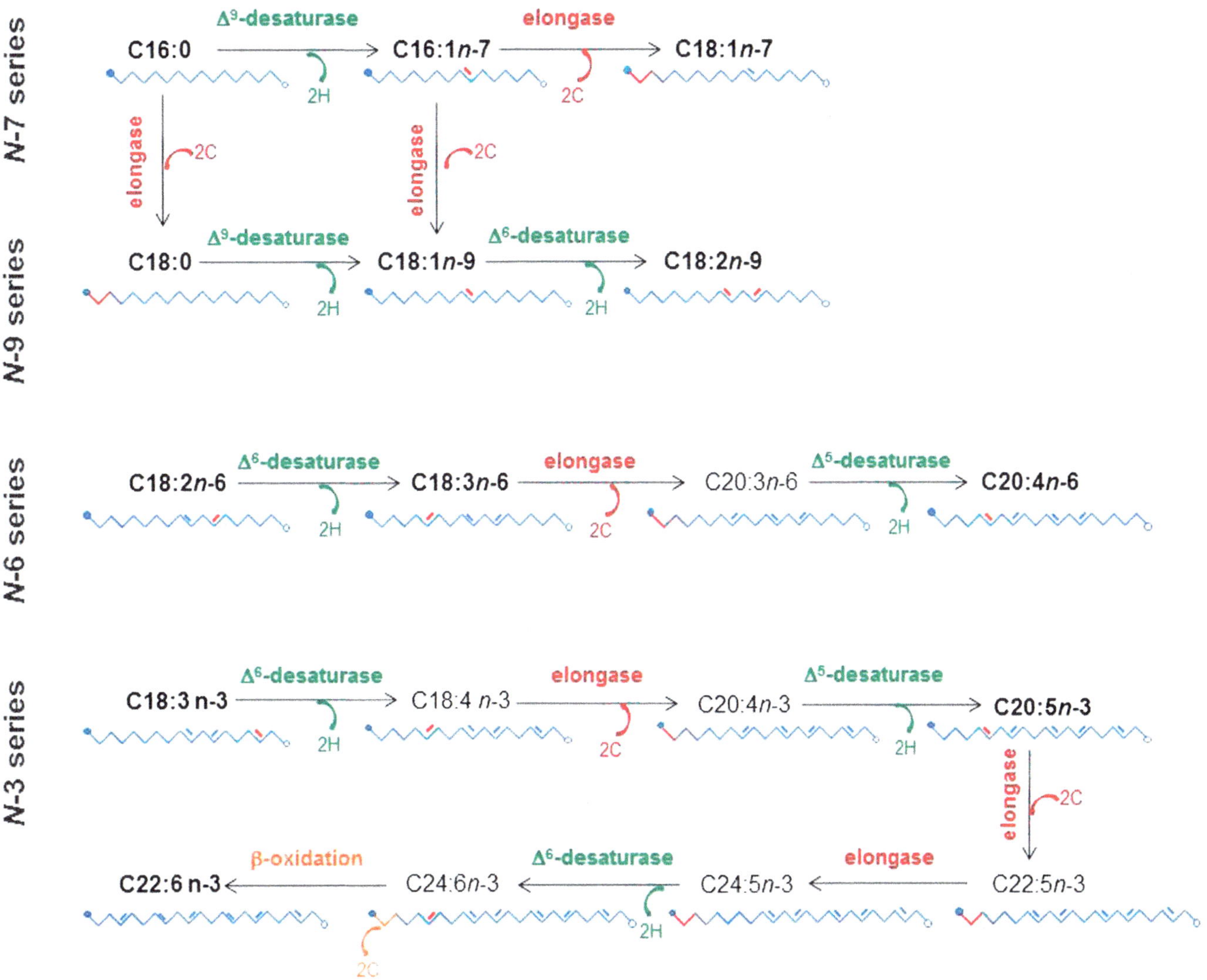

FIGURE 41.1 The main representatives of the different fatty acid families and their metabolic interconversions. $\triangle^5$, delta-5; $\triangle^6$, delta-6; $\triangle^9$, delta-9.

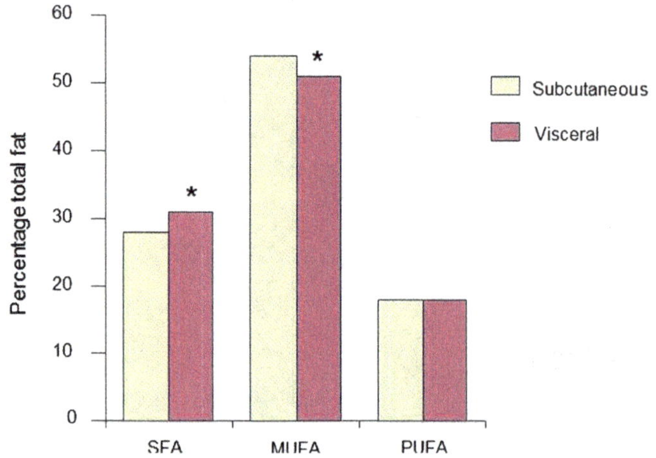

FIGURE 41.3 Differences in fat composition between subcutaneous and visceral fat in a Mediterranean Spanish population. MUFA, monounsaturated fatty acid; PUFA, polyunsaturated fatty acid; SFA, saturated fatty acid. *, $P < 0.05$ for differences in fatty acid percentages between adipose depots. *Source: Garaulet et al. [14].*

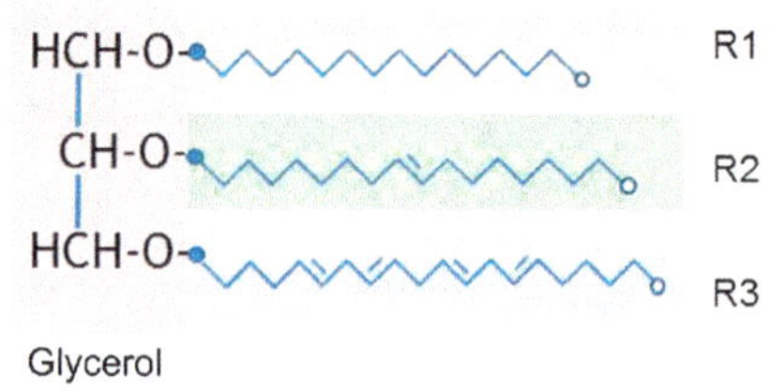

FIGURE 41.4 Structure of a trygliceride, showing the glycerol molecule esterified to different fatty acids.Most commonly, the first position (R1) is occupied by a saturated acid, the second (R2) by an unsaturated acid, and third (R3) position usually by a long-chain highly unsaturated fatty acid.

Edwards Brothers Malloy
Ann Arbor MI. USA
June 5, 2014